The Essentials of
FORENSIC MEDICINE AND TOXICOLOGY

In Loving Memory of

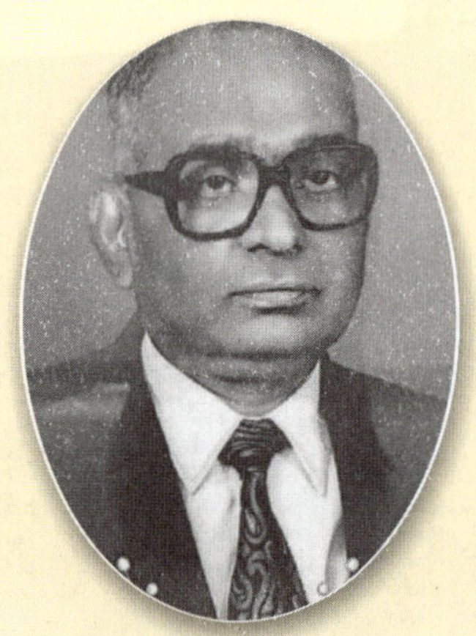

Dr KS Narayan Reddy

Retd. Principal and Professor of Forensic Medicine, Osmania Medical College

(July 17, 1930–April 9, 2021)

An inspiration to all who knew him

Forever alive in the hearts and minds of his family, friends, students, the medical fraternity, and the countless people who read and revered his books

—Pradhyumna Reddy—

(S/o Dr KS Narayan Reddy)

THE ESSENTIALS OF FORENSIC MEDICINE AND TOXICOLOGY

As per the Competency-based Medical Education Curriculum (NMC)

By

KS NARAYAN REDDY

M.D., D.C.P., Ph.D., F.A.M.S.,
F.I.M.S.A., F.A.F.Sc., F.I.A.M.S., F.A.F.M.

Retired Principal
Osmania Medical College
Hyderabad, Telangana, India

OP MURTY M.D.

Professor of Forensic Medicine and Toxicology
All India Institute of Medical Sciences
New Delhi, India

Advisors

Mahender Reddy
Professor of Forensic Medicine
Kamineni Medical College
Hyderabad, Telangana, India

Singi Yatiraj
Assistant Professor of Forensic Medicine
Bilaspur, Himachal Pradesh, India

Thirty-fifth Edition
2022

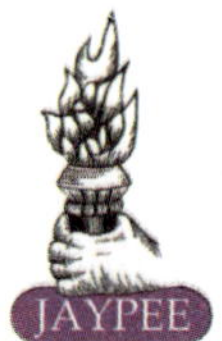

JAYPEE BROTHERS MEDICAL PUBLISHERS
The Health Sciences Publisher
New Delhi | London

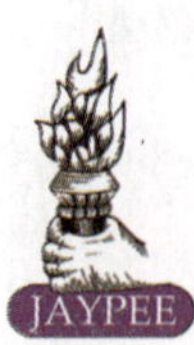

Jaypee Brothers Medical Publishers (P) Ltd.

Headquarters
Jaypee Brothers Medical Publishers (P) Ltd
EMCA House
23/23-B, Ansari Road, Daryaganj
New Delhi - 110 002, India
Landline: +91-11-23272143, +91-11-23272703
+91-11-23282021, +91-11-23245672
Email: jaypee@jaypeebrothers.com

Corporate Office
Jaypee Brothers Medical Publishers (P) Ltd
4838/24, Ansari Road, Daryaganj
New Delhi 110 002, India
Phone: +91-11-43574357
Fax: +91-11-43574314
Email: jaypee@jaypeebrothers.com

Overseas Office
J.P. Medical Ltd
83 Victoria Street, London
SW1H 0HW (UK)
Phone: +44 20 3170 8910
Fax: +44 (0)20 3008 6180
Email: info@jpmedpub.com

Website: www.jaypeebrothers.com

Website: www.jaypeedigital.com

Inquiries for bulk sales may be solicited at: jaypee@jaypeebrothers.com

The Essentials of Forensic Medicine and Toxicology

First Edition: 1973

Thirty-fifth Edition: 2022

Reprint **2024**

ISBN: 978-93-5465-321-6

Printed at: Sterling Graphics Pvt. Ltd.

PREFACE

"To study disease without books is to sail an uncharted sea, while to study books alone is not to go to sea at all."—William Osler.

"Some books are to be tasted, others to be swallowed and some few to be chewed and digested."—Bacon.

This treatise is designed to provide a brief and essentially practical guide to current teaching in Forensic Medicine with particular reference to India. The subject matter has been dealt with concisely, which is easy to grasp and simplified in presentation, and wherever necessary illustrations, tables and points have been inserted to help the students. The aim is to provide reasonable coverage of the subject as a whole. An attempt has been made to maintain the practical character of the book. We hope the reader will find it of immense help while dealing with any medicolegal case. Over and above, the book has been entirely revised and special additions and alterations have also been made and the overall text brought up-to-date.

It is intended primarily to meet the needs of the undergraduate medical students, to have clear grasp of this subject. Certain topics, such as forensic ballistics, regional injuries, anaesthetic and operative deaths, DNA fingerprinting and blood stains have been dealt with in detail to meet the requirements of medical officers involved in medicolegal work and postgraduate students. Even where less attention is given to some topics, sufficient has been included to meet the requirements of medicolegal experts. Every endeavour has been made to preclude the identification of the deceased from the photographs. Amendments in HOTA, sexual offences, domestic violence, toxicology have been incorporated. The book has been revised according to new curriculum of National Medical Commission (NMC). **The undergraduate medical students may omit the text printed in smaller type, except tables, which is meant only for medical officers**. It is important to have a clear idea of what the doctor may reasonably be expected to be able to do in any contingency. It is also important for the doctor to know what facts and opinions he/she may be expected to give. It is our aim to present in readable style, an authoritative text embracing all aspects of medicolegal problems witnessed daily by law enforcement officers, interpreted by doctors, and finally used by lawyers involved in the prosecution and defence in criminal cases, and also those engaged in civil litigation. We have consulted various textbooks and periodicals in the preparation of this book, to the authors of which, we are grateful. The opinions expressed in the text are entirely ours. We are also grateful to many friends and professional colleagues for their help and advice and to all those whose comments and criticisms have helped to keep revisions of this book accurate and up-to-date, which is hereby acknowledged wholeheartedly. It is requested that the discrepancies, if any noticed may please be intimated to us, so that it may be taken care of in the next edition. Suggestions for improvement are welcome.

The physical pathology of trauma alters little over the years, but academic and practical approaches to the subject do evolve. Accordingly, we have attempted to introduce new ideas. Advances in laboratory investigations have required considerable reappraisal. It is said that the proof of the pudding lies in the eating. The popularity of the previous editions of this title prompted the publication of this edition. It is hoped that this edition will be warmly welcomed just like the previous editions of this treatise.

We are grateful to all those working for M/s Jaypee Brothers Medical Publishers (P) Ltd., New Delhi, India, and in particular to Shri Jitendar P Vij (Group Chairman) and Mr Ankit Vij (Managing Director).

Unfortunately after completing this edition Professor KSN Reddy left for heavenly abode on 09-04-2021. He will always remain dear to readers through his concept building classical books.

KSN REDDY
OP MURTY

SOME OPINIONS

(1) Journal of Forensic Medicine and Toxicology

Vol. 15, No. 1, Jan–June, 1998

The author, a well-known and reputed medical teacher with long experience, has been very successful in giving a comprehensive account of all aspects of Forensic Medicine and Toxicology in this book, which in the opinion of this reviewer is one among the best textbooks that has so far been published by Indian authors. It provides up-to-date and reasonable material on the subject, and is well suited to undergraduate and postgraduate students, medical teachers and officers, and lawyers.

OP MURTY

(2) Journal of Indian Medical Association

Vol. 70, No. 12, 16th June, 1981

The book is a short and concise treatise on Forensic Medicine but providing reasonable coverage of the subject as a whole. This will be found well suited and very helpful not only for the undergraduates for whom this is primarily meant, but also for the postgraduate students and medical officers undertaking medicolegal works.

The author, a reputed professor with long experience, has been very successful in giving a comprehensive account of all aspects of legal medicine in this book, which in the opinion of the reviewer, is the best that has so far been published by Indian authors.

D BANERJEE

(3) Journal of Indian Academy of Forensic Sciences

Vol. 19, No. 2, 1980

The book is well written in a clear and concise style. It is designed to provide to-the-point practical guidance to teaching of forensic medicine in India. Apart from medical officers, lawyers and members of law enforcement agencies would find this book useful; the undergraduate medical students, if study texts like this, could learn a great deal of the pros and cons of the subject. But for the minor fail of perfection, Dr Reddy has succeeded in his aim of covering a vast subject in a compendium. On the whole, this is a commendable work, especially for students and specialists in this field.

B BATTACHARYA

(4) Criminal Law Journal, August, 1989

This is a very useful and exhaustive work on the subject. It is designed for the use of students and teachers of Forensic Medicine and Toxicology. It will serve as a useful practical guide to those who are dealing with medicolegal cases at the investigation stages or in the court rooms while arguing for the criminal prosecution or for providing successful defense to an accused. The medical practitioners would find a fund of information in the book during their work in medicolegal involvement. The book provides sufficient coverage on the subject. It is very well illustrated, contains useful charts and tables on various aspects of the subject matter for making the points discussed easily understandable.

LKK

(5) Medical Books News—A Guide to New Books

This is one of the most comprehensive volumes on the subject written by an Indian author and in fact contains more details than required by an undergraduate. It would, therefore, be helpful when a reference on any topic becomes necessary.

OTHER BOOKS BY THE SAME AUTHOR

(1) **THE SYNOPSIS OF FORENSIC MEDICINE AND TOXICOLOGY**
Twenty-ninth Edition, 2017, 24 cm × 18 cm, pp VIII + 390

(2) **MEDICAL JURISPRUDENCE AND TOXICOLOGY**
Fourth Edition, 2016, 24 cm × 18 cm, pp LXXX + 1374, Price ₹ 2250/-
Published by Andhra Law Times, Hyderabad

(3) **CONCISE FORENSIC MEDICINE AND TOXICOLOGY**
Fourth Edition, 2015, 17 cm × 11 cm, pp IV + 238

(4) **MCQs IN FORENSIC MEDICINE**
Sixth Edition, 2011, 24 cm × 18 cm, pp VIII + 300, Price ₹ 270/-

(5) **MEDICOLEGAL MANUAL**
Fifth Edition, 2015, 24 cm × 18 cm, pp IV + 300, Price ₹ 250/-

(6) **MEDICOLEGAL MANUAL FOR POLICE OFFICERS**
Third Edition, 2017, 24 cm × 18 cm, pp IV + 261

(7) **THE HANDBOOK OF FORENSIC MEDICINE AND TOXICOLOGY**
(Out of Print)

(8) **LEGAL MEDICINE FOR LAWYERS AND DOCTORS**
(Out of Print)

(9) **SELF-STUDY GUIDE IN FORENSIC MEDICINE AND TOXICOLOGY**
(Out of Print)

(10) **న్యాయ వైద్యశాస్త్రము**
Second Edition, 2013, 24 cm × 118 cm, pp. 243, Price ₹ 200/-

(11) **न्यायालय-संबंधी चिकित्सा की रूप रेखा तथा विषविज्ञान**
First Edition, 2007, 24 cm × 18 cm, pp. 230, Price ₹ 200/-

CONTENTS

SECTION I: FORENSIC MEDICINE

SECTION II: TOXICOLOGY

COMPETENCY TABLE

Number	COMPETENCY The student should be able to	Domain K/S/A/C	Level K/KH/ SH/P	Core (Y/N)	Suggested teaching learning method	Suggested assessment method	Chapter number
FM1.1	Demonstrate knowledge of basics of forensic medicine like definitions of forensic medicine, clinical forensic medicine, forensic pathology, state medicine, legal medicine and medical jurisprudence	K	KH	N	Lecture, small group discussion	Written/ viva voce	1
FM1.2	Describe history of forensic medicine	K	KH	N	Lecture, small group discussion	Written/ viva voce	1
FM1.3	Describe legal procedures including Criminal Procedure Code, Indian Penal Code, Indian Evidence Act, Civil and Criminal Cases, Inquest(Police Inquest and Magistrate's Inquest), cognizable and non-cognizable offences	K	KH	N	Lecture, small group discussion	Written/ viva voce	2
FM1.4	Describe Courts in India and their powers: Supreme Court, High Court, Sessions Court, Magistrate's Court, Labour Court, Family Court, Executive Magistrate Court and Juvenile Justice Board	K	KH	N	Lecture, small group discussion	Written/ viva voce	2
FM1.5	Describe court procedures including issue of summons, conduct money, types of witnesses, recording of evidence oath, affirmation, examination in chief, cross examination, re-examination and court questions, recording of evidence and conduct of doctor in witness box	K	KH	N	Lecture, small group discussion, Moot Court	Written/ viva voce	2
FM1.6	Describe offenses in court including perjury; court strictures vis-a- vis medical officer	K	KH	N	Lecture, small group discussion	Written/ viva voce	2
FM1.7	Describe dying declaration and dying deposition	K	KH	Y	Lecture, small group discussion	Written/ viva voce	2
FM1.9	Describe the importance of documentation in medical practice in regard to medicolegal examinations, medical certificates and medicolegal reports especially: • Maintenance of patient case records, discharge summary, prescribed registers to be maintained in health centres • Maintenance of medicolegal register like accident register • Documents of issuance of wound certificate • Documents of issuance of drunkenness certificate • Documents of issuance of sickness and fitness certificate • Documents for issuance of death certificate—documents of Medical Certification of Cause of Death—Form Number 4 and 4A • Documents for estimation of age by physical, dental and radiological examination and issuance of certificate	K	KH	Y	Lecture, small group discussion	Written/ viva voce	3
FM2.1	Define, describe and discuss death and its types including somatic/clinical/cellular, molecular and brain-death, cortical death and brainstem death	K	KH	Y	Lecture/small group discussion	Written/ viva voce	6
FM2.2	Describe and discuss natural and unnatural deaths	K	KH	Y	Lecture, small group discussion	Written/ viva voce	6
FM2.3	Describe and discuss issues related to sudden natural deaths	K	KH	Y	Lecture, small group discussion	Written/ viva voce	6

Number	COMPETENCY The student should be able to	Domain K/S/A/C	Level K/KH/SH/P	Core (Y/N)	Suggested teaching learning method	Suggested assessment method	Chapter number
FM2.5	Discuss moment of death, modes of death—coma, asphyxia and syncope	K	KH	Y	Lecture, small group discussion	Written/ viva voce	6
FM2.6	Discuss presumption of death and survivorship	K	KH	Y	Lecture, small group discussion	Written/ viva voce	7
FM2.7	Describe and discuss suspended animation	K	KH	Y	Lecture, small group discussion	Written/ viva voce	7
FM2.8	Describe and discuss postmortem changes including signs of death, cooling of body, postmortem lividity, rigor mortis, cadaveric spasm, cold stiffening and heat stiffening	K	KH	Y	Lecture, small group discussion, autopsy, DOAP session	Written/ viva voce/ OSPE	7
FM2.9	Describe putrefaction, mummification, adipocere and maceration	K	KH	Y	Lecture, small group discussion, autopsy, DOAP session	Written/ viva voce/ OSPE	7
FM2.10	Discuss estimation of time since death	K	KH	Y	Lecture, small group discussion, autopsy, DOAP session	Written/ viva voce/ OSPE	7
FM2.11	Describe and discuss autopsy procedures including postmortem examination, different types of autopsies, aims and objectives of postmortem examination	K	KH	Y	Lecture, small group discussion, autopsy, DOAP session	Written/ viva voce/ OSPE	5
FM2.12	Describe the legal requirements to conduct postmortem examination and procedures to conduct medicolegal postmortem examination	K	KH	Y	Lecture, small group discussion, autopsy, DOAP session	Written/ viva voce/ OSPE	5
FM2.13	Describe and discuss obscure autopsy	K	KH	Y	Lecture, small group discussion	Written/ viva voce	6
FM2.14	Describe and discuss examination of clothing, preservation of viscera on postmortem examination for chemical analysis and other medicolegal purposes, postmortem artefacts	K	KH	Y	Lecture, small group discussion, autopsy, DOAP session	Written/ viva voce/ OSPE	5, 21
FM2.15	Describe special protocols for conduction of medicolegal autopsies in cases of death in custody or following violation of human rights as per National Human Rights Commission Guidelines	K	KH	Y	Lecture, small group discussion, autopsy, DOAP session	Written/ viva voce/ OSPE	10
FM2.16	Describe and discuss examination of mutilated bodies or fragments, charred bones and bundle of bones	K	KH	Y	Lecture, small group discussion, DOAP session	Written/ viva voce/ OSPE	5
FM2.17	Describe and discuss exhumation	K	KH	Y	Lecture, small group discussion	Written/ viva voce	5
FM2.18	Crime scene investigation: Describe and discuss the objectives of crime scene visit, the duties and responsibilities of doctors on crime scene and the reconstruction of sequence of events after crime scene investigation	K	KH	Y	Lecture, small group discussion	Written/ viva voce	2
FM2.19	Investigation of anaesthetic, operative deaths: Describe and discuss special protocols for conduction of autopsy and for collection, preservation and dispatch of related material evidences	K	KH	Y	Lecture, small group discussion	Written/ viva voce	14
FM2.20	Mechanical asphyxia: Define, classify and describe asphyxia and medicolegal interpretation of postmortem findings in asphyxial deaths	K	KH	Y	Lecture, small group discussion, autopsy, DOAP session	Written/ viva voce/ OSPE	13

Number	COMPETENCY The student should be able to	Domain K/S/A/C	Level K/KH/ SH/P	Core (Y/N)	Suggested teaching learning method	Suggested assessment method	Chapter number
FM2.21	Mechanical asphyxia: Describe and discuss different types of hanging and strangulation including clinical findings, causes of death, postmortem findings and medicolegal aspects of death due to hanging and strangulation including examination, preservation and dispatch of ligature material	K	KH	Y	Lecture/small group discussion, autopsy DOAP session	Written/ viva voce/ OSPE	13
FM2.22	Mechanical asphyxia: Describe and discuss pathophysiology, clinical features, postmortem findings and medicolegal aspects of traumatic asphyxia, obstruction of nose and mouth, suffocation and sexual asphyxia	K	KH	Y	Lecture, small group discussion, autopsy, DOAP session	Written/ viva voce/ OSPE	13
FM2.23	Describe and discuss types, pathophysiology, clinical features, postmortem findings and medicolegal aspects of drowning, diatom test and, gettler test	K	KH	Y	Lecture, small group discussion, autopsy, DOAP session	Written/ viva voce/ OSPE	13
FM2.24	Thermal deaths: Describe the clinical features, postmortem finding and medicolegal aspects of injuries due to physical agents like heat [heat—hyperpyrexia, heat stroke, sun stroke, heat exhaustion/prostration, heat cramps(miner's cramp) or cold(systemic and localized hypothermia, frostbite, trench foot, immersion foot)]	K	KH	Y	Lecture, small group discussion, autopsy, DOAP session	Written/ viva voce	11
FM2.25	Describe types of injuries, clinical features, pathophysiology, postmortem findings and medicolegal aspects in cases of burns, scalds, lightening, electrocution and radiations	K	KH	Y	Lecture, small group discussion, autopsy, DOAP session	Written/ viva voce/ OSPE	11
FM2.26	Describe and discuss clinical features, postmortem findings and medicolegal aspects of death due to starvation and neglect	K	KH	Y	Lecture/small group discussion	Written/ viva voce	12
FM2.27	Define and discuss infanticide, foeticide and stillbirth	K	KH	Y	Lecture, small group discussion	Written/ viva voce	19
FM2.28	Describe and discuss signs of intrauterine death, signs of live birth, viability of foetus, age determination of foetus, DOAP session of ossification centres, hydrostatic test, sudden infants death syndrome and Munchausen's syndrome by proxy	K	KH	Y	Lecture, small group discussion, autopsy, DOAP session	Written/ viva voce/ OSCE	19
FM3.1	Identification: Define and describe corpus delicti, establishment of identity of living persons including race, sex, religion, complexion, stature, age determination using morphology, teeth-eruption, decay, bite marks, bones ossification centres, medicolegal aspects of age	K	KH	Y	Lecture, small group discussion, bedside clinic, DOAP session	Written/ viva voce/ skill assessment	4
FM3.2	Identification: Describe and discuss identification of criminals, unknown persons, dead bodies from the remains—hairs, fibers, teeth, anthropometry, dactylography, foot prints, scars, tattoos, poroscopy and superimposition	K	KH	Y	Lecture, small group discussion	Written/ viva voce	4
FM3.3	Mechanical injuries and wounds: Define, describe and classify different types of mechanical injuries, abrasion, bruise, laceration, stab wound, incised wound, chop wound, defense wound, self-inflicted/fabricated wounds and their medicolegal aspects	K	KH	Y	Lecture, small group discussion, bedside clinic, DOAP session	Written/ viva voce/ OSCE	8
FM3.4	Mechanical injuries and wounds: Define injury, assault and hurt. Describe IPC pertaining to injuries	K	KH	Y	Lecture, small group discussion	Written/ viva voce	10
FM3.5	Mechanical injuries and wounds: Describe accidental, suicidal and homicidal injuries. Describe simple, grievous and dangerous injuries. Describe antemortem and postmortem injuries	K	K/KH	Y	Lecture/small group discussion	Written/ viva voce	10
FM3.6	Mechanical injuries and wounds: Describe healing of injury and fracture of bones with its medicolegal importance	K	K/KH	Y	Lecture/small group discussion	Written/ viva voce	8

Number	COMPETENCY The student should be able to	Domain K/S/A/C	Level K/KH/ SH/P	Core (Y/N)	Suggested teaching learning method	Suggested assessment method	Chapter number
FM3.7	Describe factors influencing infliction of injuries and healing, examination and certification of wounds and wound as a cause of death: Primary and secondary	K	K/KH	Y	Lecture/small group discussion	Written/ viva voce	10
FM3.8	Mechanical injuries and wounds: Describe and discuss different types of weapons including dangerous weapons and their examination	K	K/KH	Y	Lecture/small group discussion	Written/ viva voce	10
FM3.9	Firearm injuries: Describe different types of firearms including structure and components. Along with description of ammunition propellant charge and mechanism of firearms, different types of cartridges and bullets and various terminology in relation of firearm—caliber, range, choking	K	K/KH	Y	Lecture/small group discussion	Written/ viva voce	8
FM3.10	Firearm injuries: Describe and discuss wound ballistics—different types of firearm injuries, blast injuries and their interpretation, preservation and dispatch of trace evidences in cases of firearm and blast injuries, various tests related to confirmation of use of firearms	K	K/KH	Y	Lecture, small group discussion, bedside clinic, DOAP session	Written/ viva voce/ OSCE	8
FM3.11	Regional injuries: Describe and discuss regional injuries to head(scalp wounds, fracture skull, intracranial haemorrhages, coup and contrecoup injuries), neck, chest, abdomen, limbs, genital organs, spinal cord and skeleton	K	K/KH	Y	Lecture, small group discussion, bedside clinic or autopsy, DOAP session	Written/ viva voce/ OSCE/ OSPE	9
FM3.12	Regional injuries: Describe and discuss injuries related to fall from height and vehicular injuries—primary and secondary impact, secondary injuries, crush syndrome, railway spine	K	K/KH	Y	Lecture, small group discussion, bedside clinic or autopsy, DOAP session	Written/ viva voce/ OSCE/ OSPE	9
FM3.13	Describe different types of sexual offences. Describe various sections of IPC regarding rape including definition of rape(Section 375 IPC), punishment for rape(Section 376 IPC) and recent amendments notified till date	K	K/KH	Y	Lecture, small group discussion	Written/ viva voce/ OSCE/ OSPE	18
FM3.14	Sexual offences: Describe and discuss the examination of the victim of an alleged case of rape, and the preparation of report, framing the opinion and preservation and despatch of trace evidences in such cases	K	K/KH	Y	Lecture, small group discussion, bedside clinic, DOAP session	Written/ viva voce/ OSCE	18
FM3.15	Sexual offences: Describe and discuss examination of accused and victim of sodomy, preparation of report, framing of opinion, preservation and despatch of trace evidences in such cases	K	K/KH	Y	Lecture, small group discussion, bedside clinic, DOAP session	Written/ viva voce/ OSCE	18
FM3.16	Sexual offences: Describe and discuss adultery and unnatural sexual offences—sodomy, incest, lesbianism, buccal coitus, bestiality, indecent assault and preparation of report, framing the opinion and preservation and despatch of trace evidences in such cases	K	K/KH	Y	Lecture/small group discussion	Written/ viva voce	18
FM3.17	Describe and discuss the sexual perversions fetishism, transvestism, voyeurism, sadism, necrophagia, masochism, exhibitionism, frotteurism, necrophilia	K	K/KH	Y	Lecture/small group discussion	Written/ viva voce	18
FM3.18	Describe anatomy of male and female genitalia, hymen and its types. Discuss the medicolegal importance of hymen. Define virginity, defloration, legitimacy and its medicolegal importance	K	K/KH	Y	Lecture/small group discussion	Written/ viva voce	16
FM3.19	Discuss the medicolegal aspects of pregnancy and delivery, signs of pregnancy, precipitate labour superfoetation, superfecundation and signs of recent and remote delivery in living and dead	K	K/KH	Y	Lecture/small group discussion	Written/ viva voce	16

Number	COMPETENCY The student should be able to	Domain K/S/A/C	Level K/KH/ SH/P	Core (Y/N)	Suggested teaching learning method	Suggested assessment method	Chapter number
FM3.20	Discuss disputed paternity and maternity	K	K/KH	Y	Lecture/small group discussion	Written/ viva voce	20
FM3.22	Define and discuss impotence, sterility, frigidity, sexual dysfunction, premature ejaculation. Discuss the causes of impotence and sterility in male and female	K	K/KH	Y	Lecture/small group discussion	Written/ viva voce	15
FM3.23	Discuss sterilization of male and female, artificial insemination, test tube baby, surrogate mother, hormonal replacement therapy with respect to appropriate national and state laws	K	K/KH	Y	Lecture/small group discussion	Written/ viva voce	15
FM3.24	Discuss the relative importance of surgical methods of contraception(vasectomy and tubectomy) as methods of contraception in the National Family Planning Programme	K	K/KH	N	Lecture/small group discussion	Written	15
FM3.26	Discuss the national guidelines for accreditation, supervision and regulation of ART clinics in India	K	K/KH	Y	Lecture/small group discussion	Written	15
FM3.27	Define, classify and discuss abortion, methods of procuring MTP and criminal abortion and complication of abortion. MTP Act 1971	K	K/KH	Y	Lecture/small group discussion	Written/ viva voce	17
FM3.28	Describe evidences of abortion—living and dead, duties of doctor in cases of abortion, investigations of death due to criminal abortion	K	K/KH	Y	Lecture/small group discussion	Written/ viva voce	17
FM3.29	Describe and discuss child abuse and battered baby syndrome	K	K/KH	Y	Lecture/small group discussion	Written/ viva voce	19
FM3.30	Describe and discuss issues relating to torture, identification of injuries caused by torture and its sequelae, management of torture survivors	K	K/KH	Y	Lecture/small group discussion	Written/ viva voce	10
FM3.31	Torture and human rights: Describe and discuss guidelines and protocols of National Human Rights Commission regarding torture	K	K/KH	N	Lecture/small group discussion	Written/ viva voce	10
FM4.1	Describe medical ethics and explain its historical emergence	K	KH	Y	Lecture/small group discussion	Written/ viva voce	3
FM4.2	Describe the Code of Medical Ethics 2002 conduct, etiquette and ethics in medical practice and unethical practices and the dichotomy	K	KH	Y	Lecture/small group discussion	Written/ viva voce	3
FM4.3	Describe the functions and role of Medical Council of India and State Medical Councils	K	KH	Y	Lecture/small group discussion	Written/ viva voce	3
FM4.4	Describe the Indian Medical Register	K	KH	Y	Lecture/small group discussion	Written/ viva voce	3
FM4.5	Rights/privileges of a medical practitioner, penal erasure, infamous conduct, disciplinary committee, disciplinary procedures, warning notice and penal erasure	K	KH	Y	Lecture/small group discussion	Written/ viva voce	3
FM4.6	Describe the laws in relation to medical practice and the duties of a medical practitioner towards patients and society	K	K/KH	Y	Lecture/small group discussion	Written/ viva voce	3
FM4.7	Describe and discuss the ethics related to HIV patients	K	K/KH	Y	Lecture/small group discussion	Written/ viva voce	6
FM4.10	Describe communication between doctors, public and media	K	KH	Y	Lecture/small group discussion	Written/ viva voce	3
FM4.11	Describe and discuss euthanasia	K	KH	Y	Lecture/small group discussion	Written/ viva voce	3
FM4.12	Discuss legal and ethical issues in relation to stem cell research	K	KH	Y	Lecture/small group discussion	Written/ viva voce	15
FM4.14	Describe and discuss the challenges in managing medicolegal cases including development of skills in relationship management—human behaviour, communication skills, conflict resolution techniques	K	KH	Y	Lecture/small group discussion	Written/ viva voce	2

Number	COMPETENCY The student should be able to	Domain K/S/A/C	Level K/KH/ SH/P	Core (Y/N)	Suggested teaching learning method	Suggested assessment method	Chapter number
FM4.15	Describe the principles of handling pressure—definition, types, causes, sources and skills for managing the pressure while dealing with medicolegal cases by the doctor	K	KH	Y	Lecture/small group discussion	Written/ viva voce	2
FM4.17	Describe and discuss ethical principles: Respect for autonomy, non- malfeasance, beneficence and justice	K	KH	Y	Lecture/small group discussion	Written/ viva voce	1
FM4.18	Describe and discuss medical negligence including civil and criminal negligence, contributory negligence, corporate negligence, vicarious liability, res ipsa loquitur, prevention of medical negligence and defenses in medical negligence litigations	K	KH	Y	Lecture/small group discussion	Written/ viva voce	3
FM4.19	Define consent. Describe different types of consent and ingredients of informed consent. Describe the rules of consent and importance of consent in relation to age, emergency situation, mental illness and alcohol intoxication	K	KH	Y	Lecture/small group discussion	Written/ viva voce	3
FM4.20	Describe therapeutic privilege, malingering, therapeutic misadventure, professional secrecy, human experimentation	K	KH	Y	Lecture/small group discussion	Written/ viva voce	3
FM4.21	Describe products liability and medical indemnity insurance	K	KH	Y	Lecture/small group discussion	Written/ viva voce	3
FM4.22	Explain Oath—Hippocrates, Charaka and Sushruta and procedure for administration of Oath.	K	KH	Y	Lecture/small group discussion	Written/ viva voce	3
FM4.23	Describe the modified declaration of Geneva and its relevance	K	KH	Y	Lecture/small group discussion	Written/ viva voce	3
FM4.24	Enumerate rights, privileges and duties of a Registered Medical Practitioner. Discuss doctor-patient relationship: professional secrecy and privileged communication	K	KH	Y	Lecture/small group discussion	Written/ viva voce	3
FM5.1	Classify common mental illnesses including posttraumatic stress disorder(PTSD)	K	K/KH	Y	Lecture/small group discussion	Written/ viva voce	23
FM5.2	Define, classify and describe delusions, hallucinations, illusion, lucid interval and obsessions with exemplification	K	K/KH	Y	Lecture/small group discussion	Written/ viva voce	23
FM5.3	Describe civil and criminal responsibilities of a mentally ill person	K	K/KH	Y	Lecture/small group discussion	Written/ viva voce	23
FM5.4	Differentiate between true insanity from feigned insanity	K	K/KH	Y	Lecture/small group discussion	Written/ viva voce	23
FM5.5	Describe and discuss delirium tremens	K	K/KH	Y	Lecture/small group discussion	Written/ viva voce	30
FM5.6	Describe the Indian Mental Health Act, 1987 with special reference to admission, care and discharge of a mentally ill person	K	K/KH	N	Lecture/small group discussion	Written/ viva voce	23
FM6.1	Describe different types of specimen and tissues to be collected both in the living and dead: Body fluids(blood, urine, semen, faeces saliva), skin, nails, tooth pulp, vaginal smear, viscera, skull, specimen for histopathological examination, blood grouping, HLA typing and DNA fingerprinting. Describe Locard's exchange principle	K	K/KH	Y	Lecture/small group discussion	Written/ viva voce	22
FM6.2	Describe the methods of sample collection, preservation, labelling, dispatch, and interpretation of reports	K	K/KH	Y	Lecture/small group discussion	Written/ viva voce	22
FM7.1	Enumerate the indications and describe the principles and appropriate use for: • DNA profiling • Facial reconstruction • Polygraph(Lie detector) • Narcoanalysis, • Brain mapping • Digital autopsy • Virtual autopsy • Imaging technologies	K	K/KH	N	Lecture/small group discussion	Written/ viva voce	22

Number	COMPETENCY The student should be able to	Domain K/S/A/C	Level K/KH/ SH/P	Core (Y/N)	Suggested teaching learning method	Suggested assessment method	Chapter number
FM8.1	Describe the history of toxicology	K	K/KH	Y	Lecture/small group discussion	Written/ viva voce	24
FM8.2	Define the terms toxicology, forensic toxicology, clinical toxicology and poison	K	K/KH	Y	Lecture/small group discussion	Written/ viva voce	24
FM8.3	Describe the various types of poisons, toxicokinetics, and toxicodynamics and diagnosis of poisoning in living and dead	K	K/KH	Y	Lecture/small group discussion	Written/ viva voce	24
FM8.4	Describe the laws in relations to poisons including NDPS Act, medicolegal aspects of poisons	K	K/KH	Y	Lecture/small group discussion	Written/ viva voce	24, 31
FM8.5	Describe medicolegal autopsy in cases of poisoning including preservation and dispatch of viscera for chemical analysis	K	K/KH	Y	Lecture/small group discussion, autopsy, DOAP session	Written/ viva voce/ OSPE	5
FM8.8	Describe basic methodologies in treatment of poisoning: Decontamination, supportive therapy, antidote therapy, procedures of enhanced elimination	K	K/KH	Y	Lecture/small group discussion, bedside clinic, DOAP session	Written/ viva voce/ OSCE	24
FM8.9	Describe the procedure of intimation of suspicious cases or actual cases of foul play to the police, maintenance of records, preservation and despatch of relevant samples for laboratory analysis	K	K/KH	Y	Lecture/small group discussion	Written/ viva voce	24
FM9.1	Describe general principles and basic methodologies in treatment of poisoning: Decontamination, supportive therapy, antidote therapy, procedures of enhanced elimination with regard to: Caustics inorganic—sulphuric, nitric, and hydrochloric acids; organic—carboloic acid(phenol), oxalic and acetylsalicylic acids	K	K/KH	Y	Lecture/small group discussion, bedside clinic, autopsy, DOAP session	Written/ viva voce/ OSCE	26
FM9.2	Describe general principles and basic methodologies in treatment of poisoning: Decontamination, supportive therapy, antidote therapy, procedures of enhanced elimination with regard to phosphorus, Iodine, barium	K	K/KH	Y	Lecture/small group discussion, bedside clinic, autopsy, DOAP session	Written/ viva voce/ OSCE	28
FM9.3	Describe general principles and basic methodologies in treatment of poisoning: Decontamination, supportive therapy, antidote therapy, procedures of enhanced elimination with regard to arsenic, lead, mercury, copper, iron, cadmium and thallium	K	K/KH	Y	Lecture/small group discussion, bedside clinic, autopsy, DOAP session	Written/ viva voce/ OSCE	27
FM9.4	Describe general principles and basic methodologies in treatment of poisoning: Decontamination, supportive therapy, antidote therapy, procedures of enhanced elimination with regard to ethanol, methanol, ethylene glycol	K	K/KH	Y	Lecture/small group discussion, bedside clinic, autopsy, DOAP session	Written/ viva voce/ OSCE	30
FM9.5	Describe general principles and basic methodologies in treatment of poisoning: Decontamination, supportive therapy, antidote therapy, procedures of enhanced elimination with regard to organophosphates, carbamates, organochlorines, pyrethroids, paraquat, aluminium and zinc phosphide	K	K/KH	Y	Lecture/small group discussion, bedside clinic, autopsy, DOAP session	Written/ viva voce/ OSCE	25
FM9.6	Describe general principles and basic methodologies in treatment of poisoning: Decontamination, supportive therapy, antidote therapy, procedures of enhanced elimination with regard to ammonia, carbon monoxide, hydrogen cyanide and derivatives, methyl isocyanate, tear(riot control) gases	K	K/KH	Y	Lecture/small group discussion, bedside clinic, autopsy, DOAP session	Written/ viva voce/ OSCE	36

Number	COMPETENCY The student should be able to	Domain K/S/A/C	Level K/KH/ SH/P	Core (Y/N)	Suggested teaching learning method	Suggested assessment method	Chapter number
FM10.1	Describe general principles and basic methodologies in treatment of poisoning: Decontamination, supportive therapy, antidote therapy, procedures of enhanced elimination with regard to: • Antipyretics—paracetamol, salicylates • A nti-infectives(common antibiotics—an overview) • N europsychotoxicology barbiturates, benzodiazepins phenytoin, lithium, haloperidol, neuroleptics, tricyclics • N arcotic analgesics, anaesthetics, and muscle relaxants • Cardiovascular toxicology, cardiotoxic plants—oleander, odollam, aconite, digitalis • Gastrointestinal and endocrinal drugs—insulin	K	K/KH	Y	Lecture/small group discussion, bedside clinic, autopsy, DOAP session	Written/ viva voce/ OSCE	37
FM11.1	Describe features and management of snake bite, scorpion sting, bee and wasp sting and spider bite	K	K/KH	Y	Lecture/small group discussion, autopsy	Written/ viva voce	29
FM12.1	Describe features and management of abuse/poisoning with following camicals: Tobacco, cannabis, amphetamines, cocaine, hallucinogens, designer drugs and solvent	K	K/KH	Y	Lecture/small group discussion, autopsy	Written/ viva voce	32, 33
FM14.17	To identify and draw medicolegal inference from common poisons, e.g., dhatura, castor, cannabis, opium, aconite copper sulphate, pesticides compounds, marking nut, oleander, nux vomica, abrus seeds, snakes, capsicum, calotropis, lead compounds and tobacco	S	KH	Y	Small group discussion, DOAP session	Logbook/ viva voce	32, 34

CHAPTER 1

INTRODUCTION

FM 1.1: Demonstrate knowledge of basics of forensic medicine like definitions of forensic medicine, clinical forensic medicine, forensic pathology, state medicine, legal medicine and medical jurisprudence.
FM 1.2: Describe history of forensic medicine.
FM 4.17: Describe and discuss ethical principles: Respect for autonomy, non-malfeasance, beneficence and justice.

There are two distinct aspects of law–medicine relationship: (1) Forensic medicine, and (2) Medical jurisprudence. They are essentially different subjects, but are closely related.

Forensic or legal medicine (forensic = forums of or used in Courts of law) **deals with the application of medical and paramedical knowledge to aid in the administration of justice.** It is used by the legal authorities for the solution of legal problems. Some examples are: Applying the medical knowledge in deciding cases of injuries, murder, suicide, accidents, sexual offences, poisoning, etc. **In short, it deals with medical aspects of law.**

Clinical forensic medicine deals with medicolegal aspects of examination of living human beings caused by or associated with all types of violence and other cases where legal problems are involved.

State medicine deals with legal aspects of practice of medicine, regulating professional activities of medical practitioners, standard and uniformity of medical education, and health requirement of community and environmental health.

Medical jurisprudence (juris = law; prudentia = knowledge) **deals with legal responsibilities of the physician** with particular reference to those arising from physician–patient relationship, such as medical negligence cases, consent, rights and duties of doctors, serious professional misconduct, medical ethics, etc. **In short, it deals with legal aspects of practice of medicine.**

Forensic pathology deals with the study and application of the effects of violence or unnatural disease in its various forms in or on the human body, **in determining the cause and manner of death in case of violence, suspicious, unexplained, unexpected, sudden and medically unattended deaths.**

Medical ethics deals with the moral principles which should guide members of the medical profession in their dealings with each other, their patients and the State.

Medical etiquette deals with the conventional laws of courtesy observed between members of the medical profession. A doctor should behave with his colleagues as he would have them behave with himself.

Ethical behaviour is a self-imposed duty upon each doctor. A doctor should not criticise or denigrate the professional ability of another doctor, while dealing with a patient.

Forensic medicine deals almost entirely with crimes against human beings, in which medical examination and evidence are required. Forensic medicine is mostly an exercise of common sense, combined with the application of knowledge and experience, already acquired in the study of other branches of medicine, surgery, obstetrics, etc. **Its aim is to find out the truth. Its particular field of activity is judicial investigation, both civil and criminal.** All medical work is of a responsible character, especially the medicolegal work, such as issuing certificates of lunacy, ill-health, etc. In all cases of crime involving the person, e.g., homicide, suicide, assault, sexual offences, traffic accidents, poisoning, etc., the help of the medical practitioner is sought by the police. In all such cases, the doctor will be required to appear as an expert witness in a Court of law. In some cases, the doctor is the chief source of evidence upon which legal decisions are made. In cases of sudden death, the authorities will depend mostly or completely on medical evidence in establishing the cause of death, and in case of accident to determine blame.

A doctor may be called to testify (1) as an ordinary witness who saw an incident, (2) as the medical practitioner who treated the patient, (3) as an expert to give his opinion on matter of science. In the first two conditions, it is his duty and obligation to testify. In the last condition, he may refuse the request: (1) if he feels reluctant to undergo what he fears will be a painful experience, (2) if he feels that he is not sufficiently qualified to testify with any conviction in that particular case, and (3) if he feels that he cannot spare the time to prepare properly or to make long appearances in Court. **A properly prepared physician often finds his Court room experience educative and not as traumatic as he would have anticipated.** His introduction to the legal process may be unpleasant, if he is irritated by an aggressive prosecuting or defence lawyer. The reluctance of medical practitioners to become witnesses is mainly due to the pressures of their private practice. Other factors include a fear of merciless cross-examination, harassment, and even the recall.

A doctor should not become partisan. Once a theory is embraced, it is only human nature to eagerly search for facts which support that theory, and reject those which indicate some other theory. **Brouardel, the French medicolegal authority wrote,**

"if the law has made you (the physician) witness, remain a man of science; you have no victim to avenge, no guilty person to convict, and no innocent person to save. You must bear testimony within the limits of science". All forensic science expert witnesses must strive to achieve respect, understanding and credibility in Court. **They must give the appearance, the aura of being independent, non-partisan witnesses.** The appearance and projected image of neutrality, impartiality and objectivity are as important as the authentic characteristics. **Demeanour, appearance, professional manner and general behaviour of the expert witness are almost equal in importance to forensic ability during testimony.** The attitude of a scientific witness should be the same whether he is called by the prosecution or by the defence. **The doctor really testifies neither for nor against the prosecution or the defence.** The doctor's expertise is in the application of science to a legal controversy and the proper interpretation of scientific findings. **The doctor must be honest, for confidence is inspired by honesty and success depends upon confidence. His sole obligation is to present the truth as he sees it,** adding nothing, withholding nothing and distorting nothing. He should not concern himself with the previous character of the accused or with other evidence in the case. He should not be influenced in any way by emotional consideration, such as sympathy or antipathy.

The medicolegal aspects of any case must always be secondary to life saving treatment of the patient. It is advisable that the doctor should learn to look from the medicolegal standpoint upon such of his cases as are likely to become the subject matter of judicial investigation. He should acquire the habit of making a careful note of all the facts observed by him. **Alan Moritz stated "If evidence has been properly gathered and preserved, a mistake in interpretation may always be corrected. If the facts required for a correct interpretation are not preserved, the mistake is irreversible".** He should examine the facts which come to his knowledge in his special capacity, draw his conclusions logically and correctly after a detailed consideration of the pros and cons of the case, and indicate to the Court that interpretation, along with the grounds on which it is based. Vagueness and theory have no place in forensic medicine. **Presumption is not proof, and conjecture is not evidence.** The Court has no special medical knowledge. It relies on his witness for an opinion and expects him to assist it with his special knowledge and experience. The burden of presenting medical facts and medical opinions in the best possible way rests on the doctor. **Forensic pathologist testifies on so-called "fact issues", such as cause and manner of death, rather than "ultimate issue" of guilt or innocence,** so that opinion based upon reasonable medical certainty is adequate to support the testimony of the forensic pathologist. **Medical evidence is not a substantive evidence, but is a corroborative evidence. The medical evidence does not itself prove the case of prosecution. Other things being equal, the better the presentation of medical evidence, the better is the administration of justice.** A good command of language, clear presentation, and ability in expressing a relatively firm opinion are necessary for the success of the medical witness. The presentation of findings involves both writing skills and an ability to express in the courtroom while being examined by trained lawyers. The doctor should avoid talking too much, talking too soon, and talking to the wrong persons. **Prejudicial and sensational statements should not be made prior to trial.** The pathologist should never overlook an opportunity to remain silent. The doctor must be guarded in what he says and how he says it.

The medicolegal expert is not a detective. He may use his knowledge and intelligence to help the police to solve a crime. His role should be to furnish the police with specific information on matters of which he has specialised knowledge. Because of his special knowledge, a non-medical clue may have a significance to him, which even an experienced police officer has not grasped. The medical expert should be very careful when he is examining living people. **He should not encourage an accused person to talk about the crime with which he is charged, or about the events that led to his arrest. If, during a medical examination, an accused says anything that might incriminate himself, it should be neither recorded nor reported.** However, occasions may arise when a doctor may use an admission to direct the police to certain lines of inquiry and action without actually disclosing what has been said.

Three things are needed for success: (1) the power of observation, (2) a wide range of exact knowledge, (3) the power of deduction. The power of constructive imagination is also essential when there are no more facts to be observed, and no further inferences to be drawn. There is no substitute for basic intelligence and clinical competence. Experience, common sense, and willingness to consider other possibilities are as essential in the practice of forensic medicine as a wide range of theoretical knowledge. **The attributes of the physician are: (1) caution, (2) foresight, and (3) wisdom.**

The doctor should develop a fair understanding, satisfactory appraisal and high index of awareness of the medical, philosophical and legal problems related to the determination of the manner of death. **He should be thoroughly familiar with the problems of causality and manner of death.** He should realise that total complications of extraneous injuries do not change the manner of death from unnatural to natural, e.g., the victim of a homicidal attack dying with peritonitis following abdominal injuries and surgery should be certified as homicide victim and not as surgical complications. **The doctor must be alert to where evidence should be looked for, and how it should be interpreted. His failure may make the difference between life and death or between freedom and imprisonment of a suspected person.** It may deprive a widow of compensation to which she is entitled, may cause an innocent person to be prosecuted or punished, may permit a murderer to escape punishment, or may cause some person or institution to be held financially liable to damages for which they were not responsible.

William Osler wrote: "Medicine is a science of uncertainty and an art of probability. Absolute diagnoses are unsafe and are made at expense of the conscience". Medicine is a biological science with the variability inherent in biological matters. Forensic medicine is not an exact science. Unexpected results are produced due to biological variations. One thing that makes medicine so difficult is that there is no such thing as the average man. We can only say the reading is 'within the range of normal". **The most extraordinary events occur in medicolegal practice, and a careful evaluation must always**

be made to ensure that dogmatic statements by medical witnesses do not mislead the investigating officers. In every case, there is an element of uncertainty, and absolute proof is a rarity in any medical problem. There is always a possibility for a difference of opinion among the doctors. No possibility is wholly excluded in medical experience. **Doctors should bear in mind the essential difference between probability and proof. The medical witness should not be dogmatic about his opinion, and also lawyers should not expect him to be so.** They should be reasonable in their opinions and should not overstate the likelihood of a relationship between cause and effect. **The doctor should be ready to defend every finding and conclusion on the report on clinical and scientific grounds. The doctor should put before the court all the materials which are the basis of his conclusions.** He should be aware of professional and scientific viewpoints which might differ from his, and should be familiar with the latest scientific literature in relation to the subject involved. Forensic pathologists have an ethical obligation to contribute to further knowledge, research and education in their field. For the purpose of illustrating and clarifying his testimony, the medical expert may employ photographs, maps, diagrams, charts, X-rays, skeletons, models, slides, films, tapes, etc., when they are properly verified.

Medicolegal practice requires knowledge, skills and attitudes. The skills needed are: (1) Clinical: the ability to elicit a history, to examine for injuries and to perform the appropriate investigations. **(2) Precision** in recording the findings. **(3) The ability to present the findings** in a clear, concise, correct and meaningful manner. **(4) Attitudes:** (a) Proper respect to the patient. (b) Maintain objectivity in recording the findings.

Forensic medicine can be mastered only by an extensive practical experience acquired by an application and study of medicolegal problems. Courts of law are open to the public. Medical students and newly qualified doctors should attend the Courts, where they can follow the proceedings, hear the evidence given by medical witness, and note the questions put and the replies given. This will familiarize the doctor with legal procedures and help to lessen the painful experience of giving evidence.

The general public is fast becoming law conscious and the doctors are being sued from time to time in a Court of law for their acts of omission or commission. Therefore, **it is incumbent upon doctors to have good knowledge of the law governing their profession, in order not to transgress the law. Doctors should avoid special efforts to "cover up" medical negligence or intentional wrong doing.**

HISTORY: Medicine and law have been related from the earliest times and the bonds which united them were religion, superstition and magic. The Charaka Samhita (about seventh century B.C.) lays down an elaborate code regarding training, duties, privileges and social status of physicians. It gives a detailed description of various poisons and their treatment. In fourth century, B.C., Manu (King and law-giver) in his treatise, Manusmriti, laid down various laws including punishment for various sexual and other offences, and recognised mental incapacity due to intoxication, illness and age. Between fourth and third century B.C. Arthashastra of Kautilya defined penal laws and regulated medical practice. Physicians were punished for negligence. Medical knowledge was utilised for the purpose of law. It mentions about the examination of dead bodies in unnatural deaths. Abortion, sexual offences, kidnapping, etc. were punishable offences. Law-medicine problems are found in the written records in Egypt, Sumer, Babylon, India and China dating back 4000 to 3000 B.C. A Chinese materia medica of about 3000 B.C. gives information on poisons. Imhotep (27th century B.C.), Grand Vizir, Chief Justice and chief physician of King Zoser of Egypt, enacted rules for medical practice, which was brought under law. The Code of Hammurabi, King of Babylon (about 2200 B.C.), is the oldest known medicolegal Code. Rig Veda and other Vedas (3000 to 1000 B.C.) mention about crimes like incest, adultery, abduction, killing an embryo, murder, drunkenness, etc. and their punishments. Physicians were identified as professional people. Atharva Veda gives details about remedies for various conditions. Hippocrates (460 to 377 B.C.), the "Father of Western Medicine" was born and practiced in the island of Kos in Greece, discussed the lethality of wounds. His contribution to medical ethics is by far his greatest in medical field. About 300 B.C., the Rabbis of the Rabinical Court, responsible for implementing the Jewish laws, sought the aid of medical expert in the administration of justice. Later, Greek and Roman jurists and medical men collaborated in the development of the principles of forensic medicine. Shushruta (father of Indian surgery), between 200 to 300 A.D. in his treatise Shushruta Samhita dealt with various medicolegal problems. Duties of physicians were defined. Wounds and fractures were classified. Poisons and snakes were classified and treatment prescribed. Modes of administration of poisons was described. In the sixth century A.D. the Justinian Code (Roman emperor) and Institutes regulated the practice of medicine and surgery, and established the function of the medical expert for legal procedure. The first medicolegal autopsy was done in Bologna (Italy) in 1302, by Bartolomeo De Varignana. In the thirteenth century, a manual was prepared to aid in the investigation of death in China. George, Bishop of Bamberg, proclaimed a penal code in 1507, where medical evidence was a necessity in certain cases. Caroline Code was proclaimed in 1553 in Germany by Emperor Charles V. With this expert medical testimony became a requirement rather than an option to give opinions in cases of murder, wounding, poisoning, hanging, drowning, infanticide and abortion, etc. It recognised that there were several types of homicide which were not punishable under certain conditions, one of which was an offender who was 'deprived of his understanding'. The first book on Forensic Medicine was published in 1602 by an Italian physician, Fortunato Fedele. The greatest of all works was the "Questiones Medicolegales" (medicolegal questions), written by Paulus Zacchias, who was principal physician to Pope Innocent X, and Alexander VII, and an expert before the Rota Romana, the Court of Appeal. This was published in seven volumes from 1621 to 1635 and two additional volumes in 1666, at Amsterdam. This work remained an authority in medicolegal matters until the beginning of the nineteenth century. Paulus Zacchias is considered to be the Father of Legal Medicine as well as Father of Forensic Psychiatry. In Questiones Medicolegales, he declared that physicians should have exclusive competence in the field of pathological mental states, amentias. He provided a classification of mental disorders keeping in mind the legal issues at that time.

Around the end of the sixteenth century, autopsies in medicolegal cases began to be generally practised. In the eighteenth century, professorships in legal medicine were founded by the State in Germany. Orfila (1787 to 1853), professor of chemistry and legal medicine at Paris introduced precise chemical methods into toxicology. He is considered the founder of modern toxicology. In 1843, the law regarding the criminal responsibility of insane persons was established in England in Mc Naughten's case. The discovery of DNA fingerprinting in 1985 has revolutionized the field of applied forensic medicine.

CHAPTER

2 LEGAL PROCEDURE

FM 1.3: Describe legal procedures including Criminal Procedure Code, Indian Penal Code, Indian Evidence Act, civil and criminal cases, inquest (police inquest and magistrate's inquest), cognizable and non-cognizable offences.
FM 1.4: Describe Courts in India and their powers: Supreme court, high court, sessions court, magistrate's court, labour court, family court, executive magistrate court and juvenile justice board.
FM 1.5: Describe court procedures including issue of summons, conduct money, types of witnesses, recording of evidence oath, affirmation, examination in chief, cross examination, re-examination and court questions, recording of evidence and conduct of doctor in witness box.
FM 1.6: Describe offenses in court including perjury; court strictures vis-a-vis medical officer.
FM 1.7: Describe dying declaration and dying deposition.
FM 2.18: Crime scene investigation: Describe and discuss the objectives of crime scene visit, the duties and responsibilities of doctors on crime scene and the reconstruction of sequence of events after crime scene investigation.
FM 4.14: Describe and discuss the challenges in managing medicolegal cases including development of skills in relationship management—human behaviour, communication skills, conflict resolution techniques.
FM 4.15: Describe the principles of handling pressure—definition, types, causes, sources and skills for managing the pressure while dealing with medicolegal cases by the doctor.

INDIAN PENAL CODE (I.P.C.), 1860: It deals with substantive criminal law of India. It defines offences and prescribes punishments.

CRIMINAL PROCEDURE CODE (Cr.P.C.), 1973: It provides the mechanism for punishment of offences against the substantive criminal law. It deals with police duties in arresting offenders, dealing with absconders, in the production of documents, etc. and in investigating offences. It provides for different class of Courts. It deals with actual procedure in trials, appeals, references, revisions, and transfer of criminal cases.

INDIAN EVIDENCE ACT (I.E.A.), 1872: It **deals with Law of Evidence** (different categories of evidence, the procedure of collection, preservation and use of different evidences) **and applies to all judicial proceedings in any Court.** It is common to both the criminal and civil procedure.

CRIMINAL LAW deals with offences which are considered to be against the public interest, such as offences against the person, property, public safety, security of the State, etc. Here the State is a party represented by public prosecutor, and the accused is the other party.

CIVIL LAW OR CASE LAW deals with disputes between two individuals or parties. The party bringing the action in a civil case is called "plaintiff". The accused is called "defendant" in both criminal and civil cases.

COMMON LAW is made by judges when they deliver decisions in individual cases.

INQUEST: An inquest is an inquiry or investigation into the cause of death. It is conducted in cases of suicide, murder, killing by an animal or machinery, accidents, deaths due to torture or ill-treatment, occupational diseases, suspected medical negligence, suspicious (unnatural) deaths, deaths due to anaesthesia or operation and unidentified or skeletonised bodies. **Two types of inquests** are held in India.

(1) POLICE INQUEST: The **officer-in-charge (usually sub-inspector but not below the rank of head constable)** of a **police station conducts the inquest** (S.174, Cr.P.C.). The police officer making the inquest is known as Investigating Officer (I.O.). When the officer-in-charge of a police station receives information that a person has committed suicide, or has been killed by another or by an animal or by machinery or by an accident, or has died under circumstances raising a reasonable suspicion that some other person has committed an offence, he immediately gives intimation about it, to the nearest Executive Magistrate empowered to hold inquests, and proceeds to the place where the body of such deceased person is. There, in the presence of two or more respectable persons *(panchas)* makes an investigation (S.175, Cr.P.C). **He prepares a report of the apparent cause of death**, describing wounds, fractures, bruises, and other marks of injury found on the body, and stating in what manner, or by what weapon or instrument, such injuries appear to have been inflicted. The inquest report *(panchanama)* is then signed by the investigating police officer and by the *panchas*. The body is sent for postmortem examination to the nearest authorised Government doctor, without removing clothes together with a requisition (dead body challan) and a copy of the inquest. The report is forwarded to the Magistrate. If no foul play is suspected, the dead body is handed over to the relatives for disposal.

S. 175, Cr. P.C.: A police officer proceeding under S. 174, Cr. P.C., may by order in writing, summon two or more persons for purpose of said investigation and any other person who appears to be acquainted with the facts of the case to answer truly all questions.

Private medical institutions can undertake medicolegal examination and treatment of the living, but autopsies can be conducted only with the permission of the State Government.

(2) MAGISTRATE'S INQUEST: This is conducted by a District Magistrate (Collector/Deputy Commissioner), Sub-divisional Magistrate(RDO), Tahsildar or any other Executive Magistrate especially empowered by the State Government **(Executive Magistrates).** It is done in case of (1) Dowry death. (2) In case of death of a woman within 7 years of marriage, if (a) she commits sucide, (b) dies in any circumstance raising a reasonable suspicion that some other person committed an offence, (c) any relative of the women makes a request, (d) any doubt regarding cause of death, (3) Exhumation. (4) Any person dies or disappears, or rape is alleged to have been committed on any woman, while such person or woman is in the custody of the police or in any other custody authorised by the court (S.174(4), S.176 and 176, 1-A, Cr.P.C.). In any case of death, a Magistrate may conduct an inquest, instead of or in addition to the police inquest (S.176, Cr.P.C.). Death in police custody has been omitted by Cr.P.C. Amendment Act, 2005.

OTHER TYPES: (1) CORONER'S INQUEST: This is a type of inquest done in U.K., some States in U.S.A., and some other countries, but not in India. Coroner conducts inquest in all unnatural and suspicious deaths. The doctor is summoned to his Court to give evidence at the inquest. Coroner's Court is a Court of enquiry, wherein Jurors are sworn to give a true verdict according to the evidence. He has some judicial powers.

(2) MEDICAL EXAMINER'S SYSTEM: This is a type of inquest conducted in most of the States in the United States of America, Japan, Canada, etc. but not in India. A medical practitioner known as Medical Examiner is appointed to perform the functions of Coroner. He does not have any judicial functions similar to the Coroner and he has no authority to order the arrest of any person. As the doctor visits the scene of crime and conducts the inquest, it is superior to Coroner's and police inquest.

JURY: Jury is a group of responsible, educated persons of good social position called "jurors". It is composed of an uneven number of persons. Their verdict is binding on the Judge, but if the Judge differs, the matter is referred to the High Court. Trial by jury has been abolished in India.

COURTS OF LAW: Sections 6 to 25 of Cr.P.C. deal with constitution of Criminal Courts and Offices.

Types: Courts of law are of two types: (1) Civil, and (2) Criminal. The Criminal Courts in India are of four types.

(1) The **Supreme Court** is the highest judicial tribunal, and is located in New Delhi. **It has power of supervision over all Courts in India. It is purely an appellate court in criminal cases.** The law declared by it is binding on all Courts (Article 134 of Constitution of India).

(2) The **High Court** is usually located in the capital of every State and is the highest tribunal for the State (Article 214, Constitution of India). **It may try any offence and pass any sentence authorised by law** (S.28,(1) Cr.P.C.). Judges of High Court are appointed by the president of India.

Supreme Court and High Courts act as Courts of appeal only in criminal cases, and do not hold trial *prima facie*.

(3) The **Sessions Court** is established by the State Government (S.9, Cr.P.C.) and is usually located at the district headquarters. **It can only try cases which have been committed to it by a Magistrate** (S.193, Cr.P.C.). **It can pass any sentence authorised by law, but a sentence of death passed by it must be confirmed by the High Court** (S.28 (2) and S. 366, Cr.P.C.). **District Court** deals with civil cases. An **Assistant Sessions Court** can pass sentence of imprisonment up to ten years and unlimited fine (S.28 (3), Cr.P.C.).

(4) Magistrates courts: Magistrates are of three types (S.11 to 19 Cr.P.C.).

(1) Chief Judicial Magistrate (S. 12, Cr.P.C.).

(2) First Class Judicial Magistrate.

(3) Second Class Judicial Magistrate Table (2-1).

In metropolitan cities with more than one million population, the Chief Judicial Magistrate and First Class Judicial Magistrate are designated as Chief Metropolitan Magistrate and Metropolitan Magistrate respectively (S.8, 17, 18 and 19 Cr.P.C.) Table (2-1).

Sessions judges and magistrates are appointed by the High Court.

When a person is convicted at one trial for two or more offences, twice the amount of punishment, which a Magistrate is authorised can be passed (S.31, Cr.P.C.).

Any sentence awarded by a Court may be enhanced or decreased by a higher Court. State Government has power to suspend, repeal or commute any sentence passed by a Court of law. Appropriate government may commute life imprisonment ≥ (20 years) to 14 years (S.432 and 433 Cr.P.C. 5.54 and 55 I.P.C.).

JUVENILE COURTS: They are established based on the theory that children differ mentally from adults. WHO considers children to be human beings below the age of 18 years. They try offences committed by juveniles (below the age of 18 years) (S. 27Cr. P.C.). Juvenile court is usually presided by a first class woman magistrate and 2 social workers of whom at least one shall be woman.

LABOUR COURTS: Labour Courts are constituted for the purpose of disposal of any proceeding involving any question pertaining to industrial disputes or disputes arising in scope of employment.

FAMILY COURTS: Family Courts are established to promote conciliation in, and secure speedy settlement of, disputes relating to marriage and family affairs and for matters connected therewith.

Public prosecutor (PP) is the lawyer of the state and is the person in-charge of prosecutions (S.24Cr.P.C.).

Juvenile justice board: Juvenile Justice Boards are constituted under Juvenile Justice Act to deal with juveniles (child under 18 years) in conflict with law (S. 27Cr.P.C.). They are established based on theory that children differ mentally from adults.

They are presided over by first class judicial magistrate with at least 3 year experience and 2 social workers of whom at least one shall be woman.

Table (2–1). Powers of Magistrates (S.29, Cr.P.C.)

Class of Magistrate	Imprisonment	Fine
Chief Judicial Magistrate	**Up to seven years.**	**Unlimited (S.63, I.P.C.).**
I Class Judicial Magistrate	**Up to three years.**	**10,000 rupees.**
II Class Judicial Magistrate	**Up to one year.**	**5,000 rupees.**

Offence means any act or omission made punishable by any law [S.2(n) Cr.P.C. and (S.40, I.P.C.)]. Offences are classified as (1) **Bailable**. (2) **Nonbailable**. In bailable offences, the court cannot refuse bail and the police cannot keep the person in custody.

COGNISABLE OFFENCE [S.2(c) Cr.P.C.]: It is **an offence in which a police officer can arrest** a **person without warrant from the magistrate,** e.g., rape, murder, dowry death, sex offences, robbery, ragging, death due to rash or negligent act, etc. In such offences, the individual is sent by the police to the doctor for medical examination (S.2C and 154 Cr.P.C.). In non-cognisable offences [S.2(1) Cr.P.C.] the injured person may go direct to the doctor, or he may file an affidavit in the Court of a Magistrate who will send him to the doctor for examination and report (S.41, Cr.P.C.). In non-cognisable offence, the accused cannot be arrested without a warrant issued by the magistrate.

S.53, I.P.C. Punishments: The sentences authorised by law are: (1) death, (2) imprisonment for life (S.55 and 57, I.P.C.), (3) imprisonment: (a) rigorous, i.e., with hard labour, including solitary confinement (S.73, and 74, I.P.C.), (b) simple (S.60, I.P.C.), (4) fine (S.63, I.P.C.).

Capital punishment (death penalty): The various methods of carrying out death sentence are: hanging, electrocution, lethal injection (continuous i.v. injection of sodium thiopental (unconsciousness), pancuronium bromide (paralytic, stops breathing) and potassium chloride (stops heart), shooting, gas chamber, garrotting and guillotine (a method of decapitation).

According to Article 20 (2) Constitution of India, a person shall not be charged and convicted more than once for the same offence.

The President of India has the power to grant pardons, remissions of punishments and commutation of death sentence.

SUBPOENA OR SUMMONS: Sections 61 to 69 of Cr.P.C. deal with summons. Subpoena (sub = under; poena = penalty) is a **document compelling the attendance of a witness in a Court of law under penalty, on a particular day, time and place, for the purpose of giving evidence.** It may also require him to bring with him any books, documents or other things under his control, that he is bound by law to produce in evidence (subpoena duces tectum) (S.91, Cr.P.C., S.162, I.E.A., and S.175, I.P.C.). It is issued by the Court in writing, in duplicate, signed by the presiding officer of the Court and bears the seal of the Court (S.61, Cr.P.C.). Crime number and name of the accused person are mentioned. It is served on the witness by a police officer, by an officer of the Court or other public servant, by delivering to him one of the copies of the summons. The person should sign a receipt on the back of the other copy (S.62 Cr.P.C.). It can also be served by registered post, or fixed on some conspicuous part of the house in which the person resides. If the person summoned is in the active service of the Government, the Court issuing the summons shall usually send it in duplicate to the head of the office in which such person is employed. Such head shall cause the summons to be served on such person and shall return it to the Court under his signature with the endorsement required by that section (S.66, Cr.P.C.). **A summons must be obeyed, and the witness should produce documents if asked for** (S.91, Cr.P.C.). The witness will be excused from attending the Court, if he has a valid and urgent reason.

Punishment: If the witness fails to attend the Court: (1) In a civil case, he will be liable to pay damages. (2) In criminal cases, the Court may issue notice under S.350, Cr.P.C. and after hearing the witness, if it finds that the witness neglected to attend the Court without any justification, may sentence him to a fine, or imprisonment, or the Court may issue bailable or non-bailable warrants to secure the presence of the witness (S.172 to 174, I.P.C. and S.87, Cr.P.C.). **Non-attendance in obediance to an order from court of law intentionally, i.e., summons (imprisonment up to one month or fine or both** (S.174, I.P.C.).

Priority: Criminal Courts have priority over civil Courts. If a witness is summoned by two Courts on the same day, one of which is criminal and other civil, he should attend the Criminal Court and inform the Civil Court of his inability to attend, giving his reasons. **Higher Courts have priority over the lower.** If he is summoned from two Courts of same status, he must attend the Court from where he received the summons first, informing the other Court about it. He can attend the second Court after finishing his evidence in the first Court.

CONDUCT MONEY: It is the fee offered or paid to a witness in civil cases, at the time of serving the summons to meet the expenses for attending the Court. If the fee is not paid, or if he feels that the amount is less, the doctor can bring this fact to the notice of the Judge before giving evidence in the Court. The Judge will decide the amount to be paid.

In criminal cases, no fee is paid to the witness at the time of serving the summons. He must attend the Court and give evidence because of the interest of the State in securing justice; otherwise he will be charged with contempt of Court. However, in criminal cases, conveyance charges and daily allowance can be claimed by the doctor according to Government rules. Contempt means wilful disregard or disobedience of court's order.

MEDICAL EVIDENCE

Evidence means and includes: (1) all statements which the Court permits or requires to be made before it by witnesses, in relation to matters of fact under inquiry, (2) all documents produced for inspection of the Court (S.3, I.E.A.). For the evidence to be accepted by the Courts, it must be properly identified as to what it is, and where it was found. **The evidence of eye-witness is positive. The evidence of doctor or an expert is only an opinion which is corroborative.**

Types: (1) Documentary: It includes all documents produced for the inspection of the Court.

Sections 61 to 90 of Indian Evidence Act, 1872, **deal with documentary evidence. The contents of the documents may be proved either by primary or by secondary evidence** (S.61, I.E.A.). **Primary evidence means the document itself produced for inspection of the Court** (S.62, I.E.A.). **Documents must be proved by primary evidence except in certain cases** (S.64, I.E.A.). **Secondary evidence means, certified copies, copies made from the original by mechanical processes, copies made from or compared with the original, oral account of the contents of a document** (S.63, I.E.A.). **Evidence must conform to the matters in issue, and is admitted on the basis of relevance and admissibility. (2) Oral. (A) Direct:** Evidence of a fact which is actually in issue, e.g., an electric blanket that has caused injury, prescription, or a consent form. **(B) Indirect or circumstantial:** It is not the direct testimony of an eye witness, but has a bearing upon the fact of the other and subsidiary facts which are relied upon as consistent (S.6, I.E.A.), e.g., in case of alleged murder of A by B at certain place on a particular day and time, the circumstantial evidence would be that C saw B with a knife on that day at that place, a few minutes before the murder. **Circumstantial evidence requires the Court to draw logical or reasonable inferences from the information presented.** **(C) Hearsay: It is any statement made by any person about what he did not personally witness, or evidence he obtained from a third party,** which is presented in the Court in order to assert that the facts contained in the statement are true, e.g., A gives evidence in the witness box stating that B had informed him that he had seen C committing a crime. In such case direct evidence can be given only by B that he had seen C committing a crime.

DOCUMENTARY EVIDENCE: It is of three types.

(1) MEDICAL CERTIFICATES: They **refer to ill-health, insanity, age, death, etc. They are accepted in a Court of law, only when they are issued by a qualified registered medical practitioner**. The certificate of ill-health should contain exact nature of illness. Examine and issue certificate for not more than 15 days. See patient again after 15 days and reissue. Do not give fitness on advanced date or back date. Certificate must address a particular person, such as employer, head master, prinicipal, etc. Certificate is a legal document. The signature or left thumb impression of the patient should be taken at the bottom or top of the certificate. Two identification marks should be noted. **The doctor should retain a duplicate of the certificate issued for 2 years. A medical practitioner is legally bound to give a death certificate, stating the cause of death without charging fee, if a person whom he has been attending during his last illness dies** (Registration of Births and Deaths Act, 1970). **Death certificate should not be issued by a doctor without inspecting the body and satisfying himself that person is really dead.** The certificate should not be delayed, even if the doctor's fees is not paid. **The certificate should not be given if the doctor is not sure of the cause of death, or if there is the least suspicion of foul play. In such cases, the matter should be reported to the police.** Issuing or signing a false certificate is punishable under S. 197, I.P.C.

The medical certification of death: In India, the International Statistical Classification of Diseases, Injuries and Causes of Death is used. The cause of death is divided into two main sections. (1) Immediate cause. This is subdivided into three parts, namely (a), (b), (c). **If a single morbid condition completely explains death, this will be written on line (a) of part I,** and nothing more need be written in the rest of Part I or in Part II, e.g., lobar pneumonia. Next consider whether the **immediate cause is a complication or delayed result of some other cause. If so, enter the antecedent cause in Part I line (b).** Sometimes there will be three stages in the course of events leading to death. If so line (c) will be completed. The underlying cause to be tabulated is always written last in Part I. (II) Other significant conditions contributing to the death but not related to the disease or condition causing it.

(2) MEDICOLEGAL REPORTS: They are reports prepared by a doctor on the request of the investigating officer, usually in criminal cases, e.g., assault, rape, murder, etc. The examination of an injured person or a dead body is made, when there is a requisition from a police officer or Magistrate. These reports consist of two parts: (1) the facts observed on examination (all relevant, objective descriptions including important negative findings), **(2) the opinion drawn from the facts.** These reports will be attached to the file relating to the case and the file is produced in the Court. The report will be open to the scrutiny of the defence lawyer. **It will not be admitted as evidence, unless the doctor attends the Court and testifies to the facts under oath.** Great care should be taken in writing the reports to avoid any loose wording or careless statement. This gives a chance to the defence lawyer to use them to his own advantage. The report should give the date, time and place of examination and the name of individuals who identified the person or the dead body. Exaggerated terms, superlatives, etc. should not be used. **The opinion should be based on the facts observed by himself, and not on information obtained from other sources. In an injury case, if it is not possible to give an opinion immediately, the person should be kept under observation, and necessary investigations should be done before giving the report.** The report should show competence, lack of bias and offer concrete professional advice. The report should be made soon after the examination. **It should be clear, concise, complete, legible and it should avoid technical terms as far as possible. Relevant negative information should also be given. The report should be written in duplicate using carbon papers.** The first copy is sent to the investigating officer and another copy is retained for future reference. **The doctor should sign or initial at the bottom of each page, if the report exceeds one page in length.** The name and designation of the doctor should be noted on the last page of the report and signed.

Exhibits: Clothing, weapons, etc., sent for medical examination should be described in detail, sealed and returned to the police, after obtaining a receipt. An outline of the weapon may be drawn on a paper and the measurement noted or a photograph taken.

(3) DYING DECLARATION: *(Leterm mortem = Words said before death) Section 32(1) IEA.* **It is a written or oral statement of a person, who is dying as a result of some unlawful act, relating to the material facts of cause of his death or bearing on the circumstances (S.32, I.E.A.). If there is time, Executive magistrate should be called to record the declaration.** Before recording the statement, the **doctor should certify that the person is conscious and his mental faculties are normal** *(compos mentis)*. If the condition of the victim is serious, and **there is no time to call a Magistrate, the doctor should take the declaration in the presence of two witnesses.** The statement can also be recorded by the village headman, police or any other person, but its evidential value will be less. **While recording the dying declaration, oath is not administered, because of the belief that the dying person tells the truth.**

Statement: The statement should be recorded in his/her own words, without any alteration of terms or phrases. **Leading questions should not be put.** The declarant should be permitted to give his/her statement without any undue influence, outside prompting or assistance. **If a point is not clear, question may be asked to make it clear, but the actual question and the answer received should be recorded.** It should then be read over to the declarant, and his signature or thumb impression is taken. **The statement made must be of fact and not opinion.** If the declaration is made in the form of an opinion or conclusion, questions should be asked by the recorder to bring out the facts that are the basis for the conclusion. While recording the statement, if the declarant becomes unconscious, the person recording it must record as much information as he has obtained and sign it. **If the dying person is unable to speak, but is able to make signs in answer to questions put to him, this can be recorded and it is considered as a "verbal statement".** The doctor and the witness should also sign the declaration. If the statement is written by the declarant himself, it should be signed by him, the doctor and the witnesses.

Admissibility: The declaration is admissible not only against an accused who killed the declarant, but also against all other persons involved in the same incident which resulted in his death. In India, if the declarant is in a sound state of mind at the time of making the declaration, **it is admissible in Court as evidence, even if the declarant was not under expectation of death at that time.** The declaration is sent to the Magistrate in a sealed cover. **It is produced at the trial and accepted as evidence in case of death of the victim in all criminal and civil cases, where the cause of death is under enquiry.** The person recording the declaration will have to give evidence in the Court to prove it. **If the declarant survives, the declaration is not admitted, but has corroborative value, and the person is called to give oral evidence.** The statement is important to identify the offender or to clear innocent persons.

DYING DEPOSITION: It is a statement of a person on oath, recorded by the Magistrate in the presence of the accused or his lawyer, who is allowed to cross-examine the witness. This procedure is not followed in India.

ORAL EVIDENCE: It includes all statements which the Court permits, or which are required to be made before it by the witness, in relation to matters of fact under enquiry. "Fact" means: (1) any thing, state of things, or relation of things, capable of being perceived by the senses, (2) any mental condition of which any person is conscious (S.3, I.E.A.). **In all cases, oral evidence must be direct** (S.60,I.E.A). **It must be evidence of a person who saw, heard, or perceived it by that sense or in that manner.** If it refers to an opinion or to the grounds on which the opinion is held, it must be the evidence of the person who holds that opinion on those grounds. If oral evidence refers to any material thing, the Court may require the production of such a thing for its inspection, e.g., a blood stained weapon or article of clothing, a portion of eliminated poison, etc. (S.60, I.E.A.). All facts, except the contents of documents, may be proved by oral evidence (S.59, I.E.A.). **A deaf and mute witness may testify by signs, by writing or through an interpreter** (S.119, I.E.A.). **Oral evidence is more important than documentary evidence, as it permits cross-examination. Documentary evidence is accepted by the Court only on oral testimony by the person concerned.**

EXCEPTIONS TO ORAL EVIDENCE: (1) Dying declaration (S. 32, I.E.A.). Statements, verbal or written, of relevant facts made by a person who is dead, who cannot be found, who has become incapable of giving evidence, or whose attendance cannot be procured without unreasonable delay and expenditure, is admissible as evidence (S. 32, I.E.A.). (2) Expert opinion expressed in a treatise may be proved in Court by producing such book, if the author is dead or cannot be found or cannot be called as a witness without unreasonable delay or expense (S. 60, I.E.A.). (3) Evidence of a doctor recorded in a lower Court is accepted in a higher Court, provided it is recorded and attested by Magistrate in the presence of the accused. But he is liable to be summoned, if the evidence is deficient or needs further explanation (S. 291, Cr.P.C.). (4) Evidence given by a witness in a previous judicial proceeding is admissible in subsequent judicial proceeding, when the witness is dead or cannot be found, or is incapable of giving evidence, or cannot be called without undue delay or unreasonable expense (S. 33, I.E.A. and S.291 Cr.P.C.). (5) Evidence of Mint officers or an officer of the India Security Press (S. 292, Cr.P.C.). (6) Reports of certain government scientific experts: (a) Chemical Examiner or Assistant Chemical Examiner. (b) Chief Inspector of Explosives. (c) Director Fingerprint Bureau. (d) Director, Central Forensic Science Laboratories or State Forensic Science Laboratories. (e) Director, Haffkine Institute, Mumbai. (f) Serologist to the Government (S. 293(1), Cr. P.C.). The Court has the power to summon and examine any such expert. The prosecution and defence has also a right to demand the Court to summon and examine any such expert (S.293(2) Cr.P.C.). (7) Public records: A record kept in a public office, e.g., birth and death, certificates of marriage, etc., is admissible in evidence without oral testimony (S. 35, 74, 76 and 78, I.E.A.). (8) Hospital records: Routine entries, such as dates of admission and discharge, pulse, temperature, treatment given, etc., are admissible without oral evidence. But the cause of the disease or diagnosis are not accepted without oral testimony.

EXHIBTTS: (1) Receive in a sealed packet with accompanying letter. (2) Issue receipt. (3) Always touch with gloved hands. (4) Take photographs with scale. (5) Examine in detail. (6) Give reply to the questions put by I.O. (7) Attach an identifying tag. (8) If exhibit has blood stains send it to FSL in a sealed packet and obtain receipt.

Chain of Custody of Evidence: It is a method to verify the actual possession of an object from the time it was first identified until it is offered as evidence in the Court. Each specimen when obtained, should be labelled with the victim's name, the time and date, the nature of the specimen, identification number, and signed by the doctor. This information must be documented each time the material is handled by another person, and that person must give receipt for the material and be included in the chain of custody. **The evidence must not be damaged, contaminated, or altered in any significant way.** The shorter the chain the better.

WITNESSES: A witness is a person who gives evidence regarding facts. Sections 118 to 134 of I.E.A., deal with witnesses. All persons are competent to testify unless they are prevented from understanding the questions put to them, or from giving rational answers to those questions, due to tender years or extreme old age or disease (S.118, I.E.A.).

Types: Witnesses are of two types: (1) Common, and (2) Expert.

(1) COMMON WITNESS (witness of fact; occurrence witness) **is a person who gives evidence about the facts observed or perceived by him.** He must show that he was capable of perceiving the fact by one of his own senses, and that he actually observed this fact. This principle is commonly known as the **"first-hand knowledge rule"**, which may be used to establish the exact circumstances of the case for the Court, e.g., A has seen B and C, fighting with sticks on a certain road on particular day and time. In a case of traffic accident the person who witnessed the accident becomes a common witness.

(2) EXPERT WITNESS is a person who has been trained or is skilled or has knowledge, experience or education in technical or scientific subject, and capable of drawing opinions and conclusions from the facts observed by himself, or noticed by others, e.g., doctor, firearms expert, fingerprints expert, handwriting expert, etc. (S. 45, I.E.A.).

An expert witness may give his opinion (1) upon facts which are either admitted, or proved by himself or other witnesses at the trial, (2) on matters of common knowledge, and (3) on hypothetical questions (questions based on stated assumptions) based thereon. Hypothetical questions may be asked to extract an opinion from the expert, after he assumes certain facts to be true, describing a specific situation, even though he may not have first-hand knowledge of the actual case. The expert should hesitate for a moment, so as to give the opposing lawyer an opportunity to object to the question. The answer should be given only after completely understanding the question. **The main obligation of an expert is to point out professional facts. But, he may be asked to give professional estimate which his observations seem to justify,** e.g., whether or not an injury is caused in the manner alleged or from the causes assumed; the possible consequences; the reasonable estimate of damages, etc. **A doctor's testimony can only be considered evidence when he states that the conclusion he gives is based on "reasonable medical certainty" (more probable than not in a medical sense) that a fact is true or untrue.** In other words, if the likelihood of an event is more probable than not given the facts, the physician can testify with a reasonable medical certainty. **The opinion on a key question must be given in a more guarded manner using terms, such as that the findings are "consistent with" an alleged form of trauma,** such as a fall against a hard object or with the striking of the head with a blunt instrument of a particular type or a blow from a fist. It does not exclude other mechanisms which could reasonably or possibly have caused the same findings. If he is so excessively cautious as to confuse possibilities, probabilities and certainties, his testimony will become ineffective. **Conclusions must be based on facts. Conclusions are much more important than opinions.** The expert who in spite of provocation, answers questions with goodwill and accuracy, and who does not make statements that he cannot defend, will be successful under such attack. Clear presentation, and ability in expressing a relatively firm opinion are helpful for success of the expert. Facts not otherwise relevant, are relevant if they support or are inconsistent with the opinions of experts, when such opinions are relevant.

In medicolegal cases, an expert should not give opinion, unless complete information about the case is available.

The medical evidence does not itself establish the guilt or innocence of the accused. It is only corroborative evidence. In the majority of cases, it provides expert opinions based upon objective, indisputable facts, which help to evaluate the reliability and credibility of other witnesses. **The doctor is not a witness of truth. The expert evidence is of little value, when there is a conflict of opinion between experts.** In such cases, the Courts usually accept that opinion which is not in conflict with direct opinion.

If there is difference between medical evidence of two doctors, one of whom examined the injured person and the other conducted the autopsy on the injured person after his death, as to the injuries, or the weapon used, or the time of infliction of injuries, etc., **the accused gets the benefit of doubt. Where the direct evidence is not trustworthy, conviction may result on medical evidence, if that is trustworthy. An expert witness may refer to books to refresh his memory, or to correct or confirm his opinion** (S. 159, I.E.A.). Books as such are not evidence, but if an expert refers to specific passages as representing his views, they may be taken down as his own evidence. A witness may adopt the views of any authority as his own, provided he has an honest belief in them. **The opinion of an expert can be proved false by standard books on the subject.**

A doctor can be both a common and expert witness. When he describes the wounds on the body, he acts as a common witness. But when he says that the wounds were antemortem or postmortem, or they were suicidal, homicidal, or accidental, or gives opinion regarding the cause of death, he acts as an expert witness.

HOSTILE WITNESS is one who is supposed to have some interest or motive for concealing part of the truth, or for giving completely false evidence (S.191, I.P.C.). **The Court will declare a witness as hostile on the suggestion of the lawyer of the party who has summoned the witness or prosecution lawyer.** On declaration of a witness as hostile (adverse), **he can be cross-examined by the same side lawyer.** Any of the above two types of witness can be hostile.

PERJURY: Perjury means giving wilful false/fabricated evidence. Whoever, being legally bound by an oath, or by an express provision of law to state the truth, or being bound by law to make a declaration upon any subject, makes any statement which is false, and which he either knows or believes to be false or does not believe to be true, is said to give false evidence (S.191 and 192, I.P.C. 344, Cr.P.C.). **It occurs if the person's earlier statement regarding the facts on oath and subsequent statement on oath are opposed to each other, and they cannot be reconciled.** The witness is liable to be prosecuted for perjury, and the imprisonment may extend to seven years (S. 193, I.P.C.).

The medical witness is allowed to sit in the Court if the lawyers of the accused do not object.

RECORD OF EVIDENCE: The evidence of the witness is recorded as follows (S. 138 to 159, I.E.A.): Indian Oath Act 44, S.2,4, and 6, 1969.

OATH: The witness has to take an oath in the witness box before he gives his evidence. He should take the oath as follows: **"I do swear in the name of God,** that what I shall state shall be the truth, the whole truth, and nothing but the truth". If the witness is an **atheist, he has to "solemnly affirm"** instead of "swearing in the name of God." (S.51, I.P.C.).

Oath is a declaration required by the law, which is compulsory and holds the witness responsible for consequences of his evidence. A child below 12 years is not required to take an oath.

S.178 I.P.C: Refusal to take oath is punishable with imprisonment of 6 months or fine or both.

Order of examination (138, I.E.A.):

(1) EXAMINATION-IN-CHIEF (direct examination) (S.137, I.E.A.): This is the **first examination of a witness. It consists of questions put to him by the lawyer (counsel or advocate) for the side which has summoned him. In criminal acts committed by an individual or group, the State becomes a party instead of the aggrieved person, and starts criminal prosecution, which is titled as "State versus A". In a criminal trial, the burden to prove is always on the prosecution** (adversarial system of trial), and **the accused is presumed to be innocent till the contrary is proved against him.** In Government prosecution cases, the public prosecutor first examines the witness (S.24 and 25 Cr.P.C.). If witness is called by private party, he is first examined by the lawyer of that party. **The object is to elicit all relevant, convincing medical facts** (S.138, I.E.A.), **and the conclusions which the doctor has drawn from the facts**. The doctor may have to interpret the findings of non-medical ancillary investigations provided by scientific laboratories, analysts and serologists, in all cases where the medical aspects are at issue. Before giving evidence, it is advisable that the doctor meets the public prosecutor, and discuss the previously prepared report, the certificate of death, photographs, etc., that the witness intends to show in the Court, and an outline or pattern should be worked out for the best way to elicit his testimony. **If the witness intends to modify any of his findings or conclusions, these should be pointed out to the lawyer. The doctor should help the prosecutor in framing proper questions in proper sequence, so that all essential facts are elicited.** The lawyer will be able to advice the doctor in the matters that he will attempt to emphasise and about the anticipated content of cross-examination. **In this leading questions are not allowed, except in those cases, where the Judge is satisfied that a witness is hostile** (S.142 and 154, I.E.A.).

A **leading question** is one which **suggests to the witness the answer desired, or which includes a material fact, and admits of a conclusive answer by a simple "Yes" or "No"** (S.141, I.E.A.). "Was this injury caused by a sharp weapon?" Was the length of cut 3 cm?". "Was it on the front of the abdomen?". They are all leading questions, as they suggest the answer "Yes" or "No". The proper questions should be: "What type of weapon would cause this injury?" What was the length of the cut?. Where was it seen"?

The method of examination is by question and answer. The questions are usually short and demand some specific fact and short answer. But the answer can be given in narrative form, if it would be more informative and convincing. **The effect of the questions and answers is recorded indirectly and not in the form of the question and answer** (S.275 and 276, Cr.P.C.).

(2) CROSS-EXAMINATION: In this, **the witness is questioned by the lawyer for the opposite party, i.e., lawyer for the accused (defence lawyer) (S.137, I.E.A.).** In a murder trial, the defence witness is cross-examined by public prosecutor.

The **main objects are** (1) to elicit facts favourable to his case, (2) to test the accuracy of the statements made by the witness (S.146, I.E.A.), (3) to modify, or explain what has been said, (4) to develop new or old facts, (5) to discredit the witness, and (6) to remove any undue or excessive emphasis which may have been given to any of them. In doing this, the lawyer may try to weaken the evidence by showing that the evidence given is inconsistent, inaccurate, ill-founded, contradictory, and untrustworthy. He may persuade the doctor to go slightly out of his own field of expertise and thereby risk exposure to ridicule by a better qualified expert later in the hearing.

The cross-examination need not be confined to the facts to which the witness testified in his examination-in-chief. The competence and credibility of the witness is tested by questioning his qualifications, experience and the number of cases of the kind under consideration he has personally observed, and by testing his memory or powers of observation. **When material is available, the lawyer may attack the character of the witness** (S.148, I.E.A.). The witness may be asked questions on his bias or impartiality, his previous conviction, his reputation for untruthfulness and on any handicap he may have which would affect the reliability of his evidence (S.153 and 155, I.E.A.). The Court will decide whether the witness should answer any particular question, when asked for a ruling. **The Court may forbid any questions which it regards as indecent or scandalous, unless they relate to facts in issue** (S.151, I.E.A.). The Court also has the power to disallow questions which are intended to insult or harass or offensive in form (S. 152, I.E.A.), but if they are relevant to the facts in issue, the Court cannot disallow them. **The witness has to answer any question relevant to the matter in issue, even though the answer will expose or prove his guilt directly or indirectly, e.g., which would reveal that he has committed an illegal operation** (S.146, I.E.A.). **If a witness is forced to give an answer admitting his guilt, he cannot be arrested or prosecuted for it, and also it is not taken as proof against him in any criminal proceeding (S.132, I.E.A.).** A witness is completely immune from actions for defamation (libel or slander), for anything he says in the witness box.

Answers favourable to the defence side should be given as promptly as those given on examination-in-chief. There are few observations in medicine which are capable of only one explanation. If the defence puts points to the doctor which must be conceded, the doctor should reply that alternative explanations were considered, and on balance he prefers the conclusions already expressed. **The doctor cannot change his opinion while giving evidence in a court, but he can indicate other possibilities.** Admit omissions, e.g., an examination of a drunken person may not require the use of all tests described in a treatise. This can be explained to the Court. Objectivity and impartiality are important against destructive cross-examination.

If a question is not audible, the witness should ask the lawyer to repeat the question. **If the question is not understood, the witness should ask the lawyer to explain it better.** If a question contains several different questions, each requiring a separate answer, the medical witness should ask the lawyer to break the question into individual components. **The medical practitioner should not be dogmatic about his opinion and the lawyer**

should not expect him to be so. The witness should be clear, direct and precise in his answer, as far as possible. **He should not volunteer unrelated information.** The defence lawyer may ask the witness, whether he talked about this case with anyone. The answer should be "Yes". If asked with whom he talked, he should give the name of the lawyer by whom he was called to give evidence. If a further question is put, "What did you talk about?", the most effective answer would be: "He told me to tell the truth". Sometimes, a previously published statement of his own, which may be in disagreement with what he is now stating is quoted against him (S.145, I.E.A.). The effective answer should be, "medicine advances with the times, and I try to advance with its progress".

If the defence succeeds in embarrassing or humiliating the witness, he may become tense, frightened, angry, hostile or aggressive, due to which his intellectual faculties suffer, and he will not be able to think clearly and effectively. When the reply to a question appears to damage the defence case, the lawyer may attempt to interrupt doctor's answer by asking a new question. The witness should say that he has not yet completed his answer to the preceding question. If the Judge rules in favour of the new question, the lawyer for the prosecution side will usually make a note of the question and its answer and will give the doctor an opportunity to complete his reply in re-examination. **The witness must answer a hypothetical question,** but he cannot be compelled to answer a question that is based wholly or in part upon a subject, regarding which he cannot conscientiously reply. **Leading questions are permissible during cross-examination (S.143, I.E.A.). Cross-examination has no time limit,** and may last for hours or even days. The Judge can always disallow irrelevant questions.

Objection to Testimony: When a question is asked of a witness, the opposing lawyer may say, "I object", and give his reasons for the same. The witness should not answer the question until the Court gives a ruling on the objection. If the Judge says, 'Objection overruled", the answer has to be given.

The defense lawyer should not ask a question to which he does not know the answer, for the reply may strengthen the case of the opposite side and seriously hurt his own. **Sometimes, cross-examination may act as a double-edged sword, i.e., it may damage the defence as much as the prosecution,** especially if lawyer is not familiar with the subject and the witness is efficient and honest.

(3) RE-EXAMINATION (Re-direct examination): This is conducted by the lawyer for the side which has called the witness. The object is to correct any mistake or to clarify or add details to the statements the witness has made in cross-examination. It is an opportunity for the witness to explain more fully some answer which might appear damaging to his direct evidence, because of skilful questioning or tactics by the cross-examiner. **The witness should not bring in any new matter at this stage.** The opposing lawyer has right of re-cross-examination on the new point raised (S.138, I.E.A.). **Leading questions are not allowed.**

(4) QUESTIONS BY JUDGE: The Judge may ask any question, in any form, about any fact, relevant or irrelevant, at any stage of the examination to clear up doubts. **The Court is also empowered to recall and re-examine any witness already examined,** if his evidence appears to the Court to be essential to the just decision of the Court (S.165, I.E.A. and S. 311, Cr.P.C.).

The deposition of the witness is handed over to him. The witness after carefully going through it, is required to sign at the bottom of each page, and on the last page immediately below the last paragraph, and to initial any corrections (S.278, Cr.P.C.). The witness should not leave the Court without taking permission of the Judge.

CONDUCT AND DUTIES OF THE DOCTOR IN THE WITNESS BOX

The following rules help a doctor in the witness box. (1) Be well prepared with the details of your evidence before entering the box; anticipate certain likely questions on it and be prepared to answer these in advance. It may be necessary to study the literature on the subject about which he is likely to be cross-examined. (2) Take all records, and relevant reports that may have to be quoted in the box, e.g., original notes, autopsy report, photographs, X-rays, toxicology and blood grouping reports, copy of the death certificate, drawings or diagrams, special reports on swabs or smears, culture studies, serology and various receipts to prove the chain of custody of the items of evidence. The photographs are useful in the Court: (a) to refresh memory of the findings, (b) to establish the identity of the deceased, (c) to explain the findings conveniently, and (d) to provide true-to-life picture of the investigative findings. The records should be in chronological order, and the doctor should have full knowledge of the contents of his file. (3) Do not discuss the case with anyone in the Court, except the lawyer by whom you were asked to testify. (4) Be well dressed, modest and always in time. (5) Stand up straight. (6) Be relaxed and calm and not frightened or nervous. (7) Never attempt to memorise. The law allows to refresh your memory from copies of reports already submitted or from case notes and similar records made at the time of examination. An expert may refresh his memory by reference to professional treatises (S.159, I.E.A.). A writing which is used to refresh the memory of a witness must be shown to the opposite party, if he requires it. Such party may cross-examine the witness thereupon (S.161, I.E.A.). (8) Speak slowly, distinctly, and audibly so that the Judge can record your evidence. It is advisable to watch the pen of the Judge so that the Judge is able to record all the evidence, without asking the witness to pause. (9) Look people in the eye when you speak, for it gives the impression of honesty. (10) Speak with assurance. Be confident but not over-confident or arrogant. (11) Use simple language, avoiding technical terms to the best of your ability. Practice this in advance. (12) Avoid superlatives and exaggerations, e.g., very large bruise, frightful injury, savage blow, most agonising pain, etc. (13) Do not fumble in referring to case notes, records, etc. The less you fumble, the more the Court is likely to be impressed by you. (14) Address the Judge by his proper title, such as "Sir" or "Your honour". (15) Avoid difference between your record and your testimony. If an error or slight contradiction has been made in the testimony, admit and correct it. (16) Do not underestimate the medical knowledge of the lawyers. (17) Be pleasant, polite and courteous to the lawyer. Appearance, professional manner, and general behaviour are important. (18) Do not avoid a question. Say I do not know, if it is so, for no one can be expected to know everything. It indicates honesty. (19) Never become hostile, angry, rude or sarcastic during questioning. (20) Do not lose your temper. An angry witness is often a poor witness, and the effectiveness of his testimony is diminished or destroyed. (21) Defence lawyer may irritate the witness into anger by unfair questions, abuse and unfair remarks. The witness should remain calm and keep his temper. Do not argue, just disagree if you do not agree; disagree firmly and repeatedly. (22) Don't be too anxious to please or too eager to fight. (23) Retain independence of your mind. Be honest, impartial, unbiased and truthful. A biased expert is a useless expert. Be frank to admit any points in favour of the accused if that is the truth. Speak only of facts which come within your personal

knowledge. (24) Do not alter your findings to what is said in statements to be the facts. The doctor should "tell it as it is", and should not choose sides. (25) Listen carefully to the questions. Do not hesitate to ask to have the question repeated, if you do not understand it. If still it is not clear, say so frankly, for the lawyer to reframe the question. Give yourself time to think. (26) Avoid long discussion. Answer should be brief and precise and in the form of "Yes" or "No". Never nod your head to indicate "Yes" or "No". In many medical matters, the answer requires an explanation and the doctor should resist to answer with a simple 'Yes' or 'No'. The witness is not bound simply to answer yes or no, but may qualify his answer if it is necessary for accuracy and completeness, even though the lawyer may try to demand a yes or no answer. The Court usually rules that the doctor may explain his reply. (27) Consider all aspects of the question before answering it. Answer only what is asked. (28) If you believe the question is unfair or that the lawyer is teasing you excessively, look at your lawyer before answering. If he fails to object, turn to the Judge and ask whether you should answer the question. (29) Do not overemphasise replies to questions from the cross-examining lawyer. (30) You may use an opportunity to insert a positive point that you have omitted during your chief-examination; but be careful not to provoke a new line to questioning. (31) Watch for double question and questions that include an assumption of facts which have not been proven. The answer to each part of the double question may be different. This should be emphasised by the witness. He should also state that the assumed facts are not necessarily true. (32) You are an authority in this particular case, as you have examined the patient or the dead body and have specific medical knowledge about it. What applies to many cases in general may not apply to this particular case. (33) Express an opinion from your own knowledge and experience. Say, "In my opinion ...." Do not use phrase such as "I think", or "I imagine". Put before the court all the materials which are the basis of your conclusion. Be prepared to give reasons for your opinion if asked. Never express an opinion on the merits of the case. (34) When the opinion relates to quantity or number, it should be stated within certain limits, unless an exact answer can be given, e.g., the age of an individual. Keep the opinions within the limits of reasonable medical certainty. (35) Do not be drawn outside your particular field of competence. Avoid speaking on a subject in which you have little or no practical experience, e.g., pathologist is not the right person to give evidence on clinical problems or dispensing. A general practitioner is not qualified to give evidence on the pathology of a tumour or on blood group inheritance. In such cases, he should explain that this is not a matter in which he has particular knowledge, and that he is not qualified to answer it. (36) When asked to comment upon the competence of a colleague, avoid any insulting remarks. If he is competent, say so but without superlatives. If you do not wish to make any statement, say that you have "no opinion". (37) An expert may adopt the published opinion of the writers on the subject as his own opinion. The published work need not be produced in the Court. (38) When lawyer quotes a passage from a textbook, and asks the witness whether he agrees with it, the doctor must always take the precaution before answering, of reading the portion which is quoted to him and also of reading a paragraph before and after the quoted passage since it may be taken out of context, and he should satisfy himself that the edition of the book is recent and the views expressed by the author are current. Statements contained in older editions of text books need not be accepted, as the medicine advances. There is no need to accept everything that is written; do not hesitate to disagree as the medicine advances. (39) Textbooks of established repute can be produced in evidence, even though the witness refuses to recognise the authority, or to acknowledge familiarity with its contents. (40) A medical witness has no professional privilege, and therefore he must answer any question. He must first obtain a ruling from the Judge and if directed to answer, he must do so without further delay. (41) **Volunteering of information:** Information should not be volunteered beyond that asked for in the question. The answer should also be limited to the expert's knowledge. Volunteered information is often not well prepared, and is liable to cross-examination. As an expert witness, a medical practitioner may volunteer a statement, if he thinks that injustice will result if he fails to make the statement.

MEDICOLEGAL MASQUERADES: Things are not always what they seem to be at first sight. **Many cases of homicide go undetected because of the lack of suspicion and improper or inadequate investigation.** All cases of death should be regarded as unnatural, until proved otherwise. Violent deaths may show minimal or no external evidence of injury, and conversely natural deaths can occur under such circumstances as to suggest falsely that violence was used. Accidental deaths and suicides can occur under circumstances which suggest homicide. A person who appears to have died from acute alcoholic poisoning or from the combined effects of alcohol and other drugs, may have committed suicide by using drugs, or rarely he may have been poisoned criminally. In a suicide case, alterations may be made at the scene because of disgrace. In a homicide case, the scene may be altered or rigged to suggest that death resulted from suicide or accident. Upset furniture, overturned objects and other disturbances, and blood stains on walls and floors are consistent with a struggle between assailant and victim. However, similar disturbance may be seen in case of suicide committed while the victim was acutely intoxicated by alcohol or some drug, or he was possessed by some form of psychotic excitement. Persons dying from natural causes may become hypoxic and confused terminally. They may fall against furniture and knock items over, and the scene may appear ransacked. The doctor must look for any possible inconsistencies between the apparent death scene and his actual scientific findings. In a case of hanging, the manner in which a ligature is applied to the neck, or the mode of suspension of a body may determine the manner of death. In such cases, the real cause of death can be established by complete autopsy and police investigation. The investigating officer should obtain information about the circumstances of death and the background of the deceased.

INVESTIGATION OF THE SCENE OF DEATH

Basic rules: The basic rules for investigation of any scene of crime are: (1) Verify that a crime has been committed. (2) Look for signs of how it was committed. (3) Recover and preserve evidence that might lead to the arrest and conviction of the guilty.

For murder though it has no tongue, will speak with a most miraculous organ (Shakespear in Hamlet).

The dead do tell tales.

The answers to the following questions (6W's) have to be found to prove the guilt and convict the accused.

(1) Who is the victim? (identification).
(2) When the death and injuries occurred? (time of death and injuries).
(3) Where the death occurred? (scene and circumstances of death).
(4) What injuries are present? (description of injuries).
(5) Which injuries are significant? (major, minor, true, artefacts, postmortem injuries).
(6) Why and how injuries were produced? (mechanism and manner of death, i.e., natural, accidental, suicidal or homicidal). If unnatural, determine the means or agent causing death, e.g., knife, firearm, poison, etc., and if homicide assist in identifying the person responsible for death.

CONDUCT AND DUTIES OF THE DOCTOR AT THE SCENE OF CRIME: Crime scene investigation aids in identification of suspects or victims, prove or disprove alibi, identify a modus operandi, establish the corpus delicti and establish associations among victim, suspect, scene and evidence. It is the responsibility of the police to preserve and protect the scene of crime. The doctor can ask police to arrange his visit to the scene of crime. The doctor should carry with him a hand lens, measuring tape and ruler, gloves, slides, swabs, chemical thermometer, and envelopes if possible. Complete and accurate recording of the scene as it was found is very important. This can be done by accurate diagrams, notes and photography. The scene may show evidence of a struggle, and on the body vital trace evidence may be present. The examination at the scene should be limited to a search for such evidence which might be dislodged or possibly lost during the transfer of the body to the mortuary. If a doctor sees the dead body for the first time in the autopsy room, he may form incorrect opinions about the origin of various injuries. Seeing the body at the scene of crime with the various surrounding objects, helps to avoid such mistakes. The visit to the scene of death is more valuable if the body shows a patterned injury, the origin of which is in doubt. Even a retrospective visit to the scene enables the doctor to have a true appreciation of the nature of the surroundings, which are usually found to differ from the impression formed from the descriptions of other persons, and will be of help in interpretation of the findings in the victim. The scene of a violent death usually shows significant findings for understanding, reconstructing and solving problems. The finding of a dead body together with evidence of burglary indicates murder. Disturbance of furniture may be seen sometimes, if a person dying suddenly and naturally falls down and injures himself. The sequence of events preceding death must be reconstructed logically to support or contradict inferences from other areas of investigation. The fatal injuries should be evaluated to find out how much purposeful action and walking, the victim could have carried out before he became disabled and died. In every case, priority must be given to the injured, and to any action designed to prevent further casualties. Evidence to connect victim, suspect and location of the murder may be found at the scene of the incident, on the clothing or bodies of victim and suspect, or some other place to which the body was transported.

(1) He must make sure that death has occurred. (2) If the victim of an assault is living when first seen, the doctor must do everything to save the life. (3) If death is about to occur, he should obtain a dying declaration, for otherwise valuable information will be lost, e.g., in criminal abortion. (4) He must obtain all possible information regarding the crime. (5) If he suspects foul play, the police should be informed. (6) He should retain any material which is relevant, e.g., in cases of suspected poisoning, he must look for and retain any specimens, such as vomit, leftover poison, or drinking utensils. (7) He must identify the body, which should also be identified by the relatives and the police. (8) He must enquire whether the body has been moved at all before he first saw it. (9) **Never touch, change, or alter anything until identified, measured and photographed.** He should ask the investigating officer before moving anything. Photograph the scene from several angles. He should follow but not lead the police around the scene. (10) **He should not give opinions without proper thought.** (11) **He should make adequate notes which should include:** (a) Date, time, address or location. (b) Name and sex of deceased. (c) A list of all persons present. (d) General observation about the scene; any evidence of struggle, such as overturned furniture, disturbed wall hangings, broken door or window glass pieces, displaced articles or trampled ground. If outside, record the type of weather, the state of ground and the vegetation present. (e) Temperature of the surroundings, and rectal temperature of the deceased should be taken. (f) Make a sketch noting such points of importance as direction and position of blood (pools or splashes) on the body and at the scene, position of the body and any weapons. If the weapon is in the hand of the deceased, note whether it is loosely held or tightly grasped. A correlation should be attempted between injuries present and possible weapons or other objects which might have caused them. The distribution of blood stains and their shape, which may point to the site of injury should be noted. Note the amount of bleeding at the scene. It makes the evaluation of injuries more accurate and may give indication as to the length of survival after the injuries. The plan need not be scale accurate, but the relative measurements should be accurate. Describe the clothing and note any tears, cuts, missing buttons, etc. Do not put objects through defects in clothing or wounds. Examine the hands and forearms for defence wounds. Make note of injuries and record them on body diagrams. (g) Position and appearance of the body, rigor mortis, postmortem lividity, etc., which assist in estimating the time of death. (h) Free hair, fibres or other foreign matter which is likely to be dislodged when the body is moved, should be searched and removed with adhesive tape. (i) If there are any bite marks, they should be swabbed with a cotton wool swab moisted with saline. Saliva swabs may be taken after wearing gloves to prevent the soiling of the swab with sweat. (j) The pubic hair should be combed *in situ* in cases of sexual assault, and loose hair collected. (k) In cases of rape and suspected abortion, an absorbent pad should be strapped over the vulva to collect any fluid which may run out during the transfer of the body. (l) The objects on premises, e.g., dates on mail and newspapers, condition of food on table, etc. to determine the time of death. (m) Photograph any ligature before removal, cut if necessary leaving the knots intact. (n) If a weapon is found, handle it with care to preserve fingerprints, blood stains, hair, fibres, etc. (o) Leave firearms in the condition they are found. Note position of each bullet and casing. (p) Bullets, etc., should be marked for identification. (12) **Use a pencil or other objects to open doors and cabinets.** If the weapon is not found at the scene of death, advise the police about the type of weapon that is likely to have been used. (13) **He should not smoke or throw cigarette stubs, matches or anything at the place of suspected crime,** as trace evidence including small items left behind by a suspect, may play a large part in the proof of the crime. Saliva on cigarette ends may be grouped to include or exclude suspects. (14) The scene should be examined by fingerprint examiner, followed by a trace evidence specialist. (15) Transfer the body to the mortuary wrapped in a large sheet of plastic or other clean cloth so as to retain any loose objects, hairs, fibres, etc. (16) The police should be advised not to remove the clothing, etc. from the body.

BODY LIFTING AND MOVING: The dead body should be carefully lifted and placed on to a bed sheet, length of plastic or body bag and wrapped for transport. With heavy bodies, decomposed or fragile remains, the body should be rolled on to its side and the plastic stuck underneath the body. The body can then be lifted using the plastic to hold the remains intact. In case of suicide by firearms, paper bags are placed securely over the hands.

PHOTOGRAPHS: They should show (1) General relations of the scene of body to its surroundings. (2) Special relationships between the deceased and weapon or blood stains, overturned furniture, etc. (3) Means of possible entrance to and exit from the scene. (4) Position and posture of the victim.

Take a scaled photograph of the scene as it was first viewed. A second scaled photograph should be taken, locating in the field of camera with suitable markers any small objects, such as fired cartridge case, bullet holes in walls, etc. A scaled drawing of the room or the area of interest in the investigation should be made. The dead body should be photographed from different angles.

Photographs of all injuries, major and minor, are essential. The skin should be cleaned of blood, dirt or foreign material. A ruler and a case number or other identifying information must be present in the photograph of the injury. The ruler should be placed on the skin surface adjacent to the injury at the same height as the injury. The photograph must be taken with the camera perpendicular to the skin surface. Close up photograph should be taken so that injury should fill most of the picture area. To indicate important features, markers or pointers can be inserted. If the powder residues are on the victim's skin, a scaled photograph should be made, including the entire area over which the powder residues exist. Photographs help the investigating officer and the doctor to refresh their memories for giving evidence in the Court. They also convey essential facts to the Court.

DISADVANTAGES OF THE DOCTOR NOT VISITING THE SCENE: (1) When the body is transferred to mortuary, fresh abrasions may be produced on it during transit. (2) Clothing will be disarranged, blood stains will form on parts of clothes originally free from them. When the body is lying on the back with a stab wound on the front of the chest or abdomen, the external blood loss is minimal or absent. When the body is turned, large amount of blood may escape through the wound and stain the clothes. (3) Fresh tears in clothes may be produced from

rough handling. (4) Existing rigor mortis may be broken down at least partially.

Basic Rules for Preservation of Medicolegal Evidence: For evidence to be legally accepted by the Courts: (1) It must be obtained in a legal manner. (2) It must be relevant to the issue. (3) The chain of custody of the item must be intact and known. (4) It must be evaluated by qualified experts.

COLLECTION OF EVIDENCE: (1) Collect every article even remotely likely to be helpful in the investigation. Note the source and the relative location of the exhibits at the time they were recovered. (2) Collect any item likely to carry fingerprints. (3) Use separate container for each item. (4) Every article collected must bear identifying marks. Two marking methods are commonly used. (A) Direct, in which marks are put on the item of evidence itself. (B) Indirect, in which notations of identification are placed on a container in which the evidence is placed. The container should be labelled. The data to be recorded on the label are: case number, location and description of the recovered evidence, a specific number, person who recovered the evidence, date of recovery and initials. The disadvantage of attaching a tag is, it can be accidentally torn off or intentionally removed as the evidence is handled or examined forensically. (5) Exhibits must be protected against mutilation, alteration, or contamination. If any alteration has been made between the time the exhibit was recovered and the time it was offered in evidence, this must be justified by the laboratory technician.

PRESERVATION OF PHYSICAL EVIDENCE: Use: (1) Card board "pillbox" type of containers. (2) Envelopes. (3) The pharmacist fold using paper. (4) Film containers (35mm). (5) Plastic vials and jars are useful for small samples, e.g., hair, bullets, blood and organs. (6) Airtight, leakproof, unbreakable containers for liquids and volatile substances. (7) Plastic bags for organs, clothing and larger articles, and to cover the hands or other parts of the body. (8) Larger plastic bags may be used for bodies.

Avoid excessive handling of the evidence that is gathered, as it may cause contamination or loss of transitory materials.

PROCEDURE OF CRIMINAL TRIAL

TYPES OF TRIAL: (1) Adversarial system: It is for the prosecution to prove their case to the Magistrate, beyond reasonable doubt. The defence does not have to prove innocence. (2) Inquisitorial System: (applied in Europe). Both the prosecution and defence have to make their cases to the court, which then chooses which is more credible.

The proceedings of investigations by the police in criminal offences are sent to the Judicial Magistrate of the area. **All offences punishable with death, imprisonment for life, or for a term exceeding two years are tried as warrant cases. All other cases are tried as summons cases.**

Standard of proof: In criminal cases, the **prosecution must provide evidence of a sufficient quality to convince the Court "beyond reasonable doubt" that the accused is guilty.** In civil cases the standard is based on the "balance of probabilities", so that the Court should be certain of more than 50% of the defendants culpability.

SUMMONS CASES: When the accused appears before the Court, he is given the details of the charged offence and asked whether he pleads guilty or not. If the accused pleads guilty, his plea is recorded and he is convicted. If he does not plead guilty, the Magistrate takes all the evidence supporting the prosecution, and takes the evidence produced in defence. On a consideration of all this evidence, he either finds the accused guilty and convicts him, or not guilty, and acquits him (S.251 to 255, Cr.P.C.).

WARRANT CASES: In cases filed by the police, when the accused is brought before the Court, the Magistrate must make sure that the accused has received all the required documents (207, Cr.P.C). The Magistrate considers the documents, examines the accused, and hears the prosecution and defence. If he finds the charge groundless, he records his reasons and discharges the accused. If there are grounds for believing that an offence has been committed, he frames a written charge against the accused, which is read out and explained to the accused, who is asked to plead. If he pleads guilty, the plea is recorded and he may be convicted on that plea. If he pleads not guilty, a date is fixed for the examination of the witnesses, and the prosecution evidence is recorded, during which the accused is permitted to cross-examine the prosecution witnesses. Next, the defence evidence is recorded, during which the prosecution is allowed to cross-examine the defence witnesses. After this, the lawyers for prosecution and defence make oral arguments before the Court in regard to the evidence, and the conclusion therefrom, regarding the guilt or innocence of the accused. If the Magistrate finds the accused guilty, he passes the sentence, otherwise he acquits him (S.238 to 249, Cr.P.C.).

SESSIONS TRIAL: In case of grave charges like murder, rape, etc. whether the accused pleads guilty or not, the Magistrate frames a charge of the offence (228, Cr.P.C.), which is read and explained to the accused, and passes an order committing the accused to trial by Court of Sessions, and records briefly the reasons for such commitment (209, Cr.P.C.). The Magistrate should supply copy of police report and other documents to the accused free of cost (S.207, Cr.P.C.). A warrant is issued to keep the accused in custody (87, Cr.P.C.). The Magistrate sends the charge, the record of enquiry and any weapon or other thing which is to be produced in evidence, to the Court of Sessions (209, Cr.P.C.). The Magistrate has power to take bond from any witness for appearance in his Court or any other Court to which the case may be transferred for trial (S.88, Cr.P.C.). At the first hearing, the public prosecutor opens the case by describing the charge against the accused and stating the evidence by which he proposes to prove the accused guilty of the offence charged (S.226, Cr.P.C.). If after going through the record, and hearing the submissions of the defence and the prosecution, the Judge considers that there is no sufficient ground for proceeding against the accused, he discharges him, recording his reasons for doing so (S.227, Cr.P.C.). Otherwise, the Judge frames a charge which is read out and explained to the accused and his plea is recorded (S.228 Cr.P.C.). If he pleads guilty, he may be convicted, otherwise a date is fixed for hearing (S.230, Cr.P.C.). The prosecution witnesses are called. Each witness is examined by the prosecutor, and may be cross- examined by the defence, and re-examined by the prosecution, as well as questioned by the Court. If, after hearing the prosecution evidence, examining the accused, hearing the prosecution and the defence, the Judge considers that there is no evidence that the accused committed the offence, he passes an order of acquittal (S.232, Cr.P.C.). If the accused is not acquitted, he is asked to defend himself. Any written statement submitted by the accused is filed with the record. The defence witnesses are then called. Each witness is examined by the defence, and may be cross-examined by the prosecutor and re-examined by the defence, and as well as questioned by the Judge. **The evidence of all the witnesses is recorded in writing either by Judge himself or by his dictation in open Court.** At the conclusion of the evidence, the prosecution sums up the case and the accused or his lawyer is entitled to reply, and the prosecutor may enter his submissions if permitted by the Judge. If the accused is found guilty, he is convicted, otherwise he is acquitted (S.225 to 235, Cr.P.C.). The judgement in every trial shall be pronounced in open Court (S.353, Cr.P.C.). Copy of judgement is given to the accused (S.363, Cr.P.C.). **Both the prosecution and defence can appeal to a superior Court against an acquittal or conviction in a lower Court.** When the Court of Sessions passes the sentence of death, the proceedings are submitted to the High Court for confirmation of the sentence (S.366, Cr.P.C.).

EXAMINATION OF MEDICOLEGAL CASES: Medical officers while dealing with medicolegal cases should bear in mind the following points. (1) Following category of cases should be labelled as medicolegal; accidents: traffic, machinery or animal, fall from a height, etc; assault; sexual offences; criminal abortion; burns; scalds and electrical injuries; poisoning; intoxication; snake bite, etc.; comatose patients; cases brought in terminal stages; cases brought dead; sudden unexpected death; suicide, homicide and infanticide; deaths occurring during operation or under anaesthesia; drug mishaps; suspicious deaths; cases referred from police or court. It is desirable that all major accidents should be labelled as M.L.C. to avoid complications at later date. It is left to the police to investigate. **If the case brought has been registered medicolegal at some other hospital, a fresh medicolegal report is not necessary. (2) Medicolegal cases should be examined without delay at any time of day or night.** Depending on the seriousness or otherwise of illness or injury, the patient should be admitted or referred to some specialist. Cases of head injury or abdominal injury in which symptoms are obscure should be admitted for observation. **(3) A private hospital or nursing home can treat and admit medicolegal cases except victims and accused of rape cases.** (4) **Medical Officer has no jurisdiction.** He has to examine all medicolegal cases sent by the police. (5) Obtain informed consent from the patient. **(6) Note at least two identification marks which are individualistic, preferably on the exposed areas of the person. In the case of mole, colour, size, shape, hairy or not, raised or not, and the exact anatomical location should be noted. In case of scar, note colour, size, shape, site, fixed or free, smoothness or irregularity of the surface, presence or absence of glistening and tenderness, and the direction. In case of tattoo mark, note colour, design, size, and situation.** (7) In all medicolegal cases, details of examination of injured person, whether admitted into hospital or treated as outpatient have to be entered in an Accident Register. The details of examination including name, address, date and time of examination should be entered. The general condition of the patient, state of consciousness, B.P., pulse, respiration, temperature, treatment given, etc. should be recorded. This register is a confidential record and should be in safe custody of the medical officer so that it may not be tampered. When the register has been fully utilised, it should be sent to Medical Record Section. (8) **If a patient is admitted, and later it turns out to be M.L.C., such case has to be made M.L.C. by entering in the Accident Register. The certificate will have to be issued by the doctor who labels it as M.L.C.** by referring to the case sheet and consulting the treating doctor. (9) The police should be informed about all cases labelled as M.L.C. (10) **Treatment gets priority over medicolegal formalities.** If the condition of the patient is serious and it is not possible to prepare a detailed medicolegal report, adopt life-saving procedures, and admit the patient after noting the general condition. The report should be prepared later in the ward by examining the case sheet and consulting the treating doctor. (11) **General history and a specific history of the particular incident should be obtained from the victim. In case of criminally accused person, no attempt should be made to obtain any history of the specific incident. It should be limited to questions about the causation of injuries only. If the accused says anything that might incriminate him, it should be neither recorded nor reported.** The history includes past illness or injury, current medication, substance abuse and alcohol consumption prior to arrest. (12) If death is imminent, the doctor should arrange for a **dying declaration.** (13) If the patient is treated as outpatient it should be mentioned in the report. (14) **Immunisation** should be carried out when necessary. Take adequate history about drug allergy. If history of drug allergy is available, do skin sensitivity test. The doctor should be ready to deal with any adverse drug reaction. Administer a test dose in all doubtful cases. **If death occurs due to drug reaction, inform police.** Empty ampule/vial, or the drug should be preserved. (15) Carry out all the necessary investigations. (16) When the injured person is a victim of criminal assault is admitted and treated and later referred to a higher centre for expert treatment, the doctor who has examined the case first has to prepare the wound certificate. **In an emergency, first aid should be given, and if he sends the case without recording the injuries, his inability to record relevant findings must be intimated, which would enable the second medical officer to make proper records.** (17) **All the documents and the material collected as evidence,** e.g., stomach wash sample, vomit, blood, urine, etc. in poisoning cases, vaginal swabs and pubic hair in sexual offences, foreign bodies found in wounds, blood and urine samples in drunkenness, etc., **should be properly preserved, packed and sealed and kept in safe custody till they are handed over to the police after obtaining a receipt. If the clothing is removed, it should be sealed and handed over to the police.** (18) In a case of poisoning, stomach wash should be done immediately and the specific antidote administered. Admit the patient. (19) In a criminal case, obtain a second medical opinion from a senior doctor if surgery has to be performed. (20) **The doctor should seek help from appropriate sources (experts) in difficult situations to finalise any report. The person should be referred to a specialist depending on the merits of each case.** (21) In case of difference of opinion between two experts, such as a radiologist and orthopaedic surgeon, the medical officer should adopt the opinion which he considers correct. The opinions of the experts should be attached to the file and sent to the Court. (22) **Overwritings, alterations and interpolations should be avoided. Nothing should be erased or obliterated. If a correction has to be made of a prior entry in the report, it should not be totally obliterated, but a single line should be drawn through the word to be changed, and the correct information should be written above and initialled. Avoid abbreviations.** (23) **Medicolegal reports should be issued as soon as possible to help the investigation.** The injured person must be kept under observation, if the nature of a particular injury cannot be made out at the time of examination, and the report should be given after necessary X-ray and laboratory investigations. (24) **All forms filled for X-ray, laboratory examination, etc. should be labelled by the words M.L.C.** (25) **In case of discharge or death of a medicolegal case in the hospital, the police having local jurisdiction should be**

informed without delay and death certificate should not be issued. (26) **Inform the police before discharging against advice of a medicolegal case.** (27) At the time of discharge, detailed instructions should be given in writing about the treatment and general care including diet, exercise, etc. (28) **If a person is brought dead to the hospital do not examnine the wounds, inform the police and do not hand over the body to the relatives. Fill the death certificate form if available, or note it on the outpatient ticket, without giving the cause of death.** (29) **Do not issue death certificate and do not release the body to the relatives, if (a)** the injured was brought dead, (b) a crime has already been registered by police, (c) the police has already been informed about the case, (d) when the cause of death is not known. (30) **Autopsy to be conducted on a body or not is the discretion of the police, but not of the doctor.** (31) **There is no jurisdiction for the doctor, and he has to conduct autopsy on anybody brought to him.** (32) **The doctor cannot refuse to conduct autopsy if inquest report is not given.** (33) Either a male or female medical officer can conduct autopsy on a male and female body. (34) In a dead body viscera have to be preserved if the police gives requisition. (35) **Always write injuries are antemortem in autopsy report.** Note age of injuries. (36) **Do not omit to mention vital facts in the report.** The accused will get benefit of doubt if a vital fact is omitted. (37) **If a patient dies during treatment, it is better that the doctor who was treating the patient should not conduct autopsy on that body.** Similarly, if the deceased happens to be a close relative or friend of the doctor, he should not undertake the autopsy. (38) If opinions are given to police before evaluation of data are complete, they should be clearly and unmistakably labelled as preliminary impressions, subject to change if and when the facts so warrant. (39) **The medical officer can always consult an expert if needed,** in determining the cause of death. (40) If postmortem is conducted by two doctors and they do not agree as to the cause of death, they have to read a standard textbook, and if necessary consult an expert. (41) The report should be given on the same day or as early as possible, as the details cannot be accurately recorded from memory, if there is much delay. (42) Keep confidential all information about medicolegal cases. **Postmortem report is not a public document. Postmortem report should be given only to the police.** The concerned party can obtain a copy of the report from the police, or the court, which will be issued only after filing the charge sheet. **However a xerox copy of postmortem certificate can be issued to a relative of the deceased or his authorised person on a written request on payment of the cost of reproduction in accident and natural death cases for the purpose of claiming compensation.** An undertaking should be taken that the report will be used for the stated purpose only and will not be misused for any other purpose. (43) No time limit is prescribed by law for preserving medicolegal reports. (44) **If the investigating officer gives requisition for any clarifications regarding any points in the report, the answers should be given in writing** (S.161, Cr.P.C.). (45) If the investigating officer requires any documents, such as case sheet, either the original or the xerox copy, it should be given and a receipt obtained (S.91, Cr.P.C.). (46) If the Court requires X-rays, postmortem report, or any other documents, they should be deposited in the Court and a receipt obtained. (47) **The doctor can be summoned to the police station for recording a statement if the investigation demands** (S.160 Cr.P.C.). The summoned person is bound to attend and answer questions put to him. Refusal to answer questions is punishable with imprisonment up to six months (S.179, I.P.C.) (48) **Oral statements made to the police and recorded by the police should not be signed** (S.162, Cr.P.C.).

CHALLENGES IN MANAGING MEDICOLEGAL CASES

Most of the doctors fear due to the challenges faced while handling medicolegal cases such as dealing with the police, handling the patient and their attendees. Doctors dealing with medicolegal issues (or) cases feel tremendous pressure.

These challenges could be easily addressed by acquiring thorough knowledge of handling medicolegal cases through various workshops, seminars and trainings.

Dealing with conflict with patients and relatives: Conflict with patient or relatives can be best avoided with collaboration which require open communication, often requires assertiveness and creative problem solving. (1) Remain calm and composed. (2) Create a calm atmosphere to be in a position to talk to the relatives. (3) Do not let conflict situations fester: do something about the situation. (4) Do not react without thinking the situation through. (5) Maintain respect throughout. Do not personalise the dispute. (6) Be aware of the sorts of issues that can turn into conflict. (7) Choose an appropriate time where the other party is more amenable to listening and there are no time pressures. (8) Discuss the matter in a neutral location away from the patient. (9) Begin the discussion on a broader level by asking open questions and answering them clearly and precisely. (10) Focus on the issues and listen respectfully to their viewpoint. (11) Respect on both sides is likely to improve the chance of a positive outcome. (12) If there is any chance of escalation of conflict or fear of threat to life or injury initiate Code Purple.

Stress in handling medicolegal cases: Stress is the psychological and physical state that results when the resources of the individual are not sufficient to cope with the demands and pressures of the situation. Situations that are likely to cause stress are those that are unpredictable, uncontrollable, uncertain, ambiguous, non-familiar, involving conflict, loss or performance expectations and misunderstanding. Stress may be caused by time limited events, such as apprehension of dealing with police, the pressure of avoiding errors or fear of attending courts. Stress can be avoided by professional competence, avoiding confrontation, enhancing communication skills and constant upgradation of the knowledge.

CHAPTER

3 MEDICAL LAW AND ETHICS

FM 1.9: Describe the importance of documentation in medical practice in regard to medicolegal examinations, medical certificates and medicolegal reports especially.

- Maintenance of patient case records, discharge summary, prescribed registers to be maintained in health centres.
- Maintenance of medicolegal register like accidentregister.
- Documents of issuance of wound certificate.
- Documents of issuance of drunkenness certificate.
- Documents of issuance of sickness and fitness certificate.
- Documents for issuance of death certificate—documents of Medical Certification of Cause of Death—Form No. 4 and 4A.
- Documents for estimation of age by physical, dental and radiological examination and issuance of certificate.

FM 4.1: Describe medical ethics and explain its historical emergence.

FM 4.2: Describe the Code of Medical Ethics 2002 conduct, etiquette and ethics in medical practice and unethical practices and the dichotomy.

FM 4.3: Describe the functions and role of Medical Council of India and State Medical Councils.

FM 4.4: Describe the Indian Medical Register.

FM 4.5: Rights/privileges of a medical practitioner, penal erasure, infamous conduct, disciplinary committee, disciplinary procedures, warning notice and penal erasure.

FM 4.6: Describe the laws in relation to medical practice and the duties of a medical practitioner towards patients and society.

FM 4.10: Describe communication between doctors, public and media.

FM 4.11: Describe and discuss euthanasia.

FM 4.18: Describe and discuss medical negligence including civil and criminal negligence, contributory negligence, corporate negligence, vicarious liability, res ipsa loquitur, prevention of medical negligence and defenses in medical negligence litigations.

FM 4.19: Define consent. Describe different types of consent and ingredients of informed consent. Describe the rules of consent and importance of consent in relation to age, emergency situation, mental illness and alcohol intoxication.

FM 4.20: Describe therapeutic privilege, malingering, therapeutic misadventure, professional secrecy, human experimentation

FM 4.21: Describe products liability and medical indemnity insurance.

FM 4.22: Explain oath—Hippocrates, Charaka and Sushruta and procedure for administration of oath.

FM 4.23: Describe the modified Declaration of Geneva and its relevance.

FM 4.24: Enumerate rights, privileges and duties of a registered medical practitioner. Discuss doctor-patient relationship: professional secrecy and privileged communication.

The medical profession is governed by legislation and by a Code of Ethics and Etiquette. Ethics is a voluntarily self-imposed code of conduct by the medical profession. The broad principles of medical ethics are formulated by National and State Medical Councils and the World Medical Association. Enforcement of the Code is done by the Medical Councils.

NATIONAL MEDICAL COMMISSION

National Medical Commission (NMC) is a Statutory body established under The National Medical Commission Act, 2019 (NMC Act). NMC came into existence on 25th September 2020 as the country's apex regulator of medical education and profession after dissolution of 63 year old Medical Council of India (MCI).

Composition: NMC comprises of thirty-three members, including one Chairman, ten ex-officio members and twenty-two part-time members. Out of the twenty-two part-time members, a total of nineteen are nominated by States and Union Territories. The Chairperson, certain part-time members and the Secretary of the NMC are appointed by the Central Government on the recommendation of a Search Committee.

Powers/Functions: NMC has been empowered to lay down policies and regulation to ensure: (1) (a) the observance and promotion of professional ethics in the medical profession and provision of care by medical practitioners, (b) assess requirements in health care, including human resources for health and healthcare infrastructure, (c) develop a road map for meeting such requirements, (2) to frame guidelines for determination of fees and all other charges in respect of fifty percent of seats in private medical institutions and 'deemed to be universities', which are governed under the provisions of the NMC Act, (3) to grant a limited license to practice medicine at mid-level as a Community

Table (3–1). Table highlights the differences between the NMC Act and the Indian Medical Council Act (MCI Act)

S. No.	NMC Act	MCI Act
(1)	The governing body under the NMC Act is the NMC.	The governing body under the IMC Act is the MCI.
(2)	All the members of the NMC will be appointed or nominated by the Central Government.	MCI is majorly comprised of members who are elected from amongst members of the medical faculty of Universities and State Medical Registers/Council.
(3)	Section 5 of the NMC Act provides for the composition of a seven-member Search Committee, which shall include, the Chairperson, part-time Members [in terms of Section 4(1) and 4(4)(a) of the NMC Act] and the Secretary (in terms of Section 8 of the NMC Act), who shall be appointed by the Central Government upon the recommendation of the Search Committee.	No such provision is provided under the IMC Act.
(4)	Constitution of Autonomous Boards	No such boards
(5)	Introduction of exit exams for all candidates	Only for FMGE candidates

Health Provider (CHP) who is qualified as per the prescribed criteria and can prescribe specified medicines, independently, in primary and preventive health care, (4) conducting the National Eligibility-cum-Entrance Test (NEET) and regulating the manner of conducting common counselling by the designated authority for admission to undergraduate and postgraduate, super-specialty seats in all the medical institutions, (5) for conducting the National Exit Test (NEXT), a common final year undergraduate medical examination, to be known as the (NEXT), to be held for granting licenses to practice medicine as medical practitioners and for enrolment in the State Register or the National Register. The basic difference between new NMC and old MCI is given in Table (3–1).

OTHER STATUTORY BODIES

Composition: Each Autonomous Board consists of a President, two whole-time members and two part-time members.

Functions: (1) Under-Graduate Medical Education Board grants recognition to a medical qualification at the undergraduate level. It develops competency-based dynamic curriculum for addressing the needs of primary health services, community medicine and family medicine. It frames guidelines, minimum requirements and standards for setting up of medical institutions, conducting course and examinations and norms for infrastructure, faculty and quality of education. It also facilitates faculty training and development, research and the international student and faculty exchange programmes. (2) **Post-Graduate Medical Education Board** grants recognition to a medical qualification at the postgraduate and super-specialty level. It also develops competency-based dynamic curriculum to develop appropriate skill, knowledge, attitude, values and ethics. It frames guidelines, minimum requirements and standards for setting up of medical institutions, conducting course and examinations and norms for infrastructure, faculty and quality of education. It also facilitates faculty training and development, research and the international student and faculty exchange programmes. It promotes and facilitates postgraduate courses in family medicine. (3) **Medical Assessment and Rating Board** grants permission for establishment of a new medical institution, or to start any postgraduate course or to increase number of seats and carries out inspections of medical institutions for assessing and rating. (4) **Ethics and Medical Registration Board** maintains National Registers of all licensed medical practitioners. It regulates professional conduct, promotes medical ethics and exercises appellate jurisdiction with respect to the actions taken by a State Medical Council.

MEDICAL ADVISORY COUNCIL

Composition: The Chairperson and all members of the NMC (as ex-officio members), the Chairman of the University Grants Commission, the Director of the National Assessment and Accreditation Council, and various other members to be nominated by the State Governments, Ministry of Home Affairs in the Government of India, State Medical Council, and the Central Government.

Functions: It acts as the primary platform through which the States and Union Territories may put forth their views and concerns before the NMC and helps in shaping the overall agenda, policy and action relating to medical education and training. It advises the NMC on measures to determine and maintain, and to co-ordinate maintenance of the minimum standards in all matters relating to medical education, training and research, and measures to enhance equitable access to medical education.

STATE MEDICAL COUNCILS

The **State Medical Councils are autonomous bodies** established under the State Medical Council Act. Each of these Medical Councils consist of members elected by the registered medical practitioners and those nominated by the State Government. The president and the vice-president of the Council are elected by the members from among themselves.

Functions: (1) Medical Register: The Council appoints a Registrar, who keeps a Register of medical practitioners. **Any person having any of the recognised medical qualification, can get his name registered.** The name, residence, qualifications and the date on which each qualification was granted of every person who is registered under this Act are entered in the Register on payment of prescribed fees. After passing the qualifying examination, it is necessary to undergo a period of training, before such qualification is granted to him. **A provisional registration in a State Medical Register is given to such person on application to enable him to practice medicine in an approved institution for the required period. Any additional qualification obtained later, can also be registered.** The Registrar should inform the Indian Medical Council without delay of all additions and other amendments in the State Medical Register made from time to time.

The general principles mentioned in the **Hippocratic Oath** have been brought up-to-date by the World Medical Association. The modernised versions of the Hippocratic Oath are the **Declaration of Geneva,** as adopted by the Third General Assembly of World Medical Association at Geneva, Switzerland, in September, 1948, and the **International Code of Medical Ethics,** as adopted by the General Assembly of the World Medical Association held in London, in October, 1948.

THE DECLARATION OF GENEVA: At the time of registration, each applicant shall be given a copy of the following declaration by the Registrar concerned and the applicant shall read and agree to abide by the same. The applicant shall submit a duly signed declaration. (1) I solemnly pledge to consecrate my life to the service of suffering humanity. (2) I will give to my teachers the respect and gratitude which is their due. (3) I will practise my profession with conscience and dignity. (4) The health of my patient will be my first consideration. (5) I will respect the secrets that are confided to me, even after the patient has died. (6) I will maintain by all the means in my power, the honour and noble traditions of the medical profession. (7) My colleagues will be my brothers/sisters. (8) I will not permit consideration of age, disease or disability, creed, ethnic origin, gender, nationality, political affiliation, race, sexual orientation, social standing or any other factor to intervene between my duty and my patient. (9) I will maintain the utmost respect for human life. (10) I will not use my medical knowledge to violate human rights and civil liberties, even under threat, contrary to the laws of humanity. (11) I shall abide by the Code of Medical Ethics as enumerated in the Indian Medical Council (professional conduct, etiquette and ethics) Regulations, 2009. I make these promises solemnly, freely and upon my honour.

Signature, name, place, address, date.

(2) Disciplinary Control: They have the disciplinary control over the medical practitioners. **They have the power to remove the names of medical practitioners permanently or for a specific period from their Registers when after due enquiry they are found to have been guilty of serious professional misconduct.** They are also authorised to direct the restoration of name so removed.

(3) They can issue **warning notice** similar to that of the Indian Medical Council.

Judicial Procedure of State Council: These proceedings are started: (1) When information reaches the office of the Council that a registered medical practitioner has been convicted of a cognisable offence or has been censured by judicial or other competent authority in relation to his professional character, or has been found guilty of conduct which *prima facie* constitutes serious professional misconduct. (2) By a complaint being made by some person or body against the practitioner. (3) Suo moto. The Council has the same powers as Civil Courts under Code of Civil Procedure, 1908. This makes all the enquiries on the misconduct of doctors to be judicial proceedings within the meaning of S.193, 219 and 228 of I.P.C.

Complaint: The Registrar of the Council submits the complaint to its president. The matter is referred to the Sub-committee or to the Executive Committee, which considers the complaint, causes further investigation and takes legal advise. **If no prima *facie* case is made out, the complainant is informed accordingly.** If an enquiry is to be made, a notice is issued to the practitioner specifying the nature and particulars of the charge and directing him to answer the charge in writing, and to attend before the Council on the appointed day. At the hearing, the complainant or his legal adviser, and the practitioner must be present. **After the conclusion of evidence, vote is taken and the judgement given. If the majority vote confirms that the charge has been proved, the Council must vote again and decide whether the name of the practitioner should be removed from the register or he should be warned, not to repeat the offence.**

Deletion from the register shall be widely published in local press as well as in the publications of different Medical Associations/Societies, Bodies.

Erasure of Name: The name of the doctor is removed from the medical register: (1) After the death of the registered practitioner. (2) Entries which are made in error or as a result of fraud. (3) **Penal erasure:** The main cause for erasure is serious professional misconduct, and this is known as penal erasure. It is sometimes termed **"the professional death sentence".** It deprives the practitioner of all the privileges of a registered practitioner.

Serious Professional Misconduct: (Infamous conduct in professional respect): It is any conduct of the doctor which might reasonably be regarded as disgraceful or dishonourable. The conduct of the doctor is judged by professional men of good repute and competence. It involves an abuse of professional position.

WARNING NOTICE: A registered medical practitioner is required to observe certain prescribed rules of conduct contained in Code of Medical Ethics, published by the Medical Council of India, and by several State Medical Councils. **The Council gives examples of offences which constitute serious professional misconduct, but it stresses the fact that it is not a complete list. The Council can also consider any form of alleged professional misconduct,** which does not come within any of the offences contained in the Warning Notice. Each case has to be decided on its specific facts and merits. **If any one is found guilty of any of the following acts of commission or omission mentioned in the Warning Notice issued by the Medical Council of India, shall constitute professional misconduct rendering him liable for disciplinary action.** (1) **Improper conduct with a patient** or by maintaining an improper association with a patient. Adultery has been decriminalized. (2) Conviction by a Court of Law for offences involving moral turpitude/criminal acts. (3) Issuing a false, misleading or improper certificate in connection with sickness benefit, insurance, passport, attendance in court, public services, etc. (4) Contravening the provisions of the Drugs and Cosmetics Act and regulations. (a) Prescribing steroids/psychotropic drugs, when there is no absolute medical indication. (b) Selling Schedule 'H' and 'L' drugs and poisons to the public except to his patients. (5) Issuing certificates of efficiency in modern medicine to unqualified or non-medical persons. (**Note:** The foregoing does not restrict the proper training and instruction of bonafide students, midwives, dispensers, surgical attendants or skilled mechanical and technical assistants and therapy assistants under the personal supervision of physicians). (6) A physician may patent surgical instruments, appliances and medicines or copyright publication methods and procedures. The use of such patents or copyrights or the receipts of remuneration from them, which retards or inhibits research or restrict the benefit derivable therefrom are unethical. (7) Running an open shop for sale of medicines, for dispensing prescriptions of other doctors or for sale of medical or surgical appliances. Manufacturing or sale of proprietary medicine whose formulae are not displayed on the label. (8) **Advertising:** (a) A physician should not contribute to the lay press articles and give interviews regarding diseases and treatments which may have the effect of advertising himself or soliciting practices; but is open to write to the lay press under his own name on matters of public health, hygienic living or to deliver public lectures, give talks on the radio/TV/internet, chat for the same purpose. (b) He should not advertise himself through manufacturing firms directly or indirectly. (9) An institution run by a physician for a particular purpose such as a maternity home, nursing home, private hospital, rehabilitation centre or any type of training institution, etc., may be advertised in the lay press, but such advertisements should not contain anything more than the name of the institution, type of patients admitted, type of training and other facilities offered and the fees. (10) (a) It is improper for a physician to use an unusually large signboard and write on it anything other than his name, qualifications obtained from a University or a statutory body, titles and name of his speciality, registration number including the name of the State Medical Council under which registered. The same should be the contents of his prescription papers. (b) It is improper to affix a signboard on a chemist's shop or in places where he does not reside or work. (c) A physician can announce in lay or professional press, his starting of practice, interruption or restarting of it after a long interval, or a change of his address, but such an announcement shall not appear more than twice. (11) **Dichotomy or fee-splitting,** i.e. receiving or giving commission or other benefits to a professional colleague or manufacturer or trader in drugs or appliances or a chemist, dentist, etc. (12) **Covering,** i.e. **assisting someone who has no medical qualification to attend, treat or perform an operation on some person in respect of matters requiring professional discretion or skill.** (13) Association with manufacturing firms: (a) A physician should not have any personal ownership in patents for any drug, apparatus, or instrument used in medicine or surgery. He should not ask or receive rebates or commission from prescribing of any agent used therapeutically. (b) A physician must not write prescriptions in private formulae of which only he or a particular pharmacy has the key. He can keep certain lotions or mixtures as long as the formulae of the same are available. (14) Disclosing the secrets of a patient that have been learnt in the exercise of his/her profession except (i) in a court of law under orders of the presiding judge; (ii) in circumstances where there is a serious and identified risk to a specific person and/or community; and (iii) notifiable diseases. In case of communicable/notifiable diseases, concerned public health authorities should be informed immediately. (15) Refusal on religious grounds alone to give assistance in or conduct of sterility, birth control, circumcision and medical termination of pregnancy when there is medical indication, unless the medical practitioner feels himself/herself incompetent to do so. (16) Failure to obtain consent from the patient for an operation or from guardians in case of a minor. (17) Failure to obtain consent of both husband and wife for an operation which may result in sterility. (18) A registered medical practitioner shall not publish photographs or case reports of his patients without their permission, in any manner by which their identity could be made out. If the identity is not to be disclosed, the consent is not needed. (19) In the case of running of a nursing home by a physician and employing assistants to help him, the ultimate responsibility rests on the physician. (20) A physician shall not use touts or agents for procuring patients. (21) A physician shall not aid or abet torture. (22) A physician should observe the laws of the country in regulating practise of medicine and will not assist others to evade such law. (23) A physician shall not claim to be specialist unless he has special qualification in that branch. (24) Drunk and disorderly so as to interfere with proper skilled practice of medicine. (25) No act of in vitro fertilisation or artificial insemination shall be undertaken without the informed consent of the female patient and her spouse as well as the donor. Such consent shall be obtained in writing, only after the patient is provided, at her own level of comprehension, with sufficient information about the purpose, methods, risks, inconveniences, disappointments of the procedure and possible risks and hazards. (26) Clinical drug trials or other research involving patients or volunteers as per the guidelines of ICMR can be undertaken, provided ethical considerations are borne in mind. Violation of existing ICMR guidelines in this regard shall constitute misconduct. (27) If he/she does not display the registration number accorded to him/her by the State Medical Council or the Medical Council of India in his clinic, prescriptions and certificates, etc. issued by him. (28) If he/she does not maintain the medical records of indoor patients for a period of three years and refuses to provide the same within 72 hours when the patient or his authorised representative makes a request for it. (29) On no account sex determination test shall be undertaken with the intent to terminate the life of a female foetus developing in her mother's womb, unless there are other absolute indications for termination of pregnancy. Any act of termination of pregnancy of normal female foetus amounts to female foeticide.

The important offences may be described as "the 6 A's". (1) Adultery arising out of professional relationship. (2) Advertising. (3) Abortion (unlawful). (4) Association with unqualified persons in professional matters. (5) Addiction. (6) Alcohol.

Rights and Privileges of Registered Medical Practitioners: (1) Right to practice medicine. (2) Right to choose a patient. (3) Right to dispense medicines. (4) Right to possess and supply dangerous drugs to his patients. (5) Right to add title, descriptions, etc., to the name. (6) Right to recovery of fees. (7) Right for appointment to public and local hospitals. (8) Right to issue medical certificates. (9) Right to give evidence as an expert.

Physicians can suffix to their names only recognised medical degrees/diplomas and membership/honours, which confer professional knowledge or recognise any exemplary qualifications/achievements.

RED CROSS EMBLEM: It is the distinctive sign of the medical services of an army, whose members, buildings, equipment and vehicles it protects in time of war (protective sign). In war, it also covers the formations of national Red Cross Societies and other recognised relief societies assisting the medical services of an army. The sign is conferred on national Red Cross Societies in the exercise of their other humanitarian activities. This entitles them, in peace as well as in war, to mark their persons and properties with the sign. Its use is permitted to the members of Army Medical Corps and to the Red Cross Society during war and also during rendering their service to the human society in peace time. The Red Cresent embliem is used in 33 Islamic countries

and Red Crystal emblem is used in Isreal, in place of Red Cross. The Geneva Convention Act, 1960, under S.12, prohibits use of Red Cross and other allied emblems such as "Red Crescent", "Red Crystal" for any purpose without approval of the Government of India. S.13, lays down the penalty for unauthorised use with a fine up to Rs. 500/- and forfeiture of the goods upon which emblem was used. The use of the Red Cross and allied emblems by medical practitioners is prohibited.

DUTIES OF MEDICAL PRACTITIONERS

Duty refers to the obligation to act or refrain from acting in such a way that a patient's medical condition is appropriately diagnosed and managed so that a patient is not exposed to an unreasonable risk of injury.

The following are the various types of duties: **(I) Duty to Exercise a Reasonable Degree of Skill and Knowledge: The duty of care arises simply by examining someone for signs of illness or trauma or even by accepting a patient onto a list of existing patients.** As soon as a doctor gives advice and counselling over the telephone, a legal duty to the patient arises. If no advice is given, no duty arises. Exception might be made in cases of acute emergency where life-saving instructions are given over the telephone. **For hospitals, a duty will usually arise once the patient has been admitted, but in the case of an accident or emergency unit, a general duty of care is owed to the patient.** He owes this duty to the child even when engaged by his father. He owes this duty even when patient is treated free of charge. It neither guarantees cure nor an assured improvement. A practitioner is not liable because some other doctor of greater skill and knowledge would have prescribed a better treatment or operated better in the same circumstances.

Case: (1) Whiteford Vs Hunter and Gleed (1950): A consulting engineer of London was examined by a consulting surgeon who diagnosed enlarged prostate by doing rectal examination and advised operation. The surgeon did not use a cystoscope or make a biopsy. On opening the bladder, he found an inoperable carcinoma and opined the expectancy of life to be only a few months. The patient gave up his business and went to U.S.A., where a cystoscopic examination showed a prostate with a median bar, and the pathological examination revealed chronic cystitis. An operation was performed and the calcareous material was removed from the diverticulum. There was no evidence of cancer. The patient sued the doctor for negligence and was awarded damages. The surgeon appealed and the Court of Appeal held that a mistake in diagnosis was not enough to justify negligence.

(2) Wood Vs Charing Cross Hospital: A drunken person was hit by a lorry. The doctor who examined him found no clinical evidence of bone injury or any abnormality, but the stethoscope was not used. The patient died 2 days later, and the autopsy showed fracture of one clavicle and 9 ribs on each side and congestion of lungs. The Court found the doctor negligent in not exercising reasonable care in his examination.

(3) Paynee Vs Helier: A patient was kicked in the abdomen by a horse. He went to the hospital 9 hours after the injury, where he was examined by the Casualty Officer, who was qualified 2 years ago. He found a bruise in the right iliac fossa, but did not find anybody or visceral injury. The patient was sent home, who became very ill after some days and was operated but died later. The Court found the doctor negligent as he made a wrong diagnosis due to his failure to exercise reasonable skill and care.

(II) Duties with Regard to Attendance and Examination: When a practitioner agrees to attend a patient, he is under an obligation to attend to the case as long as it requires attention. He can withdraw only after giving reasonable notice or when he is asked by the patient to withdraw. **He cannot withdraw without the consent of the patient except for valid reasons,** such as: (1) That he himself becomes sick. (2) That he is convinced that the patient is malingering. (3) Remedies other than those prescribed by him are being used. (4) That his instructions are being ignored. (5) That previous financial obligations are not being fulfilled by the patient. (6) That another practitioner is also attending the patient. (7) That the patient persists in the use of intoxicants or poisons.

If a physician is unable to treat the patient when his services are needed, he may provide a qualified and competent substitute doctor to give the services. If the practitioner cannot cure a patient, he need not withdraw, if the patient desires his services. **He should not get his patient examined or operated upon by another doctor without his permission. If the doctor is called by the police to attend a case of accident, he may give first aid and advice, but here no doctor-patient relationship is established. A medical practitioner need not accept as patients all who come to him for treatment.** He may arbitrarily refuse to accept any person as a patient, even though no other physician is available. However, **he should know that the Code of Ethics requires that in an emergency, no physician should refuse to treat a patient.** There is no law to compel a doctor to attend a patient except during military necessity.

Case: Newton Vs Central Middlessex G.H.M.S.: Newton was taken to the hospital after an accident. A doctor examined him but failed to diagnose the fractured patella and wrote, 'No clinical fracture' on the hospital card. Later, the patient saw two other doctors at the hospital, who relying on the hospital card, did not examine the knee, though the patient had complained of pain in the knee. The patient sued both the doctors for negligence. The Court held that the first doctor was not guilty because the patient went to him only for a dressing. The second doctor was held negligent as he failed to examine the knee himself.

(III) Duty to Furnish Proper and Suitable Medicines: If the doctor has his own dispensary, he should furnish the patient with suitable medicines. Otherwise, **he should give a legible prescription, mentioning full and detailed instructions.** The doctor is held responsible for any temporary or permanent damage in health, caused to the patient due to wrong prescription.

(IV) Duty to Give Instructions: The doctor should give full instructions to his patients or their attendants regarding the use of medicines and diet. He should mention the exact quantities and precise timing for taking medicines. **Patients should be instructed regarding the adverse reactions and to stop the drug in case of reaction, and to approach the doctor immediately.**

Case: Ball Vs Howard: The plaintiff was operated for appendicitis. The surgeon did not call another surgeon for consultation (though the patient requested for the same as he developed some complications), and went away without leaving proper instructions as to what was to be done. The patient called another surgeon, who performed a second operation after which the patient made a good recovery. The Court held that the first surgeon was negligent in not attending to the patient with reasonable promptness and in going away without giving instructions.

(V) Duty to Control and Warn: A physician has to warn patients of the dangers involved in the use of a prescribed drug or device. If the doctor fails to inform the patient of the known or reasonably foreseeable dangerous effects of a drug or device, he becomes liable not only for the harm suffered by the patient, but also for injuries his patient may cause to third parties. **If a drug is administered which might affect a patient's functional ability, such as driving a car or operating**

machinery or equipment, the doctor should explain the danger to the patient, and/or to someone who can control the patient's activities, such as the family, an employer, or the authorities. Similarly, when a doctor detects a medical condition that may impair the patient's ability to control his activities, the doctor has a duty to warn the patient, family, employer or authorities. **The doctor has a duty to warn the patient about his medical condition and treatment that could injure others, e.g., the doctor treating epileptic patient may be liable for injury to others caused by his patient, due to failure to advice the patient of the risks of engaging in dangerous activities, under the concept of "Reasonable foreseeability".**

(VI) Duty to Third Parties: If a patient suffers from an infectious disease, the doctor should warn not only the patient, but also third parties known to be in close contact with the patient. These include relatives, friends, co-workers, and/or proper authorities who can protect these potential victims.

(VII) Duty Towards Children and Adults incapable of taking care of themselves: When applying hot water bottles to children, special care should be taken, for the child may be injured. Special precautions should be taken in case of adults who are incapable of taking care of themselves due to insanity or some physical disability. **Precautions should be taken to prevent accidents or harm.**

Case: A woman was placed in a bed after an operation in which a hot water bottle was negligently left, due to which she was severely burnt between her shoulders. The surgeon came to see her while she was recovering from the anaesthetic. She complained to the surgeon about the pain between her shoulders, but he paid no attention to her. The Court held the doctor negligent and awarded damages.

(VIII) Duty to Inform Patient of Risks: A mentally sound adult patient must be told of all the relevant facts. If the treatment or operation proposed carries special risks which are known to the doctor but are probably not known to the patient, the doctor should inform the patient of these risks and obtain his consent. The inherent risk is one of a number of known adverse effects (or injuries) that may result from the mere use of an individual drug or the mere proper performance of a diagnostic procedure or surgical operation. **A material risk is a particular inherent risk, i.e. one known adverse effect or complication associated with a drug, procedure or treatment, that physician knows would be a significant factor in a person's decision whether to reject or accept treatment. But under certain conditions arising out of psychological factors, some facts have to be withheld.**

Case: Kankan Vs Beharelal: A prescription was given to Kankan for ear trouble, which was used as directed by the doctor. The patient developed pain and acute sensation in the ear after a year, and on examination, the drum of his right ear was found destroyed. The evidence showed that the doctor has prescribed a new and dangerous mixture for a petty complaint, and if the mixture had been used after thorough shaking, no harm would have resulted. The High Court held the doctor negligent, as he failed to warn the patient of the risk involved.

(IX) Duty with Regard to Poisons: Poisons should be handled carefully. Each poison should be kept in a separate bottle, properly labelled and kept in a separate cupboard or upon a separate shelf. When a doctor is called upon to treat a case of poisoning: (1) he should give immediate treatment, and (2) **he should assist the police in determining whether the poisoning is accidental, suicidal or homicidal.**

(X) Duty to Notify Certain Diseases: A doctor is bound to give information of communicable diseases (smallpox, chickenpox, cholera, plague, typhoid, measles, diphtheria, yellow fever, food poisoning), births, deaths, etc., **to the Public Health authorities.** If a doctor fails to conform to the statutory or administrative requirements, he will be liable not only for criminal penalties, but also for negligence in civil suits brought by injured parties.

Legal and Ethical issues: (1) Informed consent autonomy of patient. (2) Poor communication. (3) Unexpected outcome. (4) Retained foreign bodies. (5) Surgery on wrong site. (6) Extended hospital stay.

(XI) Duties with Regards to Operations: (1) He should explain the nature and extent of operation and take consent of the patient. (2) He should take proper care to avoid mistakes, such as performance of operations on the wrong patient or on the wrong limb. (3) When a surgeon undertakes to operate, he must not delegate that duty to another. (4) He must not experiment. (5) He must be well-informed of current standard practice and must follow it. (6) He must operate with proper and sterilised instruments. (7) He should make sure that all the swabs, instruments, etc., put in are removed. (8) He should take proper postoperative care and should give proper directions to his patient when discharging him.

(XII) Duties Under Geneva Conventions: In Geneva, in 1949, four conventions were agreed upon. Each convention lays down that the persons it protects, whether the wounded or sick of the armed forces (first convention), ship-wrecked persons (second), prisoners of war (third), or civilians of enemy nationality (fourth), are **to be treated without any adverse distinction based on sex, race, nationality, political opinions or any other similar criteria. Priority is authorised only for urgent medical reasons.**

(XIII) Duties with Regard to Consultation: Consultation should be advised preferably with a specialist in the following conditions. (1) If the patient requests consultation. (2) In an emergency. (3) When the case is obscure or has taken a serious turn. (4) If the quality of the care or management can be considerably enhanced. (5) When an operation or a special treatment involving danger to life is to be undertaken. (6) When an operation affecting vitality of intellectual or generative functions is to be performed. (7) When an operation of mutilating or destructive nature is to be performed on an unborn child. (8) When an operation is to be performed on a patient who has received serious injuries in a criminal assault. (9) In homicidal poisoning. (10) When a therapeutic abortion is to be procured. (11) When a woman on whom criminal abortion has already been performed has sought advice for treatment.

The consent of the patient must be taken. The doctor must tell the patient, whether he is being transferred to the consulting physician or only consulting, or it will be joint participation, and whether it will be on a continuous or intermittent basis. **A referring physician is relieved of further responsibility when he completely transfers the patient to another physician. The referring physician may be held liable under the doctrine of 'negligent choice', if it can be proved that the consultant was incompetent or had a reputation as an "errant" physician. All information about the patient must be transferred to the consultant by the referring physician.** The consultant should advise the patient to return to the practitioner who has referred him. If the patient refuses, the consultant should talk to the referring doctor and settle the matter.

Case: Molseworth's Case: The patient engaged a senior surgeon for hernia operation, but he was operated upon by a house-surgeon. The Court held that the house-surgeon had operated without the plaintiff's consent; that for an unauthorised person to do, in competent manner, an act which another was authorised to do, was technical form of trespass and patient was awarded nominal damages.

(XIV) Duty in Connection with X-ray Examination: As far as possible, **all cases of accident, unless they are very minor, should be X-rayed.** The radiologist should take precautionary measures against X-ray burns, pain or scars and other complications while giving therapy to patient.

Case: Fraser Vs Vancouver General Hospital: A patient was X-rayed after a traffic accident. The casualty officer, who was not competent, gave opinion that the neck was not broken. The Court held him negligent in not diagnosing a broken neck.

DOCTORS, PUBLIC AND MEDIA: Doctors should individually and collectively influence medical content of the media since media has an important influence on the attitudes and actions of their audience. Doctors can (a) Volunteer services to media (print, radio and television) as an expert. (b) Contribute medical-related articles to local dailies. (c) Organise events to interact with public such as health camps, blood donation drives and invite media to cover them.

(XV) PROFESSIONAL SECRECY (confidentiality): It is an implied term of contract between the doctor and his patient. The relationship of doctor and patient requires utmost trust, confidence, fidelity and honesty. The doctor is obliged to keep secret, all that he comes to know concerning the patient in the course of his professional work. Everything said by a patient or his family members to a physician in the context of medical diagnosis and treatment is confidential. **Its disclosure would be a failure of trust and confidence.** It assumes that without confidentiality, patients will not reveal everything during a consultation, esp. intimate details, due to which the clinical history may be deficient or even misleading. **The patient can sue the doctor for damages** (mental suffering, shame or humiliation) **if the disclosure is voluntary, has resulted in harm to the patient and is not in the interest of the public.**

Examples: (1) A doctor should not discuss the illness of his patient with others without the consent of the patient. (2) If the patient is major, the doctor should not disclose any facts about the illness without his consent to parents or relatives even though they may be paying the doctor's fees. In the case of a minor or an insane person, guardians or parents should be informed of the nature of the illness. (3) A doctor should not answer any enquiry by third parties, even when enquired by near relatives of the patient, either with regard to the nature of the illness or with regard to any subsequent effect of such illness on the patient without the consent of the patient. (4) A doctor should not disclose any information about the illness of his patient without the consent of the patient, even when requested by a public or statutory body, except in case of notifiable diseases. If the patient is a minor or insane, consent of the guardian should be taken. (5) Even in the case of husband and wife, the facts relating to the nature of illness of the one, must not be disclosed to the other, without the consent of the concerned person. (6) In divorce and nullity cases, no information should be given without getting the consent of the person concerned. (7) Medical officers in Government service are also bound by the code of professional secrecy, even when the patient is treated free. (8) When a doctor examines a Government servant on behalf of the Government, he cannot disclose the nature of illness to the Government without the patient's consent. (9) When a domestic servant is examined at the request of the master, the doctor should not disclose any facts about the illness to the master without the consent of the servant, even though the master is paying the fees. (10) The medical officer of a firm or factory should not disclose the result of his examination of an employee to the employers without the consent of the employee. (11) A person in police custody as an undertrial prisoner has the right not to permit the doctor who has examined him, to disclose the nature of his illness to any person. If a person is convicted, he has no such right and the doctor can disclose the result to the authorities. (12) **In reporting a case in any medical journal, care should be taken that patient's identity is not revealed from the case notes or photographs.** (13) In the examination of a dead body certain facts may be found, the disclosure of which may affect the reputation of the deceased or cause mental suffering to his relatives, and as such, the doctor should maintain secrecy. (14) The medical examination for taking out life insurance policy is a voluntary act by the examinee, and therefore consent to the disclosure of the finding may be taken as implied. A doctor should not give any information to an insurance company about a person who has consulted him before, without the patient's consent. Any information regarding a dead person may be given only after obtaining the consent from the nearest relative. (15) **The sex of unborn detected during ultrasonography should not be disclosed.**

PRIVILEGED COMMUNICATION: It is a statement made bonafide upon any subject matter by a doctor to the concerned authority, due to his duty to protect the interests of the community or of the State. To be privileged, the communication must be made to a person having interest in it, or in reference of which he has a duty. If made to more than one person, or to a person who has not a direct interest in it, the plea of privilege fails. **The doctor should first persuade the patient to obtain his consent before notifying the proper authority. If the doctor discloses professional secrets for the purpose of protecting the interest of the community,** (under a moral and social obligation), **he will not be liable to damages.**

Examples: The following are the examples of privileged communication, or in other words, exceptions to the general rule of professional secrecy.

(1) Infectious Diseases: If a patient suffering from an infectious disease is employed as cook or waiter in a hotel, or a food-handler with an enteric infection, or a teacher with tuberculosis or other infective disease, or as children's nurse, etc., **he should be persuaded to leave the job until he becomes non-infectious. If the patient refuses to accept this advice, the doctor can inform the employer about the illness of his patient.**

(2) Servants and Employees: An engine driver or a bus driver or a ship's officer may be suffering from epilepsy, high blood pressure, alcoholism, drug addiction, or colour blindness. The doctor should persuade the patient to change his employment, because of the dangers of his present occupation, both to himself and to the public. If this fails, the doctor should inform the employer, that the patient is unfit for that kind of employment.

(3) Notifiable Diseases: A medical practitioner has a statutory duty to notify births, deaths, infectious diseases, etc., to the Public Health authorities.

(4) Venereal Diseases: If a person is suffering from syphilis and is about to marry, it is the duty of the doctor to advice the patient not to marry till he is cured; if the person refuses, the doctor can disclose the syphilitic condition of the patient to the woman concerned or to her parents. Swimming pools should be prohibited to those having syphilis or gonorrhoea, but if the person refuses, the authorities can be informed. The doctor can inform the warden of a hostel, if any boarder is suffering from venereal disease.

Case: A V.D. specialist saw a young man suffering from syphilis about to enter a public bath. The specialist tried to dissuade the person from entering the bath, but he refused. The physician reported the matter to the attendant who did not allow the young man to bathe. The patient brought a suit against the doctor for breach of professional confidence, but the Court dismissed the case on the ground that the doctor acted in the interest of the community.

(5) Patient's own Interest: The doctor may disclose the patient's condition to some other person, so that he may be properly treated, e.g., to warn the parents or guardians of signs in the patient of melancholia, suicidal tendencies, etc.

(6) Self-interest: Both in civil and criminal suits by the patient against the doctor, evidence about the patient's condition may be given.

(7) Negligence Suits: When a physician is employed by the opposite party to examine a patient who has filed a suit for negligence, the information thus acquired is not privileged (no physician-patient relationship), and the doctor may testify to such information.

(8) Suspected Crime: Every person, aware of the commission of, or of the intention of any other person to commit any offence shall immediately give information to the nearest Magistrate or police officer of such commission or intention (S.39, Cr.P.C.). If the doctor learns of a serious crime, such as murder, assault, rape, etc. by treating the victim or assailant, he is bound to give information to the police. Thus, if a doctor treats a person suffering from gunshot or stab wounds due to criminal assault, he must inform the police.

(9) Courts of Law: In a Court of law, a doctor cannot claim privilege concerning the facts about the illness of his patient, if it is relevant to the inquiry before the Court. The doctor should appeal to the Court if he is asked to reveal any professional secret. If the Court does not accept this plea, he may request the Court that he may be allowed to give the answer in writing so that the public may not know it. If this is denied by the Court, the doctor has to answer the questions about the patient's confidential matters to avoid risk of penalties for contempt of Court. **In all cases, the doctor should appeal to the Judge before disclosing a professional secret. The witness should not voluntarily disclose information either in Court or out of it, but for the actual evidence demanded by the Court, he is protected from civil action against breach of confidence.** Under S. 126, and 129, I.E.A., a lawyer can claim privilege in a Court of law with regard to any communication made to him by his client.

A doctor can disclose and discuss the medical facts of a case with other doctors and paramedical staff, such as nurses, radiologist, physiotherapist, etc. to provide better service to the patient.

Physician's Responsibility In Criminal Matters: In medicolegal cases treatment gets priority. Thereafter procedural criminal law will operate in order to avoid negligent death. A doctor who is aware of the commission of crimes, such as murder, dacoity, waging war against the lawful Government, helping the escape of prisoners, etc., is legally bound to report them to the nearest Magistrate or police officer (S. 39, Cr.P.C., S. 176, I.P.C.). The doctor knowing or having reason to believe that an offence has been committed by a patient whom he is treating, intentionally omits to inform the police, shall be punished with imprisonment up to 6 months (S.202, I.P.C.). But, **if he treats a person who has attempted to commit suicide, he is not legally bound to report, but if the person dies he has to inform the police.** The practitioner's responsibility in case of criminal abortion and poisoning have been described in the relevant chapters.

Special duty of a doctor in Emergency Cases: In emergency, he has moral, ethical and humanitarian duty to do his best to help the patient in saving his life. **In medicolegal injury cases, a doctor is obliged to give necessary medical aid and to save the life of the patient and render all help to see that the person reaches the proper expert/institution as early as possible.**

Duties of a Patient: (1) He should furnish the doctor with complete information about past illness, and family history of diseases and the facts and circumstances of his illness. (2) He should strictly follow the instructions of the doctor as regards diet, medicine, mode of life, etc. (3) He should pay a reasonable fee to the doctor.

PRIVILEGES AND RIGHTS OF THE PATIENTS: Every patient has right to: (1) CHOICE: To choose his own doctor freely. (2) ACCESS: (a) To health care facilities available regardless of age, sex, religion, economic and social status, (b) to emergency services. (3) DIGNITY: To be treated with care, compassion, respect and dignity without any discrimination. (4) PRIVACY: To be treated in privacy during consultation and therapy. (5) CONFIDENTIALITY: All information about his illness and any other be kept confidential. (6) INFORMATION: To receive full information about his diagnosis, investigation and treatment plans and alternative. (7) SAFETY: Right to information should also include safety of procedures/diagnosis/therapeutic modality, complications/side-effects/ expected results as well as facilities available in the institution and other places. (8) RIGHT TO KNOW: Day to day progress, line of action, diagnosis and prognosis. (9) REFUSAL: Right to consent or refuse any specific or all measures. (10) SECOND OPINION: At any time. (11) RECORDS: Access to his records and demand summary or other details pertaining to it. (12) CONTINUITY: To receive continuous care for his illness from the physician/institution. (13) COMFORT: To be treated in comfort during illness and follow up. (14) COMPLAINT: Right to complain and rectification of grievances. (15) COMPENSATION: Obtain compensation for medical injuries/negligence.

TYPES OF PHYSICIAN-PATIENT RELATIONSHIP

(I) THERAPEUTIC RELATIONSHIP: A doctor is free to accept or refuse to treat the patient subject to constraint of his professional obligations in emergencies. Some of the examples where doctor may refuse to treat the patient could be: (1) Beyond his practising hours.

(2) Not belonging to his speciality. (3) Illnesses beyond the competence and qualification of the doctor or beyond the facilities available in his set-up/institution. (4) Doctor is unwell or any other family member is ill. (5) Doctor having important social function in the family. (6) Doctor has consumed alcohol. (7) Patient has been defaulting in payment. (8) Patient or his/her relations are non-cooperative, violent or abusive. (9) Malingerer. (10) Patient refuses to give consent/accept risk. (11) Patient demanding specific drugs like amphetamine, athletics/body-builders demanding steroids, etc. (12) Patient rejecting low-cost remedies in favour of high-cost alternatives. (13) At night on grounds of security, if the patient is not brought to him. (14) An unaccompanied minor patient or female patient. (15) Any new patient, if he is not the only doctor available.

(II) FORMAL RELATIONSHIP: The formal relationship between the doctor and the patient pertains to the situations where the third party has referred the person for impartial medical examination, like pre-employment, insurance, yearly medical check-ups, cases of rape, victims of crimes, intimate body searches and other medicolegal cases, in certain psychiatric/mental illnesses referred by Courts/police.

In these situations, the doctor is not under obligation to provide any information about his report and has to comply with the directives of the party demanding such examinations. However, if a clinical fact requiring urgent treatment is detected which is not known to the patient earlier, it may be conveyed to his family physician or the third party who has sent the patient with instructions to inform the patient.

PROFESSIONAL (MEDICAL) NEGLIGENCE (MALPRAXIS)

Professional negligence is defined as absence of reasonable care and skill, or wilful negligence of a medical practitioner in the treatment of a patient, which causes bodily injury or death of the patient. Negligence is defined as doing something that one is not supposed to do, or failing to do something that one is supposed to do.

Medical negligence is a part of the law of torts. A tort is a civil wrong for which the sufferer can seek compensation through legal action.

Due Care: It **means such reasonable care and attention for the safety of patient as their mental and physical condition may require.** It should be proportionate with the known inability of the patient to take care of himself. Due care anticipates and appropriately manages known, expected or foreseeable events and complications of the patient's disease or treatment. **Breach of standard of care occurs either by omission or commission.** A physician fails to comply with the standard of care applicable to him in two situations: (1) when he improperly, i.e., unjustifiably deviates from accepted practices (methods, procedures, and treatments), and (2) when he employs accepted practices but does so unskilfully.

Types: (1) Civil. (2) Criminal. (3) Corporate. (4) Contributory.

CIVIL NEGLIGENCE: The question of civil negligence arises: (1) When a patient, or in case of death, any relative brings suit in a civil Court for getting compensation from his doctor, if he has suffered injury due to negligence. (2) When a doctor brings a civil suit for getting his fees from the patient or his relatives, who refuse to pay the same alleging professional negligence.

Elements of negligence: Liability for negligence arises if the following conditions are satisfied: (1) **Duty: Existence of a duty of care by the doctor.** (2) **Dereliction**: The physician must conform to the standard of a "prudent physician" under similar circumstances. **The failure on the part of the doctor to maintain applicable standard of care and skill.** (3) **Direct causation: The failure to exercise a duty of care must lead to damage.** The patient must show that a reasonably close and causal connection exists between the negligent act or omission and the resulting injury without any intervening cause. This is referred to as **legal cause or proximate cause.** (4) **Damage: The damage should be of a type that would have been foreseen by a reasonable physician.**

Burden of proof: The patient should prove all four elements of negligence by a preponderance of the evidence. It requires enough proof to show that it is more likely than not, that each of the four elements of a negligent claim is true.

Proof of cause in fact: (1) **"But for" test.** If it is more likely than not, that but for the doctor's breach of duty the patient would not have been injured. (2) **Increased the risk or multiplied the risk test:** If it is more likely than not, that the doctor's breach of duty increased the risk of the patient being injured.

Injury: Any **absence of proper skill or care that causes the patient's death, diminishes his chances of recovery, prolongs his illness, causes physical harm, bodily impairment, disfigurement or increases his suffering, constitutes injury in a legal sense.** Injury is a wrong done to one's person, property or rights. **Even if the doctor is negligent, patient cannot sue him for negligence if no damage has occurred.** The patient must show the existence of an actual physical, psychological or emotional or other injury. which can be measured and compensated in terms of money.

Liability: The amount of damage done is a measure of the extent of the liability. Some examples are: (1) Loss of earning, either due to absence from work or prevention or impairment of his ability to carry out his occupation. (2) Medical expenses including medical rehabilitation, vocational rehabilitation, retraining or other incidental expenses like transportation, additional surgical procedures, daily nursing care and medications for a severely brain-damaged baby for the remainder of baby's life. (3) Reduction in expectation of life. (4) Reduced enjoyment of life, such as loss of function of limb or sense. (5) Pain and suffering, either physical or mental. Suffering includes fright, humiliation, mental anguish, grief and embarrassment. (6) Loss of potency. (7) Aggravation of a preexisting condition. (8) Death.

Personal injuries include any disease or any impairment of a person's physical or mental conditions.

Instances of Medical Negligence: It is impossible to give a complete list of negligent situations in medical practice. (1) Refusal to admit patients requiring urgent hospitalisation. (2) Failure to obtain informed consent to any procedure. (3) Failure to examine patient himself. (4) Failure to inform the patient of the risks of refusal for treatment. (5) Failure to immunise and to perform sensitivity tests when indicated. (6) Not ordering X-ray examination where the history suggests the possibility of a fracture, or dislocation or presence of a foreign body in a wound. (7) Not reading the X-ray film correctly or in failing to get it read by a competent person. (8) Failure to act on radiological or laboratory reports. (9) Inadequate clinical records and failure to communicate with other doctors involved in the treatment of a patient. (10) Administration of incorrect drugs, drugs intended for another patient, especially by injection. (11) Mistakes in labelling of bottle for infusion of blood and other i.v. fluids. (12) Failure to attend the patient in time, or failure to attend altogether. (13) Failure to keep well informed of advances in medical sciences. (14) Making a wrong diagnosis due to absence of skill or care. (15) Negligent management of procedures. (16) Failure to provide a substitute during his absence. (17) To delegate his duty of treating or operating upon a patient to another doctor without the consent of the patient. (18) Failure to give proper post-operative care. (19) Failure to give proper instructions. (20) Failure to warn the patient of side-effects. (21) Failure to obtain consultation where appropriate. (22) Experimenting on patient without consent. (23) Giving overdose of medicine and giving poisonous medicines carelessly. (24) If his negligence causes others to catch a disease from his patient. (25) Continue a practice regarding which several warnings as to its dangers have been given. (26) Prescribing a drug that had previously resulted in an adverse reaction. (27) Administration of an addiction forming drug for a long period. (28) Iatrogenic medical complications during diagnosis or treatment. (29) Prematurely discharging the patient. (30) To cover up an error of judgement.

The fact that the unauthorised additional treatment or surgery is beneficial to the patient, or that it would save considerable time and expenses to the patient, or would relieve the patient from pain and suffering in future are not grounds of defence and amount to an act of assault and therefore deficiency in service.

A doctor is not liable: (1) **For an error of judgement or of diagnosis,** if he has acted with ordinary care and secured all necessary data on which to base a sound judgement. For the treatment of a disease or injury, the doctor may adopt the one which in his judgement, will be more effective and appropriate. In such case, the doctor is not liable for an injury resulting from an error in his judgement. (2) **For failure to cure or for bad result** that may follow, if he has exercised reasonable care and skill. (3) **If he exercises reasonable care and skill,** provided that his judgement conforms to the accepted medical practice, and does not result in the failure to do something or doing something contrary to accepted medical practice.

No doctor ensures success either in his diagnosis or in his treatment. There is always room for a difference of opinion among doctors. **Bad results are not necessarily due to negligence,** e.g., some patients may be keloid formers. **The law considers the doctor negligent only when (1) he did not consider the possibility that such a complication might occur, (2) that he failed to watch for it carefully or to recognise it promptly, or (3) to treat in a timely and appropriate fashion.**

In order to establish liability by a doctor, where a departure from normal practice is alleged, it must be established: (a) that there is a usual and normal practice, (b) that practice was not adopted, and (c) that the course adopted is one, no professional man of ordinary skill would have taken, if acting with ordinary care.

Inherent risks: Some risks are inherent in any form of treatment and the doctor will not be negligent if they cause damage, provided that he has taken proper precautions, e.g., broken needle during injection. If the needle breaks, the patient should be informed and arrangements made to remove the broken piece. The doctor becomes negligent, if he fails to observe that the needle has broken, or having noted this, does not inform the patient or make arrangements to prevent further damage.

Duty of care: A doctor who agrees to give medical advice and treatment, impliedly undertakes that he is possessed of skill and knowledge for the purpose. Such a person when consulted by a patient owes him certain duties, viz. a duty of care **in deciding whether to undertake the case,** a duty of care **in deciding what treatment to give**, or a duty of **care in the administration of that treatment**. A breach of any of those duties becomes negligence. The doctor no doubt has a discretion in choosing treatment, which he proposes to give to the patient, and such discretion is relatively ample in cases of emergency.

Degree of Competence: The doctors are expected to keep well-informed of changing concepts and new developments and to follow general lines of treatment, though they are not expected to be aware of every development in medical science. **The degree of competence is not a fixed quality, but varies according to the status of the doctor.** A house-surgeon is not expected to possess the same skills as a consultant surgeon, but he is expected to limit his activities (except in emergencies) to a level of medical care which is within his competence. **A general medical practitioner is expected to use only the average degree of skill and knowledge possessed by doctors with the same or similar training, experience and knowledge in the same or similar circumstances in the specific geographic location in which the physician provides medical treatment (locality rule).**

Standard of care: The practitioner must possess a reasonable degree of skill and knowledge and must exercise a reasonable degree of care. Neither the very highest nor a very low degree of care and competence, judged in the light of the particular circumstances of each case, is what the law requires. The same high degree of skill or standard of care is not expected from a doctor practising in some remote village or town, as is expected of a doctor on the staff of a hospital in a city. A specialist must maintain standards of skill in diagnosis and treatment above those of the ordinary general practitioner. **If a doctor claims to possess superior skill, knowledge, experience or training, he will be judged according to those standards even in its absence.** If a general practitioner treats as a specialist, a case that clearly lies within a specialised medical field, he will be held liable for failure to use skill equal to that of a specialist. **The standard of care while assessing the practice as adopted, is judged in the light of knowledge available at the time of the incident, and not at the time of trial.** Similarly, when the charge of negligence arises out of failure to use some particular equipment, the charge would fail, if the equipment was not generally available at that particular time, i.e. at the time of incident. In a personal injury case, the fact that the patient's injuries become serious by his own predisposition or weakness does not diminish the extent of damages.

Liability for injury to third parties: When a doctor performs an examination at the request of a third party for sole use by third party, e.g. to determine eligibility for employment, evaluation of disability, insurance, drunkenness, etc., i.e., **to examine the patient for non-therapeutic purposes, no physician - patient relationship is established. The employed physician owes no duty to the examinee other than to avoid causing an injury,** but is under a duty to use reasonable care to avoid injury. **Physician's duty is owed to his employer.**

Proof: The burden of proving negligence lies on the plaintiff (patient). Burden of proof is the need or duty to establish proof of the facts at trial. In order to establish negligence, it is not necessary to prove that the negligent party had bad motive or intention. The essential issue that decides a case of negligence is whether a reasonably competent medical man would have acted in more or less the same manner in which the doctor against whom negligence is alleged had acted.

Case: (1) Whitamore Vs Rao: A suit was filed against the doctor for negligent treatment. The charge was that the doctor injected sulphostab or sulfarsenol, though the patient was not syphilitic. Evidence was given by the defendant doctor and other doctors that patient's blood contained parasites of malignant malaria and he had sores on his face. The Court held that the doctor was not negligent.

(2) Crivon Vs Barret Group Hospital Committee: The plaintiff was operated for the removal of a small breast tumour, and the pathologist reported that it looked like cancer. Intensive radiotherapy was given to the patient, due to which the skin surface was destroyed and there was the possibility of potential hazards. The patient on knowing the diagnosis suffered great pain and worry. Later it was found that the diagnosis was not correct. An expert pathologist gave evidence that he might have also given the same diagnosis. The Court held that the pathologist was not negligent as the interpretation of the slide was difficult and debatable. It also held that surgeon was not negligent in not taking a second opinion, as the speed of treatment was essential in the case.

(3) Roe Vs Ministry of Health: Two persons were operated upon under nupercain spinal anaesthetic, who developed permanent spastic paraplegia. The nupercain was contained in glass ampoules, which was responsible for the paraplegia. At that time this risk of percolation was not known to anaesthetists in general, and the Court held that it was only a misadventure and not negligence.

THE DOCTRINE OF RES IPSA LOQUITUR: *Res ipsa loquitur* is a rule of evidence which in reality belongs to the law of torts. **Ordinarily, the professional negligence of a physician must be proved in Court by the expert evidence of another physician. The patient need not prove negligence in case where the rule of *res ipsa loquitur* applies, which means "the thing or fact speaks for itself". The patient has to merely state what according to him was the act of negligence.**

Conditions to be satisfied: (1) that in the absence of negligence the injury would not have occurred ordinarily; (2) that the doctor had exclusive control over the injury producing instrument or treatment; (3) that the patient was not guilty of contributory negligence. This enables the patient's lawyer to prove his case without medical evidence.

Examples: (1) Prescribing an overdose of medicine producing ill-effects. (2) Giving poisonous medicine carelessly. (3) Failure to give anti-tetanic serum in cases of injury causing tetanus. (4) Burns from application of hot water bottles or from X-ray therapy. (5) Breaking of needles. (6) Failure to remove the swabs during operation which may lead to complications or cause death. (7) Blood transfusion misadventure. (8) Loss of use of hand due to prolonged splinting.

Application: This doctrine is applied both to civil and criminal negligence. It does not apply where common knowledge or experience is not sufficiently extensive to know that the patient's condition would not have existed but for the doctor's negligence. It cannot be applied against several defendants only one of whom, who cannot be identified could have caused patient's injury. The doctrine is rarely used successfully by patients.

Case: Mohn. Vs Osborne: An abdominal operation was performed by resident surgeon and at its conclusion, the surgeon was informed that the swab count was correct. Two months later, a further operation was done and a swab was found under the liver. The patient died later. The mother of deceased sued the surgeon for damages. The Court held the doctor negligent on the ground that the doctrine of res ipsa loquitur applied to the case.

Many doctrines can be used as a defence plea against the negligence claim in civil cases. (1) "CALCULATED RISK" CASES: The theory of the calculated risk doctrine is that *res ipsa loquitur* should not be applied when the injury complained is of a type that may occur even though reasonable care has been taken. This doctrine is an important defence to any doctor sued for professional negligence, who can produce expert evidence or statistics to show that the accepted method of treatment he employed had unavoidable risks.

(2) DOCTRINE OF COMMON KNOWLEDGE: This doctrine is based on the assumption that the issue of negligence in the particular case is not related to technical matters, but are within the knowledge of the medical profession, e.g. the doctor will be held responsible for the lack of application of common sense, such as failure to give fluids in dehydration, or failure to give ATS in case of injuries, or failure to apply an antiseptic to an open cut. It is a variant of res ipsa loquitur. In res ipsa loquitur, the patient need not produce evidence as to both the standard of care and specific act or omission. In doctrine of common knowledge, the patient must prove the causative (negligent) act or omission, but he need not produce evidence to establish the standard of care.

COMPOSITE NEGLIGENCE: It occurs when a patient suffers from any injury due to negligent acts of more than one person without the negligence of patient. In such case, patient may claim compensation from any one negligent person. The defendant negligent person may claim contribution from other negligent persons.

ASSUMPTION OF RISK-VOLENTI NON-FIT INJURIES: The doctor will not be held responsible for the injury suffered by the patient, which is caused by some particular type of treatment given by the doctor, being compelled by the patient even after physician's warning.

MEDICAL MALOCCURRENCE: Medicine deals with human beings, and there are many biological variations which cannot always be explained, expected or prepared for. **In some cases, in spite of good medical attention and care, an individual fails to respond properly or may suffer from adverse reactions of the drug. This is called medical maloccurrence.** The injured person cannot get monetary compensation in every mishap or accident which results in injury, if the doctor was careful in selection of the drug and has taken appropriate measures to overcome the undesirable foreseeable effects. **Accident** can be defined as an unpredictable event resulting in a recognisable injury. **Inevitable accident is an accident, not avoidable by any such precautions as a reasonable man can be expected to take,** e.g., breaking of a needle during intramuscular injection due to sudden muscular spasm, or damage to the recurrent laryngeal nerve during thyroidectomy.

NOVUS ACTUS INTERVENIENS: A person is responsible not only for his actions, but also for the logical consequences of those actions. This principle applies to cases of assault and accidental injury. Sometimes, such a continuity of events is broken by an entirely new and unexpected happening, due to negligence of some other person. If the doctor is negligent, which results in a deviation from the logical sequence of events, then the responsibility for the subsequent disability or death may pass from the original incident to the later negligent action of the doctor by the

principle of "*novus actus interveniens*" (an unrelated action intervening). Most of such interventions are of a medical nature, e.g., leaving of a swab or a surgical instrument in the abdomen after the repair of an internal injury; accidental substitution of poisonous drug for therapeutic drug, etc. **For a plea of novus actus, an element of negligence is essential.** It will depend on the extent to which it comes to be regarded as causally significant in itself. In such case, the assailant will not be fully responsible for the ultimate harm. This plea is rarely accepted by the courts.

CONTRIBUTORY NEGLIGENCE: Contributory negligence is, any unreasonable conduct, or absence of ordinary care on the part of the patient, or his personal attendant, which combined with the doctor's negligence, contributed to the injury complained of, as a direct, proximate cause and without which the injury would not have occurred. These include (1) failure to give the doctor accurate medical history. If the patient provides incomplete or inadequate information, it could result in misdiagnosis, mistreatment and harm. (2) failure to cooperate with his doctor in carrying out all reasonable and proper instructions, (3) refusal to take the suggested treatment, (4) leaving the hospital against the doctor's advice, (5) failure to seek further medical assistance if symptoms persist. **As such, the doctor's negligence is not the direct, proximate cause (actual or legal cause) of the injury suffered by the patient. Proximate cause means, that which in natural and continuous sequence, unbroken by any efficient intervening cause produces the injury, and without which the result would not have occurred.** If the doctor and the patient are negligent at the same time, it is a good defence for the doctor. **The doctor cannot plead contributory negligence, if he fails to give proper instructions.**

Liability of the doctor: The extent of contributory negligence may vary and with it will vary the doctor's liability, from complete non-liability to a substantial liability for damages. Normally, **contributory negligence is only a partial defence,** and the Court has right to fix liability between the parties **(doctrine of comparative negligence),** and damages awarded may be reduced accordingly. **The burden of proof lies entirely on the doctor. If a patient consents to take the risk of the injurious event actually taking place, he cannot claim damages.** If a doctor is not negligent, but if a patient is negligent which results in injury, it is called negligence of the patient.

The term aggravation is applied to the injury that hastens death, leads to permanent disability or introduces features or complications that do not normally develop in the natural course of the disease process. In such case the doctor cannot plead contributory negligence in civil cases.

Good Samaritan doctrine: One who assists another who is in serious danger cannot be charged with contributory negligence, unless the assistance is reckless or rash.

LIMITATIONS TO CONTRIBUTORY NEGLIGENCE: (a) THE LAST CLEAR CHANCE DOCTRINE: Under this rule, a person who has negligently placed himself in a position of danger may recover damages, if the doctor discovered the danger while there was still time to avoid the injury or failed to do so. (b) THE AVOIDABLE CONSEQUENCES RULE: It is the negligence of the patient which aggravated the damage already caused by negligence of the doctor, which could have been avoided if the patient was not negligent afterwards. In such case, the doctor cannot plead contributory negligence in civil cases.

Case: A surgeon was sued for not removing a swab from the vagina of patient. The patient complained about pain in the vagina to a nurse some time after the operation. The nurse examined the vagina and removed the swab. The patient did not inform the surgeon about the swab in the vagina. The Court held that the doctor was guilty of contributory negligence.

CRIMINAL NEGLIGENCE: The question of criminal negligence may arise: (1) When a doctor shows gross absence of skill or care during treatment resulting in serious injury to or death of the patient, by acts of omission or commission. (2) When a doctor performs an illegal act. (3) When an assaulted person dies, the defence may attribute the death to the negligence or undue interference in the treatment of the deceased by the doctor.

Conditions to be satisfied: Criminal negligence occurs if any one of the following are satisfied: **(1) indifference to an obvious risk of injury to health, (2) actual foresight of the risk, but continuation of the same treatment, (3) appreciation of the risk and intention to avoid it, but showing high degree of negligence in the attempted avoidance, (4) inattention or failure to avoid, a serious risk which went beyond mere inadvertence in respect of an obvious important matter.**

Occurrence: Criminal negligence **occurs when the doctor shows gross lack of competence, or gross inattention or inaction, gross recklessness, or wanton indifference to the patient's safety,** or gross negligence in the selection and application of remedies. **It involves an extreme departure from the ordinary standard of care.** Criminal negligence cases are very rare, and **are practically limited to cases in which the patient has died.** In order to establish criminal liability, the facts must be such that the negligence of the accused went beyond a matter of compensation between persons and showed such disregard for the life and safety of others as to amount to a crime against the State, and conduct deserving punishment. **A doctor will not be criminally liable if a patient dies due to an error of judgement or carelessness or want of due caution, though he can be liable to pay compensation.** Most of such cases are associated with drunkenness or with impaired efficiency due to the use of drugs by doctors Table (3–2).

S. 304, A., I.P.C. **deals with criminal negligence.** "Whoever causes the death of any person by doing any rash or negligent act not amounting to culpable homicide shall be punished with imprisonment up to 2 years, or with fine, or with both". According to S.357, Cr.P.C., **in addition to imprisonment or other penalty prescribed by the I.P.C., compensation may also have to be paid to the victim of criminal negligence.**

Examples: (1) Amputation of wrong finger or operation on wrong limb or wrong patient. (2) Leaving instruments, tubes, sponges or swabs in abdomen. (3) Grossly incompetent administration of a general anaesthetic by a doctor addicted to the inhalation of anaesthetic. (4) Gross mismanagement of the delivery of woman especially by a doctor under the influence of drink or drugs. (5) Performing criminal abortion. (6) Administration of a wrong substance into the eye causing loss of vision. (7) Death resulting from an operation or injection of any drug producing anaphylaxis by a quack is considered criminal negligence.

Prosecution: Criminal negligence is more serious than the civil. **To prosecute a doctor for criminal negligence, it must be shown that the accused did something or failed to do something which in the given facts and circumstances no**

Table (3–2). Difference between civil and criminal negligence

	Trait	Civil negligence	Criminal negligence
(1)	Offence:	No specific and clear violation of law need be proved.	Must have specifically violated a particular criminal law in question.
(2)	Negligence:	Simple absence of care and skill.	Gross negligence, inattention or lack of competency.
(3)	Conduct of physician:	It is compared to a generally accepted simple standard of professional conduct.	Not compared to a single test.
(4)	Consent for act:	Good defence; cannot recover damages.	Not a defence; can be prosecuted.
(5)	Litigation:	Between two parties.	Between state and doctor.
(6)	Trial by:	Civil Court.	Criminal Court.
(7)	Evidence:	Strong evidence is sufficient.	Guilt should be proved beyond reasonable doubt.
(8)	Punishment:	Liable to pay damages.	Imprisonment with or without fine.

medical doctor in his ordinary senses and prudence would have done or failed to do so. For criminal negligence, the doctor may be prosecuted by the police and charged in criminal Court with having caused the death of the patient by a rash or negligent act not amounting to culpable homicide. The prosecution must prove all the facts to establish civil negligence (except monetary loss), and gross negligence and disregard for the life and safety of the patient. **Contributory negligence is not a defence in criminal negligence** Table (3–2).

Investigation: Note the circumstances in which death occurred and the facilities available for treatment. Samples of drugs and i.v. fluids should be collected and sent to the laboratory to exclude adulteration, contamination and chemical identification. Statement of witness should be recorded. A team of doctors should conduct autopsy, and all necessary laboratory investigations should be done. An impartial expert in the same field should study the case sheet.

Supreme court guidelines: According to the guidelines of supreme court of India (1) a private complaint against a doctor may not be entertained unless the complainant has produced *prima facie* evidence before the court in the form of credible opinion given by another competent doctor to support the charge of rashness or negligence. (2) The investigating officer before proceeding against the doctor accused of rash or negligent act, **should obtain an independent medical opinion preferably from a doctor in government service. A doctor accused of rashness or negligence might not be arrested routinely,** unless his arrest is necessary for furthering investigation or for collecting evidence or the I.O. is satisfied that the doctor would not make himself available to face prosecution.

Case: (1) A hakim gave a penicillin injection to a person who died due to it. The Court held that the ignorance of the hakim alone about penicillin injections, would make his act of giving treatment rash and negligent.

(2) Kobiraj Vs Empress: A quack cut the internal piles of a patient with an ordinary knife, who died of haemorrhage. He was charged under section 304-A, I.P.C. The quack contended that he had performed similar operations before, and that he was entitled to the benefit of section 88, I.P.C., as he operated in good faith, and patient had accepted the risk. The Court held the accused criminally negligent as he was not educated in surgery.

(3) Desouza Vs Emperor: The accused was in charge of a dispensary which was badly managed with mixing up of poisonous and non-poisonous medicines. To prepare a mixture of quinine hydrochloride, the accused removed a bottle from the non-poisonous medicines cupboard and tore open the wrapper without looking at it, on which the word 'poison' was printed. Then, without reading the label on the bottle, on which was printed 'Strychnine Hydrochloride', prepared a mixture and gave it to several persons, all of whom except one died within a short time. He was convicted for criminal negligence under Sec. 304-A, I.P.C.

(4) In 1958, a German doctor went on a trip to India without getting himself vaccinated against smallpox. On return to Germany, he resumed his practice, although he showed symptoms of smallpox, he did not take any precautionary measures to see that he did not infect others. 18 of the patients caught the disease and two of whom died. The doctor was charged with criminal negligence and was punished with four months imprisonment and fine.

(5) A doctor while he was drunk, operated upon a woman for eclampsia. Two days later, the woman died due to the injuries produced during operation. The doctor was sentenced to one year imprisonment for want of reasonable care and skill due to intoxication.

A physician may be liable to both civil and criminal negligence by a single professional act, e.g., if a physician performs an unauthorised operation on a patient, he may be sued in civil Court for damages and prosecuted in criminal Court for assault.

CORPORATE NEGLIGENCE: The theory of corporate liability is typically applied in cases involving hospitals and their staff physicians. Hospitals have independent duty to their patients to investigate adequacy and review the competence of staff physicians. **This theory is based on the principle that hospitals are in a far better position than their patients to supervise a physician's performance and provide quality control.** This legal theory has been used to attack the allegedly negligent selection, retention, or supervision of its participating physicians, that is negligent credentialing. **It is the failure of those persons who are responsible for providing the accommodation, facilities and treatment to follow the established standard of conduct.** It occurs when the hospital provides defective equipment or drugs, selects or retains incompetent employees, or fails in some other manner to meet the accepted standard of care, and such failure results in injury to a patient to whom the hospital owes a duty. **In the corporate sector (hospital, nursing home, etc.)., where more than one person in more than one level fails to render appropriate service to the patient, may result in some damage to patient. Here the treating doctor and also other category of persons who were negligent will be held responsible.**

If a hospital knows or should have known, that one of the patient is likely to be a victim of professional negligence by a doctor on its staff, the hospital is liable, even though that doctor

Table (3–3). **Difference between professional negligence and infamous conduct**

	Trait	Professional negligence	Infamous conduct
(1)	Offence:	Absence of proper care and skill or wilful negligence.	Violation of Code of Medical Ethics.
(2)	Duty of care:	Should be present.	Need not be present.
(3)	Damage to person:	Should be present.	Need not be present.
(4)	Trial by:	Courts; civil or criminal.	State Medical Council.
(5)	Punishment:	Fine or imprisonment.	Erasure of name or warning.
(6)	Appeal:	To higher Court.	To State and Central Governments.

is an independent with staff privilege at the hospital. If the doctor is employed by a patient in his private capacity, and the hospital only provides facilities for treatment, the doctor alone is held responsible for any negligence.

Ethical Negligence: **Ethical negligence is the violation of the Code of Medical Ethics.** In this, no financial compensation is payable unless there is also civil negligence. If a complaint is made and the facts proved, the name of the doctor may be erased from the Medical Register Table (3–3). **This term should be better avoided.**

CAUSES OF TAKING NEGLIGENT ACTION AGAINST THE PHYSICIAN BY THE PATIENT/ RELATIONS: They are: (I) PHYSICIAN RELATED: (1) Breakdown in physician-patient relationship; or utter disregard for the life and safety of the patient (poor and ineffective communication with the patient and his relatives). (2) Rude behaviour of the physician. (3) Less frequent house calls. (4) Complex invasive procedures for diagnosis and treatment with resulting death or disability. (II) PATIENT RELATED: (1) Unrealistic expectations of cure. (2) Poor compliance with medical recommendations. (3) Frequent self-destructive behaviour (heavy smoking, drinking, use of drugs, poor dietary management). (4) Increasing awareness of rights. (5) Comments on the treatment by another doctor. (6) Lack of consent. (7) Lack of documentation, such as provisional diagnosis, relevant findings, etc. (8) Not taking second opinion whenever there is a problem and not informing relatives if patient is serious. (9) Misperception of physician's role in the society, or his affluence. (III) MEDIA RELATED: Biased publicity of negligent suits and the size of awards. (IV) ATTORNEY RELATED: (1) Lack of experience. (2) Monetary considerations. (V) ECONOMIC: (1) Increased cost of medical care. (2) Payment by insurance companies. (VI) SOCIAL: (1) Mobile population. (2) Consumers rights. (3) General increase in litigation.

Defensive Medicine: **Defensive medicine is ordering every test or X-ray on a patient to have a good background of hard data, and avoiding using a potentially risky treatment which may offer much benefit to the patient.** This may lead to withholding of beneficial treatment to the majority of patients, because of a statistical risk to the minority. The physician must not practice "defense by denial", and claim that the patient is not his, which becomes abandonment.

Precautions Against Negligence: To prove that reasonable care and skill has been exercised, the following precautions should be taken.

(1) Obtain informed consent of the patient. (2) Establish good rapport (relationship or communication) with the patient. (3) Keep full and accurate and legible medical records. (4) Employ ordinary skill and care at all times. (5) Confirm diagnosis by laboratory tests. (6) Take skiagrams in bone or joint injuries, or when diagnosis is doubtful. (7) Immunisation should be done whenever necessary, particularly for tetanus. (8) Sensitivity tests should be done before injecting preparations which are likely to produce anaphylactic shock. (9) In suspected cases of cancer, all laboratory investigations should be done without delay to establish early diagnosis. (10) No female patient should be examined unless a third person is present. (11) Keep yourself informed of technical advances and use standard procedures of treatment. (12) Seek consultation where appropriate. (13) Do not criticise or condemn the professional ability of another doctor, especially in the presence of the patient. (14) Do not exaggerate nor minimise the gravity of the patient's condition. Avoid from overconfident prognoses and promising too much to patient. (15) Never guarantee a cure. (16) Do not make a statement admitting fault on your part. (17) Do not fail to exercise care in the selection of assistants and allotting duties to them. (18) The patient must not be abandoned. (19) Do not leave patient unattended during labour. (20) Inform the patient of any intended absence from practice, or recommend or make available, a qualified substitute. (21) Transfer the patient if facilities are inadequate to handle his problem. (22) Do not order a prescription over telephone, because of possibility of misunderstanding as to the drugs or their dosage. (23) The drug should be identified before being injected or used otherwise. (24) Obtain consent for an operation or giving anaesthesia and to use discretion in obscure cases. (25) Frequently check the condition of equipment, and use available safety installations. (26) In a criminal wounding, operation should not be performed unless it is absolutely necessary. (27) Proper instructions should be given to the patient, and proper postoperative care should be taken. (28) In the case of death from an anaesthesia or during operation, the matter should be reported to the police authorities for holding a public inquiry. (29) Anaesthesia should be given by a qualified person. Only generally accepted anaesthesia should be given after clinical and laboratory examinations of the patient. The patient should be watched until he fully recovers from its effect. (30) No experimental method should be adopted without the consent of the patient. (31) No procedure should be undertaken beyond one's skill. (32) Do not fail to secure the consent of both husband and wife, if an operation on either is likely to result in sterility. (33) Establish a hospital injury prevention program. (34) Insist on continuing education of physicians. (35) Participate in medicolegal seminars.

MALPRACTICE LITIGATION INVOLVING VARIOUS SPECIALITIES: Different medical specialities have greatly different risks. The highly vulnerable specialities are: orthopaedic, obstetrics, anaesthesia, neurosurgery, plastic surgery, and accident medicine. **Following is a brief list of some of the more important examples, apart from general errors, giving rise to malpractice litigation.**

(I) Anaesthesiology: (1) Giving anaesthesia without the consent of adult patient or a child without consent of the guardian. (2) Failure to conduct physical examination or take patient's history. (3) Explosion (gaseous inhalation anaesthetic agents only). (4) Contamination of anaesthetic agent. (5) Substitution of toxic chemical for anaesthetic agent. (6) Breakage of hypodermic needle. (7) Failure to produce total anaesthesia. (8) Incorrect or excessive use of anaesthetic agents. (9) Toxic properties of anaesthetic agents: (halothane (hepatitis) and methoxyflurane (nephrotoxicity). (10) Brain damage due to hypoxia. (11) Asphyxiation from exhaustion of oxygen supply. (12)Neurological damage from spinal or epidural injections. (13) Peripheral nerve damage from splinting during infusion. (14) Incompatible blood transfusion. (15) Allowing awareness of pain during anaesthesia. (16) Paralysis following spinal anaesthesia. (17) Leaving broken spinal needle in the spinal canal. (18) Cardiac arrest occurring during surgery precipitated by improper administration of anaesthesia, e.g., improper airways, inadequate ventilation, excessive general anaesthetic agents, or muscle relaxants.

(II) General Surgery: (1) Leaving of instruments, swabs, sponges, etc. within the body cavities. (2) Operating on the wrong patient. (3) Operating on the wrong limb, digit or organ. (4) Operating on wrong side of the body. (5) Delayed diagnosis of acute abdominal lesions. (6) Failure to diagnose diabetes in complicated surgeries. (7) Failure to have a biopsy of a tumour. (8) Failed vasectomy, without warning of lack of total certainty of subsequent sterility. (9) Injection causing peripheral nerve damage. (10) Accidental ligation of vessels and ducts, such as suturing of the common bile ducts during partial gastrectomy. (11) Perforation of intestines or organs. (12) Diathermy and cautery may cause skin burns and electrocution. (13) Cardiac monitors and defibrillators may cause damage and death. (14) Leaving catheters in place too long causing infection.

The complications produced by various powders used to lubricate the inside of surgical gloves are: intestinal obstruction and peritonitis, draining sinus tracts, fistulae and granulomatous masses at the operation site simulating tumour.

(III) Orthopaedics and Accident Surgery: (1) Failure to admit in hospital when required. (2) Missed fractures, especially of the scaphoid, skull, neck of femur and cervical spine. (3) Overtight plaster casts causing tissue and nerve damage. (4) Unnecessary surgery of fractures in children resulting in growth disturbances. (5) Inadequately treated hand injuries, especially tendons. (6) Undiagnosed intracranial haemorrhage. (7) Missed foreign bodies in eyes and wounds, especially glass. (8) Sciatic paralysis from operation on the hip. (9) Leaving a broken drill tip in the bone, with subsequent infection.

(IV) Obstetrics and Gynaecology: (1) Brain damage in the newborn due to hypoxia from prolonged labour. These cases involve most expensive claims. This fear has resulted in high rate of caesarian births. (2) Failed sterilisation by unsuccessful tubal ligation resulting in unwanted pregnancies. (3) Complications of hysterectomy, such as ureteric ligation and vesicovaginal fistula. (4) Management of delivery under the influence of alcohol/drugs. (5) Performing abortion without indication (criminal abortion). (6) Foetal and maternal deaths by certain drugs. (7) Haemorrhage during delivery. (8) Amniotic fluid embolism, pulmonary thromboembolism, cerebral thrombosis, sepsis. (9) Hypersensitive disease of pregnancy, cardiac conditions, diabetes, etc. can complicate pregnancy and cause death during advanced pregnancy or delivery. (10) Perinatal foetal death. (11) Cerebral palsy (12) Foetal trauma such as fractures.

(V) General Medical Practice: (1) Failure to diagnose myocardial infarcts or other medical conditions. (2) Toxic results of drug administration. (3) Failure to take complete history resulting in wrong diagnosis and treatment. (4) Failure to take action on laboratory and other reports. (5) Allowing suicidally inclined patients in psychiatric wards to commit suicide. (6) Administration of incorrect type of drugs, especially by injection. (7) Fall from wheel chair, examination table or bed causing injuries. (8) Injection of a drug resulting in infection or tissue necrosis. (9) Prescribing of a drug known to cause reactions.

(VI) Radiology: (1) During arteriography, damage to vessel walls may result in thrombosis or embolism. (2) Air embolism may occur, especially in carotid angiography. (3) Nerve damage may occur during axillary arteriography. (4) During barium enema, inflatable balloon catheters used to retain barium, may cause perforation of rectum. (5) Defective X-ray equipment may cause electric shock. (6) X-ray and radium burns.

MEDICAL NEGLIGENCE PREVENTION: The following help to decrease the incidence of medical negligence.

(1) Rapport: Maintain healthy rapport and communication with the patient and with patient's families, with fellow physicians, nurses and paramedical personnel who may commit errors. Lack of communication, and lack of thorough understanding of a diagnostic or therapeutic problems by all parties contribute to errors. If a patient or his family does not understand or feels that the doctor is careless and if there is a bad result, he will sue the doctor. An alert, responsible team member can spot a complication early.

(2) Rationale: The doctor should use all reliable and relevant information (history, physical examination, laboratory tests, x-rays, etc.) to make diagnosis and formulate the treatment. The physician will be negligent when he relies on inadequate data or uses that data to form unsupportable or untenable conclusion with respect to diagnosis or treatment. Diagnostic and therapeutic rationale should be adequately documented in the medical record. Seek consultation where appropriate.

(3) Records: The record should be carefully prepared: complete, accurate, legible, relevant, timely and generously informative. A bad result with bad records equals liability. In a professional negligence trial, the record will be the most important evidence, regardless of the facts and the standard of care practised.

(4) Remarks: Do not reprimand the patient and his family. Do not criticise any nurse or laboratory or x-ray technician or any other health care personnel within the hearing of the patient. If necessary, take the involved person aside and be constructive in your comments. If a patient or his family overhears these remarks, they will sue the doctor. Do not criticise or condemn the professional ability of another doctor.

(5) Recipe: Do not prescribe any medicine unless there is an appropriate therapeutic indication for it. The doctor should be aware of side-effects of the prescribed drug and caution the patient appropriately. The physician must be aware of potential risks or complications, and must watch them carefully, diagnose them promptly when they occur and treat them in a timely and appropriate manner. He must be aware of possible contraindications to use of any drug associated with the patient's other diagnoses or other medications he may be using. He should inform the patient whether the drug should be taken in the fasting state or after food.

(6) Res ipsa Loquitur: If an untoward result occurs and it is thought to be due to negligence or deviation from the usual and customary standards of care, the doctor should admit the problem. Denial may cause the patient to become worse or to develop complications that may be irreversible or result in disability. Explain carefully to the patient and the family just what the problem is and why it has occurred. Assure the patient that he will solve the problem by further care or referral to another physician or medical centre. When settlement is indicated, it should be prompt and adequate in amount. He should not charge

for further medical care or charge additional fees if a second surgical operation is required or decrease the cost of hospitalisation.

(7) Respect: An attitude of care and concern, a relationship that suggests thoughtful professionalism and a humanistic approach many times solves problems. Treat the patient as the physician would wish himself or a member of his family to be treated.

(8) Results: Obtain informed consent from the patient. If a bad result occurs, sincere close attention should be given.

(9) Risks: The patient and his family must be informed of all anticipated risks: (a) serious risks or risks of serious disability or death which may occur rarely, (b) lesser risks of short duration, but greater chance of occurrence. He should be able to manage risks. Risks must be (a) identified carefully, (b) controlled and managed to prevent injury to the patient, (c) eliminated completely if possible, i.e. (i) good patient care, (ii) desirable patient care, (iii) achievable patient care. The reward for achievable patient care will be: (a) fewer damages paid, (b) cheaper medical indemnity premiums, (c) emotional and psychological benefits to the patient and satisfaction of practising a noble profession and doing it well.

(10) Review: Routinely review cases involving morbidity and mortality. Review medical malpractice cases and the testimony by medical experts.

SUPREME COURT OF INDIA GUIDELINES ON MEDICAL NEGLIGENCE

The Court collated a 11-point guidelines for the courts to adjudicate complaints against doctors. They are: (1) Negligence is a breach of duty or an act which a prudent and reasonable man will not do. (2) Negligence to be established by the prosecution must be culpable or gross and not merely based upon an error of judgment. (3) Medical professional is expected to bring a reasonable degree of skill and knowledge along with a reasonable degree of care but neither the highest nor the lowest degree of care and competence. (4) A doctor would be liable only where his conduct fell below the standard of a reasonably competent practitioner. (5) Difference of opinion cannot be cited as negligence. (6) Just because a professional looking at the gravity of illness had taken a higher element of risk to redeem the patient out of his suffering which did not yield the desired result, it may not amount to negligence. (7) Merely because a doctor chooses one course of action in preference to the other one available, he would not be liable if the action chosen by him was acceptable to the medical profession. (8) It would not be conducive to the efficiency of the medical profession, if no doctor could administer medicine without a halter round his neck. (9) It is our duty not to harass or humiliate medical professionals unnecessarily, so as to allow them to perform their duties without fear and apprehension. (10) Doctors at times have to be saved from such class complaints who use criminal process as a tool for pressurising them or hospitals and clinics for extracting uncalled for compensation. (11) Doctors are entitled to get protection so long as they perform their duties with reasonable skill and competence and in the interest of the patients.

Defences Against Negligence: (1) No duty owed to the plaintiff. (2) Duty discharged according to prevailing standards. (3) Misadventure. (4) Error of judgement. (5) Contributory negligence. (6) **Res judicata** (S. 300, Cr.P.C.). **If a question of negligence against a doctor has already been decided by a Court in a dispute between the doctor and his patient, the patient will not be allowed to contest the same question in another proceeding between himself and the doctor on the same set of facts in a different court. Only appeal can be made.** (7) **Limitation:** A suit for damages for negligence against the doctor should be filed within two years from the date of alleged negligence. A suit filed after two years will be dismissed as being beyond the period of limitation. Where breach of duty to provide care as per a particular contract between a patient and a doctor is committed, legal action can be initiated up to three years from the date of alleged negligence.

THERAPEUTIC MISADVENTURE: A **misadventure is mischance or accident or disaster.** Misadventure is of three types: (1) Therapeutic (when treatment is being given). (2) Diagnostic (where diagnosis only is the objective at the time). (3) Experimental (where the patient has agreed to serve as a subject in an experimental study). **Therapeutic misadventure is a case in which an individual has been injured or had died due to some unintentional act by a doctor or agent of the doctor or the hospital.**

Almost every therapeutic drug and every therapeutic procedure can cause death. Injection of serum, antibiotics, etc. may cause anaphylaxis in sensitive persons. History of sensitivity should be obtained before injecting such substances. **Negative history and negative test does not rule out rare possibility of anaphylactoid reaction and even death. A physician is not liable for injuries resulting from adverse reaction to drug, unless some negligence on his part contributed to cause the injury. Ignorance of the possibility of a reaction, or continuation in the prescribing of a drug with adverse reaction amounts to negligence.** While prescribing a drug that has adverse side-effects, the doctor must be certain that the prescribed drug was the proper one for the disease. If there is any other drug which would be effective in treating the disease and is less likely to cause an allergic reaction, it should be prescribed.

Examples: (1) Hypersensitivity reaction, sometimes serious or fatal, may be caused by penicillin, aspirin, tetracycline, etc. (2) Excessive administration of an antidote to a poisoned patient, may cause death. (3) Prolonged use of stilboesterol may cause breast cancer. (4) I^{131} therapy may cause thyroid cancer. (5) Electric equipment, hot water pads, and heating pads may produce burns. (6) Blood transfusion may cause serious or fatal complications from bleeding resulting from haemolytic reaction due to hypofibrinogenaemia, hypothrombinaemia and thrombocytopaenia. Other complications are haemosiderosis, viral hepatitis, hyperkalaemia and hypocalcaemia. (7) Radiological procedures used for diagnostic purposes may prove fatal, e.g., poisoning by barium enema, traumatic rupture of the rectum and chemical peritonitis during barium enema. (8) Foetal and neonatal deaths in utero may occur from drugs administered to the mother during pregnancy, e.g., dicumarol, diabenese, serpasil, iodides, synthetic vitamin K, thiazide diuretics, etc.

Precautions: To avoid a therapeutic misadventure in prescribing drugs, the following points should be noted. (1) Before prescribing any drug known to cause any adverse reaction, the doctor should make a reasonable effort to determine if any adverse reaction is likely to occur. (2) Sensitivity tests should be done before injecting preparations which are likely to produce anaphylactic shock. (3) The doctor should warn the patient of side-effects particularly possible drowsiness or similar accident-producing reaction, which may occur while he is taking the drug. (4) The doctor should inform the patient about the possibilities of permanent side-effects.

NEOPLASIA INDUCED BY MEDICAL TREATMENT: It is difficult to prove a cause and effect relationship between the therapy and trauma. (1) Haemangioendothelioma of liver induced by thorium

dioxide is the classic example. (2) Radiation will cause leukaemia. (3) X-radiation or radium application to the head, neck or upper thorax for various non-malignant conditions during childhood have an increased risk of developing thyroid gland cancer and also of the salivary glands and other head and neck structures. (4) Chlornaphazine and phenacetin may cause urinary tract carcinoma. (5) Contraceptive steroids can cause adenomas of the liver in females, and if continued unintentionally during pregnancy, the infant may develop a benign liver tumour. (6) Diethylstilboesterol causes vaginal adenosis and clear cell carcinoma of the vagina. (7) Exposure to pesticides cause skin and vulvar carcinoma.

VICARIOUS LIABILITY (liability for act of another) (vicarious = substituted): An employer is responsible not only for his own negligence, but also for the negligence of his employees, if such acts occur in the course of the employment and within its scope, by the principle of *respondeat superior* (let the master answer).

Conditions to be satisfied: (1) There must be an employer-employee relationship, (2) the employee's conduct must occur within the scope of his employment, and (3) while on the job.

Examples: (1) In general practice, the principal doctor becomes responsible for any negligence of his assistant. Both may be sued by the patient, even though the principal has no part in the negligent act. The same applies where the principal employs non-medical servants. (2) When two doctors practice as partners, each is liable for negligence of the other, even though he may have no part in the negligent act. (3) When two or more independent doctors are attending on a patient, each may be held liable for the negligence of others that he observes, or in the ordinary course should have observed and allows it to continue without objection. (4) **"Borrowed servant doctrine":** An employee may serve more than one employer, e.g., the nurse employed by a hospital to assist in operations may be the "borrowed servant" of the operating surgeon during the operation, and the servant of the hospital for all other purposes. In this case, the lending employer temporarily surrenders control over his worker and the borrowing employer temporarily takes over control. (5) A doctor may be associated temporarily with another doctor with the establishment of an employee-employer relationship between them. Thus, if one doctor assists another in the operating room for a fee, the assistant is considered as an employee of the principal surgeon. (6) If a physician has supervisory control and the right to give orders to a hospital employee in regard to the particular act, in the performance of which the employee is negligent, the physician becomes legally liable for the harm caused by the employee. (7) If a swab, sponge, instrument, etc., is left in the patient's body after the operation, the surgeon is liable for damages. (8) A hospital, as an employer, is responsible for negligence of its employees who are acting under its supervision and control. It does not matter whether they are full-time or part-time, resident or visiting, permanent or temporary, because even if they are not servants, they are the agents of the hospital to give the treatment. (9) Hospital management will be held responsible for the mistakes of resident physicians and interns in training, who are considered employees when performing their normal duties. (10) A physician is responsible for the acts of the interns and residents carried out under his direct supervision and control. (11) When employers provide medical services to their employees, or conduct pre-employment examination of prospective employees, they may be liable for the negligence of their doctors. (12) Insurers who have contracted to provide medical services may be liable for the negligence of their physicians. (13) The employer or the insurer of employees covered by Workmen's Compensation Act, may be liable for the negligence of their doctors. (14) Ordinarily, a surgeon is not liable for the negligence of anaesthetist, and the anaesthetist is not liable for the negligence of the operating surgeon. (15) Physicians and surgeons are not responsible for the negligent acts of competent nurse or other hospital personnel, unless such acts are carried out under their direct supervision and control. (16) When a doctor recommends another doctor to his patient after due care, he is not liable for the negligence of the new doctor, but he becomes liable if he knowingly refers his patient to an incompetent doctor. (17) When a sick or injured person consults his own doctor for diagnosis and treatment, and the latter recommends hospitalisation, the hospital to which the patient is admitted is not liable for the doctor's negligence resulting in injury to the patient. (18) Hospitals cannot be held responsible for the negligent acts of members of the superior medical staff in the treatment of patients, if it can be proved that the managers exercised the due care and skill, in selecting properly qualified and experienced staff. (19) If a physician has written a prescription properly, he is not liable for a pharmacist's negligence in preparing it, but he may be liable when he orders a prescription over the telephone resulting in misunderstanding as to the drugs or their dosage.

Liability: Both the employer and employee are sued by the patient, because the employee may lack funds for paying the damages. **Usually, liability will be fixed upon those actually at fault, and those whose control over the negligent is proved. The employer may be ordered by the Court to pay compensation to the injured patient. In such cases, the employer can engage in "third party proceeding", against the negligent doctor or employee asking for repayment.**

PRODUCTS LIABILITY

Products liability refers to the physical agent which caused the injury or death of the patient during treatment by the doctor. The injury or death of the patient may result from the unexpected by-product of faulty, defective, or negligently designed medical or surgical instruments or inadequate operating instructions. In such cases, the manufacturer becomes responsible for injury or death.

Proof: The doctor must prove that the manufacturer departed from standards of due care, with respect to negligent design, manufacture, assembly, packaging, failure to test and inspect for defects, or failure to warn or give adequate instructions. If the instrument functioned satisfactorily in previous operations or for several previous years in the hospital's possession, it is a proof that it was not defective at the time of supplying. Later, if the instrument develops a defect through ordinary and gradual wear and tear, or if the physician or the hospital misuses the manufacturer's medical products, the hospital or physician owner are liable for the failure to inspect, test and repair such defects. But the manufacturer becomes responsible, if the doctor can prove that the subsequent development of this defect was due to negligent design, structurally inferior component material, or improper assembly. An adequate warning cautions the user to follow directions, and may also notify the risk of disregarding directions.

Drugs: The manufacturer of medicines has a legal duty to use care in research and development of drugs. The manufacturer is liable, if a patient is injured due to a drug reaction due to the negligence or breach of warranty on the part of manufacturer. The manufacturer is also liable due to the harm caused by the contamination, adulteration, incorrect dosage or mistaken labelling of a drug. **Once the physician has been warned about possible side-effects, the manufacturer has no duty to ensure that the warning reaches the patient under normal circumstances.** From the information received from the manufacturer, and other medical sources, the doctor is required to inform the patient of those reasonably expected side-effects likely to occur in the particular circumstances. The manufacturer is responsible for performing studies of its product when adverse reactions are reported in articles in scientific journals. The result of these studies must be reported to the physicians. **The manufacturer is not responsible for unforeseeable or unknown dangers, it is unable to discover with reasonable care.** If the doctor has or should have information, knowledge, or suspicion from any source that a certain drug is likely to produce serious side-effects, he may become legally liable for prescribing it, if any substituted drug would have been adequate and satisfactory.

The manufacturer of a drug keeps a "package insert" in the drug carton or attaches it to the label of the immediate container. It bears adequate information for its use, including indications, effects, dosages, routes, methods and frequency and duration of administration, and any relevant side-effects, hazards, contraindications and precautions under which registered practitioners can use the drug safely and for the purposes for which it is intended, including all purposes for which it is advertised or represented. The burden of proving the safety and effectiveness of a new drug or new uses of an approved drug rests with the manufacturer.

Liability: The manufacturer, seller or anyone in the chain of sale, may be sued by the buyer, by another user of the product or by some third party, whose bodily injury is caused by the product. The patient has to prove that a defect in production and testing in the product existed, before it left the manufacturer's hands and that the defect was the proximate cause of the patient's injury. Evidence will have to be produced as to the drug's physical and chemical qualities, so as to show a need to warnings. **The product would be defective, if a drug manufacturer knew or should have known the presence of certain adverse effects and then failed to warn.** Causal connection should be established between the lack of warning and resulting harm.

MEDICAL INDEMNITY INSURANCE: It is a contract under which the insurance company agrees, in exchange for the payment of premiums, to indemnify (reimburse to compensate) the insured doctor as a result of his claimed professional negligence.

Objects: (1) To look after and protect the professional interests of the insured doctor. (2) To arrange, conduct and pay for the defence of such doctors. (3) To arrange all other professional assistance including pre-litigation advice. (4) To indemnify the insured doctor in respect of any loss or expense directly arising from actions, claims and demands against him on grounds of professional negligence, misconduct, etc. **When any dispute or allegation of negligence arises, the society must be contacted before any admissions or correspondence are entered into.**

MEDICAL RECORDS (M.R.)

Objects: (1) To serve as the basis for the patient's care and for continuity in the evaluation of the patient's treatment. (2) To serve as documentation for reimbursement. (3) To provide data for use in medical education and clinical research. (4) To document communication between the doctor treating the patient and any other health care professional who contributes to the patient's care. (5) To assist in protecting the legal interests of the patient, the hospital and the practitioner responsible for the patient. (6) To follow-up the patients, evaluation of drug therapy and cost accounting. (7) Medical records may be required in cases of professional negligence, for claims of third party payment under health and accident insurance, life insurance policies, policies for disability, accidental deaths, Workmen's Compensation Act, traffic accidents, etc.

Requirements: The minimum requirements of accurate medical records are: (1) Name, father's name, age, sex, occupation and address. (2) Date and hour of visiting the doctor/nursing home/hospital. (3) Evidence of informed consent. (4) Brief history of present illness, relevant past history and family history. (5) Findings of general physical and systemic examination showing objective findings and subjective complaints. (6) Diagnostic aids used and any reports received concerning the patient. (7) Date and hour of consultation with details and opinion of consultant. (8) Clinical impression with provisional and final diagnosis. (9) Progress notes including clinical observations. (10) Instructions given to the patient including diet. (11) Complications, if any. (12) Notations concerning lack of co-operation by the patient. (13) Failure of the patient to follow advice or failure to keep appointments. (14) Details of treatment including any procedures/operations recommended or performed. (15) In emergency cases, specific clinical data, and observations should be noted periodically. (16) In in-patients, the condition at the time of discharge, i.e. whether cured or relieved of complaints or referred to any other hospital or discharged on request or absconded should be noted.

The medical records must be accurate, appropriate, chronological, factual, relevant and complete. Nothing should be altered, deleted, substituted or added from the record, i.e. tampering should not be done. If tampering is done patient may be awarded large sums, even though there has been no negligence. The omission of essential details from the notes may cast a doubt on the truthfulness of the witness. If a correction has to be made of a prior entry on the record, it should not be totally obliterated, but a single line should be drawn through the word to be changed, and the correct information should be written above with the date of the change and the person's signature or legible initials. Further, an explanation as to why the record is being altered should be noted.

Good notes are of great value, not only when handing a patient over to another doctor, but also in meeting any criticism that may arise. If a patient refuses to accept the advice of his doctor, this fact should be recorded in writing. When there is a conflict of evidence, the Court will attach importance to the notes written at the time. Good notes may be of the greatest importance in supporting the doctor's evidence as against that of the plaintiff and his witnesses.

Patient has the right to know what is in his records and is entitled to a brief report of his hospital record on discharge. The next of kin can get the record in case of patient's death. Hospital has the responsibility

to supervise the maintenance of appropriate, accurate, timely and up-to-date patient's records. The rights of patients to have their hospital medical records regarded as confidential must be respected. If in the doctor's judgement making the record available to the patient would be harmful or dangerous to the patient, or not in his best interest (professional or therapeutic discretion"), the hospital can avoid to issue the record to the patient. The medical records of a patient (in-patient or out-patient) should not be given to any person without the consent of the patient. The police do not have a right to demand medical records except when there is statutory provision for such requisitions. The patient's record cannot be used in educational or diagnostic conferences or clinics or for publications, without the patient's consent. Hospitals have right to use the medical records without the consent of patient for statistical purposes and quality of care determinations. In the absence of agreement to the contrary, X-ray plates are the property of the treating doctor as part of his case record. The patient buys the skill and treatment rather than the X-ray films.

Regarding M.R. Medical Council states that: (a) A registered medical practitioner shall maintain a register of medical certificates giving full details of certificates issued with signature of patients and with at least one identification mark. (b) To maintain an MR pertaining to his/her indoor patients for a period of 3 years from the date of commencement of treatment. (c) Routine case records should be preserved up to 6 years after completion of treatment and up to 3 years after death of the patient. (d) Where there is a chance of litigation arising for medical purpose of negligence, record should be preserved for at least 25 years specially in case of minors. (e) Medicolegally important record should be preserved up to 10 years, after which they can be destroyed after making index and summary of the case. (f) There are certain records of hospital which are of public interest and are transferred to public record library after 50 years for release to public and those involve confidentiality of the individuals are released only after 100 years.

Format for Medical Record

(Regulation 3.1 of M.C.I.)

(1) Name of the patient
(2) Age
(3) Sex
(4) Address
(5) Occupation
(6) Date of first visit
(7) Clinical note (summary) of the case
(8) Provisional diagnosis
(9) Investigations advised with reports
(10) Diagnosis after investigation
(11) Advice
(12) Follow up
(13) Date
(14) Observations

Signature in full
Name of treating physician

DOCTORS, PUBLIC AND MEDIA: Doctors should individually and collectively influence medical content of the media since media has an important influence on the attitudes and actions of their audience. Doctors can (a) Volunteer services to media (print, radio and television) as an expert (b) Contribute medical-related articles to local dailies. (c) Organise events to interact with public such as health camps, blood donation drives and invite media to cover them.

CONSENT IN MEDICAL PRACTICE

Consent means voluntary agreement, compliance or permission. Consent signifies acceptance by a person of the consequences of an act that is being carried out. To be legally valid, it must be given after understanding what it is given for, and of risks involved.

Reasons for obtaining Consent: (1) To examine, treat or operate upon a patient without consent is assault in law, even if it is beneficial and done in good faith. The patient may recover damages. (2) If a doctor fails to give the required information to patient before asking for his consent to a particular operation or treatment, he may be charged for negligence.

Kinds of Consent: Consent may be: **(1) Express,** i.e, specifically stated by the patient, or **(2) Implied. Express consent may be (a) verbal, or (b) written.**

Implied Consent: An adult patient of sound mind who (1) knows that he can either agree or refuse to submit to treatment or an operation, (2) knows or has been fully or fairly informed by his doctor as to what is to be done, and (3) then cooperated with the physician, has impliedly consented in words. **The fact that a patient attends the hospital or calls the doctor to his house complaining of illness, implies that he consents to a general physical examination, to determine the nature of the illness. Consent is implied when a patient holds out his arm for an injection.** Such implied consent is the consent usually given in routine practice.

Full Disclosure: The facts which a doctor must disclose depends on the normal practice in his community, and on the circumstances of the case. In general, the patient should ordinarily be told everything. The doctor has to decide, after taking into consideration all aspects of the patient's personality, physical and mental state, how much can be safely disclosed. **The doctor need not disclose risks of which he himself is unaware. A physician need not inform the patient of risks that a person of average intelligence would be aware of, or in an emergency situation. The physician need not give information to those patients who waive their rights, but the waiver should be clearly written in the record.**

Therapeutic privilege: This is an exception to the rule of "full disclosure". Full disclosure of remote or theoretical risks involved could result in frightening a patient who is already fearful or who is an emotionally disturbed individual, and who may refuse the treatment when there is really little risk. It is only in the case of frank psychosis or extreme psycho-neurosis that the patient will be incapable of accepting the information. In these cases, the doctor may use discretion as to the facts which he discloses. The doctor should carefully note his decision in the patient's record, explaining his intentions and the reasons. He should request a consultation to establish that the patient is emotionally disturbed. The presence of a malignancy, or an unavoidable fatal lesion may not be disclosed, if the doctor feels the patient is not able to tolerate the knowledge. **If possible, the physician should explain the risks to the patient's spouse or next of kin.**

Prudent patient rule, i.e. what a prudent (reasonable) person in the patient's position would have decided, if adequately informed about all the reasonably foreseeable risks.

Informed Consent: Informed consent implies an understanding by the patient of (1) the nature of his condition, (2) the nature of the proposed treatment or procedure, (3) expectations of the recommended treatment and the likelihood of success, (4) the details of the alternative courses of treatment that are available, (5) the risks and benefits involved in both the proposed and alternative procedure, (6) the potential risks of not receiving treatment, (7) particular known inherent risks that are material to the informed dicision, so that he may accept or reject the procedure. **All disclosures must be in language the patient can understand. Physicians have a legal, moral and ethical duty to provide all relevant information that enables a patient to either accept or reject treatment.** This disclosure will very much reduce litigation, when the results are unsatisfactory or unexpected. **The patient must show that the doctor did not adhere to accepted medical standards to prove liability for lack of informed consent.**

Exceptions to informed consent: (1) Emergency. (2) Therapeutic privilege. (3) When a patient waives his right to informed consent and delegates the right to the doctor or a close relative.

Informed Refusal: The physician has a duty to disclose adequately and appropriately to the patient, the risks or possible consequences of refusal to undergo a test or treatment. After understanding all the facts, the patient can refuse to submit to treatment or an operation.

Examination may reveal findings which when used in the process of investigation can damage the party examined. If later on, the party is proved to be innocent, the damage sustained cannot be undone. This is why the right to deny consent to examination is generally given to the party.

Paternalism is an abuse of medical knowledge so as to distort the doctor-patient relationship in such a way that the patient is deprived of his autonomy, or of his ability to make a rational choice. The doctor does not disclose the nature of the illness and the proposed treatment depriving the right of patient to accept or reject treatment. The doctor may be sued under S.350, I.P.C. If patient complains to medical council, it can take action against the doctor.

RULES OF CONSENT: (1) **Consent is necessary for every medical examination.** Ordinarily, formal consent to medical examination is not required, because the patient behaves in a manner which implies consent.

(2) Oral consent should be obtained in the presence of a disinterested third party, e.g., nurse.

(3) **Written consent is not necessary in any case. However, it should be taken for proving the same in the Court if necessity arises. Written consent should refer to one specific procedure, and not blanket permission on admission to hospital. Written consent should be in proper form and suitably drafted for the circumstances.** The consent form should include specific consent to the administration of a general anaesthetic. The nature of the operation should be entered on the form as precisely as is consistent with the best interests of the patients. The wording should include a phrase to confirm that the patient has been informed of the nature of the procedure, before signing takes place. The written consent should be witnessed by another person, present at the signing to prevent any allegation that the consent was forged or obtained under pressure or compulsion.

(4) **Any procedure beyond routine physical examination,** such as operation, blood transfusion, collection of blood, etc. **requires express consent.** It must be taken before the act, but not at the time of admission into the hospital. It should be ongoing process extending overtime.

(5) The doctor should explain the object of the examination to the patient, and patient should be informed that the findings will be included in a medical report.

(6) **In medicolegal cases the doctor should inform the patient that he has right to refuse to submit to examination and that the result may go against him. If the patient refuses, he cannot be examined.**

(7) **The consent should be free, voluntary, clear, intelligent, informed, direct, and personal.** There should be no fraud, misrepresentation of facts, undue influence, compulsion, threat of physical injury, death or other consequences.

(8) **In criminal cases, the victim cannot be examined without his/her consent. The Court also cannot force a person to get medically examined, against his will.** (A) In cases of rape, the victim should not be examined without written consent. (B) In medicolegal cases of pregnancy, delivery and abortion, the woman should not be examined without her consent.

(9) **S.53, Cr.P.C.** (1) **A person is arrested on** a charge of committing an offence, and there may be reasons for believing that an examination of his person will provide evidence as to the commission of an offence. **A registered medical practitioner can examine such person, even by using reasonable force, if the examination is requested by a police officer not below the rank of sub-inspector** (or any other officer acting under his direction and good faith). **"Examination" includes,** examination of blood, blood stains, semen, swabs in case of sexual offences, sputum, sweat, hair samples, fingernail clippings, etc. by the use of modern and scientific techniques including DNA profiling and such other tests that a medical practitioner thinks necessary in that particular case. If the accused refuses examination, this may go against him in criminal proceedings. (2) **In the case of a female, the examination should be made only by or under the supervision of a female registered medical practitioner [S.53,(2) Cr.P.C].**

S.54, Cr.P.C. (1) It mandates compulsory medical examination in all cases of arrest by the police. (2) A copy of the report of such examination is to be furnished by the medical practitioner to the arrested person or the person nominated by such arrested person.

(10) In cases of **drunkenness,** the person should not be examined and blood, urine, or breath should not be collected without his written consent. But, if the person becomes unconscious or incapable of giving consent, examination and treatment can be carried out. The consent of guardian or of relatives if available, should be taken. **The person can be examined without consent, if requested by the sub-inspector of police.**

(11) **Sec. 87, I.P.C. A person above 18 years of age can give valid consent to suffer any harm,** which may result from an act not intended or not known to cause death or grievous hurt.

A person may be suffering from a disease which is certain to shorten his life. He can give free and informed consent to take the risk of operation, which though fatal in the majority of cases is the only available treatment. The surgeon cannot be held responsible, if the patient dies.

(12) **Sec. 88, I.P.C.** A person can give valid consent to suffer any harm which may result from an act, not intended or not known to cause death, done in good faith and for its benefit.

If a surgeon operates on a patient in good faith and for his benefit, even though the operation is a risk, he cannot be held responsible if the patient dies.

S. 88, I.P.C. is ambiguous and is not specific for medical treatment. The implication is that consent of parents or guardians is necessary for surgical or medical procedures if the patient is a minor.

(13) Sec. 89, I.P.C. **A child under 12 years of age and an insane person cannot give valid consent to suffer any harm which may result from an act done in good faith and for its benefit.** The consent of the parent or guardian should be taken. If they refuse, the doctor cannot treat the patient even to save the life.

A father giving consent for an operation on the child in good faith and for the child's benefit, even though the operation is risky, cannot be held responsible if the child dies.

Loco Parentis (in place of a parent): **In an emergency involving children,** when their parents or guardians are not available, **consent is taken from the person-in-charge of the child,** e.g., a school teacher can give consent for treating a child who becomes sick during a picnic away from home town, or the consent of the headmaster of a residential school.

(14) Sec. 90, I.P.C. **A consent given by a person under fear of injury, or due to misunderstanding of a fact is not valid.** The consent given by an insane or intoxicated person, who is unable to understand the nature and consequences of that to which he gives his consent is invalid.

To represent to a patient that an operation is necessary to save life or to preserve health, when that is not the case or to indicate that it will give greater relief than there is any reasonable prospect of obtaining is to perpetrate a fraud on the patient that vitiates his consent.

(15) S. 92, I.P.C. **Any harm caused to a person in good faith, even without that person's consent is not an offence, if the circumstances are such, that it is impossible for that person to signify consent,** and has no guardian or other person in lawful charge of him from whom it is possible to obtain consent in time for the thing to be done in benefit. **Nothing is said to be done in good faith which is done without due care and attention.**

A person may be involved in an accident, which may necessitate an amputation; if it is done without his consent, it is not an offence. In an emergency, the law implies consent. An emergency is defined as a medical situation, such as to render immediate treatment advisable either to save life or to safeguard health.

In an emergency, a comatose patient requiring immediate treatment, a mentally incompetent patient requiring treatment when a legal guardian is not available, an intoxicated patient who temporarily lacks the capacity to consent but requires treatment, consent is implied. A doctor may extend a procedure beyond the scope of consent to treat an emergency.

(16) S.93, I.P.C. Any communication made in good faith for the benefit of a person is not an offence, if it causes harm to that person to whom it is made.

A physician in good faith tells a patient that he cannot live. The patient dies in consequence of the shock. The physician has not committed any offence.

(17) The doctor should inform reasonably to the patient about the nature, consequences and risks of the examination or operation before taking the consent. **In an obscure case, the doctor should obtain an open consent to use his discretion for additional procedures needed to cope with unanticipated situations that endanger his health** (extension doctrine). It is not applicable to non-essential procedures. **When there are two or more methods of treatment, the patient should be allowed to choose and give consent for any method.**

If in the course of an operation to which the patient has consented, the physician discovers conditions that had not been anticipated before the operation began, and which would endanger the life or health of the patient if not corrected, the doctor would be justified in extending the operation to correct them, even though no express consent was obtained. If an anaesthetist administers a type of anaesthetic expressly prohibited by the patient, he will be responsible for damages resulting from an unfortunate occurrence caused by the anaesthetic, even though there is no negligence in its administration.

(18) Consent of the inmates of the hostel, etc., is necessary if they are above 12 years. Within 12 years, the head master or warden can give consent. If an inmate above 12 years refuses treatment, and he is likely to spread the disease, he can be asked to leave the hostel. However, if he stays in hostel, he can be treated without his consent.

(19) **When an operation is made compulsory by law, e.g., vaccination, the law provides the consent.**

(20) A prisoner can be treated forcibly without consent in the interest of the society.

(21) **Consent given for committing a crime or an illegal act, such as criminal abortion is invalid.**

(22) Consent is not a defence in cases of professional negligence.

(23) The nature of illness of a patient should not be disclosed to any third party without the consent of the patient.

(24) **For contraceptive sterilisation, consent of both the husband and wife should be obtained.**

(25) **The consent of one spouse is not necessary for an operation or treatment of other.** A husband has no right to refuse consent to any operation, including a gynaecological operation, which is required to safeguard the health of his wife. The consent of wife is enough. **It is advisable to take the consent of the spouse whenever practicable, especially if the operation involves danger to life, may destroy or limit sex functions, or may result in the death of an unborn child.**

(26) **It is unlawful to detain an adult patient in hospital against his will.** If a patient demands discharge against medical advice, this should be recorded and his signature obtained.

(27) A living adult person can give consent for donating one of his kidneys to be grafted into another person. The donor must be informed of the procedure involved and possible risks. **The donation should not be accepted, if there is any risk of life of donor.**

(28) If any person has donated his eyes to be used for therapeutic purpose after his death, **the eyes can be removed only with the consent of guardian or legal heirs.**

(29) **If any person has donated his body to be used for therapeutic or research purposes after his death, it is not binding on his spouse or next of kin.** For organ transplantation, the organs of the dead person, such as heart, kidney, liver, etc. should not be removed without the consent of the guardian or legal heirs. Precautions should be taken to preserve the anonymity of both donor and recipient.

(30) **Pathological autopsy should not be conducted without the consent of the guardian or legal heirs of the deceased.** If the autopsy is done without consent, the doctor is liable for damages for the mental anguish suffered by heirs due to the mutilation of the body. Specific authorisation should be obtained for retention of organs and parts of the body. **In medicolegal autopsies (statutory authorisation), consent is not required and the doctor can remove from the cadaver anything that is essential for purposes of examination.**

CASE: (1) MOSS Vs RISHWORTH: An 11-year-old girl was taken to surgeon for removal of tonsils and adenoids by her two adult sisters. The child died under anaesthetic. The Court held that there was no emergency which would excuse the need for parental consent, and the father could recover damages.

(2) JOCKOVACH Vs YOCUM: The arm of a 7 year old boy was crushed by a train. The boy's arm was amputated immediately as the doctors could not contact parents. The consent of the parents was implied by the emergency.

(3) WELLS Vs MC GEHEE: A 7 year old child died under anaesthesia for treatment of a broken arm, which was given without the consent of the mother as she could not be contacted. The Court held that an emergency existed.

(4) DRUMMOND'S CASE: Drummond sued a woman patient for recovery of fees. The patient counterclaimed damages as a drug was administered to her, without her consent. She alleged that phenobarbitone, which she refused to take, was mixed in soup and meat and given to her daily, which prolonged her stay in the nursing home, as a psychological consequence for 16 weeks. The Court held that the administration of a drug to a person without that person's knowledge and consent was assault, and awarded nominal damages as the drug did not cause substantial harm.

EUTHANASIA (mercy killing): (Eu = good; thanatos = death): It means producing painless death of a person suffering from hopelessly incurable and painful disease.

Types: (1) Active or positive. (2) Passive or negative. **Active euthanasia** is a positive merciful act, to end useless suffering or a meaningless existence. It is an act of commission, e.g., by giving large doses of drugs to hasten death. **Passive euthanasia means discontinuing or not using extraordinary life-sustaining measures to prolong life.** This includes acts of omission, such as failure to resuscitate a terminally ill or hopelessly incapacitated patient or a severely defective newborn infant. It is not using measures that would probably delay death, such as turning off a respirator, stopping medications or food and water and allowing the person to dehydrate or starve or not delivering cardio-pulmonary resuscitation, which permits natural death to occur.

Voluntary euthanasia means at the will of the person, and **involuntary** means against the will of the person, i.e., compulsory. **Non-voluntary refers to cases of persons incapable of making their wishes known,** e.g., in persons with irreversible coma or severely defective infants. **Euthanasia advocates the administration of lethal doses of opium or other narcotic drugs.**

Passive euthanasia: The supreme court held that 'right to die with dignity' is a part of right to life, a fundamentals right under Article 21 of the Constitution, and allowed "living will" where, an ailing adult in his conscious mind, is permitted to refuse medical treatment or voluntarily decide not to take medical treatment to embrace death in a natural way.

Guidelines: (1) The will can be executed only by an adult with a sound and healthy mind. (2) It should be voluntarily executed based on informed consent. (3) It should be expressed in clear and unambiguous terms. (4) The will should be signed by the executor before a first class judicial magistrate. (5) The will should mention the circumstances in which the treatment should be withdrawn and the name of the guardian or close relative who can authorize for starting passive euthanasia. (6) The treating physician should ascentain the genuineness from the jurisdictional first class magistrate. (7) The hospital medical board should authorize withdrawal or treatment.

The Netherlands was the first country to legalise passive voluntary euthanasia and assisted suicide in 2002, if the following conditions were met: (1) The disease is incurable. (2) The patient's suffering is unbearable. (3) Patient's condition is terminal. (4) Patient requests death. Another physician must be consulted first and life must be ended in a medically appropriate way. Other countries which have joined this select group are Belgium, Luxemburg, Switzerland, Thailand.

Assisted Suicide: A person providing information to another with information, guidance and means to take his own life with the intention that it will be used for this purpose is assisted suicide

Terminal sedation: It includes the administration of morphine and similar medications, which has a dual effect of relieving of pain and hastening the death **(aid-in-dying).** If the patient requests the same medical treatment with its known dual effects, and if the physician knowingly provides that medication by prescription so that patient can end his life, it is considered **physician-assisted suicide.**

Article 21 of the constitution of India guarntees "right to live", but does not imply "right to die".

Iatrogenic Diseases: Iatrogenic disease can be defined as a disease that results from administration of a drug, or medical or surgical acts for prophylaxis, diagnosis or treatment.

DEATHS DUE TO MEDICAL CARE: Deaths may occur due to: (1) Complications of anaesthesia. (2) Complications of surgery. (3) Nosocomial infections. The use and/or misuse of urinary catheters, techniques and equipment employed in intravenous therapy; hyperalimentation, and respiratory therapy cause most of these infections. (4) Therapeutic misadventure. (5) Professional negligence. (a) Administration of wrong dose. (b) Pharmacist dispensing wrong medicine due to illegible prescription. (c) Abbreviations of drugs. (d) Confusing patients with similar names and to administer the correct dose to the wrong patient. (e) Susceptibility of children to medication errors. (f) New approved drugs may result in death from side-effects undetected in the study population. (g) Patient or specimen misidentification in laboratory testing can lead to inappropriate and potentially life-threatening therapy. (h) Errors in reporting abnormal values in electrolyte analysis. (i) Mismatched blood transfusion.

PENAL PROVISIONS APPLICABLE TO MEDICAL PRACTICE:

S. 52, I.P.C.: Nothing is said to be done in good faith which is done without due care and attention.

S. 80, I.P.C.: Refusing to sign a statement (imprisonment up to 3 months, or with fine, or with both).

S. 118, I.P.C.: Concealing design to commit offence punishable with death or imprisonment for life. (imprisonment for 3 months if the offence is not committed and 7 years if the offence is committed).

S. 174, I.P.C.: Non-attendance in obedience to an order from public servant (imprisonment up to one month, or with fine or both).

S. 175, I.P.C.: Omission to produce document to public servant by person legally bound to produce it (one month imprisonment).

S. 176, I.P.C.: Omission to give notice or information to public servant by person legally bound to give it (imprisonment up to one month or fine or both).

S. 177, I.P.C.: Furnishing false information (imprisonment up to six months or fine or both).

S. 178, I.P.C.: Refusing oath or affirmation when duly required by public servant to make it (imprisonment up to six month or fine or both).

S. 179, I.P.C.: Refusing to answer public servant authorised to question (imprisonment up to six months or fine or both).

S. 181, I.P.C.: False statement on oath or affirmation to public servant or person authorised to administer an oath or affirmation (imprisonment up to 3 years and fine).

S. 182, I.P.C.: False information with intent to cause public servant to use his lawful power to the injury of another person (imprisonment up to six months or fine or both).

S. 191, I.P.C.: Giving false evidence.

S. 192, I.P.C.: Fabricating false evidence.

S. 193, I.P.C.: Punishment for false evidence (imprisonment up to seven years or life).

S. 194, I.P.C.: Giving or fabricating false evidence with intent to procure conviction of capital offence (imprisonment up to ten years).

S. 195, I.P.C.: Giving or fabricating false evidence with intent to procure conviction of offence punishable with imprisonment up to 10 years or life.

S. 197, I.P.C.: Issuing or signing false certificate (imprisonment up to seven years).

S. 198, I.P.C.: Using as true, a certificate known to be false (imprisonment up to 10 years and fine).

S. 201, I.P.C.: Causing disappearance of evidence of offence, or giving false information to screen offenders (imprisonment up to ten years).

S. 202, I.P.C.: Intentional omission to give information of offence by person bound to inform (imprisonment up to six months or fine or both).

S. 203, I.P.C.: Giving false information respecting an offence committed (imprisonment up to two years or fine or both).

S. 204, I.P.C.: Destruction of document to prevent its production as evidence (imprisonment up to two years or fine or both).

S. 269, I.P.C.: Negligent act likely to spread infection of disease dangerous to life (imprisonment up to six months or fine or both).

S. 270, I.P.C.: Malignant act likely to spread infection of disease dangerous to life (imprisonment up to two years or fine or both).

S. 284, I.P.C.: Negligent conduct with respect to poisonous substances (imprisonment up to 6 months or fine or both).

S. 304A, I.P.C.: Causing death by negligence (imprisonment up to 2 years or with fine or both).

S. 336 to S. 338, I.P.C.: Rash and negligent acts that endanger human life, or the personal safety of others (imprisonment from 3 months to 2 years, or fine, or both).

S. 39, Cr. P.C.: Every person, aware of the commission of, or of the intention of any other person to commit any offence punishable under I.P.C. shall forthwith give information to the nearest Magistrate or police officer of such commission or intention.

S. 160, Cr.P.C.: Police officer has the power to summon any witness (doctor) to police station for recording a statement.

S. 161, Cr.P.C.: The police has the power to examine witnesses.

S. 162, Cr.P.C.: Oral statements made to the police and recorded by the police should not be signed.

Legal protection to medical doctors is provided by S. 87 to 93, I.P.C.

MALINGERING: Malingering or shamming means conscious, planned feigning or pretending a disease for the sake of gain.

Reasons: Diseases may be feigned for several reasons, such as by soldiers or policemen to avoid their duties, by prisoners to avoid hard work, by businessmen to avoid business contracts, by workmen to claim compensation, by beggars to attract public sympathy, by criminals to avoid legal responsibility, etc. **The diseases that may be feigned are** many, e.g., dyspepsia, intestinal colic, ulcers, spitting of blood, ophthalmia, diabetes, rheumatism, lumbago, neurasthenia, aphasia, sciatica, pain in the back, blindness, deafness, vertigo, epilepsy, insanity, paralysis of the limbs, burns, artificial bruises, etc. **Patients can distort or exaggerate their symptoms but true simulation is very rare.**

Examples: (1) The patient may injure his nasopharynx with a sharp instrument, swallow the blood and regurgitate it in front of the doctor to mimic haematemesis. (2) A skilful puncturing of the anal or vaginal mucosa, may produce bleeding. (3) Excessive intake of digitalis may simulate a heart condition. (4) Eating of large amount of carrot will produce carotinaemia and may simulate jaundice. (5) Chronic ingestion of coumarin will induce a haemorrhagic diathesis. In many cases detection is easy, but in some cases it is difficult.

Diagnosis: The history of the case should be taken from the person himself, and his relatives or friends, and any inconsistencies in his description of the symptoms noted. Usually, the signs and symptoms do not conform to any known disease. **Malingering can be diagnosed by keeping the patient under observation and watching him without his knowledge.** A complete examination is essential after removing the bandages if any, and washing the part. Rarely an anaesthetic may be given to detect malingering.

CHAPTER

4 IDENTIFICATION

FM 3.1: Define and describe Corpus Delicti, establishment of identity of living persons including race, sex, religion, complexion, stature, age determination using morphology, teeth-eruption, decay, bite marks, bones-ossification centres, medicolegal aspects of age.

FM 3.2: Describe and discuss identification of criminals, unknown persons, dead bodies from the remains—hairs, fibers, teeth, anthropometry, dactylography, foot prints, scars, tattoos, poroscopy and superimposition.

Identification is the determination of the individuality of a person based on certain physical characteristics, i.e., exact fixation of personality. In partial or incomplete identification, certain facts are determined, e.g., race, age, sex, stature, etc., while other characters are not known.

IDENTIFICATION IS NECESSARY IN: (1) Living persons. (2) Recently dead persons. (3) Decomposed bodies. (4) Mutilated and burnt bodies, and (5) Skeleton. It is necessary: (1) In criminal cases like persons accused of assault, murder, rape, etc., interchange of newborn babies in hospitals, impersonation, etc. (2) In civil cases like marriage, inheritance, passport, insurance claims, disputed sex, missing persons, etc. At least two identification marks should be noted by the doctor in all medicolegal cases. Before identifying the accused person in the Court, the doctor should verify the identification marks noted by him.

The police have to establish the identity of a person. In some cases, the doctor may be able to supply the police with certain facts about an individual, a dead body or fragmentary remains, which help the police to complete identification.

Visual identification becomes difficult or impossible in cases of fires, explosions, advanced decomposition, mutilation, aircraft accidents, earthquakes, etc.

THE CORPUS DELICTI: The corpus delicti (delicti = fault; offence)(the body of offence; the essence of crime) means, the facts of any criminal offence, e.g., murder. The corpus delicti of murder is the fact that a person died from unlawful violence. It includes the body of the victim and other facts which are conclusive of death by foul play, such as a bullet or a broken knife-blade found in the body and responsible for death. **Clothings showing marks of the weapon, and drawings and photographs of the deceased showing fatal injuries** are also included in this term. **The main part of corpus delicti is the establishment of identity of the dead body, and infliction of violence in a particular way, at a particular time and place, by the person or persons charged with the crime and none other.** The case against the accused cannot be established unless there is convincing proof of these points.

Identification of a dead victim often helps the police to trace the victim's movements, to know his background, talk to his friends and find out his enemies. If the victim's identity is not known, it becomes difficult for the police to solve the crime. The identification of a dead body and proof of corpus delicti is important before a sentence is passed in murder trials, as unclaimed, decomposed bodies, or portions of a dead body, or bones are sometimes produced to support false charge. However, a conviction for an offence does not necessarily depend upon the corpus delicti, if there are eye-witnesses or strong corroborative evidence.

IDENTIFICATION DATA Fig. (4–1): (1) Race and religion. (2) Sex. (3) Age. (4) General development and stature. (5) Complexion and features.(6) External peculiarities, such as moles, birthmarks, malformations, scars, tattoo marks, wounds, occupation marks, etc.

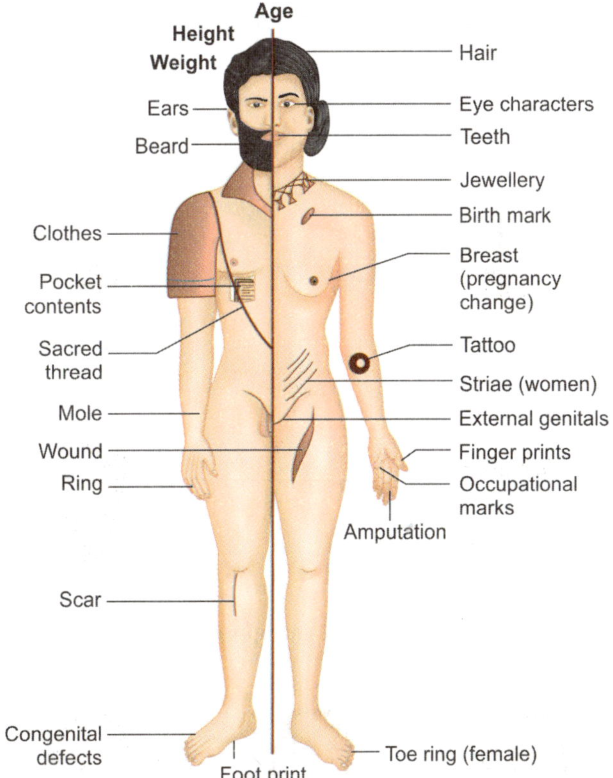

Fig. (4–1). Identification data.

(7) Anthropometric measurements. (8) Fingerprints and footprints. (9) Teeth. (10) Personal effects: clothes, pocket contents, jewellery, etc. (11) Handwriting. (12) Speech and voice. (13) Gait, tricks of manner and habit. (14) Memory and education. 11 to 14 are useful only in the living Fig. (4–1). **As no single feature is reliable for identification, a combination of features** is taken.

Sex, age, and stature are primary characteristics of identification.

RACE Figs. (4–2 to 4–5): It can be determined by:

(1) **COMPLEXION:** It is of limited value. The skin is brown in Indians, fair in Europeans and black in Negroes. Skin colour is changed by decomposition, burning, etc.

(2) **EYES:** Indians have dark eyes, a few have brown eyes. Europeans have blue or grey eyes.

(3) **HAIR:** Indians have black, thin hair. Europeans fair or light brown or reddish. Indians, Mongolians and Europeans have straight or wavy hair. Negroes have wooly hair (i.e., arranged in tight spirals). Mongolian hair is coarse and dark and usually circular on cross-section, and has a dense uniform pigmentation and dark medulla. Negro hair is elongated, oval on cross-section and has a dense pigment with an irregular distribution. Caucasian hair has round or oval shape on cross-section, with uniform distribution of fine or coarse pigment.

(4) **CLOTHES:** The dress may be helpful sometimes.

(5) **SKELETON:** The **Cephalic Index (C.I.)** or Index of Breadth is important Table (4–1).

$$\text{C.I.} = \frac{\text{Maximum breadth of skull}}{\text{Maximum length of skull}} \times 100$$

The breadth and length are measured by calipers between both parietal eminences, and between glabella and external occipital protuberance, and not by measuring tape. From the various measurements of the skull, race can be determined in 85 to 90% of cases. Because of racial mixing, all the skulls may not be correctly differentiated into the three races. Even between the skulls of same race, there will be a considerable overlap of features with those of another race.

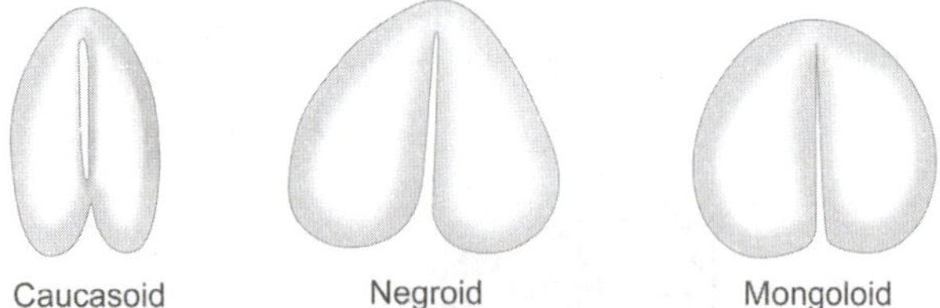

Fig. (4–2). Shape of the nasal aperture.

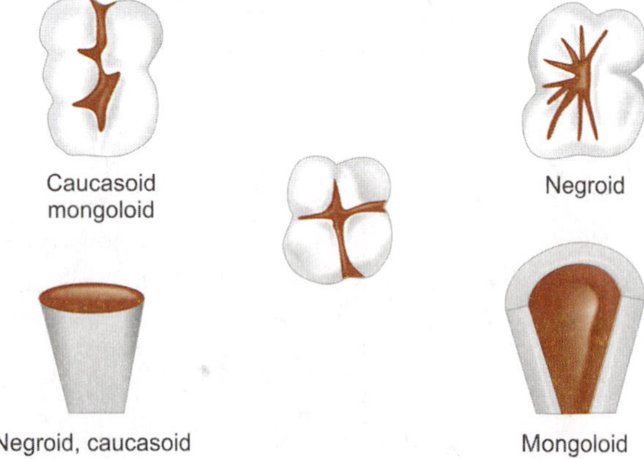

Fig. (4–3). The molars and upper incisor teeth.

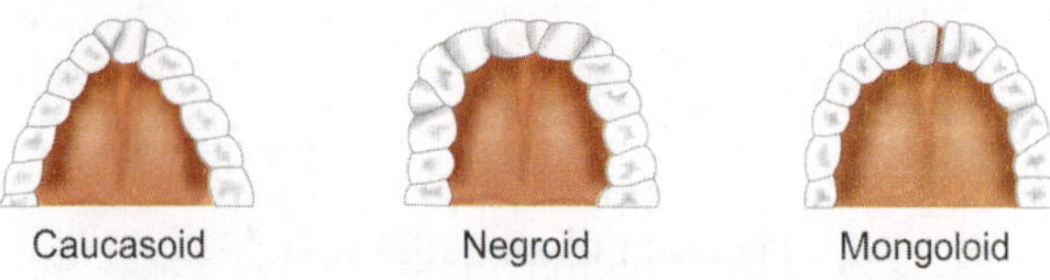

Fig. (4–4). Diagram of the shapes of upper jaw.

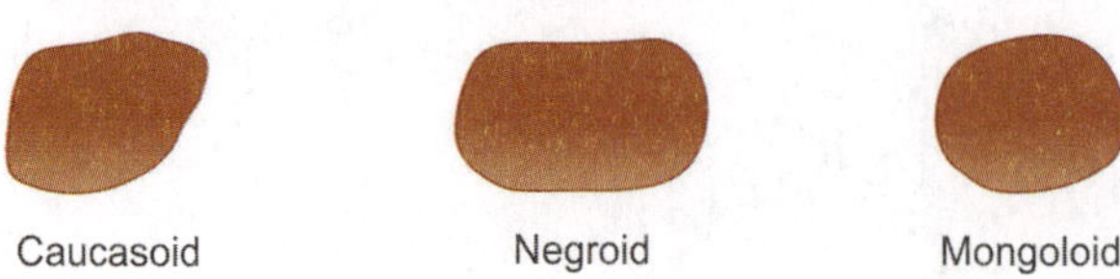

Fig. (4–5). Diagram of the shapes of orbits.

Table (4–1). Racial difference in the skull

Type of skull	Cephalic index	Race
(1) Dolicocephalic (long-headed):	70 to75	Pure Aryans, Aborigines and Negroes.
(2) Mesaticephalic (medium-headed):	75 to 80	Europeans Chinese and Indians.
(3) Brachycephalic (short-headed):	80 to 85	Mongolian.

The skull of an Indian is Caucasian with a few Negroid characters.

CAUCASIAN (WHITE): (Europeans, West Asians, Asian Indians and some Americans). Skull tends to be high with almost completely straight lower face (orthognathism). Skull rounded, orbits triangular, nasal aperture elongated, and nasal sill very sharp-edged, palate triangular, upper and lower limbs normal in proportion to body.

MONGOLIAN (YELLOW): They have in the malar and midnasal area an anterior projection, giving the appearance of a somewhat flatter facial skeleton than that of the caucasoids. Skull square, orbits rounded, nasal aperture rounded, palate rounded, upper and lower limbs smaller.

NEGRO (BLACK): The lower face projects forward (facial prognathism), skull narrow and elongated, orbits square, nasal aperture broad, and nasal sill guttered, palate rectangular, upper and lower limbs longer.

Brachycephaly is due to fusion of coronal suture. Dolicocephaly is due to fusion of sagittal suture.

Racial mixing has been and is constant, and as such pure races are uncommon. The Mongoloids include native Americans, Asiatic orientals, such as Koreans, Japanese, Chinese and Southeast Asians.

RELIGION: Hindu males are not circumcised. *Sacred thread*, necklace of wooden beads, caste marks on forehead, tuft of hair on back of head, and piercing of ear lobes if present are helpful. **Hindu females** may have vermilion (cinnabar) on head, silver toe ornaments, *thali,* tattoo marks, nose-ring aperture in left nostril, few openings for ear-rings along the helix. **Muslim females** may have nose-ring aperture in septum only, several openings in the ears along helix and usually no tattoo marks. **Muslim males** are circumcised and may have marks of corns and callosities on lateral aspects of knees and feet.

SEX

Sex has to be determined in cases of (1) heirship, (2) marriage, (3) divorce, (4) legitimacy, (5) impotence, (6) rape, etc.

In normal cases, sex determination is easy from external examination only Table (4–2), but it is difficult in cases of (1) hermaphroditism, (2) concealed sex, (3) advanced decomposition, and (4) skeleton.

A normal person has 46 chromosomes. The chromatin pattern in male is XY and in female XX. Masculine and feminine characteristics most directly depend on the level of circulating sex hormones.

Table (4–2). Sex characteristics

	Trait	Male	Female
(1)	Gonads:	A functioning testis. The penis, prostate, etc., are only appendages.	A functioning ovary. The uterus, vagina, etc., are only appendages.
(2)	Build:	Larger with greater muscular development.	Smaller with less muscular development.
(3)	Shoulders:	Broader than hips.	Narrower than hips.
(4)	Waist:	Ill-defined.	Well-defined.
(5)	Trunk:	Abdominal segment smaller.	Abdominal segment longer.
(6)	Thorax:	Dimensions more.	Shorter and rounded.
(7)	Limbs:	Longer.	Shorter.
(8)	Arms:	Flat on section.	Cylindrical on section.
(9)	Thighs:	Cylindrical.	Conical, due to shorter femur and greater deposition of fat.
(10)	Gluteal region:	Flatter.	Full and rounded.
(11)	Wrists and ankles:	Not delicate.	Delicate.
(12)	Breasts:	Not developed.	Developed.
(13)	Pubic hair:	Thick and extends upward to the umbilicus (rhomboidal).	Thin, horizontal and covers mons veneris only (triangular).
(14)	Body hair:	Present on face and chest.	Absent on face and chest.
(15)	Head hair:	Shorter, thicker and coarser.	Longer, thinner and finer.
(16)	Larynx:	Prominent. Length 4.8 cm.	Not prominent. Length 3.8 cm.

Sex chromatin: It is a small planoconvex mass [about one micron in diameter lying near nuclear membrane **(Barr body)** demonstrated by Dixon and Tarr]. In the buccal smear, the percentage of nuclei containing chromatin body ranges from zero to four in males and 20 to 80 in females.

In females, neutrophil leucocytes contain a small nuclear attachment of drumstick form **(Davidson body)** in about 3% of cells. This is absent in males.

Exact sex determination can be made using a single specimen of buccal smear, saliva or hair follicle, by the combined treatment of quinacrine dihydrochloride staining for Y chromosome which is seen as bright fluorescent body in the nuclei of male cells, and fluorescent Feulgen reaction using acriflavin Schiff reagent for X chromosomes, which is seen as bright yellow spot in the nuclei Fig. (4–6). The percentage of quinacrine positive bodies ranges from 45 to 80% in males, and 0 to 4% in females. With Feulgen reaction technique, fluorescent bodies are found in 50 to 70% of cells in females, and 0 to 2% in males. IN DECOMPOSED BODIES SEX CHROMATIN CANNOT BE MADE OUT.

By using fluorescent dyes Y chromosome can be demonstrated in dental pulp tissue up to one year. F-bodies are seen in 30 to 70% of cells in males and 0 to 4% in females.

Sex can be determined from dental pulp, bone marrow and amniotic fluid. Karyotyping (study of chromosomal constitution of the nucleus of a cell for sex determination) of foetus may be done from lymphocytes, amniocytes and fibroblasts.

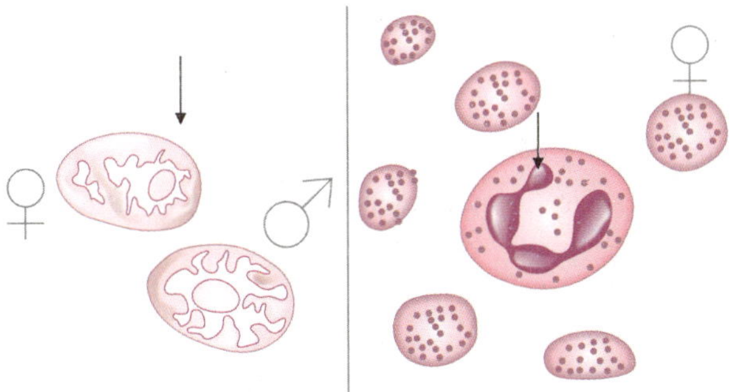

Fig. (4–6). The sex chromatin.

INTERSEX: It is an intermingling in one individual of characters of both sexes in varying degrees, including physical form, reproductive organs and sexual behaviour. It results from some defect in the embryonic development. It can be divided into four groups.

(1) Gonadal Agenesis: In this condition, the **testes or ovaries have never developed**. The nuclear sex is negative.

(2) Gonadal Dysgenesis: In this condition, the external sexual structures are present, but **at puberty the testes or the ovaries fail to develop.**

(A) KLINEFELTER'S SYNDROME: In this condition, the anatomical structure is male, but the nuclear sexing is female. The sex chromosome pattern is XXY (47 chromosomes). It is usually diagnosed when there is a delay in onset of puberty, behavioural disorders and mental retardation. Axillary and pubic hair are absent, and hair on chest and chin are reduced. Gynaecomastia, azoospermia, low levels of testosterone, sterility, increased urinary gonadotrophins, signs of eunachoidism and increased height are common. Testicular atrophy with hyalinisation of seminiferous tubules is seen histologically. Hypergonadotropic hypogonadism (defective development of testes or ovaries and excess pituitary gonadotropin secretion) is seen.

(B) TURNER'S SYNDROME: It is the most common sex chromosome abnormality of human females. Its incidence in newborn is about 1 in 2500. In this condition, the anatomical structure is female, but the nuclear sexing is male. The ovaries do not contain primordial follicles (ovarian dysgenesis). The sex chromosome pattern is XO (45 chromosomes). It can be recognised at birth by oedema of the dorsum of the hands and feet, loose skin folds in the nape of the neck, low birth weight and short stature. It is characterised by primary amenorrhoea, sterility, lack of development of primary and secondary sexual characteristics, increased urinary gonadotrophin excretion, pigmented naevi, a short fourth metatarsal, webbed-neck, shield-chest, wide-set nipples, high-arched palate, low-set ears, slow growth, learning problems, spina bifida, coarctation of aorta, septal defects, renal defects, Cushing's syndrome and a high incidence of diabetes mellitus. Most common heart

defects are bicuspid aortic valve (30%) coarcation of aorta (5 to 10%), septal defects and aortic dissection.

(3) True Hermaphroditism: This is a very rare condition of **bisexuality in which an ovary and a testicle or two ovotestis are present with the external genitalia of both sexes**. The gonad may be abdominal, inguinal or labio-scrotal in position. There may be uterus. Phallus may be penile or clitoral; the labia may be bifid as in female or fused resembling the scrotum of the male. Neither gonad is completely functional. The somatic sex chromatin may be male or female.

(4) Pseudo-hermaphroditism: In this condition gonadal tissue of only one sex is seen internally, but external appearance is of the opposite sex. **(A) Male pseudohermaphroditism: Nuclear sex is XY, but sex organs and sexual characteristics deviate to female form, because of testicular feminisation.** It is characterised by primary amenorrhoea, female external genitalia, normal size breasts, scanty or absent axillary and pubic hair. Testes are in the abdomen or inguinal canal; 5-a reductase deficiency occurs. **(B) Female pseudohermaphroditism:** Nuclear sex is **XX, but deviation of sex organs and sexual characters towards male are seen, due to adrenal hyperplasia.** 21 hydroxylase deficiency is most common.

Concealed Sex: Criminals may conceal their sex to avoid detection by changing dress or by other methods. This can be detected by physical examination.

In advanced putrefaction, sex can be determined by identifying uterus or prostate which resist putrefaction for a long time. Biopsy of the gonads will confirm the diagnosis.

SKELETON: Human skeleton is both exo- and endoskeleton. **Recognisable sex differences do not appear until after puberty except in the pelvis, and the accuracy from this bone is about 75 to 80% and without pelvis only 50%. Sex determination is rarely based on any one skeletal feature alone.** Comparative features of few bones of both sexes are summarised for reference [**Table (4–3)** (skull and mandible); **Figs. (4–7, 4–14, and 4–16)**; **Table (4–4)** (pelvis, thorax, femur); **Figs. (4–8 to 4–13, 4–15, and 4–17 to 4–19)**]. The determination of sex is based mainly upon the appearances of the pelvis, skull, mandible, clavicle, scapula, sternum and the long bones. In the skull, sexual features are

Table (4–3). Traits diagnostic of sex from skeleton

	Trait	Male	Female
		GENERAL	
(1)	General size:	Larger, more massive.	Smaller, slender.
(2)	Long bones:	Ridges, depressions and processes more prominent. Bones of arms and legs are 8% longer.	Less prominent.
(3)	Shaft:	Rougher.	Smoother, thinner with relatively wider medullary cavity.
(4)	Articular surfaces :	Larger.	Smaller.
(5)	Metacarpal bones:	Longer and broader.	Shorter and narrower.
(6)	Weight:	4.5 kg.	2.75 kg.
		SKULL (Figs 4–7 and 4–14)	
(1)	General appearance:	Larger, longer (dolichocrania).	Smaller, lighter, walls thinner; rounder (brachycrania), and smoother.
(2)	Capacity:	1500 to 1550 ml.	1350 to 1400 ml.
(3)	Architecture:	Rugged; muscle ridges more marked, esp. in occipital and temporal areas.	Smooth.
(4)	Forehead:	Steeper, (sloping), less rounded.	Vertical, round, full, infantile.
(5)	Glabella:	Rough and more prominent.	Smooth, small or absent.
(6)	Frontonasal junction:	Distinct angulation.	Smoothly curved.
(7)	Orbits:	Square, set lower on the face, relatively smaller, rounded margins.	Rounded, higher, relatively larger, sharp margins.
(8)	Supraorbital ridges:	Prominent and rounded.	Less prominent, sharper or absent.
(9)	Cheek bones:	Heavier, laterally arched.	Lighter, more compressed.
(10)	Zygomatic arch:	More prominent.	Less prominent.
(11)	Nasal aperture:	Higher and narrower. Margins sharp.	Lower and broader.
(12)	External auditory meatus:	Bony ridge along the upper border is prominent.	Often absent.
(13)	Frontal eminences:	Small.	Large.
(14)	Parietal eminences:	Small.	Large.
(15)	Frontal sinuses:	Much developed.	Less developed.
(16)	Occipital area:	Muscle lines and protuberance prominent.	Not prominent.

Contd...

Contd...

	Trait	Male	Female
(17)	Mastoid process:	Wider, longer, round, blunt.	Narrow, short, smooth, pointed.
(18)	Base:	Sites of muscular insertions more marked.	Less marked.
(19)	Digastric groove:	More deep.	Less deep.
(20)	Condylar facet:	Long and slender.	Short and broad.
(21)	Occipital condyles:	Large.	Small.
(22)	Palate:	Larger, broader, tends more to U-shape.	Smaller, tends more to parabola.
(23)	Foramina:	Larger.	Smaller.
(24)	Foramen magnum:	Relatively large and long.	Relatively small and round.
(25)	Teeth:	Larger.	Smaller.
		MANDIBLE (Fig. 4–16)	
(1)	General size:	Larger and thicker.	Smaller and thinner.
(2)	Chin:	Square (U-shaped).	Rounded.
(3)	Body height:	At symphysis greater.	At symphysis smaller.
(4)	Ascending ramus:	Greater breadth.	Smaller breadth.
(5)	Angle of body and ramus (Gonion):	Less obtuse (under 125°); prominent, and everted.	More obtuse; not prominent, inverted.
(6)	Condyles:	Larger.	Smaller.
(7)	Mental tubercle:	Large and prominent.	Insignificant.

Table (4–4). Traits diagnostic of sex from skeleton (Figs 4–8 to 4–13 and 4–17 and 4–18)

	Trait	Male	Female
		PELVIS	
(1)	Bony framework:	Massive, rougher, marked muscle sites. Stands higher and more erect.	Less massive, slender, smoother.
(2)	General:	Deep funnel.	Flat bowl.
(3)	Ilium:	Less vertical; curve of iliac crest reaches higher level and is more prominent.	More vertical; distance between iliac crests is less; iliac fossae shallow; curves of crest well marked.
(4)	Preauricular sulcus: (attachment of anterior sacroiliac ligament).	Not frequent; narrow, shallow.	More frequent, broad and deep.
(5)	Acetabulum:	Large, 52 mm. in diameter; directed laterally; wider, deeper.	Small, 46 mm. in diameter; directed anterolaterally; narrower.
(6)	Obturator foramen:	Large, often oval with base upwards.	Small, triangular with apex forwards.
(7)	Greater sciatic notch:	Smaller, narrower, deeper.	Larger, wider, shallower.
(8)	Illeo-pectineal line:	Well marked and rough.	Rounded and smooth.
(9)	Ischial tuberosity:	Inverted.	Everted; more widely separated.
(10)	Body of pubis:	Narrow, triangular, thick.	Broad, square; pits on posterior surface if borne children.
(11)	Ramus of pubis:	It is like continuation of body of pubis.	Has a constricted or narrowed appearance and is short and thick.
(12)	Ischiopubic rami:	More everted, thicker and rougher.	Less everted, thinner and smoother.
(13)	Symphysis:	Higher, bigger and narrow in width. Margins of pubic arch everted.	Lower, wider and rounded. Margins of pubic arch not everted; distance between two pubic tubercles greater. The dorsal border is irregular and shows depressions or pits (scars of parturition).
(14)	Subpubic angle:	V-shaped, sharp angle 70° to 75°.	U-shaped, rounded, broader angle, 90° to 100°.
(15)	Pelvic brim or inlet:	Heart-shaped.	Circular or elliptical; more spacious; diameters longer.
(16)	Pelvic cavity:	Conical and funnel-shaped.	Broad and round.

Contd...

Contd...

Trait		Male	Female
(17)	Pelvic outlet:	Smaller.	Larger.
(18)	Sacroiliac articulation:	Large, extends to 2½ to 3 vertebrae.	Small, oblique, extends to 2 to 2½ vertebrae.
(19)	Sacroiliac joint surface:	Large and less sharply angulated.	L-shaped and elevated anteriorly.
(20)	Sacrum:	Longer, narrower, with more evenly distributed curvature; promontory well marked. Body of first sacral vertebra larger.	Shorter, wider; upper half almost straight, curve forward in lower half; promontory less marked. Body of first sacral vertebra small.
(21)	Coccyx:	Less movable.	More movable.
(22)	Ischiopubic index: $\frac{\text{Pubic length in mm.}}{\text{Ischial length in mm.}} \times 100$	73 to 94.	91 to 115.
(23)	Sciatic notch index: $\frac{\text{Width of sciatic notch}}{\text{Depth of sciatic notch}} \times 100$	65 ± 8.	54 ± 9.
(24)	Pubic ramus ratio:	1: 1.	2: 1 or greater.
(25)	Sacral index $= \frac{\text{Breadth of base of sacrum}}{\text{Anterior length of sacrum}} \times 100$	112	116
	THORAX Fig. (4–19)		
(1)	General:	Longer and narrower.	Shorter and wider.
(2)	Sternum:	Body longer and more than twice the length of the manubrium (Hyrtl's law); upper margin is in level with lower part of the body of second thoracic vertebra; breadth more. Length more than 149 mm. (Ashley's rule).	Shorter and less than twice the length of the manubrium; upper margin in level with lower part of the body of third thoracic vertebra; breadth less. Length less than 149 mm. (Ashley's rule).
(3)	Sternal index: $\frac{\text{Length of manubrium}}{\text{Length of body}} \times 100$	46.2	54.3
(4)	Ribs:	Thicker; larger; heavier; lesser curvature and are less oblique.	Thinner; shorter; greater curvature and more oblique.
(5)	Clavicle:	Longer (151 to 153 cm.) broader, heavier, less curved.	Smaller, narrower (138 cm) lighter, more curved.
	VERTEBRAL COLUMN		
(1)	Atlas, breadth:	7.4 to 9.9 cm; mean 8.3 cm	6.5 to 7.6 cm. (mean 7.2 cm)
(2)	Length of vertebral column:	70 to 73 cm.	60 cm.
(3)	Corporobasal index of sacrum: $\frac{\text{Breadth of first sacral vertebra}}{\text{Breadth of the base of sacrum}} \times 100$	45	40.5
	FEMUR Fig. (4–15)		
(1)	Head:	Larger and forms about 2/3 of a sphere. Vertical diameter more than 47 mm.	Smaller and forms less than 2/3 of a sphere. Vertical diameter less than 45 mm.
(2)	Neck:	Obtuse angle with the shaft, about 125°.	Less obtuse angle with the shaft.
(3)	Bicondylar width:	74 to 89 mm.	67 to 76 mm.
(4)	Angulation of shaft with condyles:	Around 80°	Around 76°
	HUMERUS		
(1)	Diameter of head:	More than 47 mm.	Less than 43 mm.
	SCIATIC NOTCH INDEX ACCORDING TO KROGMANN		
(1)	Sciatic notch (Indians)	Range: 62–94 Mean: 77 SD: 7.6	Range: 76–114 Mean: 96.2 SD: 7.9

Contd...

Contd...

Trait	Male	Female
	RADIUS	
(1) Diameter of head:	More than 24 mm.	Less than 21 mm.
(2) Circumference of head:	More than 69 mm.	Less than 55 mm.
	SCAPULA	
(1) Height:	More than 157 mm.	Less than 144 mm.
(2) Glenoid cavity:	Height greater (39.2 mm).	Height less (32.6 mm).

modified by senility. **In the pelvis, sex features are independent of each other and one may even contradict the other in the same pelvis. The male pelvis stands higher and more erect than the female pelvis.** Perforated olecranon fossa is more common in females on the left side. Additional information may be obtained from the scapula and metacarpal bones.

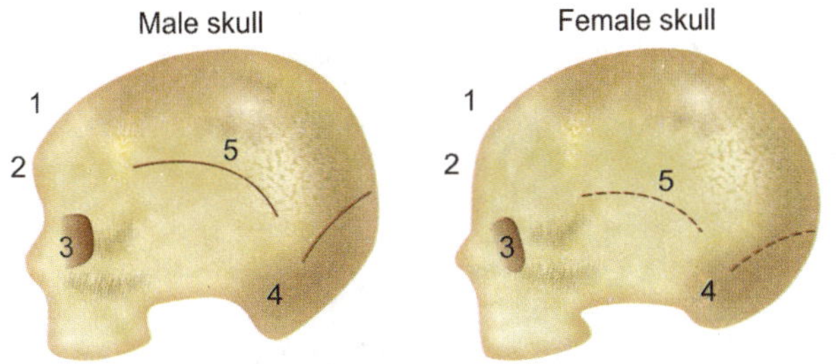

Fig. (4–7). Male Skull: (1) Forehead—receding. (2) Orbital ridges — prominent. (3) Orbits—square. (4) Mastoid process— large. (5) Muscle ridges—marked. Female Skull: (1) Forehead —high. (2) Orbital ridges—not marked. (3) Orbits—rounded. (4) Mastoid process—small. (5) Muscle ridges— faint.

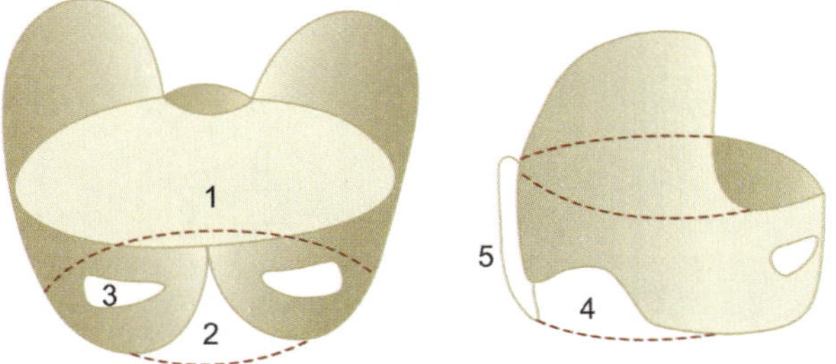

Fig. (4–8). Female pelvis: (1) General pelvic shape—flat bowl. (2) Subpelvic arch—obtuse. (3) Obturator foramen—triangular. (4) Sciatic notch—obtuse. (5) Sacrum—short and flat.

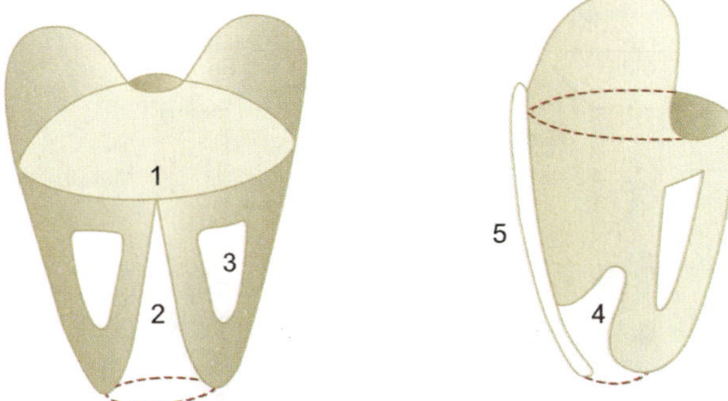

Fig. (4–9). Male pelvis: (1) General pelvic shape—deep funnel. (2) Subpelvic arch—acute. (3) Obturator foramen—oval. (4) Sciatic notch—acute. (5) Sacrum—long and curved.

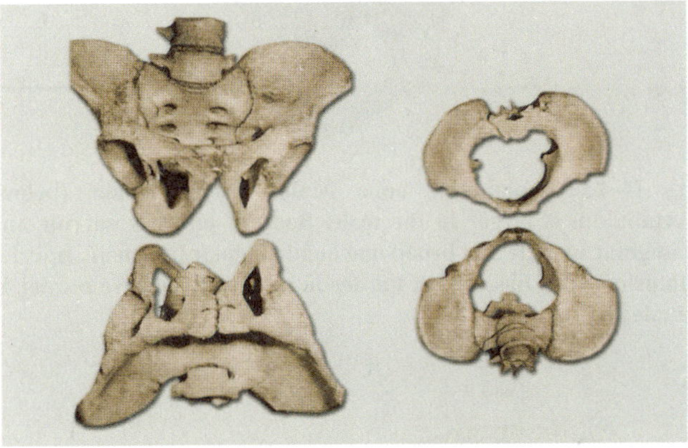

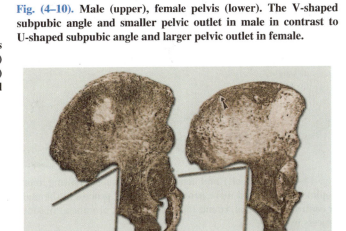

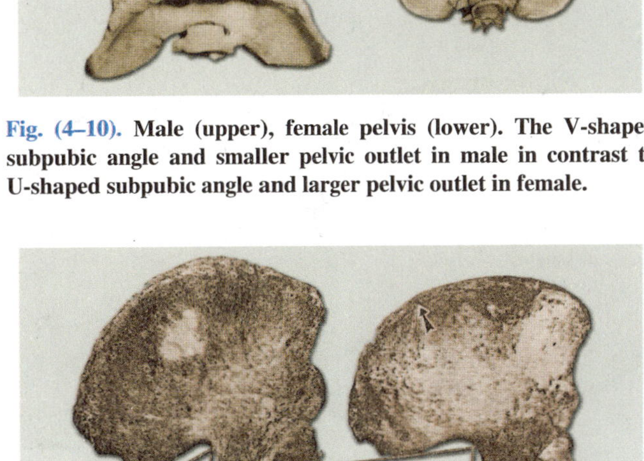

Fig. (4–10). Male (upper), female pelvis (lower). The V-shaped subpubic angle and smaller pelvic outlet in male in contrast to U-shaped subpubic angle and larger pelvic outlet in female.

Fig. (4–11). Innominate bone. The angle formed by the greater sciatic notch is more acute in the male (left) than the female (right).

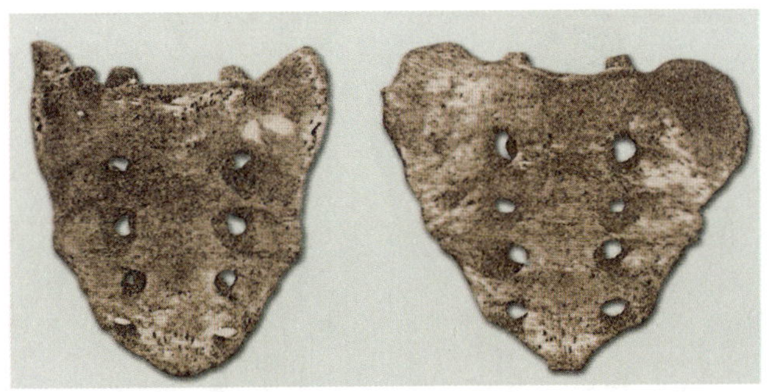

Fig. (4–12). Sacrum. It is narrower in the male (left) than in the female (right).

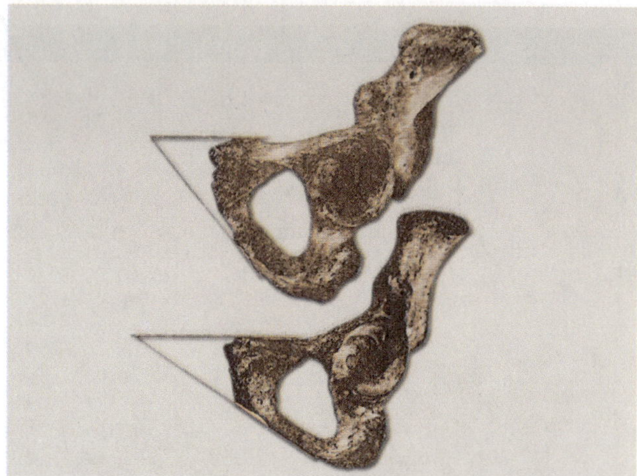

Fig. (4–13). Innominate bone. Male (above), female (below) Acetabulum is larger in the male. Body of pubis is narrow and triangular in male and broad and quadrangular in female. Inferior ramus of pubis has convex border in male and concave border in female.

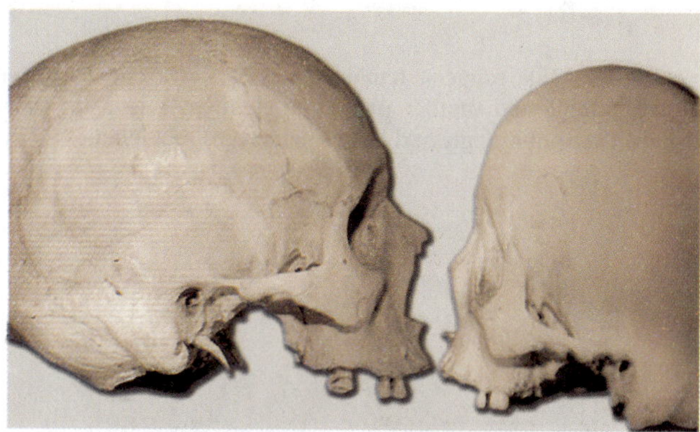

Fig. (4–14). Male (left) and female (right) skulls, showing more sloping forehead and more prominent mastoid process in the male in contrast to vertical, round forehead and less prominent mastoid process in female.

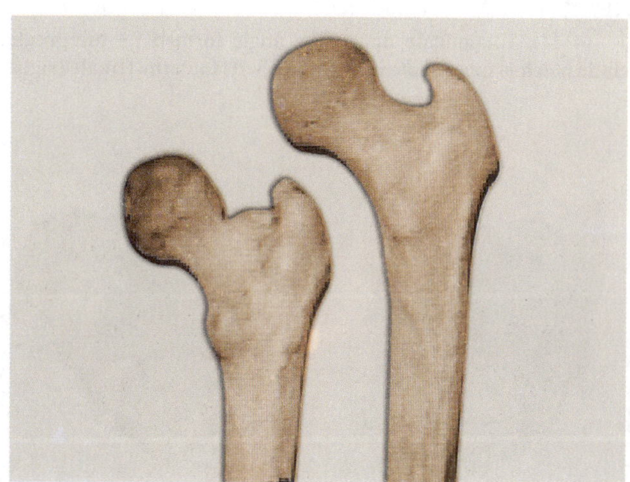

Fig. (4–15). Male (right) and female (left) femurs. The angle of the neck of femur is more obtuse in the male.

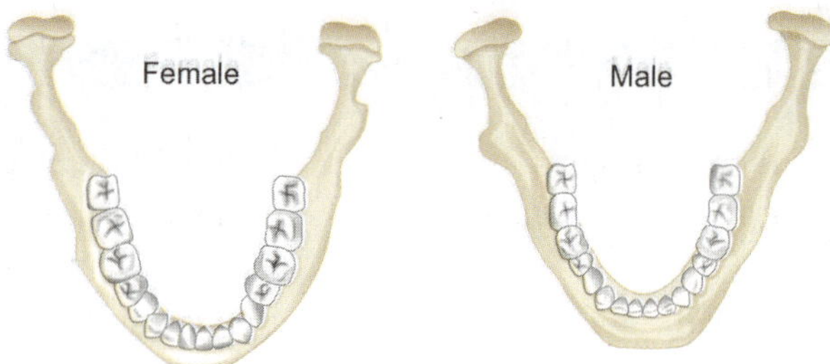

Fig. (4–16). Male and female mandibles.

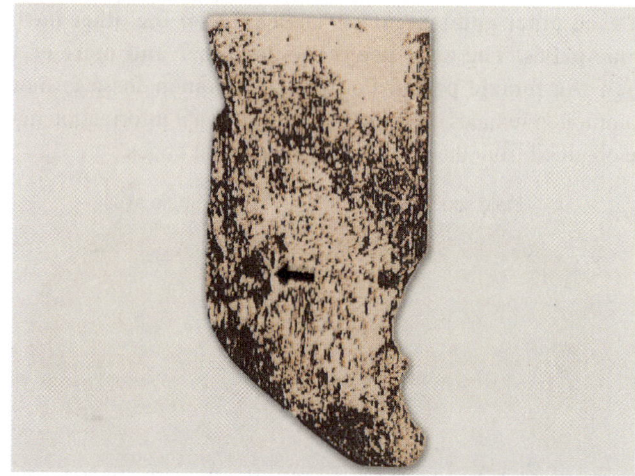

Fig. (4–17). A parturition pit (arrow) on the dorsal surface of pubic bone adjacent to pubic symphysis.

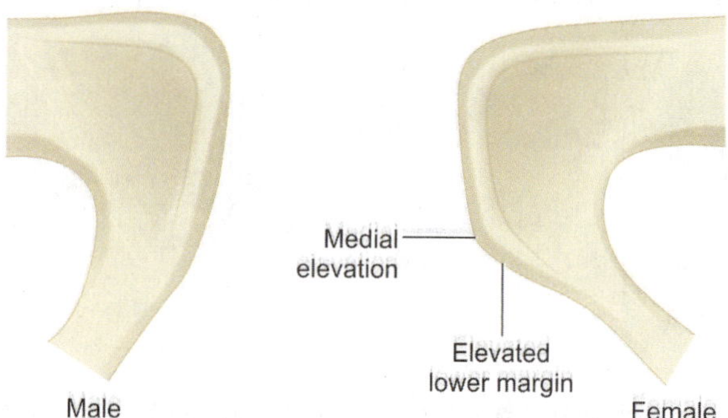

Fig. (4–18). The symphyseal block is triangular in male and rectangular in female.

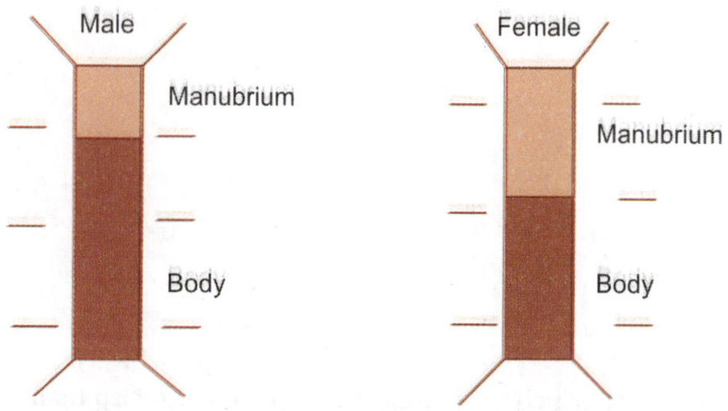

Fig. (4–19). Ratio of manubrium to body of sternum in male and female.

Table (4–5). Pfitner's table of bodily dimensions in the female compared with the male (per cent of male dimensions). The common generalization that the female is 94 per cent of the male size varies in different areas of the body

Stature	93.5	Arm length	91.5
Head breadth	98.0	Sitting height	94.5
Face breadth	94.0	Head circumference	96.0
Face height	90.0	Head height	96.0
Head length	95.5	Leg length	93.0

In females, subpubic angle, greater sciatic notch, pelvic inlet and outlet are more than in male, but obturator foramen is smaller and curve of ilium is less. The sternal index, ischiopubic index and sciatic notch index are more in females. **Greater sciatic notch is the ideal feature to determine the sex of a female child.**

Chilotic line is an anthropometric line in pelvis, the index of which is used in identifying the sex.

Medullary index of bones: The sex of the long bones can be determined on the basis of their medullary index (Diameter of medulla ÷ diameter of whole bone × 100) from tibia, humerus, ulna and radius.

In general adult female skeletal measurements are about 94% that of the male of the same race, but different measurements may vary from 91 to 98% **Table (4–5).**

According to Krogman, the degree of **accuracy in sexing adult skeletal remains** is:

Entire skeleton	100%
Pelvis alone	95%
Skull alone	90%
Pelvis plus skull	98%
Long bones alone	80%

Most anatomists do not claim 100% accuracy even where entire skeleton is available.

AGE

The age of an individual especially in earlier years can be determined from: (1) teeth, (2) ossification of bones, (3) secondary sex characters, and (4) general development in case of children.

TEETH: TOOTH DEVELOPMENT AND ERUPTION: The alveolar cavities which contain teeth are formed around the third or fourth month of intrauterine life. Development of the tooth begins with the formation of cellular tooth germ within the alveolar bone, in the shape of the crown. Apposition and calcification of enamel and dentin take place within this germ, and the crown is completely formed and calcified before any positional changes occur. At birth, the rudiments of all the temporary teeth and of the first permanent molars may be found in the jaws. Root formation begins after completion of the crown, and as the root becomes longer, the crown erupts through the bone, and finally comes out of the jaws. Neonatal line is well-formed on teeth at birth. The root is completed some time after the tooth is in full functional occlusion. The teeth calcify from crown to neck to roots. During eruption of a permanent tooth, the overlying root of its deciduous predecessor simultaneously undergoes absorption until only the crown remains. The unsupported crown then falls off.

Teeth are useful for age determination (a) by the state of development, and (b) by secondary changes.

Temporary Teeth: Temporary, deciduous or milk teeth are 20 in number: 4 incisors, 2 canines, and 4 molars in each jaw. In ill-nourished children, and especially in rickets, and in hypothyroidism, dentition may be delayed, while in syphilis, teeth may be premature or even present at birth. At about four years, there is usually spacing between the deciduous teeth. About the sixth or seventh year, first permanent molar teeth erupt behind the second temporary molars. After this, the temporary teeth begin to fall off. Between 7 to 12 years, 24 teeth are present. **At age nine, 12 permanent teeth are in the mouth; 8 incisors and 4 first molars. Deciduous molars and canines are present. At the age 10, there are 16 permanent teeth (8 incisors, 4 premolars, 4 molars) and 8 deciduous teeth (4 molars, 4 canines). At the age 11, there are 20 permanent teeth: 8 incisors, 8 premolars and 4 molars and 4 deciduous teeth (second molars). Mixed dentition is seen up to 12 years. At the age 14, there are 28 permanent teeth, and no deciduous teeth** Tables (4–7 and 4–8).

If there is doubt whether a particular tooth is temporary, take an X-ray. If it is temporary tooth, germ of the permanent tooth can be seen underneath.

Permanent teeth are 32 in number: 4 incisors, 2 canines, 4 premolars, and 6 molars in each jaw. Developmentally, teeth are divided into two sets: **(1) SUPERADDED PERMANENT TEETH are those which do not have deciduous predecessors. They erupt behind the temporary teeth. All the permanent molars are superadded permanent teeth. The first permanent molar tooth of each side erupts, while all the other deciduous teeth are present in the jaw. Superadded permanent teeth are six in each jaw. (2) SUCCESSIONAL PERMANENT TEETH are those which erupt in place of deciduous teeth. Permanent premolars erupt in place of deciduous molars. Successional teeth are ten in each jaw.**

MORPHOLOGY OF PERMANENT TEETH: Each tooth has a crown, a neck and a root embedded in the jaw bone. Teeth are composed of dentin, covered on the crown by enamel and on the root by cementum, which is attached to the alveolar bone by periodontal membrane.

INCISORS: The crown is shaped like chisel and is convex on its labial surface and concave on its lingual surface, except near the neck, where the surface becomes convex. The neck is slightly constricted. The root is single.

CANINES: They are larger than the incisors. The crown is large and conical, very concave on its labial surface and slightly concave on its lingual surface. Its masticatory edge tapers to a blunt point, which projects slightly beyond the level of the other teeth. The root is single, larger and thicker than that of an incisor.

PREMOLARS OR BICUSPIDS: They are smaller and shorter than the canines. The crown of each is nearly circular in cross-section and slightly compressed mesiodistally. The chewing surface has two cusps. The root is usually single, but may be double.

MOLARS: They are largest with broad crown. The crown is cubical; convex on its labial and lingual surfaces, and flattened on its mesial and distal surfaces. It has three, four or five cusps. Each upper molar has three roots and lower two Table (4–6).

DECIDUOUS TEETH: They resemble in form the teeth which bear the same names in the permanent set.

ERUPTION OF TEETH: Eruption is defined as the superior part of the crown of the tooth appearing level with the surface of the alveolar bone Figs. (4–20 and 4–21). **In both deciduous and permanent teeth, dentition occurs earlier in lower jaw except for the lateral incisors which erupt earlier in upper jaw.** The lower permanent incisors, premolars and molars erupt about one year earlier than do the corresponding teeth in the upper jaw. **Wisdom tooth first erupts in the lower and on the left side and then on the right side. The number and eruption of deciduous teeth is more regular than the permanent dentition. Eruption is not always bilaterally symmetrical. Tooth eruption in female may be one year before that of males.** Females have smaller teeth (esp. lower canines)

Table (4–6). Difference between temporary and permanent teeth

	Trait	Temporary teeth	Permanent teeth
(1)	Size:	Smaller, lighter, narrower, except temporary molars which are longer than permanent premolars replacing them.	Heavier, stronger, broader, except permanent premolars replacing temporary molars which are smaller.
(2)	Direction:	Anterior teeth are vertical.	Anterior teeth are usually inclined a little forward.
(3)	Crown:	China-white colour.	Ivory-white colour.
(4)	Neck:	More constricted.	Less constricted.
(5)	Root:	Roots of molar are smaller and more divergent.	Roots of molars are larger and less divergent.
(6)	Ridge:	A ridge or thick edge at the junction of the crown with the fangs present.	No ridge.

than males Tables (4–7 and 4–8). **In general, the dental and skeletal ages, correspond closely in the male, but in the female the skeletal age is generally one year ahead of the dental age.**

The ethnic, cultural, hereditary, environmental, endocrine reactions, and nutrition, all play a part in the eruption and calcification of teeth. Eruption tends to occur earlier in warmer climates and in urban areas.

From birth to fourteen years of age, the degree of formation of root and crown structures, the stage of eruption and the intermixture of temporary and permanent teeth are useful in age estimation. It is generally accepted that in a child estimation of age from teeth gives better results than skeleton. Dental X-rays show the developmental status of unerupted teeth and the degree of root completion in erupted teeth. From 14 to 20 years, dental age estimation is based upon the stage of development of the third molar. There is much variation in these, and the accuracy of dental age estimation during this period varies by about plus/minus three years. The body of the jaw grows posteriorly, and the ramus is elongated after eruption of second molar teeth. If third molars are absent, it should be noted whether there is a space in the jaw behind the second molar teeth. **If third molars are fully erupted, it indicates that an individual is above 17 years of age.** In some persons due to inadequate jaw space, the third molars never erupt into the oral cavity, particularly the mandibular third molars. Such trapped teeth are known as **impacted teeth.** All the teeth can be visualised by single X-ray by dental panoramic tomograph **(orthopantogram).**

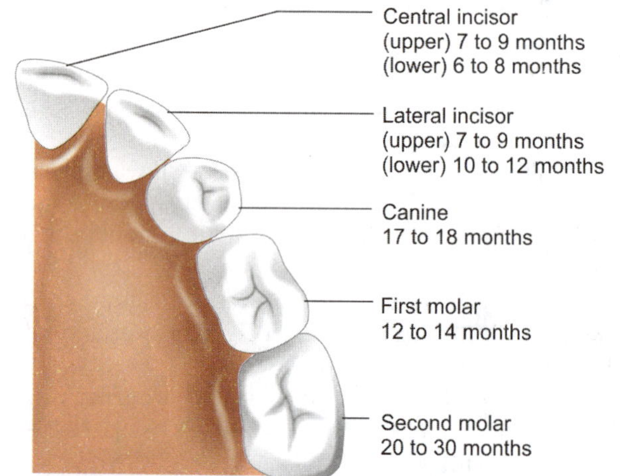

Fig. (4–20). **Eruption of temporary teeth.**

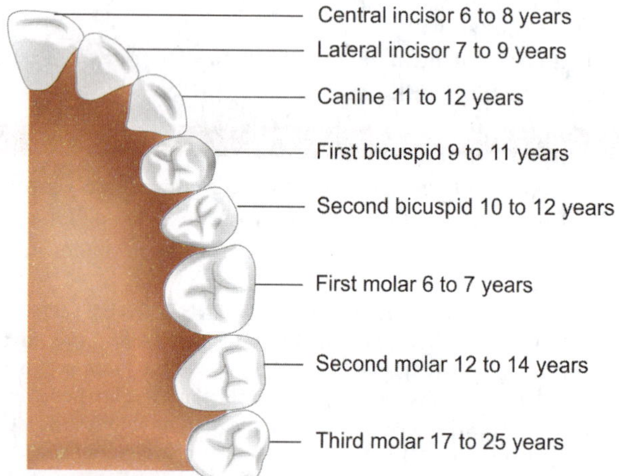

Fig. (4–21). **Eruption of permanent teeth.**

GUSTAFSON'S METHOD: The age estimation of adult over 21 years depends on the physiologic age changes in each of the dental tissues Fig. (4–22).

(1) Attrition: Due to wear and tear from mastication, **occlusal (upper) surface of the teeth is destroyed gradually,** first involving the enamel, then dentin, and at last pulp is exposed in old age. It depends on the functional use of teeth and also upon the hardness of the enamel.

(2) Periodontosis: Regression of the gums and periodontal tissues surrounding the teeth takes place in advancing age, gradually exposing the necks and the adjacent part of roots, due to which the teeth become loose and fall off. Poor oral hygiene increases periodontosis. There may be deposition of hardened debris which occurs gradually over a long period.

(3) Secondary dentin: It may develop from the walls within the pulp cavity, and decrease the size of the cavity. First it is deposited at the pulp chamber and gradually extends downwards to the apex, and may completely fill the pulp cavity. This is partly due to ageing and partly due to pathological conditions like caries, and periodontosis.

(4) Cementum apposition: The cementum increases in thickness particularly due to changes in the tooth position, especially near the end of the root. **Secondary cementum is slowly and continuously deposited throughout life, and forms incremental lines. Incremental lines appear as cross-striations on the enamel of teeth due to cementum apposition, and are thought to represent daily increments of growth.** They can be seen on histological section. The age can be calculated by

Table (4–7). Calcification and eruption of deciduous teeth

Tooth		Calcification begins	Eruption	Calcification of root completed	Resorption of root begins
Central incisor	:				
Lower	:	5 to 6 months	6 to 8 months	1½ to 2 years	4th year
Upper	:	"	7 to 9 months	1½ to 2 years	5th year
Lateral incisor	:	"			
Upper	:	"	7 to 9 months	1½ to 2 years	5th year
Lower	:	"	10 to 12 months	1½ to 2 years	5th year
First molar	:	"	12 to 14 months	2 to 2½ years	6th year
Canine	:	"	17 to 18 months	2½ to 3 years	8th year
Second molar	:	"	20 to 30 months	3 years	7th year

Table (4–8). Calcification and eruption of permanent teeth

Tooth		Calcification begins	Eruption	Calcification complete
First molar	:	At birth	6 to 7 years	9 to 10 years
Central incisor	:	3 to 4 months	6 to 8 years	10 years
Lateral incisor	:	1 year	7 to 9 years	11 years
First bicuspid	:	1½ years	9 to 11 years	12 to 13 years
Second bicuspid	:	2 years	10 to 12 years	12 to 14 years
Canine	:	4 to 5 months	11 to 12 years	12 to 13 years
Second molar	:	2 ½ to 3 years	12 to 14 years	14 to 16 years
Third molar	:	8 to 10 years	17 to 25 years	18 to 25 years

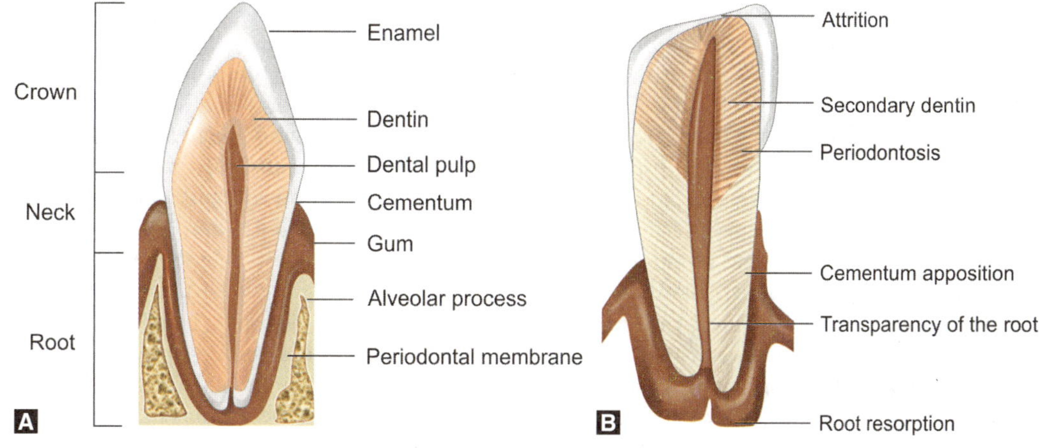

Fig. (4–22). (A) Vertical section of an incisor tooth. (B) Physiological age-processes in teeth.

counting the number of lines from the neonatal line onwards. This is mainly applicable to infants.

(5) Root resorption: It involves both cementum and dentin which show characteristically sharp grooves. **Absorption of the root starts first at the apex and extends upwards.** It usually occurs in late age. It may be due to pathological process.

(6) Transparency of the root: It is not seen until about 30 years of age. The canals in the dentin are at first wide. With age they are filled by mineral, so that they become translucent gradually and the dentine becomes transparent due to rarefaction (osteoporosis). Transparency of root occurs from below upwards in lower jaw and from above downwards in upper jaw. It is the most reliable of all criteria.

Before the tooth is extracted from a body, the degree of periodontosis is estimated. The tooth is ground down on glass slabs from both sides of the tooth to about one mm. which allows the estimation of transparency. Then the section is ground further down to about one-fourth mm. for microscopic examination. **Anterior teeth are more suitable than the posterior teeth, and the merit decreases from incisors to premolars, while third molar is quite unsuitable.** All changes are absent at 15 years. Arbitrarily, 0 to 3 points are alloted to indicate the degree of any of these changes. Stage 0 indicates no change; 1 beginning of change; 2 obvious change; and stage 3 maximum change, occurring in the dental tissues. The result corrected for standard deviation, gives an estimate of the age of the person. The error is said to be ± 4 to 7 years. The limit of error increases above 50 years of age. Age can also be determined by directly reading from the graph on which the regression line is plotted. Further modification by Johanson is said to give greater accuracy.

Boyde's Method: Cross striations develop in the enamel of teeth, till the complete formation of enamel. They represent daily incremental lines. **The age of an individual can be calculated in terms of days by counting the number of lines from the neonatal line onwards.** Neonatal line is formed very soon after birth and can be seen in about three weeks or by electron microscopy within one to two days after birth. It is useful to estimate the age of a dead infant.

Stack's Method: Stack evolved a **method to know the age of infants from the weight and height of the erupting teeth of child.** This method can be used on both deciduous and permanent teeth during their erupting phase.

GROWTH IN INDIVIDUAL BONES (OSSIFICATION OF BONES): The bones of the human skeleton are performed in hyaline cartilage. This soft tissue model is gradually converted into hard osseous tissue by the development of osteogenesis, frequently in a central position, from which the process of transformation spreads, until the whole skeleton is ossified. The appearance of such centres of ossification is spread over a long period of time. A large number are first seen in embryonic life, some appear much later in prenatal life, and others appear after birth. **The earliest centres of ossification appear at the end of second month of pregnancy. At the eleventh intrauterine week, there are 806 centres of bone growth; at birth about 450; while the adult skeleton has 206 bones.** This shows that 600 centres of bone growth have disappeared, i.e., they have united with the adjacent centres to form the adult bone. **The process of appearance and union has a sequence and a time. As a rule, ossification begins centrally in an epiphysis and spreads peripherally as it gets bigger.** At first it is entirely amorphous, rounded and pinhead sized. As it grows, it takes on the osteological details of the bone. Some bones are ossified from a single centre, e.g. carpus and tarsus. The ossification centres in carpal bones appear as follows: capitate 2 to 3 months, hamate first year; triquitrum 3, lunate 4, scaphoid and trapezoid 5, trapezium 6, pisiform 11 years. **At the end of one year two carpal bones are seen in X-ray of the wrist. Between 2 to 6 years, the number of carpal bones present on X-ray indicates the approximate age in years. Most bones are ossified from several separate centres, one of which appears near the middle of the future bone.** This centre is concerned with progressive ossification towards the bone ends. In all such bones, their ends are cartilaginous at birth. These terminal regions are ossified by separate centres, sometimes multiple; they are said to be secondary centres.

EPIPHYSEAL PLATE: Typically, a long bone such as the tibia has become ossified throughout its shaft (diaphysis) at birth; whereas its two ends (epiphyses), are later ossified by secondary centres. A layer of hyaline cartilage (epiphyseal plate) persists between the diaphysis and epiphysis. The bone increases in length at this epiphyseal plate or disc (growth plate or growth cartilage), until its final dimensions are attained. The process of union of epiphysis and diaphysis is called fusion. **Union is a process, not an event. Union of bone can be divided into various stages from stage 0- no union, stage I-starting union to stage V-completely united.** The union in long bones is interpreted as non-united, uniting (1/4, 1/2, 3/4, etc.), recently united and united, depending on the stage of union. The long limb bones show epiphyseal arrangements at both ends, while metacarpals, metatarsals, phalanges, clavicles and ribs possess an epiphysis at one end only. In some bones, the epiphyseal centres at one or both ends are more complex, e.g., in the proximal end of the humerus, which is wholly cartilaginous at birth, three separate centres appear during childhood. They soon unite to form a single epiphyseal mass, which later fuses to the diaphysis.

Growth cartilages do not grow at the same rate at all points throughout their substance. By differential rates of growth, the two bony surfaces usually become reciprocally curved, commonly in such a way that the epiphysis fits like a shallow cap over the convex end of the shaft. **There may be maturity imbalance between bones from different parts of the same individual.**

For determining the age, skiagrams of the shoulder, elbow, wrist, hip, knee, ankle, pelvis and skull should be taken in anteroposterior direction.

Variability: In biology, stability is the exception, variability is the rule, i.e., there really is no average. There is only a central tendency with a normal range of variability. The variability increases with age. **As a general rule, the ageing of bones is more accurate with respect to the appearance of centres of ossification than it is with respect to the union of epiphyses. A study of various anatomical authorities shows that there is a considerable variation regarding the ages at which the various centres of ossification in the epiphyses fuse with their respective diaphyses.**

As a general rule, the secondary centres of the limb bones that appear first are the last to fuse, whereas the late-forming epiphyses reach union with their primary centres in a shorter time period. In the long bones of upper limbs, the union occurs earlier in the elbow joint and later at the wrist. Head of the humerus is the last long bone epiphysis to unite. In the long bones of the lower limbs, the union occurs later at the knee joint and earlier at the hip and ankle joints.

Figures (4–23 to 4–43) and Table (4–9) show the process of ossification in males. They only indicate an average. Too much reliance should not be placed on them, as variations occur depending on the health, hereditary, nutritional, infectious diseases, metabolic disorders, physical activity, race, sex, endocrine and environmental factors. **Multiple criteria of skeletal age should be employed whenever possible.** The dentition may be used as a check during the first two decades of life. An estimated skeletal age based on appearance of ossification centres and union of epiphyses must always be expressed in plus or minus terms, e.g., 10 ±1 (ten years, plus or minus one year). **Skeletal development in the female can be in advance of the male up to one year, while dental development may differ only from one to four months. In males, dental and osseous ages are almost similar, but in females osseous age is in advance of**

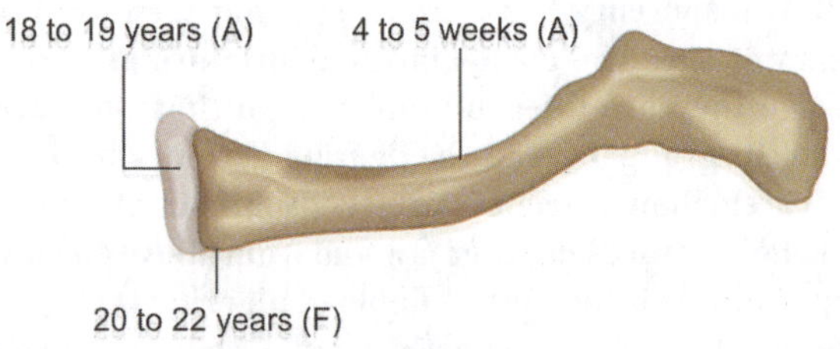

Fig. (4–23). **Appearance and fusion of epiphyses in clavicle.**

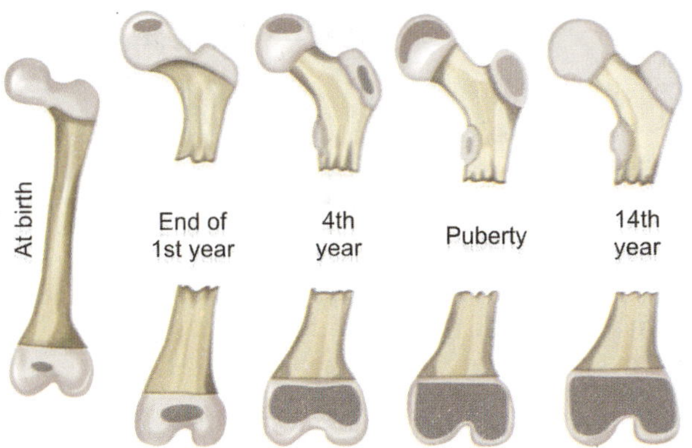

Fig. (4–24). Stages of calcification of femur.

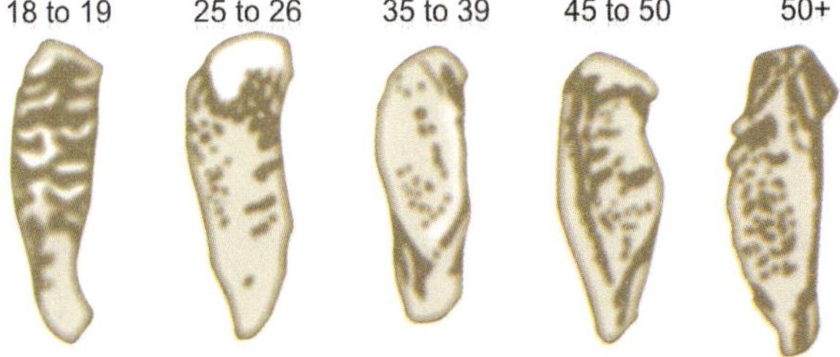

Fig. (4–25). Age changes in symphysis pubis.

the dental age. In tropical climates, ossification centres appear and epiphyseal union takes place about 2 years earlier than in temperate zones.

Union of epiphyses in cartilaginous bone occurs slightly earlier (by about one year) in the female than in the male, but the reverse is seen in the closure of the sutures of the skull.

Radiography: The epiphyseal lines on the long bones of a young individual appear as circular grooves around the ends of the bones, and on radiographs as irregular lines resembling a fracture. In skeletal remains of a young person where the bones have become completely dry, the epiphyses often separate from the shaft, which should not be mistaken for fractures.

The union of epiphyses as seen in radiographs appear earlier approximately about plus or minus six months than the periods of fusion indicated by anatomical evidence. This is due to the fact, that towards the end of the growth period, the epiphyseal plate of the cartilages becomes very thin and irregular in outline and may not show on radiograph. In a film, a persistent scar is not evidence of incomplete union or even of recent union. **In an individual bone, once union has begun, it will be completed in about 12 to 18 months.** In radiographs of growing long bones, one or more transverse lines are often observed at the diaphyseal ends. This is thought to be evidence of growth disturbance (e.g., scurvy, rickets), and are called **"scars of arrested growth".**

SYMPHYSIS PUBIS: The pubic symphysis is probably the best single criterion for determining age from third to fifth decades. It requires bones that are free of cartilage. The surface features are blurred, if there is erosion by drying and damage. The symphysial surface before 20 years has a layer of compact bone near its surface. At about 20 years, it is markedly irregular or uneven, and the ridges run transversely across the articular surface. Between 24 and 36 years, the ridges gradually disappear and the surface has a granular appearance and ventral (outer) and dorsal (inner) margins are completely defined. Early in the fifth decade, the symphysial face has an oval, smooth surface with raised upper and lower ends. Towards the end of the fifth decade, a narrow beaded rim develops on the margins. During the sixth decade, erosion of surface and breakdown of ventral margin begins. In the seventh decade, the surface becomes irregularly eroded Fig. (4–25). If the male criteria are used for females, the age would be under-estimated by about ten years as the female pubis reaches full maturity about 10 years later than the male.

Sternum: The four pieces of the body of the sternum fuse with one another from below upwards between 14 to 25 years. At about 40 years, the xiphoid unites with the body. The manubrium fuses with the body in old age at about 60 years Fig. (4–41).

Ribs: Progressive ossification of sternal rib ends of the costal cartilages correlate with increasing age within 5 to 8 years of real age.

Hyoid Bone: The greater cornu of the hyoid bone unites with the body between 40 to 60 years.

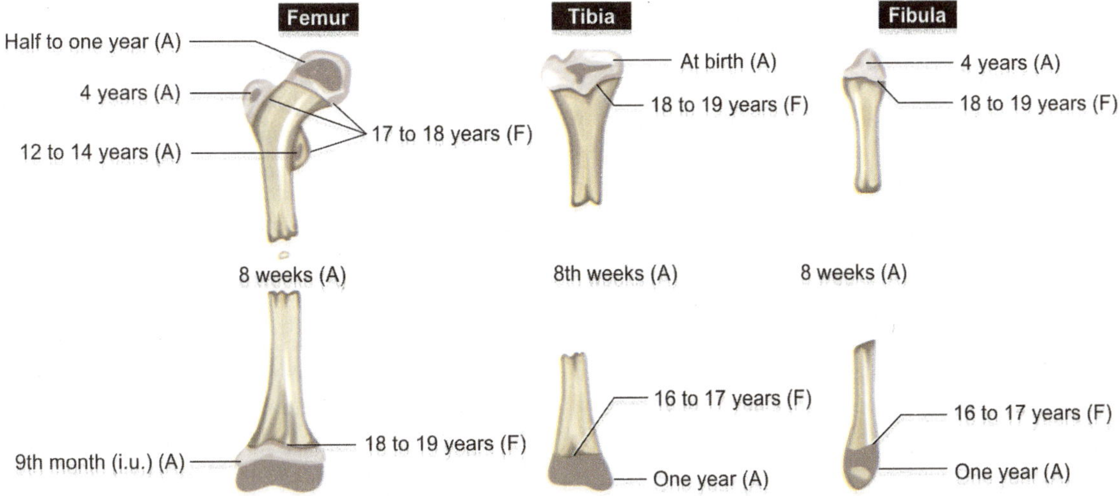

Fig. (4–26). Appearance and fusion of epiphyses in femur, tibia and fibula.

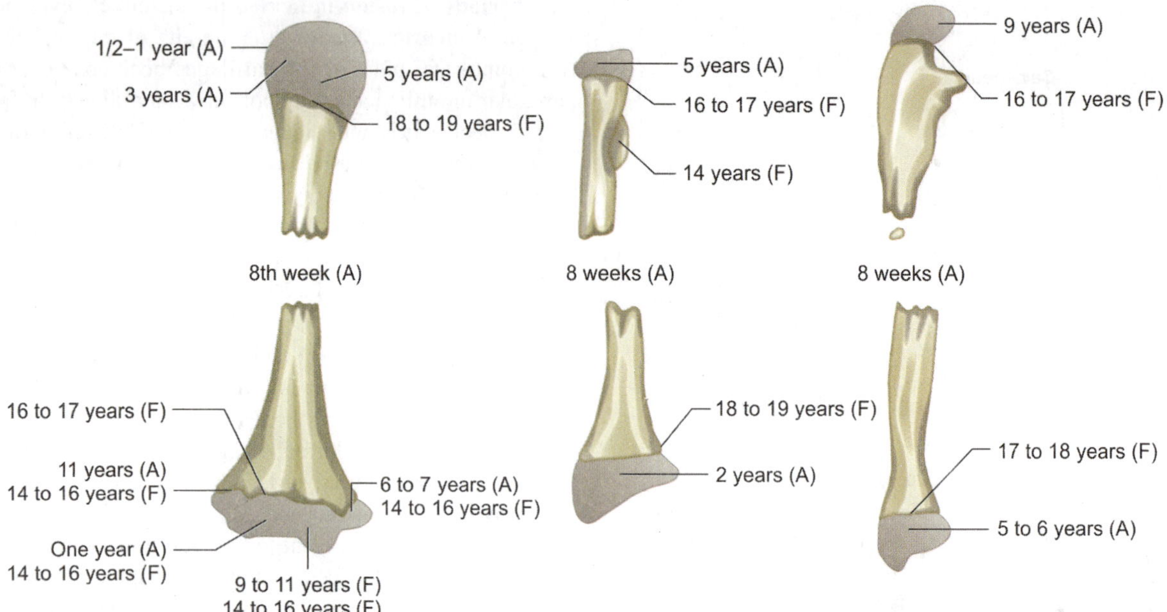

Fig. (4–27). **Appearance and fusion of epiphyses in humerus, radius and ulna.**

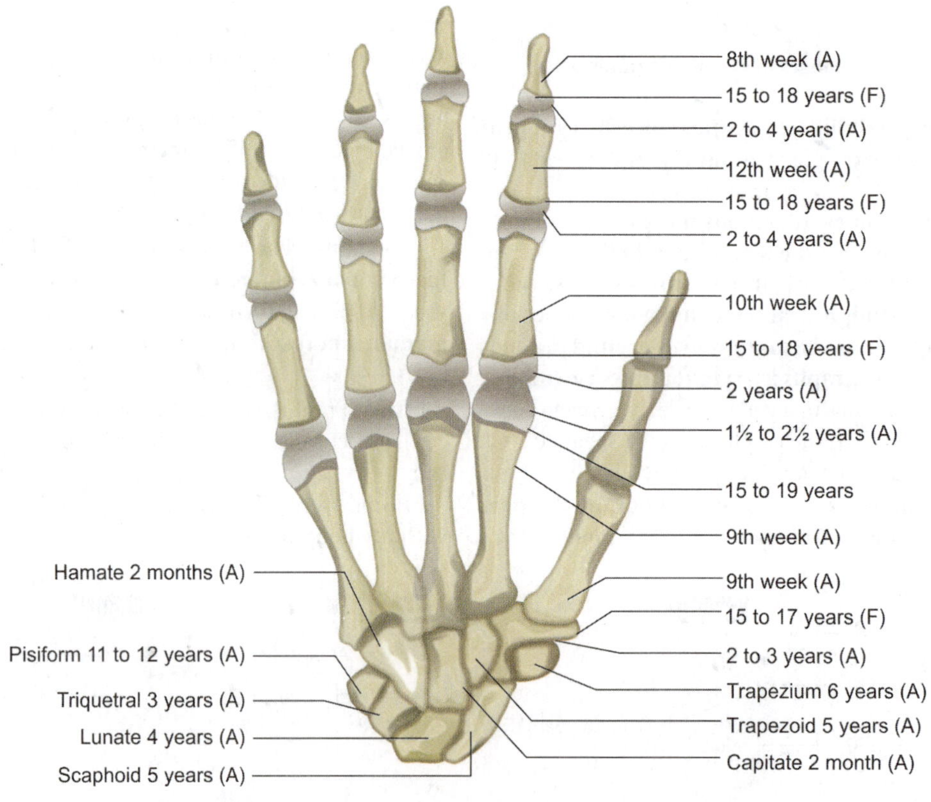

Fig. (4–28). **Appearance and fusion of epiphyses in bones of hand.**

SKULL: Bones of the calvaria are 8 in number: parietal 2, frontal one, temporal 2, occipital one, sphenoid one, and ethmoid one. Bones of the face and jaws are 14 in number: maxilla 2, zygomatic 2, nasal 2, lacrimal 2, palatine 2, inferior nasal concha 2, mandible one, and vomer one. The flexible cartilaginous joints of early life are replaced with interlocking connections between bones in maturity.

Fontanelles: Lateral and occipital fontanelles usually close within the first two months. **Posterior fontanelle closes in 6 to 8 months. The anterior fontanelle closes between 1.5 to 2 years.**

Suture closure: The condylar portions of occipital bone fuse with the squama at the third year, and with the basioccipital at the fifth year. The metopic suture closes about the third year, but in 5 to 10% cases it persists. **The basioccipital fuses with the basisphenoid at about 18 to 21 years. In the vault of the skull, closure of the sutures begins on the inner side 5 to 10 years earlier than on the outer side. The coronal, sagittal, and**

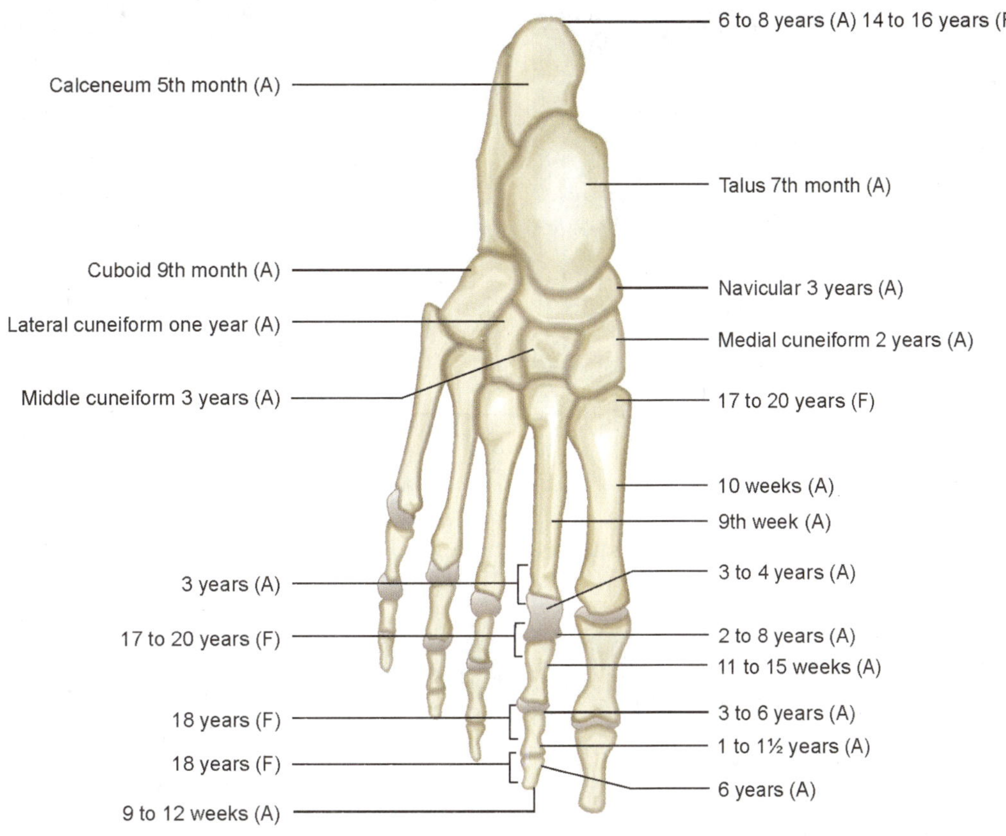

Fig. (4–29). **Appearance and fusion of epiphyses in bones of foot.**

lambdoid sutures start to close on their inner side at about the age of 25 years. On the outer side, fusion occurs in the following order: posterior one-third of the sagittal suture at about 30 to 40 years; anterior one-third of the sagittal and lower half of the coronal at about 40 to 50 years; and middle sagittal and upper half of the coronal at about 50 to 60 years. The lambdoid suture starts closing near the lambda and the union is often completed at about 45 years. **The squamous part of the temporal bone usually fuses with its neighbour by age of 60 years** Fig. (4–43). **Suture closure in skull occurs later in females than in males.** Estimation of age of skull from suture closure is not reliable. It can be given only in a range of decade. Beginning union in the vault sutures may be identified by irregular radio-opacity on each side of the suture. **The most successful estimate is done from sagittal suture, next lambdoid and then coronal.** A lateral head film is preferable for the observation of coronal and lambdoid sutures. Ectocranial suture closure is very variable. Sometimes, there may not be ectocranial suture closure. This is called **"lapsed union".** This occurs most often in the sagittal suture. With lapsing there is slight bony elevation on either side of the incompletely closed suture. Ossification centre in the mandible appears at second month of intrauterine life and the two halves of the mandible unite at the second years Table (4–10) and Fig. (4–38).

OTHER AGE CRITERIA IN THE SKULL: **A young adult skull is smooth and ivorine on both inner and outer surfaces. At about 40± 5 years, the surface begins to assume a "matted" granular, rough appearance. From 25 years onwards muscular markings become increasingly evident, especially on the side of the skull (temporal line), on the occiput (nuchal lines), and on the lateral side of the mandible (masseteric attachment). On the inside of the skull, on either side of the sagittal suture, certain pits or depressions (pacchionian depressions) become more marked with age, both in depth and in frequency. The grooves of the middle meningeal artery become deeper. After 50 years, the diploe becomes less vascularly channelled and there is increasing replacement by bone. There is no consistent age change in the thickness of the vault bones.**

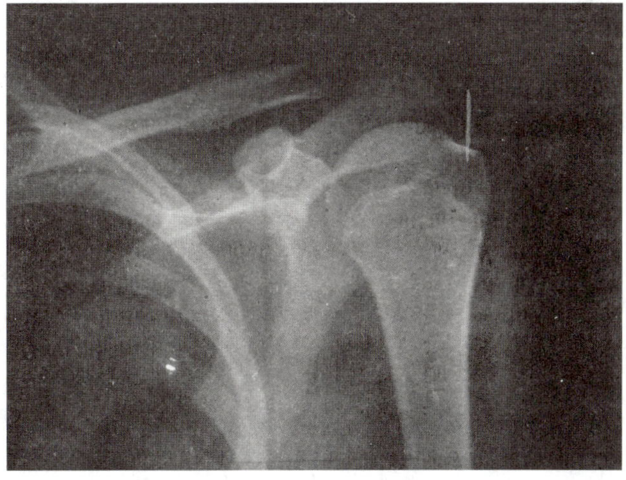

Fig. (4–30). **X-ray photograph of the shoulder. The acromion, coracoid and head of the humerus not united with the shaft. Age 15 to 18 years.**

Sacrum: Centres appear in upper segments in third month. **The five sacral vertebrae are separated by cartilage until puberty, when the lateral portions grow together.** After this, fusion of epiphyses takes place and ossification of intervertebral discs extends from below upwards. **The sacrum becomes a single**

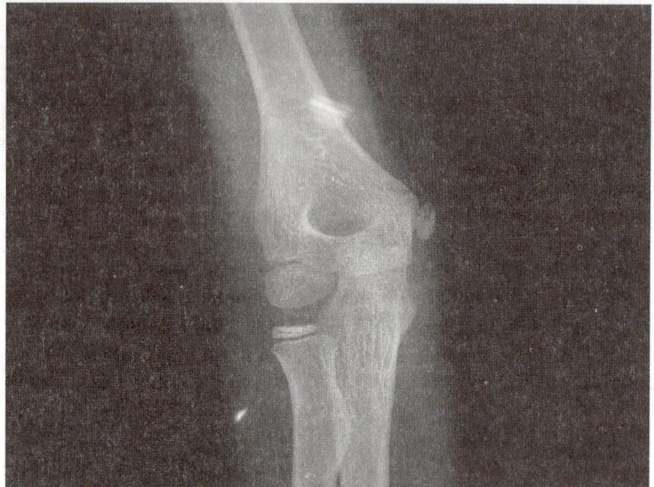

Fig. (4–31). X-ray photograph of elbow. The medial and lateral epicondyles of the humerus, olecranon and head of the radius are not united. Age between 11 to 14 years.

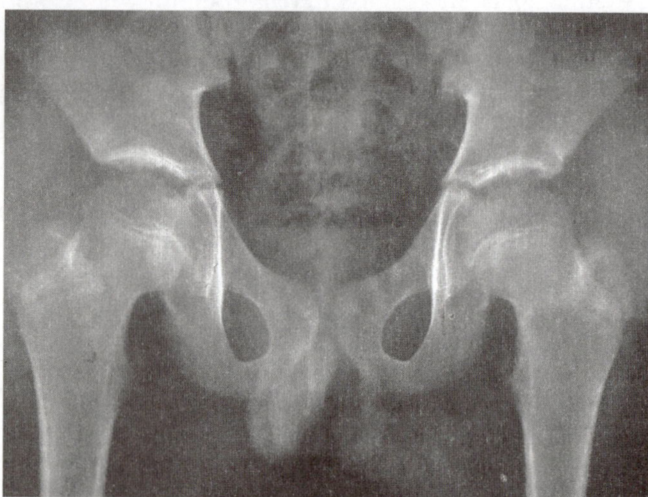

Fig. (4–34). X-ray photograph of the pelvis and hip. Ischial tuberosity and iliac crest have appeared but not fused. Upper end of the femur has united. Age 17 to 18 years.

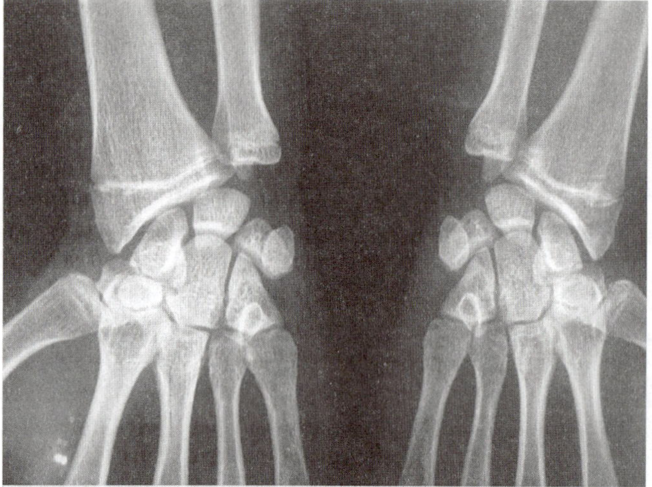

Fig. (4–32). X-ray photograph of the wrist and hand. All the carpal bones are seen. The lower epiphyses of first metacarpal not united with the shaft. Age between 12 to 15 years.

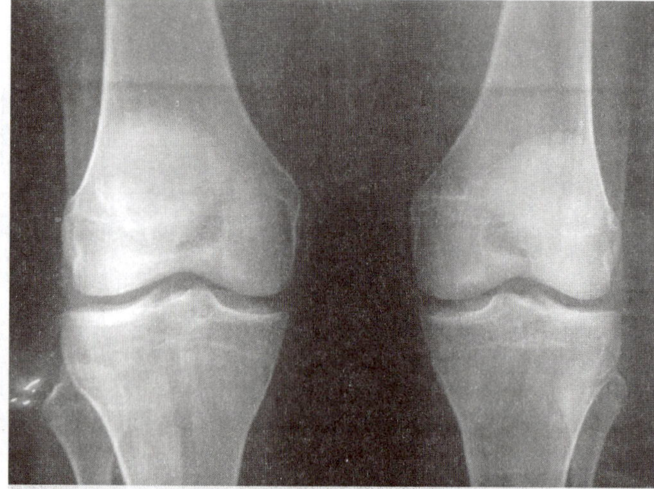

Fig. (4–35). X-ray photographs of the knee. Fusion of the epiphyses of the lower end of femur and upper end of the tibia nearing completion. Age about 18 to 19 years.

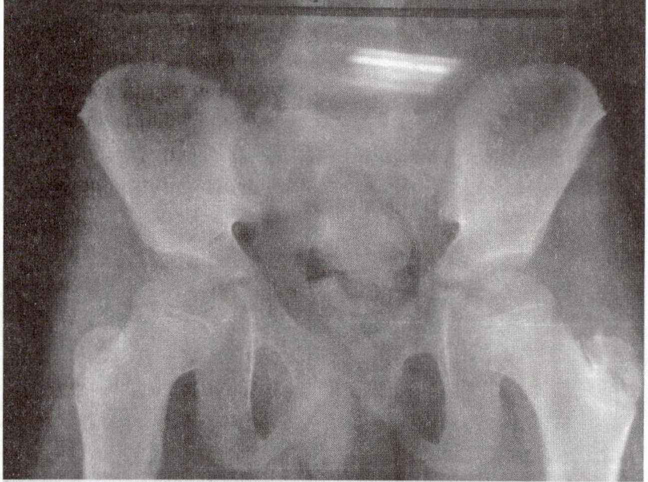

Fig. (4–33). X-ray photograph of the hip. Triradiate cartilage not obliterated. Greater trochanter of femur not united with upper end. Age below 14 years.

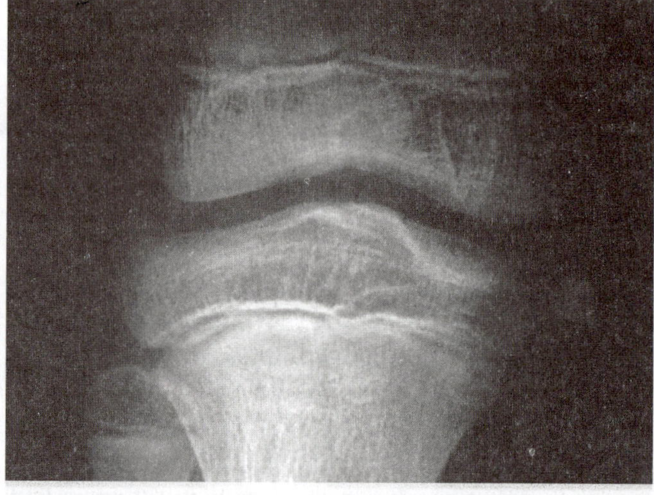

Fig. (4–36). X-ray photograph of the knee. The epiphyses of the lower end of femur and upper ends of the tibia and fibula not united with the shafts. Age about 17 years.

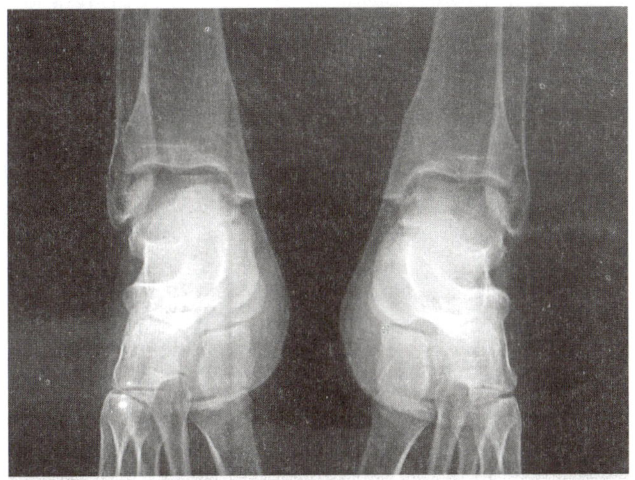

Fig. (4–37). X-ray photograph of the ankle. Secondary centre for the calcaneum appeared but not fused. The epiphyses of the lower ends of tibia and fibula not united with the shafts. Age between 6 to 14 years.

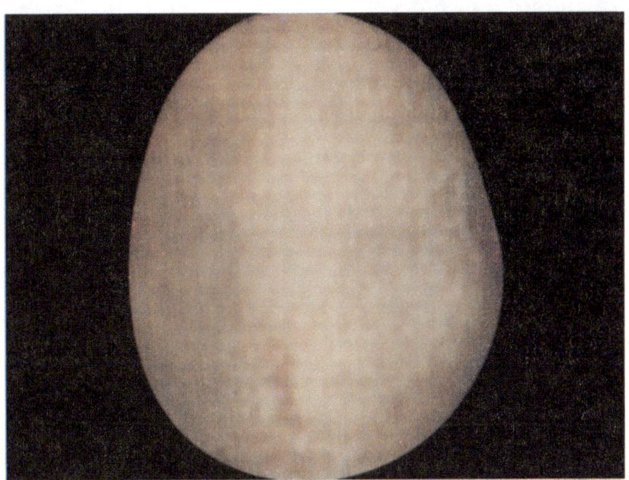

Fig. (4–38). Completed function of the sutures of the skull.

Table (4–9). Appearance of centres of ossification and union of bones and epiphyses

Age		Appearance of centre of ossification	Union of bone and epiphyses
5th year	:	Head of radius, trapezoid, scaphoid.	Greater tubercle fuses with head of humerus.
6th year	:	Lower end of ulna, trapezium.	Rami of pubis and ischium unite.
6th to 7th year	:	Medial epicondyle of the humerus.	
9th year	:	Olecranon.	
9th to 11th year	:	Trochlea of humerus.	
10th to 11th year	:	Pisiform.	
11th year	:	Lateral epicondyle of humerus.	
13th year	:	Separate centres in triradiate cartilage of acetabulum.	
12th to 14th year	:	Lesser trochanter of femur.	
14th year	:	Crest of ilium; head and tubercles of ribs.	Medial epicondyle of humerus: lateral epicondyle with trochlea; patella complete.
15th year	:	Acromion.	Coracoid with scapula; triradiate cartilage of acetabulum.
16th year	:	Ischial tuberosity.	Lower end of humerus; olecranon to ulna; upper end of radius; metacarpals; proximal phalanges.
17th to 18th year	:		Head of femur; lesser and greater trochanter of femur; acromion; lower end of ulna.
18th to 19th year	:	Inner end of clavicle.	Lower end of femur; upper end of tibia and fibula; head of humerus; lower end of radius.
20th to 21st year	:		Iliac crest; inner end of clavicle; ischial tuberosity, head of the ribs.

bone between 21 and 25 years. A gap may persist between S1 and S2, until 32 years due to "lapsed union".

VERTEBRAE: There is a close relationship between the development of cervical vertebrae and age. The immature vertebral body has a series of deep radial furrows both on the upper and lower surfaces. This feature increases in prominence up to the age of ten, and then gradually fades at from 21 to 25 years. After 45 years, osteoarthritic changes in the form of lipping of the vertebrae are seen.

SCAPULA: Between 30 to 35 years, lipping starts on the ventral margin of the glenoid cavity. By 35 to 40 years, irregular lipping occurs around the clavicular facet and inferior surface of the acromion process. By 45 years, localised bony atrophy can be seen. Cristae scapulae occur by 50 years.

Sternal end of fourth rib is an accurate and reliable method of estimating age.

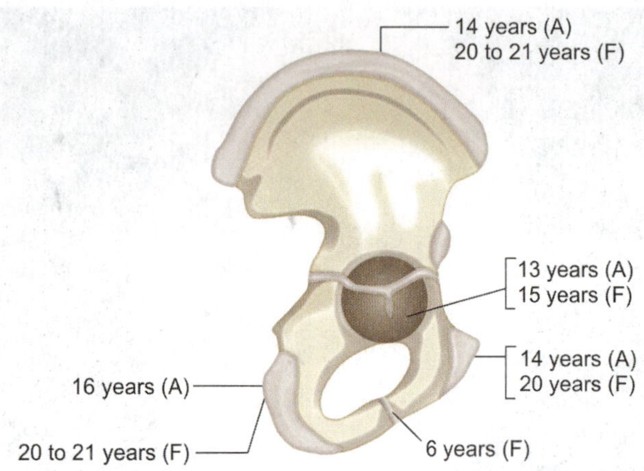

Fig. (4–39). Appearance and fusion of epiphyses in hip bone.

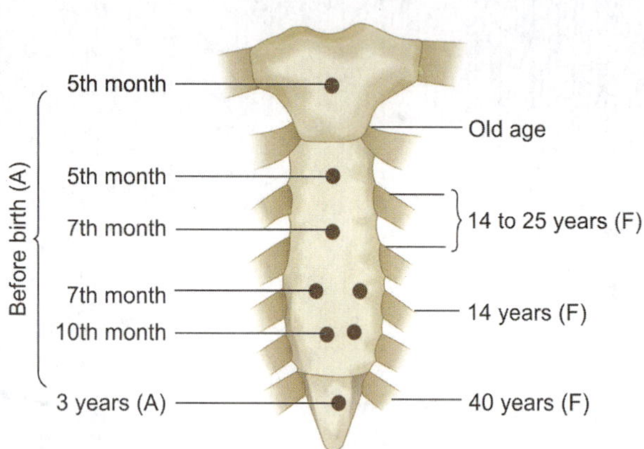

Fig. (4–41). Appearance and fusion of epiphyses in sternum.

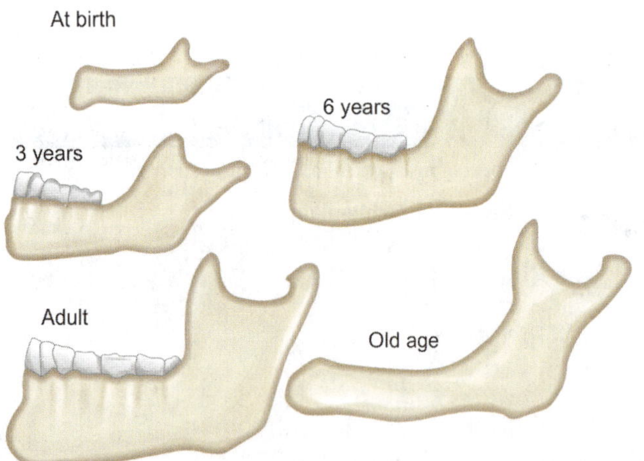

Fig. (4–40). The mandible at different periods of life and Table (4–10).

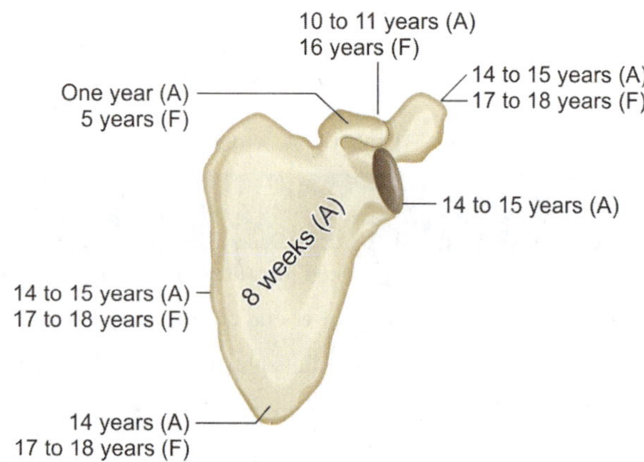

Fig. (4–42). Appearance and fusion of epiphyses in scapula.

SECONDARY SEX CHARACTERS: In the male, at about 13 to 14 years, fine hair begins to appear on pubis, the testes become larger and firmer and the penis begins to enlarge. At about fifteen years, hair is moderately grown on pubis, and hair begins to grow in axilla. At about 16 years, hair on pubis is well grown and the external genitals have an adult appearance. Hair begins to appear on the face between 16 to 18 years and voice becomes hoarse.

In the female, the breasts begin to develop about 12 to 13 years, the vulva becomes more horizontal due to forward tilting of the pelvis, the labia minora develop and some fine, pale, downy hair appears on mons

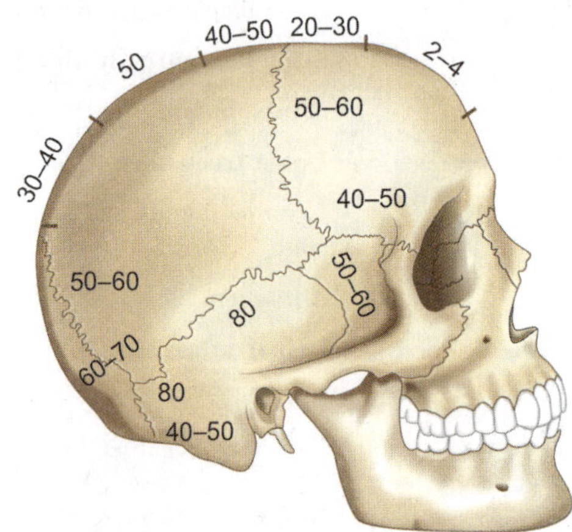

Fig. (4–43). Age of closure of cranial vault.

Table (4–10). Difference between mandible in infancy, adult life and old age, Fig. (4–40).

Trait		Infancy	Adult	Old age
(1)	Body:	Shallow.	Thick and long.	Shallow.
(2)	Ramus:	Short and oblique; forms obtuse angle with body.	Less obtuse angle (almost straight) with the body.	Obtuse angle with the body, about 140°.
(3)	Mental foramen:	Opens near the lower margin.	Opens midway between upper and lower margins.	Opens near the alveolar margin.
(4)	Condyloid process:	At a lower level than coronoid process.	Elongated and projects above coronoid process.	At a lower level than coronoid process.

veneris two months later. The labia develop and menstruation starts. At about 14 to 15 years the pubic hair is well grown and hair appears in the axilla.

ESTIMATION OF AGE AS A WHOLE

For the approximate estimation of age, the following paragraphs should be correlated with what has already been described. DOCTOR'S ESTIMATE ABOUT AGE IS NOT PROOF BUT MERELY AN OPINION.

FIRST FORTNIGHT: The changes in the umbilical cord and the skin.

FIRST SIX MONTHS: Weight and height, partial closure of anterior fontanelle and fusion of the two halves of the mandible. Ossification centres in capitate appears during second month after birth.

SIX MONTHS TO TWO YEARS: The eruption and calcification of temporary teeth is the best guide and the appearance of certain ossific centres and their size in heads of humerus, femur, tarsus and carpus.

TWO TO SIX YEARS: Ossification of tarsus and carpus and appearance of centres in epiphyses of long bones. The number of carpal bones seen on X-ray indicate the approximate age in years.

SIX TO THIRTEEN YEARS: Eruption and calcification of permanent teeth is very helpful. Alterations occur in the centres that have already appeared and additional centres appear.

THIRTEEN TO SIXTEEN YEARS: The changes of puberty and ossification of bones, especially in the region of the elbow joint.

SIXTEEN TO TWENTY-FIVE YEARS: The union of epiphyses of most of the long bones with the shafts take place. The union of epiphyses of clavicles, ends of ribs and iliac crest occur during this period. Between 20 to 30 years, incisors, tips of canines and cusps of premolars show slight to moderate wear. In the early twenties, the sternal rib shows a scalloped rim around a deepening V-shaped pit in both sexes.

TWENTY-FIVE TO THIRTY-FIVE YEARS: The coronal, sagittal and lambdoid sutures of the skull start to close. The changes in the symphysis pubis are very important.

THIRTY-FIVE TO FIFTY YEARS: There is further progress in the changes in the symphysis pubis. Between 30 to 40 years, tooth cusp wear may be moderate to severe. The medullary cavity of the humerus may have increased upward to the level of the lower end of the tuberosity. Wrinkles about the eyes, eyebrows and in front of ears appear about 35 to 40 years. Xiphoid process unites with the sternum at about forty years. Between 40 to 50 years, the vault sutures are all united both endocranially and ectocranially. The cortex of the long bones becomes thinner and less dense. In the humerus, the medullary cavity may extend upward to almost the surgical neck. Atrophic areas in the scapula and iliac fossa are of moderate to almost large size. The margins of the bodies of the lumbar vertebrae, and the inner borders of the ischial tuberosities show lipping by 40 years, which becomes well marked by 45 years. Later, it becomes more marked here and in the joints of the extremities. By the end of fifth decade, bony projections from the superior and/or inferior margins of the rib is fairly well marked in males, and the pit deepens and widens. In females, the pit is relatively shallow and the bone itself is thinner. Ossification of laryngeal and costal cartilages and hyoid bone usually begin. Early changes in the articular surfaces of many bones may appear; they include lipping, reduction of joint space, and the presence of punched-out areas of osteoporosis on X-ray examination. The skull bones gradually change from an ivory-like to granular appearance and feel.

ARCUS SENILIS: A grey opaque ring surrounds the margin of the cornea, due to degenerative changes, but is separated from the margin by an area of clear cornea. It may appear as a result of lipoid degeneration about fifty years or later, but is not complete before sixty years. When it occurs in young adults (below 40 years) due to hyperlipidaemia, it is called **arcus juveniles.**

GREYING of the hair is variable and not of much value. Scalp hair may become grey after forty years, first at the temples. Later it involves the beard and chest hair and eyebrows, but pubic hair, does not become grey before 50 to 55 years.

FIFTY TO SIXTY YEARS: The external tables of the vault become slightly thinner. The molar crowns of the teeth are usually worn flat to a single plane. If all molar cusps are so worn that the crown is a flat plane, an age of fifty plus may be concluded.

AFTER SIXTY YEARS: Further sutural closure of skull occurs. The linea and tuberosities of muscle attachment may show small osteophytic "spurs" or "spikes" in the fifties and sixties and are well advanced in the seventies. Joint changes become more extreme in character and osteoporosis is more marked. The joint between the manubrium and the body of the sternum may fuse, and calcification of the laryngeal and costal cartilages becomes more visible. The predominant features of this period are pathological skeletal changes. The hair may become silvery-white. A completely edentulous upper and lower jaws usually indicate an age of over 70 years.

Loss of collagenous stroma occurs in old age due to which the bone becomes lighter. The stroma is lost first in the outer cortex and the zone around the marrow cavity. The ends of long bones adjacent to the joints are the first to appear fragile and brittle. Radiological thinning of the cortex and progressive rarefaction of the apex of the medullary cavity in the head of the humerus and femur are helpful in the determination of age. Microradiographs of bone are useful. It is based on the correlation between increasing age and loss of bone through natural remodelling processes.

Loss of elasticity of skin, wrinkling and discolouration of the skin of buttocks and abdomen, atrophy of uterus and ovaries, brown atrophy of the heart, and atherosclerotic change in the arteries give an indication of old age.

Due to long continued ingestion of fluorides, there occurs mottling of teeth, increase in density and weight of bones, lipping of bony margins of vertebrae, which sometimes produce pressure on spinal cord leading to paraplegia.

The estimation of age becomes more uncertain after the age of 25 years. It is difficult to achieve an accuracy of even five years. A careful examination of all factors may enable the doctor to make a fair approximation to the decade within which a person may be. Any closer approximation must be made with considerable reservation.

Premature ageing may be produced due to illness, malnutrition, suffering, anxiety or worry. White hair may be produced in quite young people from grief or shock.

PROCEDURE FOR DETERMINATION OF AGE: In medicolegal cases, the age of a person is determined by medical officer on requisition from the police officer or Magistrate. Written consent of the person should be taken. The following particulars should be noted. (1) Name, father's name, age alleged by the person, sex, occupation, and address. (2) Date, time and place of examination. (3) Name of the police constable accompanying the person. (4) Marks of identification. (5) Name of the nurse or attendant present at the medical examination. (6) Height, and weight. (7) General build and changes of puberty. (8) Radiological examination of the bones.

Radiology: For estimation of age between: **6 to 12 years:** take X-rays of (1) Elbow joint. (2) Wrist joint. 6 years: Centre for lower end of ulna (A); **6 to 9 years:** medial epicondyle of the humerus (A): **9 years:** olecranon (A); **9 to 11 years:** trochlea of humerus (A); **10th to 11th year:** pisiform (A): **11th year:** lateral epicondyle of humerus (A) **13 to 16 years:** X-ray of (1) Elbow joint. (2) Pelvis. **13th year:** Separate centres in triradiate cartilage of acetabulum (A); **12 to 14 years:** lesser tronchanter of fremur (A); **14th year:** crest of ilium (A) ; fusion of medial epicondyle of humerus, lateral epicondyle with trochlea. **15th year:** fusion of triradiate cartilage of acetabulum. **16th year:** ischial tuberosity (A); fusion of lower end of humerus; olecranon to ulna, and upper end of radius.

Fusion of bones/joints in males

16 years: elbow joint.

16 to 17 years: ankle joint.

17 to 18 years: hip joint.

18 to 19 years: knee, shoulder and wrist joints.

20 to 21 years: fusion of iliac crest, ischial tuberosity and inner end of clavicle.

In females fusion of bones occurs one year earlier than in males.

The opinion about the age should be given based on the findings of physical, dental and radiological examination. Multiple criteria of skeletal age should be used.

MEDICOLEGAL IMPORTANCE OF AGE

(1) Criminal responsibility: (a) According to Railway Act, a child (no age prescribed) may be held responsible for wrecking a train or endangering the safety of commuters of train. **(b) Any act which is done by a child under seven years of age is not an offence (Sec. 82, I.P.C.).** (c) **A child between seven and 12 years is presumed to be capable of committing an offence, if he attained "sufficient maturity of understanding to judge the nature and consequences of his conduct on that occasion"** (Sec. 83, I.P.C.). This maturity is presumed in a child, unless proved otherwise by the defence. (d) A child under 12 years cannot give valid consent to suffer any harm which may occur from an act done in good faith and for its benefit (Sec. 89, I.P.C.). (e) A person above 18 years can give valid consent to suffer any harm which may result from an act not intended or not known to cause death or grievous hurt (Sec. 87, I.P.C.). (f) Persons with XYY chromosomal pattern are of aggressive and of criminal nature.

(2) Judicial punishment: According to the Juvenile Justice (Care and protection of children) Act, 2000 **"juvenile or boy" means a person (boy or girl) who has not completed eighteenth year of age.** "Juvenile in conflict with law" would mean a juvenile alleged to have committed an offence and not completed 18 years of age on the date of commission of such an offence (Juvenile Justice Care and Protection of Children Amendment Act, 2006). Juvenile Justice Boards exercise powers in relation to juveniles in conflict with law. The board may advice or warn the juvenile, or order to participate in group counselling or perform community service, or to be released on probation of conduct or to pay a fine, or to make an order directing the juvenile to be sent to a reformatory school or special home for the period until he becomes major. **No juvenile in conflict with law shall be sentenced to death or life imprisonment, or committed to prison.**

Juveniles aged between 16 to 18 years who commit heinous offences like rape or murder (punishable with imprisonment of seven years or more) will be tried as adults. However, there will be no death penalty or life term (2015 amendment).

(3) Rape: Sexual intercourse by a man with a girl under 15 years even if she is his own wife, or with any other girl under 18 years even with her consent is rape (S.375, I.P.C.).

(4) Kidnapping: S. 359 to 369, I.P.C. deal with kidnapping. **Kidnapping means taking away a person by illegal means.** It is an offence (a) to kidnap a child with the intention of taking dishonestly any movable property, if the age of child is under ten years (Sec. 369, I.P.C.); (b) to kidnap a minor from lawful guardianship, if the age of a boy is under 16 and that of a girl under 18 years (Sec. 361, I.P.C.); (c) to kidnap or maim a minor for purposes of begging (363-A, I.P.C.). (d) kidnapping, abducting or inducing woman to compel her marriage (366, I.P.C.), (e) to procure a girl for prostitution, if her age is under 18 years (Sec. 366-A, I.P.C.); and (f) to import into India from a foreign country a female for purposes of illicit intercourse, if her age is less than 21 years (366-B, I.P.C.).

(5) Employment: A child below 14 years cannot be employed for any type of work. A person completing 15 years (adolescent) is allowed to work in a factory as an adult, if a fitness certificate is issued by a certifying surgeon.

(6) Attainment of majority: A person attains majority on the completion of 18 years, but when a person is under the guardianship of Court of Wards, or is under a guardian appointed by the Court, he attains majority on the completion of 21 years (Sec. 3, Ind. Majority Act, 1875).

(7) Evidence: All persons will be competent to testify, unless they are prevented from understanding the questions put to them, or from giving rational answers due to tender years, extreme old age or disease of body or mind (S. 118, I.E.A.).

(8) Marriage contract: A female under 18 years and a male under 21 years, cannot contract marriage (Child Marriage Restraint Act, 1978). The age for female is likely to be increased to 21 years shortly.

(9) Infanticide: The charge of infanticide cannot be supported, if the infant can be proved under the age of seven months of intrauterine life.

(10) Criminal abortion: A woman who has passed the child-bearing age cannot be charged of procuring criminal abortion.

(11) Identification: An approximate age is important in any chain of identity data, e.g., when a few days old child is alleged to be the newborn child.

(12) Impotence and sterility: A boy is sterile though not impotent before puberty. Women become sterile after menopause.

AGE OF THE FOETUS

The term **developing ovum** is used for the first seven to ten days after conception, i.e., until the implantation occurs . It is called an **'embryo'** from one week to the end of 8th week, and later it is called **'foetus'**. It becomes an **infant** when it is completely born.

Gestational age can be determined from maturation of chorionic villi; foot length and ossification centres.

END OF FIRST MONTH: Length one cm; weight two-and-half g. The eyes are seen as two dark spots, and the mouth as a cleft.

END OF SECOND MONTH: Length four cm; weight ten g. The hands and feet are webbed. The placenta begins to form. The anus is seen as a dark spot. First ossification centre in a foetus appears in clavicle (4 to 5 weeks), followed by maxilla (6 weeks). Ossification centres are present in the upper segments of sacrum and mandible.

END OF THIRD MONTH: Length nine cm; weight thirty g. The eyes are closed and the pupillary membrane appears. Nails appear and the neck is formed

END OF FOURTH MONTH: Length 16 cm; weight 120 g. Sex can be recognised. Lanugo hair is seen on the body. Convolutions begin to develop in brain. Meconium is found in the duodenum.

It is not possible to draw hard and fast lines between second and third months and between third and fourth months.

END OF FIFTH MONTH: Length 25 cm; weight 400 g. Nails are distinct and soft. Light hair appears on head. Skin is covered with vernix caseosa. Meconium is seen at the beginning of the large intestine. Ossification centres are present in the middle segments of sacrum.

END OF SIXTH MONTH: Length 30 cm; weight 700 g. Eyebrows and eyelashes appear. Skin is red and wrinkled and subcutaneous fat begins to be deposited. Vernix caseosa is present. Meconium in transverse colon. The testes are seen close to the kidneys.

END OF SEVENTH MONTH: Length 35 cm; crown-rump length 23 cm; foot length 8 cm; weight 900 to 1200 g. Nails are thick. Eyelids open and pupillary membrane disappears. Skin is dusky-red, thick and fibrous. Meconium is found in the entire large intestine. **Testes are found at external inguinal ring. Gallbladder contains** bile and caecum is seen in the right iliac fossa. **Ossification centre is present in the talus.**

END OF EIGHTH MONTH: Length 40 cm; weight one-and-half to two kg. Nails reach the tips of fingers. Scalp hair is thicker, 1.5 cm. in length. Skin is not wrinkled. Left testis is present in the scrotum. Placenta weighs 500 g. Ossification centre is present in lower segment of sacrum.

END OF NINTH MONTH: Length 45 cm; weight 2.2 to three kg. Scalp hair is dark and 4 cm. long. Meconium is seen at the end of large intestine. Scrotum is wrinkled and contains both testes. Placenta weighs 500 g. Ossification centres are usually present in the lower end of the femur.

END OF TENTH MONTH (FULL-TERM CHILD): Length 48 to 52 cm; crown-rump length 28 to 32 cm; **weight 2.5 to 5 kg; average about 3.4 kg.** The length is much less variable than the weight. The male infant weighs about 100 g. more than the female. **The circumference of the head is 33 to 38 cm**. Head circumference is measured by positioning the tape at the frontal and occipital prominence. **Six fontanels are usually present in the neonatal skull.** The anterior fontanel (bregma) is located at the junction of sagittal and coronal sutures. The posterior fontanel (occipital) lies at the junction of sagittal and lambdoid sutures. At each sphenoparietal junction, a lateral fontanel is present. The posterolateral fontanels (mastoid) are located at the mastoid-occipital junctions. Anterior fontanel is 4 x 2.5 cm. At full term the head of a child is nearly one-fourth of the whole length of the body. **The surface of the brain shows convolutions,** and the grey matter begins to form. The scalp hair is dark, 3 to 5 cm long. **The face is not wrinkled. Lanugo is absent** except on the shoulders. The skin is pale and covered with vernix caseosa. The nails project beyond the end of fingers, but reach only the tip of the toes. **The cartilages have formed in the nose and ears. The testes are present in the scrotum; vulva is closed and labia minora are covered by fully developed labia majora. The rectum contains dark brownish, green or black meconium. The umbilicus is situated midway between pubis and xiphoid cartilage.** The umbilical cord is 50 to 55 cm. long, and one cm. thick. The limbs are firm, hard and rounded. **The centre of ossification is found in the lower end of femur and sometimes in the cuboid and in the upper end of the tibia.** The placenta is 22 cm. in diameter, one-and-half cm. thick at the centre, and weighs about 500 gm.

Ossification Centres: (1) Sternum: It is placed flat on a wooden board and cut with the cartilage knife in its long axis in midline.

(2) Lower end of femur and upper end of tibia: The leg is flexed against the thigh and a transverse or vertical incision is made into the knee joint. The patella is removed. The end of the femur is pushed forward through the wound, and a number of parallel cross-sections are made through the epiphysis starting from its articular surface and continuing until the largest part of ossific centre is reached. **The centre is seen as a brownish-red nucleus surrounded by bluish-white cartilage.** Further sections are made through plain cartilage above it, until the diaphyseal centre is reached. **The centre appears about the 36th week.** Its diameter is about four to five mm. at 37 to 38 weeks, and 6 to 8 mm. at full term. The upper end of tibia is similarly examined. **In 80 percent of full term infants, a centre is present in the upper end of tibia,** but in other cases it appears after birth.

(3) Bones of the foot: The foot is grasped in the left hand behind the heel, the toes pointing towards the dissector. **An incision is made between the interspace of third and fourth toes with a long knife,** backwards through the sole of the foot and heel. If centre in calcaneum and talus are not exposed, thin slices of cartilage of these bones should be cut until the presence or absence has been shown. **Centre in the calcaneum appears at the end of the fifth and in talus at the end of seventh month of intrauterine life.** A centre may be present in cuboid at birth, or it may appear shortly afterwards.

RULE OF HAASE (1895): This is a rough method of calculating the age of the foetus. The length of the foetus is measured from the crown to the heel in centimetres. **During the first five months of pregnancy the square root of the length gives the approximate age of the foetus in months, e.g. a foetus of 16 cm. is four months.**

Haase's Modification of Morisson's Law: During the last five months, the length in cm. divided by five gives the age in months, e.g., foetus of 35 cm. is 7 months.

After birth, the length of an infant is 50 cm; 60 cm. at the end of six months; 68 cm. at the end of first year, and 100 cm. (double its length at birth) at the end of fourth year and tripled by 13 years. From age two to the beginning of adolescence, the average child will grow 5 cm. per year. Birth weight doubles by four to five months of age and triples by about one year and quadruples at 24 months. After age two, average weight gain until adolescence is 2 to 3 kg annually. Head circumference increases by about twelve cm. in the first year of life. 90% of adult head size occurs by end of second year. The brain at birth is about 80% of its adult weight, and 90% by age six. In infants and children, height and weight may be compared with standard tables.

STATURE

Variations in stature: Stature varies at different times of the day by one-and-half to two cm. It is less in the afternoon and evening due to the reduced elasticity of the intervertebral discs and the longitudinal vertebral muscles. Both malnutrition and advancing years reduce stature. **After the age of thirty,** the natural processes of senile degeneration (gradual atrophy and loss of elasticity of the vertebral disks, and the individual changes of posture due to ageing processes in general) cause **gradual decrease in stature by about 0.6 mm. per year on an average. The stature is greater by one to three cm. on lying.**

On an average, the body lengthens after death by about two cm. due to complete loss of muscle tone, relaxation of large joints (hip and knee) and vertebral discs and loss of tensioning effect of paraspinal muscles on intervertebral discs, causing flattening of vertebral curvature. As decomposition sets in, joints become lax and loss of tension in intervertebral discs tends to shorten the spinal column and total height by one centimetre.

DETERMINATION OF STATURE FROM DISMEMBERED BODY: If the body has been dismembered, the approximate stature may be determined by: (1) The length from the tip of the middle finger to the tip of the opposite middle finger, when arms are fully extended, closely equals the height. (2) Twice the length of one arm, with 30 cm. added for two clavicles, and four cm. for the sternum, is equal to the height. (3) The length of forearm measured from tip of olecranon process to tip of the middle finger is equal to 5/19 of the stature. (4) The length from the vertex to the symphysis pubis is roughly half of stature. After14 years of age the symphysis pubis lies about halfway up the body. Before 14 years the trunk is longer than the lower limbs. (5) The height of head measured by the vertical distance from the top of the head to the tip of the chin is about one-seventh and the length of skull is about one-eighth of the total height. (6) The length from the sternal notch to symphysis pubis multiplied by 3.3 gives the stature. (7) The length of vertebral column is 35/100 of the height. (8) To the length of entire skeleton, add two-and-half cm. to four cm. for the thickness of the soft parts. (9) Maximum foot length divided by 0.15 gives stature.

ANTHROPOMETRY (Bertillon system): Principle: It is based on the principle that after the age of 21 years, the dimensions of the skeleton remain unchanged and also that the ratio in size of different parts to one another varies considerably in different individuals. As such, this is applicable only to adults. Data to be recorded: (1) Descriptive data: such as colour of hair, eyes, complexion, shape of nose, ears, chin, etc. (2) Body marks: such as moles, scars, tattoo marks. (3) Body measurements: such as height, anteroposterior diameter of head and trunk, the span of outstretched arms, the length of left middle finger, left little finger, left forearm, left foot, length and breadth of right ear and colour of left iris. The photographs of a front view of the head and a profile view of the right side of head are also taken. This system has now been replaced by dactylography. As a sole means of identification, photographs are not always reliable, and they may be a source of error even when they are inspected by experts.

DACTYLOGRAPHY (fingerprint system; dermatoglyphics; Galton-Henry system): **Dermatoglyphics is the study of ridge patterns in the skin**. This system was first used in India in 1858, by Sir William Herschel in Bengal. Sir Francis Galton systematised this method in 1892. Fingerprint Bureau was first established in Kolkata.

Principle: Fingerprints are impressions of patterns formed by the papillary or epidermal ridges of the fingertips. The ridge pattern of fingers appear between 12 to 16 weeks of intrauterine life and the formation is completed by 24 weeks. At birth a fine pattern of ridges is seen on the skin of the bulbs of the fingers and thumbs, parts of the palms and the soles of the feet.

Classification Fig. (4–44): (1) Loops (about 60 to 70 percent), (a) radial, (b) ulnar. (2) Whorls (about 25 to 35 percent), (a) concentric, (b) spiral, (c) double spiral, (d) almond-shaped. (3) Arches (about 6 to 7 percent). (a) plain, (b) tented, (c) exceptional. (4) Composite (about one to two percent). (a) central pocket loops, (b) lateral pocket loops, (c) twinned loops, (d) accidentals.

In a whorl, the ridges form a series of circles or spirals around the core. In a composite, there are a combination of two or more of the types, namely arches, loops or whorls.

Identification: The final identification of any fingerprint is made by comparison of many details of characteristics which occur throughout the ridge areas and by the sequence in which these characteristics occur, but not by comparing the patterns. The characteristics may take the form of ridge endings, bifurcations, lake formations, or island formations. **In practice 16 to 20 points of fine comparison are accepted as proof of identity.** The **patterns are not inherited and paternity cannot be proved through fingerprint patterns.** The **pattern is different even in identical twins**. **The fingerprint patterns are distinctive and permanent in individuals. The fingerprint system is the only guide to identity, which is unfailing in practice.** The details of these can be accurately teleprinted. Palm and footprints also provide similar material.

POROSCOPY: This is further study of fingerprints, described by Locard. **The ridges on fingers and hands are studded with microscopic pores, formed by mouths of ducts of subepidermal sweat glands.** Each millimetre of a ridge contains 9 to 18 pores. These pores number in thousands per square centimetre. **These pores are permanent and unchanged during life and vary in size, shape, width, starting and stopping on occasion and branching at points, position, extent and number, distribution and arrangement of the pores over a given length of ridge in each individual.** This method of examining pores is called poroscopy, and is **useful when only fragments of fingerprints are available in which there is no specific pattern.**

Ridgeology is the study of friction ridges which are composed of the edges of ridge units which vary in size, shape and alignment.

Edgeoscopy is the study of edges of friction ridges which normally show seven characteristic features.

The Individuality of Fingerprints: The fingerprints are capable of endless variation so that it has been speculated that there is one chance in sixty-four billions of two persons having identical fingerprints.

Quetlet's rule states that every nature-made objects present infinite variation in forms and no patterns are ever alike.

Mode of Production: A constant stream of sweat covers the skin and when the person is excited, the output of sweat increases. **Sweat contains about 99% water and one% solids,** which include salt, sulphates, carbamates, lactic acid, urea, fatty

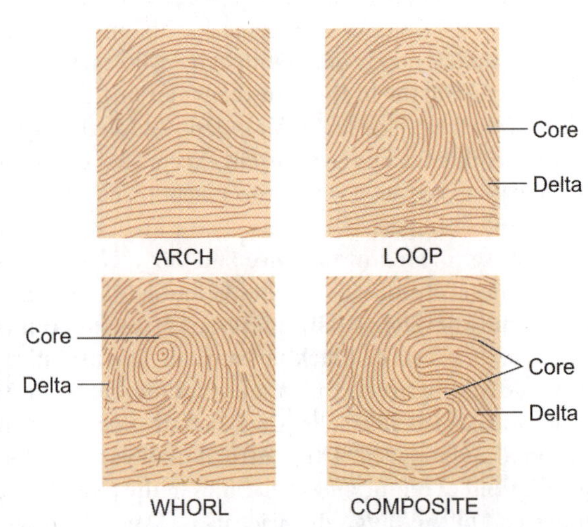

Fig. (4–44). Four main fingerprint patterns.

acids, formic acid, acetic acid, butyric acid and sometimes a little albumin. **The fingerprint may also contain oil exuded by the sebaceous glands,** which is present on the fingertips through touching the face, neck, hair, scalp, etc. **If any part of finger is applied to a smooth surface, a greasy impression of its pattern is made on it.**

TECHNIQUES OF FINGERPRINTING: The hands are washed, cleaned and dried, as otherwise the print will be blurred. The fingerprints are recorded on unglazed white paper using printer's ink. (1) A plain print is taken by applying ink to the tips of the fingers and placing the fingers directly on paper. (2) The rolled fingerprint is taken by rolling the fingers on paper from outward to inward in such a way as to obtain an impression of the whole tip. If rigor mortis is well developed, incision into the palmar surface of the fingers at the proximal interphalangeal joint will enable the fingers to be straightened, and printing can be carried out.

Types: (1) The **latent print (chance print)** is an invisible or barely visible impression left on a smooth surface. (2) **Visible prints** (patent prints) are formed by fingers stained with blood or ink or other medium. (3) The **plastic print** is an impression made on a soft surface, such as soap, cheese, mud, pitch, candles, thick dried blood, adhesives, etc.

RIDGE IMPRESSIONS: Burnt skin of the fingers on healing shows its original pattern. In manual labourers working with lime, sand, and cement the ridges on the bulbs get unduly rubbed and become broken and indistinct. Ridge impressions get malformed if the quality of ink is poor, when the ink is too liquid and spreads into the depressions, if the digit is rolled often or pulled, and when the paper is placed upon an uneven or rough surface.

DEVELOPMENT OF LATENT PRINTS: Fingerprints may be taken from almost any surface with which the fingers come in contact, including certain fabrics and human skin. A latent print may be developed by dusting the area with coloured powders to provide a contrast, and its pattern is recorded by photography. It can also be examined by oblique lighting. The commonly used powder is 'grey' powder (chalk and mercury), but white powders (lead carbonate or French chalk) are used for dusting dark surfaces. Fingerprints on paper, wood and fabrics are developed by treating them with 5% silver nitrate solution and then fixing them with sodium thiosulphate. Fingerprints on paper can also be developed by exposing it to the vapours of iodine or osmium tetroxide. Electron autoradiography method uses a high energy beam of X-rays to irradiate the lead dust on fingermarks. The scanning electron microscope visualises latent fingerprints on metal and glass. Using a continuous wave argon ion laser and observing through suitable filters, latent fingerprints show luminescence. Even ten years old fingerprints can be developed.

LIFTING OF FINGERPRINTS: Fingerprints on a large immovable hard surface is developed, photographed and then adhesive surface of cellophane tape is pressed on the print, taken out gently and pasted against a cardboard sheet for permanent preservation.

Assailant's Fingerprints: The fingerprints of an assailant will remain on the victim only after death. During pre-death struggle both the assailant and the victim will sweat due to nervous tension, and one exudate will cancel out the other. After death, the victim will not sweat, due to which the fingerprints will be left on the body. Electronographic method is used to develop latent fingerprints on skin of living persons or dead bodies. Sweating from exertion is seen on the forehead, axilla, small of the back, etc. whereas nervous sweating is almost confined to the hands and feet.

Fingerprints in Decomposed Bodies: Ridges are present both in dermis and epidermis. In advanced putrefaction and in cases of drowning, the skin is frequently found loose like a glove, which should be removed, preserved in formalin and used for impressions. Prints can be obtained from the dermis after epidermis is lost. **Histological sections up to a depth of 0.6 mm. from the surface of the skin give satisfactory fingerprints. In dead bodies, the palmar skin of the terminal phalanx of each finger should be removed separately from both hands, and after labelling, placed in separate containers, containing 10% formalin, and sent to the fingerprint bureau, if it is not possible to take the prints.**

If the fingers are shrivelled, they should be immersed in 20% acetic acid for 24 to 48 hours, or air, glycerin or liquid paraffin is injected into the bulb, which will cause the shrivelling to swell to normal size. If the skin is dehydrated, the finger is soaked in 3% solution of potassium hydroxide in warm water for a short period, until the fingers regain normal size. If the skin is fragile lead carbonate mixed with paraffin is applied on the skin and X-rayed. If the fingers are sodden, wrinkled or mummified, their outine can be made level by injecting liquid paraffin, or even formalin, within the tissues of the palmar aspects of the terminal phalanx of each finger.

Persistence of Impression at Scene of Crime: Impressions may persist for years, if undisturbed by cleaning. Even outside the house, they may persist for weeks. On glazed paper they persist for more than three years.

MUTILATION OF FINGERPRINTS: Criminals sometimes attempt to mutilate the pattern by self-inflicted wounds or burns, application of corrosives or erosion against a hard surface, but they are not destroyed unless the true skin is completely destroyed. They produce additional characteristics. It leaves some part of the skin undamaged, unless skin grafts are made. In most cases of coeliac disease, there is moderate epidermal ridge atrophy and even loss of pattern. Incomplete atrophy of the ridges is usually seen in dermatitis. Ridge alteration occurs in eczema, acanthosis nigricans, scleroderma, and dry or atrophic skin. Permanent impairment of the fingerprint pattern occurs in leprosy, electric injury and after exposure to radiation. In infantile paralysis, rickets and acromegaly, though the pattern is not altered, the distance between the ridges can be changed. Fingerprints are better protected than other parts of the body, e.g. in case of burns they are bent inwards against the palm of the hand.

Computerisation: Fingerprint reader (FINDER) is a computerised automatic fingerprint reading system which **can record each fingerprint data in half second. Prints of eight fingers are recorded excluding little fingers.** The light reflected from a fingerprint can be measured and converted to digital data which is classified, codified and stored in the computer.

Medicolegal Importance: (1) The recognition of impressions left at a scene of crime, e.g., on weapons, furniture, doors, utensils, clothes, etc., establish the identity of the criminal. (2) The identification of suicides, deserters, persons suffering from loss of memory or those dead or unconscious after being involved in an accident and of decomposing bodies. (3) Identification in case of accidental exchange of newborn infants. (4) The prevention of impersonation. (5) To maintain identity records. (6) Cheques, bank notes and other legal documents can bear a fingerprint. Rough idea about the age of a finger print can be made by studying the migration of chloride ions from the fingerprint.

In criminals, impressions of all the ten fingers are taken, but for civil purposes, the left thumb impression only is taken.

FOOTPRINTS (Podogram): The skin patterns of toes and heels are as distinct and permanent as those of the fingers. Footprints of newborn infants are used in some maternity hospitals to prevent exchange or substitution of infants. A fresh footprint of suspected person is taken and compared with the original. Any peculiarities in the foot, such as a flat foot, supernumerary toes, scars or callosities are likely to be found in the footprint. In case of bootmark, the pattern and arrangement of nails or holes in the sole may be useful. A footprint produced by walking

is usually larger than one produced by standing. The imprint on soft and loose material like sand is smaller than the foot, and the imprint produced on mud or clay is larger.

A footmark expert may identify a shoe with a mark made at the scene of crime, and by general examination may find out the number of persons involved, their actual movements at the scene and their point of entry. Individual impressions, especially in yielding soil, will indicate the shoe size and approximate weight of the person and any peculiarity of gait. A partial footmark may be quite sufficient to positively identify a shoe. Footmarks are recorded by photography, casts or lifting or by a combination. Casts can only be taken when there is a footmark in depth. As they are three dimensional, they can be easily compared with the suspect's shoes even by lay persons. Crime scene footprints are compared with the comparison prints made on similar surface by the suspect. Prints are taken in normal standing position, standing position with pressure on inner side and outer side, when walking and when jumping. It may be possible to know whether the track marks are that of a young or old person. Step length of an adult woman is 45 to 55 cm. and that of an adult male 63 to 70 cm.

PALATOPRINTS: In the anterior part of the palate, the structural details like the rugae are individual specific and permanent. The palatoprints can be used in the same way as fingerprints. Rugae are categorised as (a) primary rugae (>5 mm), (b) secondary rugae (3–5 mm) and (c) fragmented rugae (2–3 mm) (Lysell)

LIPPRINTS: (Cheiloscopy): The fissures and grooves on the lips are claimed to be characteristic of the individual. Lipprints are divided into six patterns (SUZUKI) which are specific to the individual; vertical, branched, intersected, reticular patterns, etc. 24 characteristic details have been identified. Identification is established if 7 to 9 characteristics tally. Minor differences can be noted between the right and the left and upper and lower lips. Lip prints, are seen on crockery, cloth, paper, window panes, cigarette ends, etc.

EAR PRINTS: Ears have four basic shapes: oval, round, rectangular and triangular. The shapes of ear lobes and the tips of ears are of various types. Most of the ear prints are found on doors or windows. From the suspect three prints are taken (1) functional pressure, (2) gentle pressure, (3) more pressure, on a glass pane. The print is made visible as in the case of fingerprints and a photograph of the print is taken. The same process is applied to the ear prints from the scene. Photocopies of both known and unknown ear prints are produced on plain and transparency overlays. The transparency overlay is put on the top of the unknown print and taped to the top of a light box. If the tragus point, crus of the helix points and antitragus point fit, look at the lower and upper crura of the antihelix and the helix rim. If all details coincide the prints are from the same source. The opinion can be positive, highly probable, probable, possible or no basis for comparison.

NOSE PRINTS: The lines on the nose and the shape of the tip are helpful in identification. Chance impressions may be found over door, wall, etc.

RETINA SCAN IN IDENTIFICATION: Each person's retina has an unique pattern which is not changed from birth until death. The pattern is different even in identical twins. As such, **it appears to be the most precise and reliable biometric.** A retinal scan is performed by casting an undetectable ray of low-energy infrared light into a person's eye as he looks through the scanner's eyepiece focussing on a single point for a duration of 15 seconds, which outlines a circular path on the retina. Retinal blood vessels absorb light more readily than the surrounding tissue, but the amount of reflection fluctuates. The results of the scan are converted to computer code and stored in a data base. Using suitable cameras and infrared illumination, image of cornea is copied and converted into digital templates. **The retinal template is one of the smallest of any biometric technology.** An enrolled person can be identified with a retinal scan process in seconds. **They are about 70 times more accurate than iris scans.** They are nearly impossible to fake. After death, retina decays quickly. **Retinal patterns may be altered in cataracts, glaucoma, retinal degeneration and diabetes.**

IRIS SCAN: The iris is a muscle within the eye that regulates the size of the pupil controlling the amount of light that enters the eye. It is the coloured portion of the eye, and the colouring is based on the amount of melatonin pigment within the muscle. Although the colouration and structure of iris are genetically linked, an individual's irides are unique and structurally distinct, which allows for them to be used for recognition purposes. The iris is located using landmark features. The distinct shape of iris allows for imaging feature isolation and extraction.

SKULL-PHOTO SUPERIMPOSITION: This technique was applied by Glaister and Brash in 1935 in Ruxton case. **Superimposition is the technique applied to determine whether the skull is that of the person in the photograph Fig. (4–45).** The photograph need not be front view of the face; even lateral and semi-lateral view of face can be used. A recent photograph is better. If the negative of photograph is not available, negative of the available photograph is prepared by recopying it. **The photograph is enlarged to natural size from the presence of some standard thing in the photograph of the missing person to indicate the scale.** In the absence of a standard for the measurement of face in the photograph, **photographs of the skull and face are superimposed by adjusting the magnifications until the interpupillary distances correspond,** on the assumption that the interpupillary distance in one individual is the same always when the eyes move in different directions. The negative is placed under the ground-glass of camera and salient features of the face are marked out carefully on the glass. The soft parts are removed from the skull. A comparison can be made even in the absence of the lower jaw. The skull is mounted on an appropriate skull rest, so as to align as accurately as possible with the outline of the head on the ground-glass in the corresponding portrait, making due allowance for the soft tissues covering the bone. The distance of the camera is adjusted so that the one inch scale on the ground-glass of the camera is exactly equal to the scale on the skull. This, when photographed, gives a life-sized negative of the skull. **The negatives of the photographs and the skull are superimposed by aligning the characteristic points in the negatives.**

Points for comparison: The following points are then compared. (1) The eyes within the orbital plates, with the two pairs of canthuses properly aligned. (2) The nasion. (3) The prosthion in the central line. (4) The nasal spine in the centre which is a little above the tip of the nose. (5) The lower border of the nose. (6) The lower border of the upper jaw, i.e., below the tip of the nose. (7) The zygomas below the eyes. (8) Supraorbital ridges. (9) Angle of the jaw. (10) External auditory meatus. (11) Teeth.

The two superimposed negatives are then photographed on bromide paper. The resulting superimposed photograph brings out the points of similarity or dissimilarity between the photograph and the skull. The superimposition is correct, if the

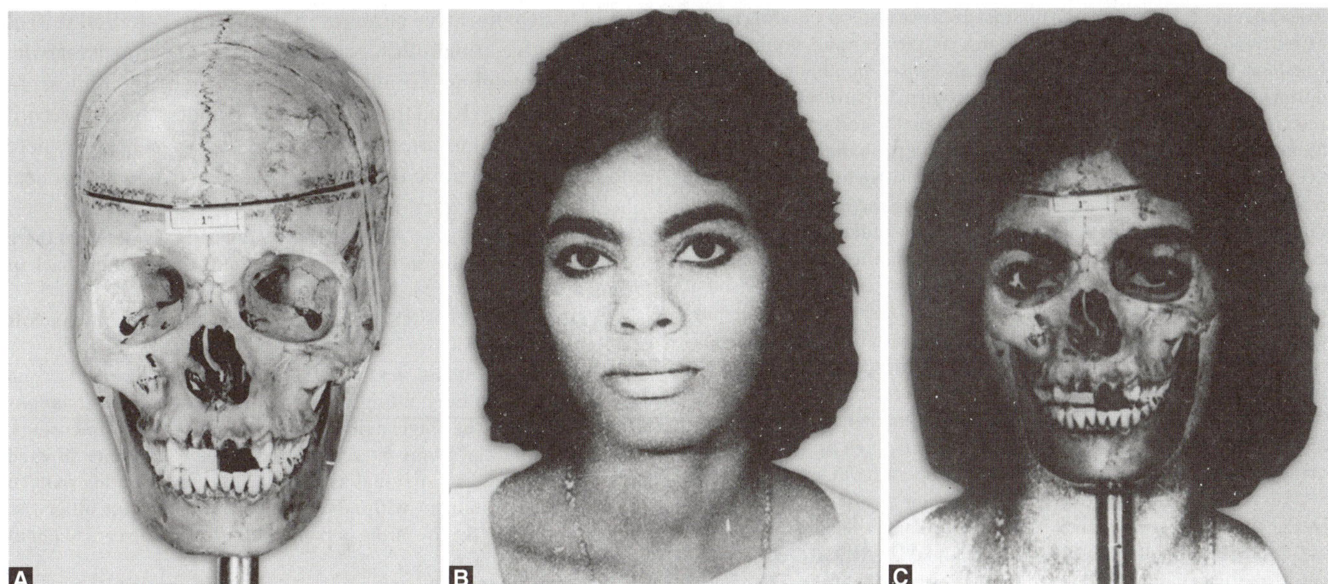

Fig. (4–45). Superimposition technique. (A) Skull photograph in the same position as face in B. (B) Photograph of missing person. (C) Result when photograph B is superimposed on the photograph A, showing resemblance in the contour of the face and skull.

outlines and the size of the skull accurately correspond to the face in the photograph. **A clear effect of the superimposed area can be obtained by combining the negative of the skull with the positive of the portrait.** For this, positive portrait and negative of the skull are rephotographed on X-ray film, thus producing a transparent positive of the skull. Finally, the two films are bound together in register and thus superimposed; they are then re-photographed on X-ray film by transmitted light Fig. (4–45).

This test is of a more negative value, because it can definitely be stated that the skull and the photograph are not those of the same person. If they tally, it can only be stated that the skull could be that of the person in the photograph, because of the possibility that another skull of that size and contour may tally with the photograph.

VIDEO SUPERIMPOSITION: The skull is fixed on a rotatable universal stand or on a cork ring placed on the floor. The photograph is also fixed with the same orientation parallel to the skull. One camera is directed at the skull and a second camera directed at the photograph of the face. Images of the skull and photograph are projected on a monitor placed near the skull. By performing a series of blending, fading and sweeping (vertical, horizontal and diagonal), the image of the skull and photograph are superimposed and analysed for conformity. All the anatomical landmarks are compared. This is an exclusionary method.

COMPUTER-ASSISTED SUPERIMPOSITION: The skull and facial photograph are digitized using a computer. The two images are compared morphologically by image processing. A scale for the digitized skull image is established by converting the actual measurement between the anthropological landmarks into the number of pixels in the monitor. For assessing the anatomical consistency between the digitized skull and face, the distance between anatomical and anthropological landmarks and the tissue thickness are measured by means of pair dots by the computer mouse. Fade in and fade out, wiping and sweeping the face and skull in a vertical or horizontal plane for comparing them is done by the computer. If the anterior teeth are present in the skull and images of the same are seen in the photograph, a positive comparison of these will provide definite consistency between the skull and photograph.

IDENTIFICATION BY RECONSTRUCTION OF FACIAL FEATURES: (1) His, determined the average thickness of the soft parts of the face at a series of fifteen, i.e., nine median and six lateral pre-determined points. Using these data, attempts at reconstruction have involved the application of clay or plastic in appropriate thickness over the landmarks, contouring the facial outlines and building up the soft features of the nose, mouth and ears. The restorer must rely on various artistic cannons, personal experience, skill and intuition. It may help to eliminate certain suspected persons, or support an identification based on other skeletal evidence. A major problem is that features which give individuality to a face, such as the eyes, lips and facial hair, are not very dependent upon the underlying bone structure. (2) 20,000 measurements of a skull can be taken using video and laser equipment, which can be stored in 30 seconds. The data from an unknown skull are then electronically 'clothed' with standard soft tissues from the memory bank and modified on screen to produce various images, which can be rotated electronically to produce various profiles. To recognise a missing person by a viewer, a variety of stored eyes, ears and noses can be added, and any feature altered instantaneously.

COMPUTER PICTURES: Several curves for each of facial creases, prominences, shape of forehead, eyes, ears, nose, cheek, lips, teeth projections, scalp hair, moustache and beard are stored in a computer. Depending on the descriptions of the different features by the persons who have seen the criminal, hundreds of varieties of face can be drawn on the screen of the computer within a few minutes. An almost exact appearance of the face can be drawn by additions and alterations of curves, which can be printed out.

PHYSIOGNOMIC RESTORATION: (1) Sculptural to give a three-dimensional bust, and (2) artistic to give drawing in two views, facial and profile, to show cephalic and facial details. Both methods try to achieve an individual likeness which will lead to identification of the suspect.

NORMAL AND ABNORMAL BONE COMPARISONS: When previous X-ray films of the skull are available for comparison with postmortem films, measurements of the skull and a detailed comparison of the frontal, sphenoidal and maxillary sinuses, sella turcica and mastoid area are useful for identification in adults. No two pairs of sinuses are the same. The frontal sinuses are individual specific and are useful even in mutilated and burnt bodies. They are unique in that no two persons (not even identical twins) have the same profile of these air spaces. They appear in second year of life and increase in size for the first two decades. They are absent in about 5% of persons and unilateral in 1%. The scalloped upper margins of the sinuses are used for comparison, these being smaller and more numerous in the female.

The sphenoid complex and the mastoid area are also very useful criteria of individuality. Abnormal bones, such as cervical and lumbar ribs, wormian bones (small bones in the skull caused by abnormal suture patterns leaving islands of bone surrounded by sutures, sometimes referred to as ('sutural' or 'intrasutural bones'), and sesamoid bones (bones included in tendons, frequently seen in the hands and feet) may provide definite points for comparison and positive identification. The trabecular fine structure of all bones (excluding the bones of the skull) may be defined with enough precision by xero-radiography to permit comparisons. Congenital or acquired abnormalities, e.g., absence of bones, displacement and malformations are very rare. Comparison of the lateral skull X-ray and X-rays of the upper ribs, humeri and femurs can provide useful information based on the pattern of the concellous bone, when previous radiographs are available. The contours of the second rib are unique. Fusion of the ribs or vertebrae may be noted. Radiographs of the carpal bones show individual details. The presence of surgical prostheses or of supportive implants, such as plates, pins or orthopaedic screws and of trephine or other operative defects of the skull are very useful. Dental radiography may show significant root shapes, socket outlines or abnormalities of tooth eruption, development or decay.

SKULL SUTURE PATTERN AND VASCULAR GROOVES: The suture patterns of the skull appear to be quite individualistic. The sagittal and lambdoid sutures are especially complicated and quite different from one person to another. However, the suture patterns are not useful for comparison because (1) the sutures close, and the pattern obliterated with age, and (2) the suture patterns are not well demonstrated in those postmortem X-ray films most commonly available.

The vascular grooves, such as those related to the middle meningeal vessels, are much more apt to be visible in X-ray films than are the suture lines, are useful for comparison to establish identity.

X-RAYS IN IDENTIFICATION: (1) **They are useful in identification** by determining the sex, age Fig. (4–46), superimposition, and identification of the person by detecting old fractures, plates, nails and screws from surgical procedures, diseases, or congenital bony changes. (2) In investigation of cases of battered baby syndrome, burns, drowning and decomposition. (3) To detect air embolism, and pneumothorax. (4) To locate missiles in the body, direction of firing, depth of the wound and type of firearm. (5) To detect parts of the mechanism of bombs and explosive devices that are embedded in the tissues. (6) To locate foreign bodies, bullet emboli, etc. (7) To detect fractures. (8) To detect pregnancy, foetal death or abnormality, hydatidiform mole, etc. (9) Electrocution. (10) Lead poisoning. (11) **Unusual calcification of tuberculous origin in the lungs or lymph nodes, or due to degenerative changes in the uterus, calcified mitral or aortic valve, phlebolith, granuloma, etc. are characteristic.** (12) Drug smuggling through sealed packets in body cavities, gut and genitalia. (13) Road traffic accidents to understand and record pattern of skeletal injuries. (14) Medical negligence cases where embolism (air, amniotic fluid), wrong placement of endotracheal tube, leaving of surgical instruments is suspected.

VEINS ON THE BACK OF HANDS: Tamassia suggests that there is complete individuality in the arrangement of the veins of the back of the hands.

STOMACH PICTURES: Barium meal X-ray of the stomach is said to be individual.

NAILS: Longitudinal striations are present on both the convex and concave surfaces of human fingernails and toenails. Parallel striations on the surface of the fingernail (numbers, distribution, dimensions, depressions and elevations, etc.) are specific for each finger of each individual and are as individual as fingerprints. The striation pattern becomes more prominent with advancing age, but remains otherwise unchanged during the life of the person. Nails grow at the rate of about 3.2 mm. per month.

DEFORMITIES: They may be congenital or acquired. Congenital deformities, such as hare-lip, cleft palate, talipes, polydactylism, web-fingers or toes, undescended testicles, etc. are frequently treated surgically, and are therefore losing some of their past importance. Old amputations, spinal defects, old fractures and deformities of the bones and nails, either from injuries or disease and surgical prostheses, such as implanted artificial heart valves, plates in the skull, etc., should be described.

Mongolian spots (congenital marks) appear as dark blue or violet, single or multiple macules in the lumbosacral region in some young children of Asiatic and African origin.

Moles (intradermal naevus) are usually round, brown or black, raised or flat with or without hair. The size and exact anatomical position also should be noted.

SCARS

A scar is a fibrous tissue covered by epithelium without hair follicles, sweat glands or pigment, produced from the healing of a wound. **Injury to the dermis produces a scar**, while superficial injuries involving only the epidermis do not produce a scar. Scars are permanent Fig. (4–47).

Examination: Good lighting is essential. **The description should include their number, site, size, and shape, the level it bears to the body surface, fixed or free, smoothness or**

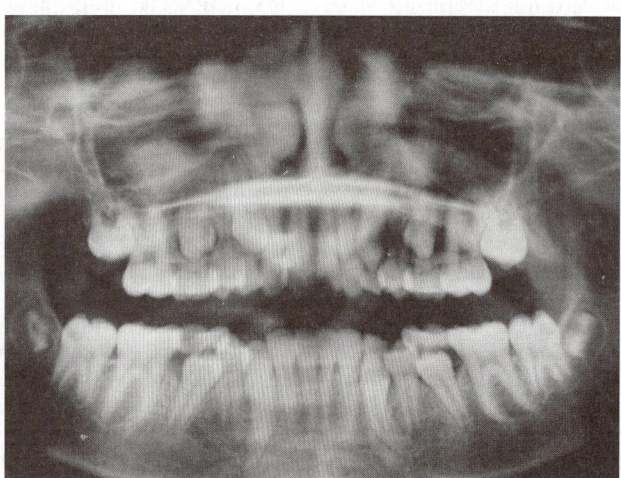

Fig. (4–46). Orthopantomogram showing mixed dentition is useful to determine age.

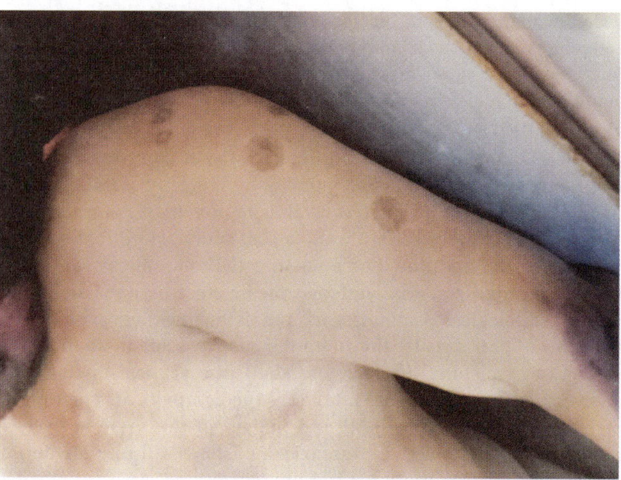

Fig. (4–47). Vaccination scars on left upper arm.

irregularity of the surface, colour, and the presence or absence of glistening and tenderness. The condition of the ends, whether tapering or not, and the probable direction of original wound should be determined. The application of heat, filtered ultraviolet light or surface friction, makes faint scars readily visible. Old scars may become unrecognisable. A magnifying glass is very useful. Suspected scars in the dead body can be proved by microscopy, by a **section stained to show the elastic tissue, which is absent in a scar.** Elastic tissue is present in striae gravidarum.

Characters: Scars may indicate the type of injury which produced them. (1) Incised wounds produce linear scars. If healing is secondary, the scar is wider and thicker in the centre than in the periphery. (2) Scars from lacerated wounds, and from wounds which have suppurated are firmer, irregular, more prominent, and are adherent to the deeper tissues. (3) Stab wound due to a knife-blade produces oval, elliptical, triangular, or irregular scars which are depressed, but may be elevated due to keloid formation. (4) A bullet wound causes a circular depressed scar. (5) Scars from scalds are spotted in appearance, tend to be continuous, often run downwards and show evidence of splashing about the main injury. (6) Scars due to corrosive acids, burns or radiation, cause irregular scars, and keloid may develop in the scar tissue, especially in Negroes. (7) Vaccination scars are circular or oval, flat or slightly depressed. (8) Many skin diseases, smallpox, syphilis, etc., cause multiple scars on the skin.

Growth: Scars produced in childhood grow in size with the natural development of the individual, especially if situated on the chest or limbs.

Age of Scars: Firm union occurs in from five to six days, producing a reddish or bluish "angry" scar. By the end of 14 days, the scar becomes pale. soft, tender and sensitive; there is no further change up to the end of second month. In about two to six months, the scar becomes white, glistening, and tenderness is slowly lost. After 6 months scar becomes tough, and there is no further change.

Erasure: The scar can be erased by excision and skin grafting, or suture of the edges of the excised area. This results in a scar which is less clearly seen.

Medicolegal Importance: (1) They form important marks for identification of a person. (2) The shape of the scar may indicate the nature of weapon or agent that caused the injury. (3) The age of the scar is important in a criminal offence. If the age of a wound corresponds with the date of the attack it may have value as circumstantial evidence. (4) Linea albicantes may indicate previous pregnancy. (5) If a person is disfigured due to scars, it becomes a grievous hurt. (6) Scar causing contracture at or around a joint restricting movement or functions of the joint becomes grievous hurt. (7) The accused may attribute scars of wounds to disease or therapeutic procedures. (8) Scar of various operative procedures also help in identification. (9) To charge an enemy with assault, a person may claim that scars due to disease are those of wounds.

TATTOO MARKS

Mode of production: Tattoo marks are designs made manually in the skin (upper dermis) by multiple small puncture wounds with needles or an electric vibrator dipped in colouring matter.

The dyes commonly used are Indian ink, carbon (black); cinnabar or vermilion (mercuric sulphide) red; chromic acid (green); indigo, cobalt, Prussian blue (ferric ferrocyanide), ultramarine (blue). Techniques and dyes vary from country to country. **The most permanent pictures are made when the dye penetrates the dermis.** Most of the marks are found on the arms, forearms and chest, but may be present on any part of the body.

Natural disappearance: If the pigment has been deposited below the epidermis, it will very slowly become fainter and certain pigments, such as vermilion, and ultramarine may disappear after about ten years. **If the dye is deposited into deeper layers of dermis, it will be removed by phagocytes. The rate of fading depends not only on the composition of the pigment, but also on the depth to which it penetrates the skin, and the site which is tattooed.** Parts protected by clothing retain the design for longer period than the exposed parts of the body. Tattoos on the hands disappear early due to constant friction Figs. (4–48 and 4–49).

Recognition: A faded tattoo mark becomes visible by the use of ultraviolet lamp or rubbing the part and examining with magnifying lens. Infrared photography makes old tattoos readily

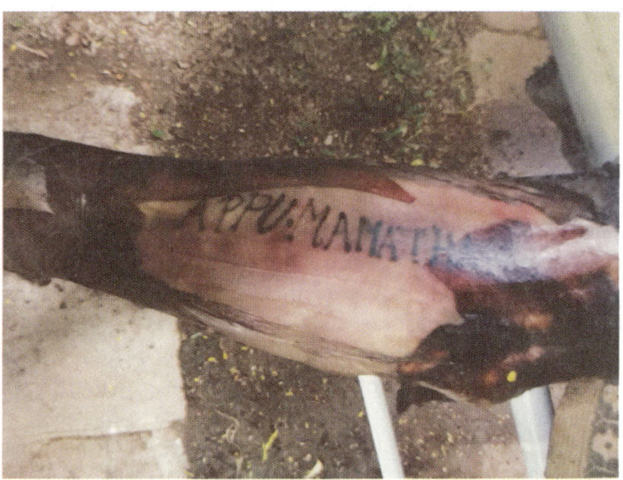

Fig. (4–48). Tatto mark seen in a decomposed body.

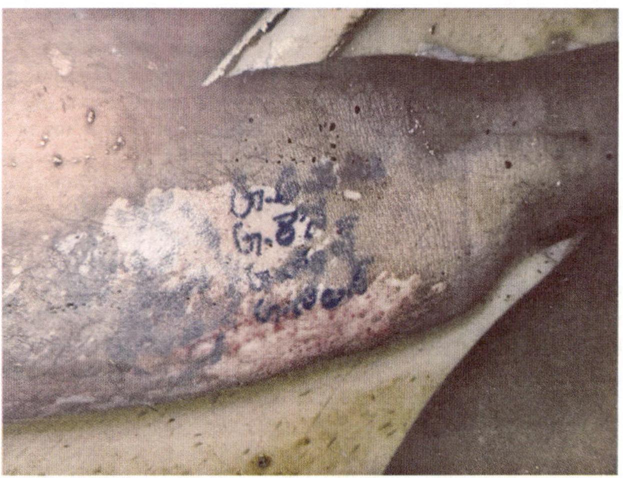

Fig. (4–49). Tattoo mark seen in superficial burns.

visible. **The marks are recognised even in decomposed bodies when the epidermis is removed by wiping the area** with a moist paper towel or a piece of cloth. Lymph nodes near a tattoo mark show a deposit of a pigment. **The colour, design, size and situation of tattoo marks should be noted.** Drawing or photography is more useful.

CASE: Sydney Shark Case: James Smith disappeared on April 8, 1935. A shark was caught alive 14 days later, which vomited a human arm at the aquarium where it was kept. Medical examination revealed that the arm was severed from a dead body by a sharp weapon. Smith's wife and brother identified the arm from the tattoo of two men boxing. The identity was also confirmed by fingerprints. Later, Patric Brady was tried for his murder at Sydney.

Complications: Septic inflammation, erysipelas, abscess, gangrene, syphilis, AIDS, leprosy and tuberculosis may occur.

ERASURE: (1) SURGICAL METHODS: (a) Complete excision and skin grafting, (b) production of burn by means of red hot iron, (c) scarification with sand paper, and (d) carbon dioxide snow. (2) ELECTROLYSIS. (3) CAUSTIC SUBSTANCES remove pigment by producing inflammatory reaction and a superficial scar, e.g., mixture of papain in glycerine, zinc chloride and tannic acid. (4) LASER BEAM: By exposure to laser beams, the particles of the dye get vapourised and expelled from the tissues in gaseous form. (5) Confluent smallpox and sometimes chronic eczema in children can obliterate tattoo marks.

Medicolegal Importance: Tattooing is useful in identity. (1) If there are large number of tattoos, positive identification can be made by tattoos alone. Initials and dates, regimental or nautical details, identity numerals, one's own name, etc., provide more scientific basis for identification. (2) Religion. (3) God of worship. (4) Indicate culture or life-style. (5) The distribution of tattooing and the nature of designs and figures may indicate a particular country or region. (6) The presence of indecent figures points to definite perversion in the individual. (7) They reflect travel, history, war, occupation, sex interest, etc. (8) Gang members may wear a tattoo of allegiance and symbolism to indicate status or other aspects relevant to their particular group. (9) Illicit drug users may have tattoos that identify them as belonging to a particular group or to obscure injection sites. (10) Homosexuals may tattoo on the back of hand between base of thumb and forefinger.

WOUNDS: Sometimes, the presence of wounds on the body may assist in connecting a suspected criminal with a given crime, e.g. a piece of skin adherent to a window glass may correspond with the wound on the thief, or rupture of fraenum of penis may be present in a person accused of rape. Dust, sand, etc., may be recovered from wounds and identified.

DISEASE: The finding of disease, e.g. gallstones, renal stones, calcified leiomyomata, silicosis, asbestosis and congenital anomalies like horseshoe kidney, are helpful. The unidentified body should be checked for amputations, body deformities, pacemakers, implanted heart valves, teeth, their fillings and restorations, degenerative changes, infection, enlarged joints of the fingers due to arthritis, immovable joints due to disease, bowed-legs and curvature of the spine. X-rays will show the presence of healed fractures, metal pins, plates, or screws used in treating fractures. Commonly found missing organs at autopsy are tonsils, appendix, gallbladder, kidney, prostate, uterus and ovaries. Surgical scars may indicate hernia repair, circumcision or an operation upon the thyroid gland.

STAINS: Stains found on body or clothing of the accused and the victim may be the same and may be derived from the walls , doors, furniture, etc., at the scene of crime.

OCCUPATION MARKS: (1) RECENT AND TEMPORARY: Contact traces of some solid or liquid the person is working with may be found on the skin, beneath the nails, in the hair, ears or on clothing. They include paint spots on painters, grease on engineers and mechanics, flour on bakers and millers, dyes on dye workers, saw dust on those engaged in timber cutting, etc. The microscopical examination of dust and debris on clothing, in the pockets and trouser turnups, under the fingernails and in the ear wax, is important in identification of unknown bodies. They may also connect the body with a specific place where a crime was committed.

(2) PERMANENT: Thickening of the palmar skin of fingers are seen on the right hands of butchers. Cuts, scars, callosities and hyperkeratosis of the hands indicate manual labourers. Tailors have marks of needle punctures on their left index finger. Coal miners have multiple 'blue scars' on the face and arms due to coal-dust contamination of small lacerations. Blacksmiths have scars on the back of the hand caused by burns from hot fragments. Opticians have small cuts on the tips of index finger and thumb. Workers in chemicals and photography usually have discoloured, distorted fingernails. Carpenters have callosities on the thumb and index finger, on the palms, and one shoulder is usually higher than the other. Bricklayers have a flattening of the thumb and index finger of the left hand due to constant picking up of bricks. The violinist has hardened tips on the fingers of the left hand.

COMPLEXION AND FEATURES: The complexion may be fair, wheat-coloured, dark, brown, pale-brown or pale-yellow. Details of the features regarding eyes, nose, ears, lips, chin, and teeth should be noted. The face may be oval, round, square or long, and eyes may be black, grey, blue or brown. The features may change considerably from disease or even from worries of a long duration. Few persons can cleverly alter their features by changing the expression of their face. Expression is altered after death.

CASE: Bhowal Sanyasi Case: Kumar Ramendra Narayan Roy, the second son of Raja Rajendra Narayan Roy of Bhowal estate in Dhaka, died in Darjeeling in 1909. In 1921, a Sadhu came to Dhaka and claimed one-third share of the Bhowal Raj Estate. He declared that he was Ramendra Narayan Roy, that after he went to Darjeeling, he was administered arsenic with the intention of killing him, due to which he became comatose and taken to be dead. His body was taken to cremation ground at night, but the funeral party left the cremation ground without lighting the pyre due to heavy storm. Some Naga Sanyasis revived him and carried him with them. He suffered from complete amnesia until 1921. After failing to regain his share of properties, he filed a suit in the Dhaka Court in 1930. Bibhabati Devi, the wife of the second son of the Raja Bahadur, and others contested the suit, on the ground that the plaintiff was an imposter. The hearing lasted for more than two years. About 1,069 witnesses on the plaintiff side and 470 on the defence side were examined, and more than 2000 photographs and documents were exhibited. The Court declared the plaintiff as Kumar Ramendra Narayan Roy and granted one-third of the property. Later, this judgement was upheld by the Calcutta High Court and by the Privy Council.

In deciding the case, complexion and features, hair, eyes, syphilitic ulcers, broken tooth, photographs, boil marks, operation scar, tiger claw mark, mole on the dorsum of the penis, the gait, voice and expression, were taken into consideration to establish the identity.

Beck Case: Adolf Beck was imprisoned for impersonation and fraud on women, after being identified by 15 out of 17 of the women. His handwriting also closely resembled that on some incriminating documents. After some years, he was released and rearrested. He was identified by 19 women. Another man was arrested for similar swindles whose handwriting was similar to that of Beck. Later, it was proved that Beck was innocent and was discharged and compensated.

EYES: MEDICOLEGAL IMPORTANCE: (1) IDENTIFICATION: (a) artificial eyes, (b) absence of one or both eyes, (c) shape, (d) colour of iris, (e) setting: deep set, bulging or prominent, (f) squint, (g) nystagmus, (h) cataract. The look of the person will show whether he is conscious, unconscious, frightened, confused, etc.

(2) ASPHYXIA: (a) proptosis, (b) congestion, (c) petechial haemorrhages.

(3) INJURIES: (a) Black eye (contusion of lids), (b) in fracture of anterior cranial fossa involving orbits, there may be effusion of

blood into the orbits, proptosis, limitation of movement of eyeball and subconjunctival haemorrhage, (c) gouging of eyes, (d) lacerated wounds, (e) penetrating wounds, (f) foreign bodies, (g) chemical burns, (h) ulceration and opacity of cornea, (i) vitreous haemorrhages are likely to affect vision, (j) rupture of choroid and retina, (k) subluxation of lens and post-traumatic cataract.

(4) Poisoning: (a) **Dilated pupils:** datura, atropine, belladonna, cannabis, cocaine, alcohol, CO, ergot, endrin, calotropis, strychnine, oleanders, HCN antihistamines, cyclic antidepressants, amphetamines. (b) **Contracted pupils:** opium, phenol, organophosphorus compounds, physostigmine, neostigmine, pilocarpine, strophanthin, nicotine, carbamates, barbiturates, benzodiazipines, caffeine, muscarine. (c) **Alternate contraction and dilation:** aconite. (d) **Large and fixed:** anticholenergic drugs, anoxia. (e) **Small and fixed:** opioids, cholinergic drugs. (f) **Variable size and fixed:** barbiturates, glutethimide, hypothermia. (g) **Nystagmus:** ethanol, phenytoin, carbamazepine, barbiturates, benzodiazipines, phencyclidine.

(5) NATURAL DISEASE: Blue sclerotics of osteogenesis imperfecta and odontogenesis imperfecta.

(6) ACUITY OF VISION: for crimes committed during night.

(7) WORKMEN'S COMPENSATION ACT.

HAIR

Trichology is the study of hair. Hair grows at the rate of 0.4 mm/day.

The examination of the hair is undertaken to find out:

(1) HAIR OR SOME OTHER FIBRE? Hair consists of bulb or root and a shaft. Considerable force is required to pluck out a lot of healthy growing hair from scalp. An adult can be lifted or dragged by the hair and the scalp may even be torn from the skull.

ANATOMY: In most hair, there are three well-defined layers. (1) CUTICLE: This is the outer layer and consists of thin, non-pigmented scales. (2) CORTEX: This is the middle layer and consists of longitudinally arranged, elongated cells without nuclei. Within these cells are fibrils on which there may be granules of pigment. (3) MEDULLA: This is the inner layer composed of keratinised remains of cells.

FIBRES: COTTON fibres are flattened and twisted tubes. They consist of long tubular cells, with thickened edges and blunt-pointed ends. LINEN fibres show cross lines or folds about which the fibre is often swollen and has a narrow lumen. Fibres are straight and taper to a point. JUTE fibres are smooth without transverse lines. The cell cavity is not uniform. The ends are blunt. SILK consists of long clear threads without any cells. They are smooth and finely striated. WOOL fibres show an outer layer of flattened cells and overlapping margins. The interior are composed of fibrous tissue but sometimes medulla is present.

(2) Human or animal: Table (4–11); Figs. (4–50 and 4–51)

Colour changes along the hair shaft called "banding" is seen in some animals.

Medullary Index of Hair: It is the ratio of diameter of medulla and diameter of the whole hair shaft. In humans it is less than 0.3 and in animals more than 0.5 The value varies in the hair of different parts of the body and as such it is also helpful to know the part of the body from which it is derived.

(3) FROM WHAT PART OF THE BODY DERIVED? Hair from the head is usually long and soft and taper gradually from the root to the tip. The beard and moustache hair are usually thicker than the hair of any other part of the body. Hair of the eyebrows, eyelashes and nostrils

Table (4–11). Difference between human and animal hair

	Trait	Human hair	Animal hair
(1)	Character:	Fine and thin.	Coarse and thick.
(2)	Cuticle:	Cuticular scales are short, broad, thin and irregularly annular.	Cuticular scales are very large and have step-like or wavy projections.
(3)	Cortex:	Thick, well-striated, and 4 to 10 times as broad as medulla.	Thin, rarely more than twice as broad as medulla.
(4)	Medulla:	Varies considerably, usually narrow; continuous, fragmented, or entirely absent.	Continuous and wider.
(5)	Pigment:	Evenly distributed.	Mostly present in the medulla.
(6)	Precipitin test:	Specific for human.	Specific for different animals.
(7)	Medullary index: Diameter of medulla / Diameter of shaft	Below 0.3	Above 0.5

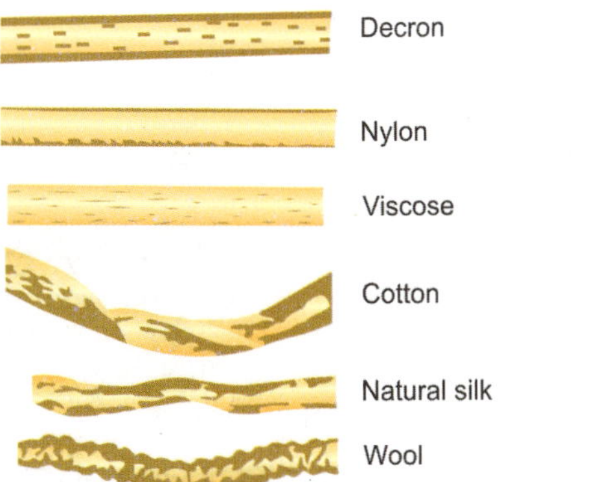

Fig. (4–50). Microscopic appearance of fibres.

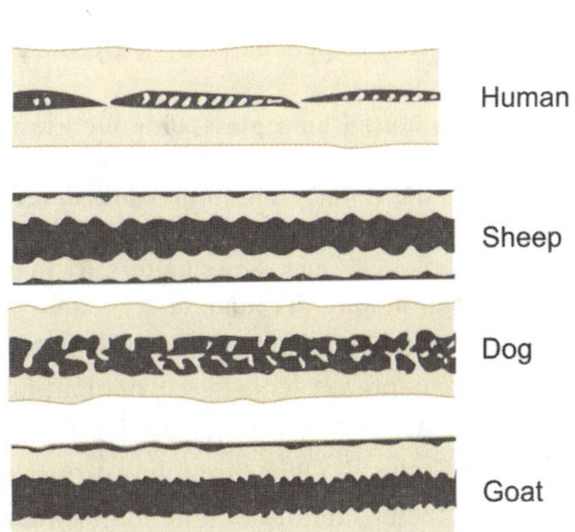

Fig. (4–51). Various hair.

is stiff, thick and taper to a point. The hair on the chest, axillae and pubic region is short, stout and curly. Hair from the axillae and pubic region also show split ends. The hair on the other parts of the body is fine, short, and flexible and does not show pigment cells in the cortex.

(4) Sex: Sexing of human hair is difficult, except that of the beard and moustache. Male hair is usually thicker, coarser and darker. In human head hair, **Barr bodies** are found in hair follicles in a proportion of 29 ± 5 percent in females and 6 ± 2 percent in males.

(5) Age: Age can be determined sometimes from the hair, but only within wide limits, as between that of an infant or an adult. Roots of hair from children will dissolve rapidly in a solution of caustic potash, but in older people roots will resist the treatment.

Age	Diameter
Twelve days	0.024 mm
Six months	0.036 mm
Fifteen years	0.053 mm
Adults	0.07 mm

The body hair of the human foetus and the newlyborn child is fine, soft, non-pigmented (colourless) and non-medullated. This **lanugo hair is replaced by hair which is coarser, pigmented, medullated, and has a more complex scale pattern.** At puberty axillary and pubic hair grows which is at first fine, soft and curly and later becomes coarse, and pigmented. Adult hair have maximum pigmentation. Loss of scalp hair in men starts from the third decade. In women, there is often loss of axillary hair and an increase of facial hair, at about the menopause. **Grey hair usually appears after forty years.**

(6) Has the hair been altered by dyeing, bleaching or disease? **Bleached hair is brittle, dry, and straw-yellow.** If the hair is coloured, the colour will not be uniform, the roots are of different colour and the hair rough, brittle and lustreless. The scalp will also be coloured. The colour of head hair will be different from the colour of hair on other parts of the body. The length of extra-follicular part of an uncoloured zone is used to determine the time of the colour last applied. Scalp hair grows at the rate of two to three mm. a week, average being two and half mm; beard hair has a slightly faster and other hair a slightly slower growth rate. Some hair can be examined chemically to find out any metal contained in the paint. Dyed hair shows characteristic fluorescence with ultraviolet light. With polarised light microscope, the undyed part appears much brighter than the rest.

(7) Is the hair identical with the hair of the victim or the suspect? By careful comparison, one can say that the hair could have come from a particular person. Debris, grease, etc., adherent to the hair is very important.

Hair is usually mounted on a glass slide for examination in a comparison microscope. For preparing cross-section, it is embedded in a wax or resin block and sliced finely. The impressions of the cuticle scales are made on cellulose acetate. Microscopically, the intimate structure of the dyed hair appears hazy, and shows uniformity in general shade which is not seen in hair of natural colour.

Because of diet and drug intake and atmospheric conditions, traces of eighteen elements are deposited in our hair in proportions quite different from other persons, which can be measured through neutron activation analysis. Only three out of one lakh persons will have comparable amount of the nine major trace elements.

When hair is irradiated in a nuclear reactor, elements are converted to radioactive isotopes. Comparison of the radiation emitted from the hair with known standards provides quantitative comparison. Electrophoretic and electrofocusing methods to study proteins and enzymes in hair root sheath and matrix proteins are of considerable importance.

(8) Did it fall naturally or was it forcibly removed? The base must be examined to see whether the root is present. If the hair has fallen naturally, the root will be distorted and atrophied, and the root sheath absent. If the hair is forcibly pulled out, the hair bulb will be larger, irregular and the sheath will be ruptured.

(9) What is the cause of the injury? If the hair has not been cut, the tip is pointed and non-medullated, but repeated injury to the tip damages the cuticle, due to which the exposed and unprotected cortex splits and frays Fig. (4–52). The hair of axilla, pubis and frequently brushed hair has ragged ends. Blows with blunt objects crushes the shaft with flattening and splitting. A sharp weapon produces a clean uniform cut surface. Recently cut hair shows a sharply cut edge with a projecting cuticle. After a week, the end becomes square, smooth and later rounded but blunt. After three to four months, the end becomes elongated, but the medulla is absent. Hair may get singed due to burns or firearm injury. **Singed hair is swollen, black, fragile, twisted or curled and has a peculiar odour; carbon may be found deposited on it.** The tip is swollen like a bulb.

Identification: Hair cannot provide a permanent record for identification, because the distribution and concentration of trace elements along the shaft of a hair varies as the hair grows. The colour of the hair may alter with disease. It is lighter in patients with malnutrition, ulcerative colitis, and Kwashiorkor; the normal colour appears when health is restored. The hair of copper smelters may be greenish, indigo workers and cobalt miners blue, aniline workers bluish and picric acid poisoning yellow. The colour of hair alters sometimes after burial.

Blood Groups: ABO groups can be determined in a single hair if hair blub is present, from any part of the body by a modified absorption-elution technique or mixed agglutination technique with hundred percent accuracy.

Medicolegal Importance: (1) Hair is important in crime investigation, for it remains identifiable on the clothes, body and the alleged weapons in crimes committed long before. It often provides the only connection between a weapon or even the accused and the victim of an assault. (a) Motor vehicles responsible for injuries may be identified by the detection of hair on the vehicle. (b) In rape and sodomy, the pubic hair of the accused may be found on the victim or vice versa. In bestiality,

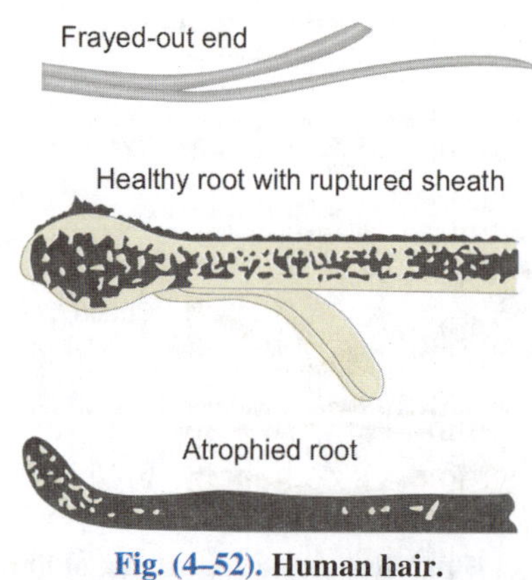

Fig. (4–52). Human hair.

animal hair may be found on the body or underclothing of the accused, or his pubic hair may be found about the genitals of the animal. (c) Stains on the hair may indicate the nature of the assault, e.g., mud stains in struggle, seminal stains in sexual offences, salivary stains in asphyxial deaths, blood stains in injury, etc. Stains may be got from the walls, doors, furniture, etc., and may indicate the scene of crime. (2) Nature of weapon can be made out from the injuries to the hair, and hair bulb. (3) Hair is useful in identification especially when there has been some known peculiarity of the hair, dyeing, bleaching or artificial waving. (4) Age of a person may be determined from the growth of hair on different parts of body. (5) Sex may be determined from their distribution on body, texture and from Barr bodies. (6) Singeing of the hair indicates burns or a close range firearm injury. (7) It is helpful in differentiating scalds from burns. (8) In chronic poisoning with heavy metals, e.g., arsenic, the poison can be detected in the hair. (9) The time of death can sometimes be determined from the length of the hair on the face.

FORENSIC ODONTOLOGY

Forensic odontology deals with the science of dentistry to aid in the administration of justice. It involves the analysis, interpretation and comparison of bitemarks, personal injuries and malpractice.

Dental identification: It depends mainly upon comparison between records of the missing persons and the findings in the bodies in relation to: (1) Restorative work. (2) Unusual features. (3) Comparison of antemortem with postmortem X-rays.

INDENTIFICATION OF AN INDIVIDUAL: The following particulars should be noted: (i) The number, spacing and situation of the teeth present, with special note of (a) unerupted and deciduous teeth, (b) permanent teeth (surface and configuration), (c) decayed teeth, (d) undersized or oversized teeth. (2) The number and situation of absent teeth. (3) Extraction: evidence of old or recent, healed or unhealed. (4) The general condition of teeth: (a) erosion, (b) cleanliness, (c) conservation, fillings and cavities, (d) colour, (e) periodontosis. (5) Peculiarities of arrangement: (a) prominence or reverse, (b) crowded or ectopic teeth, (c) overlapping, (d) malposition, (e) deformities, (f) rotation. (6) Supenumerary teeth. (7) Denture: full, partial, upper or lower, type, shape, restorative materials used. (8) Mesiodistal width of the teeth. (9) Any recognisable peculiarity of jaws, e.g., prognathism (prominence of the lower jaw). (10) Old injury or disease. Recently dislodged, loosened, chipped or broken teeth. (11) Special features, incisal edges, fractures, ridges, caries, etc. (12) Restoration and prostheses (surfaces, morphology, configuration and material). (13) Root canal therapy on X-ray examination. (14) Bone pattern on X-ray examination. (15) Oral pathology (tori, gingival hyperplasia).

Most dentists believe that no two persons have identical dentitions. Adult teeth have 160 surfaces with which dental treatments, root formation, bone patterns, tooth position, etc. can positively identify a person. Conservative dental work or fillings is most reliable in identification and includes fillings of various materials, root fillings, inlays and crown and bridge work. These can be compared with dental records and radiographs if available. In some persons the lower teeth protrude beyond the upper incisors which is known as over-bite.

Pink Teeth: In a decomposed or skeletonised body, pink teeth may be noted especially near the gum-line, due to deposition of protoporphyrin, the cause of which is not known. Asphyxia or CO poisoning as a cause of pink teeth has been disproved.

Mottled Teeth: This is the state of regional chronic dental fluorosis which exhibits opalescent pattern on the enamel surface of permanent teeth during the period of tooth calcification.

RADIOGRAPHY: X-rays accurately reveal root shape, shape of pulpal canal, shape of fillings, abnormalities, bone trabeculation patterns, caries, tooth formation and fractures. They are widely used in antemortem and postmortem comparisons. In mass disasters, a list of the possible persons involved is necessary. The more recent the antemortem record, the more reliable the evidence. If antemortem records are not available, dental information must be obtained from relatives and friends.

Medicolegal Importance: (1) **Dental identification is the most sophisticated method of comparative identification, except dactylography, if there are some features to compare and some record of those features in a missing person.** It is not of much help in developing countries as dentists often do not keep records. Teeth and jaws are usually protected from fire and mechanical trauma, and are highly resistant to postmortem destruction and decomposition Table (4–12). Dental findings establish the identification of single individuals after accidental death or homicide, and differential identification of large numbers of individuals after mass disasters, such as explosions, house fires, aircraft accidents, earthquakes and shipwrecks. Identifications have been made from intact, mutilated, decomposed, skeletonised or even burnt material Table (4–12). Diseases such as caries, syphilis (Hutchinson's teeth) help in identification. (2) Teeth are useful in estimating the age of an individual. (3) Sex and blood group can be determined from cells of pulp cavity. (4) Loss of tooth due to assault is grievous hurt. (5) Dentures, partial or complete, are useful in identification, especially if they have the patient's name or code number included in them. (6) Criminals can be identified through bite marks left either in human tissues or in food stuffs. (7) Poisons (arsenic, mercury) can be detected. (8) Colour change occurs in sulphuric and nitric acid poisoning. (9) In fluorosis, yellowish-brown discolouration or mottling is seen on the enamels.

Antemortem tooth loss or extraction. The bony rim or the alveolus is sharp and feathered. A blood clot forms within the alveolar cavity and in one to two days there is early organisation. In about a week, socket is filled with organised clot, which is replaced by fibrous tissue in 2 weeks. In two to three weeks, soft tissues are healed and the socket is partially filled with new bone. Reparative bone resorption of the alveolar rim results in a smooth rounded rim of socket. In six months, the socket is filled with new bone, but the location of the root outline is visible. In one year, the whole socket is filled with a new bone and there is depression of the bone outline. **If the entire tooth was knocked out, irregular edges of remaining bone, splintering of buccal or**

Table (4–12). Advantages and disadvantages of comparisons of teeth and fingerprints

	Trait	Teeth	Fingerprints
(1)	Burns:	Fire resistant.	Destroyed by fire.
(2)	Putrefaction:	No changes.	Subject to putrefaction.
(3)	Changes:	Compatible inconsistencies.	Unchanged.
(4)	Proof:	No acknowledged criteria of proof.	Well established criteria.
(5)	Records:	Useless without records.	Possible use of possessions.

lingual plates, areas of compressed bone, or fracture of roots or crowns of adjacent teeth are seen. It is difficult to dislodge **a healthy tooth without fracturing or loosening neighbouring teeth.** These changes can be demonstrated by X-ray of the jaw adjacent to the dislodged teeth.

BITE MARKS: Appearance: Human bites are usually semicircular or crescentic, caused by the front teeth (incisors and canines), with a gap at either side due to the separation of upper and lower jaw. The teeth may cause clear, separate marks or form a continuous or intermittently broken line. Bite marks may be abrasions, contusions or lacerations or a combination of any two or three. In forcible bite, the appearance is of two 'bows' with their concavities facing each other, and a gap at each end. The sucking action reduces the air pressure over the centre and produces multiple petechial haemorrhages, due to rupture of capillaries and small venules in the subcutaneous tissues. If the bite is forcible, the petechiae are confluent and produce a contusion. If the bitten area is irregular or markedly curved, only part of the dental arch comes in contact with the tissues. The skin may be twisted or distorted during the act of biting causing distortion of the pattern. Rarely, the bite mark may be linear in pattern, due to the scraping of the skin by the upper incisors, causing parallel tracks. Faint teeth marks become visible when examined under ultraviolet light in a dark room.

In sexual bites, the teeth are used to grip during sucking; the resulting central or peripheral suck marks are seen as petechiae, producing reddening. In many such bites teeth marks are not seen. Love bites are usually seen on breast, neck, cheek, abdomen, arms, thighs and genitalia. In sexual bites, especially of the breast or nipple, the tissue may be actually sucked into the mouth, before the jaws close upon it. This will affect the shape of the bite mark when the skin is released and flattens out once more. In child abuse, bite marks can be found anywhere on the body. Self-inflicted bite marks are usually seen on the shoulders and arms. In the living, these marks are seen from one to twentyfour hours after infliction.

Swabs of the bite mark should be taken immediately, using a swab moistened with sterile water. A swab of control area adjacent to the mark, and a swab of victim's saliva should also be taken using swabs moistened with sterile water. If there is a delay in sending the swabs to the laboratory, they should be kept in the freezer compartment of the fridge. The whole area of skin carrying the bite is removed and preserved in formalin.

RECORDING AND REPRODUCING METHOD OF BITE MARKS: (1) PHOTOGRAPHIC METHOD FIGS. (4–53 AND 4–54) : The bite mark is fully photographed with two scales at right angle to one another in the horizontal plane. Photographs of the teeth are taken by using special mirrors which allow the inclusion of all the teeth in the upper or lower jaws in one photograph. The photographs of the teeth are matched with photographs or tracings of the teeth. Tracings can be made from positive casts of a bite impression, inking the cutting edges of the front teeth. These are transferred to transparent sheets, and superimposed over the photographs, or a negative photograph of the teeth is superimposed over the positive photograph of the bite. Exclusion is easier than positive matching. As human tissues and foodstuffs do not reproduce exactly the character of the teeth biting into them, it is not always possible to relate teeth measurements to bitemarks with accuracy.

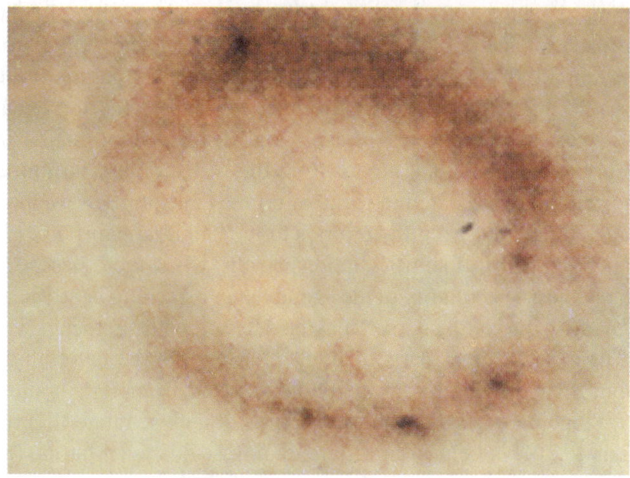

Fig. (4–53). **Bite mark.**

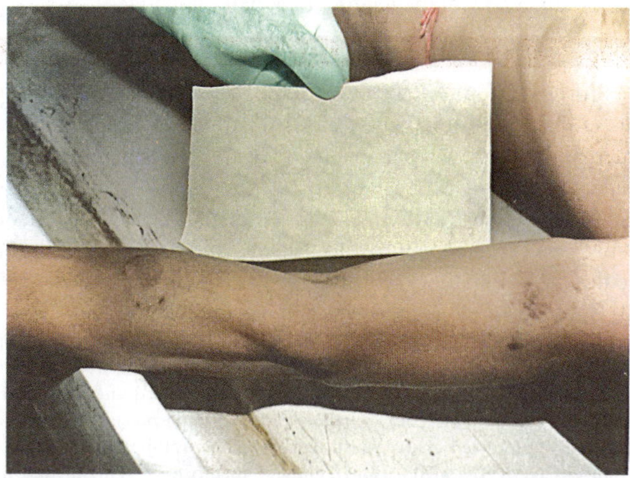

Fig. (4–54). **Teeth bite marks on upper arm and forearm.**

(2) CASTS: A plastic substance, such as a rubber or silicone based medium containing catalytic hardener is laid over the bite mark, which produces a permanent negative cast. Plaster of Paris modelling clay, plasticine or bees wax also can be used. Impressions of the upper and lower teeth of the suspect are taken.

(3) DIGITAL IMAGING of the bite marks and rendering it as a 3D data set is possible. The image is measurable to high precision and accurately compared with measurements of the case of the dentition of the suspect.

They are useful in identification because the alignment of teeth is peculiar to the individual.

ML importance: Bite marks may be found in materials left at the place of crime, e.g., foodstuffs, such as cheese, bread, butter, sandwiches, fruit, or in humans involved in assaults, when either the victim or the accused may show the marks, usually on the hands, fingers, forearms, nose and ears.

CHARTING OF TEETH: There are more than 150 different methods of identifying, numbering, and charting of teeth. The most widely used systems for permanent teeth are:

(1) Universal System: Teeth are numbered 1 to 16 from upper right to upper left, and 17 to 32 from lower left to lower right. This follows the plan advocated by the American and International Society of Forensic Odontology.

Right	1 2 3 4 5 6 7 8	9 10 11 12 13 14 15 16	Left
	32 31 30 29 28 27 26 25	24 23 22 21 20 19 18 17	

(2) Palmer's notation:

Right	87654321	12345678	Left
	87654321	12345678	

(3) Haderup System: It is similar to Palmer's notation except that it uses a plus sign(+) to designate upper teeth, and a minus sign (–) for the lower.

(4) FDI (Federation Dentaire Internationale) two-digit System: It bears a slight resemblance to Palmer's system in that both utilise the same numbers, but the F.D.I. system substitutes a number for the quadrant side and that number is placed before the tooth number. Thus the lower right canine will be number 43 in this system.

Right	1	2	Left
	4	3	

(5) Modified FDI system:

Right	1	2	Left
	3	4	

(6) Diagrammatic or anatomical chart: In this each tooth is represented by a pictorial symbol that gives the same number of teeth surfaces as those on the same teeth in the mouth. The incisors and canines are represented by four surfaces, and the premolars and molars by five (due to the occlusal surface). The positions of crowns, caries, fillings, or other abnormalities are marked on these diagrams. The diagram also includes deciduous teeth.

ANIMAL BITES: Rodents gnaw (bite persistently) away tissue over fairly limited areas. They produce shallow craters of the borders of the areas by nibbling and leave long grooves. The bites by dogs which attack suddenly are usually clear-cut, showing narrow squarish arch anteriorly, as the animal bites to hold on to the attacked person. Teeth impressions are usually deep resembling stab wounds, and small in area. These animals have long canines and six incisors. Cat bites show small rounded arch with puncture marks made by canines, and are usually associated with scratch marks from claws. Rat bites are usually very small and round. Intercanine distance can be measured to differentiate between human and animal bites, but not very useful. Distance between the upper canines in an adult ranges from 25 to 40 mm. and in children <25 mm.

RACE: In Caucasians, small nodules on lingual surface of maxillary molars (Carbelli's cusps) are most common, but rare in other racial groups. Lateral incisors in upper jaw are smaller than the central, especially in females. In Mongoloids upper incisors are shovel-shaped, canine roots are long and pointed, enamel pearls are frequent, pulp cavity of molars is wide and deep and the roots are fused and bent; a congenital lack of third upper molar is most common in Mongoloids, but can occur in any race. In Negroids teeth are large with more cusps in their molars with two lingual cusps on mandibular first premolars.

SEX: In the male, the upper central and upper lateral incisors are equal in size, but in the female, the size varies. The canines are usually smaller and more pointed in the female, compared to male, especially in the lower jaw. In the female, the mandibular first molar has four cusps.

Y chromosome may be isolated in the tooth pulp cells up to three to five months post-extraction or postmortem. Quinacrine staining is useful for this purpose.

The teeth are markedly resistant to heat Table (4–12). If heated suddenly or severely, they may disintegrate and fracture. If a dead body is burnt, the oral cavity and teeth have a better chance of remaining intact, but in a living person the lips may be drawn back exposing the anterior teeth. Depending on the temperature, intensity and duration of the fire, the crowns of anterior teeth may be scorched, ashed or explode at the gum line.

OCCUPATION, HABITS AND SOCIAL POSITION: Cobblers, carpenters, seamstresses, electricians, dress-makers, etc. have central notches in the incisal edge of the front teeth, due to the holding of the thread, needle, nails, etc. Musicians have localised attrition of their teeth. Some of them have wide defects on the front of the teeth, while others have defects on the incisal edges. In pipe smokers and cigarette smokers who use holders, there is a visible loss of material on the incisal edges of the teeth, mostly at the angle of the mouth. In heavy smokers, a black stain is deposited upon teeth. Loosening of certain teeth can be found in almost all those who habitually bite various objects or hold them in their teeth. The labial enamel and later the exposed dentin are dissolved in workers exposed to corrosive acids. Excessive chewing of acid foods causes erosion of all surfaces of teeth. Copper causes a green, silver a black, and lead, aniline and bismuth a bluish colour, particularly at the neck of the teeth or at the marginal part of the gum. Social position and sometimes the country of origin can be ascertained from the quality and type of restorations.

CASE: (1) Prinz (1915) reported the murder of a banker. A cigar holder with a mouth piece of amber which had a tip worn down in a characteristic way was found near the body. The lesion was thought to have been caused by the teeth of the owner of the mouthpiece. The Judge saw this mouthpiece. During the trial when the Judge was questioning a witness, he noticed a deformity in the teeth of that man which reminded him of the defect in the cigar-holder. The witness, a cousin of the deceased, and his heir was shown how well the mouthpiece fitted the deformity in his own teeth and he finally admitted to being a murderer.

(2) A train loaded with petrol, and a passenger train ran into each other in Norway in 1944. The first carriage of the passenger train was engulfed in burning petrol for 12 hours, due to which only burnt remains of bodies were left. The teeth and dental restorations were little affected in some cases.

(3) Ried (1884) reported the murder of a doctor and his mother. The bodies were found in the kitchen. A few dislocated teeth were found, two of which did not belong to those murdered, which were later proved to belong to the murderer, who had lost them during the fight with his victims.

(4) Paulick (1949) reported the murder of an old man by whose side was found an apple with characteristic bite marks. The marks showed three teeth close to each other, two of which were broad and the third small, irregular, probably due to a carious tooth. The bite did not correspond to the teeth of the victim. A prostitute was arrested, and dental examination proved that the bite marks were produced by her teeth.

(5) Euler (1925) reported the investigation of multiple murders, in which a large number of extracted teeth were found. An insane person had collected only caries-free teeth from his victims. Out of the 351 teeth, Euler found 20 left lower canines. Considering all the teeth in relation to the curve for caries development, he arrived at the number of 29 individuals. Later, a note book was found which contained the names and ages of all the murdered numbering from one to 31.

CLOTHES AND ORNAMENTS: The clothing may indicate the social status to a certain extent from the texture and value. Any variety of uniform is very valuable for identification. Clothing may also indicate the occupation. The examination of clothing and personal effects is helpful in the identification of victims in mass disasters, such as fires, explosions and aircraft crashes. A detailed description of the size, colour, condition and type of each garment and a record of laundry marks, name tags and labels of tailors should be given. Photographs and examination for invisible laundry marks by ultraviolet light are useful. The clothing may contain keys, letters, bank books, visiting cards, licenses or other documents which may give a clue to the name and address of the individual. Other personal effects like watches, rings, keys, belt buckles, etc., may be engraved with initials, names or dates. Eyeglasses may also be helpful. Bullet holes, tears, cuts or tyre marks found on clothing may give information regarding the cause and manner of death. The design of the ornaments varies from region to region. General cleanliness of the person and the state of the teeth, hands and feet give some idea of social status. If shoes are worn, the epidermis of the soles of the feet is thin and smooth without any fissures and cracks. A criminal may interchange his identity with that of another person by clothing and personal effects.

HANDWRITING (Calligraphy): Handwriting is characteristic of the individual, especially if it is written rapidly, but it may be disguised or forged. Mental and nervous disease and rheumatism alter the character. Evidence of handwriting experts is not conclusive, because it is opinion evidence.

SPEECH AND VOICE: Certain peculiarities of speech, e.g., stammering, stuttering, lisping and nasal twang become more evident when the individual is talking excitedly. Speech is also affected by nervous disease. To recognise a person from the voice is risky. It is possible for a person to alter his voice at will. Tape recording is useful. No two voices are really alike. All the frequencies produced by the utterance of a single syllable can be plotted on a time baseline, which gives an acoustic "Spectrogram", characteristic of the speaker. This is helpful in trapping anonymous telephone callers.

GAIT: Any identification based on recollection of physical characteristics (lameness, particular body postures or movements) of person in question by friends and relatives is unreliable. The gait may be altered by an accident or by design.

TRICKS OF MANNER AND HABIT: They are frequently hereditary, e.g., left-handedness. Jerky movement of shoulders or muscles of face is an individual characteristic.

MEMORY AND EDUCATION: They are sometimes useful, especially in cases of imposture.

CHAPTER 5

MEDICOLEGAL AUTOPSY

FM 2.11: Describe and discuss autopsy procedures including postmortem examination, different types of autopsies, aims and objectives of postmortem examination.
FM 2.12: Describe the legal requirements to conduct postmortem examination and procedures to conduct medicolegal postmortem examination.
FM 2.14: Describe and discuss examination of clothing, preservation of viscera on postmortem examination for chemical analysis and other medicolegal purposes, postmortem artefacts.
FM 2.16: Describe and discuss examination of mutilated bodies or fragments, charred bones and bundle of bones.
FM 2.17: Describe and discuss exhumation.
FM 8.5: Describe medicolegal autopsy in cases of poisoning including preservation and dispatch of viscera for chemical analysis.

Introduction: **Autopsy or necropsy means, postmortem examination of a body. In each and every case the autopsy must be complete, all the body cavities should be opened, and every organ must be examined, because evidence contributory to the cause of death may be found in more than one organ.** Partial autopsies have no place in forensic pathologic practice. **A complete autopsy is necessary to substantiate the truth of the evidence of eyewitnesses. A poor autopsy is worse than no autopsy at all, as it is more likely to lead to a miscarriage of justice.**

The autopsy should be carried out by the doctor, and not left to a mortuary attendant. The doctor should remove the organs himself. The attendant should prepare the body and help the doctor where required, such as sawing the skull cap, reconstruct the body, etc.

Types: The approach of the **forensic pathologist** to the investigation of death is different from that of the hospital pathologist. **(1) Pathological Autopsy:** The hospital pathologist has easy access to relevant information about the history, physical condition and course of the disease leading to death. The history directs the pathologist to the appropriate ancillary investigations. His main aim is to find morphologic changes (extent of a known disease) explaining signs or symptoms of the disease and the effectiveness of treatment. It helps to determine cause of death, the extent of natural disease, or the combination of comorbidities that led to death. It detects previously unrecognised disease. It helps the family to know of inheritable conditions present in the deceased. It often relies on histologic assessment. It is academically oriented.

(2) Medicolegal Autopsy: In medicolegal autopsies, often the clinical history is absent, sketchy, doubtful or misleading. In some cases, identity may not be known. He has to determine time of death and age of injuries. He has also to determine the cause, manner and mechanism of death. If there are any inconsistencies between the apparent death scene and his actual findings, he has to visit scene of crime. He has to carry out careful external examination including clothing, in the determination of the pattern of injuries and their relationship to the object or weapon causing them and collect trace evidence. **It has evidentiary and confirmatory value for public interest.**

Objects: (1) To find out the **cause of death,** whether natural or unnatural. This is done by detecting, describing and recording any external or internal injuries, abnormalities and diseases. (2) To find out **how the injuries occurred.** (3) To find out the **manner of death,** whether accidental, suicidal or homicidal. (4) To find out the **time since death.** (5) To **establish identity** when not known. (6) To **collect physical evidence** in order to identify the object causing death and to identify the criminal. (7) To **retain relevant organs and tissues** as evidence. (8) In newborn infants to determine the **question of livebirth and viability.** (9) To find factual and objective information for police and court

If autopsy is not done, the exact cause of death, the presence and extent of disease or injury, the incapacitation produced by them, and whether there was any pain or suffering becomes only speculation.

Rules for Medicolegal Autopsies: (1) The body should be labelled as soon as it arrives in the mortuary. (2) **The autopsy should be conducted in a mortuary and never in a private room.** However, it may become necessary to do an autopsy at the site, when the body is in an advanced state of putrefaction, and its transportation is difficult, and materials of evidential value may be lost in transport and when immediate examination of the body without its removal to hospital is essential due to any special reason. (3) **It should be conducted only when there is an official order authorising the autopsy, from the police or Magistrate.**

(4) It should be performed as soon as possible after receiving requisition, without undue delay. (5) **The medical officer should first read the inquest report carefully and find out the apparent cause of death, and obtain all the available details of the case from case sheet, accident register, etc., so that attention may be directed to the significant points,** while doing the postmortem examination and to carry out appropriate investigations, e.g. toxicology, microbiology, virology, radiology, etc. Lack of such information may result in loss of vital evidence. **Case sheet helps to know** (i) Nature of wound if sutured or if the patient survives for few days. (ii) If surgical incision passes through an injury during operation. (iii) Therapeutic wounds, e.g. surgical stab wounds of chest or abdomen for insertion of drainage tubes, tracheostomy, venesection, etc. and operative procedures. (iv) A drainage tube may be introduced through stab of chest or abdomen. (v) Resuscitation injuries (artefacts) due to artificial respiration or cardiac massage. (vi) In firearm wounds to know the wound of entrance and exit, if there was surgical intervention. (vii) Not to mistake collection of blood in chest and abdominal cavities due to operation from that due to trauma. (viii) Areas of tenderness for the detection of contusions. (ix) If after head injury, the patient is maintained on respirator, lung shows areas of collapse, haemorrhages and hyaline membrane (respirator lung; an artefact). (x) To detect greenstick fractures or fissured fractures. (xi) The cause of death e.g. diabetes, asthma, epilepsy, uraemia, renal failure, etc., in negative autopsy. (xii) The actual poison consumed or to suspect a particular poison from the signs and symptoms observed during life. (6) **The examination should be conducted in daylight as far as possible,** because colour changes, such as jaundice, changes in bruises, changes in postmortem staining, etc. cannot be appreciated in the artificial light. If the body is received late in the evening, a preliminary examination is done to note the external appearances, the body temperature, extent of postmortem lividity and rigor mortis, etc. The actual postmortem may be conducted on the next day as early as possible. **There is no law, which prevents autopsy being conducted during night.** (7) **The body must be identified by the police constable who accompanies it and relatives of the deceased.** The names of those who identify the body must be recorded. In unidentified bodies, the marks of identification, photographs, and fingerprints should be taken. (8) **No unauthorised person should be present at the autopsy.** The investigating police officer may be present. (9) If the doctor does not find the injuries recorded in inquest report, he should state that such injuries are not present, or are misinterpretations or PM changes and not injuries. Difference in injuries in wound certificate and autopsy report benefits accused (as to weapon used, injuries and time of injuries). (10) As the autopsy is conducted, details of examination should be noted verbatim by an assistant or use a voice-activated tape recorder and sketches made of all the important injuries. (11) **Nothing should be erased and all alterations should be initialled in the report. (12) Even if the body is decomposed, autopsy should be performed as certain important lesions may still be found.** (13) **Both positive and negative findings should be recorded.** (14) After completion of autopsy, the body is handed over to the police constable. (15) **P.M. report should not be issued to the party.**

Autopsy Room: It should be properly ventilated, illuminated and clean with plenty of running water. Daily cleaning and disinfection must be done with weekly fumigation. Phenol, savlon or glutaraldehyde 2% can be used for disinfection. During autopsy care must be taken to prevent unnecessary soiling of floor, walls and instruments and splashing of body fluids and water. All instruments must be washed with disinfectant after use. Biomedical and other materials must be disinfected and disposed according to Biomedical waste management rules, 2016. Universal work precautions should be followed. Staff must be immunised for tetanus, tuberculosis, hepatitis B, etc.

AUTOPSY ROOM PHOTOGRAPHY: OBJECTS: (1) to provide a visual record for the pathologist to refer to at a later time, (2) to allow other professionals to review the pathologists findings and to formulate their own opinions, (3) to show to the judge in trial, and (4) for teaching purpose.

PROCEDURE: (1) Photographs should be taken from above, and at right angles to the body to avoid perspective distortion. All objects, such as scalpels and scissors should be excluded. (2) The case number should be placed in a corner or along one edge of the photograph. A pointer, e.g. a narrow triangle of thin cardboard, may be used if a lesion is not readily visible. (3) In violent deaths, front and back views of the uncleaned body with its clothes and also after removal of the clothes should be taken. Then the body should be washed and in the naked body, a distant shot to indicate the location of injuries and close-up shots of major wounds to show details should be taken, keeping a scale to show the dimensions of the wound. (4) In an unknown body photograph of the face should be taken. (5) Victim's hands should be photographed to demonstrate electrical burns, defence cuts, etc. (6) Ligatures, gags and bindings should be photographed before removal from the body. (7) For potographing viscera, the shot should be vertical to the lesion. (8) Isolated organs should be cleaned with a sponge and placed on a green cloth and photographed.

THE AUTOPSY PROTOCOL: A protocol is a signed document containing a written record which serves as proof of something. Autopsy protocol is used in two basic forms: (1) narrative (in story form), (2) numerical (by the numbers). The advantages of numerical protocol are: (1) It provides a guide for an orderly description of all autopsy findings and tends to prevent the omissions of minor details. (2) It is objective and impersonal.

AUTOPSY REPORT: It consists of: (1) The preamble: This should mention the authority ordering the examination, time of arrival of the body at the mortuary, the date and place of examination, the name, age and sex of the deceased and the means by which the body was identified. (2) The body of the report: This consists of a complete description of the external and internal examination of the body. It should contain a description of the nature, direction, exact situation and dimensions of the wounds. Number should be assigned to each of the wounds that are described. Diagrams are often of value. The report should include all of the positive findings and all the relevant negative findings, because it may be taken to mean that it was not examined or specifically looked for. (3) Conclusions: The conclusion as to the cause of death must be given, based on the postmortem findings. Conciseness and clear language are of high value in the expression of the opinion. The report should be detailed, comprehensive, honest, objective and scientific. This is followed by the signature and qualifications of the doctor.

A properly performed autopsy furnishes objective facts which can disprove the weight and worth of misleading statements.

EXTERNAL EXAMINATION: The external examination will provide most of the substance of the report, where death occurred due to trauma. It is important in interpretation, e.g. in a case of a pedestrian involved in a traffic accident, in which the vehicle involved has not been identified or where due to lack of witnesses, the circumstances of the accident are obscure. Both the issues might be clarified by a good description of the surface injuries. The body should not be embalmed

prior to autopsy. Embalming changes the appearance of wounds and can produce artefacts.

The following should be noted: (1) Clothes: The clothing should be listed and examined, and described with regard to type of garment, its colour and consistence, size, manufacturer's label, laundry marks, uniforms or uniform logos, tears, loss of buttons or disarrangement indicating a struggle, as each item is removed from the body. Clothing should be removed gently, taking care to avoid contamination, or loss of any trace evidence, such as hair, fibres, paint fragments, glass, sand, vegetable matter, etc., which should be collected, mentioning the site, sealed and handed over to the police. Hair, fibres, vegetation, etc. can be picked with forceps, packed and labelled. The clothes should be removed carefully without any tearing to avoid confusion of signs of struggle. The clothing can be removed by unbuttoning, unzippering or unhooking if possible. If they cannot be removed intact, they should be cut in an area away from any bullet hole or objects, along a seam in the garment. **Clothing removed from the victim should not be thrown on the ground or floor or otherwise discarded or destroyed.** They should be handled as little as possible and without any deliberate shaking or dusting. Cuts, holes or blackening from firearm discharges should be noted and compared with the injuries on the body. No object should be put through defects in clothing or wounds. Blood stains, seminal stains, grease stains, etc., should be described. **Stains due to poison, vomit, etc. should be kept for analysis. Wet clothing should be hung up to dry, but should not be heat dried. Packing of wet clothes may promote growth of fungus. Stained and unstained areas of clothes should not be allowed to come in contact to avoid additional soiling, and as such clothes should not be folded while stains are wet. The clothes should be placed into clean plastic bags or other suitable clean containers. Separate bags or containers should be used for each article. Document all clothing of the deceased in PM report. They should be handed over to the police in sealed packet.**

List the ornaments. (1) Describe the type, design and colour of each (yellow or white metal; white, red or green stones, etc.). (2) **Nail scraping** should be taken. Any visible fibres or other matter in the hand or adherent to it should be removed and placed in envelopes. Ten small envelopes are labelled, one for each finger. A matchstick is cut, or the apex of a twice-folded filter paper is run under the nail. The finger is held over the envelope marked with its number as the material is removed, and then the scraper is dropped into the envelope, which is sealed. Contamination of the specimen with the epithelium or blood of the deceased should be avoided. (3) **Vaginal and anal swabs** are taken and also swabs from areas of suspected seminal staining in all cases of sexual assault. Pubic hair should be combed through. Matted pubic hair should be cut out with scissors and samples of pubic hair taken. (4) **Height and weight Fig. (5–1)** of the body, and general state, body build, (fat, strong, medium, thin), development and nourishment. If a weighing machine is not available, approximate estimate of the weight of an adult body can be made by measuring the stature and girth of chest and waist. (5) **General condition of the skin** (rash, petechiae, colour, looseness, turgor), asymmetry of any part of the body or muscular wasting. (6) **General description:** This includes stature, sex, age, colour, race, build, deformities, nutrition, hair, scars, tattoo marks, moles, pupils, skin disease, circumcision, amputations, deformities, etc. (7) Note the **presence of stains** on the skin from blood, mud, vomit, faeces, corrosive or other poisons, or gunpowder. They should be described precisely and in detail. (8) The presence of **signs of disease**, e.g., oedema of legs, dropsy, surgical emphysema about the chest, skin disease, eruptions, etc., are to be noted. (9) The **head hair** should be examined. Any foreign matter should be removed with forceps, and the hair combed through for trace evidence. Samples of both cut and pulled hair from at least six different areas of the scalp should be taken and labelled as to their origin. (10) **The face** should be examined for frothy fluid at the mouth and nose, cyanosis, petechial haemorrhages, pallor, etc. (11) The eyes should be examined for the condition of the eyelids, conjunctivae, softening of the eyeball, colour of sclerae, opacity of the cornea and lens, state and colour of pupils, artificial eyes, contact lenses, petechiae, and periorbital tissues for extravasation of blood. (12) **The ears** should be examined for leakage of blood, or CSF. (13) **The neck** must be examined for bruises, fingernail abrasions, ligature marks or other abnormalities. Observe degree of distention of neck vessels. (14) **Thyroid:** size, nodularity. (15) **Lymph nodes:** cervical, axillary, inguinal. (16) **Thorax:** symmetry, general outline. (17) **Breasts:** size, masses. (18) **Abdomen:** presence or absence of distension or retraction, striae gravidarum. (19) Back: bedsores, spinal deformity. (20) **External genitalia:** general development, oedema, local infection, position of testes. (21) **The natural orifices**, i.e., mouth, nostrils, ears, vagina, etc. should be examined for injuries, foreign matter, blood, etc. If the mouth cannot be opened, the masseter and temporalis muscles are divided above their insertion into the mandible, to allow the jaw to become mobile. The state of the lips, gums and teeth, marks of corrosion, and injuries to inside of the lips and cheeks should be noted. The state of the tongue, position with relation to the teeth, and the presence or absence of bruising or bite marks should be noted. The presence of froth about the mouth and nostrils and smell of alcohol, phenol, etc., should be noted. (22) Note the **position of all the limbs** and particularly of the arms, hands and fingers. The hands should be examined for injuries, defence wounds, electric marks, etc., and if clenched to find out if anything is grasped in them. To open the hand completely, the flexor tendons of the fingers are cut at the wrist. The fingernails must also be carefully examined for the presence of any blood, dust or other foreign matter, indicative of struggle. Note for oedema, needle marks, ulcers, gangrene, tumours, digital clubbing, etc. (23) Needle puncture marks in the arms, buttocks, etc. should be looked for. (24) **External wounds should be systematically examined taking up each part of the body in turn**. The description of wounds should include nature, site, length, breadth, depth, direction, position, margins, base and extremities. The condition of their edges, presence of foreign matter, coagulated blood and evidence of bleeding into nearby tissues noted. Determine whether they were caused before or after death, and their time of infliction. Collect foreign materials, e.g., hair, grass, fibres, etc., that may be in the wound. **If the injuries are obscured by hair, as on the scalp, the area should be shaved.** Deep or penetrating wounds should not be probed until the body is opened. In burns, their character, position, extent and degree should be mentioned. The use of printed body sketches is very useful. Each injury can be drawn in, and measurement noted alongside each and distances from anatomical landmarks recorded. Injuries should be numbered and related to written notes. Photographs are useful. There is no substitute for a good colour photograph to preserve the appearance of a wound or injury. If the blood spots or smears on the skin are important, the area should be photographed before and after the skin is cleaned. **Excluding stab and firearm wounds, all the injuries should be divided into two broad areas: external and internal.** For recording injuries, the use of text can be greatly helped by the addition of body charts, sketches and photographs (25). The limbs and other parts should be examined for fractures and dislocations by suitable movements and by palpation and confirmed by dissection. (26)

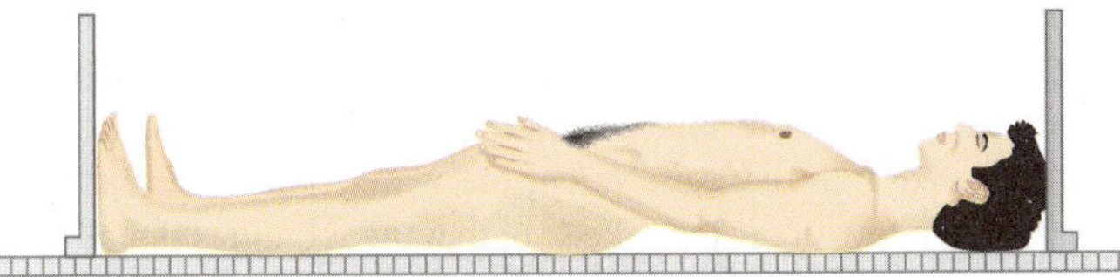

Fig. (5–1). Method of measuring the length of a dead body.

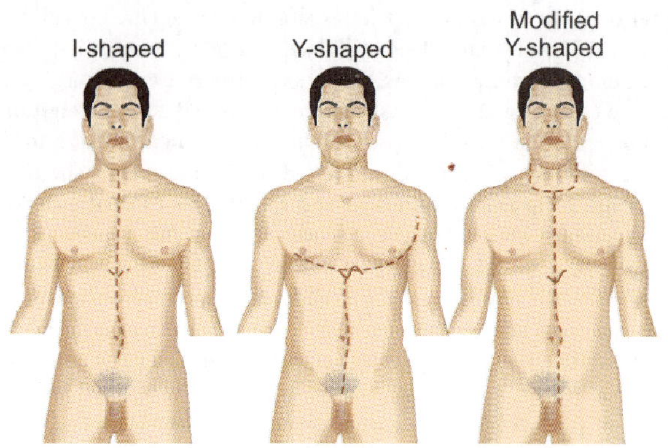

Fig. (5–2). Primary skin incisions.

The time since death should be noted from rectal temperature, rigor mortis, postmortem hypostasis, putrefaction, etc. (27) **A list should be made of all articles removed from the body, e.g., clothes, jewellery, bullets, etc.** They should be labelled, mentioned in the report and handed over to the police constable in a sealed cover after obtaining receipt. (28) **The report should include all of the surgical procedures, applied dressings and other diagnostic and therapeutic measures (drainage tubes, catheters, etc.) found on external examination.**

Cardiac pacemaker if present should be removed because the mercury batteries cause an explosion if body is burnt or will cause environmental pollution if buried.

Skin Incisions: Primary incisions are of three types **Fig. (5–2)**.

(1) The **"I"-shaped incision,** extending from the chin straight down to the symphysis pubis, passing either to the left or right of the umbilicus. The umbilicus is avoided because the dense fibrous tissue is difficult to penetrate with a needle, when the body is stitched after autopsy.

(2) "Y"-shaped incision begins at a point close to the acromial process. It extends down below the breast and across to the xiphoid process. A similar incision is then made on the opposite side of the body. From the xiphoid process, the incision is carried downwards to the symphysis pubis.

(3) Modified "Y"-shaped incision: An incision is made in midline from suprasternal notch to symphysis pubis. The incision extends from suprasternal notch over the clavicle to its centre on both sides and then passes upwards over the neck behind the ear.

The incision must be adopted according to the special condition of the case, e.g., in stab wounds of the chest or abdomen, the usual incision may have to be altered to avoid such wounds.

INTERNAL EXAMINATION: It is convenient to start the examination with the cavity chiefly affected. **In a case of suspected cranial injury, the skull should not be opened until the blood has been drained out by opening the heart.**

OPENING OF BODY CAVITIES: ABDOMEN: The pathologist should stand on the right side of the body, if he is right-handed On one side of autopsy table there should be instrument trolley with instruments shown in **Fig. (5–3)**. The recti muscles of the abdomen are divided about 5 cm. above symphysis. A small cut is made in the fascia big enough to admit the left index and middle fingers, palmar surfaces up. The fingers are separated in a V (to protect the underlying structures) and a sharp-bladed knife is inserted between them, and the peritoneum is cut up to the xiphoid. The thickness of the fat in the abdominal wall is noted. In fatty people, a few transverse incisions can be made on the inner side of the abdominal wall to divide muscle and fat, which allows lateral flaps to gape widely, and a full view of the abdomen can be had. The condition of the abdominal cavity and organs is observed before anything is disturbed or altered, to find out if there is any blood, pus or fluid in the cavity, or perforation or damage to any organ. If blood, pus or any other fluid is present, its quantity is measured. If this precaution is not taken, the examiner will be frequently in doubt, as to whether any blood or damage to organs found at a later stage is a result of the opening of the body, or whether it was already present. Note the amount of fat in the mesentery and omentum. Note abnormalities and position of abdominal organs, adhesions, old operations, pathological processes, injuries and height of diaphragm in relation to the ribs. The peritoneum is examined for adhesions, congestion, inflammation or exudation, Describe the course, direction and depth of injuries and enumerate structures involved by the injury. Identify and label any foreign object, bullets, fragments of knives, etc. and specify its relation to a given injury. Photograph injuries to document their location. Include a scale to show their size. Photographs can be used to demonstrate and correlate external injuries and internal injuries.

NECK: A block 12 to 20 cm. high, should be placed under the shoulders, to allow the head to fall back and thus extend the neck. The skin is held with a toothed forceps and with a sharp, long-handled scalpel, the dissection is carried out immediately deep to the skin through the platysma. The subcutaneous dissection should be carried up to the lower border of the lower jaw, well laterally on the side of the neck and clavicle. The deep cervical fascia is incised and reflected from the cervical muscles and the submandibular gland. The sternomastoid muscle is freed from its clavicular and sternal attachments, separated from its underlying fascia and reflected on each side. The omohyoid, sternothyroid, and thyrohyoid muscles are exposed, inspected and reflected on each side. The thyroid gland and the carotid sheaths are freed by blunt dissection from their investing connective tissue. The larynx, trachea, pharynx and oesophagus are mobilised and pulled away from the prevertebral tissue by blunt dissection.

MOUTH: The mouth is opened, and the tip of the tongue pushed upwards and backwards with a forceps. The knife is inserted under the chin through the floor of the mouth. Cut along the sides of the mandible to the angle of the mandible, dividing the neck muscles attached to the lower jaw. At the angles of the mandible, turn the blade inward to avoid cutting the carotid artery. The tongue is pushed down under the mandibular arch with the index and middle fingers. The soft palate is then cut to include the uvula and tonsils with tongue and neck organs to be removed. The knife is carried backwards and laterally on both sides of the midline to divide the posterior pharyngeal wall. The middle finger of the left hand is passed into the larynx and with the scalpel, the pharyngeal tissues are dissected from behind forwards and laterally, and the pharynx is pulled down to the upper part of the neck. The dissection is then carried distally through the prevertebral muscles on the anterior surface of the cervical vertebrae, until the whole of the neck structures are free to the level of suprasternal notch. The great vessels including the carotids should be divided in the neck.

PNEUMOTHORAX: Cases of pneumothorax are demonstrated before the chest wall is opened by various methods: (1) A pocket is dissected on the affected side between the chest wall and the skin, and is filled with water, and the wall is punctured with the knife under the water. The scalpel should be twisted a few times to make sure that the wound is open. If air under pressure is present, it will bubble out of the opening through the water. (2) A wide-bore needle (16-gauge) attached to a 50 ml syringe without the plunger is introduced into subcutaneous tissue

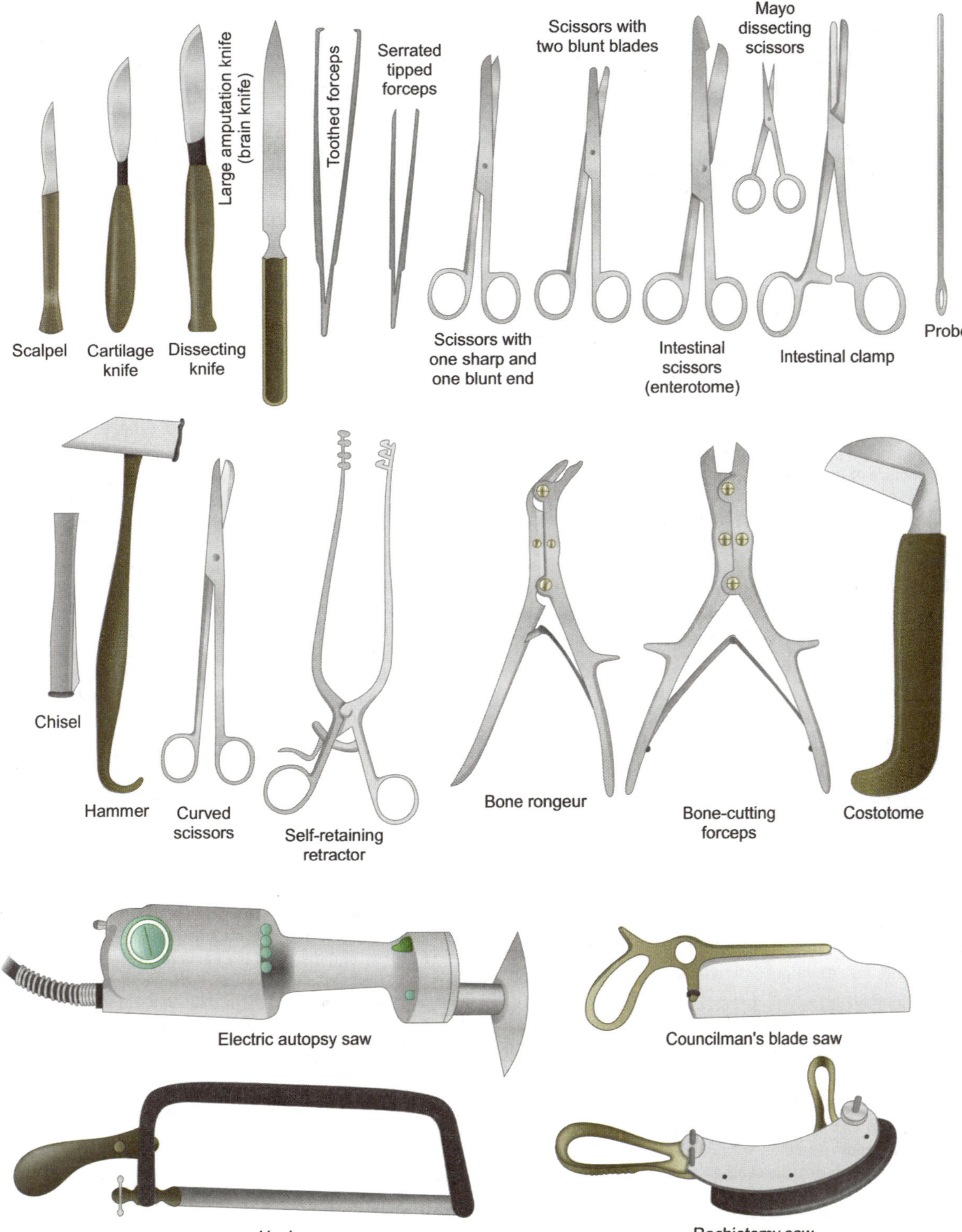

Fig. (5–3). Autopsy instruments.

over an intercostal space and the syringe is then filled with water. The needle is pushed to enter the pleural cavity. If air is present it will bubble out through the water. (3) One of the intercostal muscle is carefully removed until the underlying parietal pleura is seen. If there is no pneumothorax, visceral pleura of lung will be seen immediately below the parietal pleura. If there is a pneumothorax visceral pleura will not be seen. (4) Chest X-ray.

CHEST: The muscles of the chest are dissected away, keeping the edge of the knife directed inwards towards the ribs, carried back to the midaxillary line, down to the costal margin and up over the clavicles.

The ribs, sternum and spine should be examined for fractures, and the chest is opened by cutting the costal cartilages with a cartilage knife. Begin at the upper border of the second cartilage, keeping very close to the costochondral junctions. The knife should be inclined about 30° to

the vertical. In old persons where the rib cartilages are calcified, a pair of rib shears or handsaw are used. Then, disarticulate the sternoclavicular joint on each side by holding the knife vertically and inserting the point into the semicircular joint. The position of this joint can be made out by moving the shoulder tip with the left hand, which causes the joint capsule to move. To divide the joint capsule, the knife is put in vertically and turned in a circular manner. The diaphragm is divided at its attachment to the lower ribs and sternum up to the spine.

The pleural cavity should be examined before complete removal of the sternum, to prevent leakage of blood from subclavian and jugular veins into the pleural cavity before inspection. Do not pull the sternum and ribs to avoid negative pressure resulting in aspiration of air into the vessels. Before removal of the thoracic organs, *in situ* inspection should include: (1) observation of the lumen of the main pulmonary vessels, (2) observation of the right atrium and ventricle for air embolism, (3) the state of distension or collapse of the lungs, (4) pleural cavities for the presence of fluid, blood or pus and pleural adhesions, (5) pericardium for cardiac tamponade, and (6) collection of blood sample from the heart for toxicological examination.

The pericardial sac normally contains 20 to 50 ml. of straw-coloured fluid and the pericardium is smooth and glistening. White spots (milk spots) on the surface of the heart indicate healed pericarditis. In acute pericarditis, the sac contains large collections of serous or purulent fluid and fibrin deposits (bread-and-butter pericardium). Haemorrhagic fluid in the sac is seen in malignancy and rarely in tuberculosis, uraemia, bleeding diseases and secondary to myocardial infarction.

AIR EMBOLISM: If air embolism is suspected, the head should be opened first and the surface vessels of the brain examined for gas bubbles, which must be prominent and definite, but not segmental breakup of the blood in the vessels with collapsed segments between. Care should be taken to avoid pulling the sternum and ribs to avoid creating negative pressure in the tissues which may result in aspiration of air into vessels. Air embolism can be demonstrated by: (1) Before handling the thoracic organs, the pericardium is opened, heart is lifted upwards and the apex is cut with a knife. The left ventricle is filled with frothy blood, if air is present in sufficient quantity to cause death. (2) If the right ventricle contains air, the heart will float in water. (3) Another method of demonstrating air embolism is by cutting the pericardium anteriorly and grasping the edges with haemostat on each side. The pericardial sac is filled with water and right heart is punctured with a scalpel and twisted a few times. Bubbles of air will escape if air is present. (4) A wide-bore needle attached to a 50 ml syringe filled with water is inserted into the right ventricle. If air is present it will bubble out through the water. (5) Air in inferior vena cava can be demonstrated by puncturing it under water, and looking for escape of bubbles of gas. (6) Chest x-ray. **(7) Pyrogallol test: 4 ml. of a 2% freshly prepared pyrogallol solution is collected into two 10 ml syringes. To the first syringe four drops of 0.5 M sodium hydroxide solution is added. Gas is aspirated from the right side of the heart. The needle is removed and replaced with a stopper, and the syringe shaken. If air (oxygen) is present, the mixture turns brown. In the second syringe some air is introduced and the test repeated as a control. The solution should turn brown. This test helps to differentiate gas present in the heart from gas formed due to decomposition.**

If fat embolism is suspected, the pulmonary artery should be dissected under water and the escape of fat droplets noted.

METHOD OF REMOVAL OF ORGANS: (1) **Virchow's technique:** Individual organs are removed one by one. Cranial cavity is exposed first, followed by thoracic, cervical and abdominal organs. Spinal cord is removed from the back. In this the anatomico-pathologic relations are not preserved. (2) **Rokitansky's technique:** It involves *in situ* dissection in part, combined with *en block* removal. It is preferred choice in patients with highly transmissible diseases, such as HIV, hepatitis B. (3) **Lettulle's technique:** Cervical, thoracic, abdominal and pelvic organs are removed *en masse* and dissected as organ block. It has the advantage of leaving all attachments intact. (4) **Ghon's Technique:** Cervical, thoracic, abdominal organs and urogenital system are removed as organ blocks. Neuronal system is removed as another block.

The greater omentum lying across the small intestine is pushed upwards across the liver. The upper part of the small intestine is grasped in the left hand, and followed upwards until it disappears retroperitoneally to become the duodenum. The mesentery is penetrated with the point of the knife at the duodenojejunal flexure, and two pieces of string are passed through the hole. They are then brought upwards and tied separately and tightly around the gut. The gut is divided between these two ligatures. The coils of the intestine are pulled forwards by the left hand and the mesentery is cut close to the mesenteric border of the gut until the ileocaecal valve is reached. The caecum is mobilised, and the ascending colon pulled forwards and medially by the left hand, and its attachments with the posterior abdominal wall are cut with the knife up to the hepatic flexure. The omentum is pulled down and the transverse mesocolon is cut through with a knife, until the splenic flexure is reached. Then descending colon is freed in a similar manner until the sigmoid is also free. The upper part of the rectum is mobilised and cut through between two ligatures below the brim of the pelvis. The whole of the small and large intestine is removed from the abdominal cavity.

Next, the axillary bundles which lie behind the clavicles and first rib are cut, by passing the knife upwards on each side from the thoracic cavity into the neck. Pleural adhesions between the lungs and the chest wall if any, should be cleared of by fingers or knife. Slip the fingers of both hands between the lateral portion of one lung and the inner side of the chest wall. The left hand works up to the apex, the right down to the base, and they meet at hilum. The neck structures are grasped *en masse* in the left hand and pulled downwards, cutting the structures on the front of the spinal column to the level of the diaphragm. After this, the thoracic organs are put back in the thorax. The stomach and spleen are pulled medially by the left hand and the diaphragm is removed by cutting through its attachment to the ribs on both sides. The thoracic organs are pulled down by gentle traction on the neck structures and the cruciate ligament which attaches the diaphragm to the spine is cut. The organs are then put back into the thorax.

The spleen and the tail of the pancreas are held in the left hand, and dissection is carried behind them to the midline. The diaphragmatic surface of the spleen is held in the palm, and the vessels at the hilum are cut after they have been inspected. The liver is pulled medially and the knife is passed behind it to free it from attachments. The peritoneum and fat are cut just outside the lateral border of the kidney, which is then grasped in the left hand and mobilised by dissection behind it to the midline, freeing it from the anterior surface of the iliopsoas muscle. The ureter is identified and freed all the way down to its entry to the bladder. Both kidneys are then taken in the left hand, and the knife is carried down the midline behind the aorta to the pelvis. The knife is passed around the side wall of the pelvis, dividing the lateral attachments of the bladder, each side of the pelvis being dissected downwards to the midline. The anterior surface of the bladder is freed with the fingers from the pubic bone. The femoral vessels are cut at the level of the brim of the pelvis. The contents are pulled upwards and the urethra and vagina divided as low as possible. The whole block of thoracic and abdominal organs are pulled forward and removed *en masse*.

The atlanto-occipital joint should be examined by moving the head on the spine, to note any fracture- dislocation. Examine the cervical spine for fractures. The so-called "UNDERTAKER'S FRACTURE" is caused due to the head falling backwards forcibly after death, which tears open one of the intervertebral disc usually around C-6 and C-7, due to which subluxation of the lower cervical spine occurs. The thoracic and lumbar spine should be examined by pushing a hand under the body to raise up

the spine forward, which will show any abnormal movement at the site of fracture. The cervical spine can be tested by manual manipulation. To detect fractures of the sacroiliac joints or of the pelvic bones, the pelvis should be squeezed from side to side by pressure on each iliac crest.

EXAMINATION OF ORGANS: The *en masse* chest and abdominal organs are kept on a wooden board with posterior surface upwards and the tongue facing the operator.

DESCRIPTION OF AN ORGAN: A description of the organ systems should be limited to a clear, concise, objective description of shape, colour, and consistency and the presence or absence of any lesions other than those systematically described under trauma. The microscopic description may be limited to the positive findings. The pathologist should indicate those tissues he had examined and the number of sections he has taken in any one tissue.

(1) SIZE: Measure by tape. In the liver, blunting of the inferior border points to enlargement, and sharpness to atrophy. A usually tense capsule is in favour of enlargement, and loose capsule with laxness. A straight course of superficial vessels as on heart shows increased size, while undue tortuosity means decrease.

(2) SHAPE: Note any departure from normal.

(3) SURFACE: Most organs have a delicate, smooth, glistening, transparent capsule of serosa. Look for any thickening, roughening, dullness or opacity.

(4) CONSISTENCY: The softness or firmness as measured by pressure of the finger.

(5) COHESION: It is the strength within the tissue that holds it together. It is judged by the resistance of the cut surface to tearing, pressure or pulling. An organ with reduced cohesion is friable, while when it is increased, the tissue seems to be tough or leathery. If a small toothed forceps bites into a testis it should pull away threads composed of tubules if it is normal.

(6) CUT SURFACE: (A) Colour: Every organ (except brain) is basically some shade of grey, but this is altered by the red contributed by its blood supply. Other colours can be added by jaundice or fatty infiltration (yellow), lipofuscin or haemosiderin (brown), malarial pigment (grey-brown). Anaemia causes pallor, while congestion adds a blue tinge. (B) Structure: This is a factor of the particular organ, e.g., cortex and medulla in the kidney. In disease these may become indistinct or greatly exaggerated.

ORAL CAVITY: Examination of organs should be done systematically from above downward so that nothing is missed. Examine the tongue for any disease or injuries, especially bite marks which are usually seen along the sides, and less commonly at the tip. A small haemorrhage is seen under intact mucosa in bite marks. Serial incisions should be made through the tongue for the presence of bruises. The pharynx, epiglottis and glottis should be examined, especially for a foreign object. The condition of the tonsils should be noted.

NECK STRUCTURES: A large blunt-pointed scissors is used to cut open the oesophagus from the posterior surface up to the cardiac end of the stomach. The lower end often shows postmortem erosion, due to the regurgitation of gastric juice through the relaxed cardiac sphincter. Note for the presence of any capsules, tablets, powders, etc. , which should be preserved. Special precaution should be taken in case of varices. If the oesophagus is cut at the lower end, blood will drain from varices, which would then collapse and may be missed. When death occurs from rupture of oesophageal varices, the break should be demonstrated. A blunt-ended fine probe is helpful in cases where milking of the veins does not force a little blood through the tear. Injection of saline or coloured fluid into a varix is useful to find the leak from the tear.

The larynx lies opposite third to sixth cervical vertebrae in the adult male and little higher in the adult female and children. Laryngeal prominence is 2 to 5 cm. below the hyoid bone when the chin is held up. The larynx, trachea and bronchi are examined by cutting them open from the posterior surface. The presence of blood, mucus, foreign bodies, vomited matter, tumours, inflammation, mucopus, etc., in them should be noted. The thyroid is removed and examined. Sections are made in both lateral lobes along their longest diameter. The parathyroids are examined. The carotid arteries must be examined for the presence of thrombosis particularly at the bifurcation near the skull. The hyoid bone, thyroid and cricoid cartilage are examined for any fracture or contusions.

JAWS: If rigor is present, to remove mandible, autopsy incision is extended into a neck "V" and the skin of the lower part of the face is dissected. The masseter and temporalis muscles are divided above their insertion into the mandible, to allow the jaw to become mobile. The maxilla, palate and inferior part of facial skeleton is removed by sawing horizontally across the maxilla at the level of lower margin of nasal aperture, taking care to saw above tooth roots.

LUNGS: Place the lungs with the anterior surfaces uppermost and open the pulmonary artery and continue into the lung tissue as far as small scissors will allow one to go. Look for thrombi, emboli and atherosclerosis. Trace the course of pulmonary veins into the lung, looking for evidence of thrombosis. An antemortem embolus may sometimes be coiled, and when straightened out resembles a cast of the vessel from which the thrombus originated, usually in the leg. There may be side-branches but it does not fit the vessel in the lung. Massive pulmonary emboli completely block either the main trunk of the pulmonary artery or impact in one of the major pulmonary vessels, more commonly the right side and is always fatal.

To separate the lungs, the long-bladed knife is placed blunt-edge upwards under the hilum of each lung and turned around so that the sharp edge is upward. Then with a short sawing motion, the hilum is completely cut through. The lung is held on the upper surface by the left hand (or by an interposed sponge) and the organ cut across from apex to base with the large brain knife, held parallel to the board. This produces an anteroposterior slice. The lungs are examined for consolidation, oedema, emphysema, atelectasis, congestion, Tardieu spots, emboli, tumour, infarction, etc. The smaller bronchi are examined for mucosal thickening, infection and blockage. The smaller pulmonary arteries are examined for thrombosis or embolism.

For fixation of lungs, a cannula is held or tied into the bronchus and 10% formal-saline is perfused through a tube from a reservoir held one metre above the lung. The lung is then put in formalin solution.

AORTA: The scissors is passed into the iliac vessels, and the whole length of the aorta is cut on its posterior surface around the arch, up to the aortic valve. Note for any chronic aortitis with plaque formation which obstructs the mouths of the coronary arteries.

HEART: Remove the heart with great vessels attached, at least one cm beyond the pericardial fold. Examine the pericardium while the heart is still *in situ* for adhesions, pericarditis, discolouration of an underlying infarct, aneurysms, injuries and any fluid or blood. Open with inverted T-shaped incision. Measure height from the base of aorta to the apex and width at the level of valvular region, and circumference one cm. below A-V sulcus, Examine surface for any visible fibrosis or recent infarcts. The pulmonary arteries should be palpated before they are cut for the presence of thrombus or embolus. **If thrombus is felt, right ventricle and pulmonary trunk are opened in situ and the size and extent of thrombus noted. The size varies from clots to massive coiled thick structures. In the pulmonary trunk the larger ones will be saddle-shaped, bifurcating into pulmonary arteries. They are pink in colour and firmly adherent to the vessel wall. Postmortem clots are soft, friable and yellow or red in colour.** Superior and inferior vena cavae should be examined for the presence of thrombi and emboli. The heart is held at the apex and lifted upwards and pulmonary vessels, superior and inferior vena cavae, and the ascending aorta are cut as far away as possible from the base of the heart. The isolated heart is studied as follows **It is opened in the direction of the flow of blood (inflow-outflow method), with the enterotome Fig. (5–4).** The right atrium is cut between the openings of superior and inferior vena cavae. A small secondary incision is

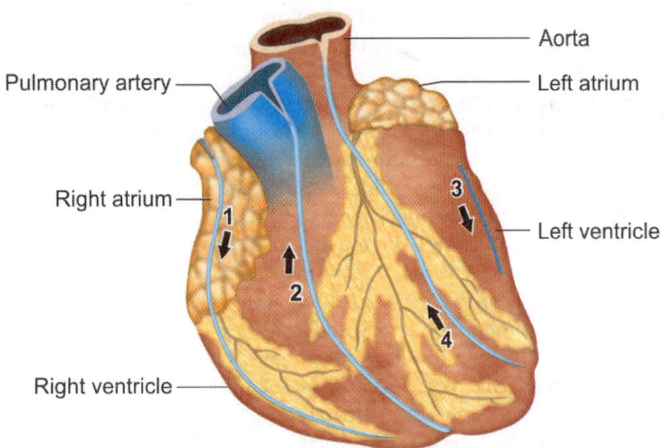

Fig. (5–4). **Incisions into the isolated heart.**

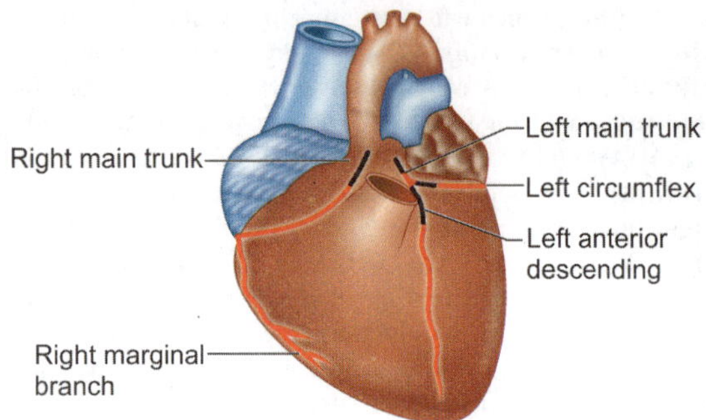

Fig. (5–5). **The main coronary arteries with the most frequent sites of occlusion.**

made to open the auricular appendage to detect thrombi. While opening the right ventricle, the lateral margin of right ventricle faces the dissector, the atria being directed towards him. The enterotome introduced into the right atrium, cuts through the tricuspid orifice, and opens the right ventricle along the lateral margin. **The circumference of an intact valve of heart can be measured by inserting specially made graduated cones, marked at various levels with the circumference after opening the atrium. To demonstrate the competence of the pulmonary valve** the heart is held in the palm of hand so that the pulmonary valve is horizontal and neither collapsed nor stretched. A gentle stream of water is directed on to the valve. After the blood is washed away, it can be observed how well the cusps come into apposition, and whether water leaks into the already opened ventricle. **The competence of tricuspid and mitral valve cannot be satisfactorily tested postmortem.** In opening the pulmonary valve, the heart is placed so that the apex is directed towards the examiner. The enterotome is introduced into the right ventricle close to the apex, and the conus pulmonalis and pulmonary valve are cut about 10 mm. to the right of, and parallel to the interventricular septum in the anterior wall of the right ventricle. **The interventricular septum is identified by the anterior descending branches of the coronary vessels crossing down the epicardium.** The incision should extend into the pulmonary trunks and the left pulmonary artery. Note whether the contents of the right ventricle and auricle are fluid blood, currant-jelly clot or chicken-fat clot. The left atrium is cut between the openings of the pulmonary veins. Then, the left atrium is cut along its lateral wall. This incision extends through the mitral orifice, and passes along lateral margin of the left ventricle up to the apex. The circumference of mitral valve should be measured. The next incision extends from the apex along the interventricular septum into the aorta, opening the aortic valve. The water competency of the aortic valve can be tested after cutting the aorta transversely. Both auricular appendages should be examined for the presence of thrombi. Examine interatrial septum, and for patency of foramen ovale. Examine chordae tendinae and papillary muscles for infarction, adherence to each other or rupture and chambers for any visible fibrosis or recent infarcts. The heart should be weighed, after the blood clots in the cavities are removed, and measurements of the circumference of valves and of thickness of right and left ventricle should be taken. The muscle of the right and left ventricles is incised in a plane parallel to epicardial and endocardial surfaces, which reveals infarction and fibrosis most clearly. **In death due to ventricular fibrillation heart is flabby**.

Coronary arteries: The anatomy of coronary arteries varies considerably. Usually, there is a short main trunk of the left coronary artery, which soon bifurcates into the circumflex branch, and the anterior descending branch. Ostia of coronary arteries should be examined for patency of lumen, thrombus and any narrowing Fig. (5–5). **The coronary arteries** are examined before opening the heart by making **serial cross-sections along the entire course of the major vessels about 2 to 3 mm. apart, using a scalpel.** This method demonstrates narrowing (percentage stenosis) of the vessel, and any antemortem thrombus in its lumen, without danger of dislodging it. The coronaries should not be opened by passing a scissors through them from the ostia, as they have a crushing and cutting action and produce so much distortion that any thrombus is obscured, and also the thrombus may be pushed along with the point of the scissors. **The most common site of thrombus in 1 cm away from the origin of left coronary artery.** The anterior descending branch of the left coronary artery is cut downwards along the front of the septum, then the circumflex branch on the opposite side of the mitral valve. The right coronary artery is followed from the aorta to the cut near the pulmonary valve, and then above the tricuspid valve. The presence of acute coronary lesions, e.g., plaque rupture, plaque haemorrhage, or thrombus should be noted. Calcified coronary vessels that cannot be cut with a scalpel should be stripped off the heart and decalcified for at least 24 hours before cutting.

Subendocardial Haemorrhages Figs. (5–6 and 5–7): The haemorrhages are **seen in the left ventricle,** on the upper part of the left side of the interventricular septum and on the opposing papillary muscles and adjacent columnae carnae. The haemorrhages are flame-shaped, confluent and tend to occur in one continuous sheet rather than patches. When the bleeding is severe, it may raise the endocardium into a flat blister. The mechanism of production is obscure. **They are nonspecific finding and are seen:** (1) after sudden severe hypotension due to severe loss of blood or from shock, (2) after intracranial damage, such as head injury, cerebral oedema, surgical craniotomy or tumours, (3) death from ectopic pregnancy, ruptured uterus, antepartum or postpartum haemorrhage, abortion, (4) various types of poisoning, especially arsenic.

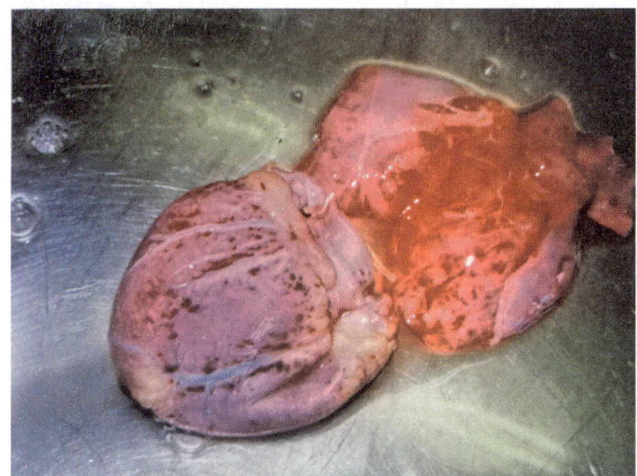

Fig. (5–6). Epicardial haemorrhages.

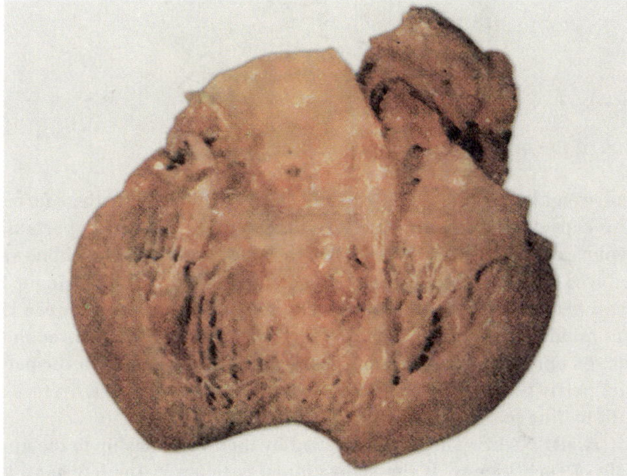

Figs. (5–7). Subendocardial haemorrhages on the interventricular septum.

ANTEMORTEM THROMBI: They are dark red, firm but friable, dry, pale, granular, adherent to vessel wall and on section show alternate layers of platelets and fibrin (coralline platelet thrombus). Dark lines are composed of red cells and a network of fine white lines of fibrin. Older thrombus is greyish-red and varies in colour from place to place. When lung is sliced, emboli slightly project above the surface. The postmortem thrombus is dark-red, glistening, soft, jelly-like and very friable.

AGONAL THROMBI: In case of a person dying slowly with circulatory failure, a firm, stringy, tough, pale-yellow thrombus forms in the cavities, usually on the right side of the heart. The process may begin in the atrial appendage, in the apex of the ventricle or in the angles of the ventricular surfaces of tricuspid valve. It extends and fills the right auricle and ventricle and spreads into the pulmonary artery and its branches like a tree-like cast. In the left ventricle, agonal thrombi are not so big.

POSTMORTEM CLOTS: Two types are seen: (1) when blood clots rapidly, a soft, lumpy, uniformly dark-red, slippery, moist clot is produced ("red currant-jelly"). (2) When red cells sediment before blood coagulates, the red cells produce a clot similar to the first type. Above this, a pale or bright-yellow layer of serum and fibrin is seen ("chicken-fat"). The fibrin clot may be soft or jelly-like, but is elastic, when the amount of fibrin is greater. Usually, a mixture of the two types of clot is seen. Postmortem clots are moist, smooth, shiny, rubbery, homogeneous, loosely or not at all attached to the underlying wall, and there are no fine white lines of fibrin (striae of Zahn). When pulled out of the vessels it forms cast of the branches. When the lung is sliced, clot does not pour out of cut small vessels. Postmortem fibrinous clots in heart are known as cardiac polyps.

POSTMORTEM FLUIDITY OF THE BLOOD: Shortly after death the blood is usually fluid, and when it is removed from the body, it undergoes spontaneous coagulation. If the autopsy is done a few hours after death, the blood may be partly clotted and partly fluid. Uncoagulable fluid blood is normally present in the limb vessels and often in the heart of any healthy person who dies suddenly from any cause. It does not give any indication of the cause of death. In most deaths from asphyxia, the blood is fluid and incoagulable. The postmortem fluidity of the blood is due to presence of fibrinolysins, liberated from the vascular endothelium. Fibrinolysin activation occurs due to release of plasminogen activator, through the receptors on the vascular wall for various vasoactive materials that increase during the agonal period. Fibrinolysis is also activated by the leakage of plasminogen-activator due to increased permeability, and to degeneration and necrosis of the cell membrane, as a result of excessive acidosis after death. It is considered that the lysin is adsorbed on to the thrombi, and released into solution when the fibrin is lysed. Under certain conditions, the fibrinolysin may be so active that fibrin is destroyed as rapidly as it is produced, and postmortem clots never develop in the vessels. In other cases, thrombi are formed, but they undergo lysis. In deaths associated with infection and cachexia, and slow natural death, fibrinolysins may fail to develop and abundant clots are seen in the heart and in the limb vessels. The concentration of circulating fibrinolysins is more in healthy persons, which is further increased during exercise and also due to emotional stress. Therefore, blood is fluid in young persons dying of unnatural causes.

UNCLOTTED BLOOD: In sudden death, the clots are greatly reduced in amount. The blood remains fluid in certain cases of septicaemia, in CO poisoning, in rapid death from asphyxia, with large doses of anticoagulants, in hypofibrinogenaemia due to amniotic fluid embolism, retained abortion or puerperal sepsis.

ABDOMEN: For examining the abdominal organs, keep the organs on the board with the liver away from the operator and the anterior surface upwards.

STOMACH: The stomach is removed after applying double ligatures at each end, and is placed in a clean dish. **It is opened along its greater curvature, from the cardiac to pyloric end.** Note the size of pyloric ring with a finger, and open the duodenum along the anterior wall. The contents are examined for nature of any food which may be present, and its state of digestion, smell, colour, character and also for the presence of foreign or suspicious matter. The contents are washed out if not required for chemical analysis, and mucous membrane is examined for the presence of congestion, haemorrhage, ulceration or other abnormal conditions.

Stomach contents: The gastric contents are yellow or yellow-green in regurgitation of bile from the duodenum. In paralytic ileus, a foul-smelling, copious, thick fluid, dirty-green, brown or black is found. In gastrocolic fistula, faecal material may be found. In massive haemorrhage, the stomach is filled with large soft clots which may take the form of a cast of the gastric outline. Small haemorrhages are partially digested and have "coffee-ground" appearance. Blood may be swallowed from the lungs, oronasopharynx or oesophagus.

INTESTINES: Examine the small and large intestine for serosa, diameter of the various portions, colour, consistency of wall, adhesions, herniae or other abnormalities. The superior mesenteric vessels are examined for any disease, thrombi or emboli. Hold the upper cut end in the left hand and apply the sharp edge of knife against the attachment of the mesentery to the jejunum. Long, sweeping, to-and-fro movements will separate the intestine due to the mere weight of the knife. The inferior mesenteric vessels are examined and the transverse colon and

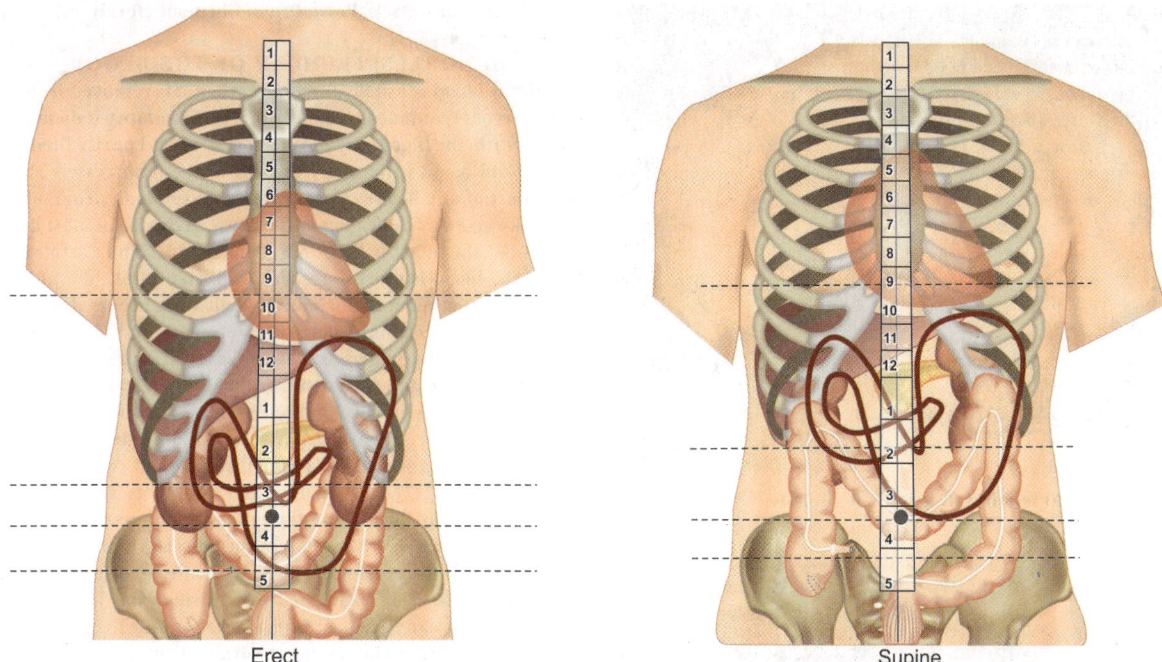

Fig. (5–8). Changes in positions and interrelationships of the organs in erect and supine positions.

pelvic mesocolon are separated from the mesentery. The small intestine is opened along the line of mesenteric attachment, and the large intestine along the anterior taenia. They are examined for congestion, inflammation, erosion, ulcers, perforation, etc. The contents are also examined Fig. (5–8).

LIVER: It is removed by itself or attached to the stomach and the duodenum when bile ducts are to be examined. Its weight, size, colour, consistency and the presence of any pathologic process or injury is noted. It is cut into 2 cm. thick slices which run in the long axis.

In chronic venous congestion, the cut-section has a granular (nutmeg) appearance. Amoebic abscesses are usually single, large and confined to the right lobe. Pyogenic abscesses are multiple. In fatty liver, the cut-section is greasy. In portal cirrhosis, the liver is studded with nodules, 1 to 3 mm. in diameter. In post-hepatic cirrhosis, nodules of varyig sizes, 4 to 10 mm. or more are seen. In biliary cirrhosis, the liver is granular and olive-green in colour.

The anterior wall of the second part of the duodenum is opened and the ampulla of Vater is identified. Squeeze the gall bladder gently and note if bile enters the duodenum. The common bile duct is opened with a fine scissors. Look for tumours, calculi and strictures. The portal vein and hepatic artery are opened. The condition and nature of lymph nodes in the neighbourhood are noted.

SPLEEN: The spleen is removed by cutting through its pedicle. Note size, weight, consistency, condition of capsule, rupture, injuries or disease. It is sectioned in its long axis, and the character of parenchyma, follicles and septa noted. Look for accessory spleens.

In congestive splenomegaly, the pulp is very soft and can be scraped easily. In portal hypertension, it is greatly enlarged and firm. It is also enlarged in malaria, Kala-Azar, portal vein thrombosis, leukaemia, reticulosis, schistosomiasis, etc.

PANCREAS: The pancreas is usually removed together with the stomach and duodenum. It is sliced by a series of cuts at right angles to the long axis, which gives the best exposure of the ductal system. The duct can be probed and opened by scissors in its full length before any cuts are made. In acute haemorrhagic pancreatitis, areas of fat necrosis will be seen as small, round, opaque areas around the pancreas and in the mesentery.

KIDNEYS: The abdominal aorta is opened along its anterior midline. The renal artery ostia are examined for thrombi, emboli or atherosclerosis. Renal veins are also examined for thrombus. Note size and weight of kidney. The capsule is stripped with toothed forceps. The capsule strips with difficulty in chronic nephritis, hypertensive nephrosclerosis and pyelonephritis. In these conditions, the kidneys are reduced in size, and their surface is granular. Hold the kidney in the left hand between the thumb and fingers, the ureter passing between ring and middle fingers. The kidney is sectioned longitudinally through the convex border into the hilum so as to split in half and open the pelvis. The pelvis is examined for calculi and inflammation. The ureters are split by fine scissors.

ADRENALS: They are identified by their relationship to the upper pole of each kidney. If the right kidney is taken in the left hand and pulled forward, the adrenal will be projected forwards in the tissues between the upper pole and the undersurface of the liver, which tends to fall backwards when the kidney is pulled forward. The left adrenal lies much more medially in relation to the kidney, and can be found by pushing the medial border of the left kidney forwards, and cutting into the tissues between the kidney and spleen. The periadrenal fat is gripped with a forceps and cut, and adrenal removed. Cut the gland gently with a scalpel without applying undue pressure. Haemorrhage is seen in meningococcal septicaemia, bleeding disease, hypertension, birth trauma, pregnancy, etc.

BLADDER: It is opened from the fundus and incision extended into the urethra. The condition of the wall and amount and character of urine are noted. In acute cystitis, the mucosa is red, swollen and covered with fibrin and pus. In chronic cystitis, the mucosa is covered with much mucus and pus and may show ulcerations.

PROSTATE: It is examined for enlargement or malignancy. Vertical cross-section through the lateral and median lobes are made with knife. In prostatitis the organ is firm, and in carcinoma it is hard and granular.

TESTES: Incise the inguinal canal from the peritoneal aspect and pull out a loop of vas with finger. Free the vas to the internal inguinal ring. Push the testis up out of the scrotum with the right hand, and pull the vas with the left hand. The testis usually comes out without difficulty or damage. The testis and epididymis are held with the left hand and are cut longitudinally with knife. Note for the presence of any clotted blood inside the scrotum and around the testis. Normal seminal tubules can be lifted like thin long filaments by toothless pointed forceps. In acute orchitis and epididymitis, the organ is swollen and firm and may show small abscesses. In chronic orchitis, the organ is firm, nodular and reduced in size.

FEMALE GENITALIA: **The tubes, ovaries and uterus are freed from the pelvis and are removed. The anterior vaginal wall is cut from below upwards, exposing the cervix. The fornices are examined. The uterus is opened from the external os to the fundus. Two short incisions are made in the fundus from main longitudinal incision towards each cornu, to expose endometrium. The ovaries are sectioned longitudinally, and the tubes are cut across at intervals. If the uterus contains a foetus, its age should be determined.**

HEAD: **A wooden block is placed under the shoulders so that the neck is extended and the head is fixed by a head rest, which should have a semicircular groove to hold the back of the neck.**

Scalp incision: A coronal incision is made in the scalp, which **starts from the mastoid process just behind one ear, Fig. (5–9) and is carried over the vertex of the scalp to the back of the opposite ear (intermastoidal incision).** The incision should penetrate to the periosteum. The scalp is reflected forwards to the superciliary ridges, and backwards to a point just below to the occipital protuberance. Any bruising of the deeper tissues of the scalp or injury to the bone should be noted.

Removal of skull cap: The temporal and masseter muscles are cut on either side, for sawing the skull. **The saw-line is made in slightly V-shaped direction, so that the skull cap will fit** Fig. (5–10) **exactly back into the correct position.** The saw-line should go through the bones along a line extending horizontally on both sides, from about the centre of the forehead to the base of the mastoid process, and from these latter points backwards, and upwards to a point a little above the external protuberance. **Thickness of the skull varies in different parts,** being thinner where protected by thick muscles. **The average thickness is 3 to 5 mm.** Care should be taken to avoid sawing through the meninges and brain. To avoid this, stop when saw meets little resistance. A chisel and hammer should not be used to loosen the

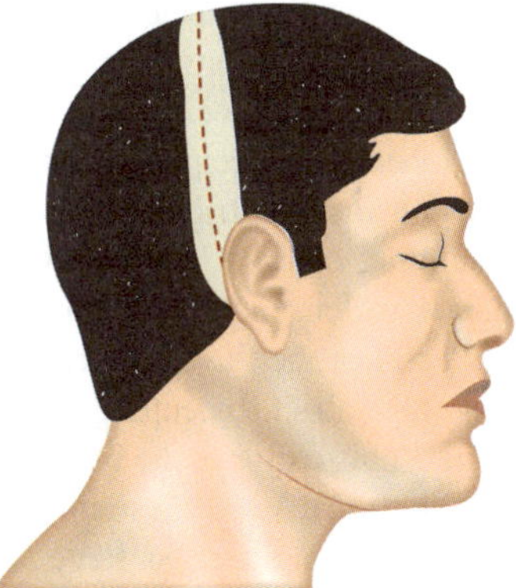

Fig. (5–9). Primary scalp incision.

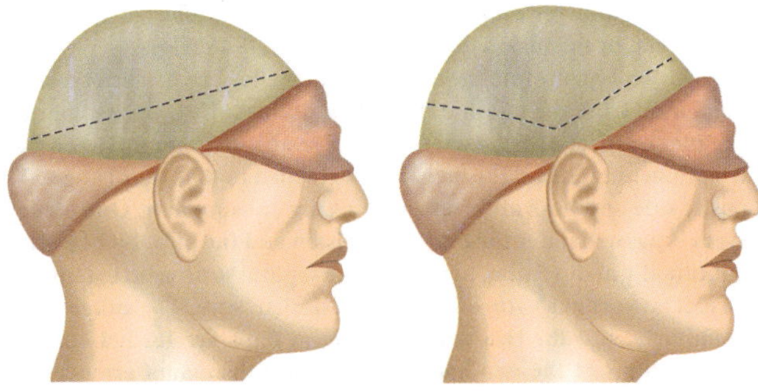

Fig. (5–10). Common method of removing the skull cap.

skull completely. Heavy hammering may cause false fractures, or extend any existing fractures. Skull fractures can be elicited by tapping of the skull which gives a "cracked pot" sound. Skull cap is removed by gently inserting and twisting the chisel at various places through the cut. Fixation of dura to bone is much firmer in children, in whom it tends to dip into the sutures.

Meninges: The meninges are examined for congestion, disease, etc. In old persons, the meninges over the vertex are often white and thickened, with little calcified patches (arachnoid granulations). A note should be made of extradural or subdural haemorrhage, which should be measured, and also of intracranial tension. If they are solid, express in terms of grams of weight, or area covered over the superior portion of the brain. Describe variation in thickness if the material is semi-liquid and cannot be easily collected. **The superior longitudinal sinus is opened along its length with a scalpel, and carefully examined for an antemortem thrombus.** This is of medicolegal importance, as antemortem thrombus in this situation can lead to back-pressure in the bridging veins crossing the subdural space, and cause subdural haemorrhage.

Removal of dura mater: The dura mater is grasped anteriorly with a forceps, and with a scissors or scalpel, the dura mater is divided from before backwards at the level of the skull division on both sides. The scalpel is now passed vertically downwards alongside the falx cerebri at its anterior end, and the knife turned medially to divide the falx. With the forceps, the dura and the falx are now pulled backwards, and the surface of the brain examined.

The dura is stripped from the base of the skull with forceps to look for basal fractures. The bones of the skull must be tested for any signs of abnormal mobility. Subdural haemorrhage can be washed, whereas subarachnoid haemorrhage cannot be washed.

If the skull is crushed or broken into pieces, replacement and fixation of the bone fragments may be carried out by using an electric drill and copper wire, for personal identification and determination of type of violence.

REMOVAL OF BRAIN: Free the falx cerebri from the cribriform plate and pull dura and falx backwards. The brain is removed by inserting the four fingers of left hand between frontal lobes and skull, and drawing frontal lobes backwards and cutting the vessels and nerves at the base. The tentorium is cut along the posterior border of the petrous bone. The brain is supported by the left hand. The knife is passed into occipital foramen and cervical cord, first cervical nerves and cerebral arteries cut as far below as possible. The right hand grasps the cerebellum and the brain is removed from the cranial vault. If any intracranial haemorrhage is present, the blood should be collected and measured. The child's brain attains mature size and weight at about six years of age.

Examination: The surface and base are examined for haemorrhage, injury or disease. The condition of the cerebral vessels, especially the vessels in the circle of Willis **Fig. (5–11)** is noted for the presence of arteriosclerosis, minute aneurysms, etc. In the fixed brain, cortical contusions and haemorrhages are much more distinct, but it becomes difficult to dissect out ruptured Berry aneurysms or small haemangiomas. Ruptured Berry aneurysms may be more easily dissected under a flow of running water, by a careful blunt dissection from the origin of the greater intracerebral vessels, around the circle of Willis, to the major branches of the circle. Berry aneurysms (size varies from few mm. to few cm.) are usually present at the junction of vessels

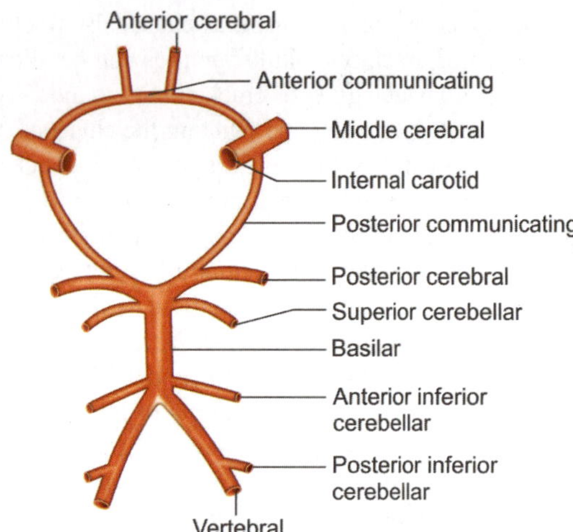

Fig. (5–11). **Circle of Willis.**

especially at the junction of the posterior cerebral arteries, the posterior communicating vessels, the middle cerebral arteries and the anterior communicating arteries. Note for cerebral infarction which may occur due to a thrombus or atheroma or due to raised intracranial pressure causing obstruction to venous outflow. Haemorrhagic infarction appears as a pinkish-purple discolouration of the cortex with stippled haemorrhages.

Fixation of Brain: For complete examination of the brain, it is fixed in 10 percent formalin for one week. In foetuses and infants, acetic acid may be added to formalin which makes the tissues firmer. To facilitate penetration of formalin, the lateral fissures are opened with the fingers which tear open the pia-arachnoid, and a long sagittal cut is made through the corpus callosum to allow formalin to pass into the ventricles. The brain can also be perfused with fixative through the arterial stumps before further fixation by immersion. **To keep the organ in its natural form, the brain is suspended upside down, supported by a string passed under the basal vessels and attaching the ends of the thread to the two sides of the jar.** Gauze should not be put beneath or around the brain, as it imprints an ugly pattern. The weight of the brain is increased by about 8% due to fixation in formalin.

Dissection of brain: The brain is placed in its normal anatomical position, and with a long knife the two halves of the brain are separated by a single incision which passes through corpus callosum, and through the midline of the midbrain, pons and medulla. If the incision passes through the median plane, it will pass through the cavity of the septum lucidum and expose the internal surfaces of its two laminae which form part of the medial walls of the lateral ventricles on each side. The incision passes through the third ventricle, the aqueduct of Sylvius and the fourth ventricle. The lateral ventricles are opened by dissection of the anterior, posterior and inferior horns, and the ependymal lining examined. Turn the cerebellum over and cut straight down through the vermis to expose the fourth ventricle Fig. (5–12). To expose the dentate nucleus, cut obliquely through each hemisphere. Whole of the stem is sectioned transversely at intervals of a few millimetres, to demonstrate haemorrhages or other abnormalities. The cerebral hemispheres are placed base down on a board, and serial sections made in the coronal plane, beginning at the frontal

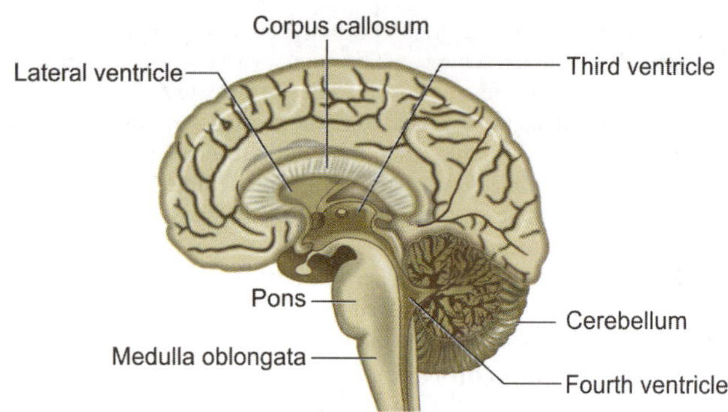

Fig. (5–12). **Median section of the brain.**

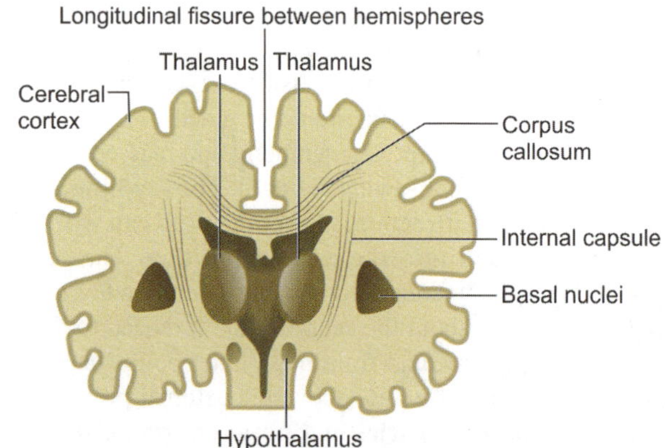

Fig. (5–13). **Cross-section of the brain.**

pole passing backwards to the occiput, at intervals of about one cm. The slices should be moved aside in sequence and placed on the cutting board so that they can be identified consecutively later. Other method is to make a horizontal cut through the cerebrum, parallel to the cutting board at a level through the tips of the frontal lobes and temporal lobes to the occipital lobes. Inspect the choroid plexus and locate the interventricular foramen. The fornices and corpus callosum are cut and bent backwards. Examine the thalamus and caudate nucleus Fig. (5–13). The third ventricle will now be exposed. Pass a probe through the aqueduct of Sylvius. Now expose the fourth ventricle by cutting along the vermis in the midline with scalpel. This exposes the basal ganglia and lateral ventricles. Expose the third ventricles and trace the aqueduct. If there are injuries to the brain, successive sections parallel to the wounded surfaces should be made till the whole depth of the lesion is seen.

DISSECTION OF HEAD IN INFANTS: Rokitansky's method is autopsy technique for infants. The scalp flaps are reflected as in adult. The skull can be opened as described by Baar (1946) Fig. (5–14). With a knife, incision is made into the anterior fontanelle at its posterior margin, about 5 mm. from the midline. The point of the knife is pushed parallel to the inner aspect of the parietal bone for one to 2 mm. between dura and leptomeninges, and the incision is extended to the lateral angle. The opposite side and both anterior margins are cut similarly. One blade of scissors is passed under the original incision and the parietal bone is cut longitudinally about 5 mm. parallel to the sagittal suture, up to lambdoid suture. The coronal suture is cut in a similar way. The other side is cut similarly, and the two parietotemporal flaps are turned outward. Similarly, flaps of the two halves of the frontal squama are prepared and turned outward. Usually, a horizontal fronto-medial extension is required with the help of a bone forceps, which leaves only short bridge

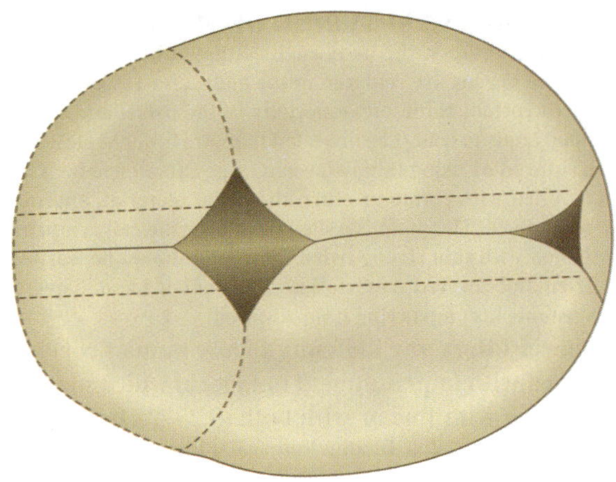

Fig. (5–14). Technique for opening the skull of a newborn infant.

for outward reflection of the flaps. This leaves a medial strip about one cm. in width with the intact underlying superior longitudinal sinus.

After reflecting the flaps, the vertex of the brain and the terminations of the pial veins into the superior longitudinal sinus are examined for haemorrhage. The hemispheres are gently pushed sideward and falx cerebri is examined. Haematoma may be found between the falx and the medial aspect of the hemispheres or between the two dural layers of the falx. The superior longitudinal sinus is opened and examined for thrombi. The falx is separated at its antero-inferior insertion, and the brain is removed as in the case of an adult. The tentorium is examined for tears and for haematoma between its layers. The dural sinuses are opened and the dura is detached from the base and sides of the skull with a pair of forceps, or a part of the dura is held with a towel and is pulled.

CEREBRAL OEDEMA: In generalised oedema of the brain, flattening of the cerebral convolutions with obliteration of the sulci, and a herniation of the inner portions of the temporal poles through the tentorial hiatus, and of portions of the cerebellar lobe and cerebellar tonsils through the foramen magnum are found. In true "coning" the cerebellar tonsils will be discoloured or even necrotic. Gross changes are not present when oedema is present in minor degree. When it is of severe degree and widespread, the convolutions are flattened, lateral ventricles are reduced to mere slits, and the white matter appears glistening, smooth and shiny. The cerebral hemispheres are pressed hard against the dura. The increased bulk of the hemispheres causes tentorial herniation and the uncus is pushed down the tentorial orifice. The brain may weigh up to 1750 g. Histologically, the white matter is vacuolated and in severe cases shows pools or lakes of pale staining fluid. In head injury, the oedema is seen in the white matter around or deep to contusions, lacerations or ischaemic lesions.

The middle ear can be examined by chiselling out wedge-shaped portion of petrous temporal bone. The mastoid is examined by nipping away the bone with a pair of bone forceps. The orbits can be examined by removing the orbital plates in the base of the skull. The sphenoid and frontal sinuses are opened from the inside of the skull by a chisel. The pituitary is removed by chiselling the posterior clinoid process and incising the diaphragm of the sella turcica around its periphery. Abscess formation in or septic condition, etc., about the jaws and teeth should be looked for.

VERTEBRAL COLUMN: The atlanto-occipital joint should be examined for any fracture-dislocation by moving the head on the spine. The cervical spine should also be examined. If there is excess mobility, look for haemorrhage on the anterior surface of the spinal ligaments and cut into the bodies of the vertebrae. The thoracic and lumbar spine should be examined by pushing the spine forwards with the hand under the body, which will show abnormal movement at the site of any fracture. The pelvis should be squeezed from side to side by pressure on each iliac crest. Mobility of the pelvis indicates fractures of the sacro-iliac joints or of the pelvic bones. The thorax should be examined for recent or old fractures of the ribs.

REMOVAL OF SPINAL CORD: It is not examined routinely, unless there is an indication of disease or injury. The body is placed prone on the table, face downwards. A wooden block is placed under the chest, and the head is bent downwards. This stretches cervical spine. An incision is made on the back in midline extending from the occipital protuberance to the lower end of sacrum and the muscles are dissected away from the top of the spinal column, noting their condition. The atlanto-occipital joint capsules are incised and articular surfaces examined. The atlas is disarticulated. The laminae are sawed close to the transverse processes through the entire length of spine on each side of the spinous process, by means of an adjustable double blade saw, and are separated with the chisel. It is easier to cut through the arches of the atlas and the axis with a pair of bone shears. The lumbar end of the freed spinous processes are grasped with bone forceps and spinous processes lifted upwards in one piece. The dura is slit open along the midline with scissors and the presence of haemorrhage, inflammation, suppuration, infarction, degeneration, crushing or tumour is noted. The nerves are cut from below up as they pass through spinal foramina. The cord is separated at the foramen magnum. The cord is sectioned transversely and serially. The vertebral column is examined for fractures or dislocations. The empty spinal canal must be examined for disc protrusion, tumours, fractures, dislocations and vertebral collapse.

EXTREMITIES: The femoral vessels are examined by a longitudinal incision down the centre of the upper anterior half of the thigh, starting below the inguinal ligament. They should be examined in continuation with iliac vessels. For examination of popliteal and calf veins, a vertical midline incision is given over the back of the knee joint and leg and skin flaps are reflected. The tendon of Achilles is divided. The calf muscles are then separated from the bones from the heel upward. Transverse sections about two cm. apart are then made in the calf muscles. If thrombi are present, they protrude as firm, solid, tube-like masses. The major arteries of the calf pass between the tibia and fibula. For removal of the marrow from the femur, the incision for the femoral vessels can be employed. In the upper end of the shaft, a rectangle of cortex is cut out, using a rotary saw, and the marrow is scooped out.

All the organs and parts removed from the body should be returned to the dead body for the purpose of burial, except when they are required for further studies or to be produced as evidence in subsequent trial. If the organs are retained by the doctor for his department, without consent of next of kin, he can be sued by any relative of the deceased.

ENDOSCOPIC TECHNIQUE OF POSTMORTEM DIAGNOSIS: The method requires the use of rigid Hopkins-endoscope of 4 mm and 8 mm diameters with 0°, 90°, and 130° view angles having a light source from fibreglass cable. The endoscope is fitted with zoom lens camera for photographic documentation.

Sinuses, fundus, external auditory meatus, larynx, etc. can be directly visualised. Bullet tracts in the body can be traced accurately. Hepatic, splenic and diaphragmatic injuries and intraperitoneal and thoracic haemorrhages can be visualised. Natural orifices can be clearly examined.

VIRTUAL AUTOPSY (VIRTOPSY): It is a non-invasive technique of examining dead bodies to find out the cause of death. It does not destroy some important evidence which may be destroyed in the usual autopsy. It is a combination of CT and MR imaging, photogrammetry and 3D optical measuring technique, CT images give information about morbid anatomical findings and MR imaging demonstrates soft tissue injury, organ trauma, state of blood vessels, tissue and bones. Multi-slice compound tomography (MSCT), multi-planar reconstruction (MPR) and volume rendering technique (VRT) done in injuries by firearms, explosions, charred bodies, decomposed bodies, child abuse, bones for fractures, sex and age can be determined. MR spectroscopy measures metabolites formed due to decomposition, which help to estimate time since death. Two dimensional and three dimensional imaging is done with multislice CT. Emphysema, air embolism, pneumothorax, hyperbaric trauma and decompression effects can be better appreciated. When an injury is caused by a weapon, using a computer software, virtual model of an injury with the 3D image of a simulation can be created by using a similar weapon. In a firearm injury entrance and exit wounds can be determined based on fracture pattern with inward and outward bevelling of the bone. The track of the projectile inside the brain or other internal organs with haemorrhage and damage to tissues can be viewed with CT scanning. Biopsy of organs can be done.

At present it is not a practical alternative due to cost factor and more so X-ray machine is good enough for forensic students. It has certain inherent disadvantages of misinterpretations and inability to detect organ lesions.

PSYCHOLOGICAL AUTOPSY: Psychological autopsy is a set of postmortem investigative procedures that help ascertain and evaluate the role that physical and psychological factors play in the death of a victim of suicide, thus to determine the manner of death to as high a degree of certainty as possible. In some cases of suicide, police reports may be incomplete as sources of information. Description of scene of death, position of body, evidence at the scene, such as weapons, poison and notes, etc. are necessary. Equivocal deaths are those that do not indicate the manner of death, e.g. they were not witnessed or involved conflicting data. **It involves systematic collection of psychological data through structured interviews of the deceased's family members, friends, coworkers, employers and fellow students, who had dealt with the deceased.** Data are sought about his medical, educational, sexual, marital, employment, alcohol, drugs, phobias, moods, interpersonal relationship, friends and colleagues, personality coping style, psychiatric history and general emotional life, judging abilities, concentration, I.Q. and chronology of events leading up to the time of committing suicide. **When it is combined with first person accounts of the deceased's last days of life, i.e. evidence from the site of death, police investigation reports and archival documents, e.g. medical and mental health records, school and occupational records, previous suicide attempts and financial records, conclusions can be drawn as to the intention of the deceased, and therefore his role in causing his own death.**

It has four main functions: (1) determination of mode of death; (2) to determine the state of mind at the time of death; (3) to retrieve the most honest information possible in a way that will be healing for survivors, and (4) to gain information that will be helpful in treating future patients.

The psychological autopsy is most commonly introduced in those involving custodial care taking (police custody and prisons) and those of contested life insurance claims. They have also been introduced in criminal cases (suicide or homicide), worker's compensation (unsafe job conditions), product manufacturer's (depressants) and professional negligence (proximate cause of suicide) **cannot validly inform an expert that a suicide definitely occurred, as the information gathered may be biased, but it significantly improves manner of death determination.**

This procedure also has therapeutic value, leading to bereavement counselling, the relieving of guilt feelings and the answers to other questions.

CLEANING AND SUTURING OF THE CADAVER: After completing the autopsy, the body cavities should be cleaned of blood, fluid, etc. The organs are replaced in the body, and any excess space is packed with cotton, cloth, etc. especially in the pelvis and the throat, where blood tends to leak. The dissected flaps are brought close together and well sutured by using thin twine and large curved needle. The skull should be filled with cotton or other absorbent material, and the skull cap fitted in place. The scalp is pulled back over the calvarium and the scalp stitched with thin strong twine. The body should be washed with water, dried and covered with clothes. The body is handed over to the police constable accompanying it for disposal.

Whoever offers any indignity to any human corpse shall be punished with imprisonment for a term which may extend to one year or with fine or with both (S.297, I.P.C.).

Autopsy in Custodial Death: National Human Rights Commission (NHRC) has laid down protocol in cases of deaths in police action, custodial deaths, and death prison. While conducting PM of the deceased photographs should be taken and the PM examination should be video filmed: (i) to record the detailed findings of PM examination, especially for marks of injury and violence, (ii) to supplement the findings of PM examination so as to rule out any undue influence or suppression of material information, (iii) to facilitate an independent review of the PM report at later stage if required.

Protocol for Video Filming and photography of PM examination: (i) At the time of video filming of the PM examination, the voice of the doctor conducting the PM should be recorded. The doctor should narrate his prima-facie observations while conducting PM examination. (ii) 20-25 coloured photographs covering the whole body should be taken. Some photographs of the body should be taken without removing clothes. The photographs should include the following: (a) Profile photo-face (front, right lateral, and left lateral views), back of head. (b) Front of body (up to torso-chest and abdomen), and back. (c) Upper extremity—front and back. (d) Lower extremity—front and back. (e) Focusing on each injury/lesion after properly numbering the injuries. (f) Internal examination findings. (2) Photographs on soles and palms each, after making incision to show absence/evidence of any old/deep seated injury. In case of firearm injuries, the distance from heel as well as midline must be taken in respect of each injury. (iii) Photographs should be taken by holding the camera at right angle to the objects after incorporating postmortem number, date of examination, and a scale for dimensions in the frame of photographs itself.

(i) Both hands of the deceased should be wrapped in white paper bags and dead body should be covered in special body bags for proper transportation, (ii) Clothing on the body of deceased should be collected, examined, preserved and sealed by the doctor and sent to the concerned FSL. A detailed note regarding examination of the clothing should be included and subjected to radiological examinations (X-rays/CT scan) prior autopsy.

The PM report along with the recorded video film and photographs should be sent to the commission within 2 months of the incident. If the viscera are sent for examination, PM report and other documents should be sent to the commission without waiting for the viscera report. The viscera report should be sent subsequently as soon as it received.

AUTOPSY OF A CASE OF AIDS AND INFECTIONS: Highly infectious diseases transmitted by direct contact or contact with infected materials, clothing, discharges, vomit, etc. are cholera, rabies, tetanus, anthrax, poliomyelitis, mumps, septicaemia, typhoid, tuberculosis, hepatitis B & C, diphtheria, C.S.F. meningitis, smallpox, plague, tick-borne encephalitis, equine encephalomyelitis, T-cell lymphotropic viruses I and II, and HIV. Patients with presenile dementia may have Creutzfeldt-Jakob disease (CJD) caused by virus, which is present in highest concentration in nervous and lymphoid tissues. It appears that the CJD agent can be acquired only by ingestion, inoculation or transplantation. Hepatitis B and C viruses are present in blood stream and concentrated in hepatic tissue.

Inoculation tuberculosis of skin (prosector's wart) is seen in persons engaged in postmortem examinations. There is a risk of transmission of HIV through needle prick injury during collection of blood and other body fluids, and mucosal splashes and skin contact with superficial injury during autopsy on a HIV infected dead body. HIV in high concentrations

has been found to remain viable for three weeks and from liquid blood after two months. HIV and hepatitis viruses are not associated with air-borne transmission. HIV is present mostly in lymphoid tissue and brain, and also in colon and lungs.

It is better to leave some organs in situ in the cadaver rather than eviscerating *en masse.* Another method is to fix lungs and other organs whole after removal rather than slicing them before fixation.

UNIVERSAL WORK PRECAUTIONS: (1) All infected bodies should be wrapped and tied in double layer tough plastic bag, with a red colour tag mentioning "Biologically Hazardous". The label should mention the name, age, sex, registration number, etc. (2) Workers who have exudative lesions or weeping dermatitis or external injury should not handle AIDS victims. (3) Proper protective clothing, full sleeves overalls instead of simple surgical gowns, water-proof plastic apron, head cap, face mask, goggles if eye glasses are not worn, double gloves (heavy autopsy gloves over surgical gloves), waterproof rubber gumboots of knee length with shoe covers. A plastic visor will protect eyes and mucosal surfaces from splash injury. A high efficiency particulate air-filled respirator or a powered air-purifying respirator should be worn. (4) Handling sharp instruments: Avoid accidental pricks and cuts from needles, scalpels, etc. If a cut is made in the rubber gloves or needle injury occurs they should be removed immediately and replaced with new ones. Hands and other skin surfaces should be washed immediately and thoroughly if contaminated with blood or other body fluids. Infection of AIDS can be acquired by transdermal inoculation through cuts and needle punctures. About 0.3 to 0.5% of individuals will become seropositive. Transmission rates from contaminated needle punctures or close contact are 10 to 30 times higher for serum hepatitis than for AIDS. The incident should be reported to proper authority to get their blood check for HIV seropositivity. (5) Handling specimens for laboratory examination: Mucocutaneous contact with the body fluids, and aerosol inhalation should be avoided. They should be properly labelled and filled with 10% formalin solution and should be handled with gloved hands. (6) Disposal of used instruments: They should be dipped in 2% glutaraldehyde (cider) for half-an-hour, washed with soap or detergent and water, dried and then rinsed in methylated spirit and air dried. (7) All soiled gauze and cotton, etc. should be collected in a double plastic bag for incineration. (8) Laundry material, such as aprons, towels, etc. should be soaked in one percent bleach for half-an-hour, washed with detergent and hot water, and autoclaved. (9) Clean-up procedure: Wear new intact disposable gloves. Small spatters and spills of blood and other body fluids can be wiped up with disposable tissues or towels which are discarded in special bio-hazard bags and properly disposed. The autopsy table and floor should be cleaned with one percent bleach solution, followed by washing with soap and water. (10) Disinfectants: 1:10 dilution of common household bleach or a freshly prepared sodium hypochlorite solution are recommended. Liquid chemical germicides commonly used in health care facilities and laboratories are effective against HIV and viruses. (11) In case of accidental injuries or cuts with sharp instruments, contaminated with blood or body fluids or not, while working on a body, the wound should be immediately washed thoroughly under running water, bleeding encouraged and disinfected. (12) To minimise aerosol splatter, skull can be opened with an electrical oscillating saw attached to a vacuum dust exhaust and filter or with a band saw under a transparent anti-slash cover. After autopsy all body orifices should be packed and the body should be wrapped in double layer heavy plastic sheet bag and secured properly, so that there is no leakage. A tag should be attached for identification. (13) After completing autopsy, hands and face should be washed with soap and water and rinsed in 70% methylated spirit. (14) The body should be burnt or incinerated.

Universal precautions apply to blood, semen and vaginal secretions as well as to CSF, synovial fluid, pleural fluid, peritoneal fluid, pericardial fluid and amniotic fluid. Universal precautions do not apply to faeces, nasal secretions, sputum, sweat, tears, urine and vomitus unless they contain visible blood. If the recommended guidelines are adhered to, there is no risk to the staff conducting autopsies on AIDS patients.

CORONA VIRUS (COVID-19)

The corona virus disease, also known as COVID-19 infection, is caused by the SARS-CoV-2 virus and spreads through the respiratory route, via aerosols, droplets, etc., that are generated when an infected person coughs, and causes infection when another person inhales the same. The pandemic started towards the end of the year 2019 and has spread to all countries of the world within a span of few months. The spread of the disease happens in waves, in terms of the number of people affected, with an increasing trend, a peak, followed by a decline and persistence in low numbers. Multiple such waves have occurred since the onset of the pandemic, with different regions affected differently.

Since the onset of the pandemic, the SARS-CoV-2 virus has undergone multiple mutations, which have resulted in wider spread and possible evasion from the protective effects of the vaccine. Multiple variants have been detected and isolated, the important ones being Alpha, Beta, Gamma, Delta and Omicron variants, which are also labelled by WHO as variants of concern (VOC). A VOC must satisfy one of the following criteria, for it to be labelled as such:

(i) Increase in transmissibility or detrimental change in COVID-19 epidemiology

(ii) Increase in virulence or change in clinical disease presentation

(iii) Decrease in effectiveness of public health and social measures or available diagnostics, vaccines, therapeutics.

SARS-Co-2 has developed several mutations in its genome, these are termed as variants among these variant of concern (VOC), the Delta and Omicron variants have caught attention due to their rapid spread and severity of disease. Many of them are associated with rapid transmissibility. The B. 11 .7 (Alpha), B-1.351 (Beta, P.1 (Gamma), B-1 .427 (Epsilon), B1.429 (Epsilon), B.1 .617.2 Delta and B.1 .1 .529 (Omicron) (WHO, ICMR).

Delta variant: The Delta variant (B.1.617.2) was first detected in India in October 2020, and was labelled as a VOC because of increased transmissibility and capability to cause a serious infection. It was responsible for the second wave of the COVID pandemic in India as well as multiple infections across the world, with just the US and UK recording nearly 2.5 million cases. CDC, USA had reported that the Delta variant is more contagious, causing more severe illness in unvaccinated people as well as causing breakthrough infections in vaccinated people, which can spread the virus to others. In Delta variant wave there was a large number of mucormycosis cases with high fatality rate. Mucormycosis of brain, ears and skin were there. A total number of 2,50,000/- died in India in second wave (UN Report). It had a peak in the month April and May, 2021 where AIIMS alone 962 people died in one month due to this variant.

Omicron variant: The Omicron variant (B.1.1.529) was first identified in South Africa in November 2021, although it had spread to multiple countries by then. In comparison to the Delta variant, infection due to the Omicron variant is much less severe. And mainly confines to upper respiratory track. However, transmissibility is higher 70% more than Delta variant which can result in higher number of infections and hospitalizations. It lacks power to penetrate deeper t012bb.

The Omicron variant is also capable of evading immunity that has developed due to previous infection or vaccination, which further expedites the rate of transmission.

Preventive measures suggested by WHO include the use of face masks, social distancing and hand sanitization. Vaccination against COVID-19 is also in practice, which according to experts have aided in limiting the number of infections and fatalities. The first vaccine was approved in August 2021, following which multiple vaccines have come up globally. It caused third wave where incidence was present in the month of January, 2022 but was less fatal as only 35 deaths were seen at AIIMS in one month period.

SRS-CoV2 is appositive stranded RNA virus. The viral genome is surrounded by: Nucleocapsid (N) protein, spike (S) protein, envelope (E), membrane (M) proteins and haemagglutinin esterase (HE) glycoprotein.

Diagnostic testing:

(1) Nasopharyngeal swabs

(2) Chest X-ray (CXR) may not any worth noting fining in beginning phase. I moderate cases reveal consolidation and ground glass opacities in bilateral, lower and peripheral zones. Such findings can also be seen in viral infection in COVID-19 these are more prominent and faster.

(3) **Chest CT** is very informative and can detected better than X-ray.

CT severity score: Each of the five lung lobes is scored on a scale of 0 to 5. Total score is the sum of lobar scores. Score of less than eight is considered mild, 9-15 moderate and more than 15 is labeled as severe. Maximum score is 25.

(4) Clinical investigation during hospitalization: Complete blood count—lymphopenia is common: Liver function test—elevated transaminase levels; Renal function test; D-dimers; inflammatory markers like ferritin, C-reactive protein, and erythrocyte sedimentation rate (ESR).

AUTOPSY IN COVID-19 DEATHS (STANDARD GUIDELINES BY ICMR)

Coronavirus Disease-2019 (COVID-19) is caused by the novel coronavirus, a RNA virus. First reported in 2019 in Wuhan, China, has caused a major pandemic worldwide in 2020. It has been classified under risk group 3 of biological agents.

The **deaths in hospital and under medical care due to COVID-19 is a non-medicolegal case** and does not require postmortem examination and the required certification of death is being done by treating doctors. **Even embalming of such bodies should be avoided.** SARS-CoV-2 RNA may still be **detected up to 3 days postmortem** and possibly longer based on available data from experiences with MERS-CoV and SARS-CoV; however sensitivity may be reduced with a longer postmortem interval. Forensic Postmortem Examination is an inquest based medical examination vide S. 174, Cr.P.C. and 176, Cr.P.C. and inquest itself contains panchanama, statements from witness and all other allied circumstantial evidence details. Dissection of bones and tissues generates aerosol which may lead to spread of infection. Thus it is recommended that general examination, external examination, examination of clothing, multiple photographs and verbal autopsy (as depicted by WHO) and criteria of elimination and exclusion, the postmortem should be conducted strictly avoiding any invasive surgical procedures and avoiding splashing of body fluids contact for staffs, body handlers and doctors conducting postmortem. Use of an oscillating bone saw should be avoided for known or suspected COVID-19 cases. Use chisel and hammer, hand shears as an alternative cutting tool. If an oscillating saw is used, attach a vacuum shroud to contain aerosols. **Limit the number of personnel during autopsy.** Mortuary staff should apply standard precautions (i.e., perform proper hand hygiene and use appropriate PPE, including long sleeved gown, gloves and facial protection if there is a risk of splashes from the patient's body fluids or secretions onto the body or face of the staff member).

After autopsy, the body should be packed in a body bag and the body bag should be disinfected with 1% hypochlorite solution from outside. After storage of body in storage chambers or autopsy, all the surfaces, instruments, storage chambers and transport trolleys should be properly disinfected with **1% Hypochlorite solution for a minimum period of 10 minutes.**

No viscera will be preserved in any suspected COVID-19 positive case. However, collection of the following postmortem specimens is recommended (i) Upper respiratory tract swabs: nasopharyngeal swab AND oropharyngeal swab. (ii) Lower respiratory tract swab: Lung swab from each lung. (iii) Separate clinical specimens for testing of other respiratory pathogens and other postmortem testing as indicated. (iv) Formalin-fixed autopsy tissues from lung, upper airway, and other major organs

Autopsies should be conducted in an adequately ventilated room, i.e. at least natural ventilation with at least 160L/s/patient air flow or negative pressure rooms with at least 12 air changes per hour (ACH) and controlled direction of air flow when using mechanical ventilation.

THE AUTOPSY AND DISPOSAL OF RADIOACTIVE CORPSE: If the amount of radioactivity is less than 5 millicuries, no extra precautions are necessary. If the body contains between 5 to 30 millicuries of radioactive material, the doctor must wear heavy rubber gloves, plastic aprons, plastic shoe covers and spectacles to reduce contamination. Instruments with long handles should be used during the autopsy. Organs and fluids that are most radioactive should be removed first and placed in covered glass jars, labelled and examined for radioactivity from time to time. Fluid of the pleural and peritoneal cavity should be flushed copiously with running water and disposed off directly into the sewer. Contaminated wearing dress should be thoroughly cleaned with soap and water, and stored for suitable decay of the radioactive material before being sent to laundry. Instruments can be brought to a safe level by soaking them in water with soap or a detergent. Contamination of the floor of the autopsy room should be avoided. Spilled fluid should be cleaned with dry disposable water, held with forceps and put into a suitable vessel. If the radiation level is high, a team may be required to complete the autopsy. Special organs may be removed first, and detailed dissection done away from the body, or after a period of cold storage, or fixation to permit radioactive decay. If the body contains more than 300 millicuries of activity after autopsy, it should be embalmed in the hospital morgue. The presence of a cardiac pacemaker must be recorded, especially if it is one which might contain mercury or a radioactive substance, as explosions in crematoria from the heating of mercury batteries have proved hazardous.

Occupational hazards in medicolegal autopsies: (1) Infections can be transmitted through percutaneous contact or puncture by autopsy instruments. (2) Aerosol/droplet inhalation can cause tuberculosis, rabies, anthrax, plague, etc. (3) Eye contact can cause localised or generalised infection. (4) Exposure to noxious agents such as, formaldehyde, pesticides, corrosives, etc. (5) Exposure to radiation due to autopsy on a victim of radiation. (6) Constant exposure to traumatized, mutilated and decomposed dead bodies can cause depression, personality disorders, alcohol abuse, etc.

Preventive measures: Vaccination against tetanus, polio, tuberculosis, hepatitis, etc., and adoption of universal work precautions.

LABORATORY PROCEDURES

(1) HISTOPATHOLOGY: Various internal organs are examined routinely. A typical portion of affected area as seen by gross examination should be removed along with a portion of normal borderline tissue. It should be cut into pieces of 20 mm × 12 mm × 5 mm for proper preservation. The specimens can be fixed in ten percent neutral formalin or 95% alcohol. The amount of preservative should be 6 to 10 times the volume of the tissue to be fixed. Specimens must be rinsed before fixation to remove blood clots.

(2) BACTERIOLOGICAL EXAMINATION: All specimens must be collected under sterile conditions. Blood for culture must be obtained before organs are disturbed. After opening the pericardial sac, the anterior surface of the right ventricle is seared with heated knife, and 10 ml of blood aspirated using a sterile needle and syringe. The same technique may be used to remove material from other organs. The sample should be placed in sterile stoppered containers. The subarachnoid space is opened with a sterile scalpel and a specimen is taken from the space by sterile swabs from which smears and cultures may be made. The samples should be placed in sterile stoppered containers. For culture of splenic tissue, the surface of the organ (2x2cm) is seared with a hot spatula, and the area is punctured with a sterile instrument and pulp is scraped. In deaths due to septicaemia, spleen is the best organ for culture, or blood is collected from a peripheral vein.

(3) SMEARS OF BRAIN CORTEX, SPLEEN AND LIVER may be stained for malarial parasites. Smears of bone marrow from ribs or sternum is stained and examined for blood dyscrasias. Smears from chancres and mucous patches are examined fresh by dark field method or stained.

(4) VIROLOGICAL EXAMINATION: A piece of appropriate tissue is collected under sterile conditions and the sample freezed or preserved in 80% glycerol in buffered saline. The specimen should be placed in a sterile container and sealed tightly.

(5) BLOOD: Before autopsy, 10 to 20 ml. of blood can be drawn from the femoral or external iliac vein in the groin by a syringe. The flow may be increased by massaging the leg to drive blood proximally. The jugular or subclavian vein can also be used. After removal of the viscera, blood can be collected by raising the arm, and holding a small container under the cut end of a subclavian vein. The arm can be elevated and massaged towards the shoulder, if the flow is slow. Similarly, blood

can be collected from cutting the iliac veins at the brim of the pelvis, or from the jugular vein. Blood should never be collected from the pleural or the abdominal cavities, as it can be contaminated with gastric or intestinal contents, lymph, mucus, urine, pus, or serous fluid. Blood should not be collected from heart cavities, inferior vena cava or portal or hepatic veins. In case of cocaine, plastic bottles should be avoided. In case of CN and CO airtight cap should be used. In cases of volatile poisons a thin layer of liquid paraffin is advised over the top of fluid to avoid evaporation. Alcohol and barbiturates can diffuse passively after death from the stomach and intestines into adjacent organs or cavities leading to erroneous results. Blood should be collected from the femoral vessels. Other sites, in descending order of preference are the subclavain vessels, root of aorta, pulmonary artery, superior vena cava and the heart. When blood samples are collected for volatile substances, small glass bottles with aluminium foil-lined should be used, which should be filled to the top to avoid loss of volatile substances into the head space and stored at 4°C. For blood grouping, a piece of filter paper or a clean cotton gauze can be used to soak up some blood and dried.

(6) C.S.F.: It is collected by lumbar puncture or from the cisterna magna by inserting a long needle between the atlas and the occipital bone. Direct aspiration of CSF can be done from the lateral ventricles or third ventricle after removal of the brain.

(7) VITREOUS HUMOUR: A fine hypodermic needle is inserted through the outer canthus into the posterior chamber of the eye, (centre of the globe), after pulling the eyelid aside followed by aspiration with a syringe. One to two ml. of fluid can be aspirated from each eye. Water can be re-introduced through the needle to restore the tension in the globe for cosmetic reasons.

(8) LUNGS: In solvent abuse and death from gaseous or volatile substances, a lung is mobilised and the main bronchus tied off tightly with a ligature. The hilum is then divided and immediately the lung is put into a nylon bag, which is sealed. Plastic (polythene) bags are not suitable as they are permeable to volatile substances.

(9) ENZYMES: Small pieces of tissues are collected into a thermos flask containing liquid nitrogen.

(10) FAECES is examined for protozoa and helminths. Five to ten gm. without any preservative should be sent for bacteriologic examinations.

(11) URINE: It can be obtained by catheter or suprapubic puncture with syringe and long needle before autopsy, or by making an incision on the anterior surface of the bladder during autopsy.

(12) CYST FLUID is examined for ecchinococcus hooklets.

(13) BITE MARKS: Swab the bite site with a saline-moistened cotton swab, dry and place in a test tube and plug with cotton.

(14) VAGINAL AND ANAL SWABS.

(15) URETHRAL DISCHARGE.

(16) RECTAL SWABS: For bacteriological examination swabs taken from the mucosa of rectum are suitable.

PRESERVATION OF VISCERA IN CASES OF SUSPECTED POISONING: Viscera should be preserved: (1) If death is suspected to be due to poisoning either by the police or the doctor. (2) Deceased was intoxicated or used to drugs. (3) Cause of death not found after autopsy. (4) In cases where an unusual smell, colour or an unidentifiable material is detected in stomach contents. (5) Anaphylactic deaths. (6) Death due to burns. (7) Advanced decomposition. (8) Accidental death involving driver of a vehicle or machine operator. The following must be preserved in all fatal cases of suspected poisoning.

(1) **Stomach** and its contents. If the stomach is empty, the wall should be preserved.

(2) The upper part of **small intestine** (about 30 cm.length) and its contents.

(3) **Liver** 200 to 300 gm.

(4) **Kidney** half of each. as one kidney may be dysfunctional.

(5) **Blood** 30 ml. Minimum 10 ml.

(6) **Urine** 30 ml.

As most poisons are taken orally, the poison is most likely to be present in the stomach and intestinal contents and in their wall. **After absorption all poisons pass through the liver, which is the major detoxicating organ and has the power of concentrating many poisons** making them identifiable when the blood and urine concentrations may have declined to very low levels. **The kidney being the organ of excretion contains large amounts of poison,** which is excreted into the urine. **Levels of drugs in the muscle more accurately reflect blood levels than the liver or kidney.**

The cellular barrier of mucous and serous membranes breakdown after death, due to which substances in the stomach and intestine can migrate to the organs in the thorax and abdomen, causing false rise in the blood level. After death most variation in concentration of a substance is caused by uneven distribution by enzymatic and microbiological activity and by diffusion from sites of higher concentration.

It is essential to prevent contamination of the solid viscera with the contents of the gastrointestinal tract, because an idea of the length of time since ingestion may be had from the relative amounts of poison in the stomach, intestines and the solid organs. **If the poison is only found in the contents of the stomach, and none in the solid viscera and is not an irritant, doubts may occur about the actual proof of absorption.** Therefore, it is important to keep the contents of the alimentary canal in separate bottles. **Poison found in urine, unless added with evil intention is a proof of absorption and excretion.** If the poison is also found in the food or medicine preserved, this would be very strong additional evidence. **The stomach contents are of primary value for estimating the quantity ingested in acute overdoses, and qualitatively in identifying substances which have been recently ingested.**

Containers: For preservation of viscera, the glass bottles used should be of one litre capacity, clean, wide-mouthed, white and fitted with glass stoppers. **Rubber inserts should not be used under caps, because it can extract from the contents certain poisons, such as chloroform and phenols.** Glass containers should be cleaned with sulphuric acid-chromate solution, rinsed with distilled water and dried. **Polyethylene bags or containers can be used, but volatile poison may diffuse through plastic.** When lungs or other tissues are to be preserved for analysis for volatile substances, nylon bags should be used, as they are not permeable to such substances. Blood should be collected in screw-capped bottle of about 30 ml.

Preservatives: (1) Saturated **sodium chloride** solution, except in poisoning from corrosive acids (except phenol), alkalis, corrosive sublimate, and aconite. (2) **Rectified spirit,** except in cases of suspected poisoning by (a) alcohol, kerosene, (b) chloroform, ether, (c) chloral hydrate, (d) formic acid, (e) formaldehyde, acetic acid, (f) phenol, (g) phosphorus, and (h) paraldehyde, because the organic acids and paraldehyde are soluble in alcohol and the phosphorescence of phosphorus is diminished by alcohol. (3) **Ten. mg./ml of sodium or potassium fluoride (prevents glycolysis, inhibits enzyme enolase and inhibits bacterial growth), and 3 mg. potassium oxalate (anti-coagulant) should be used for preserving blood.** Fluoride should also be added to urine, CSF, and vitreous humour if alcohol estimation is required, and also to samples for analysis for cocaine, cyanide and CO. In poisoning by oxalic acid, ethyleneglycol, fluoride and CO, 30 mg. sodium citrate should be added for 10 ml. of blood as preservative. In case of cocaine, plastic bottle should be avoided. In case of CO and CN, airtight caps should be used. In case of volatile poisons, a thin layer of liquid paraffin is put over the top of fluid to avoid evaporation. **One ml of concentrated hydrochloric acid or 100 mg. of thymol or 100 mg. of sodium fluoride can be used for 10 ml urine as a preservative. Toluene is better.** Equal quantity of saturated solution of sodium chloride or rectified spirit can also be used.

Preservative is not necessary if (1) viscera can be analysed within 24 hours, (2) if sample can be kept in a refrigerator or ice box, (3) bone, hair, nails, (4) lung for detecting inhaled poisons.

N.B: The viscera should not be preserved in formaldehyde because extraction of poison, especially non-volatile organic compounds becomes difficult. **For blood grouping and DNA profiling a piece of filter paper or clean cotton gauze can be used to soak up some blood and dried.**

INSTRUCTIONS FOR PRESERVATION AND DESPATCH OF VISCERA: (1) The stomach and its contents, and the small intestine and its contents are preserved in one bottle, and the liver and kidney in another bottle. The blood and urine are preserved separately. (2) **The stomach and intestines are opened before they are preserved. The liver and kidney are cut into small pieces of 0.5 to 1 cm. thickness** or they can be minced in a grinder or mixer. so that they are well-preserved. (3) **The quantity of preservative should be equal to or more than the viscera in bulk.** (4) **Only two-thirds of the capacity of the bottle should be filled with the viscera and preservative** to avoid bursting of bottle if gases of decomposition are formed. (5) The stoppers of bottles should be well-fitted, covered with a piece of cloth, and tied by tape or string and the ends sealed. **The bottles should be sealed as soon as possible to prevent loss of volatile substances and possible contamination by external material.** (6) **The bottles should be labelled** which should contain the name of the victim, age, sex, autopsy number, police station, crime number, the organs it contains, the date and place of autopsy, preservative used and signature. If the contents are infectious, a clearly visible warning should be put on the label. (7) **A sample of the preservative used, i.e., 25 ml of rectified spirit or 25 g of sodium chloride is separately kept in a bottle and sent for analysis, to exclude the possibility of any poison being present as a contaminant.** (8) The sealed bottles containing the viscera and preservative are put into a box which is locked and the lock is sealed using personal or departmental seal. (9) A copy of the inquest report, postmortem report and the authorisation from the Magistrate are sent to the Forensic Science Laboratory along with the viscera. The viscera are not analysed unless there is an authorisation letter from the Magistrate or a police officer not below the rank of Deputy Superintendent, which is issued on an application by the investigating police officer. (10) The key of the box and a sample seal on a piece of paper, corresponding to the seal used on bottles and lock are kept in an envelope, which is sealed and sent with viscera box. (11) The viscera box is handed over to the police constable after taking a receipt, who delivers it personally in the office of the FSL, after obtaining a receipt for the same.

Preservation of additional viscera: In certain cases of poisoning, the following articles are preserved. **(1) Heart:** strychnine, digitalis, yellow oleander. **(2) Brain:** 100 gm. of cerebrum or cerebellum: alkaloids, organophosphorus compounds, opiates, CO, cyanide, strychnine, barbiturates, anaesthetics and volatile organic poisons. **(3) Spinal cord** entire length: strychnine and gelsemium. **(4)** Gallbladder, morphine, cocaine, methadone, glutathione, major tranqulizers. **(5) Fatty tissue from abdominal wall:** Pesticides. **(6) Bile:** It is best removed by puncturing the gall bladder *in situ*. Narcotic drugs, cocaine, urea, creatinine, morphine, glutathione, barbiturates and some tranquilisers. **(7) C.S.F.:** alcohol. **(8) Vitreous humour:** alcohol, chloroform, cocaine, morphine, tricyclic antidepressants, urea creatinine, etc., and for sugar and electrolytes. **(9) Lung:** one lung in gaseous poisons, hydrocyanic acid, alcohol, chloroform, etc. Tie trachea and collect bronchial air. Use a nylon bag which should be heat-sealed. **(10) Skin:** In deaths where hypodermic injection marks, or areas where absorption of poison through the skin may have occurred and in corrosive poisons, an area of 10 cm. radius about the site, with as much underlying fat and muscle as possible, and the whole needle track is removed. Control specimens should be taken from the opposite side of the body. The usual substances injected are insulin, morphine, heroin, cocaine and other illicit drugs. **(11) Bone:** 10 cm. of the shaft of the femur is taken in cases of subacute or chronic poisoning by arsenic, antimony, thallium or radium. **(12) Hair:** An adequate sample (20 to 30) of head hair should be removed with tweezers to remove the roots, and tied in locks. **(13) Nails:** All the nails should be removed entire by inserting the blade of a Spencer-Wells forceps under the nail-plate, grasping it and twisting. Nails also be can removed by dissecting the lateral margins and proximal base. **(14) Uterus:** Uterus and appendages and upper part of vagina are preserved in cases of criminal abortion. Sticks and foreign bodies found in the genital tract are preserved separately. **(15) Muscle:** If the internal organs are badly putrefied, muscle tissue (3x3 cm 50 to 100 g) especially of thigh which is well preserved can be analysed. **In embalmed body the best specimen may be skeletal muscle from the buttock.** **(16) Fat:** 10 g. from abdominal wall or perinephric region in cases of poisoning by pesticides and insecticides.

N.B.: If the contents are infectious, e.g., hepatitis B virus, HIV, tuberculosis, tetanus, anthrax, gas gangrene, etc. or contain radioactives, this must be communicated to the chemical examiner.

The viscera should be refrigerated at about 4°C. if not forwarded to the laboratory. They can be destroyed either after getting the permission from the Magistrate, or when the investigating police officer informs that the case has been closed.

INFORMATION SUPPLIED TO THE LABORATORY: The pathologist should provide all available information to the toxicologist, i.e. (1) brief details of symptoms if any, and length of illness, (2) if poison taken is not known, drugs or poisons to which the deceased was known to have access, including medication being taken, (3) history obtained from family members and friends, (4) postmortem interval before samples were obtained, (5) list of samples provided and sampling site for each and preservatives used, (6) empty containers or medications found at the scene, (7) autopsy findings, and (8) any special risk with the samples, e.g.

hepatitis B virus, AIDS, etc. It is very important to recover and send the container in which the toxic substance had been kept, which narrows the toxicologist's search to one or more specific compounds. The pathologist should not ask the toxiocologist to look for a "general unknown poison" in the viscera preserved.

CAUSE OF DEATH: **The doctor must consider history, description of the fatal environment and circumstances optimally provided by primary sources, treatment leading up to death and manipulation of the body after death which can cause injuries, before arriving an autopsy interpretation.** If the victim was admitted in the hospital, the clinical record must be correlated with the autopsy findings. **He should not confuse effects of therapy with significant trauma.** After completing the postmortem examination, a complete but concise report should be written in duplicate using carbon papers. The first copy is sent to the investigating officer in a sealed cover, and another copy is retained for future reference. Autopsy report should contain a list of specimens and samples retained for further examination. The report should be given on the same day, as the details cannot be accurately recorded from memory, if there is much delay. If laboratory tests have to be carried out, an interim report should be written and later, after obtaining the reports, a supplementary report, modified if necessary is written. It has been said with a considerable measure of truth, that **autopsy reveals the diseases and lesions that the person lived with, and not necessarily those which killed him.** A definite opinion should be given whenever possible, but if the cause of death cannot be found out, it should be mentioned in the report. In such cases, viscera should be preserved and histological and bacteriological examinations carried out. **While giving cause of death, the word 'probably' should be avoided.** In suspected cases of poisoning, the opinion should be kept reserved until the Chemical Examiner's report is received. **The conclusion that death was caused by poison depends on evaluation of clinical, autopsy, toxicologic and circumstantial evidence. If opinions are given to police before evaluation of data are complete, they should be clearly and unmistakably labelled as preliminary impressions, subject to change if and when the facts so warrant.** Further medical or police investigation, chemical analysis, histological and bacteriological examinations, etc. will all modify the interpretation of autopsy findings. **When the findings are less clear-cut, or are multiple, probability of various alternatives can be offered. It must be recognised that the determination of cause and manner of death are opinions, not facts.** The opinion of one medicolegal officer can differ from another. **If the cause of death is not found on autopsy, the opinion as to the cause of death should be given as " undetermined" or "unascertained" and the manner of death as "unknown".** When there are no positive postmortem findings, the cause of death can be inferred from the accurate observations by reliable witnesses, concerning the circumstances of death.

Medical opinions are conclusions based on facts. Some facts, such as gross autopsy findings do not change. Opinions are based on the facts and findings as they are known at the time the opinion is given. If the facts which form the basis for the opinion change, the opinion can and often will change.

Autopsy of Decomposed Bodies: It is a fundamental rule of forensic pathology that **all human remains should be examined, even when they are not likely to provide information. Even when the body shows advanced decomposition, a thorough examination may show a gross traumatic or pathological lesion.** Period of declaring a body as unclaimed is 48 hours. Localised areas of redness may indicate antemortem injury. Incision into the discoloured area may confirm dark-red ecchymoses in the subcutaneous fat and muscle, in contrast to adjacent uninjured yellow or pale-red fat. The skin though discoloured, may show the presence of a gross external injury, e.g., a bullet wound, lacerated wound or incised wound. Fractures are easily detected. Gross pathological lesions may be found, e.g., valvular lesions of the heart. Antemortem thrombi may persist. Calcification of cartilages, changes in sacrum, symphysial surface of pubic bone, changes in joints, colour of hair.

EFFACEMENT OR OBLITERATION OF IDENTITY: The identity of a dead body may be destroyed by the following methods.

(1) Purposive removal of the identifying features, e.g, fingerprints, tattoo marks, scars, moles, teeth, hair, etc. and articles of clothing.

(2) Animals, e.g., rats, dogs, jackals and hyenas and birds, such as vultures may attack a dead body and mutilate it in a very short time, when the body is exposed in an open place.

(3) Burning or incineration.

(4) Advanced putrefaction.

(5) Dismemberment and burying or throwing different parts in different places.

(6) Biocremation or chemical hydrolysis: The body is placed in a stainless steel cremation chamber (similar to pressure cooker), **A mixture of 95% water and 5% of potassium hydroxide is added. 150°C heat and 60 pounds of pressure a square inch is applied. The average adult body takes about 2 to 3 hours to complete a biocremation.** The bones are dried, powdered, placed in an urn and given back to family. The sterile solution is recycled to the earth. It is an environmentally friendly option as it uses less energy and releases less carbon dioxide.

(7) Dismemberment by moving vehicles, like trains or by machinery.

(8) Bomb explosions, which may disintegrate the body.

DNA profiling: DNA profile should be compared by single probe analysis with that of parents, children, siblings and if necessary other relatives from autopsy derived tissues for identification of missing persons.

EXAMINATION OF MUTILATED BODIES OR FRAGMENTS: **Mutilated bodies are those which are extensively disfigured, or in which a limb or a part is lost but the soft tissues, muscles and skin are attached to the bones.** Sometimes, only a part of the body, such as head, trunk or a limb may be found. The scene should be photographed before anything is disturbed. The body parts should be arranged in anatomic order. Appropriate specimens should be obtained for toxicologic analysis and DNA profiling, such as muscle, a piece of long bone, plucked hair.

(1) Human or Animal: Recognition may be made by shape, structure and weight of the objects. This is easy if the head, trunk or limbs are available, but when pieces of muscle only are available without attached skin or viscera, it is very difficult. In such cases, definite opinion can be given by performing

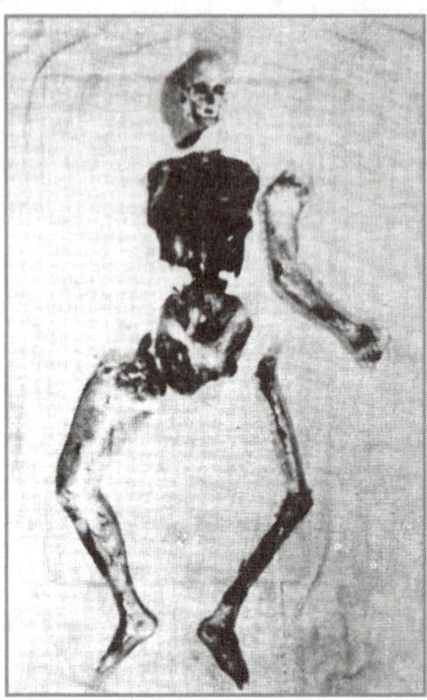

Fig. (5–15). **Reconstruction of dismembered human remains.**

precipitin test, or anti-globulin inhibition test using blood, or any other soft tissue, if the tissue is not severely decomposed.

(2) One or more Bodies: This is determined by fitting together all separate parts. If there is no disparity or reduplication, and if the colour of the skin is same in all parts, they belong to one body. Testing for similarity of blood groups and haemoglobin from different parts is helpful Fig. (5–15).

(3) Sex: It can be determined if the head or trunk is available, from the presence and distribution or absence of hair, characters of the pelvis, skull, etc. It can also be determined from the recognition of prostatic or uterine tissue under a microscope which resist putrefaction, and are found even in advanced state of putrefaction.

(4) Age: Age can be determined from general development, skull, teeth and ossification of bones. Calcification of cartilages, changes in sacrum, symphysial surface of pubic bone, changes in joints, colour of hair.

(5) Stature: It can be determined from the measurement of long bones.

(6) Identity: It can be determined from fingerprints, tattoo marks, scars, moles, hair, teeth, deformities, any disease, absence of any internal organ, etc., articles of clothing and superimposition technique.

(7) Race: It can be determined from hair, skin and skull.

(8) Manner of Separation of Parts: This is determined by examining the margins of the parts, whether they had been cleanly cut, sawn, hacked, lacerated, disarticulated at the joints or gnawed through by animals.

(9) Time since Death: Time since death may be inferred from the progressive changes in the body after death and entomology of cadaver.

(10) Cause of Death: The cause of death can be made out if there is evidence of fatal injury to some vital organ or large blood vessel, or marks of burning or deep cuts or fractures of bones, especially of the skull or the cervical vertebrae, hyoid bone or of several ribs.

(11) Antemortem or Postmortem: This may be determined by examining the margins of parts for evidence of vital reaction. In decomposing bodies, haemorrhage along the wound track on dissection indicates antemortem nature.

EXAMINATION OF BONES

Forensic anthropology is that branch of physical anthropology which for forensic purposes deals with the identification and analysis of skeletonised remains known to be or suspected of being human. The skeletal remains should be examined only by an expert in an institution, where necessary facilities are available.

Sometimes, bones are found disposed off in jungle, in the open, in the ditches or rubbish dumps, etc., or may be found while digging foundations for buildings or skeleton may be exhumed. In case of mass disaster, where many persons die in the same area at the same time from fire, air crashes, etc., the help of the anthropologist is sought in identification, if the remains are skeletonised, badly burned or mostly destroyed.

General Description: Keep the bones in anatomic arrangement and draw a skeletal chart, indicating which bones are present. A complete list of all the bones sent for examination should be prepared, and photographs of all the bones are taken. The sand, dust or earth present on the bones is removed with brushes and wooden picks and scrapers. **Light applications of acetone help to remove tight dirt.** Note the attachment of soft tissues to bones if any, and their stage of putrefaction. The skeletal remains should be first examined in the condition in which they were found with whatever soft tissues present. **Note whether the bones are moist and humid, or dry and their smell.** The bones are then washed by brushing with lukewarm water, and are placed under shelter to dry slowly. If soft tissues are attached, the bones are boiled in water for five to six hours in the case of young bones, and for twelve hours or more in the case of adult bones, or they can be immersed in a dilute aqueous solution of trisodium phosphate and household detergent (sodium hypochlorite 5 to 6%) for several days. With this, the soft parts, including tendon attachments and the periosteum can be removed easily with an ordinary scrubbing brush. It is very difficult to disarticulate a dry skull through outside pressure. The disarticulation is usually done by filling the cranial cavity with a substance that swells when moistened and forces the bones apart through expansion. The specific gravity of a bone, which forms the densest part in the human body is two. Many of the procedures and techniques employed have already been discussed in the chapter on "Identity".

(1) Are the remains actually bones? Sometimes stones or even pieces of wood are mistaken by the public for bones. Anatomical shape and structure will help.

(2) Human or Animal: The knowledge of human as well as comparative anatomy is necessary to find out whether particular bones are human or not. It is easy when whole skeleton or entire bones are available. Difficulties arise when there is marked fragmentation, burnt bones and with smaller bones of some animals, such as digits, metacarpal and metatarsal bones. If the bone is fairly fresh, and some of the blood constituents are still present, the precipitin test is useful. **If the bones are fresh, DNA analysis can be done from the marrow cells for identification of species. Serological tests are not useful in case of bones not having extractable plasma proteins (5 to 15 years old bones), and burnt and cremated bones. Bones of the hand and wrist of bears may be confused with human hands. Microscopic**

structure is also useful, but bones of great apes cannot be distinguished from those of man. Non-human bones contain sheets of plexiform structures in cross-section. **Human and animal bones can also be distinguished by chemical analysis of bone-ash.**

(3) One or more Individuals: This can be determined by reconstructing the skeleton. If there is no disproportion in the size of various bones, or reduplication, articulation is correct, and if the age, sex and race of all the bones is same, they belong to one individual.

If commingling (mixing) of bones from more than one skeleton is suspected, they can be separated by the use of a short wave ultraviolet lamp. When the surface of bones are exposed to ultraviolet radiation, they reflect a variety of colours. The radiated colour is derived from fluorescence of organic elements in the bones, inorganic substances on the surface of the bones, and to a lesser extent reflected light. **The bones of different persons can be segregated by the difference in the colour emissions.**

(4) Sex: Recognisable sex differences are not present before puberty. After puberty, the sex can be determined by examination of the pelvis, skull, manubrium-gladiolus ratio, diameter of head of femur and humerus and measurements of femur, tibia, humerus and radius. In parous women, the dorsal border of pubic symphysis becomes irregular and/or undermined by depression or pits believed to be caused due to trauma during child-bearing. These are called scars of parturition.

(5) Age at Death: It can be determined from examination of teeth, ossific centres, amount of wear and tear in teeth, length of long bones, epiphyseal union, pubic symphysis, closure of skull sutures, cortical resorption, bony lipping, osteoporosis, calcification, osteoarthritic changes, etc. After the completion of bony union, age cannot be determined in an exact number of years. Foetal age can be determined by measuring the length of the ossified portions of the long bones. In case of broken bones, a rough estimate of the age can be made by measuring the external diameter of the long bones at midshaft. Ancient bones are light, brittle and often red-brown.

The general age can also be estimated by the resorption patterns in the cortex of the long bones. In infancy, most resorptive activity is found in the medullary third of the cortex. In childhood, it is scattered throughout the thickness of the cortex, and during adolescence is most marked just under the periosteal surface. In young adulthood, there is very little resorption. Beginning in the sixties in men and earlier in women, the medullary third of the cortex undergoes increasing resorption, with thinning of the cortex from within. These changes in the cortical tissue are microscopic. Kerley has described for the quantifying four cortical elements for estimating age, i.e., osteons, osteon fragments, lamellar bone, and non-haversian canals. With the loss of cancellous tissue, the proximal end of the medullary cavity of humerus assumes a cone-shape, the tip of which gradually ascends and reaches the surgical neck between 41 to 50 years, and the epiphyseal lines between 61 to 74 years. With advancing age, there is gradual fatty replacement of red bone marrow.

(6) Race: There are certain racial differences in the skeleton, chiefly in the skull and face measurements, teeth and lower extremities.

(7) Stature: When the skeleton is incomplete, or severely disintegrated, the stature may be calculated by applying mathematical formulae to the length of the long bones. Long bones must be measured by means of osteometric board; measurement by the use of tapes or calipers are not accurate. **Pearson's formulae (1899)** were used for a number of years. **Trotter and Gleser formulae (1958)** are more satisfactory. **Harrison and Dupertuid** and **Hadder** also published their tables. These formulae have been constructed using skeletons of Europeans and North Americans, and as such are not accurate for Indians. Moreover, there is considerable variation between the different ethnic and geographical groups in India. **The principle of these formulae is to measure the length of long bone and multiply it with a given factor, and then adding a fixed factor. The formulae are different for dry bones and wet bones, for white persons and Negroes, and for males and females.** A single formula cannot suit all parts of India due to different morphological features and racial characters. Steele (1970) has devised a method for estimating stature from fragmented pieces of major long bones. **Formulae for stature are not valid for children, giants or dwarfs.** In Negroes, the femora are proportionally longer and less curved than of other races.

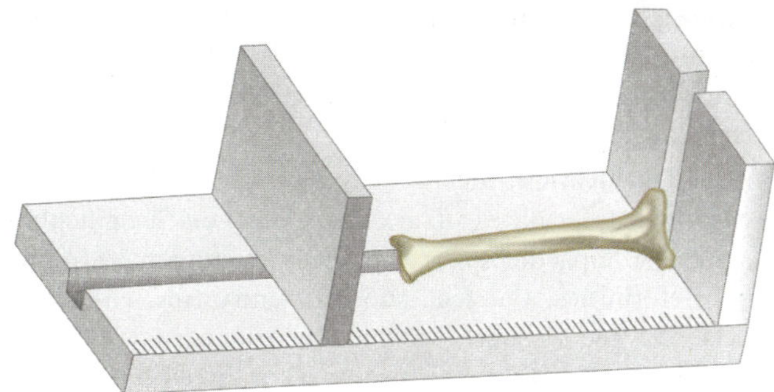

Fig. (5–16). Osteometric board.

Osteometric Board: This has a rectangular base with a ruler fixed along one of its long sides. An upright is fixed at one end of the board, and a second one slides along the board. The bone is placed with one of its ends against the fixed upright and the movable upright is brought up to the other end of the bone. The distance between the uprights is then shown on the ruler. Hepburn osteometric board modified by Trevor is commonly used Fig. (5–16).

If osteometric board is not available, the bones should be measured on a flat bench with the maximum lengths taken between two vertical, parallel boards placed in contact with the bone ends. If the bones are covered with articular cartilage, subtract for radius and humerus 3 mm. each, tibia 5 mm. and femur 7 mm. before applying the formulae.

Weight-bearing long bones are used for applying these formulae. Femur and tibia give more accurate results than humerus or radius. The average stature obtained from a measurement of more than one long bone gives a more accurate result than when calculated for a single bone. Right side bones are normally measured in the dry state without cartilage. **The results obtained are not quite accurate, and the error may be up to 2.5 cm.** Measurements of femur, tibia, humerus and radius are useful. Long bone lengths are measured as follows: (1) Femur: Head to medial condlye. (2) Tibia: Lateral condyle to tip of medial malleolus. (3) Fibula: Tip of head to tip of lateral malleolus. (4) Radius: Medial margin of head to tip of styloid process. (5) Ulna: Top of head to tip of styloid process. (6) Humerus: Trochlea to the head. **A useful rule of thumb is that the humerus is 20%,**

the tibia 22%, the femur 27%, and the spine 35%, of the individual's height in life. In the absence of long bones, adult stature can be calculated from the articular length of the five metacarpals.

(8) Identification: Identity may be established from teeth, disease and deformities of the bone, old healed or healing fractures, orthopaedic surgical procedures, regional atrophy, spinal deformities, flat feet, supernumerary ribs, congenital defects, etc., and by superimposition technique using the skull. **In the skull, all major dimensions are reduced by 1 to 2% by drying. In the vertebral column, total length is reduced by 2.7% by drying.** If previous X-rays are available, it may be possible to make positive identification on the basis of contours and cancellous patterns of various bones and the profile of the pituitary fossa. Dental charts and dental radiographs are also useful. Other methods include X-ray comparison of trabecular patterns and neutron activation analysis to distinguish the relative mineral contents. Certain diseases and developmental problems can lead to asymmetry of human skeleton from side to side, such as poliomyelitis, Paget's disease, neurofibromatosis. **It may be possible to identify the ABO group of skeletal material.** Identity can be established by DNA typing of tooth pulp, soft tissue, bone marrow of sternum or femur and compared with DNA profile of parents, children or siblings of the deceased. **In anatomically dissected bodies bones smell of formalin and red lead is present in blood vessels.**

(9) Nature of Injury: The ends of the long bones should be examined carefully to find out if they have been cut by sharp cutting instruments or hacked or sawn or gnawed through by animals. If the body disintegrates naturally, articular surfaces are smooth.

ANIMAL BITES: Rodents cause characteristic parallel grooves "chisel marks" due to gnawing. Dog, fox and wolf cause heavy damage by gnawing, beginning with softer cancellous articular regions and flat bones, moving to shafts of long bones and skull. Carnivora tooth marks include puncture through thin bones, pits or indentations when penetration did not occur and furrows from molars scraping the bone. Spiral fractures of long bones occur with strong jawed larger canids. Deer and sheep hold bones with back teeth which may be partially broken to give "fork-shaped" or "double-pronged" fragment. Crabs, fish and turtle may leave shallow marks.

In a skeleton, usually the inside of the skull is filled with earth. As the earth dries, it forms a hard ball which can cause fragmentation of skull in transit. Postmortem conditions may cause fractures and fragmentation due to continued and repeated freezing and thawing and from the pressures of shifting soil weight.

Burnt bones: Depending upon the degree of heat applied, the bone will be more or less destroyed. Heat makes the bones brittle, so that breakage may occur during collection. **The shape of burnt bone is preserved, but it becomes powder when pressed between the fingers. In a burnt skull, the cracking often has a circular pattern with sharp edges, which look like cuts. Whether the bones have been burned with flesh covering them or in the dried state can be made out from their appearance.** This is important to know whether the body was disposed off imme-diately after death, or after the decomposition of the soft parts. Unprotected bone when burnt undergoes charring, cracking (usually transverse), splintering and may be reduced to ashes, whereas bone embedded in thick, soft tissue shows the melted, guttered condition characteristic of fusion by heat. A bone burnt in the open is white, but when burnt in a closed fire, black or ash-grey.

(10) Time since Death: Determination of the time of death by the appearance of the skeletal remains, such as presence or absence of ligaments, cartilages, etc. is very difficult due to the various factors, such as burial or non-burial, the type of soil, climatic conditions, particularly temperature and humidity, accessibility of insects, carnivorous animals, etc. Due to bleaching by the sun, the bones appear pale ivory. **The answer depends upon the circumstances under which the bones have been found, e.g., burial and cold weather will diminish decomposition.** When force is applied on living or recently dead bone, particularly those of skull, bending, twisting and distortion are possible, referred to as plastic deformation. When force is applied to dry, dehydrated, brittle bone, it will fracture and fragment. **After the soft tissues disappear, pieces of cartilage and ligaments remain attached to bone for 3 to 4 months or more. Traces of marrow and periosteum may remain in, or attached to the bones for several months.** A fairly recent bone is slightly greasy to the touch and is heavy. **Odour is a good indication of relatively recent death.** After the bones have lost the covering tissue, and the odour of decomposition is lost, the bones still appear fresh. Repeated freezing and thawing of the bones when buried superficially may cause a bone to expand and crack within a few years. In older burials, the cancellous bone at the metaphyses and epiphyses may be eroded away by weathering. Ground-water seepage may leach the normal calcium phosphate out of bone in non-biological distributions, or may deposit excess calcium carbonate, depending on the nature of the ground water. In mineral-rich areas, leached areas are found in some parts of the skeleton and heavily mineralised bone in others. This can be detected by examining histological ground-section of long bones or by microradiographs of un-decalcified ground-section of these bones. **A fairly recent bone is slightly greasy to the touch, and is heavy** due to the persistence of collagen and the normal apatite matrix. Bones tend to absorb iron salts, pigments and fine sand from the percolation of water and may become heavily impregnated, so that after many years they are dark in colour and weigh more than the original dry bone.

DATING OF BONES: The date of a bone can be corroborated by following methods (Knight). (1) A recent bone will have about 4 to 5 g.% of nitrogen which gradually diminishes with decay. Between 50 to 100 years, the nitrogen content is more than 3.5 g. %, and if it is more than 2.5 g.%, the age will be less than 350 years. (2) A fresh bone shows about 15 amino acids mostly derived from collagen. Glycine and analine are predominant. A bone more than 100 years old will contain 7 amino acids. Proline and hydroxyproline tend to disappear after 50 years. (3) A bone less than 100 years old fluoresces in ultraviolet light over most of its cut surface. There is progressive loss, and it is absent in 500 to 800 years. (4) Blood pigments persist up to 100 years since death in temperate zones. (5) Precipitin tests are negative after about 10 years. (6) There is no significant fall in the C^{14} content of bones during the first century after death. After prolonged burial, probably over 50 years, histological examination of ground-sections of bone may show globular pockets of resorption, which result from the acid balance of the bacteria and their byproducts. Ancient bones tend to be dry, brittle, chalky and the marrow cavity is dry, free of fat and often contains particles of earth or sand. Minerals in the bone may be replaced chemically by minerals in the sediments, while maintaining the original shape of the bones, a process termed diagenesis. This occurs over a long time periods and leads to fossilisation.

(11) Cause of Death: The cause of death cannot be made out unless there is evidence of fracture or injuries which usually cause death, e.g., fractures of skull bones, upper cervical vertebrae, hyoid bone, several ribs or marks of deep cuts in long bones or marks of burning. The bones should be examined for foreign bodies, knife-blade, firearm injuries or any disease, e.g., caries or necrosis. The type of the weapon can be known from the type and depth of the cut in the bone. Metallic poisons, e.g., arsenic, antimony, lead or mercury can be found in bones long after death. Arsenic can be detected even in burnt bones. Presence of diatoms in bone marrow indicates death from drowning.

CASE: (1) ALAVANDER MURDER CASE: Alavander, aged 42 years was murdered on 28th August, 1952, by Prabhakar Menon, with the help of his wife Devaki, who had confessed to the husband of having been seduced by Alavander. The next day, his headless trunk with arms and legs was found in the third class compartment of Indo-Ceylon Express at Manamadura station. Two days later, his head was found at Royapuram sea beach, Chennai. The identity was established from the fingerprints, circumcised penis, socks, waist thread, overriding canine teeth and pierced earlobes.

(2) THE ACID-BATH MURDER CASE: John George Haigh took Mrs. Olive Durand Deacon, a rich widow to Crawlye in his car, on 18-2-1949. There, he took her into a store shed, shot her through the back of the head, removed her Persian lamb coat and jewellery and put her fully clothed in a steel tank and filled it with strong sulphuric acid. After 3 days, he removed some fat and bones floating in sludge in the tank, and then pumped some more acid into the tank. On the next day, he poured off the contents of the tank on the ground opposite the door. A number of fragments of tissues, bones, intact upper and lower acrylic dentures and gallstones, were found in the acid sludge. A London dentist recognised the dentures as made for Mrs. Durand Deacon. Bloodstained lamb coat and jewellery were also identified. Haigh was arrested, charged with murder and convicted.

(3) PARKMAN-WEBSTER CASE: Dr. Parkman, who had loaned money to Professor Webster was lured into the chemistry laboratory of Dr. Webster on 2-11-1949, where he was killed with a knife. The body was mutilated, then destroyed in a furnace and by chemical agents. A week later, an entire trunk of a human body with left thigh and some artificial teeth were recovered from Webster's laboratory. The age, sex and stature tallied with those of Dr. Parkman. The dentist, Mr. Keep, who had attended Dr. Parkman, identified the blocks of mineral teeth recovered from the furnace. He demonstrated that mandibular mineral blocks fitted the original plaster model which he had preserved. Webster was tried and convicted.

(4) THE RUXTON CASE: Two women, Mrs. Isabella Ruxton, wife of Dr. Ruxton, aged 35 years and Mary Rogerson, their maid, aged 20 years, disappeared from the house of Dr. Ruxton in Lancaster on 15-9-1935. A quantity of human remains (70 portions) were found in a ravine near Moffat, about 107 miles from Lancaster. The remains consisted chiefly of two heads, thorax, pelvis, segments of the upper and lower limbs, three breasts, portions of female external genitals, and the uterus and its appendages. The disarticulation had been carried out without damage suggesting the anatomical knowledge of the person. Both bodies had been mutilated to remove all evidence of identity and sex. All the remains were assembled and found to represent two female bodies, aged about 35 to 45 years and 18 to 22 years, respectively. Casts of the left feet of the two women fitted perfectly shoes belonging to Mrs. Ruxton and her maid. Superimposition of photographs of the skull on life-size photographs of the heads of two women were found to tally in every respect. The fingernails of the younger were scratched and her finger prints tallied with prints found on many articles in the house of Dr. Ruxton. The newspapers and certain garments found with the bodies were useful in identification. Entomologist was able to show that the parts were thrown in the ravine 12–14 days prior to discovery. The parts assigned to Mrs. Ruxton showed signs of asphyxia and fracture of the hyoid bone, suggesting strangulation. In the body assigned to Mary Rogerson, there was a fracture on the top of skull. A number of human blood stains were found in the bathroom and on the stair carpets and pads, in the house of the accused. Fragments of human tissue were found in the drain traps and a suit of clothes of the accused was contaminated with blood. Dr. Ruxton was found guilty of murder and sentenced to death.

(5) NAGARAJU CASE: A doctor in the Indian Army, killed his wife and daughter by manual strangulation in a train during their journey from Delhi to Secunderabad. In a hotel bathroom at Secunderabad, he neatly dismembered his wife's body into portions convenient for transport, and dumped them at various places in a nearby tank, tied in pieces of a saree, house coat and hand bag, to cover up the crime. The left lower limb was carried by a stray dog to nearby residential quarters, which was the starting point of the police investigation. The search of the bank led to the recovery of upper and lower trunk portions in two pieces, right lower limb, left upper limb, the skull devoid of soft tissues and brain, and mandible. The intact body of female child 14 months old, fully clothed was also found along with the human remains. The disarticulation had been carried out without damage, suggesting the anatomical knowledge of the culprit. All the remains were assembled and found to represent a female body aged between 20 to 25 years, 158 to 159 cm. in stature. Superimposition of the photographs of the skull on life-size photograph of the head of the woman were found to tally in every respect. The police investigation and the medical examination established the identity of the deceased and culprit. Faced with the evidence and to cheat the gallows, the culprit committed suicide.

EXHUMATION

Exhumation is the digging out of an already buried body legally from the grave. There is no time limit for exhumation in India.

Legal issues: Autopsies are performed on exhumed bodies: (1) In criminal cases, such as homicide, suspected homicide disguised as suicide or other types of death, suspicious poisoning, death as a result of criminal abortion and criminal negligence. (2) In civil cases, such as accidental death claim, insurance, workmen's compensation claim, liability for professional negligence, survivorship and inheritance claims or disputed identity.

Authorisation: The body is exhumed only when, there is a **written order from the Executive Magistrate** (S. 176, Cr.P.C). The body can be exhumed by any government doctor.

Procedure: Detailed information about the alleged deceased and the clothes worn at the time of burial is necessary before starting exhumation. The body is exhumed under the supervision of a medical officer and Magistrate in the presence of a police officer. Wherever practicable, the Magistrate should inform the relatives of the deceased, and allow them to remain present at the enquiry (176(4) Cr.P.C.). **The grave site should be positively identified** with identifying features, such as location of burial plot, the headstone, and gravemarker. The distance of the grave from some of the permanent objects like trees, rocks, road or fence should be noted. **It should be conducted in natural light.** If the grave is in an open place with lot of spectators, the area should be screened off by holding up sheets around the body or vehicles may be used to block visibility from the public. The burial should be uncovered 10 to 15 cm. at a time, and notes should be made about the condition of the soil, water content and vegetable growth. Measure the depth of the grave from the surface to the skull and from the surface to the feet. If possible, the burial pit should be opened up to 30 cm. on all sides of the body. Expose the body with the use of a soft brush or whisk broom. After the dirt has been removed from above and around the corpse, it should be photographed in the position in which it was found. A drawing of the grave and body or skeleton should be made noting all the details, e.g., if the face is up, or to the right, arms are extended, or the lower limbs are flexed. **If decomposition is not advanced, a plank or a plastic or canvas sheet should then be lowered to the level of the earth on which the body rests, the body gently shifted on to planks or sheet and then removed from the grave.** If skeletonisation is advanced, then it may become necessary to dig down beside and then beneath the body so that some firm material, such as a sheet of hardboard may gradually be inserted under the body, which can then be lifted and transported on it. Record the condition of the remains, e.g., fully intact and solid, eroding and friable, charred. If the body is disintegrated, remove all elements and place them in bags or boxes. If the body is skeletonised, after removing the remains, the soil must be sifted in a finely-meshed screen to recover smaller objects, e.g., teeth, epiphyses, bullets, etc.

The condition of the burial clothes and the surface of the body should be noted. In cases of suspected mineral poisoning, samples of the earth (about half kg.) in actual contact with the body and also from above, below and from each side should be collected. Any fluid or debris in the coffin should also be collected. A portion of the coffin and burial clothes must be removed in order to exclude any possibility of contamination from external sources. The body should be identified by close relatives and friends. All personal effects, clothing, hair, nails, etc., should be picked up for examination.

Autopsy: Disinfectants should not be sprinkled on the body. If the body has been buried recently, the postmortem examination is conducted in the usual manner. **Various artifacts have to be interpreted correctly.** In much putrefied bodies, an attempt should be made to establish the identity. All the viscera should be preserved for chemical analysis. If the body is reduced to skeleton, the bones should be examined.

SECOND AUTOPSY: Before performing the second autopsy, the doctor should obtain all the available documents relating to the case, especially the first autopsy report, photographs of the scene of death of the body taken during first autopsy, inquest papers of first PM, hospital records, police investigative reports, X-rays, etc. **If possible the first autopsy pathologist should be called to correlate all the findings. Contusions become visible when the blood is drained from the tissues following the first autopsy.** Decomposition causes merger of the contusions with blurring of their patterns. The interpretation of the findings of a second autopsy performed on a previously autopsied exhumed body is difficult due to the progressive decomposition changes, various artifacts of burial and exhumation, previous removal and dissection of viscera, and serious alterations resulting from the first autopsy. Videograph the autopsy. The findings should be documented in great detail, whether the findings are confirmatory or contradictory from the result of first autopsy. It is possible that valuable results may be obtained. **Even if no new information is obtained from the second autopsy, it will help in putting an end to rumours or suspicions.**

CHAPTER

6 DEATH AND ITS CAUSE

FM 2.1: Define, describe and discuss death and its types including somatic/clinical and cellular molecular death, and brain-death, cortical death and brainstem death.
FM 2.2: Describe and discuss natural and unnatural deaths.
FM 2.3: Describe and discuss issues related to sudden natural deaths.
FM 2.5: Discuss moment of death, modes of death— coma, asphyxia and syncope.
FM 2.13: Describe and discuss obscure autopsy.
FM 4.7: Describe and discuss the ethics related to HIV patients.

Thanatology (thanatos = death) deals with death in all its aspects, including changes that occur with and after death. There is a progression from clinical death to brain death, biological death and then cellular death. Brain death follows clinical death immediately due to lack of oxygen. First the cerebral cortex, then cerebellum and then lower brain centres die. Ultimately the brain stem and the vital centres die. Thereafter the process of cellular death begins.

S.46, I.P.C.: Death denotes death of a human being unless the contrary appears from the context. Registration of Births and Deaths Act, Sec. 2(b) defines death as permanent disappearance of all evidence of life at any time after livebirth has taken place.

Types: (1) somatic, systemic or clinical, and (2) molecular or cellular.

SOMATIC DEATH: It is the complete and irreversible stoppage of the circulation, respiration and brain functions (Bishop's triad of life), but there is no legal definition of death. Nicolas Bishop's triad of life (1638–1686) is circulation, respiration and brain function. Another is Bichat's mode of death (1771–1802) is asphyxia (stoppage of respiration), coma (stoppage of brain function), syncope (stoppage of circulation). According to current concept, somatic death is death of brainstem. The question of death is important in resuscitation and organ transplantation. **As long as circulation of oxygenated blood is maintained to the brain stem, life exists.** Whether the person is alive or dead can only be tested by withdrawal of artificial maintenance. **A person who cannot survive upon withdrawal of artificial maintenance is dead.**

Organ transplantation: The success of a homograft mainly depends upon the type of tissue involved, and the rapidity of its removal after circulation has stopped in the donor. Cornea can be removed from the dead body within 6 hours, skin in 24 hours, bone in 48 hours and blood vessels within 72 hours for transplanatation. Kidneys, heart, lungs, pancreas, intestines, and liver must be obtained soon after circulation has stopped as they deteriorate rapidly. The recipient body does not reject a transplanted cornea. Cornea donors range in age from newborn to 70 years or older. Most bone transplants last the life of the individual.

THE MOMENT OF DEATH: Death is not an event, it is a process. Historically (medically and legally), the concept of death was that of "heart and respiration death", i.e. spontaneous stoppage of heart and lung functions. Heart-lung bypass machines, mechanical respirators and other devices, however have changed this medically in favour of a new concept "brain death", that is, irreversible loss of cerebral function.

BRAIN DEATH: It is of three types: (1) CORTICAL OR CEREBRAL DEATH with an intact brain stem. This produces a vegetative state in which respiration continues, but there is total loss of power of perception by the senses. This state of deep coma can be produced by cerebral hypoxia, toxic conditions or widespread brain injury. (2) BRAINSTEM DEATH, where the cerebrum may be intact, though cut off functionally by the stem lesion. The tissue in the floor of the aqueduct, between the third and fourth ventricles of the brain contains ascending reticular activating system, which extends throughout the brainstem from the spinal cord to the subthalamus, determines arousal. The loss of the vital centres that control respiration, and of the ascending reticular activating system that sustains consciousness, cause the victim to be irreversibly comatose and incapable of spontaneous breathing. This can be produced by raised intracranial pressure, cerebral oedema, intracranial haemorrhage, etc. It is well recognised that brainstem death is compatible with aspects of "brain life". For example, neurological regulation of hormonal secretion, an electroencephalographic activity possibly representing cortical function, commonly exist even when the formal criteria for diagnosing brain death are satisfied. (3) WHOLE BRAIN DEATH, i.e. permanent cessation of functions of cerebrum, cerebellum and brainstem.

FUNCTIONS OF BRAINSTEM: A properly functioning paramedian tegmental area of the brain stem is a precondition for full consciousness which enables the cerebral hemispheres to work in an integrated way. Lesions of this part are associated with profound coma. The brainstem is also responsible for the respiratory drive, and in large measure (but not exclusively) for the maintenance of blood pressure. All motor output from the brain travel through the brainstem. Apart from vision and smell, all the sensory traffic coming into the brain arrives through the brainstem. The brainstem also mediates the cranial nerve reflexes.

If the brainstem is damaged due to trauma, cerebral oedema, haemorrhage, hypoxia or infection, such as poliomyelitis, respiratory motor system fails and damage to the ascending reticular activating system causes permanent loss of consciousness, and higher centres in the cortex are also irreversibly damaged causing **'whole brain death'.**

Harvard Criteria For Determining Brainstem Death: **(1) Unreceptivity and unresponsivity:** Total unawareness to externally applied stimuli and inner need and complete unresponsiveness to even the most intense painful stimuli. **(2) No movements:** No spontaneous muscular movements in response to stimuli such as pain, touch, sound or light for a period of at least one hour. **(3) Apnoea:** Absence of spontaneous breathing for at least one hour. **(4) Absence of elicitable reflexes. (5) Irreversible coma** with abolition of central nervous system activity is evidenced in part by the absence of elicitable reflexes. The pupils are fixed and dilated and do not respond to a direct source of bright light. **(6) Isoelectric EEG:** It has confirmatory value.

All these tests should be repeated after 24 hours with no change. Further it is stressed that the patient be declared dead before any effort is made to take him off the ventilator, if he is then on a ventilator. This declaration should not be delayed until he has been taken off the respirator and all artificially stimulated signs have ceased.

Diagnosis of Brainstem Death: Exclusions: (1) Where the patient may be under the effects of drugs, e.g. therapeutic drugs or overdoses. (2) Where the core temperature of the body is below 35°C. (3) Where the patient is suffering from severe metabolic or endocrine disturbances which may lead to severe but reversible coma, e.g., diabetes.

Preconditions of diagnosis: (i) Patient must be deeply comatose. (ii) Patient must be maintained on a ventilator. (iii) Cause of the coma must be known.

Personnel who should perform the tests: (1) Brainstem death tests must be performed by two medical practitioners. (2) Doctors involved should be experts in this field. Under no circumstances are brainstem death tests performed by transplant surgeons. (3) At least one of the doctors should be of consultant status. Junior doctors are not permitted to perform these tests. (4) Each doctor should perform the tests twice.

TESTS TO BE PERFORMED: Before the tests are performed the core temperature of the body is taken to ensure that it is above 35°C. The diagnosis of brainstem death is established by testing the function of the cranial nerves which pass through the brainstem, such as (pupillary response to light, corneal reflex, vestibulo-ocular reflex, gag or cough reflex, grimacing). If there is no response to these tests, the brainstem is considered to be irreversibly dead.

Certification: When two doctors have performed these tests twice with negative results, the patient is pronounced dead and a death certificate can be issued.

There are two distinct schools of diagnosing death: (1) French and English schools that are similar to Harvard. (2) Austro-German school that includes Harvard criteria and bilateral serial angiography of internal carotid and vertebral artery criteria. A negative angiogram for more than 15 minutes proves death.

VEGETATIVE STATE: Whole or part of the brain can be irreversibly damaged due to hypoxia, cardiac arrest, intracranial haemorrhage, poisoning and trauma to the brain. If the cortex alone is damaged, the patient passes into deep coma, but the brainstem will function to maintain spontaneous respiration. This is called "persistent vegetative state" and death may occur months or years later due to extension of cerebral damage or from intercurrent infection. They are not in need of life-sustaining treatment but require nutrition and hydration. In this the patient breathes spontaneously, has a stable circulation and shows cycles of eye opening and closing which may simulate sleep and waking, but is unaware of the self and the environment. Commonest causes are diffuse axonal injury and diffuse ischaemic brain damage. There is widespread bilateral damage to the neocortex, diffuse damage to white matter, and bilateral damage to the thalami.

TISSUE AND ORGAN TRANSPLANTATION: (1) **Homologous donation** means grafting of the tissue from one part of the body to another in the same patient, such as skin or bone. **(2) Live donation** includes blood and bone marrow transfusion. Live organ donation include kidney and parts of the liver. **(3) Cadaveric donation:** Most organs must be obtained while the donor heart is still beating to improve chances of success.

Xenograft is grafting of animal tissue into humans, which has limited success. **Zoonoses** are transmission of animal diseases.

THE BEATING-HEART DONOR: After brainstem death has been established, the retention of the patient on the ventilator facilitates a fully oxygenated cadaver transplant, the so-called "beating-heart donor". The results of the transplant are much improved. This has no legal sanction.

'Supravital period' or 'intermediary life' is the period of survival of some tissues after irreversible circulatory arrest.

The latency period is an undisturbed period characterised by continuing aerobic energy production which is limited by the oxygen reserve.

The **resuscitation period** is the duration of complete ischaemia after which the ability to recover expires, during which there is a breakdown of ATP to below 60% of the normal value and a steep increase of lactic acid. The resuscitation period of the heart is 3 to 4 minutes.

MOLECULAR DEATH: It **means the death of cells and tissues individually, which takes place usually one to two hours after the stoppage of the vital functions. Molecular death occurs piecemeal.** Individual cells will live on their residual oxygen for a variable time after the circulation has stopped, depending on the metabolic activity of the cell. The subsequent changes occur due to metabolic dysfunction and later from structural disintegration. Nervous tissues die rapidly, the vital centres of the brain in about five minutes, but the muscles live up to one to two hours.

Mechanical excitability of skeletal muscle: (1) Tendon reaction or Zasko's phenomenon: Striking the lower third of the quadriceps femoris muscle about 10 cm. above the patella with a reflex hammer causes an upward movement of the patella because of contraction of the whole muscle. This can be seen up to 1 to 2 hours after death. It seems to be a propogated excitation of muscle fibres.

(2) Idiomuscular contraction or bulge: Striking at the biceps brachii muscle with the back of a knife causes a muscular bulge at the point of contact due to local contraction of the muscle. In the second phase lasting for 4 to 5 hours, a strong and typically reversible idiomuscular pad develops. In the last phase, a weak idiomuscular pad develops between 8 to 12 hours, which may persist up to 24 hours.

Electrical excitability of skeletal muscles of the face may be observed for few hours after death.

ANOXIA: According to Gordon (1944) the stoppage of vital functions depend upon tissue anoxia. **Anoxia means "lack of oxygen".** It may be: **(1) Anoxic anoxia: In this type, oxygen cannot reach the blood, because of lack of oxygen in the lungs.** This occurs: (a) from breathing in a contaminated atmosphere, e.g., from exposure to the fumes in wells and tanks, or from exposure to sewer gas, (b) from mechanical interference with the passage of air into or down the respiratory tract, e.g., in smothering, choking, hanging, strangulation, drowning, traumatic asphyxia and certain forms of acute poisoning. **(2) Anaemic anoxia:** In this type, **oxygen-carrying capacity of the blood is reduced,** e.g., acute massive haemorrhage, poisoning by carbon monoxide, chlorates, nitrates, coal-tar derivatives. **(3) Stagnant anoxia:** In this type, **impaired circulation results in a reduction of oxygen delivery to the tissues,** e.g., heart failure, embolism and shock. **(4) Histotoxic anoxia:** In this type, the **enzymatic processes** by which the oxygen in the blood is used by the tissues **are blocked,** e.g., acute cyanide poisoning.

Anoxic anoxia due to lack of oxygen in the inspired air or mechanical obstruction to respiration is usually known as asphyxia or mechanical asphyxia. **These four types of anoxia ultimately lead to cardiac failure and death.**

Modes of Death: The mode of death refers to the abnormal physiological state that pertained at the time of death. According to Bichat, there are three modes of death, depending on whether death begins in one or other of the three systems, irrespective of what the remote causes of death may be. These modes are: (1) Asphyxia, (2) Coma, and (3) Syncope.

ASPHYXIA

Asphyxia is a condition caused by interference with respiration, or due to lack of oxygen in respired air, due to which the organs and tissues are deprived of oxygen (together with failure to eliminate CO_2), causing unconsciousness or death. The term asphyxia indicates a mode of dying, rather than a cause of death. Young and middle-aged adults have almost complete saturation of their arterial blood with oxygen, at a level of 90–100 mm Hg (12–13.5 KPa), while in persons above 60 years, it is between 60–85 mm Hg (8–10 KPa). In severe to fatal asphyxia it falls to between 20–40 mm Hg (3–5 KPa), which results in hypoxia even though haemoglobin is 90% saturated. **The brain weight is about 1.4% of body weight, but it uses 20% of total available oxygen.** Nervous tissues are affected first by deficiency of oxygen and their functions are disturbed even by a mild oxygen deficiencies. In total ischaemia of brain, cessation of nerve cell function in the cerebral cortex starts after 8 to 15 seconds and in the brainstem ganglia after 25 to 30 seconds. Irreparable damage occurs in the cells of cortex after about 3 minutes; in basal ganglia after 6 to 7 minutes and in vagal centre after about 9 to 10 minutes. **Subnormal oxygen in the blood supply to the brain causes rapid unconsciousness. In all forms of asphyxia, heart may continue to beat for several minutes after stoppage of respiration. The Rule of thumb is: breathing stops within twenty seconds of cardiac arrest, and heart stops within twenty minutes of stopping of breathing.** If the heart functions for several minutes after stoppage of breathing, the weight of the lungs may increase to 450 to 500 g.

Types and Causes: (1) Mechanical: In this the **air-passages are blocked mechanically.** (a) Closure of the external respiratory orifices, as by closing the nose and mouth with the hand or a cloth or by filling these openings with mud or other substance, as in smothering. (b) Closure of the air passages by external pressure on the neck, as in hanging, strangulation, throttling, etc. (c) Closure of the air-passages by the impaction of foreign bodies in the larynx or pharynx as in choking. (d) Prevention of entry of air due to the air-passages being filled with fluid, as in drowning. (e) External compression of the chest and abdominal walls interfering with respiratory movements, as in traumatic asphyxia.

(2) Pathological: In this, the **entry of oxygen to the lungs is prevented by disease of the upper respiratory tract or of the lungs,** e.g., bronchitis, acute oedema of the glottis, laryngeal spasm, tumours and abscess. Paralysis of the respiratory muscles may result from acute poliomyelitis.

(3) Toxic: Poisonous substances prevent the use of oxygen. (a) The capacity of haemoglobin to bind oxygen is reduced, e.g., poisoning by CO. (b) The enzymatic processes, by which the oxygen in the blood is utilised by the tissues are blocked, e.g., cyanides. (c) Respiratory centre may be paralysed in poisoning by opium, barbiturates, strychnine, etc. (d) The muscles of respiration may be paralysed by poisoning by gelsemium.

(4) Environmental: (a) **Insufficiency of oxygen in the inspired air,** e.g., enclosed places, trapping in a disused refrigerator or trunk. (b) **Exposure to irrespirable gases** in the atmosphere, e.g. sewer gas, CO, CO_2. (c) Exposure to high altitude.

(5) Traumatic: (a) **Pulmonary thromboembolism** from femoral vein thrombosis due to an injury to the lower limb. (b) **Pulmonary fat embolism** from fracture of long bones. (c) **Pulmonary air embolism** from an incised wound of internal jugular vein. (d) **Bilateral pneumothorax** from injuries to the chest wall or lungs.

(6) Postural asphyxia: This is seen where an **unconscious or stuporous person,** either from alcohol, drugs or disease, **lies with the upper half of the body lower than the remainder.**

(7) Iatrogenic is mainly associated with anaesthesia.

Pathology: Compression of neck: When the neck is compressed, occlusion of jugular veins prevents venous drainage from the head, but the arterial supply continues through the carotid and vertebral arteries. When the air-passages are occluded, the impaired oxygenation in the lungs causes decrease in the oxygen content of arterial blood. **Reduction in oxygen tension causes capillary dilation which is followed by stasis of blood in the dilated capillaries and venules, which produces capillo-venous engorgement. This blood stasis causes congestion of organs,** and venous return to the heart is diminished leading to anoxia, which causes capillary dilatation and the vicious cycle goes on **Fig. (6–1).**

(1) Petechial haemorrhages are caused due to **raised venous pressure from impaired venous return resulting in overdistension and rupture of venules, especially in lax tissues and not due to hypoxia of the vessel walls. A minimum of 15 to 30 seconds is required to produce congestion and petechiae. Petechiae vary in size from 0.1 to 2 mm. If larger than this they are called ecchymoses.** Sometimes, large haemorrhages

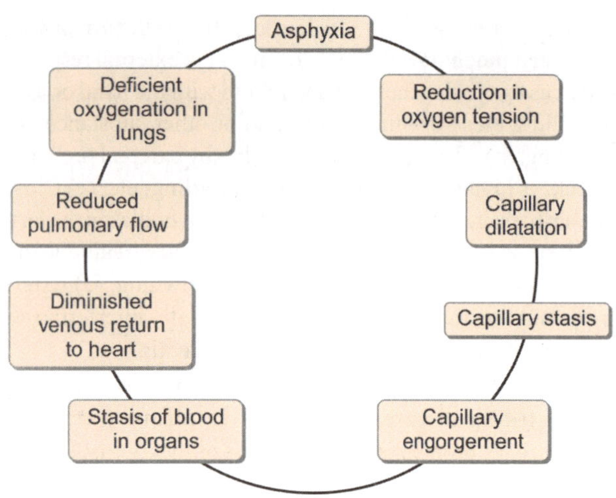

Fig. (6–1). Vicious cycle of asphyxia.

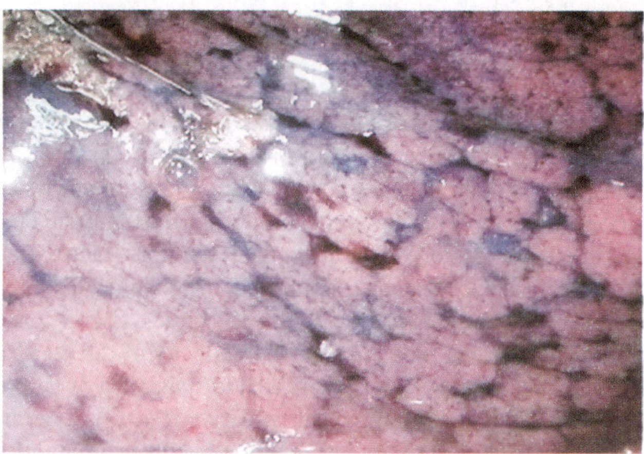

Fig. (6–4). Tardieu spots present over subpleural surface (petechial haemorrhages—true Tardieu sports mostly seen over visceral surface of pleura).

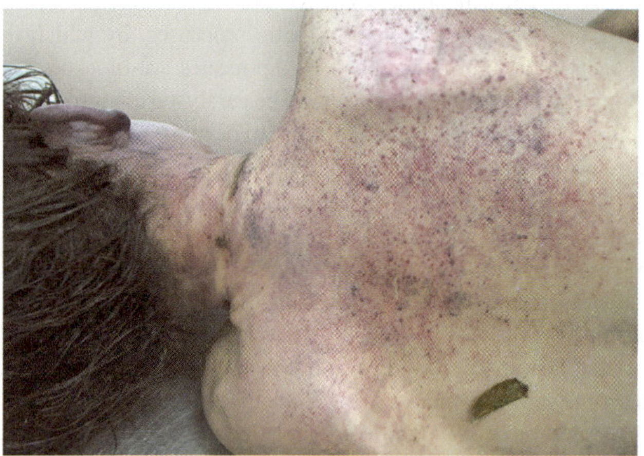

Fig. (6–2). Petechial haemorrhages over the back of chest.

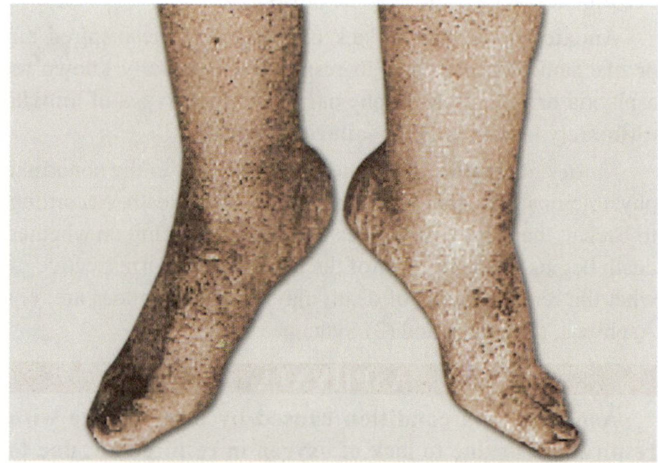

Fig. (6–5). Tardieu spots on feet and legs (dependent areas) in a case of hanging.

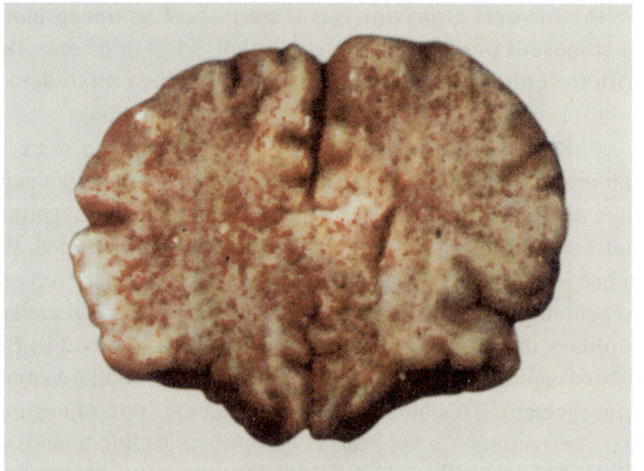

Fig. (6–3). Petechial haemorrhages in the brain.

are seen on upper chest and back of the body Fig. (6–2). **Petechiae are seen in the skin, sclerae, conjunctivae, outer and inner surfaces of the eyelids and on the mucosal surfaces in the mouth. Petechial haemorrhages may be found in the substance of the viscera, such as brain** Fig. (6–3) **but they are readily seen in serous membranes, particularly in the visceral pleura** Fig. (6–4) in the interlobar fissures and around the hilum and pericardium. In infants and children, thymus may show numerous petechiae. In the brain, they are seen in white matter and there may be larger patches of bleeding in the subarachnoid space where superficial vessels have ruptured due to acute venous engorgement. **When carotid arteries are obstructed, intensity of cerebral, facial, and orbital petechiae are much less prominent,** than what is seen in cases where venous obstruction predominates. In sudden complete carotid obstruction, facial pallor can be striking. Bleeding from the ear and nose occurs when the back-pressure is severe to rupture small superficial vessels. **Numerous petechiae may be produced as a common autopsy artefact during reflection of scalp flaps in all types of death and are of no significance. They are often present in normal postmortem hypostasis, especially where the mode of death was congestive, as in heart disease. Petechiae can develop after death in dependent areas of the body** Fig. (6–5). Petechiae are rarely seen in the parietal pleura and peritoneum except in haemorrhagic diatheses.

(2) Congestion occurs due to obstructed venous return and capillo-venous distention. When the neck is compressed, face, lips and tongue become swollen and reddened. **The colour change of congestion is usually darkened by the onset of cyanosis.** The increased CO_2 tension in blood causes capillary dilatation and loss of tonicity of vascular walls, leading to stasis of blood. Internal organs are also congested. **Increased capillary permeability probably results from a combination of stasis and hypoxia.** The increased capillary and venous permeability causes transudation of fluid into tissues. In the early stages, the transudation is followed by increased lymph drainage and oedema does not develop. If the hypoxia continues, oedema of the tissues develops. **Oedema of the lungs is common, and is usually caused due to combination of hypoxia and raised pulmonary vessel pressure,** and its presence indicates struggle for survival for a time. Oedema of the brain occurs due to back-pressure and hypoxia. Generalised oedema is not prominent. **Congestion and oedema are non-specific and result due to obstructed venous return.** When the neck is compressed, the face, lips, and tongue become swollen and reddened.

(3) Cyanosis (**bluish colour of the skin,** mucous membranes and internal organs) follows congestion of the face, as venous blood containing much reduced haemoglobin after perfusing the head and neck becomes more blue. **In constriction of the neck, cyanosis follows congestion of the face. Cyanosis produced during life may be partly or wholly overshadowed by hypostasis which may be a deep-purple or blue and may be mistaken for true cyanosis.** If the airway is blocked, the impaired oxygenation in the lungs causes decrease in the oxygen content of the arterial blood, which causes darkening of all organs and tissues and will increase the cyanosis of the face. **About 24 hours after death, oxygen will be dissociated from the blood and cyanosis will appear in any dead body.** Oxygenated blood is bright-red. It becomes purplish-blue when oxygen is given up. Cyanosis is marked in the skin where hypostatic livid stains develop, and lips, ears, tip of nose, fingernails, cheeks, and internally the lungs, liver, spleen, kidneys and meninges are cyanosed. **More than 5 g/100 ml of whole blood should be in the form of reduced haemoglobin to produce cyanosis regardless of the total haemoglobin concentration.** The essential cause of cyanosis is diminished oxygen tension in the blood with a rise in proportion of the reduced haemoglobin. Methaemoglobin and sulphhaemoglobin also cause cyanosis.

When the deceased is found with the head lower than the body, marked congestion, cyanosis and petechial haemorrhages are common.

Heart: Dilatation of the heart chambers on the right side and fluidity of the blood in deaths due to asphyxia are absolete and should be disregarded. This is seen in any type of congestive death, including primary heart failure from many diseases, and is due to the generalised rise in venous and intracardiac pressure. Distension of the atria and ventricles is a common postmortem finding and may result from secondary muscular flaccidity.

Lungs: The light lungs (about 300 gm.) are more compatible with sudden rhythm disturbance and cessation of the action of the heart. **Heavier lungs (450 to 500 gm. or more) indicate cessation of respiration with continuance of the heartbeat for several minutes.**

HISTOLOGY: (1) Partial disruption of alveolar septa with distinctive haemorrhage within the alveoli and intra-alveolar oedema fluid. (2) Brick-red discolouration of nerve cells in cerebral cortex seen in stained neurological sections. Pallor and vacuolar degeneration of Purkinje cells in the cerebellum. (3) Vacuolar degeneration of liver cells in prolonged suffocation.

Asphyxial Stigmata: Asphyxia is not a pathological entity, and cannot be clearly recognised from morbid anatomical findings alone. **The triad of (1) cyanosis, (2) facial, palpebral, bulbar, subpleural and subepicardial petechiae, (3) visceral congestion, are all due to raised venous pressure. They are merely consistent with, but not diagnostic of asphyxia from anoxic anoxia. Reliable local indications of fatal obstructing trauma must be demonstrated to establish that death occurred from mechanical asphyxia.** Parenchymatous degenerative changes develop in rapid hypoxic and rapid anoxic deaths, but they are non-specific.

SYMPTOMS: (1) STAGE OF DYSPNOEA: The excess of carbon dioxide in the blood stimulates the respiratory centre. The respiratory movements become increased in rate and amplitude, blood pressure is increased, pulse rate increases and there is slight cyanosis.

(2) STAGE OF CONVULSIONS: The effort to breathe is mostly expiratory, the face is deeply congested, blood pressure is increased, pulse is fast, veins in the neck become swollen. There are frequently convulsions which cease as the victim becomes insensible and the reflexes are abolished.

(3) STAGE OF EXHAUSTION: The respiratory centre is paralysed, the muscles become flaccid. There is complete insensibility, reflexes are lost and the pupils are widely dilated. The breathing is gasping, mostly inspiratory with long intervals between the gasps. The blood pressure falls, muscles relax, respiration ceases, and death takes place. The pulse is imperceptible, but the heart may continue to beat for some minutes after respirations have ceased. The three stages last for 3 to 5 minutes before death takes place.

Postmortem Appearances: External: Postmortem hypostasis is well developed. The face is either pale in slow asphyxia, or distorted, congested, often cyanosed and purple, and sometimes swollen and oedematous. Ears and fingernails are bluish. The eyes are prominent, the conjunctivae are congested and the pupils are dilated. The tongue is protruded in most cases, and frothy and bloody mucus escapes from the mouth and nostrils. Postmortem discharge of semen from the meatus is common in any type of death, not only in asphyxia. **Petechial haemorrhages, known as Tardieu spots are most marked where for mechanical reasons, capillary congestion is most prominent. Their distribution lies above the level of obstruction in strangulation cases, but in long-standing hanging cases als, these can be seen Fig. (6–5).** They appear commonly in the scalp, eyelids and face in hanging and strangulation and in the zone above the level of compression in traumatic asphyxia. A hand lens is useful to identify petechial haemorrhages. **They are produced by simple mechanical obstruction to the venous return of blood from the parts, resulting in acute rise in venous pressure and overdistension and rupture of thinwalled peripheral venules, especially in lax, unsupported tissues, such as forehead, skin behind the ears, eyelids, circumoral skin, conjunctivae and sclerae, neck, buccal mucosa, epiglottis, visceral pleura, pericardium, thymus and rarely in the serosa of the bowel** Figs (6–3 to 6–5). They may occur in many non-asphyxial states. In some asphyxial deaths petechiae are seldom found. In many cases unconsciousness can occur in several seconds.

Internal: **The blood is fluid and dark, because of increased amount of CO_2.** The large veins are full of blood. Vessels may burst in the eardrum and in the nose causing bleeding. The larynx and trachea are usually congested, and contain a varying amount of slightly frothy mucus. **The lungs are dark and purple. If the backpressure persists, there is exudation of serous or serosanguineous fluid in the alveoli, producing oedema.** The amount of pulmonary oedema does not indicate the time interval between injury and death. Accumulation of fluid in the posterior and dependent parts of the lungs after death, should not be mistaken for pulmonary oedema. Some of the marginal portions of the lungs may show emphysematous changes. **The abdominal viscera show marked venous congestion.** The brain is often congested. The cranial sinuses are usually filled with dark blood.

Petechial haemorrhages are numerous where the capillaries are least firmly supported, as in subconjunctival tissues and under the pleural and pericardial membranes Fig. (6–4) **but they can appear almost anywhere if the degree of congestion and cyanosis is sufficient. The petechiae are usually round, dark, and well-defined, varying in size from a pin's head to two mm.** They may occur as isolated minute haemorrhages or present in large numbers, and at times fuse to form patches of red colour, especially at the back of the heart. They are numerous in the region of auriculoventricular junction of heart and the lower lobes and the interlobar fissure of the lungs and thymus. In the brain, petechiae occur in the white matter, and there may be larger patches of bleeding in the subarachnoid space, because of acute venous engorgement. Often profuse petechiae and ecchymoses are seen under the scalp due to the same mechanism. When present over the visceral pleura of lungs, these petechiae are also referred to as Tardieu spots **Fig. (6–4)**. The time taken for these various signs to occur depends on the circumstances, from a few seconds to several minutes. **Petechiae and ecchymoses are common non-specific autopsy findings and may be seen in many non-asphyxial deaths** beneath the pericardium, pleura, interlobar fissures and around the hilum. Petechiae are likely to occur in association with cyanotic congestion and may not be visible until the area is drained of blood during autopsy. **Sometimes, it is difficult to distinguish petechiae from the cut ends of congested vessels, especially in the brain.** Microscopic examination will confirm the nature of haemorrhage. **Cutaneous and visceral petechiae, especially the latter can appear and enlarge as a postmortem phenomenon.** They are seen on the front or back of corpses who have died from causes other than mechanical asphyxia. They are often seen in normal postmortem hypostasis, especially where the mode of death was congestive as in many types of natural heart disease. **As such petechiae are highly unreliable indicators of an asphyxial process.**

Natural diseases: The natural disease which produce haemorrhages in the skin include bacterial endocarditis, meningococcal septicaemia and blood dyscrasias, especially purpura and haemophilia, and also in deaths from coronary thrombosis, acute heart failure, secondary shock, and rapid anoxia. Petechiae can be seen following any severe increase in intrathoracic pressure including asthmatic attack, heart failure, respiratory failure, straining at stool, and soon after delivery. These conditions produce relatively large haemorrhages which tend to combine. **Their distribution is general, whereas petechiae due to asphyxia are present above the level of obstruction.**

Asphyxia causes vomiting due to medullary suboxia, due to which the air-passages may be filled at the end of asphyxial event by the inhaled vomit. This finding especially in infants, should not be assumed to be the cause of asphyxia as it is more likely the result of asphyxia. **About 20 to 25% of all individuals aspirate food agonally whatever may be the cause of death,** probably due to lack of normal protective mechanisms of air passages at or about the time of death.

Variations in the intensity of asphyxial signs: The intensity of asphyxial signs can vary depending on the duration of contact. If, during the process of asphyxia, heart failure occurs before respiratory failure, the asphyxial signs may be less marked, depending at which stage in the asphyxial process, the cardiac arrest occurred. In many cases of foetal hypoxia, asphyxial signs are absent, such as sudden blockage of trachea by food, plastic bag pulled over the head or when victim enters a space devoid of oxygen. **Sometimes, the findings are not sufficient to use an accurate term, and the cause of death has to be given within a broad framework, such as "consistent with asphyxia".**

In the presence of putrefaction, mechanical asphyxia is indicated by presence of petechial haemorrhages under the eyelids, conjunctivae, sclerae and facial skin.

DELAYED DEATHS: In asphyxia the higher cortical centres suffer first from hypoxic injury, followed by basal ganglia and ultimately the vital centres, which explains delayed deaths. Such delayed deaths usually follow periods of unconsciousness, resulting from anoxic cerebral damage and subsequent hypostatic pneumonia. Other lethal sequelae include, massive subcutaneous and mediastinal emphysema from tracheal and laryngeal lacerations, or occlusion of airway due to oedematous or haemorrhagic swelling of pharyngeal tissues or the aryepiglottic folds. When death occurs hours, days or weeks after the asphyxial episode, the proximate cause of death is the traumatic incident.

COMA: It is a state of unarousable unconsciousness determined by the absence of any psychologically understandable response to external stimuli or inner need. It involves the central portion of the brain stem. Coma is a clinical symptom and not a cause of death.

CAUSES: (1) Compression of the brain, e.g., effusion of blood on or in the brain, inflammation, abscess or neoplasm of brain. (2) Drugs: opium, hypnotics, cocaine, alcohol, anaesthetics, cyanide, atropine, phenol, oxalic acid, CO, etc. (3) Metabolic disorders and infections: uraemia, cholaemia, eclampsia, diabetes, pneumonia, infectious fevers, heat stroke, etc. (4) Other causes: embolism and thrombosis in the cerebral vessels, epilepsy, hysteria, etc.

AUTOPSY: Injuries or disease of the brain may be present as noted in the causes of coma. The lungs, brain and the meninges are congested. Splanchnic pooling of blood occurs.

SYNCOPE: Syncope is sudden stoppage of action of the heart, which may prove fatal. This term is also not used as a cause of death. Syncope or fainting is due to vasovagal attacks resulting from reflex parasympathetic stimulation. Syncope is caused by reflex bradycardia or asystole, or by reflex splanchnic vasodilation. Due to the acute reflex circulatory changes, blood pressure falls suddenly causing cerebral anaemia and rapid unconsciousness. Recovery is common.

CAUSES: (1) Anaemia due to sudden and excessive haemorrhage. (2) Asthenia from deficient power of heart muscle as in fatty degeneration

of the heart, myocardial infarction and certain poisons. (3) Vagal inhibition. (4) Exhausting diseases.

AUTOPSY: The heart is contracted and the chambers are empty when death has occurred from anaemia, but chambers contain blood when death occurs due to asthenia. The lungs, brain and abdominal organs are usually pale. Splanchnic pooling of blood occurs.

CAUSE OF DEATH: The cause of death is the disease or injury responsible for starting the sequence of events, which are brief or prolonged and which produce death. It may be divided into: (1) IMMEDIATE CAUSE, i.e., the injury or disease present at the time of terminal event, e.g., bronchopneumonia, peritonitis, trauma, etc. (2) BASIC CAUSE, i.e., pathological processes responsible for the death at the time of the terminal event or prior to or leading to the event, e.g., gunshot wound of abdomen complicated by generalised peritonitis. (3) CONTRIBUTORY CAUSE, i.e, the pathological process involved in or complicating, but not causing the terminal event. In some cases, the basic and the immediate cause may be identical.

Determination of the cause of death following autopsy is an interpretive and intelligent procedure, and depends upon sound evaluation of all data, circumstances surrounding the death, morphological evidence of disease and injury and additional laboratory investigations. In fact, the more a forensic pathologist knows about the total investigation, the more he can contribute from his autopsy. The effectiveness of the doctor would be greatly diminished if he had to work alone, and receives bodies for autopsy without clothing, or a knowledge of the circumstances surrounding death. The recognition of the structural organic changes or chemical abnormalities, which cause stoppage of the vital functions is the first step. Understanding the mechanism by which the anatomical and chemical deviations from normal actually caused death, i.e. how they produced or initiated the sequence of functional disturbance which were sufficient to cause respiratory or cardiac arrest, which are the two ultimate lethal processes, is the second step.

The MANNER OF DEATH: It indicates the circumstances under which the person died. It is established from the personal and family history, circumstantial information from the scene of death, witnesses of the event, information from family members and others and by the autopsy findings. If death occurs exclusively from disease, the manner of death is natural. If death occurs exclusively by injury or is hastened due to injury in a person suffering from natural disease, the manner of death is unnatural or violent. Violence may be suicidal, homicidal, accidental or of undetermined or unexplained origin.

MECHANISM OF DEATH: It is the physiological or biochemical disturbance, produced by the cause of death which is incompatible with life, e.g., shock, sepsis, toxaemia, severe metabolic acidosis and alkalosis, ventricular fibrillation, respiratory paralysis, etc.

AGONAL PERIOD is the time between a lethal occurrence and death.

CLASSIFICATION OF THE CAUSE OF DEATH: According to the autopsy findings, the cause of death may be grouped as follows.

(I) NATURAL CAUSES: (a) Where a lesion is found at autopsy which is incompatible with life. (b) Where a lesion is found at autopsy which is known to cause death.

(II) UNNATURAL CAUSES: (a) Where a lesion is found at autopsy which is incompatible with life. (b) Where a lesion is found which may have caused death or which may have precipitated death, but which is also known to be compatible with continued life.

(III) OBSCURE CAUSES: Where no lesion is found at autopsy, or if a lesion is found it is of a minimal or indefinite nature.

NATURAL CAUSES: WHERE A LESION IS FOUND AT AUTOPSY WHICH IS NOT COMPATIBLE WITH LIFE: In this category, the structural abnormalities establish beyond any doubt the identity of the disease which caused death. It is apparent that the lesions observed are incompatible with life because of its nature, site or extent, and they are antemortem in origin. The examples are: massive pulmonary thromboembolism, spontaneous intracerebral haemorrhage, ruptured myocardial infarct, rupture of an aortic aneurysm.

(B) WHERE A LESION IS FOUND AT AUTOPSY WHICH IS KNOWN TO CAUSE DEATH: This category includes deaths in which some lesion is found at autopsy which may have caused death, but which is also compatible with continued life, e.g., arteriosclerosis of the coronary arteries, advanced chronic heart diseases, lobar pneumonia, etc. The autopsy does not reveal any other reasonable explanation for death, and the location, nature, severity and extent of the anatomical changes are sufficient to cause death, but it is not a conclusive proof. In such cases, the clinical history is important. In the case of coronary arteriosclerosis, if the deceased had several attacks of angina pectoris before his death, it can be reasonably assumed to be the cause of death. If the clinical history is unusual, the possibilities suggested by the history should be excluded before the death is attributed to the lesion.

Stenosing coronary atherosclerosis can cause sudden death, in which the autopsy may reveal a few scattered foci or only a single site of significant luminal narrowing, and there may be no recent vascular occlusive lesion. In most cases of sudden coronary death, a fresh thrombus or a recent myocardial infarct is not found at autopsy. In these cases, correlation of the morbid anatomy with the suddenness of death must be based on hypotheses. Emotional stress, e.g., anger, fear, joy, apprehension, etc., can precipitate acute failure in persons with organic heart disease, especially of the coronary atherosclerotic type. Emotional excitement significantly increases the workload of the heart which can overtax the limits of tolerance of damaged, labouring heart.

In a normal person sudden release of adrenaline due to extreme terror can initiate ventricular fibrillation and death. Sudden deaths following assaults or even threats may occur due to existing heart disease.

Such events may be encountered in criminal charges arising out of collapse during fights, in minor assaults upon old persons, in litigation related to death from workstress, etc.

Sufferers from asthma and epilepsy can die suddenly and unexpectedly for no obvious reasons.

UNNATURAL CAUSES: (A) WHERE A LESION IS FOUND AT AUTOPSY WHICH IS NOT COMPATIBLE WITH LIFE: In some deaths, injuries may be found at autopsy which are incompatible with life in any person, e.g., decapitation, crushing of the head, avulsion of the heart from the large blood vessels. If they are antemortem, they are the definite cause of death.

(B) A LESION IS FOUND AT AUTOPSY WHICH MAY HAVE CAUSED OR PRECIPITATED DEATH, BUT IS COMPATIBLE WITH LIFE: At autopsy certain injuries may be found which from their nature, site or extent may not appear to be sufficient to cause death in a healthy person. But such injury may be the cause of death due to some complication resulting directly from the injury, but which is not demonstrable at autopsy. The degree of shock or the extent of haemorrhage following an injury cannot be assessed at autopsy. In such cases, the absence of any other adequate cause of death, and a consideration of the circumstances of the injury and of the symptoms found, may enable the doctor to attribute death to the injury with reasonable certainty.

In some cases, an injury may not appear to be sufficient to cause death, but some natural disease may be present which is known to cause death, e.g., coronary arteriosclerosis. In such cases, the circumstances of death and the symptoms found at the time of collapse may suggest that the death was precipitated by the injury.

NEGATIVE AUTOPSY: When gross and microscopic examination, toxicological analyses and laboratory investigations fail to reveal a cause of death, the autopsy is considered to be negative. 2 to 5% of all autopsies are negative. In teenagers and young adults, up to the age of about 35 years, there is a higher proportion of negative autopsies than in older group. A negative autopsy may be due to: **(1) Inadequate history:** Deaths from vagal inhibition, status epilepticus, hypersensitivity reaction, laryngeal spasm in drowning, etc. may not show any anatomical findings. **(2) Inadequate external examination:** The presence of fresh and old needle marks may be missed on cursory examination in a drug addict. Death from snake bites and insect bites cannot be explained unless the bite marks are identified. The burn may be missed in electrocution. **(3) Inadequate or improper internal examination:** Air embolism and pneumothorax are often missed. **(4) Insufficient laboratory examinations. (5) Lack of toxicological analysis. (6) Lack of training of the doctor.**

OBSCURE AUTOPSIES are those which do not show a definite cause for death, in which there are minimal, indefinite or obscure findings, or even no positive findings at all. They are a source of confusion to any pathologist. Frequently, these deaths are due to obscure natural causes, but they may be due to certain types of injury or complications of injury, or to poisoning. Mild degrees of natural disease should not be implicated unless other possibilities are most carefully eliminated.

The obscure causes are: (1) Natural diseases: (a) With obscure or some microscopic findings. (b) Death precipitated by emotion, work-stress, and (c) Functional failure, such as epilepsy, paroxysmal fibrillation.

(2) Biochemical disturbances: (a) Uraemia, diabetes, potassium deficiency. (b) Respiratory pigment disorders, such as anaemic anoxia, porphyria.

(3) Endocrine dysfunction: (a) Adrenal insufficiency. (b) Thyrotoxicosis or myxoedema.

(4) Concealed trauma: (a) Cerebral concussion. (b) Self-reduced neck injury. (c) Blunt injury to the heart. (d) Reflex vagal inhibition.

(5) Poisoning: Without macroscopic change: (a) Delayed suboxic or narcotic poisoning. (b) Anaesthetic overdosage or maladministration. (c) Neurotoxic or cytotoxic poisons. (d) Plant poisoning.

(6) Miscellaneous: Allergy, drug idiosyncrasy.

Obscure autopsies are usually seen in a younger, healthy person who dies suddenly and unexpectedly. Non-medical persons believe that the cause of death can always be determined by autopsy. The police may press the doctor for giving a positive statement with regard to the cause of death. In such cases, the doctor should admit his inability to give a positive opinion. **Such obscure cases require clinical and laboratory investigations and interview with persons who had observed the deceased before he died, to know the signs and symptoms shown by the deceased before his death.** Laboratory investigations may be bacteriological, virological, histological, biochemical and toxicological. In these cases, re-examine the body and look for tongue bite, foreign body in respiratory tract, fat or air embolism, sepsis, cardiac hypertrophy, coronary ostia patency, atherosclerosis, severe narrowing of coronary arteries, coronary thrombosis, fatty liver, pancytopaenia or leukaemia, sickle cell thrombi in the brain, myocarditis, electrolyte imbalance, anaphylaxis, drug reaction, small electrical burns, needle marks, etc. Common obscure deaths are hypoglycaemia, hyperkalaemia, cardiac arrhythmias, conduction system disorders, epilepsy, vagal inhibition, snake bites, etc. Review available history and obtain more if possible. **In cases where general senile atrophy of most organs is present without any other positive finding and the history is not helpful for a specific cause of death and natural causes are excluded, cause of death can be certified as "myocardial degeneration due to senility". When circumstances are unequivocally those of a natural death, the cause of death can be given as "undetermined natural circumstances". When circumstances are equivocal, the cause and manner of death should be given as "undetermined". In the absence of positive findings from these sources, a careful assessment of possible functional causes of death must be made, before any cause of death is given as undetermined.** The presence of infectious, malignant, occupational and other diseases are also excluded. Even in these disappointing cases, the negative morbid anatomical and chemical examination is of great value in excluding injuries or poisons, which may have been alleged to have caused or played some part in the death. **Though the pathologist cannot establish the cause of death, he can exclude many conditions which have been incorrectly attributed to have caused death.**

(1) NATURAL CAUSES: CARDIAC LESIONS: Acute rheumatic carditis may cause sudden death in a young adult. In some such cases, naked-eye changes may be absent, but typical Aschoff bodies of rheumatic fever are found in the myocardium on microscopic examination. Acute toxic myocarditis of diphtheria may cause sudden death, in which the primary lesion in the nose or throat may be overlooked. Idiopathic myocarditis may cause sudden death. Brown atrophy of the heart and senile heart may prematurely fail suddenly. Myocarditis, fibrosis, and necrosis of conducting tissue may escape detection. Small coronary thrombosis and easily dislodged emboli may be overlooked.

Acute occlusion of coronary artery may result from thrombosis or haemorrhage within the wall of the artery. Zones of occlusion are usually less than five mm. in length, and most of the occlusions occur within three cm. of the orifices of the vessels. **First part of the anterior descending branch of left coronary artery within two cm. of its origin is commonly affected,** followed by the proximal part of the right coronary artery, first part of the circumflex branch of left coronary artery, and the short main trunk of left coronary artery. Fresh thrombi are dark-brown, and attached to the vessel walls. Old thrombi appear as homogeneous yellowish or grey, firm plugs blocking the vessels. **Most infarcts occur in the left ventricle in the anterior wall.** Posterior infarcts may be due to blockage of either the right vessel or the circumflex branch of the left artery. **Infarction usually occurs when the lumen is reduced to twenty percent or less.** Right ventricle is involved in less than ten percent cases. Coronary insufficiency from narrowing of the lumen of major vessels may lead to chronic ischaemia and hypoxia of the muscle distal to the stenosis. **Hypoxic myocardium is electrically unstable and liable to arrhythmias and ventricular fibrillation, especially at moments of sudden stress, such as exercise or an adrenaline response, such as anger or emotion.**

MYOCARDIAL INFARCTION: (1) A laminar infarct in which the subendocardial region of much or even all of the left ventricle is involved, sometimes extending through half or more of the thickness of the wall. It produces less well-defined gross changes than the transmural infarct. It occurs due to generalised stenosis in the major branches of coronary vessels. (2) A regional or focal infarct is more common caused by localised occlusion or severe stenosis in a coronary artery. It is a well demarcated zone of necrosis. There is usually a thin rim of preserved subendocardial myocardium which is perfused directly by the blood in the ventricular chamber. Right ventricle and atria are involved in less than 10% of cases. The papillary muscles are usually involved. There is no need for the ischaemia to be severe enough to produce a myocardial infarct. **At autopsy, no naked eye changes are seen for the first 12 to 18 hours.** After this period, there is oedema and pallor of the affected area which is the first sign, and the cut surface looks granular and dull. After 24 hours to third day, the area becomes better demarcated, and turns yellow and is surrounded by an area of hyperaemia. In one to three days there is a progressive softening and thinning of infarcted area, which is maximum about the tenth day, and rupture may occur during this period. With breakdown of myocytes, red streaks appear due to dilated vascular channels and area of interfibre haemorrhage, giving rise to "tigroid" appearance, though sometimes the yellow element is virtually uniform or red streaks may fade after a few days. There may be a red zone in the less damaged muscle around the periphery. From the third week and later, the centre of the infarct becomes gelatinous and the colour become grey. By the end of first week, the entire infarct is bright yellow or yellow-green, soft and has a thin hyperaemic border. By ten days, the periphery of the infarct appears reddish-purple due to growth of granulation tissue. Later, the necrotic muscle is resorbed and the infarct shrinks and becomes pale grey. By the end of 6 weeks, the infarcted area is replaced by a thin grey-white, hard, shrunken fibrous scar which is well developed in about three months. During the next month or two, fibrosis replaces the dead muscle to form a scar.

Severe narrowing of coronary arteries (at least 75%) without thrombosis or myocardial infarction is a common cause of sudden death. A physical or emotional stimulus may demand sudden increase in cardiac effort, and if the circulation of the deceased is unable to satisfy the immediate need for increased oxygen, death may result (acute coronary insufficiency). Fresh thrombotic lesions are seen in less than 25% of the cases. Transitory coronary artery spasm can cause death in persons suffering from angina without narrowing of the coronary arteries and without significant atherosclerosis or congenital anomalies. Spasm of the coronaries may lead to cardiac arrhythmia and death. A thrombus or an occlusive lesion in the terminal part of the artery may be overlooked. **The ostia of the coronary arteries may be occluded by atherosclerosis of the aorta.** A ventricle which is overworked and under-nourished may suddenly go into ventricular fibrillation or asystole. This can occur even if the arteries are not completely blocked and is often precipitated by a sudden demand for an increased cardiac output. The lesions of the conducting system of the heart may sometimes cause arrhythmias and death. **Any person with a heart in excess of 420 gm. is at risk of sudden death, even though the coronary arteries are normal.** In these cases a state of electrical instability occurs from chronic hypoxia, so that sudden stresses, such as exercise or emotion can suddenly cause the arrhythmias.

Sympathetico-adrenal stimulation causes increased myocardial irritability resulting in ventricular extrasystoles and ventricular fibrillation and death occurs after several minutes. At autopsy, coronary artery sclerosis, fatty heart, chronic valvular disease, etc. may be seen. Lungs are congested and oedematous with pleural petechial haemorrhages.

Concealed Trauma: (a) Cerebral Concussion: This may cause death without any external or internal marks of injury.

(b) Neck Injury: Cervical spinal fracture-dislocation may occur in diving, fall on head, impact downstair with a wall-facing, from oblique impact or by fall of some object on the head, in such a way as to cause the dislocation especially with the head thrown back. The dislocation may be associated with tears of the ligaments and with the displacement of the skull from the spine. Sudden movements of the head over the spine with displacement may cause contusion and laceration of the spinal cord and rapid death. If death is delayed, there may be oedema, softening and necrosis of the cord. **Injury to the spinal cord causes spinal concussion and may cause death.** Unconsciousness is not seen in all persons, but all get up with residual tingling, numbness, weakness of arms or legs and gait defects. Routine autopsy and X-ray may not show any abnormality. The dislocation of the cervical segments is often self-reducing, and externally there may not be any injury, or there may be abrasions on the brow or chin. Complete dissection of spine is essential. The spinal cord, cut longitudinally, may show internal bruising. Death may be instantaneous.

(c) Blunt Injury to the Heart: Contusion of the chest as in steering-wheel impacts, head-on collisions, from blast or heavy punching, may temporarily or permanently derange the heart without much evidence of trauma. **Contusion of the heart may cause death.** Trauma may cause arterial spasm and it is likely that a functional inhibition or coronary spasm may cause sudden death that sometimes follow upon blows to the chest.

(D) INHIBITION OF THE HEART: (Vagal Inhibition; vasovagal shock; reflex cardiac arrest; nervous apoplexy or **Instantaneous physiological death): Instantaneous physiological death means death of a person with no abnormality sufficient to be presumed to have caused death and where death occurs within few seconds. Sudden death occurring within seconds or a minute or two due to minor trauma or relatively simple and harmless peripheral stimulation are caused by vagal inhibition.**

Mechanism: Pressure on the baroreceptors situated in the carotid sinuses, carotid sheaths, and the carotid body (located in the dilated part of the wall of internal carotid artery just above the bifurcation of common carotid artery, and situated about the level of angle of mandible and at the level of upper border of thyroid cartilage) causes an increase in blood pressure in these sinuses with resultant slowing of the heart rate, dilatation of blood vessels and a fall in blood pressure. Carotid sinus contains numerous nerve endings from the glossopharyngeal nerve. It communicates with the medullary cardiovascular centre in the brain and the dorsal motor nucleus of the vagus. It is intimately connected with the control of blood pressure and heart rate. **In normal persons, pressure on the carotid sinus causes minimal effects** with a decrease in heart rate of less than six beats per minute, and only a slight reduction (less than 10 mm Hg) in blood pressure. **Some individuals show marked hypersensitivity to stimulation of the carotid sinuses, characterised by bradycardia and cardiac arrhythmias ranging from ventricular arrhythmias to cardiac arrest.** Stimulation of the corotid sinus baroreceptors causes impulses to pass via Hering's nerve to the afferent fibres of the glossopharyngeal nerve (9th cranial nerve); these in turn link

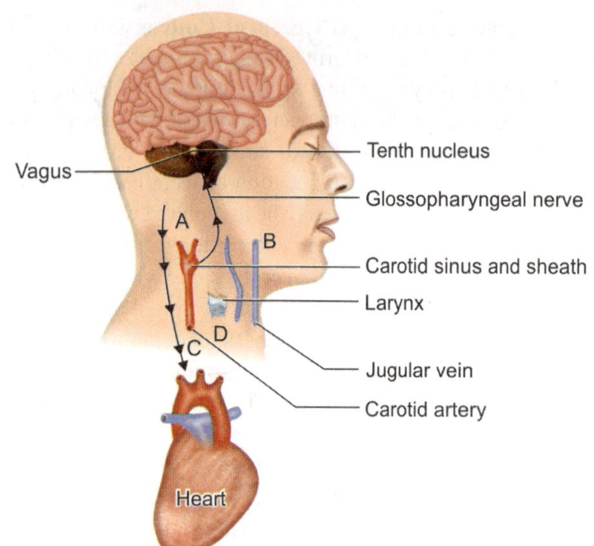

Fig. (6–6). The coarse distribution of the receptor system in vagal inhibition reflexes.

in the brainstem to the nucleus of the vagus nerve (10th cranial nerve). **Parasympathetic efferent impulses, then pass to the heart via the cardiac branches of the vagus nerve. Stimulation of these fibres causes a profound bradycardia.** This reflex arc is independent of the main motor and sensory nerve pathways. There is wide network of sensory nerves in the skin, pharynx, glottis, pleura, peritoneum covering viscera or extending into the spermatic cord, cervix, urethra, perineum and coeliac plexus. Afferent fibres from these tissues pass into the lateral tracts of the spinal cord, effect local reflex connections over several segments and also pass to the brain. The vagal nucleus is controlled by the synaptic connections in the spinal cord, which may be facilitated from both the sensory central cortex and from the thalamic centres. The latter may be responsible for emotional tone noted in the vagal reflex **Fig. (6–6).**

Parasympathetic stimulation of the heart can be initiated by high neck compression, pressure on carotid sinus or sometimes by direct pressure over the trunk of the vagus nerve.

Causes: (1) **The commonest cause of such inhibition is pressure on the neck particularly on the carotid sinuses as in hanging or strangulation.** (2) Impaction of food in larynx or unexpected inhalation of fluid into the upper respiratory tract. (3) Sudden immersion of body in cold water. (4) Unexpected blows to the larynx, chest, abdomen, or genital organs. (5) Extensive injuries to the spine or other parts of the body. (6) The insertion of an instrument into the bronchus, uterus, bladder or rectum. (7) Puncture of a pleural cavity usually for producing a pneumothorax. (8) Sudden evacuation of pathological fluids, e.g., ascitic or pleural. (9) Sudden distension of hollow muscular organs, e.g., during attempts at criminal abortion, when instruments are passed through the cervix or fluids are injected into the uterus. (10) In degenerative diseases of the heart, e.g., sinus bradycardia and partial or complete A-V block; parasympathetic stimulation further depress the heart rate and may induce a Stokes-Adams attack which may be fatal.

Variation: There is great variation in individual susceptibility. Death from inhibition is accidental and caused by microtrauma. The stimulus should be sudden and abnormal for the reflex to occur. The reflex is exaggerated by fear, apprehension, struggling, a high state of emotional tension, and also any condition which lowers voluntary cerebral control of reflex responses, such as a mild alcoholic intoxication, a degree of hypoxia or partial narcosis due to incomplete anaesthesia. The release of catecholamines during such adrenal responses may well sensitise the myocardium to such neurogenic stimulation. The victims are usually young adolescents of nervous temperament.

Autopsy: When death results from inhibition, **there are no characteristic postmortem appearances.** The cause of death can be inferred only by exclusion of other pathological conditions, and from the accurate observations by reliable witnesses, concerning the circumstance of death.

CASE: A soldier was dancing with his girlfriend in the presence of many others in a hall. While dancing, he playfully "tweaked" (pinched) her neck. She dropped down dead on the spot. There were no injuries or signs of asphyxia. Death was as a result of vagal inhibition.

ANAPHYLACTIC DEATHS: Anaphylaxis is an acute immunologic reaction characterised by cutaneous, gastrointestinal, respiratory and cardiovascular signs and symptoms that can rapidly progress to shock and death. Deaths due to allergic reactions are rare. Most deaths occur within 1 to 2 hours and are preceded by signs and symptoms suggesting hyperacute bronchial asthma. Sometimes, deaths are delayed for several hours with nervous symptoms, such as coma or with symptoms of circulatory failure resembling traumatic shock.

AETIOLOGY: Allergic reactions may occur due to: (1) Drugs: penicillin, aspirin, horse-serum products, vaccines, iodine-containing agents. (2) Insect bites. (3) Foods: fish, sehll-fish, eggs, nuts, fruits. (4) Hormones: insulin, ACTH. (5) Enzymes; trypsin.

The anaphylactic syndrome is caused by local and systemic release of endogenous active substances. These include leukotrienes, C, D, E or histamine, eosinophilic chemotactic factor and other vasoactive substances, such as bradykinin and kallikrein. Anaphylactic shock is due to bronchospasm with contraction of the smooth muscle of the lungs, vasodilation, and increased capillary permeability. Death occurs due to laryngeal oedema, bronchospasm and vasodilation. Serum tryptase levels are an indicator of mast cell activation and if elevated suggest, an allergic mediator release, particularly in anaphylaxis. Peak levels of tryptase occur 1 to 2 hours after anaphylaxis and then decline with halflife of about two hours.

SIGNS AND SYMPTOMS: The onset of symptoms is within 15 to 20 min. General: malaise, weakness, sense of illness, oedema of face. Dermal: injection marks with surrounding wheals, skin rashes, urticaria, pruritus, erythema. Mucosal: periorbital oedema, nasal congestion, angio-oedema, cyanosis. R.S.: sneezing, rhinorrhoea, dyspnoea. Upper airway: laryngeal oedema, hoarseness, stridor, oedema of tongue and pharynx. Lower airway: dyspnoea, acute emphysema, asthma, bronchospasm. G.I: nausea, vomiting, dysphagia, abdominal cramps, diarrhoea C.V.S: tachycardia, palpitation, shock. C.N.S.: anxiety, convulsions. Death may occur due to anaphylactic shock, asphyxia due to oedema of glottis, bronchospasm or cardiovascular collapse.

AUTOPSY: History is very important. Search for injection sites or sting marks. The sting area should be excised and frozen at -70°C and submitted for antigen-antibody reactions. Findings are non-specific. There is usually oedema of the larynx (recedes soon after death), oedema of epiglottis, trachea and bronchi, emphysema, cyanosis, petechial haemorrhages, congestion and oedema of the lungs, focal pulmonary distension alternating with collapse and bronchiolar constriction, froth in the mouth and nostrils, visceral congestion, and infiltration of bronchial walls with eosinophils.

DRUG IDIOSYNCRASY: The administration of drugs in amounts which are known to be harmless to normal person may cause death due

to drug idiosyncrasy, e.g., many persons are hypersensitive to cocaine. The diagnosis is based mainly on clinical history.

DIABETES: An elevated vitreous glucose level is an accurate reflection of an elevated antemortem blood glucose level. Glucose levels above 200 mg% are diagnostic of diabetes mellitus even if i.v., glucose infusions were administered. Glucose level in vitreous falls gradually as the time after death increases.

ASTHMA: Decreased airflow occurs due to allergic release of histamine and other vasoactive compounds, which cause contraction of smooth muscles of bronchi. If airflow obstruction is not relieved, there will be steady progression to elevated CO_2, metabolic acidosis, exhaustion and death. **Asthma can cause sudden death without being in status asthmaticus or even an acute attack.** The mechanism is obscure.

At autopsy, the lungs appear overexpanded, and completely occupy the chest cavity. A sticky tenacious white mucus deposit fills the bronchi. Microscopically, chronic inflammatory infiltrate with numerous eosinophils are seen around the bronchi. The basement membrane of the bronchi is thickened and has a wavy appearance. In chronic cases, there is protrusion of bronchi above the cut surfaces of the lungs.

EPILEPSY: Very few persons die in status epilepticus. Death is caused due to respiratory failure following acute epileptic seizure, status epilepticus, aspiration during seizures or uncontrolled dysrhythmia due to ischaemic changes in myocardium.

Sudden death due to epileptic seizures is most likely due to a lethal cardiac arrhythmia induced or propagated by the disorganised neural discharges of seizure. **Sudden death can occur without being in a status epilepticus or even without a typical fit. In such cases the mechanism is obscure.** Repetitive seizures can cause bilateral hippocampal sclerosis. Common findings are external evidence of fits, bite over sides of tongue (25%), gum thickening if on medication, injuries sustained during fall or accident during fits, oedema of brain, cerebellar atrophy, pulonamry oedema and aspiration of gastric contents.

NEGRI BODIES: They are intracytoplasmic, deeply eosinophilic inclusions found in the pyramidal cells (ganglion or nerve cells) of hippocampus and uncus and Purkinje cells of cerebellum. One to two cm. cubes of tissue should be preserved in 50% glycerol-saline.

Vaccination deaths: Adverse reactions occur in one in one lakh immunisations due to injection by wrong route, into wrong tissues or into blood vessels, breaking of cold chain, contamination at manufacturing level. There is history of sudden collapse, redness of area, high fever, persistent crying, screaming, arching of back and seizures.

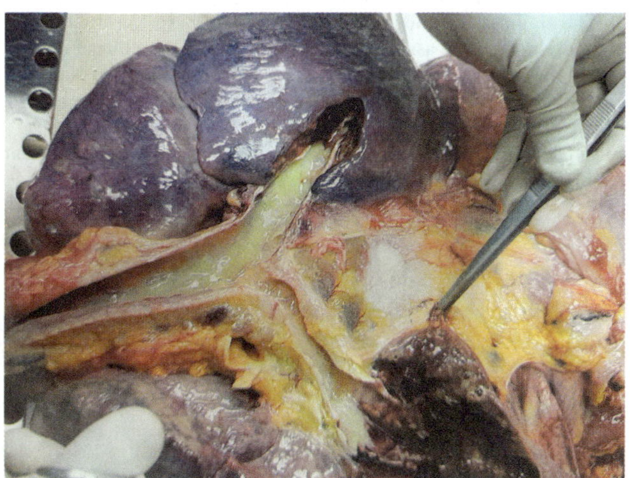

Fig. (6–7). Mucus in respiratory tract in asthma.

Autopsy: Redness, allergic skin patches, petechial haemorrhages, increased secretions in trachea and bronchi, congestion of internal organs. Death occurs due to immediate or delayed anaphylaxis.

AIDS/HIV

HIV attaches itself to the T-receptor molecule on T-helper lymphocytes in order to infect them. T-helper lymphocytes are found in most body fluids, such as semen, saliva, tears and breast milk. After infection with HIV, blood becomes positive after 2 to 18 months. HIV remains viable in blood up to 2 months and is present mostly in brain, colon, lungs and lymphoid tissue. Air-borne transmission does not occur. AIDS is usually communicated by sexual intercourse or from blood transfusion. HIV causes profound depression of cell-mediated immunity. This suppression exposes patients to a variety of opportunistic infections and malignant conditions. Mandatory testing, i.e., without consent of the person is done for screening donors for blood, semen, organs or tissues. According to guidelines laid by the Government of India, the status of HIV should not be disclosed to blood donor. The intention is to spare him of the agony of knowing the helplessness of his situation. If the blood drawn is positive, it should be discarded. Once blood sample is drawn, the register of patient identities should be kept quite separate and sample identified only with a code number. If the donor wants to know the result of HIV test, he should be referred to an accessible HIV testing centre where supplemental tests with counselling will be offered to him. HIV testing requires both pre-test and post-test counselling. Patient has to be informed face to face about the test result and not over the telephone or by a third party. HIV positivity should not be revealed to unauthorised persons.

The Centre for Disease Control (CDC), estimates that 5.5% of all HIV positive persons are employed in the health care field. According to the guidelines issued by CDC, with the exception of health care workers and personal service workers who use instruments that pierce the skin, no testing or restriction is indicated for workers known to be infected with HIV, but otherwise able to do their jobs. A person testing positive for HIV cannot be removed from service, if he is physically fit to discharge his duties. **Doctors in government service are obliged to treat AIDS cases. The treating doctor has the duty to inform the paramedical staff involved in the treatment of such patients, the mortuary staff, pathologist and the staff of the crematorium so that due precautions can be taken by these people,** who are likely to come in direct contact with the infected biological material. WHO guidelines state that there is no public health rationale to justify isolation, quarantine or discrimination based on a person's HIV status. If pregnant, they should be allowed to decide whether to continue or terminate the pregnancy. **HIV positive women should be advised to avoid pregnancy as there is one in three chance of having an infected child. Breast feeding may result in transmission of HIV from mother to child. Recently, Supreme Court of India has ruled for disclosure of the HIV positive status by the doctor to his patient's wife/spouse confidentially.**

A man suffering from AIDS, knowingly marries a woman and transmits the infection to that woman, would be guilty under S.269, I.P.C. (negligent act likely to spread infection/disease dangerous to life (imprisonment for 6 months) and S.270, I.P.C. (malignant act likely to spread infection/disease dangerous to life (imprisonment for 2 years). Non-voluntary disclosure of HIV status can be made by the counsellor to (1) healthcare worker involved in treatment or care of HIV/AIDS patients, (2) the spouse/sexual partner or injecting drug partner sharing the same needle where there is risk of transmission.

Diagnosis primarily depends on detection of HIV antibodies in serum and identification of DNA and RNA pattern in the infected cells.

Legal, Ethical, and Moral Aspects: (1) Newborn infants are highly susceptible to the disease if their mothers are infected. (2) Parental drug abuse and sex with affected persons are the source of infection. (3) Spread by blood transfusion of disease by blood donors. (4) Disposal of syringes and needles should be made compulsory. (5) Law should be enacted to protect the interests and rights of the public and general.

SUDDEN DEATH

Death is said to be sudden or unexpected when a person not known to have been suffering from any dangerous disease, injury or poisoning is found dead or dies within 24 hours after the onset of terminal illness (WHO). Some authors limit sudden deaths as those occurring instantaneously or within one hour of onset of symptoms. **Emphasis is placed more on the unexpected character, rather than suddenness of death.** The incidence is approximately 10 percent of all deaths. No period in life is exempt. **Natural death** means that the death was caused entirely by the disease, and the trauma or poison did not play any part in bringing it about.

CAUSES: (I) DISEASES OF THE CARDIOVASCULAR SYSTEM (45 to 50%): (1) Coronary atherosclerosis with coronary thrombosis. (2) Coronary atherosclerosis with haemorrhage in the wall causing occlusion of the lumen. (3) Coronary artery disease (narrowing and obliteration of the lumen by atherosclerosis). (4) Coronary artery embolism. (5) Occlusion of the ostium of the coronary artery associated with atherosclerosis or syphilitic aortitis. (6) Arterial hypertension with atherosclerosis. (7) Rupture of the fresh myocardial infarct Fig. (6–8). (8) Spontaneous rupture of aorta. (9) Angina pectoris. (10) Pulmonary embolism. (11) Systemic embolism occurring in bacterial endocarditis. (12) Rupture of aortic or other aneurysm. (13) Cardiomyopathies, alcoholic myopathy, asymmetrical hypertrophy of the heart. (14) Lesions of the conducting system: fibrosis, necrosis. (15) Valvular lesions: aortic stenosis, aortic regurgitation, mitral stenosis, rupture of the chordae, ball-valve thrombus. (16) Fatty degeneration of the heart. (17) Acute endocarditis. (18) Acute myocarditis. (19) Acute pericarditis. (20) Congenital heart disease in the newborn. (21) Senile myocardium.

(II) RESPIRATORY SYSTEM (15 to 23%): (1) Lobar pneumonia. (2) Bronchitis and bronchopneumonia. (3) Rupture of blood vessel in pulmonary tuberculosis with cavitation. (4) Pulmonary embolism and infarction. (5) Air embolism. (6) Influenza. (7) Diphtheria. (8) Acute oedema of the glottis. (9) Acute oedema of the lungs. (10) Lung abscess. (11) Massive collapse of the lung. (12) Pleural effusion. (13) Pneumothorax caused by rupture of emphysematous bleb. (14) Neoplasm of the bronchus. (15) Bronchial asthma. (16) Impaction of foreign body in the larynx and regurgitation of stomach contents into air-passages and bronchioles.

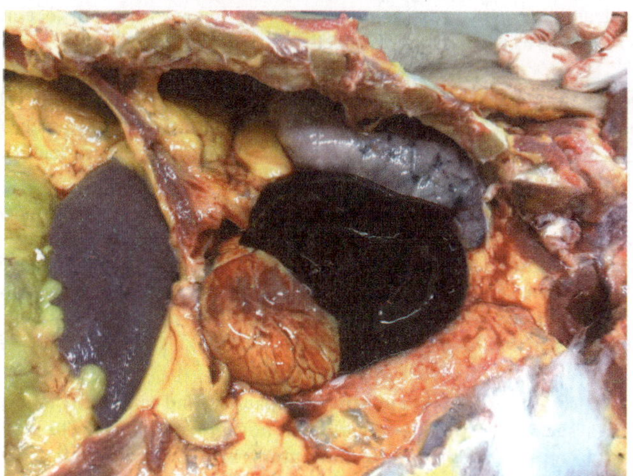

Fig. (6–8). Cardiac tamponade.

Courtesy: **Dr. Anil Kohli, UCMS, Delhi.**

(III) CENTRAL NERVOUS SYSTEM (10 to 18%): (1) Cerebral haemorrhage. (2) Cerebellar haemorrhage. (3) Pontine haemorrhage. (4) Subarachnoid haemorrhage. (5) Cerebral thrombosis and embolism. (6) Carotid artery thrombosis. (7) Brain abscess. (8) Brain tumour. (9) Meningitis. (10) Acute polioencephalitis. (11) Cysts of third or fourth ventricle. (12) Epilepsy.

(IV) ALIMENTARY SYSTEM (6 to 8%): (1) Haemorrhage into the gastrointestinal tract from peptic ulcer, oesophageal varices, cancer oesophagus, etc. (2) Perforation of ulcers, e.g., peptic, typhoid, amoebic or malignant. (3) Acute haemorrhagic pancreatitis. (4) Strangulated hernia. (5) Twisting and intussusception of the bowel. (6) Paralytic ileus. (7) Appendicitis. (8) Bursting of the liver abscess. (9) Rupture of enlarged spleen. (10) Intestinal obstruction. (11) Obstructive cholecystitis.

(V) GENITOURINARY SYSTEM (3 to 5%): (1) Chronic nephritis. (2) Nephrolithiasis. (3) Obstructive hydronephrosis and pyonephrosis. (4) Tuberculosis of the kidney. (5) Tumours of the kidney or bladder. (6) Rupture of ectopic pregnancy. (7) Toxaemia of pregnancy. (8) Uterine haemorrhage due to fibroids. (9) Cancer vulva eroding femoral vessels. (10) Twisting of ovary, ovarian cyst or fibroid tumour.

(VI) MISCELLANEOUS (5 to 10%): (1) Addison's disease. (2) Diabetes mellitus. (3) Haemochromatosis. (4) Hyperthyroidism. (5) Blood dyscrasias. (6) Cerebral malaria. (7) Shock due to emotional excitement. (8) Reflex vagal inhibition. (9) Anaphylaxis due to drugs. (10) Mismatched blood transfusion.

The majority of sudden deaths caused by atherosclerotic coronary artery disease are not associated with a coronary thrombus or an acute myocardial infarct. Coronary artery spasm can occur in persons with normal coronary arteries. Myocardial infarction and rare cases of sudden death do occur. Hypertension is the most common cause of concentric left ventricular hypertrophy which can cause sudden death even in the absence of significant atherosclerotic coronary artery disease.

CHAPTER

7 POSTMORTEM CHANGES

FM 2.6: Discuss presumption of death and survivorship.
FM 2.7: Describe and discuss suspended animation.
FM 2.8: Describe and discuss postmortem changes including signs of death, cooling of body, postmortem lividity, rigor mortis, cadaveric spasm, cold stiffening and heat stiffening.
FM 2.9: Describe putrefaction, mummification, adipocere and maceration.
FM 2.10: Discuss estimation of time since death.

SIGNS OF DEATH AND CHANGES FOLLOWING DEATH

Forensic taphonomy is the interdisciplinary study and interpretation of postmortem processes of human remains in the dispositional context, **i.e., the history of changes of a body following death.** A knowledge of the signs of death help to differentiate death from suspended animation. The changes which take place may be helpful in estimation of the approximate time of death. **Order of appearance of signs of death:**

(I) Immediate (somatic death).
(1) Insensibility and loss of voluntary power.
(2) Cessation of respiration.
(3) Cessation of circulation.
(II) Early (cellular death).
(4) Pallor and loss of elasticity of skin.
(5) Changes in the eye.
(6) Primary flaccidity of muscles.
(7) Cooling of the body.
(8) Postmortem lividity.
(9) Rigor mortis.
(III) Late (decomposition and decay).
(10) Putrefaction.
(11) Adipocere formation.
(12) Mummification.

Insensibility and Loss of Movement: This is the earliest sign of death, but it can lead to error if precautions are not taken. They are found in cases of prolonged fainting attack, vagal inhibitory phenomenon, epilepsy, trance, catalepsy, narcosis, electrocution, etc.

Cessation of Respiration: This must be complete and continuous. The stethoscope is placed over the upper portions of the lungs and larynx where the faintest breath-sounds can be heard. **Complete stoppage of respiration for more than 5 minutes usually causes death.** Respiration may stop for a very short period without causing death. It may occur. (1) as a purely voluntary act, (2) Cheyne-Stokes breathing, (3) drowning, and (4) newborn infants.

Feather test, mirror test and Winslow's test are of historical importance only.

Cessation of Circulation: The stethoscope is placed over the precordial area where the heartbeat can be heard readily. Under normal conditions, **stoppage of heartbeat for more than 5 minutes is irrecoverable and is accepted as evidence of death.**

Magnus test, Icard's test, diaphanous test, fingernail test, and heat test are of historical importance only.

SUSPENDED ANIMATION (apparent death): **In this condition signs of life are not found, as the functions are interrupted for some time, or are reduced to minimum.** However, life continues and resuscitation is successful in such cases. **The metabolic rate is so reduced that the requirement of individual cell for oxygen is satisfied through the use of oxygen dissolved in the body fluids.** In freezing of the body, or in severe drug poisoning of the brain, the activity of brain can completely stop and in some cases start again.

Types: (1) Suspended animation may be produced voluntarily. **Practitioners of yoga can pass into a trance, death-like in character.** (2) Involuntary suspension of animation **lasting from a few seconds to half-an-hour or more may be found** in vagal inhibition, severe syncopal attacks, newborn infants, drowning, electrocution, sunstroke, cholera, narcotic poisoning, after anaesthesia, shock, hypothermia, cerebral concussion, insanity, etc. The patient can be resuscitated by cardiac massage or electric stimulator and artificial respiration.

CASE: **(1) A physician was called to examine an elderly man at his home. The doctor saw the man lying in bed motionless, quickly checked the man's heart beat and pulse and declared the man dead. In the autopsy room, while the body was being placed on the table, the doctor heard a gurgling sound and noticed a slight swallowing movement. The man was rushed to a hospital and lived for two more months.**

(2) Two doctors, both experienced physicians, were driving behind an omnibus which ran over a child. They went to the scene and found the child lying under the front wheel of the bus; she was black in the face and appeared to be dead. Of this they were quite certain. It was impossible to extricate the child until the vehicle was reversed to set her free, a step which the driver took only after considerable persuasion. As soon as she was released, the child immediately showed signs of life. She was taken to an adjoining shop, and a few minutes later, she was found about to be given a drink. This the doctors forbade as they felt sure that rupture of viscera had occurred. The child was taken to hospital and after a day, made a complete and uneventful recovery.

(3) A man aged 83 years attempted suicide by smothering. He was certified to be dead and was taken to the mortuary. His relatives had come with wreaths. The undertakers also arrived, but were surprised to see the "dead man" seated on top of the coffin and complaining of hunger. He subsequently walked home unaided.

All postmortem changes are dependent on ambient temperature. High temperature accelerates the changes.

CHANGES IN THE SKIN: Skin becomes **pale and ashy-white and loses elasticity** within a few minutes of death. The lips appear dark-red to black, dry and hard due to drying.

CHANGES IN THE EYE: (1) Loss of Corneal Reflex: This is found in all cases of deep insensibility, e.g. epilepsy, narcotic poisoning, general anaesthesia and therefore not a reliable sign of death.

(2) Opacity of the Cornea: This may occur in certain diseases (cholera, wasting diseases) before death. The opacity is due to drying and is delayed for about two hours if the lids are closed after death. **If the eyelids are open for a few hours after death, a film of cell debris and mucus forms two yellow triangles on the sclera at each side of the iris, with base towards the margin of cornea and apex towards medial or lateral canthus of the eye, which become brown and then black called "tache noire" Figs. (7–1 and 7–2)** within 3 to 4 hours, upon which dust settles and the surface becomes wrinkled (artefact).

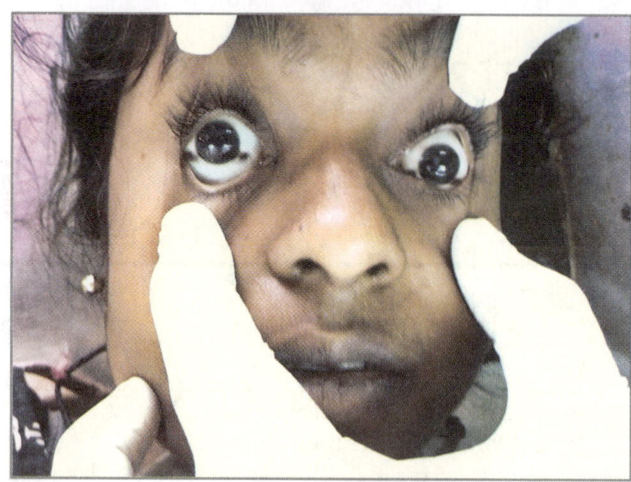

Fig. (7–1). **Tache noire.**

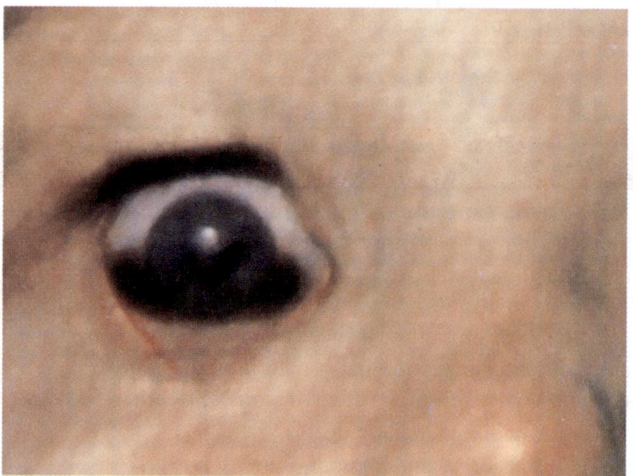

Fig. (7–2). **Tache noire.**

(3) Flaccidity of the Eyeball: The eyes look sunken and become softer within minutes due to reduction of intraocular tension. During life, the intraocular tension varies between 14 to 25 gm; soon after death it is less than 12 gm; within half an hour it is less than 3 gm., and becomes nil at the end of two hours.

(4) Pupils: **Soon after death, pupils are slightly dilated,** because of the relaxation of muscles of the iris. Later, they are constricted with the onset of rigor mortis of the constrictor muscles and evaporation of fluid. As such, their state after death is not an indication of their antemortem appearance. **Occasionally, rigor mortis may affect ciliary muscles of iris unequally, so that one pupil is larger than the other.** If different segments of the same iris are unequally affected, the pupil may be irregularly oval or have an eccentric position in the iris. **The pupils react to atropine and eserine for about an hour after death, but they do not react to strong light.** The shape of the pupil cannot be changed by pressure during life, but after death, if pressure is applied by fingers on two or more sides of the eyeball, the pupil may become oval, triangular or polygonal.

(5) Retinal Vessels: **Fragmentation or segmentation (trucking or shunting) of the blood columns (Kevorkian sign) in the retinal vessels appear within minutes after death, and persists for about an hour.** This occurs all over the body due to loss of blood pressure but **it can be seen only in retina by ophthalmoscope.** The retina is pale for the first two hours. At about six hours, the disk outline is hazy and becomes blurred in 7 to 10 hours. These changes are of little practical value.

(6) Chemical Changes: **A steady rise in the potassium values occur in the vitreous humour after death up to 100 hours.**

COOLING OF THE BODY (ALGOR MORTIS)

Loss of Body Heat: The cooling of the body ('chill of death') after death is a complex process, which **does not occur at the same rate throughout the body.** The body will not cool according to Newton's law. After stoppage of circulation, convectional transport of heat inside the body stops. **Heat is generated by residual metabolic process (glycogenolysis) of dying tissues and by metabolic activity of intestinal bacteria, due to which body temperature does not fall for some time.** With the start of cooling, a temperature gradient develops from the surface to the core of any part of the body. **Exchange of heat between the core and surface of the body occurs only by conduction. At first heat is lost from superficial layers of the body only.** Due to the low velocity of heat transport inside the body, it takes some time for heat to be conducted from the deeper layers to the more superficial layers, until finally, the temperature gradient reaches the core. **Internal organs cool primarily**

by conduction. Conductive heat exchange occurs due to the temperature difference between the body and surroundings, e.g. clothing, covering, air, water, etc. **The body heat is mostly lost by conduction (absorption of heat by objects in contact with the body) and convection (movement of air).** At non-contact areas heat exchange occurs by convectional mechanism, which exceeds that of contact surface. **Heat exchange by radiation (loss in the form of infrared heat rays) is extensive for the first hour, but decreases later,** depending on the rapid decrease in skin temperature. Only a small fraction of heat is lost by evaporation of fluid from the skin. **For about half to one hour after death, the rectal temperature falls little or not at all. (postmortem temperature plateau; isothermic phase) Fig. (7–3). This is followed by a linear rate of cooling (between 0.4 to 0.6°C per hour) for the next 12 to 16 hours.** Then the cooling rate is relatively uniform in its slope. Then it gradually becomes slower, and when the temperature is within about 4°C of the environment, rate of cooling becomes very slow. The human body rarely reaches the ambient (atmospheric) temperature unless the latter is at or near freezing, probably because enzyme and bacterial action starts during early decomposition. **The curve of cooling is sigmoid or inverted 'S' shaped in pattern,** because of some residual enzymatic activity and due to retention of heat for some time. In serious illness, circulation begins to fail before death, and hands and feet become cooler than the rest of the body; this coolness gradually extends towards the trunk. In sudden death, the cooling starts after death.

Measurement of temperature: A laboratory thermometer 25 cm. long, with a range of 0 to 50°C. which can be read in single degrees is used. **The rectum is the ideal place to record temperature except in cases of sodomy.** The thermometer should be inserted 8 to 10 cm. and left there for two minutes. The temperature can also be recorded by making a small opening into the peritoneal cavity and inserting the thermometer in contact with the inferior surface of the liver. **The external auditory meatus or the nasal passages also can be used** to record temperature. Where the nose is used, the probe or bulb should be passed up to the cribriform plate, and in the ear, should be placed on or through the tympanic membrane. A small electronic thermocouple with a digital readout is better. The time of this reading is recorded and temperature of environment is recorded at the same time. **Reading should be made at intervals of 1 to 2 hours, in order to obtain the rate of fall of temperature.**

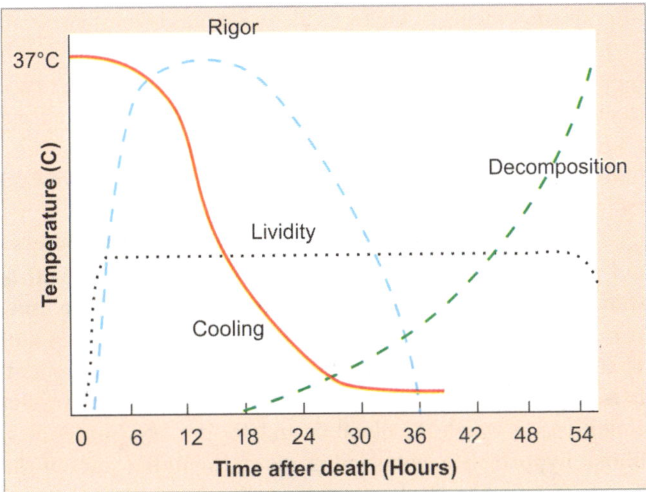

Fig. (7–3). Chart showing the major changes to estimate time since death.

A rough idea of approximate time in hours of death can be obtained by using the formula:

$$\frac{\textbf{Normal body temperature — rectal temperature}}{\textbf{Rate of temperature fall per hour}}$$

Variations in rectal temperature: The rectal temperature is between 36.5 to 37.5°C. Rectal temperature is about 0.6°C to 1°C higher than oral. **There are individual and daily variations up to 1 to 1.5°C. being lowest in the early morning and highest in the late evening. During sleep, the rectal temperature is 1/2° to 1°C. lower.** It cannot be assumed that the body temperature is normal at death. In cases of fat or air embolism, certain infections, septicaemia, heatstroke and in pontine haemorrhage, thyrotoxicosis, psychotic (emotional) stress, administration of neuroleptic medication, CO poisoning, intoxication with heroin and cocaine, drug reactions, etc. a sharp rise in temperature occurs. Exercise or struggle prior to death may raise the rectal temperature up to 1.5° to 2°C. Low temperature occurs in cases of collapse, congestive cardiac failure, hypothermia, hypothyroidism, administration of muscle relaxants, cholera, secondary shock, etc.

Factors Affecting Rate of Cooling: (1) The difference in temperature between the body and the medium: The temperature fall is rapid when the difference between body and air temperature is great. In India, during summer, the temperature of the environment may be higher than that of the body temperature, and as such the cooling is very slow. **In tropical climates the heat loss is roughly 0.4°C to 0.6°C and in temperate countries 1°C per hour. (2) The build of the cadaver**: The rate of heat loss is proportional to the weight of the body to its surface area. Thus, children and old people cool more rapidly than adults. **(3) The physique of the cadaver**: Fat is a bad conductor of heat. Fat bodies cool slowly and lean bodies rapidly. **(4) The environment of the body**: A body kept in a well-ventilated room will cool more rapidly than one in a closed room. Moist air is a better conductor of heat than dry air, so that cooling is more rapid in humid atmosphere than in dry atmosphere. Body heat is lost three times faster in water than in dry, cold area of some temperature because, water is a far better conductor of heat. **Cooling in still water is about twice as fast as in air, and in flowing water, it is about three times as fast.** Bodies cool more slowly in water containing sewage effluent or other putrefying organic material than in fresh water or sea water. **(5) Covering on or around the body:** The rate of cooling is slow when the body is clothed, as clothes are bad conductors of heat. A breadspread covering may at least halve the rate of cooling.

Because of the above external variable factors, an accurate formula cannot be devised to define rate of heat loss. The rectal temperature of an average-sized naked body reaches that of environment in about 15 to 20 hours. **If the body is exposed to a source of heat for a few hours shortly after death, its temperature will rise. A body in zero weather may undergo freezing and become stony-hard from formation of ice in**

cavities and blood vessels. The ice inside the skull may expand and cause separation of sutures.

Medicolegal Importance: Determination of temperature of the body is important only in cold and temperate climates, where more people die indoors. They are often useless in warm or tropical climate zones and outdoor deaths. In tropical zones, the postmortem fall in temperature may be minimal. It helps in the estimation of the time of death, which is not reliable.

Postmortem Caloricity: In this condition, the **temperature of the body remains raised for the first two hours or so after death. This occurs:** (1) when the regulation of heat production has been severely disturbed before death, as in sunstroke and in some nervous disorders, (2) when there has been a great increase in heat production in the muscles due to convulsions, as in tetanus and strychnine poisoning, etc., and (3) when there has been excessive bacterial activity, as in septicaemic condition, cholera and other fevers.

POSTMORTEM HYPOSTASIS

This is the bluish-purple or purplish-red (due to deoxyhaemoglobin) discolouration, which appears under the skin in the most superficial layers of the dermis (rete mucosum) of the dependent parts of the body after death, due to capillo-venous distention. It is also called **postmortem staining, subcutaneous hypostasis, livor mortis,** cadaveric lividity, suggilations, vibices and darkening of death.

Mechanism: It is caused by the stoppage of circulation, the stagnation of blood in blood vessels, and its tendency to sink by force of gravity. The blood tends to accumulate in the toneless capillaries and venules of the dependent parts of the body. Filling of these vessels produces a bluish-purple colour to the adjacent skin. The heavier red cells have a tendency to settle first imparting a deeper colour to the affected parts. **The upper portions of the body drained of blood are pale. The intensity of the colour depends upon the amount of reduced haemoglobin in the blood.** In cases of large amount of reduced haemoglobin before death, the blood has deep purplish-red colour. **The colour of the hypostasis may vary from area to area in the same body.**

In the recently dead or dying tissues, oxygen dissociation takes place, which is continued until equilibrium is reached between the tension of the oxygen in the capillaries and the surrounding tissues. There may also be backward flow of venous blood from the venular end of the capillaries, which adds to the blueness of the blood after death. **It is not possible to distinguish the postmortem discolouration from that produced by cyanosis in the living.**

Development: Postmortem lividity **begins shortly after death, but it may not be visible for about half to one hour after death in normal individuals, and from about one to four hours in anaemic persons. Dull-red patches of 1 to 2 cm. diameter appear in 20 to 30 minutes to two hours. These patches then deepen, increase in intensity and become confluent in 1 to 4 hours. In the early stage these patches can be mistaken for bruises** Table (7–1). In doubtful cases, a portion should be removed for microscopic examination.

Christison refers to two cases, in one of which two persons were convicted, and in the other three narrowly escaped conviction, upon a mistake of this kind.

Table (7–1). Hypostasis related to the time of death [hours post-mortem (hpm)]

Stage	Lower limit	Upper limit
Beginning	0.25	3
Confluence	1.0	4
Maximum	3.0	16
Thumb pressure	1.0	20
Complete shifting	2.0	6
Incomplete shifting	4.0	24

Computed by Mallach from literature data.

The areas then enlarge and combine to produce extensive discolouration. In some bodies, isolated patches of lividity remain separate from the large areas of lividity resembling contusions. Frost erythema, hypothermia induced red-purple spots seen over prominent parts of the body such as shoulder, knee or elbow joints may sometimes be mistaken for hypostatic patches. **Circulatory stasis in the aged, and sometimes the effect of cold, may resemble the effects of violence.** Such marks are usually found on ears, shins, forearms and hands, where the circulation is comparatively poor and the skin is exposed. **When lividity first develops, if the end of the finger is firmly pressed against the skin and held for a second or two, the lividity at that part will disappear and the skin will be pale or white. When the pressure is released the lividity will reappear.** The plasma tends to cause oedema of the dependent parts and contributes to the cutaneous blisters of early putrefaction. In the early stages mottled patches of hypostasis may be seen on the upper surfaces of the body, especially the legs and thighs due to uneven dilatation of the vascular bed. These patches soon join together and slide down to the dependent parts. **It is usually well developed within four hours and reaches a maximum between 6 to 12 hours (primary lividity) and persists until putrefaction sets in** Fig. (7–3). It is present in all bodies, but is more clearly seen in bodies of fair people than in those of dark. It may not be appreciated in old and anaemic persons.

Shifting of lividity: If the body is moved within few hours after death, patches of lividity will disappear and new ones will form on dependent parts, (secondary lividity), but lividity to a lighter degree remains in the original area, due to staining of the tissues by haemolysis **(complete shifting).** This may take from a few minutes to up to one hour. In **incomplete shifting,** after turning the body over, lividity appears slightly in the downward facing parts.

Intensity: It is intense in asphyxia, where the blood may not readily coagulate, and in cases of sudden death with a short agonal period and a great circulating blood volume. It is less marked in death from haemorrhage, anaemia and wasting diseases due to reduced amount of blood and pigment. It is less marked in death from lobar pneumonia, and other conditions in which the blood coagulates quickly. **Sometimes, bluish hypostasis becomes pink along the upper part of the horizontal margin, the lower parts remaining dark.** This is due to the haemoglobin being oxygenated where the erythrocytes are less densely packed in the upper layers of hypostasis.

The extent of lividity. It mainly depends upon: (1) the volume of blood in circulation at the time of death, and (2) the length of time that the blood remains fluid after death. **Hypostatic congestion resembling postmortem hypostasis may be seen a few hours before death in case of a person dying slowly with circulatory failure,** e.g. cholera, typhus, tuberculosis, uraemia, morphine and barbiturate poisoning, congestive cardiac failure, deep coma, and asphyxia. In such cases, hypostasis will be marked shortly after death. Lividity can be marked shortly after death in a person dying slowly from circulatory failure.

Petechial haemorrhages: Numerous coarse or fine petechial haemorrhages may be present in hypostatic areas in deaths during an anoxic state. They are very common in narcotic poisoning and in sudden collapse due to acute cardiac arrest. **Petechiae may be seen in hypostatic area in 18 to 24 hours due to rupture of small vessels.**

The distribution of P.M. hypostasis: The distribution of the stain depends on the position of the body. (1) **In a body lying on its back** (supine) it first appears in the neck, and then spreads over the entire back extending up the flanks and sides of the neck, with the exception of the parts directly pressed on, i.e. occipital scalp, shoulderblades, buttocks, posterior aspects of thighs, calves and heels. **Any pressure prevents the capillaries from filling, such as the collar band, waist band, belts, wrinkles in the clothes, etc. and such areas remain free from colour and are seen as strips or bands called vibices**. This is also caused by pressure of one area of the body with another; in which case "mirror image" blanching may be seen **(contact pallor, contact blanching). Such pale areas should not be mistaken for marks due to beating, or when they are present on the neck, due to strangling.** Hypostasis is usually well-marked in the lobes of the ears and in the tissues under nails of the fingers. **In asphyxial deaths, the nail beds will retain the cyanotic colour present, when the body was first refrigerated. As the vessel walls become permeable due to decomposition, blood leaks through them and stains the tissues. At this stage, hypostasis does not disappear,** if finger is firmly pressed against the skin. The pattern of lividity may be modified by local changes in the position of the body, e.g., if the head is turned to one side and slightly flexed on the neck for some hours after death blood may gravitate into a linear distribution determined by the folds formed in the skin and subcutaneous tissues. If such a body is examined after the neck has been straightened, the linear discolouration of the stains may be mistaken for marks due to beating. (2) **If the body is lying in prone position,** the lividity appears in the loose connective tissues in front, the colour is intense and Tardieu spots are common. **Sometimes, the congestion is so great that minute blood vessels are ruptured in the nose, and cause bleeding Fig. (7–4).** In persons who die in prone position, petechiae, ecchymoses and cutaneous blood blisters may develop after death, in areas of deep hypostasis especially in the shoulders or over the chest, which may be mistaken for asphyxial death. They are more common in cyanotic, congestive types of death and become more prominent as postmortem interval lengthens. (3) **If the body has been lying on one side,** the blood will settle on that side. (4) **If the body is left with the head downwards,** the confluent petechiae and ecchymoses may be so marked that they virtually blacken the face and neck. In sudden infant death syndrome and in drunken persons and epileptics who die face down on a pillow or other surface, pale areas are often seen on the face around the nose and mouth due to pressure against the supporting surface. This should not be mistaken for suffocation. (5) **If the body is inverted as in drunken persons who slide out of bed, hypostasis will appear in the head and neck. The eyes may suffuse, and numerous haemorrhages may appear in the conjunctivae and hypostatic areas.** This may give rise to suspicion of suffocation or strangulation. (6) If the body has been suspended in the vertical position as in hanging, hypostasis will be most marked in the legs, hands and external genitalia, and if suspension be prolonged for a few hours, petechial haemorrhages are seen in the skin. (7) **In drowning,** postmortem staining is usually found on the face, the upper part of chest, hands, lower arms, feet and the calves, as they are the dependent parts. If the body is constantly moving and changing its position, as after drowning in flowing water, the staining may not develop. (8) **Sometimes, blotchy areas of lividity appear on the upper surface of the limbs due to some irregularity of capillary dilatation at the time of death.** The internal jugular veins are markedly engorged due to the blood which has drained from the head. This blood cannot drain away below to the heart, as the valves in the subclavain veins prevent the drainage of blood into the upper limbs. As a result of this, the tributaries of the superficial veins in the neck cannot be effectively drained, due to which **isolated areas of lividity may develop on the front and sides of the neck resembling bruises. In certain cases, isolated patches of lividity remain separate from the large areas of lividity resembling contusions.**

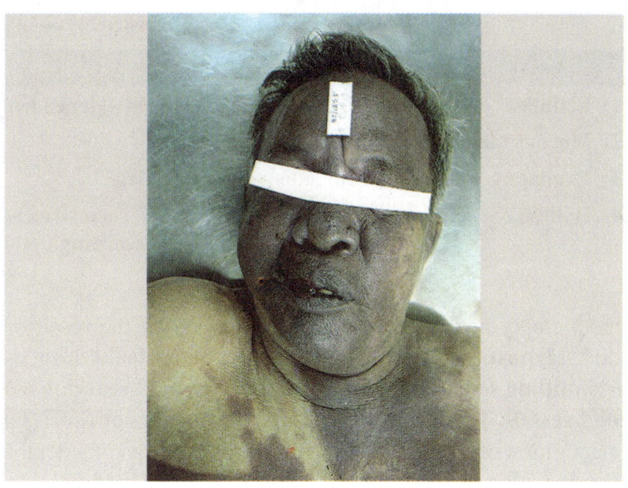

Fig. (7–4). PM hypostasis on front of body due to body lying in prone position.

Fixation: It was thought that **fixation of p.m. hypostasis** was due to clotting of blood in blood vessels, but it is not correct. **The physical factors for fixation of p.m. staining are:** (1) Blood cannot pass out of the capillaries after formation of p.m. hypostasis. (2) Rigor mortis obliterates the big vessels, and as such the blood cannot pass through these vessels to settle in venules and capillaries in a new area. (3) After full development of rigor mortis, venules and capillaries are compressed and

Table (7–2). Difference between postmortem hypostasis and congestion

Trait	Hypostasis	Congestion
(1) Redness:	Irregular and occurs on a dependent part.	Uniform all over the organ.
(2) Mucous membranes:	Dull and lusterless.	Normal.
(3) Exudate:	No inflammatory exudate.	Exudate may be seen.
(4) Hollow viscus:	Stomach and intestine when stretched show alternate stained and unstained areas according to the position of coils.	Uniform staining.

almost empty and cannot be easily distended by the resettling blood. **Hypostasis becomes fixed when blood leaks into the surrounding soft tissues due to haemolysis and breakdown of blood vessels. This usually occurs in 6 to 12 hours or more,** but the condition of blood at the time of death exerts a considerable influence. Non-displacement and non-shifting of lividity is due to haemoconcentration by loss of fluid which penetrates the wall of those vessels related to the hydrostatic pressure. Fixation occurs earlier in summer and is delayed in asphyxial deaths and in intracranial lesions. **Some authors are of the opinion that hypostasis does not get fixed.**

Calorimetry shows an increasing paleness of the hypostasis between 3 to 5 hours, from a wavelength of 575 nm at 3 hours at an average rate of 2 nm per hour. Vanezis claims that there is a linear relationship between the fading colour of the hypostasis, and time during the first 24 hours, after which the relationship in unpredictable.

Haemorrhages: Tiny, often spot-like, sometimes confluent oval to round, bluish-black haemorrhages **(death spots, postmortem ecchymoses)**, are exclusively limited to areas of hypostasis as a result of mechanical rupture of subcutaneous capillaries and venules. **They are seen commonly in the back of the shoulders and neck, and sometimes on the front of the chest, even when the body is lying on its back.** They are common in cyanotic congestive types of death, and appear more prominent with the increase in postmortem interval, and may blacken the face and skin. They are more prominent when the body lies with the head downwards.

Absence of hypostasis: Hypostasis may be sparse or even **absent in deaths where considerable blood loss of at least 65% of the circulating blood volume in adults and 45% in infants, occurs before death due to trauma. In severe anaemia lividity will be absent.**

Internal Hypostasis: Hypostasis also occurs in the dependent parts of internal organs Table (7–2). When a body is in supine position, hypostasis is seen in the posterior portions of the cerebrum and cerebellum, the dorsal portions of the lungs, posterior wall of the stomach, dorsal portions of the liver, kidneys, spleen, larynx, heart, and the lowermost coils of intestine in the pelvic cavity. **Hypostasis in the heart can simulate myocardial infarction, and in the lungs it may suggest pneumonia; dependent coils of intestine appear strangulated.**

Colour changes: In asphyxia, the colour of the stains is deeply bluish-violet or purple. A brownish hypostasis may be seen in methaemoglobinaemia and rarely a bronze colour in Clostridium perfringens septicaemia usually associated with septic abortion. In septic abortion from Cl. welchii, greenish-brown colour is seen. A bright pink colour is seen in hypothermia and bodies taken from cold water, and in refrigerated bodies as the wet skin allows atmospheric oxygen to pass through, and also at low temperatures haemoglobin has a greater affinity for oxygen. This may be most marked over large joints and dependent areas. **Refrigerated bodies may also assume a pink colour.** In mummification, lividity may turn from brown to black with drying of the body.

Infection combined with disseminated intravascular coagulation sometimes causes blotchy purplish, red or pink rashes which may be mistaken for bruises or abrasions.

Colour Changes in Poisoning: The hypostatic areas have distinct colour in certain cases of poisoning, e.g. (1) In carbon monoxide poisoning, the colour is cherry-red Fig. (7–5). (2) In hydrocyanic acid poisoning and sometimes in burns the colour is bright-red. (3) In poisoning by nitrites, potassium chlorate, potassium bicarbonate, nitrobenzene, acetanilide, bromates, and aniline (causing methaemoglobinaemia) the colour is chocolate or brownish-red Fig. (7–6). (4) In poisoning by phosphorus the colour is dark-brown or yellow. (5) In poisoning by hydrogen sulphide, the colour is bluish-green. (6) In CO_2 poisoning, the colour is deep-blue.

Colour Changes in Decomposition: Changes in postmortem lividity occur when putrefaction sets in. In early stages, there is haemolysis of blood and diffusion of blood pigment into the surrounding tissues, where it may undergo secondary changes, e.g., sulphhaemoglobin formation. The capillary endothelium and the surrounding cells show lytic changes. Microscopically, the cellular outlines are obscured and the capillaries are not identifiable.

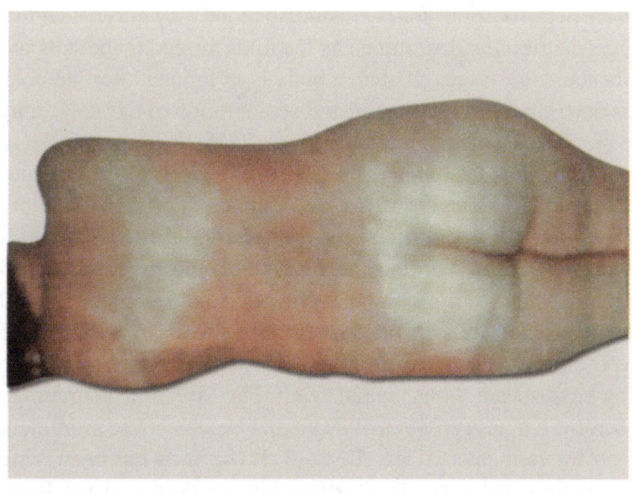

Fig. (7–5). Cherry-red PM hypostasis in CO poisoning.

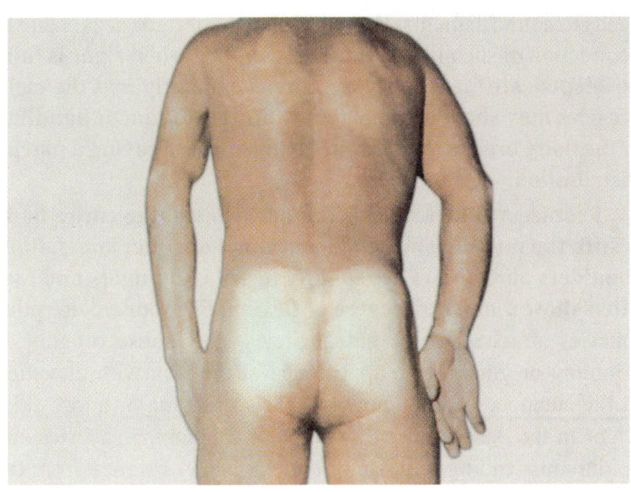

Fig. (7–6). **Chocolate-colored PM lividity in sodium chlorate poisoning.**

A contused area shows similar putrefactive changes and it becomes impossible to determine whether the pigment in a stained putrefied area originated from an intravascular (hypostasis) or/and extravascular localised collection of blood (contusion). There is diffusion of blood-stained fluid in the chest or abdominal cavities. As decomposition progresses, the lividity becomes dusky in colour and turns brown, green and back before finally disappearing with destruction of the blood.

Medicolegal Importance: (1) It is a sign of death. (2) Its extent helps in estimating the time of death, which is unreliable, because of its variability in its appearance. (3) It indicates the posture of the body at the time of death. (4) It may indicate the moving of the body to another position sometime after death. (5) Sometimes, the colour may indicate the cause of death. (6) Sometimes, distribution of lividity may suggest manner of death.

VARIOUS COLOUR MARKINGS ON DEAD BODY: Various types of colour markings may be seen on the skin or in the internal organs of dead body.

(A) ANTEMORTEM ORIGIN: (1) Trauma: Bruises and traumatic asphyxia. (2) Asphyxia: Cyanosis. (3) Inflammation: Congestion in organs or the skin. (4) Emboli: Fat embolism. (5) Physical: Exposure to severe cold, and heat.

(B) POSTMORTEM ORIGIN: (1) Hypostasis. (2) Putrefaction. (3) Poisoning: CO, HCN, nitrites, chlorate, etc.

(C) ARTIFICIAL: Paint, grease, dust, mud, coal, blood, semen, etc.

The cause of the colouration can be determined by the patterns of colour distribution, shape, relationship of clothing, etc.

Effects of Keeping Cadavers in Refrigerating Chamber: If the body is refrigerated soon after death, the onset of rigor mortis is delayed. Reddish patches appear on the surface, especially in the hypostatic region, and sometimes in internal organs. **The blood is bright-red and injuries like abrasions and contusions become prominent.** The tissues are dehydrated and become hard.

MUSCULAR CHANGES

After death, the muscles of the body pass through three stages: (1) Primary relaxation or flaccidity. (2) Rigor mortis or cadaveric rigidity. (3) Secondary flaccidity.

Primary Flaccidity: During this stage, death is only somatic (no cellular death) and **it lasts for one to two hours. All the muscles of the body begin to relax soon after death.** The lower jaw falls, eyelids loose tension, and joints are flexible. Body flattens over areas which are in contact with the surface on which it rests **(contact flattening).** Muscles are relaxed as long as the ATP content remains sufficiently high to permit the splitting of the actin-myosin cross-bridges. Muscular irritability and response to mechanical or electrical stimuli persist. Peristalsis may occur in the bowel, and ciliary movements and movements of white cells may continue. **Discharges of the dying motor neurons may stimulate small groups of muscle cells and lead to focal twitching, although these decrease with time. Anaerobic chemical processes may continue in the tissue cells,** e.g., the liver cells may dehydrogenate ethyl alcohol to acetic acid, and complex chemical changes may occur in the muscles. **Pupils react to atropine or physostigmine. but not to light.** Loss of muscle tone in the sphincters may result in emptying of bladder. Muscle protoplasm is slightly alkaline.

RIGOR MORTIS

Rigor mortis (death stiffening; cadaveric rigidity) is a state of stiffening of muscles, sometimes with slight shortening of the fibres. Individual cell death takes place in this stage.

Mechanism: Rigor mortis is a physico-chemical change that occurs within muscles. A voluntary muscle consists of bundles of long fibres. Each fibre is formed of densely packed myofibrils extending through its whole length. These myofibrils are the contractile elements, and are made up of protein filaments of two types, actin filaments (thin) and myosin filaments (thick) which form a loose physico-chemical combination called actomyosin, which is physically shorter than the two substances uncombined. In the relaxed condition, the actin filaments interdigitate with the myosin filaments only to a small extent. Under the influence of the nerve impulse, the arrays of actin filaments are drawn into the arrays of myosin filaments, rather like pistons into cylinders. This causes the muscle to contract.

During life, the separation of the actin and myosin filaments, and the energy needed for contraction are dependent on adenosinetriphosphate (ATP). Three metabolic systems are responsible for maintaining a continuous supply of ATP in the muscle: (1) Phosphagen system. (2) Glycogen-lactic acid system. (3) Aerobic system. ATP is responsible for elasticity and plasticity of the muscle. The dephosphorylation of ATP by the action of ATPase produces ADP and phosphate, and a large amount of energy, which is used for muscle contraction. The free phosphate then engages in a phosphorylation reaction that converts glycogen to lactic acid. The lactic acid enters blood stream and reconverted to glycogen in the liver. The lost ATP is replaced during life by resynthesis, which is dependent upon the supply of glycogen. **At the time of somatic death, enough ATP is present in the muscle to maintain relaxation. After death the ATP is progressively and irreversibly destroyed leading to increased accumulation of lactates and phosphates in the muscles. There is no resynthesis of ATP. The postmortem alteration of ATP is due to dephosphorylation and deamination.** Postmortem loss of integrity of the muscle cell sarcoplasmic reticulum allows calcium ions to flood the contractile units of the muscle fibres (sarcomeres) initiating the binding of actin and myosin molecules and mimicking the normal contraction process. Normal relaxation in life is achieved by energy-dependent (ATP-driven) pumping of calcium back across the membrane of the sarcoplasmic reticulum, but this fails after death because of membrane disruption and lack of ATP, due to which **increased calcium level in the sarcomeres causes muscle contraction. When the ATP is reduced to a critical level (85% of the normal), the overlapping portions of myosin and actin filaments combine as rigid link of actomyosin, which is viscous and inextensible, and causes hardness and rigidity of muscle rigor. The rigidity of the muscle is at its maximum, when the level of ATP is reduced to 15% and lactic acid level is 0.3%.** The actin-myosin complex is trapped in a state of contraction until it is physically disrupted by the onset of putrefaction. This process is characterised by proteolytic detachment of actin molecules from the ends of the sarcomeres, and consequent loss of the structural integrity of the contractile units. The muscles then soften and relax.

The Order of Appearance of Rigor: All muscles of the body, both voluntary and involuntary are affected. It does not start in all muscles simultaneously (Nysten's rule). It first appears in involuntary muscles; the myocardium becomes rigid in an hour. It begins in the eyelids, neck and lower jaw and passes upwards to the muscles of the face, and downwards to the muscles of the chest, upper limbs, abdomen and lower limbs and lastly in the fingers and toes. In individual limbs, it usually progresses from above downwards. Such a sequence is not constant, symmetrical or regular. In individual limbs, it disappears in the same order in which it has appeared. Rigor mortis always sets in, increases and decreases gradually.

Shapiro (1950) suggests that rigor mortis does not follow the anatomical sequence usually described. He suggests that as rigor mortis is a physicochemical process, it is most likely to develop simultaneously in all the muscles, although the changes are more easily first detected in the smaller masses than in the larger. The **proximo-distal progression** is more apparent than real, for the sequence is determined by the bulk and kind of muscle involved. This would explain the fixation of elbow or knee joints at an earlier stage than the shoulder or hip joints, but this does not explain why the small muscles of the fingers and toes should be the last to stiffen.

Development: The development of rigor is concerned with muscles only. It is independent of the integrity of the nervous system, though it is said to develop more slowly in paralysed limbs. Before rigor mortis develops, the body can be moved to any posture, and the rigor will fix in that posture. **When rigor is developing, the extremities can be moved and the rigor, temporarily overcome, develops later and fixes the extremities in their new position, although the rigidity will be less than other symmetrical groups,** which have not been disturbed. Skeletal muscle contains two types of fibres. (1) Type I (red) which are rich in mitochondria with dominant oxidative metabolism. (2) Type II (white) which are relatively poor in mitochondria with dominant glycolytic metabolism. Rigor occurs at different times in the above types of muscles. The fibres which are still slack and some others which are not fully contracted, retain capacity for reversible binding of myosin heads to actin filaments. Re-establishment of rigor occurs due to contraction of such fibres. **If force is applied when rigor is fully developed, stiffness is broken up permanently and the rigid muscles may show postmortem ruptures. Frequent handling of the body breaks the rigor in certain places, leaving a patchy distribution.**

Features: When rigor is fully developed, the entire body is stiff, the muscles shortened, hard and opaque; knees, hips, shoulders and elbows are slightly flexed and fingers and toes often show a marked degree of flexion. Rigor of erector pilae muscles attached to the hair follicles, may cause roughness, pimpling or goose-flesh appearance of the skin with elevation of the cutaneous hairs, known as **cutis anserina** or goose skin. Rigor in the dartos muscle of scrotum can compress testes and epididymis leading to postmortem extrusion of semen from the urethral meatus. The pupils may be partially contracted. Rarely, if the uterus is in labour at the time of death, the rigor mortis may cause the uterus to contract and expel the foetus.

Testing: Rigor is tested by trying to lift the eyelids, depressing the jaw, and gently bending the neck and various joints of the body. Note the degree (absent, minimal, moderate, advanced or complete) and distribution.

P.M. Changes caused by Rigor Mortis: In the heart, rigor causes ventricles to contract, which may be mistaken for left ventricular hypertrophy. This can be excluded by measuring weight, estimating the relative size of left side and measuring ventricular thickness. **Secondary muscular flaccidity may result in distension of the atria or ventricles,** which should not be mistaken for antemortem dilatation of the chambers, or myocardial degeneration. Because of these postmortem changes, it is not possible to determine at autopsy whether a heart has stopped in systole or diastole. Muscle relaxation immediately after death with opening of the eyes and mouth and subsequent fixation in rigor mortis often occur after death, giving the **face the appearance of grimacing,** but this does not reflect whether the individual's last moments were of fear or fright.

Time of Onset: In India, it begins one to two hours after death and takes further one to two hours to develop and gets well-established in the entire body in six hours in summer. In temperate countries, it begins in three to six hours and takes further two to three hours to develop Table (7–3). The so-called rule of 12 (march of rigor) is not applicable in tropical countries.

Duration of Rigor Mortis: In India, usually it lasts 24 to 48 hours in winter and 18 to 36 hours in summer. It may begin to disappear in about 12 hours. It lasts for 2 to 3 days in temperate regions. These times are variable, because of many extrinsic and intrinsic factors. **When rigor sets in early, it passes off quickly and vice versa.**

Table (7–3). Rigor related to time of death (hpm)

Stage	Lower limit	Upper limit
Beginning	0.5	7
Maximum	2.0	20
Re-establishment after breaking	2.0	8

Computed by Mallach from literature data.

Conditions Altering the Onset and Duration:

(1) AGE: **Rigor is commonly found in stillborn infants at full term. In healthy adults, it develops slowly but is well-marked and lasts longer, while in children and old people it is feeble and rapid.**

(2) NATURE OF DEATH: **The onset of rigor is early and duration is short in deaths from diseases causing great exhaustion and wasting, e.g., cholera, typhoid, tuberculosis, cancer, etc. and in violent death as by cut-throat, firearms, electrocution and lightning. In organophosphate poisoning rigidity appears early. CO poisoning delays disappearance. The onset is delayed in deaths from asphyxia, severe haemorrhage, apoplexy, pneumonia, and nervous disease causing paralysis of muscle. In death due to poisoning from HCN and strychnine, it starts early and persists longer. It may disappear very rapidly in case of widespread bacterial infection, especially in gas gangrene, where putrefaction begins early. Rigor mortis is frequently absent in persons dying from septicaemia.**

(3) MUSCULAR STATE: **The onset is slow and the duration long in case where muscles are healthy and at rest before death. The onset is rapid, and duration short, if there is fatigue or exhaustion (violent or heavy exercise, severe convulsions) before death. In persons who run prior to death, rigor may develop earlier and rapidly in their legs, compared to other parts. Rigor may be delayed or very weak in emaciated persons.**

(4) ATMOSPHERIC CONDITIONS: **The onset is slow and duration long in cold weather. Rigor persists longer in cold wet air than in fresh dry air. It is prolonged by dry cold air and cold water. The onset is rapid due to heat, because of the increased breakdown of ATP, but the duration is short. If the body is in an extremely hot environment and decomposition begins, rigor mortis may disappear in 12 hours after death. It may persist for 3 to 4 days in refrigerated conditions.**

Because of the number and variability of the factors which influence the development of rigor mortis, it is not possible to draw any general rule for the rate of its onset, duration and disappearance.

Medicolegal Importance: (1) It is a sign of death. (2) Its extent helps in estimating the time of death, which is not reliable. (3) It indicates the position of the body at the time of death. If the body is lying on its back with its lower limbs raised in the air, it indicates that the body reached full rigidity elsewhere while lying in a position where the legs were flexed or the feet suspended and was later moved to the latter position where the support is no longer present.

CONDITIONS SIMULATING RIGOR MORTIS

(1) Heat Stiffening: **When a body is exposed to temperatures above 65°C. a rigidity is produced, which is much more marked than that found in rigor mortis.** The degree and depth of the change depends on the intensity of the heat and the time for which it was applied. It is seen in deaths from burning, high voltage electric shock and from falling into hot liquid. Heat causes stiffening of the muscles, because the tissue proteins are denatured and coagulated as in cooking. **The muscles are contracted, dessicated or even carbonised on the surface.** A zone of brownish-pink 'cooked meat', is seen under this, overlying normal red muscle. Changes in posture, especially flexion of the limbs occur due to muscle contraction. **Heat stiffening cannot be broken down by extending the limbs as in rigor mortis.** The stiffening remains until the muscles and ligaments soften from decomposition and the **normal rigor mortis does not occur.**

(2) Cold Stiffening: **When a body is exposed to freezing temperatures (–5°C or lower) before acid metabolites appear in the muscles, the tissues become frozen and stiff, due to freezing of the body fluids and solidification of subcutaneous fat simulating rigor.** The body is extremely cold and markedly rigid. When the joints are forcibly flexed, ice breaks in the synovial fluid with a sudden sharp sound. **If the body is placed in warm atmosphere, the stiffness disappears and after a time, the normal rigor mortis occurs rapidly and passes off quickly. Hardening of the subcutaneous fat especially in infants sometimes makes the skin-folds rigid, which may be mistaken for ligature mark.**

(3) Cadaveric Spasm or Instantaneous Rigor: Mechanism: The mechanism of cadaveric spasm is **obscure but possibly may be neurogenic** and not the same chemical process as true rigor **Fig. (7–7)**. The persistence of contraction after death may be due to the failure of the chemical processes required for active muscular relaxation to occur during molecular death. **Adrenocortical exhaustion which impairs resynthesis of ATP may be a possible cause. It differs only in the speed of onset and the circumstances in which it occurs.**

Muscles involved: Cadaveric spasm (cataleptic rigidity) is a rare condition. **In this, the group of muscles which have been actively working and contracted at the moment of death become stiff and rigid immediately after death without passing into the stage of primary relaxation. As such, the change preserves the exact attitude of the person at the time of death for several hours afterwards.** The spasm is primarily vital phenomenon, in that it originates by normal nervous stimulation of the muscles. **This is usually limited to a single group of voluntary muscles and frequently involves the hands** Fig. (7–7). Occasionally, the whole body is affected as seen in soldiers shot in battle, when the body may retain the posture which it assumed at the moment of death. The difference between rigor mortis and cadaveric spasm is given in **Table (7–4)**.

Predisposing Factors: It occurs especially in cases of intense physical and/or emotional activity such as excitement, fear, severe pain, exhaustion, cerebral haemorrhage, injury to the nervous

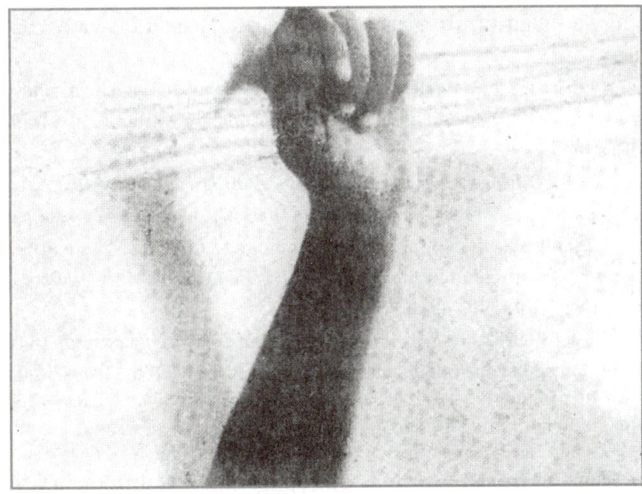

Fig. (7–7). Cadaveric spasm. The indoor aerial is seen firmly grasped in the hand causing electrocution.

Table (7–4). Difference between rigor mortis and cadaveric spasm

Trait	Rigor mortis	Cadaveric spasm
(1) Production:	Freezing and exposure to temperature above 65°C will produce rigor.	Cannot be produced by any method after death.
(2) Mechanism:	Known. Reduction of ATP.	Not clearly known.
(3) Predisposing factors:	Nil.	Sudden death, excitement, fear, exhaustion, nervous tension, etc.
(4) Time of onset:	1–2 hours after death.	Instantaneous.
(5) Muscles involved:	All the muscles of the body, both voluntary and involuntary.	Usually restricted to a single group of voluntary muscles.
(6) Muscle stiffening:	Not marked; moderate force can overcome it.	Marked; very great force is required to overcome it.
(7) Molecular death:	Occurs.	Does not occur.
(8) Body heat:	Cold.	Warm.
(9) Electrical stimuli:	Muscles do not respond.	Muscles respond.
(10) Muscular reaction:	Acidic.	Alkaline.
(11) Medicolegal importance:	Indicates time of death.	Indicates mode of death, i.e. suicide, homicide or accident.

system, firearm wound of the head, drowning, convulsant poisons, such as strychnine, etc. **No other condition simulates cadaveric spasm and it cannot be produced by any method, after death.** Very great force is required to overcome stiffness. It passes without interruption into normal rigor mortis and disappears when rigor disappears. **Coagulation of protein is seen in burns on microscopic examination but not in cadaveric spasm.**

Medicolegal importance. (1) Occasionally, in case of suicide, the weapon, e.g., pistol or knife is seen firmly grasped in the victim's hand which is a strong presumptive evidence of suicide. Attempts may be made to simulate this condition in order to conceal murder. But, ordinary rigor does not produce the same firm grip of a weapon, and the weapon may be placed in the hand in a way which could not have been used by a suicide. (2) If the deceased dies due to assault, some part of clothing, e.g., button of his assailant or some hair may be firmly grasped in the hands. (3) In case of drowning, material such as grass, weeds or leaves may be found firmly grasped in the hands, which indicates that the victim was alive on entering the water.

CASE: (1) Tidy (1882) mentioned the soldier at Balaclava whose body remained in position on his horse for some time after he had been killed by a shell.

(2) Tidy also cited the incident at Sedan, described by Rossbach (1870), when six soldiers were killed by a shell. The head of one preserved his laughing expression, present at the moment of death. The body of another, who also had his head blown off, remained in a sitting posture, with a cup still in his hand.

(3) Tidy (1882) described two lovers who, after taking cyanide were found folded in each other's arms, their bodies stiffened in this position.

(4) Spilsbury (1944) recorded the case of a woman found dead, seated upright in her bath; she held a sponge in her hand which was raised half way to her face. Death was due to cerebral haemorrhage.

Secondary Relaxation: Flaccidity following rigor mortis is caused by the action of the alkaline liquids produced by putrefaction. Another view is that rigidity disappears due to solution of myosin by excess of acid produced during rigor mortis. A third view is that enzymes are developed in dead muscle which dissolve myosin by a process of autodigestion.

DECOMPOSITION

It involves two processes: (1) Autolysis and (2) Putrefaction.

AUTOLYSIS: Autolysis is self-digestion of tissues. Soon after death, cell membranes become permeable and breakdown, with release of cytoplasm containing enzymes. Lysosomes and their digestive enzymes (mainly hydrolases) are released from the cells. The proteolytic, glycolytic and lipolytic action of ferments cause autodigestion and disintegration of organs, which occurs without bacterial influence. This chemical process is increased by heat and is stopped by freezing or inactivation of enzymes by the heat. The earliest autolytic changes occur in parenchymatous and glandular tissues and in the brain. The lining of intestines, adrenal medulla and pancreas autolyse within hours of death. Autolytic fermentation results in maceration of the dead foetus in utero, early softening and liquefaction of the brain of the newborn and infants, and softening of the internal organs. Autodigestion by acid gastric juice is a common finding in the newborn and infants, and is seen as softening and rupture of the stomach and lower oesophagus. In adults, such digestion may start before death in cases of intracranial lesions. The earliest external sign is a whitish, cloudy appearance in the cornea.

PUTREFACTION: It is the final stage following death, in which destruction of the soft tissues of the body occurs. The terms decomposition and putrefaction are used as synonyms. Putrefaction usually follows the disappearance of rigor mortis. During hot season, it may commence before rigor mortis has completely disappeared from the lower extremities.

Mechanism: Organisms enter the tissues shortly after death, mainly from the alimentary canal, and less often through the respiratory tract or through an external skin wound. Multiplication of bacteria begins within 4 hours and peak is reached within 24–30 hours. The intestines contain more than one thousand different species of bacteria. The fall in the oxygen concentration in the tissues and rise in hydrogen ion concentration after death favour bacterial growth and spread throughout the body. **Because the protective agencies of the body are absent, the bacteria spread through the blood vessels using the proteins and carbohydrates of the blood as culture media. Destruction is caused mainly by the action of bacterial enzymes, mostly anaerobic organisms derived from the intestines.** Other enzymes are derived from fungi, such as Penicillium and Aspergillus and sometimes from insects, which may be mature or in larval stage. **The chief destructive bacterial agent is Cl. welchii, which causes marked haemolysis, liquefaction of postmortem clots and of fresh thrombi and emboli, disintegration of tissue and gas formation in blood vessels and tissue spaces.** Bacteria produce a large variety of enzymes and these breakdown the various tissues of the body. **Lecithinase produced by Cl. welchii is most important.** This hydrolyses the lecithin which is present in all cell membranes including blood cells, and is responsible for the postmortem haemolysis of blood. The other organisms include Streptococci, Staphylococci, bacteroids, anaerobic lactobacilli, diphtheroids, B. proteus, B. coli., B. aerogenes capsulatus, etc. Streptococci and Staphylococci multiply 10 to 100 times and even more in blood and tissues of corpses kept at room temperatures. As body temperature falls, multiplication of bacteria is slowed and below 20°C multiplication is almost completely stopped, though most enzymes produced by bacteria will continue to act at much lower temperatures. Any factor which delays cooling of body will hasten putrefaction process. It begins immediately after death at the cellular level, which is not evident grossly. **Lipolytic enzymes are less active, but hydrolytic breakdown starts early and goes on steadily until little neutral fat remains.** There is progressive breakdown of soft tissues and the alteration of their proteins, carbohydrates and fats.

Features: The characteristic features of putrefaction are: (1) changes in the colour of the tissues, (2) the evolution of gases in the tissues, and (3) the liquefaction of tissues. The same changes seen on surface of the body occur simultaneously in internal organs.

The exact chronological order of the appearance of putrefactive changes is highly variable and depends on a broad variety of individual as well as environmental conditions.

(1) **Colour Changes: External: Bacteria spread directly from the bowel into the tissues of the abdominal wall. At an early stage of putrefaction, haemoglobin diffuses through the vessels and stains the surrounding tissues a red or reddish-brown colour Figs. (7–8 to 7–13).** In tissues, various derivatives of haemoglobin are formed including sulphur-containing compounds, and the colour of the tissues gradually changes to a greenish-black. **The first external sign of putrefaction in a body lying in air is usually a greenish discolouration of the skin over the region of the caecum Fig. (7–8)** which lies fairly superficially, and where the contents of the bowel are more fluid and full of bacteria. **Internally, this is seen on the undersurface of the liver, anterior peritoneal surface of right lobe of liver and adipose tissue around gallbladder,** where that organ is in contact with the hepatic flexure and transverse colon. **The colour results from the conversion of haemoglobin of blood into sulphmethaemoglobin by the hydrogen sulphide** formed in the large intestine and escaping into the surrounding tissues. **The colour appears in 12 to 18 hours in summer and in one to two days in winter.** Green colouration is more clearly seen on a fair skin than on a dark one. The green colouration then spreads over the entire abdomen, external genitals and then **patches appear successively on the chest, neck, face, arms and legs.** The patches become dark-green and later purple and dark-blue. They are at first scattered, but later on join together and the whole skin of the body appears discoloured. The putrefactive bacteria spread most easily in fluid and tend to colonise the venous system. Wrinkling of the fingertips occurs early which become leathery, and the nails become prominent.

Marbling of Skin: The superficial veins especially over the roots of the limb, thighs, sides of the abdomen, shoulders, chest and neck are stained greenish-brown or purplish-red depending on the total amount of sulphhaemoglobin formation within the affected vessels (linear branching pattern) due to the haemolysis of red cells, which stains the wall of the vessel and infiltrates into the tissue, giving a **marbled appearance (red, then greenish pattern in skin resembling the branches of a tree). This starts in 24 hours, but is prominent in 36 to 48 hours Fig. (7–9).** The clotted **blood becomes** fluid, and as such, the position

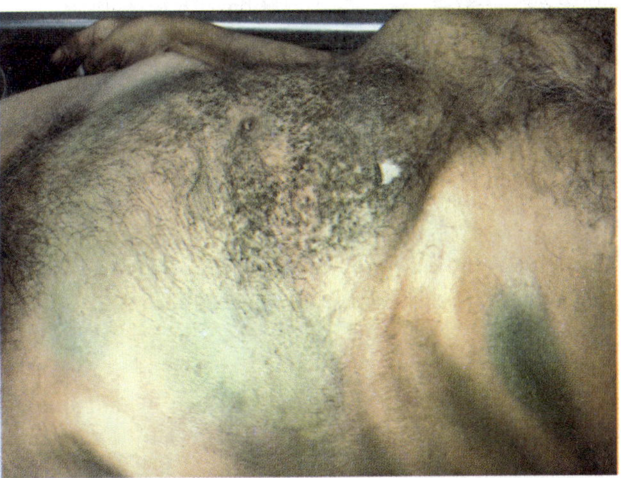

Fig. (7–8). Greenish discoluoration of right iliac fossa.

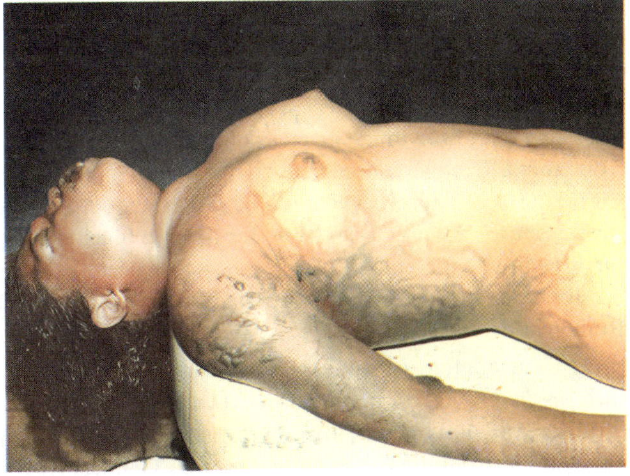

Fig. (7–9). Putrefactive network (Marbling).

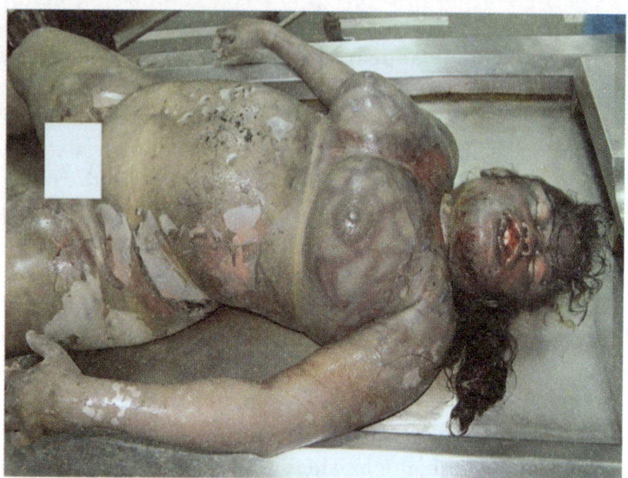

Fig. (7–10). Advanced decomposition. Marbling, bloating.

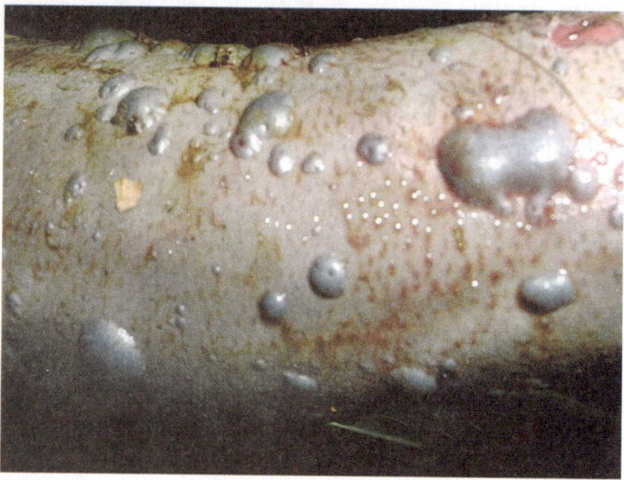

Fig. (7–11). Blisters in puterfaction.

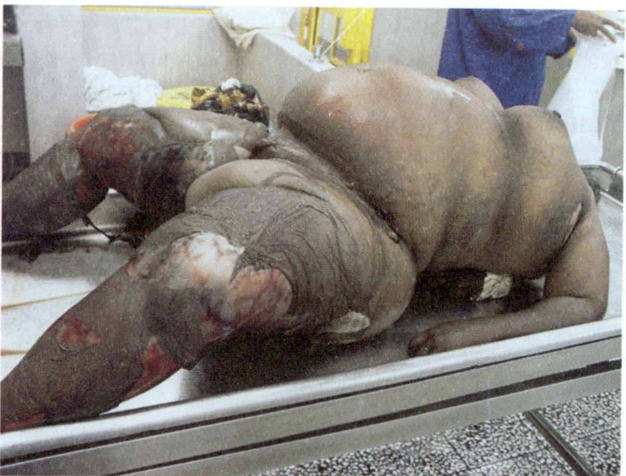

Fig. (7–12). Gaseous distension of body due to decomposition.

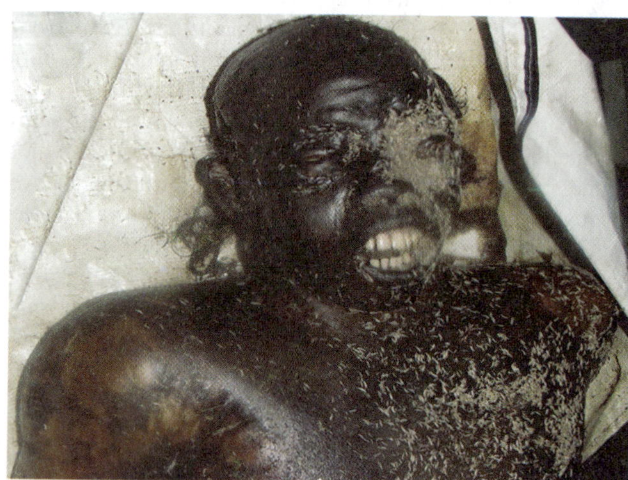

Fig. (7–13). Blackening of body and maggots in advanced.

of the postmortem staining is altered, and the fluid blood collects in the serous cavities. **Putrefactive effusion of foul-smelling bloodstained fluid** into the pleural cavities usually starts at about the time when the skin becomes macerated Fig. (7–10). Such effusions usually do not exceed 60 to 100 ml. unless death resulted from drowning, when several hundred ml. of drowning medium which oozed out through the lungs and visceral pleura, may be present in the thoracic cavities. **The reddish-green colour of the skin may become dark-green or almost black in 3 to 4 days.**

Internal: The earliest internal change is a reddish-brown discolouration of the inner surfaces of the vessels, especially of the aorta. Internally, decomposition proceeds more slowly than the surface. **The same changes of colour are seen in the viscera, but the colour varies from dark-red to black, rather than green.** With this colour change, **the viscera become softer and greasy to touch. Finally, they breakdown into a soft disintegrating mass.**

(2) Development of Foul-smelling Gases: The chemical processes in this stage are those of reduction, the **complicated proteins and carbohydrates being split into simpler compounds** of aminoacids, ammonia, CO, CO_2, hydrogen sulphide, phosphorated hydrogen, methane and mercaptans. The gases are non-inflammable in the early stages, but as the decomposition progresses, enough of hydrogen sulphide is formed, which can be ignited to burn with a blue flame. **Gases collect in the intestines in 12 to 18 hours in summer, and 1 to 2 days in winter and the abdomen becomes tense and distended.** At about the same time, the eyeballs become soft, the cornea becomes white and flattened or compressed. Later, the eyes collapse. **The gas formation in the blood vessels may force bloodstained fluid, air or liquid fat between the epidermis and dermis forming small blisters in 18 to 24 hours Fig. (7–11).** Blisters are formed first on the lower surfaces of trunk and thighs, where tissues contain more fluid due to hypostatic oedema.

Gas bubbles accumulate in the tissues, causing crepitant, sponge-like feeling which soon begins to distend the body. **From 18 to 36 hours after death, the gases collect in the tissues, cavities and hollow viscera under considerable pressure, and the features become bloated and distorted** Fig. (7–7). On opening the abdomen, the gas escapes with a loud explosive noise. Discoloured natural fluids and liquefied tissues are made frothy by gas.

Pressure effects of putrefactive gases: Due to the presence of gas in the abdomen, the diaphragm is forced upwards

compressing the lungs and heart, and bloodstained froth exudes from the mouth and nostrils (postmortem purge), which can be mistaken for the bleeding following antemortem injury. Bloodstained frothy fluid has no particular significance. It can be due to rupture of small pulmonary or pharyngeal vessels. The compression of heart, forces out its contents. Pressure of the gases may force food from the stomach into the fauces, and this may fall into the larynx.

Swelling due to gases is most marked in the face, genitalia and abdomen Fig. (7–12). Sometimes limbs are relatively free of putrefaction when changes are marked in the face and trunk. The early changes of decomposition in the face, especially when the head of the cadaver is dependent may be mistaken for signs of strangulation, especially when there is oozing of fluid from the nose. **In 24 to 48 hours, the subcutaneous tissues become emphysematous,** due to which even a thin body appears obese. In males, gas is forced from the peritoneal space down the inguinal canals and up to the scrotum, resulting in massive scrotal swelling. The breasts and penis are greatly distended. The eyes bulge from their sockets, the tongue is forced out between the swollen and discoloured lips.

Maggots are produced in 1 to 2 days which have proteolytic enzymes that dissolve the tissue **Figs. (7–13 and 7–16).** As they eat, **they may create holes that resemble gunshot wounds. An unusually large accumulation of maggots on one area of the body may indicate a pre-existing antemortem wound.** This allows air to enter under the skin and more maggots into the body cavity. The activities of maggots may raise the temperature to something near or even above that of normal body heat.

The junction of the epidermis and dermis is weakened by the release of hydrolytic enzymes, which causes the **epidermal layer to slip off the dermal layer (skin slippage) producing large, fragile sacs of clear or pink-red serous fluid.** These gradually enlarge, join together and rupture, exposing large areas of slimy, pink dermis. The exposed subdermal tissue dries with a yellow parchment appearance The skin shows "slippage", and the skin of the hands and feet may come off in a "glove and stocking" fashion. The breakdown of vessel walls and cell membranes leads to waterlogging of the tissues which helps the spread of bacteria. **The sphincters relax and urine and faeces may escape. Wounds caused before or after death bleed, due to pressure of the gases within the heart and blood vessels, and whether they are antemortem or postmortem cannot be made out. The anus and uterus may prolapse after two to three days, and postmortem delivery of a foetus may take place. Meningeal haemorrhage and haematoma persist well.** Owing to the pressure of the gas in the blood vessels, hypostatic stains may be displaced in any direction. **After three days, the face is so discoloured and bloated that identification becomes very difficult** Fig. (7–7). **Bloodstained fluid (tissue liquefaction stained by haemolysis) may leak from mouth, nostrils, rectum and vagina.** In fat people, the fat, especially omental and mesenteric may liquefy into a translucent yellow fluid. The hair becomes loose and is easily pulled out. The nails are also loose. **In 3 to 5 days or more, the sutures of skull especially of children are separated and liquid brain comes out. Teeth (anterior teeth and often premolars) become loose and may fall out.** In advanced putrefaction, conjunctival petechiae may not be distinguished due to haemolysis, and the conjunctivae have a homogeneous grayish to light-greenish appearance. **Postmortem luminescence is usually due to contamination by bacteria, e.g., Photobacterium fischeri, and the light comes from them and not from putrefying material. Luminescent fungi, Armillaria mellea, is another source of light.**

When the nutrient material is used up, the formation of gas stops, and the swelling gradually subsides. The gas leaves the tissues, usually by escaping as a result of damage to the structures or by drainage through a postmortem wound. When the putrefactive juices have drained away and the soft tissues have shrunk, the speed of decay is appreciably reduced.

Distribution: A body lying in air decomposes usually in the following order: abdomen, chest, neck, face, legs, shoulders, arms. The distribution of the putrefactive changes may be influenced by the position in which the deceased was lying after death, e.g. if a person dies with his head in a dependent position, putrefactive changes will be advanced in the head and neck compared with the remainder of the body. A person dying upon a warm electric blanket may decompose rapidly, the decomposition will be more advanced in those parts of the body in contact with the heated blanket. If only part of the body is in contact with the blanket, there may be a sharp line of demarcation between the decomposition caused by the blanket and the unheated areas of the body.

Rigidity due to Inflation of the Tissues with Gases: In this condition, changes of decomposition are well marked (2 to 3 days). The lower limbs are abducted, flexed and rigid, the arms are abducted and flexed, the hands are open and the fingers are wide apart. **False rigidity is produced due to the accumulation of gases in the tissues, because of rapid decomposition of tissues that have imbibed much fluid.** The rigidity persists till the escape of gases due to advancing decomposition. **This condition is especially seen in bodies recovered from water.**

(3) Liquefaction of Tissues: Colliquative putrefaction begins from 5 to 10 days or more after death. The abdomen bursts and the stomach and intestines protrude. In children, thorax also bursts. Blood slowly disappears from blood vessels. In obese people, the body fats, especially omental, mesenteric and perirenal may liquefy into a translucent, yellow fluid filling the body cavities between the organs. **The tissues become soft, loose and are converted into a thick, semi-fluid, black mass and are separated from the bones and fall off** Figs. (7–14 to 7–17). The cartilages and ligaments are softened in the final stage. Small foetuses rapidly disappear in putrefied blood in cases of ruptured ectopic pregnancy.

Decomposition may differ from body to body, from environment to environment and from one part of the same body to another. Differential decomposition means a situation where one body shows differential stages of decomposition in different parts of the body. **Sometimes, one part of the body may be mummified, while the rest may show liquefying putrefaction.**

Internal Phenomenon: Internally, decomposition proceeds more slowly than at the surface. Organs putrefy at markedly different rates. As the blood decomposes, its colouring matter transudes into the tissues, which **gradually change to greenish-yellow, greenish-blue and greenish black colour. The viscera**

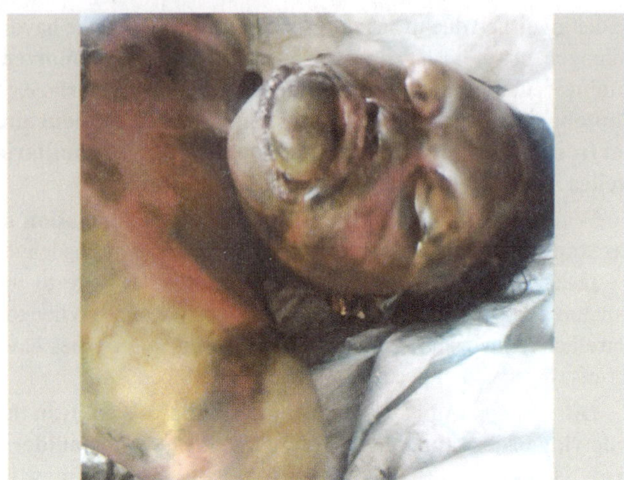

Fig. (7–14). Advanced decomposition showing bulging eyes and protruding rongue.

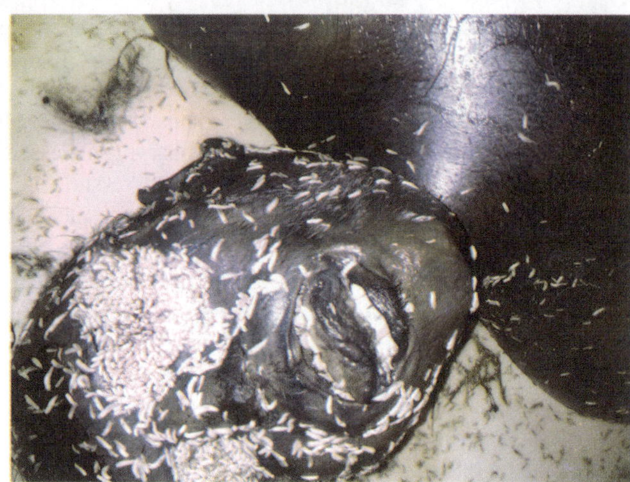

Fig. (7–16). Maggots over the face in advanced putrefaction.

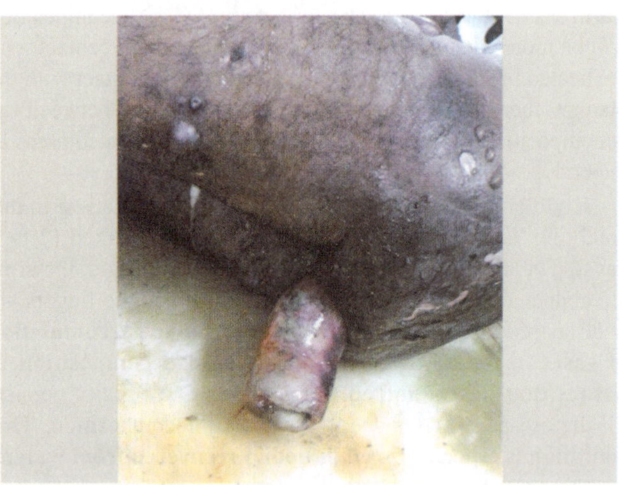

Fig. (7–15). Prolapse of rectum in highly decomposed body.

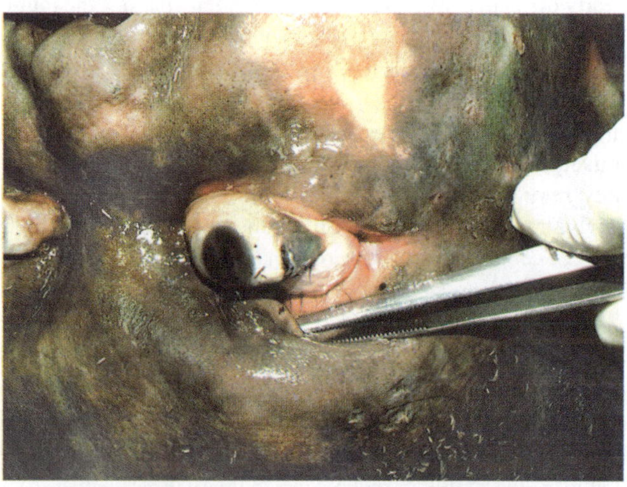

Fig. (7–17). Liquefaction of eyeball in decomposition.

become greasy and softened. The softer the organ, the more blood it contains, and the nearer to the sources of bacteria, the more rapidly it putrefies. The lining of the intestine, adrenal medulla and pancreas autolyse within hours of death. The capsules of the liver, spleen and kidney resist putrefaction longer than the parenchymatous tissues, which are usually converted into bag-like structures filled with thick, turbid fluid material. The organs composed of muscular tissues and those containing large amount of fibrous tissue resist putrefaction longer than the parenchymatous organs, with the exception of the stomach and intestine, which because of the contents at the time of death, decompose rapidly.

The various organs putrefy at different rates, depending on their structure, vascularity and access of air and bacteria Figs. (7–14, 7–15 and 7–17). As a general rule, the organs show putrefactive changes in the following order. (1) Larynx and trachea. (2) Stomach, intestines, pancreas and spleen. (3) Liver, lungs. (4) Brain. (5) Heart. (6) Kidneys, bladder. (7) Prostate, uterus. (8) Skin, muscle, tendon. (9) Bones.

LARYNX AND TRACHEA: At first the mucous membrane becomes brownish-red and later greenish, and is softened in 12 to 24 hours in summer and 2 to 3 days in winter.

STOMACH AND INTESTINES: They putrefy in 24 to 36 hours in summer, and 3 to 5 days in winter. Dark-red irregular patches involving the whole thickness of the wall are first seen on the posterior wall and then on the anterior wall. Gas blebs are formed in the submucous layer which project as small multilocular cysts of varying size into the lumen. They become softened, dark-brown and change into dark, soft, pulpy mass. The mucosa appears macerated and can be easily peeled off. The mucosa becomes brown by diffusion of blood into tissues with subsequent alteration of the haemoglobin. Other breakdown products reacting with sulphur may stain the mucosa green or black. The stomach may show perforation.

In the intestines, when there is much blood or bile pigment in the lumen, it passes into the wall and stains it. Various breakdown products of protein with sulphur produce green or black mucosa.

SPLEEN: It becomes soft, pulpy and liquefies in two to three days.

OMENTUM AND MESENTERY: They putrefy early if loaded with fat. They become greyish-green and dry in one to three days in summer.

LIVER: It becomes softened and flabby in 12 to 24 hours in summer. Multiple blisters appear in 24 to 36 hours. Cl. welchii form

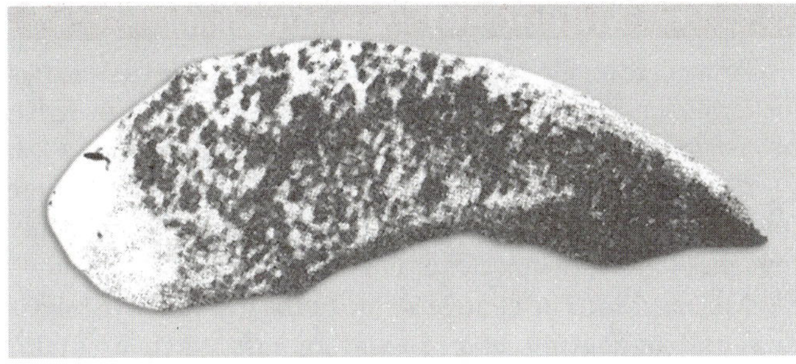

Fig. (7–18). Cross-section of liver showing honeycomb appearance due to putrefaction.

characteristic small clumps in a tissue space and produce gas, which soon increase in size. These lesions appear first as small, opaque, yellowish-grey, dendritic figures in the parenchyma. When bubbles develop, the organ has a honeycombed, vesicular or 'foamy' appearance, Fig. (7–18). The greenish discolouration extends to the whole organ, which finally becomes coal-black. In newborn children, the liver putrefies earlier than in adults. Socalled "Putrefaction Crystals", yellowish particles composed of tyrosine and leucine are formed on the surface of the internal organs, especially on the surface and bottom of the liver and the capsule of the spleen.

The liver becomes deep blue if there is much passive congestion; green if there is oozing of bile from the gall bladder, or blue-black in the subcapsular area if the pigment comes from the adjacent loops of intestine. In case of jaundice, the liver becomes green a few hours after death, if the pigment is oxidised to biliverdin. In the early stage, the discolouration is seen round the branches of the portal vein. In advanced putrefaction, the liver becomes green or black.

GALLBLADDER: The gallbladder resists putrefaction for a long time, but the bile pigments may diffuse early through adjacent tissues.

PANCREAS: It becomes softened and haemorrhagic.

HEART: It becomes soft and flabby and the cavity appears dilated. Rarely white granularity may be seen on the epicardial and endocardial surfaces of heart and below capsules of liver, kidneys and spleen. The nodules are one mm. or less in size and are called "miliary plaques". They consist of calcium and soapy material.

LUNGS: Gaseous bullae are formed under the pleura which are small, pale-red and scattered, and later join together. Later the lungs become soft, collapse and are reduced to a small black mass.

BRAIN: The leptomeninges may appear red, and the liquefying brain may be grey-green.

KIDNEYS: The renal tissue becomes flabby and the surfaces are dull and appear parboiled. The cortex darkens and later becomes green.

ADRENALS: The cortex softens from within forming a core around the softened medulla. Later, the medulla liquefies and the interior of the gland appears as a narrow slit or as a wide cyst-like cavity.

BLADDER: It resists putrefaction for a long time if it is empty and contracted. Urine may show albumin due to transudation of serum proteins from the blood, within 48 hours after death.

PROSTATE: It resists putrefaction for a very long time.

UTERUS: The virgin uterus is the last organ to putrefy. Gravid uterus or soon after delivery, it rapidly putrefies.

Body Farm: It is a research facility dedicated to the estimation of time of death. Bodies are exposed to different ways to decompose. In all stages of decay, animal activity, smell, body temperature and weather conditions are recorded, for gaining a better understanding of decomposition process. Five such facilities exist in USA. The findings are not relevant to India.

CONDITIONS AFFECTING THE RATE OF PUTREFACTION: (A) EXTERNAL: (1) TEMPERATURE: Putrefaction begins above 10°C and is optimum between 21°C and 38°C. A temperature increase of 10°C usually doubles the rate of most chemical processes and reactions. It is arrested below 0°C. and above 48°C. The rate of decomposition is about twice as rapid in summer as in winter. Advanced putrefaction may be seen within 24 to 36 hours in summer. Differences in temperature can cause varying areas in the same body to show different rates of decomposition. Pillows put over and under the deceased's head prevent circulation of air and cause much more decomposition in the face than is seen in other parts of the body.

A frozen body will not undergo decomposition until it defrosts. If decomposition has already set in, refrigeration of the body may not stop decomposition completely.

(2) MOISTURE: For putrefaction moisture is necessary, and rapid drying of the body practically inhibits it. If organic substance is dried, putrefaction is arrested. After death from general anasarca, putrefaction is very rapid, and bodies recovered from water, if left in the air decompose rapidly. Organs which contain water decompose more readily than the dry one.

(3) AIR: Free access of air hastens putrefaction, partly because the air conveys organisms to the body. In normal condition, the unbroken skin acts as an impermeable barrier to bacteria. Moist and still air helps putrefaction.

(4) CLOTHING: Initially clothing hastens putrefaction by maintaining body temperature above that at which putrefactive organisms multiply for a longer period. If the clothing is tight as under the belts, suspenders, socks, tight-fitting undergarments, and boots, the putrefaction is slow, for it causes compression of the tissues, which drives out the blood from the part, and prevents the entry of internal organisms. Clothes prevent the access of airborne organisms, flies, insects, etc., which destroy the tissues.

(5) MANNER OF BURIAL: If the body is buried soon after death, putrefaction is less. Putrefaction is delayed if body is buried in dry, sandy soil, or in a grave deeper than two metres, and when the body is covered and placed in a coffin because of exclusion of water, air and action of insects and animals. When a body is buried in lime, decomposition is delayed. Putrefaction is rapid in a body buried in a damp, marshy or shallow grave without clothes or coffin, because the body is exposed to constant changes of temperature. Putrefaction is more rapid in porous sandy soil than in soils with an excess of clay. Putrefaction is more rapid if changes of decomposition are already present at the time of burial. In acid peaty soils even the bones may be destroyed. When the bodies are buried in a common grave without coffins, those bodies lying in the centre of the grave may be better preserved.

(B) INTERNAL: (1) AGE: The bodies of newborn children who have not been fed, decompose very slowly because the bodies are normally sterile. If the child has been fed before death, or if the surface of the body has been injured in any way, decomposition tends to take place with great rapidity. Bodies of children putrefy rapidly and of old people slowly.

(2) SEX: Sex has no effect.

(3) CONDITION OF THE BODY: Fat and flabby bodies putrefy quickly than lean bodies, due to larger amount of fluid in the tissues and excess fat, and greater retention of heat.

(4) CAUSE OF DEATH: Bodies of persons dying from septicaemia, peritonitis, inflammatory and septic conditions, general anasarca, asphyxia, etc., decompose rapidly. In the case of generalised sepsis, bodies undergo rapid decomposition even if they were immediately refrigerated. Putrefaction develops very rapidly in infection due to Cl. welchii, e.g. acute intestinal obstruction, some cases of abortion and in gas gangrene. Putrefaction is delayed after death due to wasting diseases, anaemia, severe haemorrhage, debility, poisoning by carbolic acid, zinc chloride, strychnine and chronic heavy metal poisoning, due to the preservative action of such substances on the tissues or their destructive or inhibitive action on organisms, which influence decomposition.

(5) MUTILATION: Bodies in which there are wounds, or which have suffered from other forms of violence before death, putrefy rapidly owing to the ease with which organisms gain access to the damaged tissues. In case of dismemberment, especially if this has been done while the blood is still fluid, the limbs putrefy slowly, because they are

drained of the blood, and intestinal organisms do not gain entry. The trunk putrefies rapidly because of the action of intestinal bacteria, and the access of airborne organisms.

Because of the above variable factors, it is not of much use to attempt to construct a timetable for the stages of decomposition.

In advanced putrefaction, no opinion can be given as to the cause of death, except in cases of poisoning, fractures, firearm injuries, etc.

ODOUR MORTIS: About 50 volatile chemical compounds were identitied as being associated with human remains which are unique to the decomposition of human remains. Field portable analytical instruments can be used to locate human remains in shallow burial sites.

PUTREFACTION IN WATER: Casper dictum states that **a body decomposes in air twice as rapidly as in water, and eight times as rapidly as in earth.** The variations are very real, and it is not of much practical value. The rate of putrefaction is slower in water than in air. Putrefaction is more rapid in warm, fresh water than in cold, salt water. It is more rapid in stagnant water than in running water. Putrefaction is delayed when a body is lying in deep water and is well protected by clothing, while it is rapid in a body lying in water contaminated with sewage. As the submerged cadavers float face down with the head lower than the trunk, gaseous distension and postmortem discolouration are first seen on the face and then spread to the neck, upper extremities, chest, abdomen and the lower extremities in that order. Fluid gravitation in the head favours marked decomposition. When the body is removed from the water, putrefaction is hastened as the tissues have absorbed much water. The epidermis of the hands and feet becomes swollen, bleached and wrinkled after immersion, and may be removed as a cast of the extremity, after 2 to 4 days. After several weeks in water, macerated flesh may be stripped off from the body by the action of currents or the contact with the floating objects. Fish, crustacea (crabs, lobsters, shrimps, etc.) and water-rats in a sewer may destroy the body. Moulds may be located anywhere on the body, but generally are found only on the exposed surfaces. Fungus may grow on body which varies in colour from white and yellow to green and black.

SKELETONISATION: The time required for skeletonisation varies considerably and mainly depends on the ambient temperature, insect colonisation of the body and scavenger activity. In a hot humid environment with heavy insect activity a corpse can be skeletonised within a few days. In the case of an exposed body, flies, maggots, ants, cockroaches, rats, dogs, jackals, vultures, etc., may reduce the body to a skeleton within a few days. When the body is in the water, it may be attacked by fishes, crabs, etc., which reduce the body to a skeleton in a few days. In an uncoffined body buried in a shallow grave, putrefaction is delayed to a moderate extent. In a deeply buried body, the lower temperature, the exclusion of air, absence of animal life, etc., markedly delay decomposition. The important factors are seasonal, climatic variation, the amount of soil water, the access of air, and the acidity or otherwise of the soil water. In bodies placed in airtight coffins, decay process may not occur for several decades, but in a poor coffin which admits air and water, bodies will decompose quickly. In India, an uncoffined buried body is reduced to a skeleton within about 1 to 2 years. Disarticulation often occurs from the head downwards and from central to peripheral. Articulated bones are seen up to 3 weeks. In about 5 weeks some are articulated. In about one year complete disarticulation occurs and most of small bones are missing. Some bones are broken in 2 to 4 years. Bone decay occurs after 10 to 12 years. Buried bones may decay at different rates, e.g. neutral soil may not destroy the skeleton at all. Acidic soil may cause decay in about 25 to 100 years. In a hot climate, bones on the ground surface may decay in 5 to 10 years. In tropical countries, weathering of the skull may occur in 5 to 6 years. The outer table disappears irregularly, followed by inner table. The protein content of the bones decomposes. As the bones contain largely inorganic material, they will crumble, rather than decompose. Flat bones and the bones of the infants and old, breakdown faster.

ADIPOCERE (Saponification)

Adipocere (cire = wax) is a modification of putrefaction. It is the formation of soft, whitish, crumbly, waxy and greasy material, occurring in fatty or fat containing tissues of a dead body Figs. (7–19 and 7–20). In this, **the fatty tissues of the body change into a substance known as adipocere.** It is seen most commonly in bodies immersed in water or in damp, warm environment.

Mechanism: The change is due to the gradual hydrolysis and hydrogenation of pre-existing fats, such as olein, into higher fatty acids, which combine with calcium and ammonium ions to form insoluble soaps, which being acidic, inhibit putrefactive bacteria. Ultimately, the whole of the fat is converted into palmitic, oleic, stearic and hydroxystearic acid, together with some glycerol, and a mixture of these substances forms adipocere. These form a matrix for remnants of tissue fibres, nerves and muscles. Crystals with radial markings can be found in adipocere. **At the time of death, body fat contains, about half percent of fatty acids, but in adipocere they rise to 20% within a month and over 70% in three months. The process starts under the influence of intrinsic lipases, and is continued by the bacterial enzymes of the clostridia group, mainly Cl. perfringens,** as the bacteria produce lecithinase,

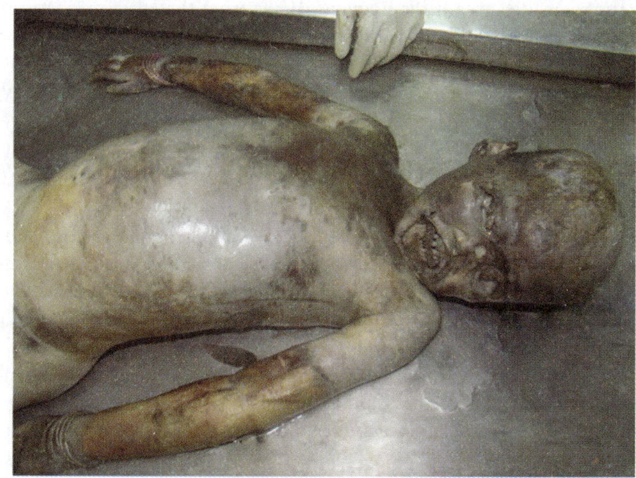

Fig. (7–19). Early stage of adipocere formation.

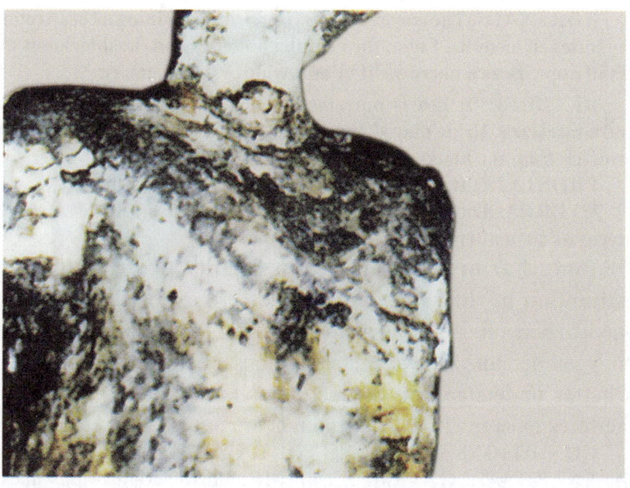

Fig. (7–20). Adipocere.

which facilitates hydrolysis and hydrogenation. **Water is essential for the bacterial and enzymatic processes involved in adipocere formation.**

Factors influencing adipocere formation: Water helps to remove glycerin which is formed during hydrolysis of the fats. **The water required for the hydrolysis is obtained mainly from the body tissues, which therefore become more and more dehydrated.** In a body immersed in water, this fluid contributes to the hydrolysis of the subcutaneous fat, but the formation of adipocere in deeper sites starts before the extraneous water enters the interior of the body. **Activation of lipid peroxidation is a significant component of the mechanism** (Manulik, et al, 1999). **Adipocere is delayed by cold and hastened by heat.** A warm, moist, anaerobic environment favours adipocere formation. **It is more frequently seen in females, the well-nourished mature newborn children, the obese and in corpses that have been submerged in water for a long period.** It is also seen in buried bodies. The bodies enclosed in a water-tight coffin for many years may be converted to adipocere even in the absence of external water.

Properties: Adipocere has a distinct offensive or sweetish smell, but during the early stages of its production, a penetrating ammoniacal odour is noticed. The smell remains in the clothing of those handling such bodies for several days. One's olfactory sense rapidly becomes accustomed to the smell of adipocere, and one cannot smell it after about two minutes exposure. The sense of smell rapidly returns after a few minutes in the open air. **Fresh adipocere is soft, moist, whitish and translucent, but old samples are dry, hard, cracked, yellowish and brittle.** It shows fragments of fibrous tissues and muscle in the fracture. It is inflammable and burns with a faint-yellow flame. It floats in water and dissolves in alcohol and ether.

Distribution: **It forms in any site where fatty tissue is present. It is formed first in the subcutaneous tissues. The face, buttocks, breasts and abdomen are the usual sites.** The limbs, chest wall, or other parts of the body may be affected, but **sometimes the entire body is converted into adipocere.** Fatty tissue between the fibres of skeletal muscle and in the myocardium and in the substance of the liver, kidney, etc., is also converted into adipocere. **The epidermis disappears as adipocere forms,** probably due to decomposition and shedding, and the dermis becomes darkened. Multiple whitish-grey, rounded outgrowths, varying from one to ten mm. in diameter are seen on the surface. They resemble moulds but are protruding clusters of crystals from the underlying adipocere. In widespread adipocere, the soft tissues are markedly dry, unless there has been prolonged immersion in water. **Small muscles are dehydrated, and become very thin, and have a uniform greyish colour.** The depths of large muscles have a pink or red colour in bodies with complete conversion of the fat to adipocere. The intestines and lungs are usually parchment-like in consistency and thinness. **The liver is prominent and retains its shape. Histologically, the gross features of the organs can sometimes be appreciated, even though the cells are lacking. Adipocere may persist for decades,** but finally either degenerates or is removed by mechanical forces or by animals.

Time Required for Adipocere Formation: The rate of adipocere formation is extremely variable depending mostly on temperature and also humidity of environment. In temperate countries, the shortest time for **its formation is about three weeks in summer, when it occurs to a certain extent** Fig. (7–8). Stiffening, hardening and swelling of the fat occurs over a period of months. **In most cases, the change is partial and irregular, but rarely the whole body may be affected. Complete conversion in an adult limb requires at least three to six months.** In India, it has been observed to begin within 4 to 5 days. Adipocere may persist for years or decades.

Medicolegal Importance: (1) When the process involves the face, the features are well preserved, which help to establish the identity. (2) The cause of death can be determined, because injuries are recognised. (3) The time since death can be estimated which is not reliable.

MUMMIFICATION

It is a modification of putrefaction. **Dehydration or drying and shrivelling of the cadaver occurs from the evaporation of water, but the natural appearances of the body and general facial features are preserved.**

Features: **It begins in the exposed parts of the body like face, hands and feet and then extends to the entire body including the internal organs** Figs. (7–21 and 7–22). **The skin may be shrunken and contracted, dry, brittle, leathery and rusty-brown to black in colour,** stretched tightly across anatomical prominences, such as the cheek bones, chin, costal margins and hips, adheres closely to the bones, and often covered with fungal growths. As the skin contracts, some of the fat cells in the subcutaneous tissues are broken, and the liquid oil is forced into the dermis which becomes translucent. **The entire body loses weight up to 60 to 70%, becomes thin, stiff and brittle.** In mummified bodies, arms are often abducted in the shoulder joints, flexed in elbow joints, and hands are clenched into fists in most cases. This flexion is often seen in lower limbs also. This is due to shrinkage of muscles and tendons. **Mummification may be partial in some cases, with only limbs or head or trunk being affected.** Mummified tissues are dry, leathery and brown in colour. **The internal organs become shrunken, hard,**

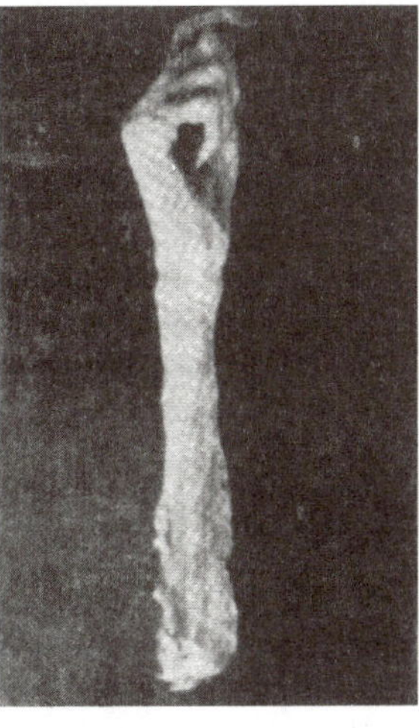

Fig. (7–21). Mummified forearm.

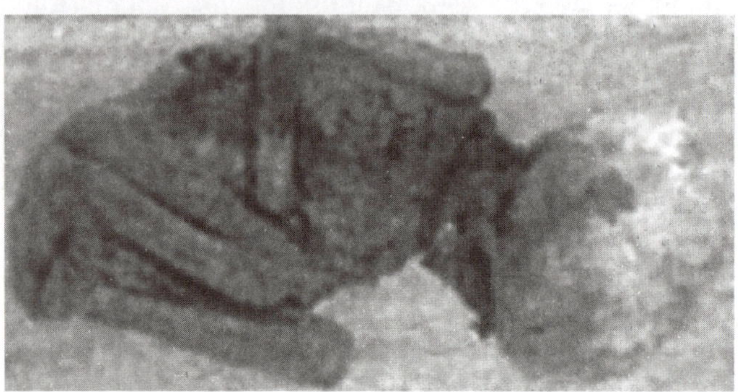

Fig. (7–22). **Mummified foetus.**

dark-brown and black and become a single mass. Later, due to putrefaction and maggot activity, they may disappear. If a mummified body is not protected, it will break into fragments gradually, and reduced to skeleton, though tough, leathery shreds of skin tendons and ligaments may persist for many years, but if protected, it may be preserved for years. Mummified bodies may be attacked by insects especially moths and larvae of various flies which destroy the body. **A mummified body is practically odourless.**

Collagen, elastic tissues, cardiac and skeletal muscle, cartilage, and bone are usually demonstrable histologically in the mummification material.

Factors necessary for the production of mummification: (1) The absence of moisture in the air, and (2) the continuous action of dry or warmed air.

Mummification of newborn children may occur if they are left in a trunk, or a kitchen cupboard, where the atmosphere is warm and dry. **Marked dehydration before death favours the development of mummification. Mummification occurs in bodies buried in shallow graves in dry sandy soils, where evaporation of body fluids is very rapid** due to the hot dry winds in summer. Chronic arsenic or antimony poisoning is said to favour the process.

Differential decomposition: Occasionally, a **body which shows evidence of mummification in certain parts may show adipocere changes in others.** Thus, there may be found some adipocere in cheeks, abdomen and buttocks, and mummification of the arms and legs.

The time required for complete mummification of a body. It varies from three months to a year and is influenced by the size of the body, atmospheric conditions and the place of disposal.

Medicolegal Importance: It is the same as that of adipocere.

CONDITIONS PRESERVING THE BODY

(1) EMBALMING: Embalming is the treatment of the dead body with antiseptics and preservatives to prevent putrefaction and preserve the body. By this process proteins are coagulated, tissues are fixed, organs are bleached and hardened and blood is converted into a brownish mass. **Embalming produces a chemical stiffening similar to rigor mortis, and normal rigor does not develop. Embalming rigidity is permanent.** Decomposition is inhibited for many months, if the injection is made shortly after death, and if done several hours after death, the body will show mixture of bacterial decomposition and mummification, and will disintegrate in a few months.

Embalming alters the appearance of the body, tissues and organs, making it difficult to interpret any injury or disease. Embalming completely destroys cyanide, alcohol and many other substances. Determination of the presence of many of the alkaloids and organic poisons becomes very difficult. The fixation process makes it difficult to extract drugs. Blood grouping cannot be made out. Extraction of DNA becomes difficult. Thrombi and emboli will be dislocated and washed away.

A body weighing 70 kg will require a fluid equivalent of ten litres Table (7–5). About 10% of it will be lost through venous drainage, purging, etc. **To be very satisfactory, embalming should be done within six hours of death.**

Embalming is required when a body has to be transported to distant places either by road, rail or air. It assures that the body is not hazardous to public health. If ascites is present, the fluid should be removed. No objection certification should be taken from police for transportation of a dead body.

Vitreous humour, synovial fluid and bile are ideal samples for screening for toxicology. Muscle mass from psoas and gluteal region can also be used.

INJECTION METHODS: Arterial injection is forcing of fluid in an artery to reach the tissues through the arterioles and capillaries. Diffusion occurs into the cells and tissues for preservation at the capillary level. Femoral artery is located in the inguinal canal, midway between the anterior superior iliac spine and pubic tubercle. Femoral vein is located one cm. medial to the artery. Various instrumental procedures are used for injecting the embalming fluid.

(1) Hand/foot pump.

(2) Stirrup pump.

(3) BULB SYRINGE: This is a variety of manual pump, similar to Higginson's syringe. It consists of a bulb-type rubber syringe and rubber tubing at either end. Valves built into the bulb allow suction on one side and ejection on the other side, when the bulb is squeezed. The injection needle is attached to the delivery end, and the suction end dips into the fluid container.

Table (7–5). **A typical embalming fluid**

Ingredient	Proportion
Formalin (Preservative)	1.5 L
Methanol (Preservative)	500 mL
Phenol (Germicide)	50 mL
Thymol (Fungicide)	5 gm
Sodium borate (Buffer)	600 gm
Sodium citrate (Anticoagulant)	900 gm
Glycerin (Wetting agent)	600 mL
Sodium chloride (Controls pH)	800 gm
Eosin (1%, Cosmetic)	30 mL
Soluble wintergreen (Perfume)	90 mL
Water (Vehicle)	up to 10 L

NB: **Sodium borate and sodium citrate should be dissolved in hot water and allowed to cool. Add rest of the components and dilute with water to make up 10 L. Allow to stand for a few hours and filter.**

(4) GRAVITY INJECTOR: It is the simplest, safest and slowest of the injection methods. The gravity bottle or percolator should hold at least ten litres of fluid. A rubber tubing (preferable to use a transparent plastic tube) with a clamp to control the rate of flow is attached to the mouth of the bottle. A needle is attached to the other end of the tube. The bottle is filled with arterial fluid and raised above the body by a pulley and tackle and fixed at a height. A rise of one metre gives a fluid pressure of 0.6 kg/sq.cm., and two metres about one kg/sq cm. This method takes a longer time and the distribution of fluid is uneven with some areas untouched by the fluid.

(5) MOTORISED INJECTORS: Fluid from an injection tank is forced into the vascular system using air from a compression tank. The pressure and flow rate are controlled by devices. About ten litres of arterial solution is injected into the vascular system within thirty minutes. The injection pressure is about 2 kg/sq cm.

METHOD OF INJECTION: (1) CONTINUOUS INJECTION AND DRAINAGE: The arterial injection is given continuously, against vein tube that is kept open throughout injection. The embalming time is much shortened. Venous drainage and tissue saturation is poor. This method is least satisfactory.

(2) CONTINUOUS INJECTION WITH DISRUPTED DRAINAGE: The injection is made continuously with vein tube closed. The blood in the veins build up a resistance for the arterial flow which helps in the better diffusion of the fluid.Thick blood is discharged when the drain tube is opened. This method is better than the continuous discharge and drainage.

(3) ALTERNATE INJECTION AND DRAINAGE: The arterial fluid is injected for some time with the drain tube closed. The injection is stopped when the superficial veins swell, and the drain tube is opened. When the flow of blood from the drain tube stops, it is closed and the injection started. This process is repeated several times till the embalming is complete.

(4) DISCONTINUOUS INJECTION AND DRAINAGE: This consists of repeated arterial injection of small quantities at two hour intervals. The total quantity of injection fluid is in excess of ordinary injection done at a time. The injection is continued for three or four times. The venous drain tube which is kept closed is opened a little before and kept open a little after starting another dose of injection. This is the best method.

The injection is given in an artery at one site and drainage occurs from a vein at another location: Commonly used combination of vessels is: (a) femoral artery (injection), right internal jugular vein which is the largest systemic vein (drainage), (b) common carotid artery (injection), and femoral vein (drainage), axillary or subclavian artery (injection) and internal jugular vein or femoral vein (drainage). This method allows thorough distribution of fluid throughout body. Injection of femoral artery will produce more even distribution of embalming fluid, and drainage from internal jugular vein will give quickest clearing of face. In obese bodies, injection of carotid artery and drainage from internal jugular vein is the best choice. A wedge or 'T' shaped incision is given on anterior wall of vessel, and cannula is inserted and ligated cannulae are left at their positions. Flexing of limbs, changing position of body, massaging intermittently during the procedure enchances the perfusion. Local injections are given in the palm, sole and dorsum of hand and foot till there is rounding up of tips of fingers and toes. High pressure and low flow rate is preferred while injecting embalming fluid. For prompt diffusion of fluid initially, the rate of injection should be one liter in 5 minutes. Later the pressure and rate of flow are reduced.

Preinjection fluid contains anticoagulants and buffers. Four to five litres should be injected and after 30 minutes arterial fluid. It loosens clots in venous system and improves drainage.

After death 85% of blood is found in capillaries, 10% in veins, and 5% in arteries. The surface area of capillary network is about six thousand sq. meters.

If bed sores or wounds are present, cavity fluid should be injected into surrounding areas. If fungal infection is present, mycostatic agent should be added to embalming fluid.

VISCERA: If the viscera are to be returned to the cavities, they should be stored in a viscera plastic bag mixed with two litres of cavity fluid for several hours, and then placed in cavities and covered with absorbent cotton and cavities closed.

DECOMPOSED BODIES: Stronger solutions have to be used. Hypodermic embalming is the method of choice. Bodies exposed to radiation: The body should be washed for several hours to reduce radioactivity level.

JAUNDICED BODIES: Greenish discolouration is seen in arterial embalming of jaundice case due to reaction of formalin with bilirubin. This can be avoided by using embalming solutions containing glutaraldehyde or polymer-formaldehyde complexes.

NORMAL EMBALMING: (1) ARTERIAL EMBALMING: The embalmer should wear impervious apron, cap, mask and gloves. Place the body supine on the table. The clothing on the body and surgical dressing if any should be removed and the body washed with an antiseptic soap and warm water. Rigor mortis, if present should be broken by bending, massaging, rotating the head, etc. The nostrils are cleaned and plugged with a wad of cotton soaked in arterial solution. The cheek may be filled out with cotton soaked in arterial solution. The mouth should be closed. The eyelids should be closed. If the eyeball is sunk arterial solution should be injected into the orbit and eyeball. The head should be elevated 8 to 10 cm. and placed on a head rest, and the feet raised to facilitate drainage. The anal orifice should be plugged with cotton wool soaked in cavity fluid. The vagina should be plugged similarly.

CHOICE OF VESSELS: The nearer the vessel to the heart, the better the result, especially for drainage. A single-point injection often leaves patches of areas unfixed by the embalming fluid. Multiple sites of injection may be required in cases of traumatic death, autopsied cases and postmortem mutilations. The 'six-point' injection involves right and left common carotid arteries for the head and neck, right and left axillary arteries for the upper limbs and the right and left femoral arteries for the lower limbs. The trunk may be injected sending the fluid through these arteries towards the heart. On completion of the injection, the cannulae are removed and vessels should be ligated to prevent leakage of embalming fluid. Each side of the face should be separately injected through the common carotid artery of the side to ensure equal distribution of the fluid and to prevent distortion of the face due to over-injection. After injection of one artery, it should be ligated before injecting into other artery.

The desired arteries and veins are dissected and raised to the surface. The vessels are cannulated with suitable tubes. It is better to drain one vessel from each of the high and low drainage points. The particular limb in relation to the artery exposed should be embalmed first and the artery is tied off. The vein is left open till the end. Discontinuous method of injection with small quantities (about 1 to 2 litres) of arterial fluid, followed by drainage is the best method. Mechanical injection is better than the gravity injector or manual pumps. The drainage tubes should be left in place, till the cavity treatment is over. All drainage points should be ligated after completion to prevent a leak.

(2) CAVITY EMBALMING: CLOSED CAVITY TREATMENT: If possible, cavity treatment should be done after half to one hour, which will allow for the hardening of the viscera, and facilitate piercing of the gut. A motorised aspirator if available is better. A 30 cm. long trocar is inserted into the abdomen through a small incision, about 5 to 6 cm above the umbilicus in the midline. The trocar is first directed upwards, backwards and to the left to pierce and aspirate the stomach. Then the trocar is slightly withdrawn and pushed up towards the right to pierce the right side of the heart. Next the right and left pleural sacs are reached by piercing the diaphragm and aspirated. Next several punctures are made in the small intestine, caecum and colon to suck out the contents. The urinary bladder, sigmoid colon and rectum should be aspirated.

Next, 1 litre of cavity fluid should be injected in abdominal and 1 liter in thoracic cavity distributing it evenly throughout the cavities. The following fluid is recommended.

Formalin	**60%**
Methanol (preservative)	**25%**
Liquefied phenol (germicide)	**10%**
Glycerin	**25%**
Sodium lauryl sulphate	**1%**
Mercuric chloride	**1%**
Eucalyptus oil	**1%**

POSTEMBALMING DRAINAGE: Much of the undrained blood stagnates in the large vessels of the trunk. This should be removed by aspiration during cavity treatment.

If the body has to be transported to a distant place, it should be securely covered and fixed with an impermeable protective cover. To absorb unexpected leakage and discharges from the body, it should be covered with sawdust.

An embalmed body, if left uncared will ultimately turn into a mummy due to dehydration. It will be shrivelled to skin and bones.

(2) MUMMIFICATION.

(3) ADIPOCERE FORMATION.

(4) FREEZING: If the body is frozen soon after death and kept in that state, it will be preserved for decades. If it is later exposed to warm temperature, more advanced putrefaction is usually seen on the outer body surface than internally.

(5) Bodies which have been in water or soil containing antiseptic substances, sometimes become impregnated with these material and do not decompose.

(6) By injection of solution of arsenic, lead sulphide and potassium carbonate into the femoral artery or into the aorta, bodies are preserved for the purpose of dissection.

ESTIMATION OF POSTMORTEM INTERVAL

The interval between death, and the time of examination of a body is known as postmortem interval.

Objectives: (1) to know when the crime was committed, (2) it gives the police a starting point for their inquiries, and allows them to deal more efficiently with the information available, (3) it might enable to exclude some suspects and the search for the likely culprits started earlier, (4) to confirm or disprove an alibi, (5) to check on a suspect's statements.

In civil cases, time of death might determine who inherits property or whether an insurance policy was in force. It is also important in criminal cases.

Time of death: The exact time of death cannot be fixed by any method, but only an approximate range of time of death can be given, because there are considerable biological variations in individual cases. One should never give a single estimate of the time since death, but use a range of times, between which the death was presumed to have taken place. The longer the postmortem interval, the wider is the range of estimate, i.e., the less accurate the estimate of the interval. **In determining time of death, the doctor should not over-interpret what he sees and should not make dogmatic, unsupportable and potentially inaccurate statement.** First, all available history should be taken, and then local physical or environmental factors at the scene of crime, such as presence of fires and domestic heating, open windows, atmospheric temperature, etc. **The range of time provided is at best an educated guess, based on knowledge and experience and subject to error.**

The points to be noted are: (1) Cooling of the body. (2) Postmortem lividity. (3) Rigor mortis. (4) Progress of decomposition, adipocere and mummification.

(5) ENTOMOLOGY OF THE CADAVER: Entomology is the study of the form and behaviour of insects. Myiasis is a condition caused by infestation of the body by fly maggots.

Flies (Musca domestica and M.vicinia) may deposit their eggs (pearly-white, one mm, long; about 120 to 150 eggs at one sitting) on the fresh corpse in any natural or traumatically created shaded orifices. These include between the lips or the eyelids, in the nostrils, genitalia, or in the margins of a fresh wound, ears, mouth, hair and the ground-body interface, within a few minutes after death, and in some cases even before death during the agonal period. When skin decomposition begins, the eggs can be deposited anywhere. In 8 to 24 hours in summer, larvae or maggots (white, segmented, 1 to 2 mm. in length at birth; 12 mm. when full grown) are produced from the eggs, which crawl into the interior of the body and produce powerful proteolytic enzymes, and destroy the soft tissues. The maggots burrow under the skin and make tunnels and sinuses which hasten putrefaction by allowing air and bacteria. The maggots become pupae (dark-brown, barrel-shaped, 6 mm. length) in 3 to 6 days, and the pupae become adult flies in three to six days. The complete life cycle from egg to adult may take 5 to 6 days in summer and 8 to 20 days in winter. Body lice usually remain alive for three to six days, after death of a person.

(6) GASTROINTESTINAL TRACT: Emptying of stomach: The amount of stomach contents and the extent of their digestion may be helpful to estimate the time of death, if the hour at which the deceased took his last meal is known. **The gastric emptying of either liquids or solids is subject to relatively wide differences in the same and different individuals even if the same meal is ingested. The quantity and digestive state of gastric contents is modified by the following factors:** (1) The total quantity of food taken at a meal. (2) Additional snacks taken between a meal. (3) The ratio of solid to liquid in the meal. (4) The carbohydrate/fat content. (5) Marked variation between individuals. (6) Variation in the same individual from day to day. (7) Dramatic variations due to psychogenic and endocrine factors.

The stomach contents do not enter the duodenum after death. Digestion of the stomach contents may continue for some time after death. This may create further difficulties. It seems that there are no significant differences in solid food emptying rates between young and old persons. The emptying rate increases directly with meal weight. The stomach empties gradually. **The stomach usually starts to empty within ten minutes after the first mouthful has entered. The bulk of the meal leaves the stomach within two hours. A light meal (small volume) usually leaves the stomach within 1 to 2 hours after being eaten, a medium-sized meal requires 3 to 4 hours and a heavy meal 5 to 8 hours.** A carbohydrate meal leaves the stomach more rapidly than a protein meal, because carbohydrates are reduced to a semi-fluid state rapidly and a protein meal leaves the stomach more rapidly than fatty meal. Fluids and semi-fluids leave the stomach very rapidly (within two hours), after being swallowed. If water is ingested with a solid meal, the water is emptied rapidly and separately and is not influenced by either the weight or total calories of the accompanying solid meal. Milk leaves rapidly, whereas meat and pulses are retained longer. **Stomach contents which are identifiable by naked eye are usually ingested within two hour period.**

Variability in gastric emptying: **A head injury, physical or mental shock or stress,** may completely inhibit the secretion of gastric juice, the motility of the stomach and the opening of the pylorus, and **undigested food may be seen after more than 24 hours. Any illness or emotional stress, may prolong the emptying time for many hours.** Digestion is delayed during sleep and during coma. Strong alcohols irritate the mucosa and tend to delay emptying. Hypermotility caused by emotional disturbance can result in rapid passage of food through the intestines causing diarrhoea. The head of the meal reaches the hepatic flexure in about six hours, splenic flexure in 9 to 12 hours, and pelvic colon in 12 to 18 hours. The state of digestion and transportation rate of food from the stomach into the duodenum depends on several factors, such as anatomical, physiological, pathological, psychological, agonal, kind of food, etc., which contribute to great intra- and interindividual variability of gastric emptying. **The actual recognition of stomach contents may be useful as it may indicate what the last meal consisted of and narrow the time of death to the interval between two meals, provided the type of meal is definitely known. Unless death was sudden and unexpected, reliance cannot be placed upon the state of digestion or the volume of stomach contents. If the stomach is full containing undigested food, it can be said that death occurred within two to four hours of the eating of the last meal. Any estimate of a postmortem interval is only an opinion based upon probabilities and is subject to limitations. It is too uncertain to have much validity.** The presence of food in the small intestine or of faecal matter in large intestine is not of much value in determining the time of death.

The presence of urine in the bladder and faeces in large intestine may indicate that death could have occurred late in the night.

(7) CEREBROSPINAL FLUID: Cisternal fluid is examined. Postmortem changes of CSF electrolytes are based mainly on the hypoxic damage of the choroid plexus. The amount of potassium increases at a constant rate in relation to the temperature of the body during the first 20 hours. The concentrations of sodium, calcium and magnesium have no obvious relationship to time since death.

(8) BLOOD: There is a progressive increase of lactic acid. The values increase by 50 to 75 fold in 12 to 24 hours, the steepest increase occurring in first 6 to 8 hours. Aminoacid nitrogen is less than 14 mg/dl up to 10 hours, but rises to 30 mg/dl by 48 hours. Acid phosphatase levels increase 20 times by 48 hours. Amylase levels increase 3 to 4 times on second day. Glutamate-oxalate transaminase (AST4) and lactate dehydrogenase (LDH) increase linearly over the first 60 hours. Sodium levels fall by 0.9 mEq/l per hour. Organic phosphorus level in serum reach 20 mEq/l at 18 hours after death.

(9) PERICARDIAL FLUID: 10 to 15 ml can be obtained, as opposed to 1 to 2 ml of vitreous humour and 5 ml of CSF. Constituents are not helpful in estimating time since death.

(10) SYNOVIAL FLUID: There is linear rise of potassium, which increases more than double within the first two days.

(11) VITREOUS HUMOUR: The potassium concentration at the time of death is 5 to 8 mmol/l. The rise of potassium concentration per hour is 0.17 to 0.238 mmol per hour. The reason for varying range may be due to electrolyte imbalances at the time of death. The variation between the two eyes may be up to 10% The relationship between potassium concentration and time after death is not completely linear, as it depends on the degree and rapidity of decomposition. The slope is 0.2 mmol/1 per hour. Madea and Henssge proposed the following formula.

$$PMI = 5.26 \times K\ conc - 30.9$$

There is a linear relationship between vitreous potassium concentration and time elapsed after death up to 120 hours. The 95% limits of confidence are ±20 hours up to 100 hours. The rise is mainly due to diffusion from the retina into the centre of the globe. Temperature, chillness and urea retention affect the range.

There is a linear rise of hypoxanthine(Hx) up to 120 hours. The rise begins immediately after death. There is a correlation between vitreous hypoxanthine and vitreous potassium values. The 95% confidence limits are ± 32 hours.

Chlorides decrease at less than 1 mmol/1/h and sodium by about 0.9 mmol/1/h. Urea exceeding 150 mmol/1 indicates uraemia. The vitreous glucose usually falls after death and can reach zero within a few hours. A vitreous glucose of more than 11.1 mmol/1 indicates diabetes, and less than 1.4 mmol/1 of hypoglycaemia.

(12) MUSCLE ENZYMES: Myofibrillar protease activity increases linearly and creatinine phosphokinase decreases linearly after death. A strong positive correlation is found between the ratio of non-protein nitrogen and total soluble protein and also creatinine concentration and time since death.

All the biochemical changes are temperature dependent. The above findings apply to cold and temperate climates. Chemical methods are of limited practical value. They are widely considered as the least reliable and the least practicable of all other methods.

(13) HAIR: Hair does not grow after death; the contraction of the skin towards the hair roots gives the illusion of growth. A sample of hair is shaved from the chin and its length measured. From this, a rough estimation of the time since the last shave can be made, for beard hair grows at the rate of 0.4 mm. per day.

(14) THE SCENE OF DEATH: The dates on mail or newspapers, sales receipts or dated slips of paper in the deceased's pockets, when the neighbours last saw the person, degree of coagulation of milk, state of food on a table, etc. may be valuable. The state of dress should be noted as regards whether the person is fully dressed or in the night dress. If the watch has stopped, the hour at which it has stopped should be noted. In drowning, the watch commonly stops shortly after immersion. If a corpse lies undisturbed on growing grass, or plant-bearing soil, underlying grass or vegetation soon dries, turns yellow or brown and dies.

RADIOACTIVE CARBON: C_{14} accumulates in living organic matter. The C_{14} content of the organism is steadily maintained as long as it lives. **After death, the radioactivity gradually weakens taking about 5,600 years to reach half its initial activity.** A simple carbon compound, such as CO_2 or acetylene, or even carbon itself is prepared from the bones, and the radioactivity is estimated. Accelerated mass spectrometer (AMS) directly counts C_{14} atoms, rather than counting rate of disintegration. **For medicolegal purposes, radiocarbon dating is not useful as the technique cannot date bones less than a century old.**

Tower of silence is used by Parsees to dispose off dead bodies.

PRESUMPTION OF DEATH: This condition has only legal importance, and medical evidence is rarely necessary. This question arises in cases of inheritance of property or in obtaining insurance money, when a person is alleged to have been dead and the body is not

found. Under the Indian Evidence Act (S107), a person is presumed to be alive, if there is nothing to suggest the probability of death within 30 years. But if proof is produced that the same person has not been heard of for seven years by his friends and relatives, death is presumed (S. 108, I.E.A.).

PRESUMPTION OF SURVIVORSHIP: The question of presumption of survivorship may arise in connection with inheritance of property, when two or more persons die in a common disaster, e.g., earthquake, shipwreck, plane-crash accident, etc. The question may arise as to who survived longest, and if no direct evidence on this is available, the question becomes one of presumption. The case is decided by the facts and evidence available. In the absence of such evidence, age, sex, constitution, nature and severity of injuries and the mode of death should be taken into consideration (S. 107, I.E.A.).

COMMORIENTES: Persons who die together on the same occasion, where it cannot be ascertained who died first.

CHAPTER

8 MECHANICAL INJURIES

FM 3.3: Mechanical injuries and wounds: Define, describe and classify different types of mechanical injuries, abrasion, bruise, laceration, stab wound, incised wound, chop wound, defense wound, self-inflicted/fabricated wounds and their medicolegal aspects.
FM 3.6: Mechanical injuries and wounds: Describe healing of injury and fracture of bones with its medicolegal importance.
FM 3.9: Firearm injuries: Describe different types of firearms including structure and components. Along with description of ammunition propellant charge and mechanism of firearms, different types of cartridges and bullets and various terminology in relation of firearm—caliber, range, choking.
FM 3.10: Firearm injuries: Describe and discuss wound ballistics—different types of firearm injuries, blast injuries and their interpretation, preservation and dispatch of trace evidences in cases of firearm and blast injuries, various tests related to confirmation of use of firearms.

Injury: **An injury is any harm, whatever illegally caused to any person in body, mind, reputation or property (Sec. 44, I.P.C.).** Medically a wound or injury is a break of the natural continuity of any of the tissues of the living body. **Mechanical injuries (wounds) are injuries produced by physical violence.** **Trauma** is an injury or wound to a living body caused by application of external force or violence.

Classification of injuries: Medical: (I) Mechanical or physical Injuries: (A) **Due to blunt force:** (1) Abrasions. (2) Contusions. (3) Lacerations. (4) Fractures and dislocations. (B) **Due to sharp force:** (1) Incised wounds. (2) Chop wounds. (3) Stab wounds. (C) **Firearms:** (1) Firearm wounds. (2) **Blast** injuries.

(II) Thermal Injuries: (1) **Due to cold:** (a) Frostbite. (b) Trench foot. (c) Immersion foot. (2) **Due to heat:** (a) Burns. (b) Scalds.

(III) Chemical Injuries: (1) Corrosive acids. (b) Corrosive alkalis.

(IV) Explosions.

(V) Miscellaneous: Electricity, lightning, X-rays, radioactive substances, etc.

Legal: (1) Simple. (2) Grievous. (3) Dangerous.

Medicolegal: (1) Suicide. (2) Homicide. (3) Accident. (4) Fabricated. (5) Self-inflicted. (6) Defence. (7) Antemortem or postmortem.

GENERAL PRINCIPLES: **A wound is caused by a mechanical force which may be either a moving weapon or object, or the movement of the body itself. In the first case, the counterforce is provided by the inertia of the body, and in the second case by the rigidity of some stationary object against which he falls. A combination of these two events is seen in most cases. Due to the impact between the forward moving force and the counterforce, energy is transferred to the tissues of the body, which causes a change in their state of rest or motion. The human body contains many complex tissues which greatly vary in their physical properties, such as state of solidity, fluidity, density and elasticity, and because of this a change in the state of rest or motion of the body produced by a forceful impact does not affect the tissues uniformly. Some of the energy is spent in moving the body as a whole, but most of the energy may cause non-uniform motion of localised parts of the body, due to which the affected tissues will be subjected to compression or to traction strains or to a combination of both. All the body tissues, except those which contain gas, are resistant to compression, i.e., they resist force tending to reduce their volumes. Mechanical force does not cause compression of the tissue but causes their displacement and deformation, and traction strains are produced in the affected tissues. Such strains may be due to forces causing simple elongation of tissues, but they may be due to more complex mechanism, such as bending, torsion or shearing. A shear strain is a strain which is produced in a body by the forceful alteration of its shape but not its volume. It causes or tends to cause two parts of a body in contact with each other to slide relatively to each other in a direction parallel to their plane of contact. Because of the great variation in the resistance of the different tissues to traction, they rupture with varying ease, as their cohesiveness is exceeded. The rigid tissues like bones resist deformation, but if the limits of their elasticity is exceeded fracture occurs. The soft tissues are plastic, and as such, mechanical force alters their shape, which is limited by the cohesion between the tissue cells, connective and vascular tissue frameworks and capsules of organs. Soft tissues rupture when they are stretched beyond the limits of their tensile strength.**

Factors governing the nature and extent of wounds: (1) The nature of the object or instrument causing the wound: **If a blow is inflicted from a sharp-edged object, the force is concentrated to a very limited area or a point or a line which causes deep penetrated or clear separation of the tissues. The hardness of the tissues will resist the passage of the object. With a blow from a blunt instrument having a flat surface, a relatively large area of body surface is involved, which dissipates the energy, due to which the damage caused to a unit mass of the tissue within that area is less than that due to a narrow object. Irregularities in the shape of the instrument, or curvature of the part of the body struck, such as at the top of head, may limit the area of the actual impact to a small size and damage will be more. A fall against a projection may produce more serious injury than a similar fall against a flat surface. When a blow is struck with a plastic instrument, some of the energy will be spent in deforming or breaking the instrument, which increases the size of the area of impact and increases the period over which the energy is discharged, due to which the damage caused is less with a rigid instrument.**

(2) Amount of energy discharged during impact: Kinetic energy is measured in a moving object by: KE = ½ mv^2, where m = mass and v = velocity. An object with definite velocity and definite weight has a definite amount of energy. When the mass doubles, kinetic energy is also doubled. However, when velocity is doubled, kinetic energy increases four times. This indicates that the velocity has far more influence on the energy compared to the mass of the object. A light bullet has a relatively great destructive power because of its high velocity.

(3) The condition under which the energy is discharged: In an impact, most of the energy may be spent in causing generalized movement of the body, due to which the person may be knocked down, but local injury may be minimal. If the body or the part of the body struck is immobilized, the greater part of the force is spent in causing localized tissue damage. If the head is free to move, a blow may cause little damage, but a similar blow to a head resting on the ground may cause marked injury to the skull. Any factor which increases the period of time over which the energy is discharged will also decrease the destructive effect of a blow, e.g., a punch with a fist if withdrawn quickly will produce more damage than one where the fist stays in place.

(4) The nature of the affected tissues: (A) The skin: The skin readily changes shape when it is struck as it is very pliable and little elastic. It is also resistant to traction forces. Because of these factors, often the skin is not damaged when struck with a blunt instrument, although underlying structures may be severely damaged. The skin may easily split when crushed against rigid bone.

(B) The subcutaneous tissues: Elasticity and plasticity: The subcutaneous tissues are very plastic due to their fat content and the pliability of connective tissue, due to which they protect the body by the cushioning effects which they have on blows. The incompressible fat of the subcutaneous tissues may be crushed and displaced between the skin and underlying structures producing bruises due to severe blows from blunt instruments (Hooke's law of elasticity).

(C) The muscles: The muscles are usually not damaged due to blows, because of their great plasticity and elasticity and their strong encapsulating sheaths. They may be crushed against bone or lacerated by fragments of displaced and broken bone. The muscles may rupture, if they are unduly stretched.

(D) The bones: When a force is applied to a bone it may bend without breaking, but it fractures when it is bent beyond the limits of its elasticity.

(E) Body fluids: Fluid is incompressible, but is readily displaced. A blow over a hollow organ which contains fluid may set up powerful hydrostatic forces in that fluid which are transmitted equally and uniformly in all directions, which may cause rupture of anatomically distant and mechanically weak tissues, e.g., a sudden compression of the chest may rupture distal venules and capillaries, as seen in traumatic asphyxia. The violent displacement of fluid in the gastrointestinal or urinary tract may cause distant ruptures of portions of these tracts.

(F) Gases: Gases are readily compressible; lungs may be extensively compressed without any structural damage but when lungs are compressed suddenly and violently, sufficiently powerful pneumostatic forces may cause damage to tissues.

Application: Different wounds may be caused from equal forces when applied to the same region of the body in different circumstances. Sometimes, minor forces may produce severe wounds, and relatively severe forces may cause minor wounds. Because of these, often on scientific grounds it is not possible to give an opinion as to the amount of force which must have been used to cause a particular wound. It is also not possible to predict the amount of damage which could be caused by the application of a certain force. The doctor should give his opinion in broad qualified terms. Sometimes injuries of internal organs do not show any sign of external damage.

ABRASIONS

An abrasion (gravel rash) is a destruction of the skin, which usually involves the superficial layers of the epidermis only. Thickness of skin is 1.6 mm.

Mechanism: They are caused by friction against a rough surface or by compression, such as a lateral rubbing action by a glancing blow, a fall on a rough surface, by being dragged in a vehicular accident, fingernails, thorns or teeth bite. Most abrasions are caused by a lateral rubbing action. **Some pressure and movement by agent on the surface of the skin is essential.** In its simplest form, the epidermal cells are flattened and their nuclei are elongated. **The rougher the surface, and the more rapid the movement of the skin over it, the deeper is the injury. If sufficient friction is applied, partial or complete removal of the epithelium may occur and the superficial layer of dermis is damaged.** Many abrasions have some deeper areas of subepidermal damage which may result in superficial scarring. Sometimes, full thickness of the skin may be damaged in places, but usually in an interrupted, irregular manner, and intact epidermis remains within the area of the abrasion. The exposed raw surface is covered by exudation of lymph and blood which produces a protective covering known as a scab or crust.

Features: Abrasions vary in size, depending on the extent of the body surface exposed to the abrading force. They are simple injuries, bleed slightly, heal rapidly and **scar is not formed.** Large abrasions can cause severe pain and bleeding. The size, situation, pattern and number of abrasions should be noted.

Types: Abrasions are of four types.

(1) Scratches: A scratch (linear abrasion) is an abrasion with length but no significant width, or a very superficial incision, depending on the agent. A scratch produced from the tip of the knife or razor can be called a **point scratch**. **They are caused by a sharp or pointed object, not sharp enough to incise, but pointed enough to gouge or scratch,** i.e. remove a portion of the skin's surface, passing across the skin, such as fingernails, pin or thorn. **The surface layers of the skin are collected in front of the object,** which leaves a clean area at the start and tags at the end.

Fingernail abrasions: When the skin is gripped in a static fashion, **fingernail abrasions may be straight or curved, one to 2 mm breadth, often about half to one cm. long, wide at the start, narrow at the end.** As the skin is put under lateral tension when it is indented by nails, it may distort, so that when the tension is released the elasticity of the skin causes it to return to its original position, carrying the nail mark with it. The curve may then reverse to form either a straight line or a convexity, but this is always not true. Pointed nails are more likely than those with straight edges to give these paradoxical results. They may be parallel vertical linear scratches that may be several millimetres wide and placed a centimetre or two apart, if the fingers are dragged down the skin.

(2) Grazes Figs. (8–1, 8–2, 8–6 to 8–8) (sliding, scraping or grinding abrasion): They are the most common type. **They occur when there is movement between the skin and some rough surface in contact with it. They show uneven, longitudinal parallel lines (grooves or furrows) with the epithelium heaped up at the ends of these lines (which does not occur to a significant degree), which indicate the direction in which the force was applied.** The furrow may be broad at one end, and narrow in the opposite direction. **Usually, the skin is uniformly denuded at the start or may be serrated. The epidermis is scraped away, destroyed or detached.** A glancing

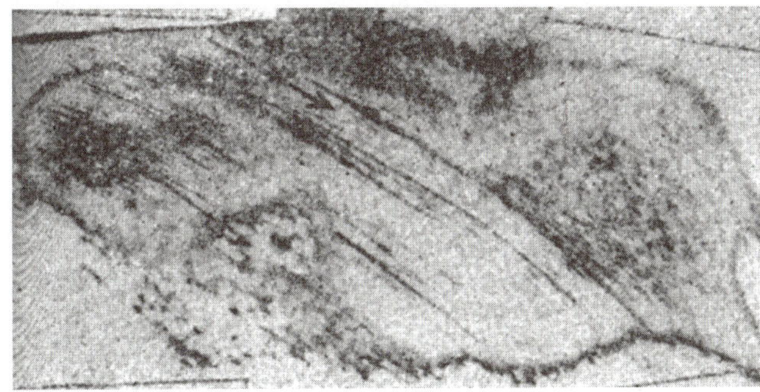

Fig. (8–1). **Abrasion indicating direction of force.**

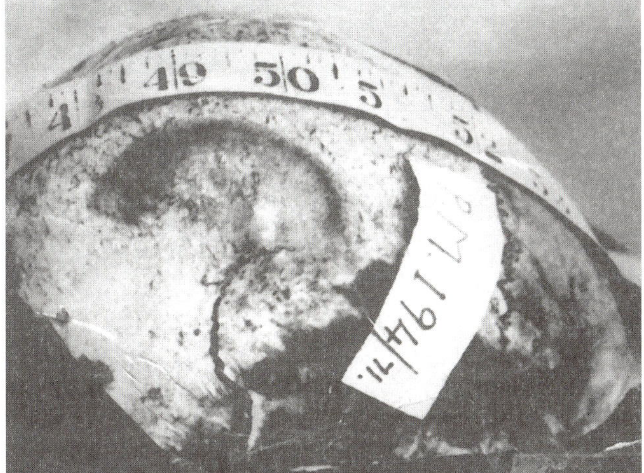

Fig. (8–2). **Abrasion of the skull due to tearing force produced by the automobile wheel also causing avulsion laceration of the scalp.**

kick with a boot also produces a graze. **These abrasions are commonly seen in a road accident.** Many abrasions extend into the dermis, because of the corrugations of the dermal papillae, and bleeding occurs. Deep abrasions have a typical punctate or spotty appearance. **An abrasion caused by violent lateral (tangential) rubbing against a surface as in dragging over the ground is called brush burn or gravel rash.** It is a scraping injury over a large area. **"Friction burn" (scuff or brush abrasion) is an extensive, superficial, reddened excoriated area without serous ooze or bleeding and with little or no linear mark Figs. (8–1 and 8–2).** It may occur due to tangential contact with a smooth surface or when the skin is covered by clothing. Brush burns and friction burns are seen in motor cyclists, persons ejected from vehicles, pedestrians, cyclists thrown forward after the primary impact from a motor vehicle. If a victim is struck a glancing blow with a rough object, such as a stone or a stick, brush burn will be caused.

(3) Pressure Abrasions (crushing or friction abrasions): They are caused by crushing of the superficial layers of the epidermis and are associated with a bruise of the surrounding area. If the movement of instrument is around 90° to the skin, a pressure type of abrasion occurs. In this type, **the movement is slight and largely directed inwards.** The **ligature mark** in cases of hanging and strangulation and the **teeth-bite marks** are the examples.

(4) **Impact Abrasions (contact or imprint abrasions): They are caused by impact with a rough object, when the force is applied at or near a right angle to the skin surface. The abrasion** is **slightly depressed below the surface,** unless there is bulging due to underlying contusion or local oedema. **If the impact is forcible, the dermis is damaged with an underlying bruise.** When a person is knocked down by a motor car, the pattern of the radiator grille, a headlamp rim or the tread of the tyre may be seen on the skin, which may contain road dirt, paint flakes, grease, etc., Figs. (8–3 to 8–8). Impact by a solid object may produce abrasion at the periphery where the skin is forced downwards. **If a person strikes a flat and relatively smooth surface, an abrasion can be produced which shows little or no linear markings, as in traffic accidents.**

Patterned abrasions Figs. (8–4, 8–5 and 8–8): Impact abrasions and pressure abrasions reproduce the pattern of the object causing it and are called patterned abrasions. **Patterned injury is any injury that suggests an inflicting instrument or unique means of its causation. Patterned abrasions are produced when the force is applied at right angle to the surface of skin Fig. (8–8).** If the skin is struck with a weapon having a patterned surface, or the body falls against a patterned surface, the abrasion of the epidermis is caused from the ridges of the object, if it has a profile of varying height. **The skin may be compressed into the cavities of the pattern with capillary**

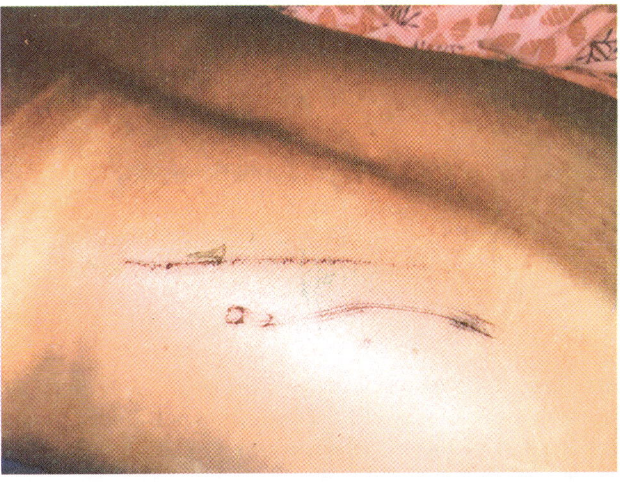

Fig. (8–3). **Scratch abrasions.**

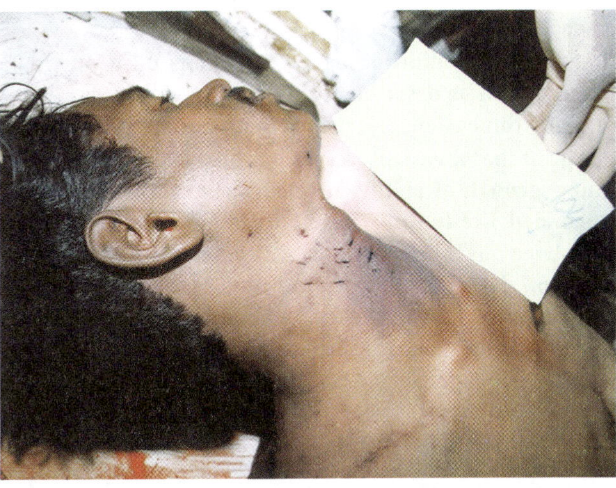

Fig. (8–4). **Finger nail abrasions.**

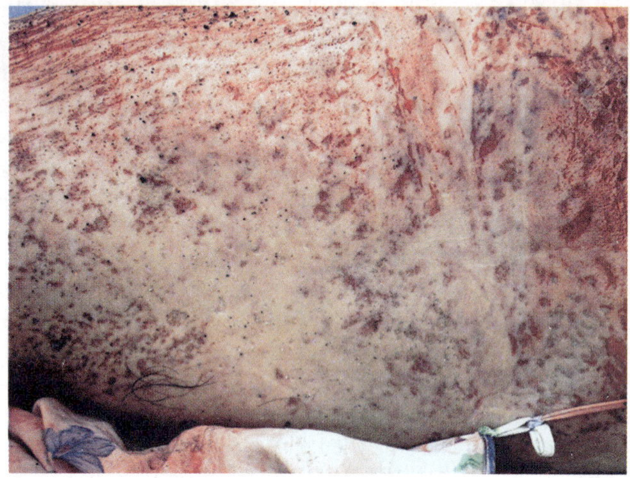

Fig. (8–5). **Gravel (imprint) abrasions due to fall from a height.**

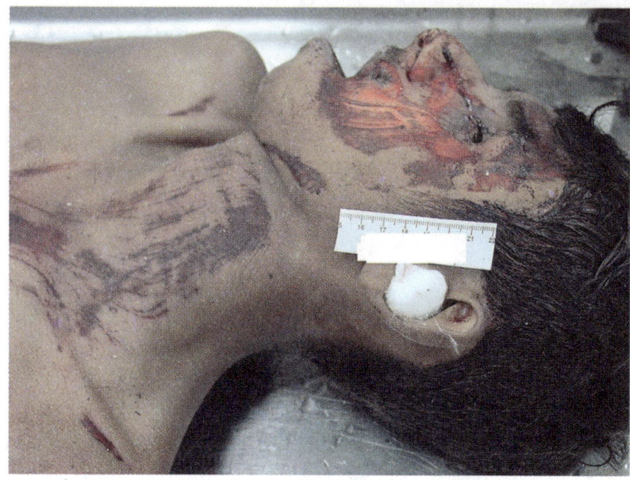

Fig. (8–6). **Grazed abrasion over face.**

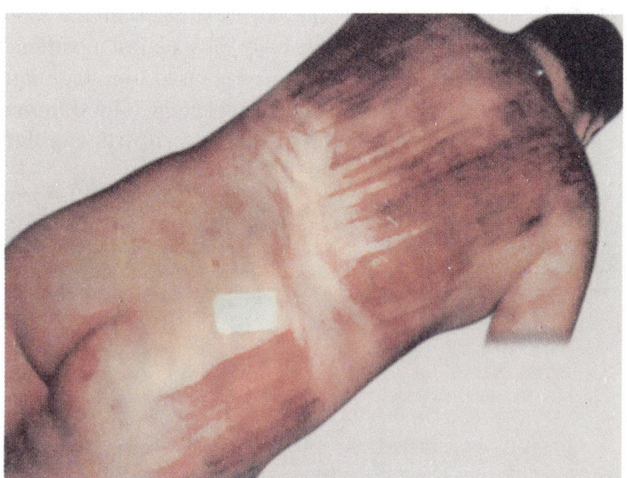

Fig. (8–7). **Brush burn on the back.**

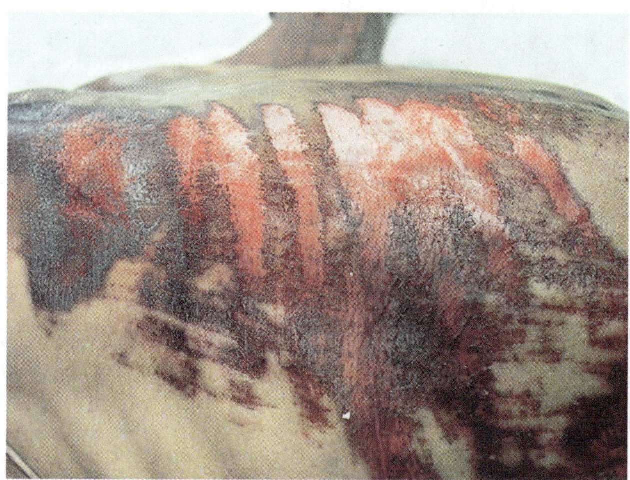

Fig. (8–8). **Injury: Graze abrasion patterned.**

damage leading to an intradermal bruise, e.g., when a motor tyre passes over the skin. **Other examples of patterned abrasion are: imprint of bicycle chain, weave of coarse fabrics, the spiral of electric wires, ropes, serrated knife,** etc. Multi-thonged whip, such as a cat-o-nine-tails, leaves a series of linear abrasions or superficial tears. Usually, the pattern and shape are non-specific.

If there are multiple minor abrasions on a particular area, they can be described together as present over an area of (giving dimensions) on the particular anatomic region.

Age of the Abrasions: **Abrasions heal from the periphery by new growth of epithelial cells. The exact age cannot be determined. Fresh:** Bright red. **12 to 24 hours:** Lymph and blood dries up leaving a bright red scab. **2 to 3 days**: Reddish-brown scab. **4 to 7 days**: Dark brown to brownish-black scab. Epithelium grows and covers defect under the scab. **After 7 days:** Scab dries, shrinks and falls off, leaving depigmented area underneath, which gets gradually pigmented.

Histologically, perivascular cellular infiltration is seen at four to six hours. At 12 hours three layers are seen: a surface zone of fibrin and red cells; a deeper zone of infiltrating polymorphs ; and a deepest layer of abnormally staining collagen. At 48 hours, scab is well-formed and epithelial regeneration is seen at the margins of the scab. By 4 to 5 days, small abrasions are completely covered by epithelium. By 5 to 8 days, subepithelial formation of granulation tissue is prominent. Reticulum fibres are seen at 8 days, and collagen fibres at 9 to 12 days. The last stage is regression which begins about 12 days. During this phase, the epithelium is remodelled and becomes thinner and even atrophic.

Antemortem and Postmortem Abrasions: **Abrasions produced slightly before or after death cannot be differentiated even by microscopic examination.** In superficial lesions or when decomposition is advanced, differentiation is difficult. **On drying, abrasions become dark-brown or even black. In a body recovered from water, abrasions may not be seen on first inspection,** but they are easily seen after the skin dries. Abrasions may be produced after death when a body is dragged away from the scene of crime. The distribution of such abrasions depends upon the position of the body while it is being dragged. Postmortem abrasions are typically found over the forehead, the prominent points of the face, anterior trunk, backs of hands and the fronts of the lower legs. Facial injuries ooze blood, mimicking antemortem wounds. **After death, the abraded epidermis becomes stiff, leathery and parchment-like, brown, more prominent and may be mistaken for burns.** This is classically seen in ligature mark of hanging and strangulation Table (8–1).

Table (8–1). Difference between antemortem and postmortem abrasions

Trait		Antemortem abrasions	Postmortem abrasions
(1)	Site:	Anywhere on the body.	Usually over bony prominences.
(2)	Colour:	Bright reddish-brown.	Yellowish, translucent, and parchment-like.
(3)	Exudation:	More; scab slightly raised.	Less; scab often lies slightly below the level of skin.
(4)	Microscopic:	Intravital reaction and congestion seen.	No intravital reaction and no congestion.

CIRCUMSTANCES OF INJURIES: Abrasions are usually seen in accidents and assaults. Suicidal abrasions are rare. Sometimes, hysterical women produce abrasions over accessible areas like the front of forearms or over the face to fabricate a false charge of assault. Abrasions on the face or body of the assailant indicate a struggle. Persons collapsing due to heart attack tend to fall forward and receive abrasions to the eyebrow, nose and cheek, but there will be no injuries on the upper limbs. A conscious person when falling puts out his hands to save himself, and abrasions may be produced on the palmar surfaces of the hands. The alcoholic tends to fall backwards and strikes his occiput on the ground.

Medicolegal Importance: (1) They give an idea about the site of impact and direction of the force. (2) They may be the only external signs of a serious internal injury. (3) Patterned abrasions are helpful in connecting the wound with the object which produced them. (4) The age of the injury can be determined, which helps to corroborate with the alleged time of assault. (5) In open wounds, dirt, dust, grease or sand are usually present, which may connect the injuries to the scene of crime. (6) Character and manner of injury may be known from its distribution. (a) In throttling, crescentic abrasions due to fingernails are found on the neck. (b) In smothering, abrasions may be seen around the mouth and nose. (c) In sexual assaults, abrasions may be found on the breasts, genitals, inner side of the thighs and around the anus. (d) Abrasions on the face of the assailant indicate a struggle. (e) Abrasions on the victim may show whether the fingernails of the assailant were long, irregular or even broken.

Differential Diagnosis: (1) Erosions of the Skin Produced by Ants: Ants and roaches produce brown erosions with minute irregular margins of the superficial layers of the skin. They are most commonly found at mucocutaneous junctions, about the eyelids, nostrils, mouth, ears, knuckles, axillae, groins, and genitalia. They are also seen in the moist folds of the skin. Sometimes they are localised, and may simulate antemortem abrasions. Examination by hand lens shows multiple crescent-shaped, sand-like bite marks. Each one is separated by normal skin. Vital reaction is not seen. **(2) Excoriations of the Skin by Excreta:** In infants, slight inflammation with excoriation may be seen in the napkin area (groin and buttocks) at the time of death. After death, these areas become dry, depressed and parchment-like and the colour varies from pale-yellow to deep-copper (Nappy abrasions). **(3) Pressure sores. (4) Drying of the skin** of the scrotum produces hardened, reddish-brown colouration resembling abrasion.

CONTUSIONS (BRUISES)

A contusion is an effusion of blood into the tissues, due to the rupture of blood vessels (veins, venules and arterioles), caused by blunt object, such as fist, stone, stick, bar, whip, hammer, axe, wooden handle, poker, shod foot, boot, etc.

Types: (1) Intradermal. (2) Subcutaneous. (3) Deep.

Situation: The bruise is usually situated in the corium and subcutaneous tissues, above the deep fascia, often in the fat layer. Contusions may be present not only in skin, but also in internal organs, such as the lung, heart, brain and muscles and any tissue.

Features: In contusion, **there is a painful swelling, and crushing or tearing of the subcutaneous tissues usually without destruction of the skin Figs. (8–9 to 8–13). The extravasated blood is diffusely distributed through the tissue spaces, and the margins are blurred.** Bruises may be seen in association with abrasions (abraded-contusion) or lacerations. Bruises in hypostatic area may show slight swelling of the area or an abrasion. When a large blood vessel is injured, a tumour-

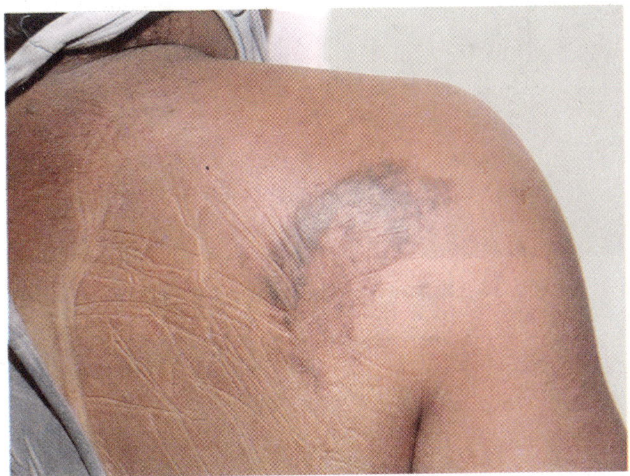

Fig. (8–9). Contusion on right upper part of back of chest.

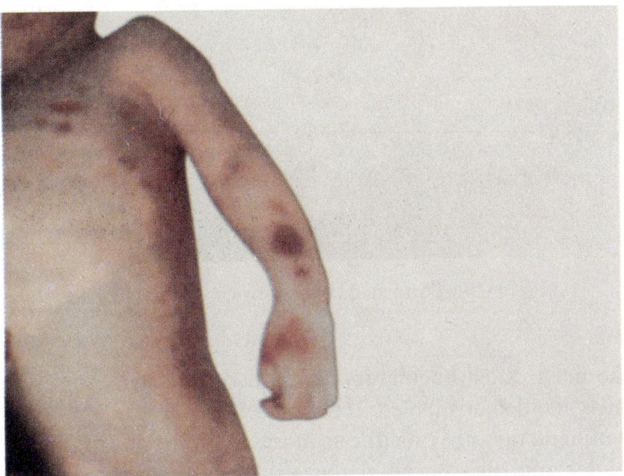

Fig. (8–10). Multiple bruises on the forearm.

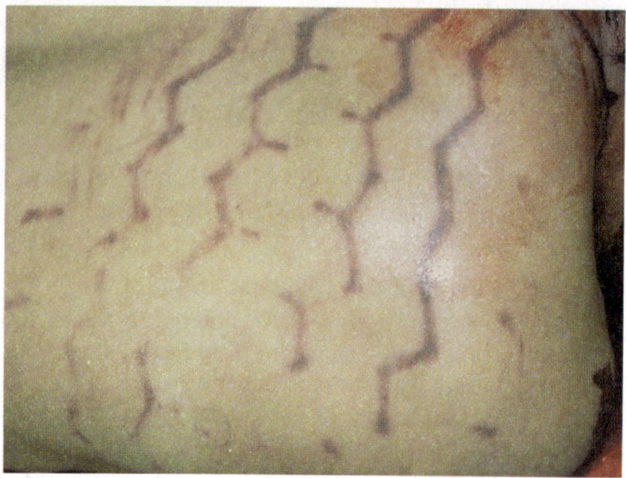

Fig. (8–11). Patterned abrasions caused by tyre tread.

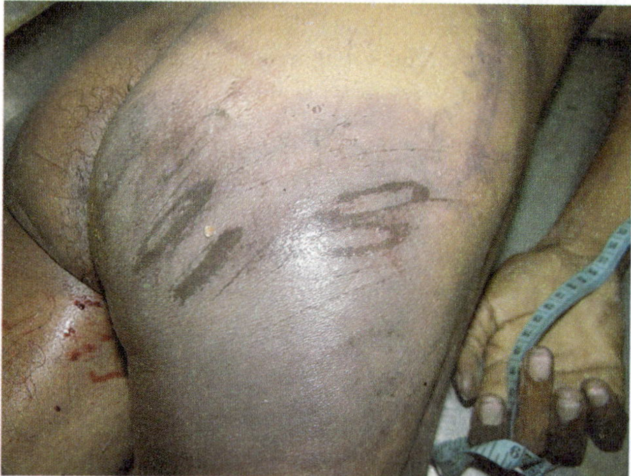

Fig. (8–12). Patterned contusions over buttock.

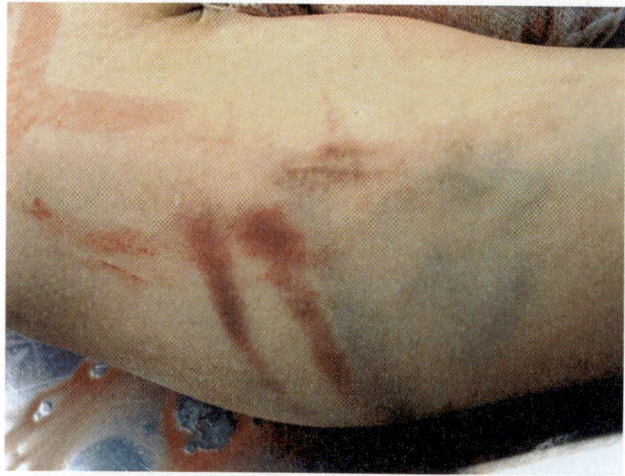

Fig. (8–13). Patterned contusions caused by a stick.

like mass called **haematoma** is formed. Petechial bruises are finely mottled or stippled. **If the petechiae become larger and confluent, they are called ecchymoses. A fresh bruise is usually tender and slightly raised above the surface of the skin,** and even a deep-seated bruise shows some swelling when compared with the opposite limb or part of the body. **A bruise has lighter colour in the centre because extravasated blood is pushed outward by the impact. Mongolian spot** (hyperpigmented skin in the lumbosacral region) should not be confused with contusion.

Size: Bruises vary in size from pinhead to large collections of blood in the tissues. **The size of a bruise is slightly larger than the surface of the agent which caused it, as blood continues to escape into the area.** Development of marked tissue swelling in the vicinity of a bruise usually results in loss of its original shape. As a general rule, the greater the force of violence used, the more extensive will be the bruise.

Factors modifying size and shape:

(1) Condition and Type of Tissue: **If the part is vascular and loose, such as face, vulva, scrotum, a slight degree of violence may cause a large bruise,** as there is sufficient space for blood to accumulate. **If the tissues are strongly supported, and contain firm fibrous tissues and covered by thick dermis,** such as abdomen, back, scalp, palms and soles, a blow of **moderate violence may produce a comparatively small bruise.** In boxers and athletes, bruising is much less, because of good muscle tone. Bruising is relatively more marked on tissues overlying bone, which acts as anvil, with the skin between the bone and the inflicting force. Chronic alcoholics bruise easily. **Bruising of the scalp is better felt than seen. Bruising of the scalp with fluctuant centres can simulate depressed fracture. Even a severe injury may produce little haemorrhage, if it was preceded by an injury which produced deep shock.** Resilient areas, such as the abdominal wall and buttock bruise less.

Bruising is not seen if the injured part is thickly covered, or if the weapon used is a yielding one, such as sand bag. Bruising may be absent if the pressure be continued until death occurs.

(2) Age: **Children bruise more easily** because of softer tissues and loose and smaller volume of protecting tissue that overlies blood vessels, and old persons bruise easily because of loss of subcutaneous tissues and flesh and cardiovascular changes.

(3) Sex: **Women bruise more easily than men,** because the tissues are more delicate and subcutaneous fat is more. Fat people bruise easily, because of greater volume of subcutaneous tissue. A slight pressure with the fingers on the arm of a woman, and especially if she is obese and not accustomed to work or exercise, may produce a definite bruise.

(4) Colour of Skin: Bruising is more clearly seen in fair-skinned persons than those with dark skin Fig. (8–9), in whom they may be better felt than seen. **The areas of extravasated blood appear darker even on heavily pigmented negroid skin.** Examination by ultraviolet light, bruises appear as darker areas, even on heavily pigmented skin. **If the body is embalmed, skin bruises become more prominent** probably (1) by forcing of additional blood into the damaged area, (2) increased transparency of overlying skin, and (3) formation of a dark pigment complex. Contusions appear much more clear in black and white photographs than by direct observation. **Colour photographs more truly reproduce contusions.**

(5) Natural Disease: When the vessels are diseased as in arteriosclerosis, bruising occurs very easily and may even result from coughing or slight exertion. **In children,** small bruises may be caused by the violent coughing as in whooping cough. Prominent bruising following minor trauma is seen in a person suffering from purpura haemorrhagica, leukaemia, haemophilia, scurvy, vitamin K and prothrombin deficiency and in phosphorus poisoning. Purpuric areas are clearly delineated from the surrounding tissue and never show swelling. Many old persons (esp. those on systemic steroids) develop senile ecchymoses all over their bodies, especially on extremities. These can occur with little force or even spontaneously.

(6) Gravity Shifting of the Blood: Bruises do not always appear at the site of impact. A deep bruise, especially that due to the crushing of tissue against the bone may take a long time to become visible and also may not appear below the actual point of impact. Blood will track along the fascial planes (or between muscle layers) which form the least resistance and may appear where the tissue layers become superficial (ectopic bruising, or percolated or migratory contusion). The site of bruise does not always indicate the site of the violence. Haemorrhages in the soft tissues around the eyes and in the eyelids (spectacle haematoma; **black eye), may be caused by** (1) direct trauma, such as a punch in the eye, (2) blunt impact to the forehead, the blood gravitating downwards over the supraorbital bridge, (3) fracture of the floor of the anterior fossa of the skull. A bruise behind the ear may indicate a basal fracture, rather than a direct blow behind the ear (Battle's sign), (4) in fracture of the jaw, a bruise may appear in the neck, (5) in fracture of the pelvis, a bruise may appear in the thigh, (6) in fracture of the femur, a bruise may appear on the outer side of the lower part of the thigh, (7) a blow to upper thigh may appear as a bruise above the knee, (8) a kick on the calf of the leg may appear as a bruise around the ankle.

Patterned Bruising: A patterned contusion is one in which the size and shape, mirror a portion of the object which caused it. With heavier impacts or objects, the tissues beneath the impacting objects are crushed, and the contusion pattern is solid rather than outlined. **(1) A bruise is usually round, but it may indicate the nature of the weapon especially when death occurs soon after infliction of injury. If the person is living, this pattern may become obscure as the area of bruising tends to extend and merge with adjacent structures.** (2) A blow from a solid body, such as a hammer, or the closed fist usually produces a rounded bruise. (3) Bruises made by the end of a thick stick may be round, but if any length of the stick hits the body, they are elongated and irregular. (4) **A blow with a rod, a stick or a whip produces two parallel, linear haemorrhages (railway line or tram line type) Figs. (8–12 and 8–13). The intervening skin appears unchanged, because the rod forcibly dents the tissues inwards and momentarily stretches each side of the dent.** This causes rupture of vessels in the marginal zones with a line of bruising, whereas the base of the dent becomes compressed and the vessels are not injured. **Blood from the base of the dent gets displaced to the sides due to the pressure by the object. When the rod is removed and the skin comes back to its normal position, the two sides of the depression remain as contused lines. In a bruise produced by a long rigid weapon, e.g., stick, the edges of the bruise may be irregular and the width may be greater due to infiltration of blood in the surrounding tissues along the edges of the bruise.** A blow with a rigid weapon like a stick on a curved surface of the body, in a region where the soft tissues are particularly pliable, e.g., the buttocks, compress the tissues under the force of impact. In such case, the contusion is not limited to the maximum convexity of the affected part, but it may extend over the whole of the curved surface. (5) When the body is struck by a broad flat weapon, such as a plank, the edges of the plank may cause parallel bruises in the skin, separated by apparently normal tissue. (6) Bruises caused by blows from whips are elongated, curve over prominences, and may partially encircle a limb or the body. They are seen as two parallel lines, the distance between which is roughly equal to the diameter of the whip. (7) Bruises made by pliable canes are similar to those due to whip, but never encircle a limb or curve round the sides of the body. (8) Bruises from straps, belts or chains, leave a definite imprint. (9) A woven, spiral or plaited ligature may sometimes produce a patterned bruise. (10) Contact injuries from firearms may produce abrasion with bruising indicating the outline of the muzzle of the weapon. (11) Patterned bruising is also seen in motor car accidents. (12) Suction or biting on sides of the neck or the breasts, during erotic love-making or sexual intercourse produces elliptical patterned bruises. They frequently consist of a shower of petechial haemorrhages, which may be confluent. They may sometimes reproduce the shape of the upper and lower lips. (13) In a bruise caused by impact with a patterned object, the haemorrhage which is relatively small, may be sharply defined if it lies in the immediate subepidermal layer, and the pattern is distinct due to translucency because of the thin layer that overlies it. Such contusions are commonly seen when the impacting object has alternating ridges and grooves (such as the tread of a motor tyre in a traffic accident, kick with ribbed, rubber soles of shoes, impact from whips), as the skin will be forced into the grooves and distorted. Intradermal bleeding will occur and the red lines may be produced not by the ridges which are pale as the pressure forces the blood from the small vessels, but by the grooves, by a squeezing or bursting effect on the cutaneous capillaries. (14) Forceful compression with the sole or the heel may imprint an intradermal bruise of the pattern of the sole or heel of the shoe. Kicking and jumping on a person combined is known as **'stomping'.** (15) If a violent blow is struck on a clothed area of the body, or if the clothing is grabbed and twisted over the skin, petechial haemorrhages occur within the skin reproducing the texture of clothing.

Delayed Bruising: A superficial bruise appears immediately as a dark-red swelling. **A deep bruise may take several hours, or one or two days to appear and deeper extravasation of blood may never appear. Therefore, one more examination should be carried out 48 hours after the first examination, to note bruises of slower development Fig. (8–12). Occasionally, when an injury is produced before death, the bruise may appear some time after death, due to further escape of blood from the ruptured vessels due to gravitation, mainly due to percolation, and rapid haemolysis of stagnant blood, the pigment diffusing locally and producing a stain on the surface (come-out bruise).** This may explain the difference of opinion between two observers, who have examined the person or the body at different times. The pressure of the gases of putrefaction may cause the extravasated blood to extend along the tissue spaces and give rise to a false impression of the extent of antemortem bruising. **Haemolysis of extravasated red cells**

and diffusion of pigment into the surrounding tissues may also cause postmortem extension of bruise. Therefore, in assessing the extent of bruising, the postmortem interval should be considered. **The examination of whole body by ultraviolet light will sometimes clearly show otherwise undetectable areas of bruising. At autopsy, when the superficial tissues are drained of blood, contusions may become more prominent and extensive than before.** Surgical removal of the corneas for transplant purposes can cause haemorrhage in the eyelids simulating antemortem trauma. Removal of the vitreous soon after death can also cause scleral haemorrhage.

Deep Tissue and Organ Contusions: All organs can be contused. **Deep contusions are clearly seen during autopsy, as the blood is drained from blood vessels and also due to postmortem autolytic changes** Fig. (8–14). A contusion of the brain may initiate enough swelling with gradual accumulation of acid byproducts of metabolism, with further swelling and impairment of function, confusion, coma and death. Contusions in vital centres, e.g., which control respiration and blood pressure can be fatal, even when very small. A small contusion of the heart can cause serious disturbance of normal rhythm or stoppage of cardiac action and death. Large contusions often prevent adequate cardiac emptying and lead to heart failure. Contusions of other organs may cause rupture of that organ with slow or rapid bleeding into the body cavity, and may cause death.

Sometimes, haemorrhages are seen in areas of lividity on the arms or shoulders of fat persons without evidence of trauma on other parts of the body. These haemorrhages are produced by tearing of small veins in the skin when the body is lifted from the scene of death. At autopsy, blood drains from blood vessels so that the deep bruises may show up against the white areas as the blood in the contusions will not drain.

The Age of Bruise: A bruise heals by destruction and removal of the extravasated blood. The more vascular the area, the smaller the contusion, and the healthier the individual, the more rapid will be the healing. The red cells disintegrate by haemolysis, and the haemoglobin is broken down into haemosiderin, haematoidin and bilirubin by the action of enzymes. Factors affecting colour of contusion include: (1) depth of bleeding, (2) amount of bleeding, (3) environmental lighting, and (4) overlying skin colour.

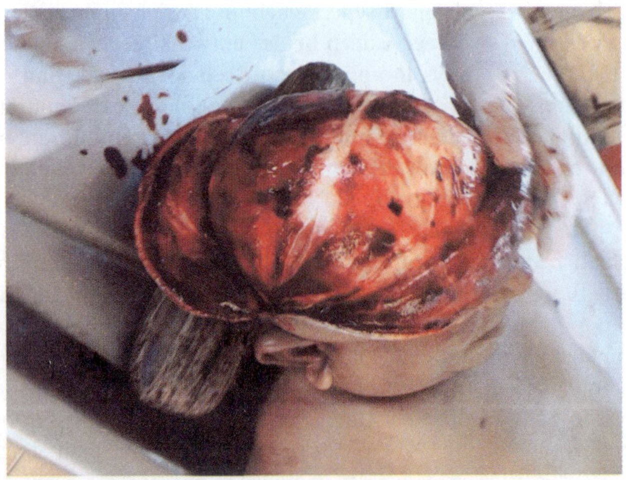

Fig. (8–14). Extensive contusion of scalp.

The colour change starts at the periphery and extends inwards to the centre.

At first: Red.

Few hours to 3 days: Blue.

4th day: Bluish-black to brown (haemosiderin).

5 to 6 days: Greenish (haematoidin).

7 to 12 days: Yellow (bilirubin).

2 weeks: Normal.

The rate of colour change is quite variable, not only between persons, but in the same person and from bruise to bruise. Bruises in children change colour rapidly and may be completely absorbed in a few days. **In interpreting the age of a bruise by colour changes, one should be very cautious. Subconjunctival ecchymoses do not undergo usual colour changes due to diffusion of atmospheric oxygen through the conjunctival tissue.** They are at first bright red, then yellow before disappearing. In old people, healing of bruise is very slow. A bruise sustained at the time of carbon monoxide poisoning is likely to have a bright-red colour.

It is difficult to estimate the exact age of a bruise with any degree of certainty even by microscopic examination.

HISTOPATHOLOGY: Contusions and abrasions produced immediately before death show a marked decrease in the acidic mucopolysaccharides of the connective tissue ground substance, as demonstrated by Alcian Blue or dialyzed iron technique. Acidic mucopolysaccharide is absent in contusions more than an hour old, but reappears in the bruises several days old showing the increase of connective tissue. On microscopic examination, the presence of tissue reaction of a degree beyond a margination and limited emigration of the white cells indicates that the contusion was probably antemortem. If the red cells have lost their shape and staining characteristics, and if iron containing pigment is found either at the site of injury or in the regional lymph nodes, probably 12 hours have passed after the injury. It is of some value in distinguishing cerebral haemorrhage occurring due to accident from natural haemorrhage, which could have been occurring for some time, and which may have caused the accident. Towards the end stage of healing process, large histiocytes containing coarse granules of haemosiderin pigment can be seen microscopically in section of contused area. The site of a bruise may contain crystals of haematoidin for a long period after the injury.

Antemortem and Postmortem Bruising: In antemortem bruising, there is swelling, damage to epithelium, extravasation, coagulation and infiltration of the tissues with blood and colour changes. These signs are absent in postmortem bruises. The margins of postmortem bruises are usually quite sharply defined, and those of antemortem bruises are less sharp or indistinct for the greater part, indicating vital reaction in the damaged tissues.

Appreciable bruising does not occur after death due to arrest of circulation, but **by using great violence, small bruises can be produced up to 2 to 3 hours after death,** in areas where the tissues can be forcibly compressed against bone and also in hypostatic area, e.g., the back of the scalp, if the body is dropped on the ground, or on trolleys or postmortem tables.

Decomposed bodies: In a body lying on its back, blood accumulates in posterior or dependent half of scalp due to gravity. **In decomposed bodies, especially in the scalp, haemolysis of red cells produces a diffuse discolouration of the soft tissues, due to which it becomes impossible to differentiate between an**

Table (8–2). Difference between hypostasis and bruise

	Trait	Hypostasis	Bruise
(1)	Cause:	Due to distension of vessels with blood in the dermis.	Due to ruptured vessels which may be superficial or deep.
(2)	Site:	Occurs over extensive area of the most dependent parts.	Occurs at the site of and surrounding the injury; may appear anywhere on the body.
(3)	Appearance:	No elevation of the involved area.	Often swollen because of extravasated blood and oedema.
(4)	Epidermis:	Not abraded.	May be abraded.
(5)	Margins:	Clearly defined.	Merge with surrounding area.
(6)	Colour:	Uniform bluish–purple in colour.	Old bruises are of different colour. Fresh bruises may appear more intense than the adjacent hypostatic area.
(7)	Incision:	On incision blood is seen in blood vessels, which can be easily washed away. Subcutaneous tissues are pale.	Shows extravasation of blood into the surrounding tissues, which is firmly clotted and cannot be washed by gentle stream of water. Subcutaneous tissues are deep reddish-black.
(8)	Effect of pressure:	Absent in areas of the body which are even under slight pressure.	Little lighter over the area of pressure or support.

antemortem contusion and an area of postmortem hypostasis. In hypostatic areas blood vessels breakdown with leakage of red cells into the soft tissue which haemolyse due to decomposition; erythrocytes in soft tissue in a contusion also haemolyse, and as such the appearances are similar.

Demonstration of Bruising: **At autopsy, bruises may not be readily detected or they may be obscured by patches of postmortem lividity, or by the dark colour of the skin** Table (8–2). Contusions of the scalp can be demonstrated by reflecting the scalp and making incisions into the scalp from the aponeurotic surface. Contusions of the neck can be demonstrated by reflecting the various structures of the neck in layers. **Contusions in the subcutaneous tissues may be detected by parallel incisions through the skin Figs. (8–15 and 8–16).** Deep bruises are detected by deep incisions made into the muscles. When in doubt, a portion must be taken for microscopy. The extent of bruising and the injury to the underlying soft tissues and muscles can be seen by dissecting the skin away from the underlying fat and muscle fascia.

Medicolegal Importance: (1) Patterned bruises may connect the victim and the object or weapon, e.g., whip, chain, cane, ligature, vehicle, etc. (2) The age of the injury can be determined by colour changes. (3) The degree of violence may be determined from their size. (4) Character and manner of injury may be known from its distribution. (a) When the arms are grasped, there may be 3 or 4 bruises on one side and one larger bruise on the opposite side, from the fingers and thumb respectively, indicating the position of the assailant in front of, or behind the victim. (b) Bruising of the arm may be a sign of restraining a person. (c) Bruising of the shoulder blades indicate firm pressure on the body against the ground or other resisting surface. (d) In manual strangulation, the position and number of bruises and nail marks may give an indication of the method of attack or the position of the assailant. (e) Bruising of thigh especially inner aspect, and of genitalia indicates rape. (5) In open wounds, dirt, dust, grease or particles of stone or sand are usually present, which may connect the injuries to the scene of crime.

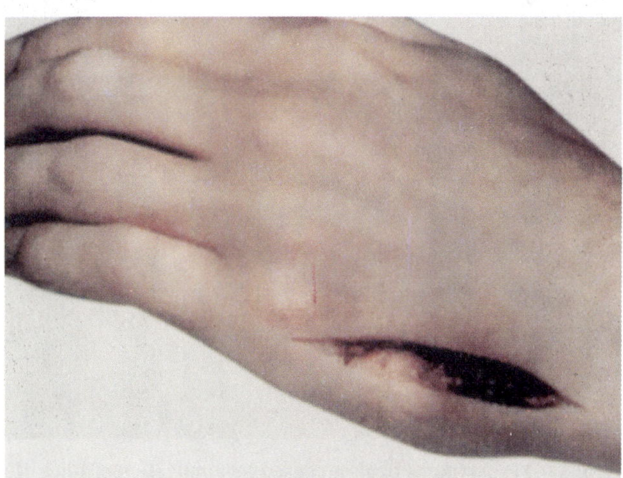

Fig. (8–16). An incision to demonstrate deep contusion on the back of the hand.

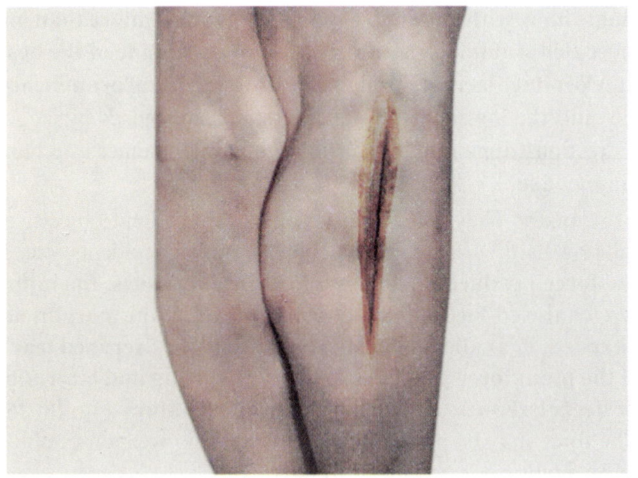

Fig. (8–15). An incision to demonstrate deep contusion on the calf muscles.

Bruises are of less value than abrasions because: (1) Their size may not correspond to the size of the weapon. (2) They may become visible several hours or even one to two days after the injury. (3) They may appear away from the actual site of injury.

Table (8–3). **Difference between true bruise and artificial bruise**

	Trait	Artificial bruise	True bruise
(1)	Cause:	Juice of marking nut.	Trauma.
(2)	Site :	Exposed accessible parts.	Anywhere.
(3)	Colour:	Dark-brown.	Typical colour changes.
(4)	Shape:	Irregular.	Usually round.
(5)	Margins:	Well-defined and regular, covered with small vesicles.	Not well-defined, diffuse and irregular; no vesicles.
(6)	Redness and inflammation:	Seen in the surrounding skin.	Seen in the site.
(7)	Contents:	Acrid serum.	Extravasated blood.
(8)	Itching:	Present.	Absent.
(9)	Vesicles:	May be found on fingertips and on other parts of the body due to scratching.	Absent.
(10)	Chemical tests:	Positive for the chemical.	Negative.

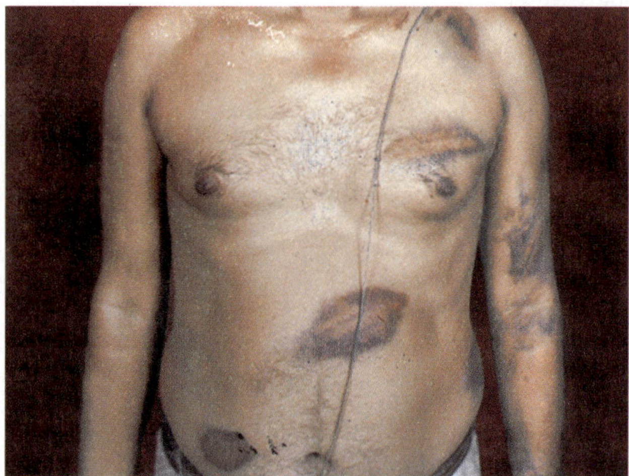

Fig. (8–17). **Artificial bruises caused by application of juice of marking nut.**

(4) They do not indicate the direction in which the force was applied.

Complications: (1) A contusion may contain 20 to 30 ml. of blood or even more. **Multiple contusions can cause death from shock and internal haemorrhage.** (2) Gangrene and death of tissue can result. (3) The pooled blood can serve as a good site for bacterial growth, especially by clostridial group. (4) Rarely, in severe sudden compression of the subcutaneous tissue, pulmonary fat embolism may occur.

Artificial Bruises: Juice of marking nut when applied to skin produces injuries, which simulate bruises **Table (8–3).** They are produced to make a false charge of assault **Fig. (8–17)**.

CIRCUMSTANCES OF INJURIES: Accidental bruises are very common and may be seen on prominences, such as the forehead, nose, elbows and knees. Presence of mud, sand, grease or oil gives an idea of the manner of causation. Multiple contusions from minor trauma are often seen in alcoholics, which may be mistaken to be caused by physical violence. Self-inflicted bruises are rare, as they are painful. They are seen over accessible areas, usually on the head, especially in a hysterical individual or the insane. Homicidal bruises may be seen on any part of the body. It is not possible to differentiate an injury caused by a fist or weapon and a fall. Contamination of the wound should be looked for. Tangential forces or glancing blows may tear large flaps of tissue, exposing the underlying skull.

LACERATIONS

Lacerations are tears or splits of skin, mucous membranes, muscle or internal organs produced by application of blunt object to broad area of the body, which crushed or stretched tissues beyond the limits of their elasticity. They are also called tears or ruptures Figs. (8–18 to 8–25).

Mechanism: Localised portions of tissue are displaced by the impact of the blunt force, which sets up traction forces and causes tearing of the tissues. Unless great force is used, most lacerations require a firm base to act as an anvil for the skin and underlying tissues to be pinned against. In lacerations of soft areas, such as buttock, thigh, calf, abdomen, upper arm, etc., the lacerating agent is either a projecting point or edge, or a completely blunt object is pulled obliquely against the tension of the skin until it tears.

The object causing a lacerated wound crushes and stretches a broad area of skin, which then splits in the centre. The edges are irregular and rough, because of the crushing and tearing nature of the blunt trauma. Frequently, the skin, at the margins is abraded due to the flatter portion of the striking object rubbing against the skin as it is indented by the forceful blow. The margins are contused due to the bleeding into the tissues caused by trauma. **A single blow with a blunt weapon may produce more than one lacerated wound, e.g., a single blow over the side of the head may produce lacerated wounds over the parietal prominence, ear and the lower jaw.** Some lacerations are caused by jagged projections ripping into the skin in the same manner as a blunt knife or axe.

Causes: They are caused by blows from blunt objects, by falls on hard surfaces, by machinery, traffic accidents, etc. **If the force produces bleeding into adjacent tissues, the injury is a 'contused-laceration' or 'bruised-tear'. If the margins are abraded, it is called "abraded laceration" or "scraped tear". If the blunt force produces extensive bruising and laceration of deeper tissues, it is called "crushing" injury** Fig. (8–25). The force may be produced by some moving weapon or object or by a fall.

Types: (1) Split Lacerations: Splitting occurs by crushing of the skin between two hard objects. Scalp lacerations occur

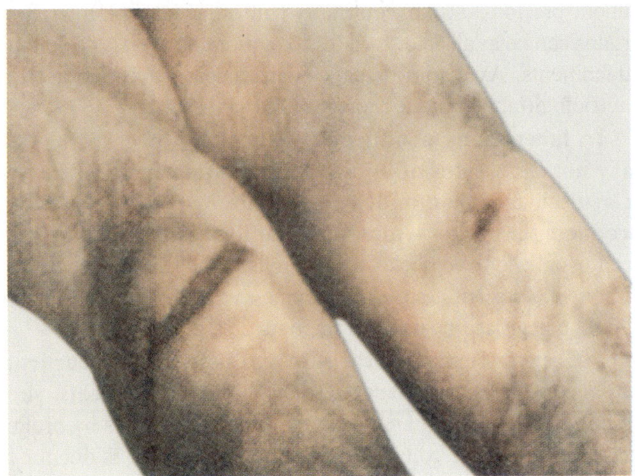

Fig. (8–18). **Lacerated wound on knees.**

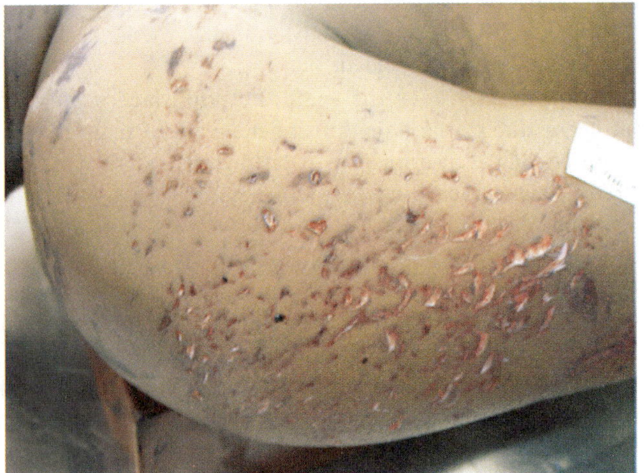

Fig. (8–19). **Multiple punctate lacerations caused by broken glass piece.**

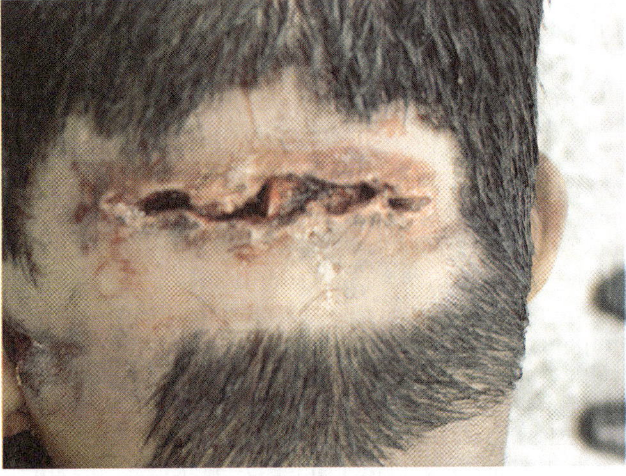

Fig. (8–20). **laceration of scalp.**

due to the tissues being crushed between skull and some hard object, such as the ground or a blunt instrument. **Splits are not undermined, but show tissue bridges.**

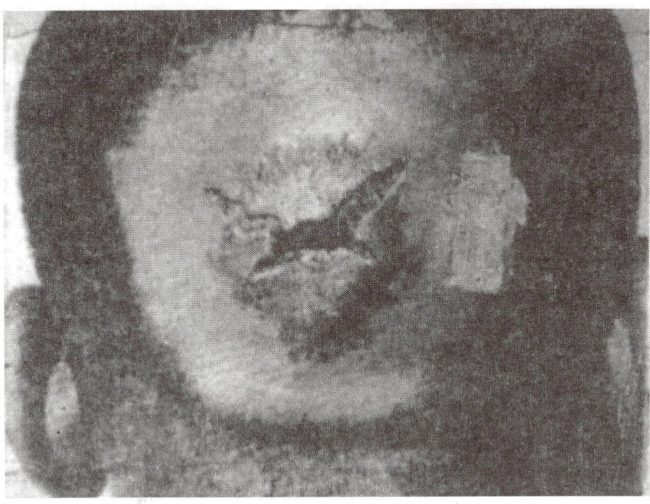

Fig. (8–21). **Laceration of scalp (star-shaped).**

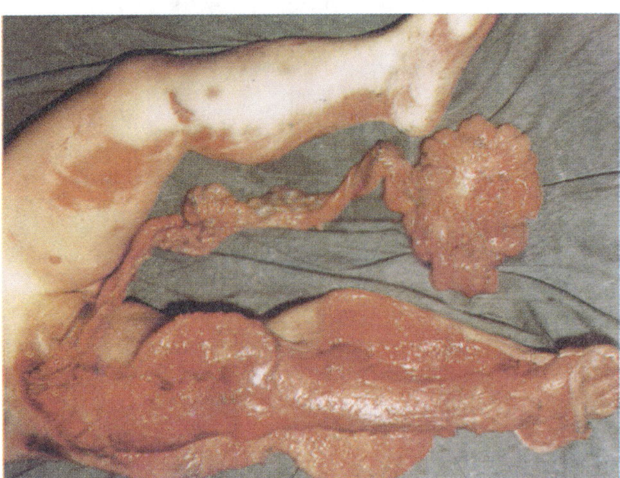

Fig. (8–22). **Avulsion of whole of front of right lower extremity caused by running over off wheel of automobile.**

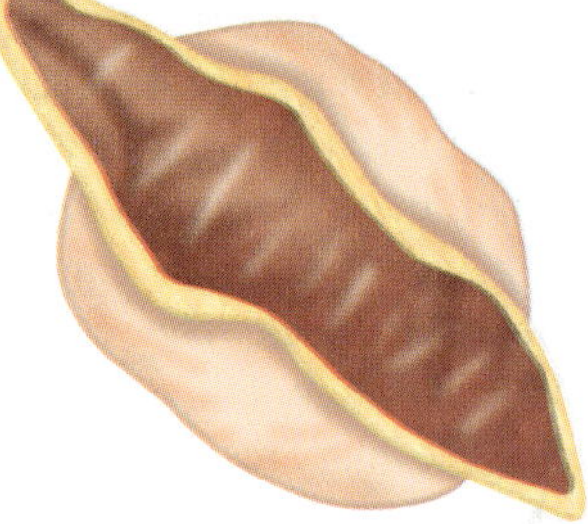

Fig. (8–23). **Lacerated wound showing tissue bridges.**

Incised-like or Incised-looking Wounds: **Lacerations produced without excessive skin crushing may have relatively sharp margins.** Blunt force on areas where the skin is close to bone, and the subcutaneous tissues are scanty, may produce a wound which by linear splitting of the tissues (as the skin is easily stretched during impact), may look like incised wound. **The sites are the scalp, eyebrows, cheek bones, lower jaw, iliac crest, perineum, and shin. A wound produced by a fall on the knee**

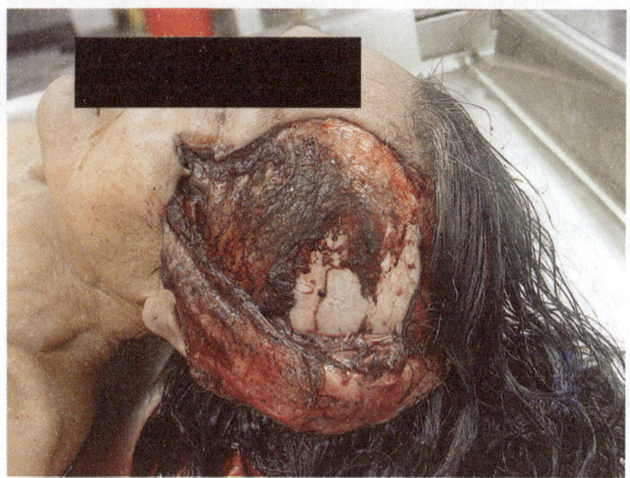

Fig. (8–24). Avulsed lacreration of scalp.

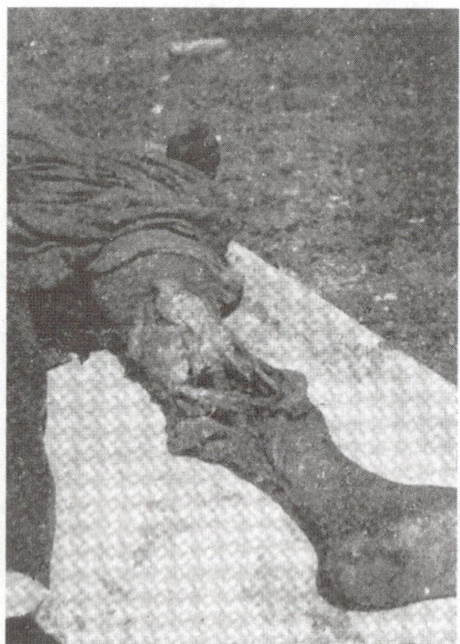

Fig. (8–25). Crush injury leg caused by run over accident.

or elbow with the limb flexed, and by a broken glass or sharp stone also simulates incised wound.

(2) Stretch Lacerations: **Overstretching of the skin, if it is fixed, will cause laceration.** There is localised pressure with pull which increases until tearing occurs and produces a flap of skin, which is peeled off the underlying bone or deep fascia. This is seen in the running over by a motor vehicle, and the flap may indicate the direction of the vehicle. They can occur from kicking, and also when sudden deformity of a bone occurs after fracture, making it compound. The injury results in irregular tearing of the skin and tissues. Foreign material may be found in the depth of the wound.

(3) Avulsion (shearing laceration): **An avulsion is a laceration produced by sufficient force (shearing force) delivered at an acute angle to detach (tear off) a portion of a traumatised surface or viscus from its attachments** Fig. (8–24). The shearing and grinding force by a weight, such as lorry wheel passing over a limb may produce separation of the skin from the underlying tissues (avulsion) over a relatively large area. This is called "flaying". **The underlying muscles are crushed, and the bones may be fractured. The separated skin may show extensive abrasions** from the rotating frictional effect of the tyre, but one portion is still in continuity with adjacent skin. Internally, organs can be avulsed or torn off in part or completely from their attachments. Avulsion of scalp is also caused by traction from hair being trapped in machinery.

In lacerations produced by shearing forces, the skin may not show signs of injury, but the underlying soft tissue is avulsed from the underlying fascia or connective tissue, producing a pocket which may be filled with blood. This is seen usually on the back of the thighs of pedestrians struck by motor vehicles. In a case of extreme avulsion, an extremity or even the head can be torn off the body.

(4) Tears: **Tearing of the skin and tissues can occur from impact by or against irregular or semi-sharp objects, such as door handle of a car.** It may be caused by blows by broken glass, or fall over a rough projected object. **A tear is deeper at the starting point than at the termination.** This is another form of overstretching.

(5) Cut Lacerations: Cut lacerations may be **produced by a heavy relatively sharp-edged instrument such as axe, hatchet, chopper, etc.** The margins are usually abraded with bruising. This term should be better avoided.

In an impact over the scalp, external laceration may not occur due to the hair, but inner layers of scalp may be lacerated. If the instrument is padded or has a broad striking surface, severe fractures of the skull may occur without external laceration.

Lacerations of the internal organs may be caused by: (1) direct injury of the viscera by fragments of fractured bone, (2) development of traction shears or strain shears in the viscera, (3) stretching of the visceral attachments, and (4) hydrostatic forces.

Characters: (1) **Margins are irregular, ragged and uneven, and their ends are pointed or blunt, and they too show minute tears in the margins. The edges of lacerations, especially over a bony area, e.g., skull are undermined due to the crushing and tearing force of the impact.** If a blunt object, e.g., a bottle strikes the skin surface, the edge at the point of impact will be sharp and turned inwards, whereas the other edge may be everted, exposing the hair follicles in the depths. Tearing at the ends of lacerations, at angles diverging from the main laceration itself, so-called swallow tails, are frequently noted. (2) **Bruising is seen either in the skin or the subcutaneous tissues around the wound.** If the force is exerted by an object with a downward course, the lower margin of the wound is likely to be bruised more and undermined than the upper. Equal undermining of all sides indicates a perpendicular impact. (3) **Deeper tissues are unevenly divided with tags of tissues at the bottom of the wound bridging across the margin because different components of soft tissue have different strengths.** Tissue bridges (bridging fibres) consist of nerves, blood vessels and elastic and connective tissue fibres Fig. (8–23). (4) Hair bulbs are crushed. (5) Hair and epidermal tags may be driven deeply into the wound. (6) **Haemorrhage is less** because the arteries are crushed and torn across irregularly, and thus retract and the blood clots readily, except in wounds of the scalp, where the temporal arteries bleed freely as they are firmly bound and unable to contract. (7) **Foreign matter may be found in the wound.** (8) Depth varies according to the thickness of the soft parts at the site of the injury and degree of force applied. The depth of the wound will contain blood clot. (9) The shape and size may not correspond with the weapon or object which produced it. A laceration is usually curved; the convexity of the curve points towards the direction of application of force. (a) A blunt round end may cause stellate laceration. (b) A blunt object with an edge, such as hammer head, may cause crescentic laceration **(patterned laceration).** (c) Long, thin objects, such as pipes, tend to produce linear lacerations, while objects with flat surfaces produce irregular, ragged, or Y-shaped lacerations. (10) If the impact is from an angle, the skin on side of wound opposite to direction of motion is usually torn free or undermined for a variable distance. The other side, i.e. the side from which the blow was delivered, will be abraded and bevelled. Gaping is seen due to the pull of elastic and muscular tissues.

Age: Age determination of laceration is difficult unless there are clear signs of healing, such as granulation tissue, fibroblast ingrowth, or organising infiltrate.

Antemortem lacerations show bruising, eversion, gaping and blood-staining of margins, greater bleeding and vital reaction.

COMPLICATIONS: (1) Laceration of an internal organ may cause severe or even fatal bleeding. Temporal arteries may bleed freely as they are firmly bound and unable to contract. Multiple lacerations, involving only the skin and subcutaneous tissue, each causing some haemorrhage, may combine to cause shock and death. (2) Infection. (3) If it is located where skin stretches or is wrinkled, e.g., over joints, repeated and continued oozing of tissue fluids and blood may cause irritation, pain and dysfunction. (4) Pulmonary or systemic fat embolism may occur due to crushing of subcutaneous tissue.

Medicolegal Importance: (1) The type of laceration may indicate the cause of the injury and the shape of the blunt weapon. (2) Foreign bodies found in the wound may indicate the circumstances in which the crime has been committed. (3) The age of the injury can be determined.

Abrasions, contusions and lacerations are the external visible evidence of blunt impact injury which may be the only external sign of deeper and sometimes fatal injury of deeper lying structures.

CIRCUMSTANCES OF INJURIES: Violent, uncoordinated muscular contractions can produce disruptive tissue stresses which produce fractures, and lacerations of tendons and muscles. Internal forces and hydrostatic pressure created by convulsions can cause mural lacerations in hollow viscera. Suicidal lacerations are usually situated on the exposed parts of the body, and mostly on the same side. In the case of a fall on the head, the abraded scalp surface will be circular and completely surrounds the laceration. A blow with a blunt, narrow object, such as the edge of an angle iron or a crowbar will produce a linear tear with finely abraded margins. Homicidal wounds are usually seen on the head.

Combinations of Abrasions, Contusions and Lacerations: Abrasions, contusions and lacerations are frequently seen together or as integral parts of one another. **The same object may cause a contusion with one blow, a laceration with second, and an abrasion with a third.** Sometimes, all three types of injury may result from a single blow. Sometimes, an imprint may result from an object, and it may be difficult to determine whether the imprint is primarily an abrasion or a contusion.

Punching: Punching, i.e. blows with the clenched fist will produce abrasions and contusions; laceration may occur over bony prominences. Punches on the face may split the lips, fracture the teeth, nose, jaw or maxilla and produce black eye.

Kicking: Kicking and stamping injuries are caused by a foot which is either swung or moved downwards (compression) with some force. They will produce abrasions, contusions and sometimes lacerations, which are more severe than punching. The feet may be used to stamp down on the recumbent body, causing deep injuries to abdominal organs and fractures of ribs and sternum. The pattern of the footwear may be imprinted on to the skin.

INCISED WOUNDS

An incised wound (cut, slice) is a clean cut through the tissues (usually the skin and subcutaneous tissues, including blood vessels), caused by sharp-edged instrument. The wound is longer than it is deep. It has length rather than depth and tends to gape Figs. (8–26 to 8–33).

Mechanism: It is produced by the pressure and friction against the tissue, by an object having a sharp-cutting edge, such as knife, razor, scalpel, scissors, sickle, cleaver, sword, etc. In this, **the force is delivered over a very narrow area, corresponding with the cutting edge of the blade.**

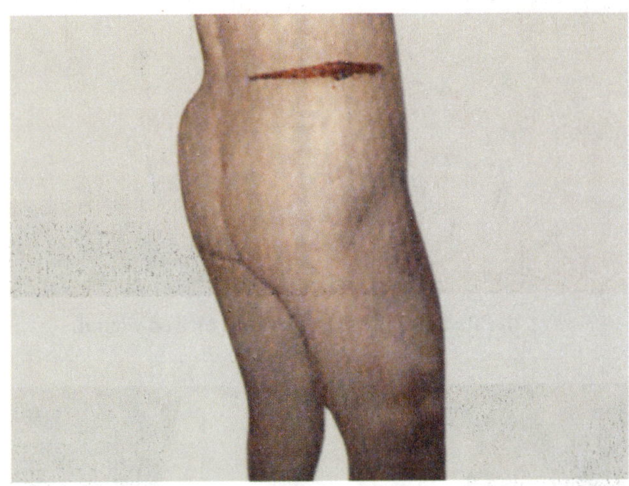

Fig. (8–26). Incised wound on the flank.

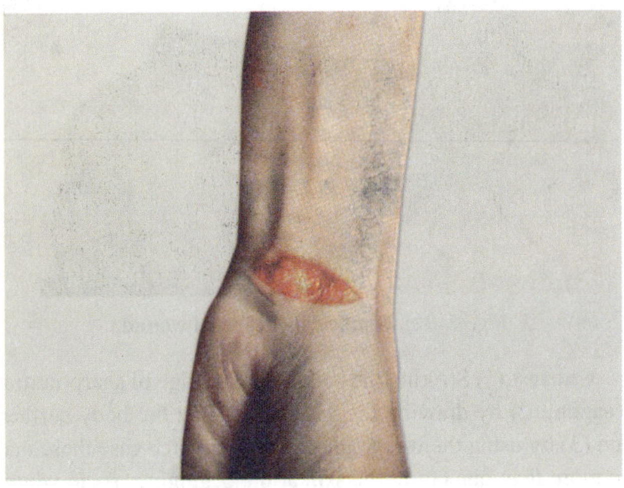

Fig. (8–27). Suicidal incised wound on the front of the wrist.

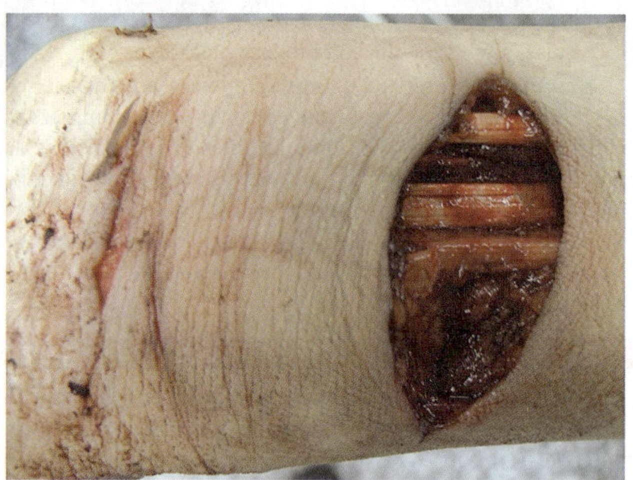

Fig. (8–28). **Multiple hesitation cuts and a gaping incised wound.**

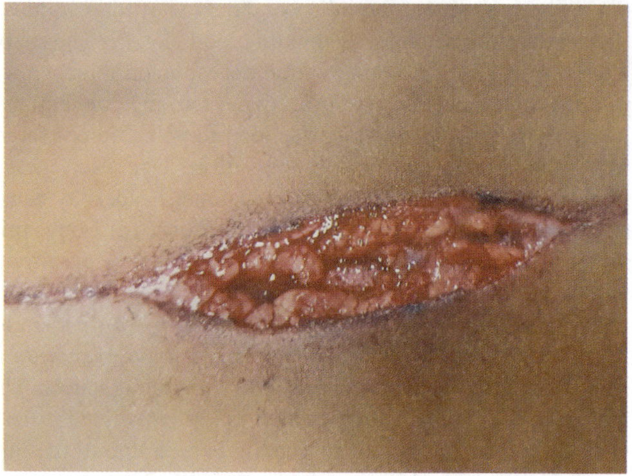

Fig. (8–29). **Gaping incised wound showing tailing.**

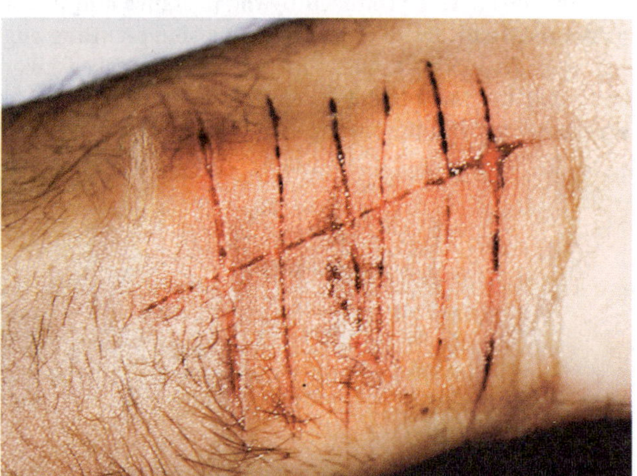

Fig. (8–30). **Self-inflicted superficial incised wound.**

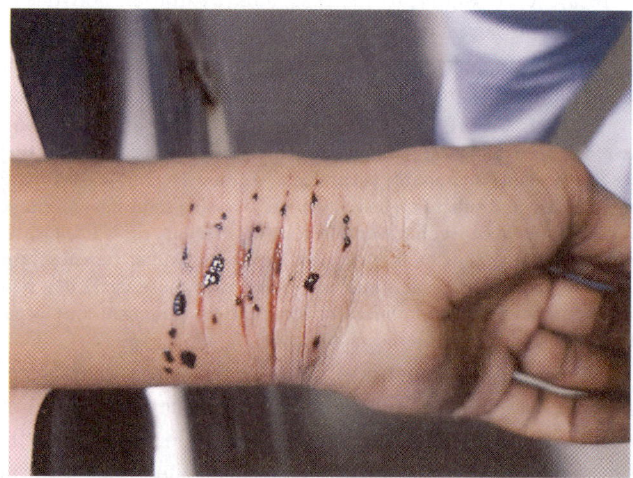

Fig. (8–31). **Suicidal incised wound on the front of wrist.**

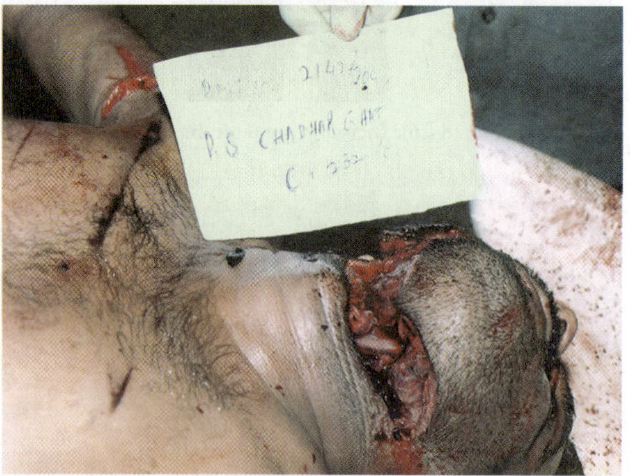

Fig. (8–32). **Homicidal cut throat wound.**

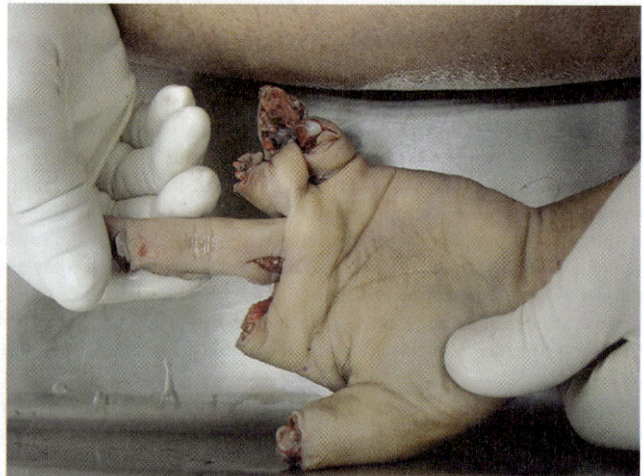

Fig. (8–33). **Chopped fingers of hand.**

Causes: (1) Striking the body with the edge of sharp-cutting weapon, (2) by drawing the weapon, against the body surface, and (3) by using the weapon like a saw in which case there may be more than one cut in the skin at the beginning of the wound which merge into one at the end.

Characters: (1) Margins: The edges are clean-cut, well-defined and usually everted. The edges may be inverted, if a thin layer of muscle fibres is adherent to the skin as in the scrotum. The edges are free from contusions and abrasions. A dull irregular-edged or nicked cutting edge may produce a wound with irregular, contused, and/or abraded margins, as the wound is caused more by the pressure applied by the weapon than by the cutting edge. A serrated knife may produce a saw-toothed cut on the body, if the blade passes obliquely or at shallow angle. **The depth of the wound will not show any bridging tissue.**

(2) Width: The width is greater than the thickness of the edge of the weapon causing it, due to retraction of the divided tissues. Shaking of the blade tends to make the wound wider than the weapon.

(3) Length: The length is greater than its width and depth, and has no relation to the cutting edge of the weapon, for it may be drawn to any distance. When the skin becomes folded under the cutting edge of the weapon, a single movement of the weapon may produce a series of incised wounds separated one from another by bridges of normal skin. **A curved weapon like a sickle, produces a stab from the pointed end, and incised wound from the blade, sometimes with an intervening intact skin.** Rarely, there may be a superficial tail (a shallow scratch) at the termination known as tailing of wound which indicates direction.

(4) Shape: It is usually spindle-shaped due to greater retraction of the edges in the centre. **Gaping is greater if the underlying muscle fibres have been cut transversely or obliquely,** and less when cut longitudinally **Figs. (8–28 and 8–29)**. Incised wounds crossing irregular surfaces may be irregular in depth, but will be linear. The wound may take zig-zag course if the skin is loosely attached as in axillary fold, because the skin is pushed in front of the blade before it is cut. If the blade is curved, the edges will be crescentic. If the surface is convex, such as the occipital region or buttocks, the straight-bladed weapon may also produce a crescentic wound.

(5) Haemorrhage: As the vessels are cut cleanly, the **haemorrhage is more.** If the artery is completely cut, the bleeding will be more due to its inability to contract or retract. Spurting of blood occurs if an artery is cut.

(6) Direction: Incised wounds are deeper at the beginning, because more pressure is exerted on the knife at this point. This is **known as the head of the wound.** Towards the end of the cut the wound becomes increasingly shallow, till finally as the knife leaves the tissues the skin alone is cut. This is known as the **tailing of the wound,** and indicates the direction in which the cut was made **Fig. (8–29)**.

(7) Bevelling cut: If the blade of weapon enters obliquely, the wound will have a beveled margin on one side with undermining (undercut) on the other side so that subcutaneous tissue is visible, indicating the direction from which the blade entered, and if the blade is nearly horizontal, a flap wound is caused. **Bevelling can be produced by sharp weapon only. It is usually homicidal** and may indicate the relative position of the assailant and the victim.

Age of Incised Wound: In an uncomplicated wound, healing occurs as follows: **Fresh:** Haematoma formation. **12 hours:** The edges are red, swollen and adherent with blood and lymph; leucocytic infiltration. **24 hours**: A continuous layer of endothelial cells covers the surface; overlying this a crust or scab of dried clot is seen. Scar tissue is formed in 1–2 weeks. A gaping wound heals by formation of granulation tissues after a variable period.

HISTOPATHOLOGY: Few minutes: Dilatation of capillaries and margination and emigration of neutrophils, reactive changes in the tissue histiocytes and swelling of the vascular endothelium. 12 hours: Reactive changes occur in the fibroblasts at the site of injury within few hours; monocytes appear in the exudate. Leucocytic infiltration is appreciable. 15 hours: Monocytes begin to undergo mitotic division. 24 hours: Epithelium begins to grow at the edges. Vascular buds begin to form. 72 hours: Neutrophils are largely replaced by macrophages. Vascularised granulation tissue is formed. 4 to 5 days: New fibrils are formed. Epithelial cell proliferation continues, forming a thickened layer. One week: Soft, reddish scar formation in small wounds. The above changes are considerably modified if infection of the wound occurs.

In healing by second intention, inflammatory reaction is more intense and much larger amounts of granulation tissue are formed resulting in greater mass of scar tissue.

WOUNDS BY GLASS: Wounds produced by glass are lacerated, but can resemble incised and stab wounds. If a sharp-pointed piece of glass enters by its point, the wound has a stab-like appearance. **Margins of the wound will almost always show tiny side cuts due to irregularities of the glass.** Particles of glass may be found in the wound **Fig. (8–19)**. Assault with broken glasses or bottles show multiple irregular incised-type wounds of variable depth and severity. Glass is almost invariably radio-opaque.

Medicolegal Importance: (1) They indicate the nature of weapon (sharp-edged). (2) The age of the injury can be determined. (3) They give an idea about the direction of the force. (4) Position and character of wounds may indicate mode of production, i.e., suicide, accident, homicide.

Features of self-inflicted wounds: (1) They are multiple and parallel or nearly so, in any one area. (2) They are uniform in depth and direction. (3) They are relatively minor. (4) The fatal wounds are present on several limited accessible areas of the body, such as front of the neck, wrists, groin, and occasionally on the back of legs or on chest. (5) They avoid vital and sensitive areas like eyes, lips, nose and ears. **(6) Hesitation marks or tentative cuts or trial wounds:** They are cuts which are multiple, small and superficial often involving only the skin and are seen at the beginning of the incised wound.

The sites of election of suicidal incised wounds are: throat, wrist and front of chest Table (8–4). When preliminary incisions are inflicted with some violence they may be few, but commonly they are superficial and multiple. The fatal incisions are usually made with great violence, and the large gaping wound produced by suicide should not be mistaken for homicidal wounds. **When a safety razor blade is used, unintentional cuts are found on the fingers,** where the blade has been gripped.

SUICIDAL incised wounds of extremities are usually found on the flexor surface of the wrists, outer side of the left arm, and forearm, the front and outer side of the thighs, and the front of the abdomen and chest Figs. (8–28, 8–30 to 8–32 and 8–34). Fatal incised wounds of the arms are almost always suicidal. Suicidal wounds of chest are usually on the left side and directed downwards and inwards. A wound caused by running on knife tends to be more horizontal in direction. A person who commits suicide usually exposes the portion of the body to be incised, e.g., he may open his collar before cutting his throat, or pull up his shirt before cutting his chest or abdomen. Usually the victim hyperextends the wrist before making the cut, which causes the radial artery to slip at the lower end of the radius, which escapes injury. Flexor tendons may be cut. Suicides usually do not injure the face.

Some mentally disordered persons may inflict hundreds of small wounds upon themselves. A knife, razor or broken glass may be used

Table (8–4). Difference between suicidal and homicidal cut-throat wounds Fig. (8–34)

	Trait	Suicidal wounds	Homicidal wounds
(1)	Situation:	Left side of the neck and passing across the front of the throat; rarely on both sides.	Usually on both sides.
(2)	Level:	High; above the thyroid cartilage.	Low; on or below the thyroid cartilage Fig. (8–48).
(3)	Direction:	Above downwards and from left to right in right–handed person. Sometimes horizontal cuts across the front of the neck are seen which do not show variation in depth at either end.	Transverse or from below upwards. If attacked from the right side of victim, the wound runs from left to right; if from behind, it may resemble suicidal wound.
(4)	Number of wounds:	Multiple, may be 20 to 30, superficial, parallel and merged with the main wound; rarely single.	Multiple, cross each other at a deep level; not repeated in depths of the main wound.
(5)	Edges :	Usually ragged due to overlapping of multiple superficial incisions.	Sharp and clean-cut; bevelling may be seen.
(6)	Hesitation cuts:	Present.	Absent.
(7)	Tailing :	Present.	Absent.
(8)	Severity:	Usually less severe. One wound may be extremely deep, extending up to cervical vertebrae, but sometimes 2 or 3.	More severe; all the tissues including the vertebrae may be cut.
(9)	Wounds in other parts of the body :	Often present across wrists, groin, thighs, ankles, or knees; and rarely on the back of neck.	No wounds on wrists, etc. but severe injuries usually on the head and neck.
(10)	Defence wounds:	Absent; unintentional cuts may be found on the fingers if a blade has been used.	Present.
(11)	Hands:	Weapon may be firmly grasped due to cadaveric spasm.	Fragments of clothing, hair, etc., may be grasped.
(12)	Weapon:	Usually present.	Usually absent.
(13)	Vessels:	As head is thrown back, carotid artery is drawn beneath sternomastoid and against the spine and usually escapes injury.	Jugular vein and carotid artery are likely to be cut.
(14)	Blood stains:	If standing, stains on the mirror and on front of body and clothes running from above downwards and splashes on feet.	If asleep, blood runs down on both sides of the neck and collects behind the neck and shoulder; stains found on both palms, for the victim attempts to cover the wound.
(15)	Clothes:	Not cut or damaged.	May be cut corresponding in position to those in the body; disarrangement, tears and loss of buttons.
(16)	Circumstantial evidence:	Quiet place, such as bedroom or locked bath-room; usually stands in front of a mirror in order to direct the hand better; suicidal note or farewell letter may be found.	Disturbance at the scene, such as disarrangement of furniture in a room; trampling and crushing of vegetable matter and shrubs, or confused foot prints outside.

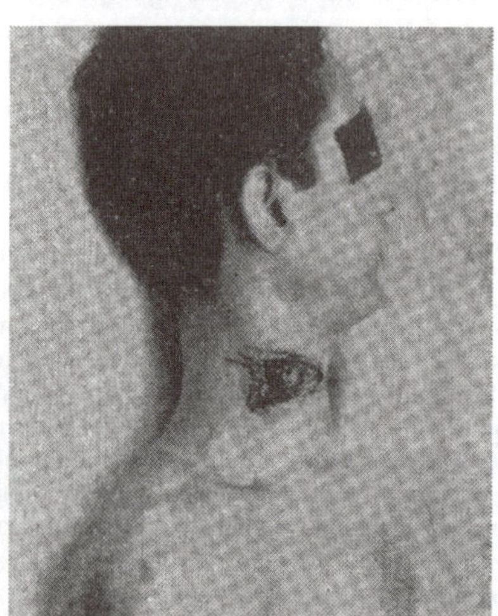

Fig. (8–34). Suicidal cut-throat with hesitation marks.

and a large number of cuts produced on the arms which may cross each other. Small stabs may be produced on the chest or temples. Paranoid schizophrenics with a strong religious flavour to their delusions may remove penis, scrotum, and testes. Ears and nose may be mutilated.

HOMICIDAL WOUNDS: They are usually multiple and can occur in any region of the body. Wounds of the chest are usually present over a wider area and are more horizontal. They may be directed from below upwards which is rarely seen in suicidal wounds. Incised wounds situated on the back, or in such a position as cannot be easily reached by a suicide, are homicidal. Incised wounds on nose, ears and genitals are usually homicidal, and are inflicted on account of jealousy or revenge in cases of adultery, causing disfiguration. Cut-throat wounds cause immediate death from haemorrhage, air embolism, or inhalation of effused blood into the respiratory tract Table (8–1).

ACCIDENTAL incised wounds are common usually in the home or workshop, and are of a minor nature. They may be caused by falling upon a sharp-cutting weapon held in the hand, or upon a sharp-pointed object or by a sharp piece of broken glass. They may be situated anywhere on the body, but are commonly seen about the hands.

In a decomposed body, it is difficult to differentiate a laceration from an incised wound. When a body with incised wounds, stab wounds, or lacerations is immersed in water soon after infliction of injuries, the blood in the wounds is lysed by water and passes into the water, and whether the injuries are antemortem or postmortem cannot be made out.

CHOP WOUNDS (Slash wounds): They are deep gaping wounds caused by a blow with the sharp-cutting edge of a fairly heavy weapon, like a hatchet, an axe, sword, broad heavy knife, chopper, saber, or meat cleaver. **The dimensions of the wound correspond to cross section of penetrating portion of the blade Figs. (8–2, 8–35 to 8–37).** The margins are sharp and may show slight abrasion and bruising with marked destruction of underlying organs. If the edge is blunt, the margins are ragged and bruised. **Undermining occurs in the direction towards which the chop is made.** When the whole blade strikes the body at the same time, the depth may be same throughout the wound. **Usually the lower end (heel) of the axe strikes the surface first, which produces a deeper wound than the upper (toe) end. The deeper end indicates the position of the assailant.** In the skull, the undermined edge of the fracture defect is the direction in which the force is exerted, and the slanted edge is the side from which the force was directed. In case of long bones, the bone fragments get loosened on the opposite side of the force. **With axe and heavy cutting weapons, the initial impact slices cleanly through the bone on one edge.** The rebound removal of the weapon is at a slightly different angle, either from deliberate intention or from relative movements between bone and blade. This cracks off an irregular fragment of bone of the opposite side so that the defect has one smooth and one rough edge particularly near the ends of the chop wound. If the extremities are attacked, there may be complete or incomplete amputation of the fingers or other bones, and the joints may be separated or disarticulated. Wounds on the head and trunk are usually associated with injuries to important structures and are fatal. The cranium may be depressed, but if the weapon strikes obliquely, a piece of the skull may be removed. If the chopping blow is tangential, a disk-shaped portion of bone or skin or soft tissue may be cut away. The neck may be almost completely separated.

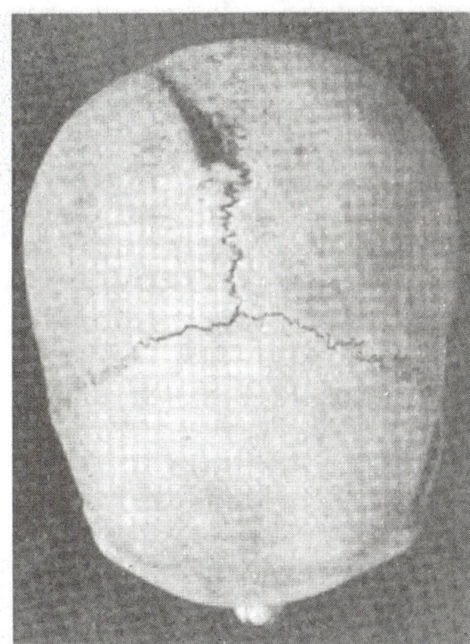

Fig. (8–37). Cut injury of the skull. The wide gap anteriorly is caused by the heel of the axe in a frontal attack.

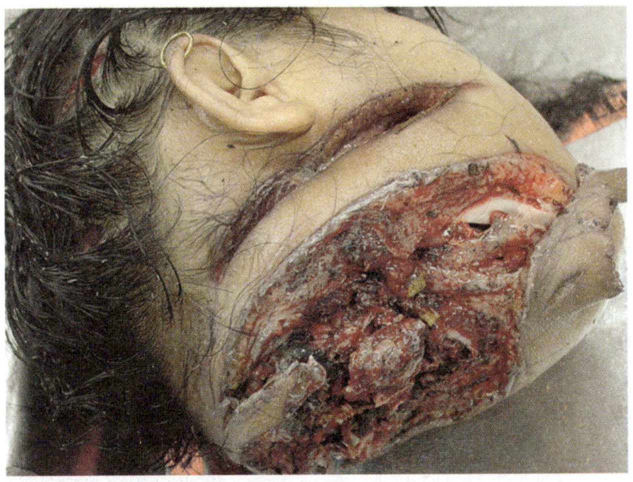

Fig. (8–35). Decapitation and above a chop wound.

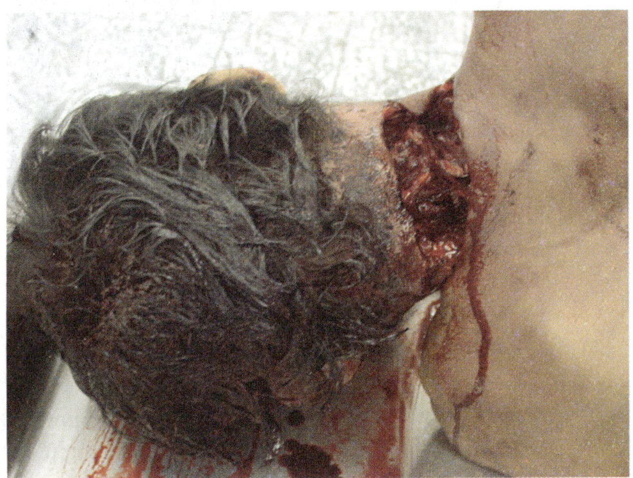

Fig. (8–36). Chop wound on back of neck.

Most of these injuries are homicidal and usually inflicted on the exposed parts of the body like the head, face, neck, shoulders and extremities. Accidental injuries are caused by power fans, band saws or ship or airplane propellers, which may lacerate the soft tissues extensively or amputate parts of the body. Suicidal chop injuries are very rare.

STAB OR PUNCTURED WOUNDS

A stab wound is produced when force is delivered along the long axis of a narrow or pointed object, such as knife, dagger, sword, chisel, scissors, nail, needle, spear, arrow, screw driver, etc. into the depths of the body Figs. (8–38 to 8–48). The wound is deeper than its length and width on the surface of skin Table (8–6). This can occur by driving the object into the body, or from the body's pressing or falling against the object. The most common stabbing instruments are kitchen knives, sheath knives or pen-knives.

Types: (1) **Puncture wounds** When soft tissues are involved. (2) **Penetrating wounds,** when they enter a cavity of body or a viscus. (3) **Perforating wounds** or through-and-through puncture wounds are produced when the weapon enters the body on one side and comes out from the other side. **The wound of entry is**

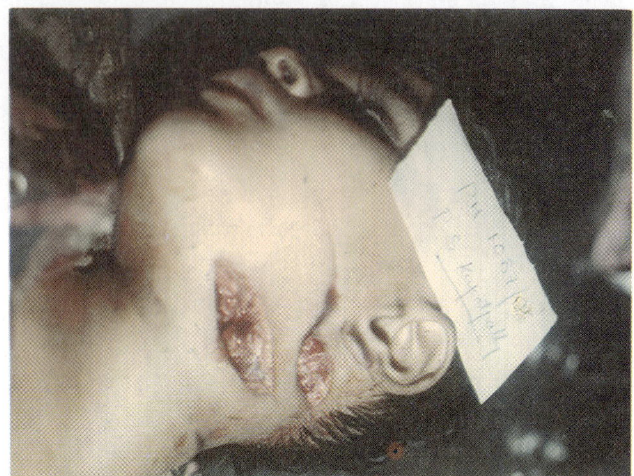

Fig. (8–38). **Stab wounds showing tailing.**

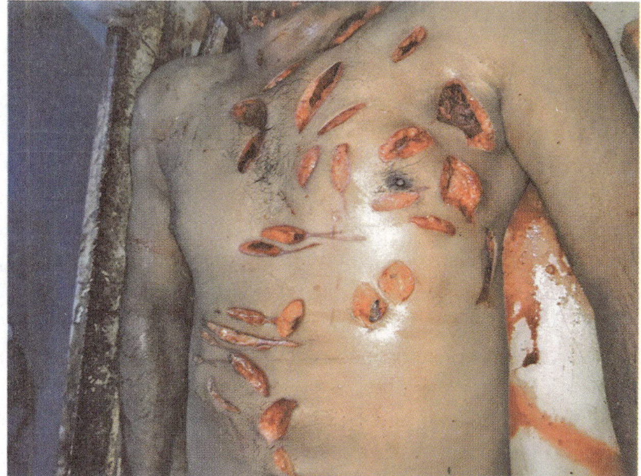

Fig. (8–39). **Homicidal stab wound on front of chest and abdomen some of them showing tailing.**

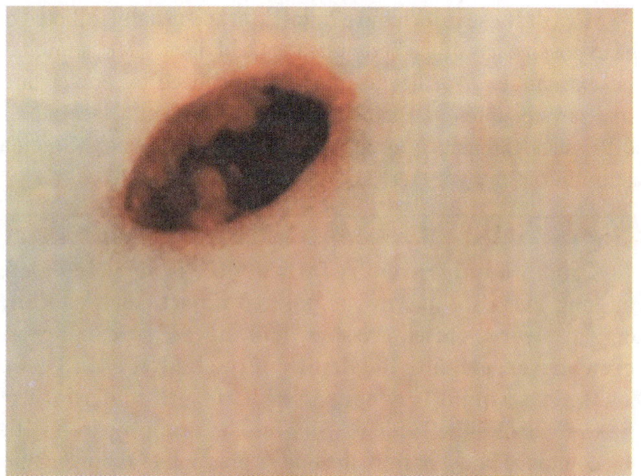

Fig. (8–40). **Stab wound showing gaping.**

larger with inverted edges, and the wound of exit is smaller with everted edges, due to tapering of blade. The victim of a fatal penetrating injury may not show signs and symptoms of injury until many hours have passed.

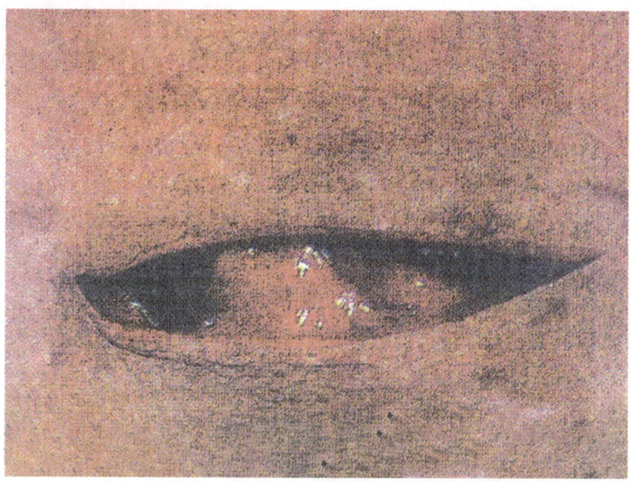

Fig. (8–41). **Stab wound with a single-edged weapon.**

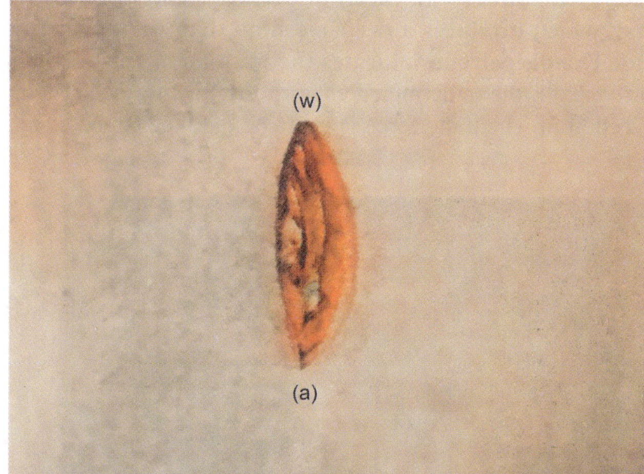

Fig. (8–42). **Stab wound with a single-edged weapon, one end acute (a) while other end is wedge shaped (w).**

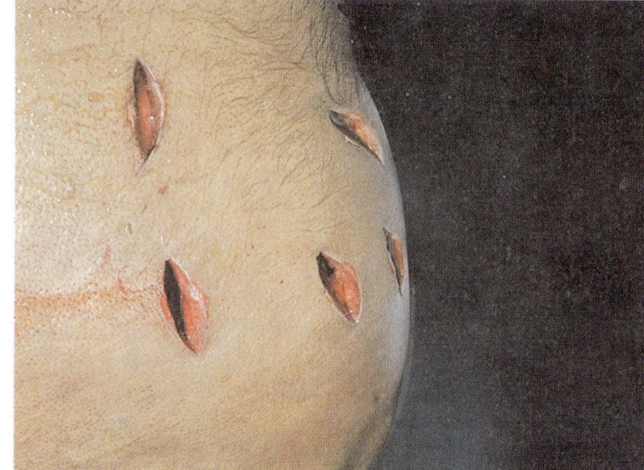

Fig. (8–43). **Stab wounds caused by double-edged weapon.**

Characters: (1) Margins: The edges of the wound are clean-cut and inverted Figs. (8–38 and 8–40). The margins can be everted when the wound is situated over the fatty area, such as protuberant abdomen or gluteal region. **There is usually no**

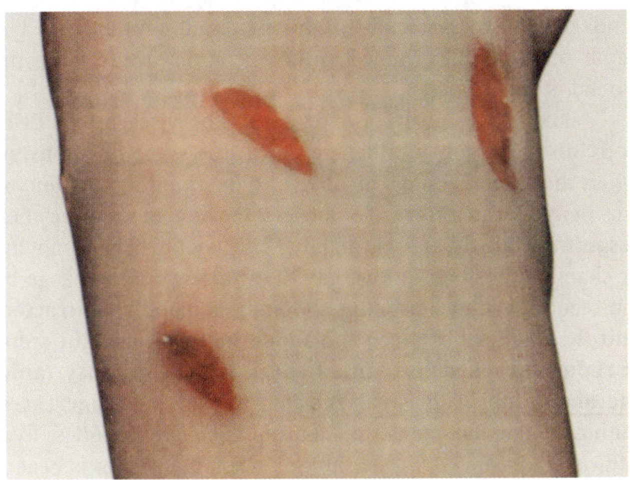

Fig. (8–44). **Multiple stab wound.**

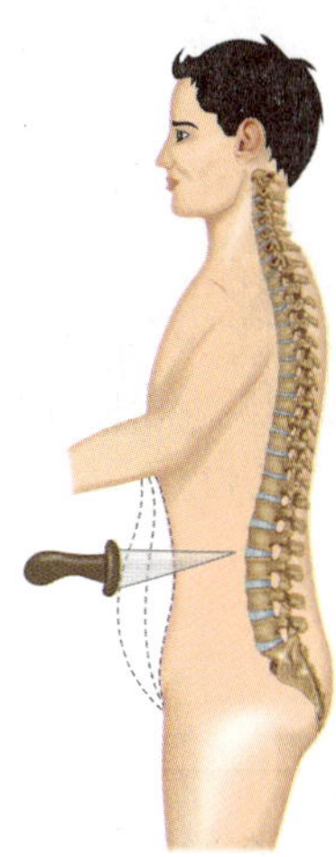

Fig. (8–45). **Assessment of depth of penetration of a stab wound.**

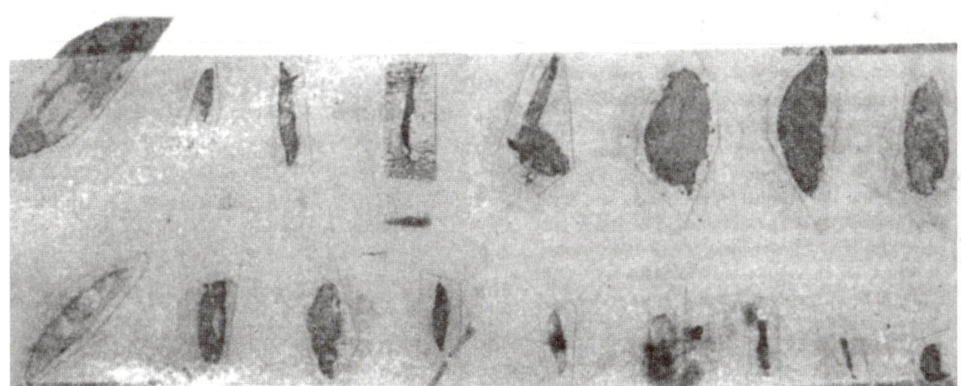

Fig. (8–46). **Appearances of stab wounds on the skin by different types of weapons.**

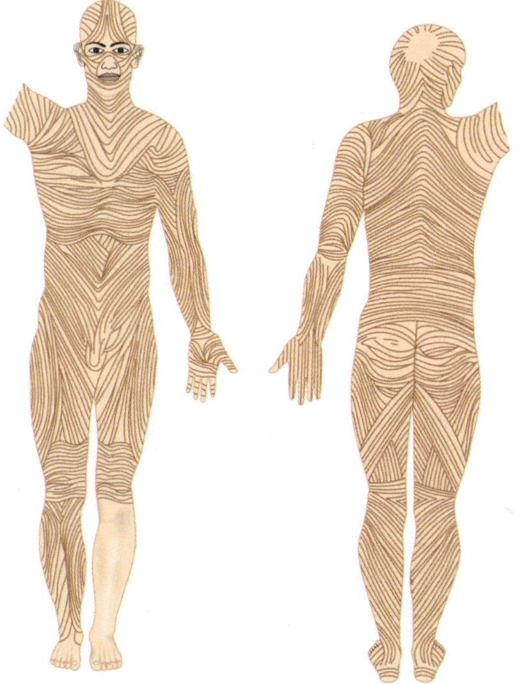

Fig. (8–47). **Cleavage lines of Langer.**

abrasion or bruising of the margins, but in full penetration of the blade, abrasion and bruising (hilt mark) may be produced by the hilt-guard (metal piece between the blade and handle) striking the skin. The margins may be abraded and ragged if the cutting edge is blunt. The mark will be symmetrical, if the knife strikes the skin at right angle. If the knife strikes in a downward angle, the mark will be prominent above the stab wound, and if the knife strikes in an upward angle, the abrasion will be below the stab wound. **In oblique stab wounds, a knife striking from the right will have an abrasion on the right side and vice versa.** In such cases, the suspected knife should be examined to determine the compatibility of the shape of the abrasion around the stab wound, with the handle of the knife in question.

(2) Length: **The length of the wound is slightly less than the width of the weapon up to which it has been driven in, because of stretching of the skin** Fig. (8–45). **For measuring the length of stab wound, the edges of the wound should be brought together.** Deliberate lateral, forward, or backward movement of the weapon during its withdrawal from the body tends to widen the wound, and the length will be more than the maximum width of the blade. **If the instrument is thrust in, and is then completely withdrawn with the cutting edge dragging against one end, the wound would be extended superficially, producing a tail.**

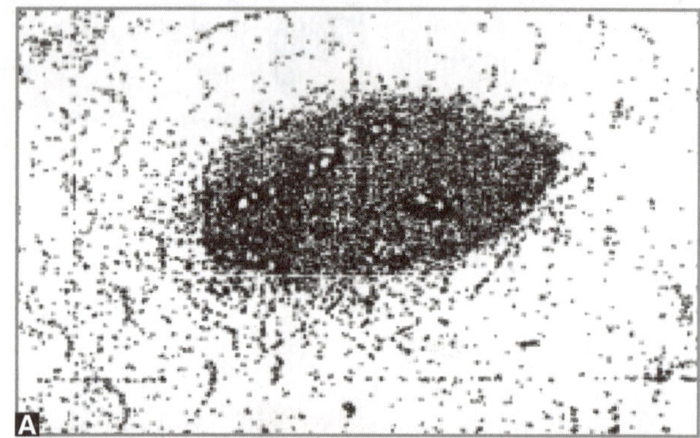

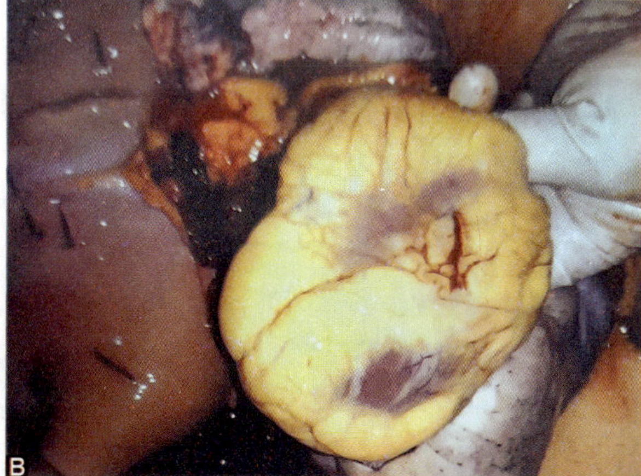

Fig. (8–48). (A) Boat-shaped stab wound produced by a single-edged blade. (B) Stab injuries over heart and liver.

(3) Width: By examining multiple stab wounds in the body, the length and width of the knife blade can be determined approximately. In most cases, the wound gapes across the centre, to form a long ellipse. **The maximum possible width of the knife blade can be approximately determined if the edges of a gaping wound are brought together.** Elasticity or laxness of the skin can change the width by one to two millimetres. **A stab wound inflicted when the skin is stretched will be long and thin, which becomes shorter and broader when the skin is relaxed.** The opening may be enlarged by backward, forward or a lateral movement of the weapon.

(4) Depth: The depth (length of track) is greater than the width and length of the external injury Fig. (8–45). It is not safe to find out the depth of a stab wound by introducing a probe, because it may disturb a loose clot and may lead to fatal haemorrhage, or cause serious damage and may produce multiple false wound tracks. **The depth of a stab wound is usually equal to, or less than the length of the blade that was used in producing it, but on yielding surfaces like the anterior abdominal wall, the depth of the wound may be greater, because the force of the thrust may press the tissues underneath.** In young persons, the chest is mobile and may be compressed during the stabbing. The breast, buttocks and thigh are indented by a full thrust, and the depth of wound may exceed the length of the weapon. Expansion and retraction of the chest during breathing must also be considered. **Many of the internal organs are not fixed but have a variable degree of mobility.** This should be taken into account when estimating the depth of the wounds. **After the withdrawal of the weapon, the wound tends to close by expansion of the tissues along the track.** The depth should be determined in the operation theatre when the wound is repaired.

Variations in position of viscera: The viscera of a dead body on the autopsy table are not in the same positions, as when the same person was alive and in standing position, or was bent over in a state of emotional tension, at the time of an assault. During fight, fright and flight, the victim may be moving or changing position in a variety of postures, which change by the second. **When tense, the abdomen is usually contracted, and the distance between the abdominal wall and the spine is reduced. When the same body is on the autopsy table, the abdominal wall is relaxed and this distance increases.** Similarly, the anatomical relationship between the lungs, liver and other viscera is not the same as when the person is bent at the hips and when lying flat. In a stab wound on the anterior wall of the chest, the postmortem depth is greater than it was during life, because of the collapse of the lung. If the stab is on the back of the chest, the depth of the wound will be less, as the lungs will collapse posteriorly (Fig. 5–8, autopsy chapter).

The force required to inflict stab wound: It is subjective, and can only be stated in comparative terms, such as slight force, moderate force, considerable force, and extreme force. **The depth of stab depends on:** (1) **Condition of the knife: The sharpness of the extreme tip of the knife is the most important factor in skin penetration.** Once the tip has perforated the skin, the cutting edge is of little importance, and the rest of the blade will pass into the body with ease, without any further force being applied unless obstructed by bone or cartilage. **A thin, slender, double-edged knife will penetrate more deeply than an equally sharp, wide, single-edged blade inserted with the same force. A blunt-pointed** instrument requires considerable force to puncture the skin and penetrate the soft tissues. **(2) The resistance offered by the tissues or organs: Apart from bone and calcified cartilage, the skin followed by muscle is most resistant to knife penetration.** Uncalcified cartilage is easily penetrated by a sharp knife, though more force is required. Forcible stab from a strong, sharp knife can penetrate rib, sternum or skull. **(3) Clothing:** The amount of clothing and its composition, e.g., multiple layers of tough cloth, leather belts, thick leather jackets, or coats, etc. require greater force. (4) The speed of thrust of the knife. (5) **Stretched skin is easier to penetrate than lax skin,** e.g., chest wall. (6) **When the knife strikes the skin at right angle, it usually penetrates more deeply** than when it strikes from some acute angle. (7) When the knife penetrates the skin rapidly, e.g., if the body falls or runs on to the blade, **the momentum of the forward moving body is sufficient to cause fatal injury.** However, the knife must be sharp-pointed and held firmly so as to penetrate easily, as a blunt knife held loosely will be turned aside by the approaching body. If the tip of knife has been turned by striking bone, it will tend to pull tissue out through the external wound, as it is being withdrawn, especially in abdominal injuries where omentum may be found protruding through the wound.

Track of stab wound: A piece of pliable tubing may be introduced gently, and if it goes in easily may reveal the true track. Later, the tubing can be made more rigid and straight by inserting a probe into it. **Dissection in the tissues parallel to, but away from the wound, will reveal the track.** Radio-opaque

Table (8–5). Difference between suicidal, homicidal and accidental stab wounds

Trait	Suicidal wounds	Homicidal wounds	Accidental wounds
(1) Number:	Often single.	Frequently multiple.	Usually single.
(2) Site:	Accessible precordial area or upper abdomen.	May be anywhere.	May be anywhere.
(3) Tentative wounds:	May be present around site of fatal wound.	May be present rarely but away from fatal wound.	Absent.
(4) Clothing:	Removed from injured area.	Normally not disturbed.	Not disturbed.
(5) Defence wounds:	Absent.	Often present.	Absent.

Table (8–6). Difference between incised, lacerated and stab wounds

Trait	Incised wound	Lacerated wound	Stab wound
(1) Manner of production:	By sharp objects or weapons.	By blunt objects or weapons.	By pointed sharp or blunt weapons.
(2) Site:	Anywhere.	Usually over bony prominences.	Anywhere; usually chest and abdomen.
(3) Margins:	Smooth, even, clean-cut and everted.	Irregular and often undermined.	Clean-cut, parallel edges. Lacerated if weapon is blunt-pointed.
(4) Abrasion on edges:	Absent.	Usually present.	Absent.
(5) Bruising:	No adjacent bruising of soft tissues.	Bruising of surrounding and underlying tissues.	Rare.
(6) Shape:	Linear or spindle-shaped.	Varies; usually irregular.	Linear or irregular.
(7) Dimensions:	Usually longer than deep; often gaping.	Usually longer than deep.	Depth greater than length and breadth.
(8) Depth of wound:	Structures cleanly cut to the depth of wound.	Small strands of tissue at the bottom bridge across margins.	Structures cleanly cut.
(9) Haemorrhage:	Usually profuse and external. Spurting of blood may be seen.	Slight except scalp and external.	Varies; usually internal.
(10) Hair bulbs:	Cleanly cut.	Crushed or torn.	Usually clean cut.
(11) Bones:	May be cut.	May be fractured.	May be punctured.
(12) Foreign bodies:	Absent.	Usually present.	Usually absent.
(13) Clothes:	May be cut.	May be torn.	May be cut.

material or dyes can be injected into stab wound to demonstrate the wound track by X-rays.

Rarely, a single stab may produce multiple skin wounds: (a) a tangential stab of the arm, which passes through superficial tissues and then re-enters the chest wall, (b) a knife passing through the edge of a sagging female breast re-entering thorax.

(5) Shape: The size and shape of a stab wound in the skin is **dependent on the type of implement, cutting surface, sharpness, width and shape of the weapon, body region stabbed, the depth of insertion, the angle of withdrawal, the direction of thrust,** the movement of the blade in the wound, cleavage direction, the movement of the person stabbed, and the condition of tension or relaxation of the skin.

Cleavage lines of Langer: Stab wounds and incised wounds are slit-shaped with two acute angles, or gape open depending on their location and their orientation, with regard to the so-called **cleavage lines of Langer Fig. (8–47). The pattern of fibre arrangement of the dense feltwork of intimately intermingled dermal collagen and elastic fibres is called the cleavage direction or lines of cleavage of the skin, and their linear representation on the skin are called Langer's lines, which is almost same in all persons.** Cleavage lines in the dermal layers of skin are mostly arranged in parallel rows. In the extremities they tend to run longitudinally; in the neck and trunk circumferentially. **A stab wound which runs parallel to the cleavage lines will remain slit-shaped and narrow** and the dimensions of the blade will be represented with considerable accuracy. **A stab wound which cuts through the cleavage lines transversely will gape.** If the knife is inserted in an oblique plane, the skin defect is wider and the wound may gape asymmetrically and assume a semicircular or crescentic shape. **To ascertain the shape of the instrument, the edges of a wound may be manually approximated with slight twisting or they may be held together with a transparent adhesive tape.** The resulting slit is considerably longer than the original oval-shaped wound. This will counter the claim of the defence that the suggested knife could not have produced a stab wound of the type as seen before reconstruction. The dimensions of the gaping wound are not useful to assess the shape of the blade.

Weapons causing stab wounds: The shape of the wound usually corresponds to the weapon used, but the shape of the

wounds made by the same weapon may differ on different parts of the body Fig. (8–46). (1) If a single-edged weapon is used, the surface wound will be triangular or wedge-shaped, and one angle of the wound will be sharp, the other rounded, blunt or squared off. Blunt end of the wound may have small splits in the skin at each end of the corner, so-called **"fishtailing"**, if the back edge of the blade is stout. Some stab wounds caused by single-edged weapon have bilateral pointed ends like those due to double-edged weapons. This is due to: (a) The initial penetration by the knife point to a depth of about one cm., first produces a dermal defect with sharp angles at each end. As the knife penetrates more deeply, the end in contact with the cutting edge of the blade continues to be sharply angulated. The opposite end which is in contact with non-cutting surface of the knife, also remains sharply angulated because the dull surface does not imprint its shape to the skin defect. It merely causes further separation of the skin which continues to be torn along the course of its original direction. (b) The knife penetrating the skin at an oblique angle. As the knife perforates, it is pulled down with the cutting-edge cutting through the skin, and the blunt surface of the back of the knife does not impart its shape to the skin defect, as it does not contact it. (c) Many single-edged knives have a cutting edge on both sides at the tip. The initial thrust into the skin will produce a double-pointed wound, and as the blade passes through the skin, if it is pulled down slightly, the blunt back portion of the knife will not come in contact with the skin. The serosal planes and muscle fasciae (pleural surface, liver capsule and the pericardial sac) often clearly show the wedge-like shape of a knife. Leather and certain synthetics maintain the shape of a cut. **In some single-edged knives, both ends are blunt. This is caused if the knife penetrates to full length up to the guard, because of ricasso** (short, unsharpened section of blade between the cutting edge and guard). **By examination of a single wound, it is not possible to say, whether it was caused by a single-edged or double-edged weapon. If multiple stabs are produced by a single-edged weapon, examination of all the stab wounds will reveal the single-edged nature of the weapon.** (2) If a double-edged weapon is used, the wound will be elliptical or slit-like and both angles will be sharp or pointed coming to a fine "V" point Fig. (8–50). If the knife penetrates to full length up to the guard, one or both edges may be blunt because of ricasso. (3) **A round object** like the spear may produce a circular wound. (4) **A round blunt-pointed object,** such as a pointed stick, or metal rod may produce a circular surface wound with inverted ragged and bruised edges. Foreign material, such as dirt, rust or splinters may be found in the wound. The blunter the tip of the object, the coarser or more stellate will be the hole it makes. (5) **A pointed square weapon** may produce a cross-shaped injury, each of the 4 edges tearing its way through the tissues. (6) A fall on a pointed article, e.g., pieces of broken glass, will produce a wound with irregular and bruised margins, and fragments of glass may be found embedded in the soft tissues. (7) Stab wounds inflicted with a **broken bottle,** appear as clusters of wounds of different sizes, shapes, and depth, with irregular margins, and varying depth. (8) Stabbing with a **fork** produces clusters of 2 or 3 wounds, depending upon the number of prongs on the fork. (9) **A screwdriver** will produce a slit-like stab wound with squared ends (rectangular) and abraded margins. (10) A stab

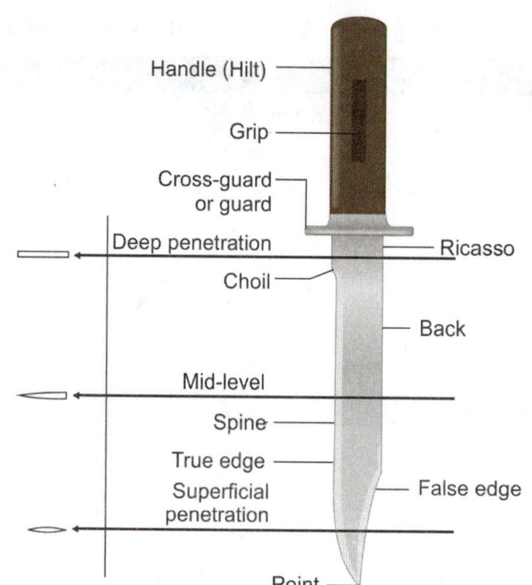

Fig. (8–49). Knife with clip-pointed blade. Differing skin wounds produced by same knife, at three different depths of penetration.

Fig. (8–50). Spear-pointed blade.

wound through a crease or fold in the skin, such as through a sagging abdomen or female breast, crease of the armpit or groin near the scrotum are likely to result in an atypical injury. (11) Thick relatively blunt-edged blades, e.g., bayonets, may produce cross-shaped stab wounds, because cutting and tearing of the skin occurs simultaneously and at right angles to each other. When a knife is twisted as it is withdrawn from the tissues, the external wound may have a cruciate appearance. (12) Ice-picks or similar instruments produce stab wounds, resembling small caliber bullet wounds. (13) **Irregularly-shaped stab wounds** such as L or V-shaped may be mistaken to be produced by two distinct stabbings in the same location. These atypical injuries are produced by stabbing, followed by simultaneous twisting and cutting (rocking), or the victim moving relative to the knife, or by a combination of the two. There will be a primary stab wound with an extension of it, due to the knife edge cutting the skin in a different direction as it exits. Small notches in margins of the skin defects or curving can be produced by the same mechanism. A great number of possibilities capable of causing atypically shaped stab wounds exist, the interpretation of which are usually difficult. (14) If the scissors is closed, the tip of the scissors splits rather than cuts the skin, producing a linear stab wound with abraded margins. Deep penetration will produce 'Z'-shaped wound. If the screw holding the two blades is projecting, there are small lateral splits in the wound centre. If the two blades of the scissors are separated, each thrust will produce two triangular stab wounds. (15) A knife with a serrated back edge will produce a stab wound, the back edge of which may be torn or ragged. If the knife enters obliquely, serrated abrasions may be seen on the skin adjacent to the end of the wound. (16) Target arrows have pointed conical ends which produce circular wounds. Hunting arrows have 2 to 5 knife-like edges which produce cross-like or X-shaped wounds with the 4 edged arrow head. The margins of the wound are incised-like, without abrasions.

(6) Direction: When the knife penetrates at an angle, the wound will have a bevelled margin on one side with undermining (undercut), so that subcutaneous tissue is visible, indicating the direction from which the knife entered. In solid organs like the liver, the track made by the weapon is better seen. **The principal direction should be noted first and other next,** e.g., backwards and to the right. If the weapon is partially withdrawn and thrust again in a new direction, two or more punctures are seen in the soft parts with only one external wound. **If the wound is perforating, it should be described in sequential order: the wound of the entrance, the path of the wound track, and the wound of exit.** If the wound is penetrating, the wound of entrance should be described first, then the depth and direction of wound track, and specific termination.

Complications: (1) External haemorrhage is slight but there may be marked internal haemorrhage or injuries to internal organs. (2) The wound may get infected due to the foreign material carried into the wound. (3) Air embolism may occur in a stab wound on the neck which penetrates jugular veins. Air is sucked into the vessels due to the negative pressure. (4) Pneumothorax. (5) Asphyxia due to inhalation of blood.

Concealed Puncture Wounds: These are puncture wounds caused **on concealed parts of the body, such as nostrils, fontanella, fornix of the upper eyelids, axilla, vagina, rectum, and nape of the neck.** Fatal penetrating injuries can be caused without leaving any readily visible external marks, e.g., thrusting a needle or pin into the brain through the fontanelles, through the inner canthus of the eye, or into the medulla through the nape of the neck. These injuries may not be detected unless searched carefully.

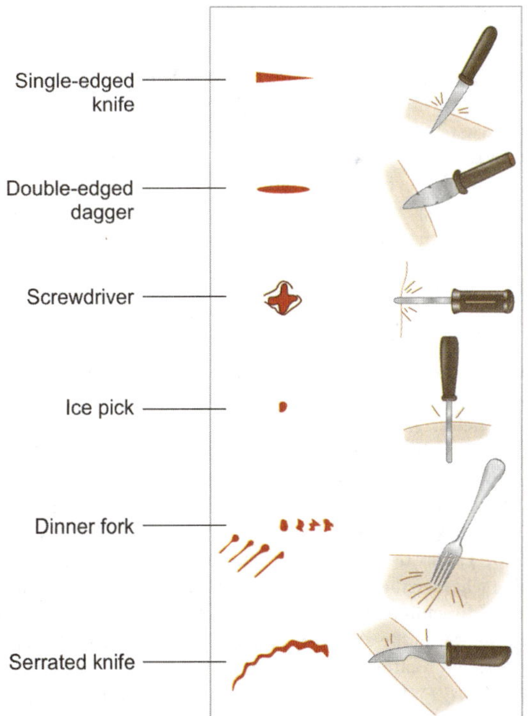

Fig. (8–51). Skin wounds produced by different weapons.

Examination: The following points should be noted : (1) Identification and labelling of cuts and damage to clothing. (2) Distribution of blood stains. (3) Removal of clothing, layer by layer. (4) Identification and labelling of wounds. (5) Wounds: (a) Position (height from heels), (b) location (measurements from fixed anatomical landmarks), (c) description including margins, size, shape, ends, extension, (d) direction, (e) depth, (f) trauma to viscera, (g) estimation of force required, (h) foreign bodies. **To indicate the general character of the instrument which inflicted the stab wound, the term "incised' or 'lacerated' should be included in the description of the stab wound, e.g., 'incised-stab wound', 'lacerated-stab wound', etc.** Probes should not be thrust into deeper tissues before examination of thoracic and abdominal organs *in situ.* **Organs should not be removed until they are examined *in situ* for injuries associated with the wound track.** To examine the length of the wound track, probe should be inserted through the skin and wound track through the injured organs and tissues to the track's termination before evisceration. The relationship between the wound and weapon can be established by the shape, width, length, and presence of blood on the weapon.

If the knife is found embedded in the body, the thumb and index finger should grasp the sides of the handle immediately adjacent to the skin to remove it, to preserve fingerprints of assailant on the handle of weapon. **When multiple stab wounds are present, they should be numbered and photographed.** A sketch or a printed body diagram should be used. When clubbing several wounds in one particular region use the words. "multiple incised/stab wounds" with minimum and maximum dimensions.

Incised-stab wound: Incised-stab wound is a wound, which starts as an incised wound and ends as a stab wound by the sudden thrust of the blade into the body, **or starts as a stab wound and becomes incised wound** as the knife is pulled out of the body at a shallow angle to the skin surface producing an incised wound. If a nick or a pork-shaped cut is present at the end of the stab wound opposite to the incised portion, then the wound has started as an incised wound and ended as a stab wound. If the fork is at the end of the stab wound where the incised wound arises, then the wound has started as a stab wound.

AN EXAMPLE OF DESCRIPTION OF STAB WOUND: Stab wound, wedge-shaped on the right upper chest, placed obliquely, with the inner end lower than the upper outer end. Length was 3 cm. The maximum width at the centre was 4 mm. The centre of the wound was just below the line joining the nipples, being 6 cm. from the midline, 6 cm. from the right nipple, and 18 cm. below right collar bone. The inner end was sharp and outer blunt. The lower margin was undermined. A track is established on the right anterior thoracic wall, passes through the fifth interspace, through upper lobe of right lung to a depth of 8 cm. A right haemothorax of 300 ml. of fluid and clotted blood is present.

The external and internal appearances of a stab wound help to give an opinion upon: (1) dimensions of the weapon, (2) the type of weapon, (3) the taper of the blade, (4) movement of the knife in the wound, (5) the depth of the wound, (6) the direction of the stab, and (7) the amount of force used.

Examination of the Weapon: The doctor should note: (1) the length, width and thickness of the blade, (2) whether single-edged or double-edged, (3) the degree of taper from hilt to tip,

(4) the nature of the back edge in a single-edged weapon, e.g., squared-off, serrated, etc., (5) the face of the hilt guard adjacent to the blade, (6) any grooving, serration or forking of the blade, and (7) sharpness of the extreme tip of the blade and the cutting edge.

The weapon should be sent to laboratory for finger prints and trace evidence. Preserve blood for comparison with blood on the suspected weapon.

Absence of blood stains on knife: **In some cases of stabbing, the blade of the knife may not be bloodstained.** (1) In solid organs, bleeding occurs only after the knife is withdrawn, because bleeding is prevented by the pressure of the knife. During the withdrawal of the knife, the muscular and elastic tissue of the solid organs, and the elastic tissue of the skin may contract about the knife, wiping off the blood present on the knife blade. In such cases, analysis of wiping of the blade might still yield sufficient tissue to perform at least limited DNA analysis and typing. (2) The clothing if present, may also wipe off the blood. **(3) An injury may cause deep shock and severe circulatory collapse. Subsequently, even if a deeply penetrating wound is produced, there may be little bleeding. (4) When a victim is stabbed multiple times and bleeds heavily, the last stab wound inflicted may appear bloodless.** This causes difficulty in deciding whether this wound was inflicted before, during, or soon after death.

Some injuries cannot be divided clearly into stab or incised wounds, but may exhibit features of both.

Medicolegal Importance: (1) The shape of the wound may indicate the class and type of the weapon which may have caused the injury. (2) The depth of the wound will indicate the force of penetration. (3) Direction and dimensions of the wound indicate the relative positions of the assailant and the victim. (4) The age of the injury can be determined. (5) Position, number and direction of wounds may indicate manner of production, i.e., suicide, accident, or homicide. (6) If a broken fragment of weapon is found, it will identify the weapon or will connect an accused person with the crime.

Autopsy: Clothes Examine clothes while still on body and its relation to injuries on the body. Sketches/photographs should be taken. Cuts in clothes should be measured and described. Describe blood stains on clothes site, size, shape, direction, margins, etc. of injuries should be described. Length of injury should be measured with and without edge opposition. Distance of injuries from heel level should be measured. Hair and blood samples should be retained.

Internal: Dissection of tissues layer by layer parallel to, but away from the wound will reveal the track. Measure blood in the cavities.

CIRCUMSTANCES OF INJURIES: SUICIDE **Suicidal stab wounds are found over accessible areas of the body. The common site is the chest over the heart region. The direction of the wound is upwards, backwards and to the right. The depth is variable, some are superficial and others enter the pericardium or heart. The suicide may not withdraw the point of the weapon from the skin, and stab himself repeatedly in different directions through the same skin wound. Rarely one stroke is fatal, and the knife may be found sticking in the wound. In many cases, even multiple stabs do not cause death and the person may resort to other methods which present a puzzling picture. Stab wounds of the head are rare. Usually, a number of stabs extending only to the bone are seen in the temporal region. Suicidal stab wounds of the spine, abdomen, neck and extremities are rare. In suicide, there are no corresponding cuts or rents on clothings on part of the body which is normally covered by clothes, as a person who commits suicide exposes his body by opening his clothes and then inflicts wounds. In some suicides, the victim may be able to conceal the weapon.**

Common methods of suicide are: poisoning, hanging, burning, drowning, jumping from a height, stabbing and cutting and railway injuries.

HARA-KIRI: It is an unusual type of suicide, in which the **victim inflicts a single large wound on the abdomen with a short sword, while in a sitting position or falls forward upon a ceremonial sword and pulls out intestines.** To produce impalement on to a knife, there should be enough momentum by the victim moving toward the knife and it would need to be fixed firmly in some way. The sudden evisceration of the internal organs causes a sudden decrease of intra-abdominal pressure and cardiac return, producing sudden cardiac collapse.

HOMICIDE: Most deaths from stab wounds are homicidal, especially if found in an inaccessible area. The wounds are multiple, widely scattered and deeply penetrating, involving the chest and abdomen. In case of a sudden surprise attack, a single wound is found at a vital spot. If there is a struggle, there may be a number of wounds, sometimes associated with defence cuts on the hands. In a few cases, a number of wounds may be found in a localised area, almost of the same depth. These occur when the assailant threatens the victim, who is held by another assailant. These wounds are usually seen on the face or neck, and may be far away from the fatal injury. Homicidal stab wounds of the chest may have any direction, but the common direction is at an angle from left to right and from above downwards. Fatal stab wounds of right chest usually injure right ventricle, aorta or right atrium. Stab wounds of the left chest usually involve the right ventricle when parasternal, and left ventricle as the stab wounds become more lateral and inferior. Severing of the left anterior descending coronary artery is rapidly fatal. Most stab wounds of the heart and lungs occur over the front of the chest, rarely the sides, and least on the back. Stab wounds of the lower chest can injure the heart and lungs and also abdominal viscera. In OVERKILL HOMICIDE, assailant continues stabbing beyond the victim's death. When a knife is thrown at a person, the skin resistance will cause significant loss of its kinetic energy and the stab may not be deep because of further resistance of the internal tissues. Postmortem stab wounds do not show bruising and are often yellow, or tan, due to absence of tissue perfusion, parchmented and sharply defined.

ACCIDENT: Accidental wounds are rare. They are caused by falling against projecting sharp objects like glass, nails, etc., or a person may be gored by the horns of a bull, buffalo, etc. An upward or downward track is quite inconsistent with an accidental stab wound. Impaling injuries are very rare and caused when a person falls or jumps from a building and lands on a fence or ornamental railings at play or mechanical catastrophe at work. When the knife penetrates the skin rapidly, e.g., if the body falls or runs on to the blade, the knife does not need to be held rigidly in order to prevent it being pushed backwards. Its inertia, if the tip is sharp, is quite sufficient to hold it in place. A moving sharp object striking the person may produce a stab wound. In accidental stabbing, the weapon should be anchored or held firmly.

ACCIDENTAL, SELF-INFLICTED OR INFLICTED BY OTHERS, Tables (8–5 and 8–7): The following factors are helpful to determine whether the wounds are suicidal, accidental or homicidal. (1) The nature, direction, extent and situation of the wounds. (2) The presence of foreign matter in the wound or adherent to the margins. (3) The nature of the suspected weapon or instrument. (4) Scene of the crime.

DEFENCE WOUNDS: Defence wounds result due to the immediate and instinctive reaction of the victim to save himself Figs. (8–33, 8–52 and 8–53).

Table (8–7). Differences between suicidal, homicidal and accidental wounds

	Trait	Suicide	Homicide	Accident
(1)	Nature of wounds:	Usually incised and stab.	Usually chop wounds, lacerations and stab.	Usually lacerations, abrasions and contusions.
(2)	Number of wounds:	Multiple.	Multiple.	Usually single, may be multiple.
(3)	Target area:	Accessible parts only, i.e., front and sides of the body, such as neck, wrists, left side of chest, groin, etc.	No fixed site; vital parts, such as head, chest, abdomen.	Anywhere; usually on exposed parts and bony prominences. Number of wounds on the same side.
(4)	Wound grouping:	Arranged.	Irregular.	Vulnerable parts.
(5)	Direction:	In right-handed persons from left to right and from above downwards.	Any direction.	Any direction.
(6)	Severity:	Mostly superficial; one or two deep wounds.	Mostly severe and extensive.	Variable severity.
(7)	Hesitation marks:	Usually present.	Absent.	Absent.
(8)	Defence wounds:	Absent.	May be present.	Absent.
(9)	Secondary injuries:	Absent.	May be connected with fight.	May be associated with accident.
(10)	Weapon:	By the side of the body or may be grasped firmly due to cadaveric spasm.	Absent.	Present.
(11)	Clothes:	Not damaged as they are usually removed.	May be damaged.	May be damaged and stained with oil, grease, mud, dirt, etc.
(12)	Scene of crime:	Usually inside closed room; no disturbances of surroundings.	Disturbed and disorderly with signs of struggle and blood stains.	Varies with the nature of the accident.
(13)	Motive:	Present, such as domestic worries, disappointment in love, chronic disease, failure in examination, etc.	Revenge, robbery, sexual offences.	Absent.

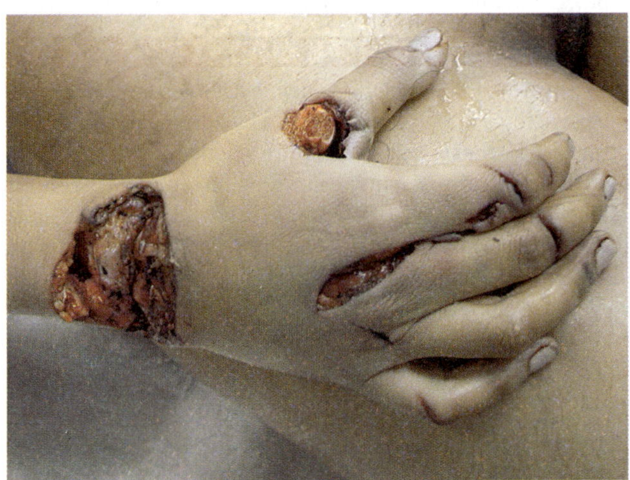

Fig. (8–52). Defence wounds on fingers and wrist.

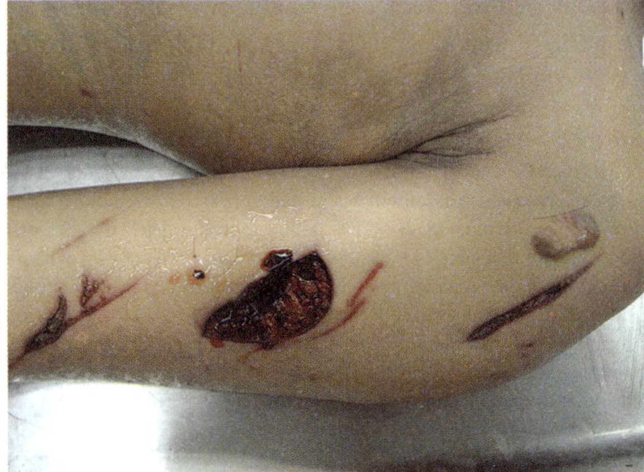

Fig. (8–53). Defence wounds on shoulder and upper arm.

Types: (1) Active defense wounds are caused when the victim tries to grasp the weapon. (2) Passive defence wounds are caused when the victim raises the hands, arms or legs.

Active: If the weapon is sharp, the injuries will depend upon the type of attack, whether stabbing or cutting. In stabbing with a single-edged weapon, if the weapon is grasped, a single cut is produced on the palm of the hand or on the bends of the fingers or thumb. If the weapon is double-edged, cuts are produced both on the palm and fingers. The cuts are usually irregular and ragged, because the skin tension is loosened by gripping of the knife. A typical knife defence wound may be seen in the web between the base of the thumb and index finger, when the blade is grasped.

Passive: When attacked with blunt object or fists most persons will attempt to protect their eyes, head and neck by raising their arms, flexing their elbows and covering the head and neck, or try to grasp the weapon. As a result bruises and abrasions are produced on the extensor or ulnar surfaces of the forearms, wrists, backs of the hands, knuckles and lateral/posterior aspects of the upper arms. Fractures of the carpal bones, metacarpals and digits may occur. Defence wounds may be found rarely on the shins and feet if the victim was lying on the ground usually face up, as he kicks at the assailant. The arms and posterior aspects of lower limbs and back may be injured as the victim curls into a ball with flexion of spine, knees and hips to protect the anterior part of the body and genitals. The leg may be brought across the other or the thigh raised, due to which outer side may receive blows and kicks. When attacked, with a sharp weapon, the victim usually holds up the hand or forearm and receives cuts on the hand, wrist, ulnar border of the forearm and on the fingers. They are often irregular in depth and distribution, markedly shelved with loose flaps of skin and copious bleeding. Defence wounds indicate homicide. In the female, they suggest sexual assault. **Defence wounds are absent** if the victim is unconscious, or is taken by surprise, or attacked from the back, or under the influence of alcohol or drugs. Defence wounds also occur in firearm injuries, where an arm is raised in an attempt to shield the trunk or head.

Offensive Manual Injuries: Abrasions and contusions over the knuckles can be sustained due to offensive efforts by the victim, or by his defensive efforts. Ragged knuckle lacerations on the victim indicate that his fist struck the assailant's anterior teeth when he struck a blow on the latter's open mouth. Fractures of the fourth and fifth metacarpals (knuckle fractures) may occur when the assailant is punched on his head or chin. In manual assault, the hands of the suspected assailant may show injuries indicative of or compatible with his involvement in assault.

SELF-INFLICTED AND FABRICATED WOUNDS:

Self-inflicted wounds are those inflicted by a person on his own body. **Fabricated wounds (fictitious, forged or invented wounds) are those which may be produced by a person on his own body (self-inflicted), or by another with his consent.**

Self-inflicted wounds are: (1) Found on accessible areas of the body. (2) Repetitive wounds may be grouped together. (3) Site of injuries are bare of unclothed. (4) May be inflicted in front of a mirror. (5) Do not involve the features.

Motive: They may be produced for the following reasons. (1) To charge an enemy with assault or attempted murder. (2) To make a simple injury appear serious. (3) By the assailant to pretend self-defence or to change the appearance of wounds, which might connect him with the crime. (4) By policemen and watchmen acting in collusion with robbers to show that they were defending the property. (5) In thefts by servants or messengers for the above reason. (6) By prisoners, to bring a charge of beating against officers. (7) By recruits to escape military service. (8) By women to bring a charge of rape against an enemy. (9) Injuries may be seen in parasuicide or in mental illness.

Types of wounds: Fabricated wounds are mostly incised wounds, and sometimes contusions, stab wounds and burns. Lacerated wounds are rarely fabricated. Incised wounds are usually superficial, multiple and parallel, are of equal depth at origin and termination. They avoid vital and sensitive areas like the eyes, lips, nose and ears. The direction is from behind forwards on the top of the head, from above downwards on the outer side of upper arm, from below upwards on the front of forearms, variable on the legs and vertical on the abdomen and chest. Some mentally disordered persons may inflict hundreds of small wounds upon themselves. Paranoid schizophrenics with a strong religious flavour to their delusions may remove penis, scrotum and testes. Stab wounds are usually multiple and superficial and seen about the left arm or shoulder and sometimes on the chest. Burns are superficial and seen usually on the left upper arm. The clothes are not cut, and if cuts are seen they are not compatible with the nature of the wounds. The history of the assault is incompatible with the injuries.

Old linear scars in sites of election suggest previous similar attempts. They are seen on the face, on the front of the trunk, on the arms and on the fronts of the legs.

CASE: A youth alleged that he had been the subject of a murderous attack and had received a number of letters over a long period threatening him with death. He had been placed under police protection. His story was that he had been followed by a man, and when he walked into a stairway he was brutally attacked with a razor. He shouted for help, and his assailant, whom he described in detail, ran away. He was in a weak and frightened state when he reported the matter to the police, and was bleeding from wounds in his back. On medical examination. The wounds consisted of a number of fine cuts just penetrating the skin between his shoulder-blades, more or less parallel to one another and apparently made from below upward by a right-handed man. They were undoubtedly self-inflicted, by means of a sharp instrument such as a razor used very carefully. On repeated questioning, he admitted he had made the cuts by fixing a razor-blade on the end of a cleft stick and doing the job by adjusting two mirrors. The various threatening letters were in his own handwriting. Later, he duly confessed to the police.

Therapeutic Wounds: These are wounds produced by doctors during the treatment of a patient, such as surgical stab wounds of the chest for insertion of chest tubes, of the abdomen for drains, thoracotomy and laparotomy incisions, incisions on the wrists, antecubital fossae and ankles, and tracheostomy incisions. Some of these wounds may be mistaken for traumatic wounds, e.g., a surgical stab wound of the chest for putting a drainage tube. Sometimes, a traumatic wound may be enlarged and included in the surgical procedure, or a drainage tube may be put in a homicidal stab wound.

FORENSIC BALLISTICS

A firearm is any weapon which discharges a missile by the expansive force of the gases produced by burning of an explosive substance. **Forensic ballistics is the science dealing with the investigation of firearms, ammunition and the problems arising from their use. Proximal (internal) ballistics** is the study of firearms and projectiles, **Intermediate (exterior) ballistics** is the study of the motion of projectile after it leaves the gun barrel till the time it hits the target. **Terminal ballistics** involves the study of behaviour of missiles once they penetrate their targets. **Wound ballistics** is the study of the effects of missiles on living tissue.

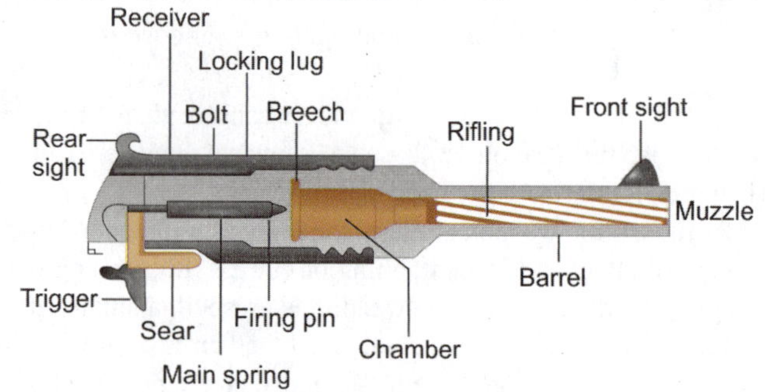

Fig. (8–54). Nomenclature of small arm.

GENERAL MAKEUP AND MECHANISM: Firearms consist of a metal barrel in the form of hollow cylinder of varying length, which is closed at the back end and is called the breech end; and the front open end is called the muzzle end. The inside of the barrel consists of three parts. (1) The chamber, at the breech end to accommodate the cartridge which is usually of large size than the bore, (2) the taper, called lead or lead in rifled arm and chamber cone in a smooth bore, connects the chamber to the bore, and (3) the bore, which lies between the taper and the muzzle. A breech action is attached to the barrel at the breech end to close the end of the barrel. It consists of a receiver which contains a bolt or block which closes and locks. The bolt or the block (consists of firing pin, spring, trigger and extractor) can be opened to insert a fresh cartridge into the chamber. Spent cartridges are removed by extractor claw. Bolt is a sliding rod that pushes a cartridge into the firing chamber as it closes and locks. When the weapon is closed for firing, the barrel comes into position against a flat block of metal called breech face, which seals the breech end of the chamber. The block is pierced in its centre to accommodate the firing pin which is actuated by a spring and moves forward when trigger is pressed. When the weapon is cocked (ready to be fired), the hammer has been pulled back against a strong spring and is held back by the end of the sear, which rests in a notch known as the bent. When the trigger is pulled, the sear is disengaged from the bent and the hammer moves forward and strikes a small pushrod (firing pin or striker). In hammerless guns, the striker is used to fire the gun and the cocking (readying of firing mechanism) is done by pulling back of the bolt action. The barrel of a "breakdown" action gun or rifle, i.e., a weapon which opens like a shotgun, has at its breech end a movable limb called extractor, which moves backwards withdrawing the cartridge, when the breech is opened Fig. (8–55). In a bolt action weapon, a small claw fitted to the front end of the bolt, pulls out the cartridge with it, when the bolt is withdrawn. The lock contains the lock and trigger mechanism, i.e. the apparatus for discharge of the weapon. The slide is the top part of semiautomatic that contains the barrel and on which the sights are mounted. A firearm is provided with sights with which one can aim, so that the bullet can strike the target accurately. The 'stock' is the supporting or handle part of the weapon, the end (rare portion) of which is the butt. The slide is the top part of semiautomatic that contains the barrel and on which the sights are mounted. The hand-arms (slide arms) are provided with grips for grasping them by hand. In long barrelled weapons, the butt is elongated to fit into shoulder. Those with long barrels (shoulder arms) are fired from the shoulder, i.e., rifle and shotgun, and those with short barrels are fired from the hand, i.e., pistol and revolver. Firearms except revolvers and hammer guns have a safety device, which locks the firing mechanism when it is applied, known as safety catch.

Classification: (I) According to the condition of barrel: (A) Rifled weapons: (1) Rifles: (a) Air and gas-operated rifles. (b) 0.22 rifles. (c) Military and sporting rifles. (2) Single-shot target-practice pistols. (3) Revolvers. (4) Automatic pistols. (5) True automatic weapons (machine guns). **(B) Smooth-bored weapons** (shotgun) **Fig. (8–55).** (1) Cylinder bore. (2) Choke bore. (3) Paradox (hammered, hammerless). (4) Breech loader. (5) Muzzle loader. (6) Country made.

(II) According to firing action: (1) Over-bolt action. (2) Under-bolt action. (3) Lever action. (4) Pump action or autoloading model.

(III) According to barrel lengths: (1) Side arms (hand-arms): They are guns with short barrel such as revolvers and pistols. (2) Shoulder arms: They are heavy long barrelled guns, which are fired from the shoulders such as shot guns or rifles.

Small Firearms: Firearms meant to propel projectiles less than 2.5 cm diameter are called small arms, such as hand arms and shoulder arms.

Rifled Arms: The bore is scored internally with a number of shallow spiral "grooves", varying from two to more than 20, the **most common being six, which run parallel to each other but twisted spirally, from breech to muzzle. These grooves are called "rifling" and the projecting ridges between these grooves are called "lands" Figs. (8–56 and 8–57).** Rifling is made by a broach. **Riflings vary in number, direction, depth and width.** The turning of spiral groove is called the twist and the angle of turning is called the pitch. When the bullet passes through the bore, its surface comes into contact with the projecting spirals which give the bullet a spinning or spiralling motion. **Rifling gives the bullet a spin, greater power of penetration, a straight course (trajectory) and prevents it from unsteady movement as it travels in the air.** A handgun bullet usually makes a single turn about its longitudinal axis in 25 to 45 cm. of forward motion. **Micro-groove system of rifling consists of 15 to 20 round grooves in bore of the barrel.** Rifled firearms are divided into: (1) Low velocity (up to 360 metres per second). (2) Medium velocity (360 to 750 m/s). (3) High velocity (750 to 1260 m/s). (4) Very high velocity (above 1260 m/s).

Caliber or gauge: It is measured by the internal dimension of the barrel and is given in decimals of inch or millimetres

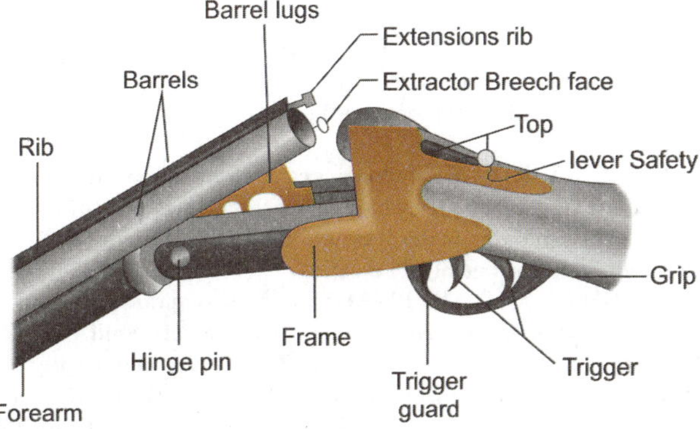

Fig. (8–55). Diagram showing details of twin-barrel (smooth-bore) shotgun.

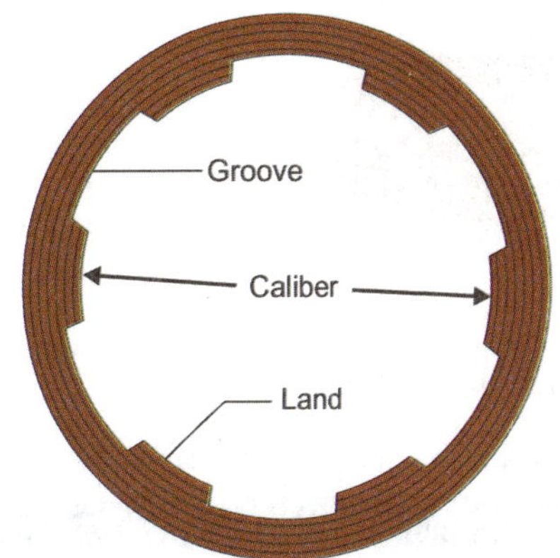

Fig. (8–56). Cross-section of rifled barrel.

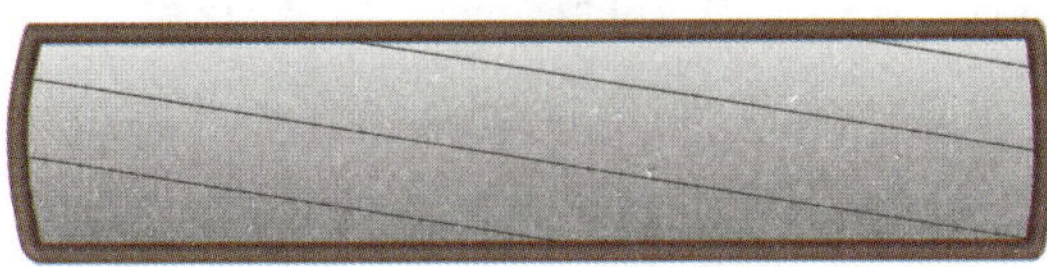

Fig. (8–57). Longitudinal section of a rifled barrel.

Fig. (8–56). **The dimension of the rifled weapon is measured between a pair of diametrically opposed lands and not grooves. In smooth-bored weapons, the bore is measured similarly up to 1.27 cm. (half inch). For larger bores, the size is determined by the size of the lead ball which will exactly fit the barrel, and by the number of such balls of equal size and weight as can be made from 454 gm. (one pound) of pure lead.** Thus the 12 bore gun is one whose diameter is that of a ball of lead of such a size that 12 balls may be made from 454 gm. The smaller the number of gauge, the greater the diameter of the barrel Table (8–9).

Helixometer is the instrument to examine the interior of the barrel.

SHOTGUN Fig. (8–55): It may be single-barrelled or double-barrelled, the barrels lying side by side, or occasionally mounted one over the other. It is intended for firing a single ball, slug or a charge of shots. The barrel varies in length from 55 to 72 cm. Shotgun bores vary from 4 to 20. The common gauges are 12, 16 and 20. The weapon is made to 'break' or open on hinge across the breech facing for the insertion and extraction of cartridge cases. The interior of the barrels is smooth. When the entire barrel from breech to muzzle is of the same diameter, it is called cylinder-bore Fig. (8–58). In choke-bore, the distal seven to ten cm. of the barrel is narrow. Different degrees are known as full-choke, half-choke and quarter-choke or improved cylinder Table (8–8). Some weapons have facility for removing the barrel and replacing it with another degree of choke. The choking lessens the rate of spread of shot after it leaves the muzzle, increases the explosive force and increases the velocity. There are some shotguns which have small portion of their bore near the muzzle end rifled, which are called "paradox guns". Some shotguns have the whole of their bore rifled with very shallow grooves. A musket is a military shoulder arm. It has a long forestock and usually takes a bayonet (pointed knife-like weapon) at the muzzle. It is smooth-bore weapon, e.g., 0.410 musket. 0.410 musket fires a single shot at high velocity and is effective up to 90 metres. Many shotguns have removable and interchangeable barrels. The muzzle velocity of shotgun is about 240 to 300 m/s and of 0.410 musket from 350 to 600 m/s. Shotguns are effective up to 30 metres. The effective range and penetrating power of a shotgun will depend upon the quantity of propellent charge, size of the shot, length of barrel and presence or absence of choking. Muzzle loading guns are loaded entirely from muzzle end with the help of a rod using gunpowder, pieces of cloth, stones, metal fragments, seeds, bolts, wood, screws, etc.

Table (8–8). Various degrees of choke

Designation	Constriction in	
	mm	inch
(1) Full choke	1.00	0.04
(2) Three-quarter choke	0.75	0.03
(3) Half choke	0.50	0.02
(4) Quarter choke	0.25	0.01
(5) True cylinder	0	0

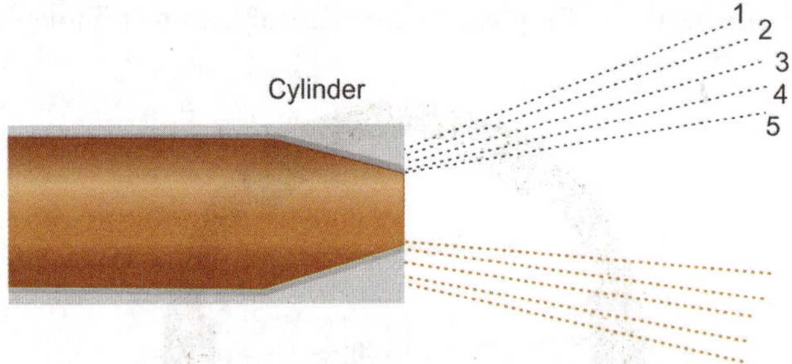

Fig. (8–58). Choking of shotgun. (1) Improved cylinder. (2) Quarter choke. (3) Half choke. (4) Three fourth choke. (5) Full choke.

Table (8–9). Shotgun gauges with decimal equivalents

Shotgun (gauge)	Bore diameter	
	Inch	mm.
10	0.775	19.69
12	0.730	18.52
16	0.670	16.81
20	0.615	15.62
28	0.550	13.97
410	0.410	10.41

RIFLE Fig. (8–59): A rifle is a gun with a long barrel, the bore of which is rifled. A carbine is a short-barrelled rifle, or a musket. Its barrel is less than 55 cm. in length and is meant for persons on horse-back. It may be self-loading or automatic or both. It is effective up to 300 metres. The bore of a rifle varies from 5.6 to 7.7 mm (0.22 to 0.303 inch). It has a firing range up to 1,000 metres. The military rifle has a magazine and bolt action, muzzle velocity of 800 metres per second and can kill at a range of 3,000 metres. The longer barrel gives an increased speed to the projectile. Velocity is the speed of the bullet or projectile at a predetermined point in its flight. The pressure in the firing chamber is about 20 tonnes per square inch. The bullet as it leaves the barrel, rotates at about 3,000 revolutions per second. The muzzle velocity is 450 to 1500 metres per second. Rifles may be single-shot, repeating, semi-automatic and automatic.

REVOLVER Fig. (8–60): Revolvers are so-called because the cartridges are put in chambers in a metal cylinder, which revolves or rotates before each shot, to bring the next cartridge opposite the barrel, ready to be fired. It has a cylindrical magazine situated at the back of the barrel, which has a revolving motion, and can accommodate 5 to 6 cartridges, each housed in a separate chamber. In the single action type, a bolt had to be moved manually to eject the spent cartridge and to bring a new round into the breech from a magazine cylinder and to bring the cartridge in the proper position for firing. In the double action type, the hammer can be cocked by hand, or by a prolonged pull on the trigger. The bores vary from 5.6 to 11.25 mm (0.22 to 0.45 inch). The muzzle velocity is 150 to 180 metres per second. They are low velocity weapons. The effective range is 100 metres.

AUTOMATIC PISTOL: It is a hand arm in which the cartridge is loaded directly into the chamber of the barrel Fig. (8–60). When a cartridge is fired, the empty cartridge case falls on the ground several metres away, and a new cartridge slips into the breech automatically by means of gas pressure developed at each discharge. The cartridges are contained in a vertical magazine in the butt, which can accommodate 6 to 10 cartridges. They are really semi-automatic or self-loading, because the trigger has to be pressed each time a round is fired. The bores vary from 6.35 to 11.25 mm (0.25 to 0.45 inch). The muzzle velocity is 300 to 360 metres per second or more. They are high-velocity weapons. Their effective range (ability for penetration in human body) is about 100 metres.

ASSAULT RIFLES: These are automatic weapons firing intermediate rifle bullets. They have a detachable magazine of 20 rounds or more. Most popular is the Russian-made AK-47 firing 600 rounds per minute over a range of 300 metres.

AIR RIFLE AND AIR PISTOL: In these, compressed air is used to fire lead slugs. Some weapons use cartridges of liquid CO_2 as the propellant. The velocity is very little (80 to 105 m/s), and usually minor injuries are caused. Their range is about 40 metres. The missile is single and fired through rifled barrel. The bores vary from 4.4 to 5.6 mm. Death can occur from injury to the head, heart and abdomen. The slug can enter the skull and pass through the whole mass of the brain, but does

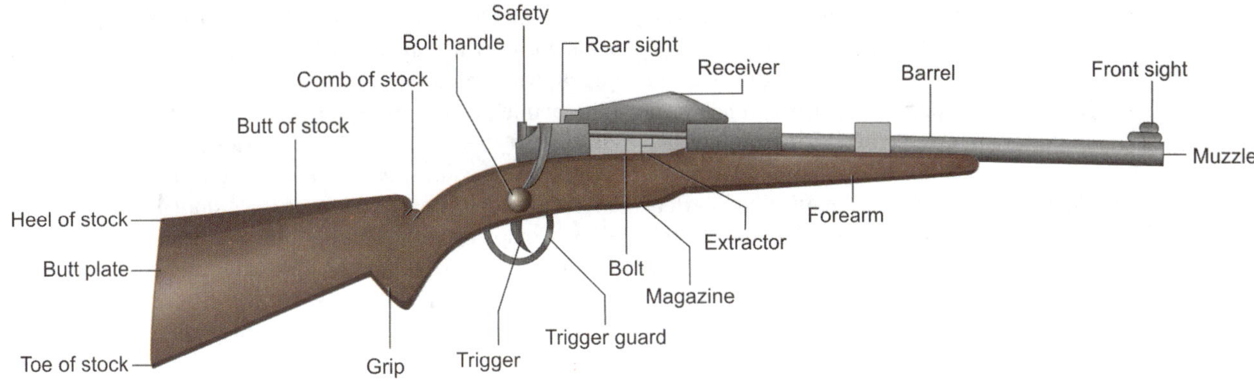

Fig. (8–59). Diagram showing general characters of a rifle.

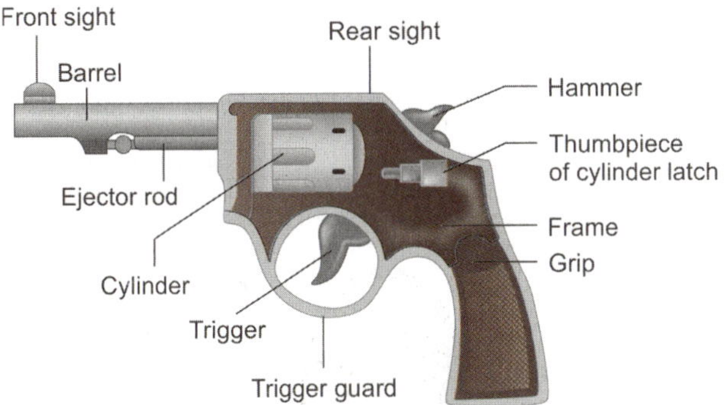

Fig. (8–60). Diagram showing general characters of a revolver.

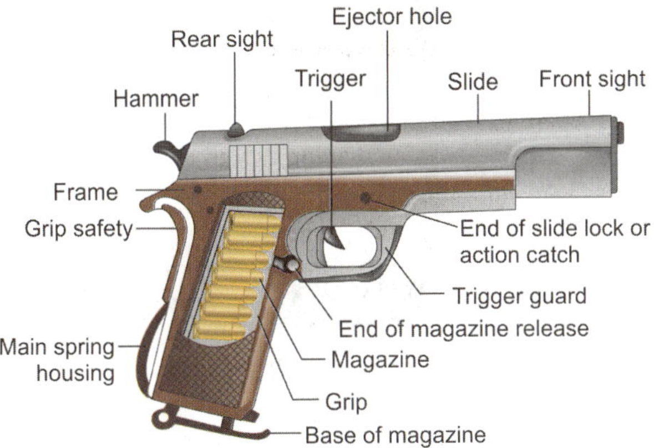

Fig. (8–61). Diagram showing general characters of a pistol.

not produce an exit wound. Abrasion ring may be present, but there is no burning, blackening and tattooing.

ROCKETS are bombs that are propelled to their target by self-contained reaction motors. MINES are hidden explosive ordinance. GRENADES are small fragmentation ammunitions either hand-thrown, fired from rifles or ejected from special grenade launchers.

ELECTRA STUN GUNS: They are electrical self-defence weapons. They deliver many thousands of volts of electricity at very low amperage. The person loses control of voluntary muscles, collapses and remains dazed and sluggish for few minutes. They leave a small red mark on the skin. They are safe and effective.

HUMANE (VETERINARY) KILLERS: They are used in abattoirs and by veterinary surgeons to kill large animals. Captive-bolt type weapon inflicts a clean, penetrating injury, about 5 cm. deep, which can be mistaken for a stab injury. Another type discharges 8 mm bullet, the injuries resemble a contact wound produced by a conventional weapon.

PEN GUNS: Tear gas pen guns may be modified so as to fire ordinary cartridge.

ZIP GUN: It is a crude home-made single shot rifled firearm.

STUD GUNS: They are tools used to fire metal studs into wood, concrete and steel.

BOOBY TRAPS are bombs which are tuned to explode in the presence of a person while he is engaged in searching premises for any incriminating object.

AUTOMATIC WEAPONS: An automatic gun is one which reloads and fires continuously as long as the trigger is depressed and the magazine is charged. Machine-guns or sub-machine guns continue to fire through the action of gases of the previous explosion and of the ejector and recoil spring. Submachine guns have a firing rate of 600 to 800 shots/minute.

IMPROVISED FIREARMS OR COUNTRY-MADE FIREARMS are common in India. They are of various calibres, but 12 bore is the commonest. They are usually smooth-bored. Some of them can be mistaken for factory-made guns, but others do not appear to be guns at all. Walking-stick guns and folding guns are single-barrelled shotguns.

CARTRIDGE: Shotgun Cartridge: The shotgun cartridge consists of a case of short metal cylinder which is continuous with a cardboard or plastic cylinder. **The case is rimmed, which helps to keep the cartridge in correct position in the chamber, and makes extraction easy. The case helps to keep the various components in place, prevents the backward escape of the gases and provides a waterproof container for the gunpowder.** The length of the cartridge varies from 5 to 7 cm. Cartridge cases are stamped at the factory to indicate type and make. **The cartridge case is filled as follows from the base: percussion cap (detonator cap; primer battery cup), which is set into the centre of the base of the cartridge cylinder, gun powder, a thick felt-wad with cardboard discs lying in front and behind it, the shot (charge or load) and finally the retaining cardboard disc, over which the edges of the cartridge cylinder walls are pressed.** Some cartridges have top wad over the lead shot to keep the shot in place. The diameter of the wadding used in the cartridge is greater than that of the bore of the gun. **Wad prevents heat from the gunpowder from fusing or distorting the pellets and acts as a piston and seals the bore completely, thus preventing the expanding gases from escaping and disturbing the shot charge.** The felt wad contains grease, which lubricates the bore after the firing of each round. The modern one piece plastic wadding tends to have greater range due to its greater weight. **The powder is protected from the grease wad by a thin grease-proof card wad.** Wads may be glazed-board, straw-board, plastic, cork, felt, etc. and may be disc-shaped Fig. (8–63 and 8–66) cup-shaped, or bizarre-shaped. **The card-wad behind the shot charge prevents the shots from getting lodged in the felt-wad and seals the bore completely. Some cartridges contain 'power piston' formed from four leaflets or petals folded so as to produce a cylindrical shape, which holds the shot inside a polythene cup, which may contribute to the wound at short range.** Some cartridges may have brightly coloured plastic granules as a filler between the shot, which may be found inside the wound.

SHOTS (PELLETS) They are of two types. (1) Soft or drop shot is made of soft lead, (2) Hard or chilled shot is made from lead and hardened by antimony. The shots may also be plated with copper. "Buckshot" is the largest and has a diameter of 6 to 8 mm. Pellets deform easily due to friction as they rub against the inside of the barrel. The heat can cause melting and fusion of pellets Figs. (8–62 and 8–63). Rifled slugs are single projectile, and are used in shotguns for big game hunting. They are similar in shape to a blunt bullet with a deep hollow cavity in the base and weigh from 23 to 33 g. The sides commonly have angularly inclined fins or ribs that resemble very coarse rifling marks on bullet. The slugs are usually a little smaller in diameter than the shotgun bore itself. The slugs have much greater range than pellets. The spiral grooves on the slugs impart spinning effect.

Rifled Cartridge: It consists of a metal cylinder with a flat base which projects as a rim except in an automatic pistol. Rimless cartridge has an extractor groove near the base. **The primer cup (percussion cap) is fitted in a circular hole, usually in the centre of the base and has a flash hole in the centre which communicates with the powder space inside. The metal cylinder or cartridge case is elongated, and its distal end tightly grips the base of the bullet** (projectile or missile). **The gunpowder lies between the detonator and the bullet. Usually there is no wad Fig. (8–64),** but sometimes one piece wad is kept. Low-power rim-fire cartridge may not contain gunpowder but only a primer compound in the circumferential hollow rim Figs. (8–64 and 8–65). As such, those cartridges cannot produce the tattooing. Many bullets have near the base, a circumferential groove called **"cannelure"**, into which the end of the case is crimped. A bullet without cannelure is held in position by stabs on the circumference of the case.

PRIMERS: Primer is the brain of the cartridge. Centrefire rifle and pistol primers are small metal cups usually held in place in the cartridge head primer pocket by friction. The primer cup contains the priming mixture and an anvil so placed that the blow of firing pin on the primer cup crushes the priming mixture against the anvil centre

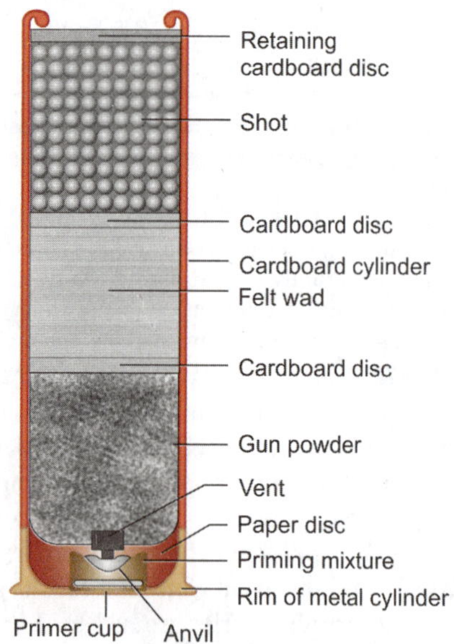

Fig. (8–62). Shotgun cartridge.

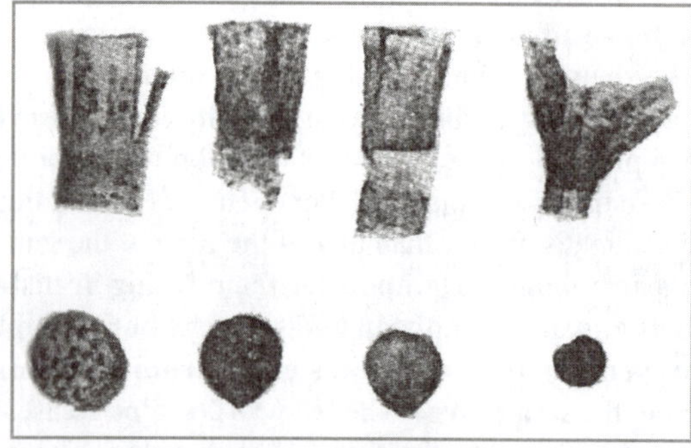

Fig. (8–63). Fired shot shell wads.

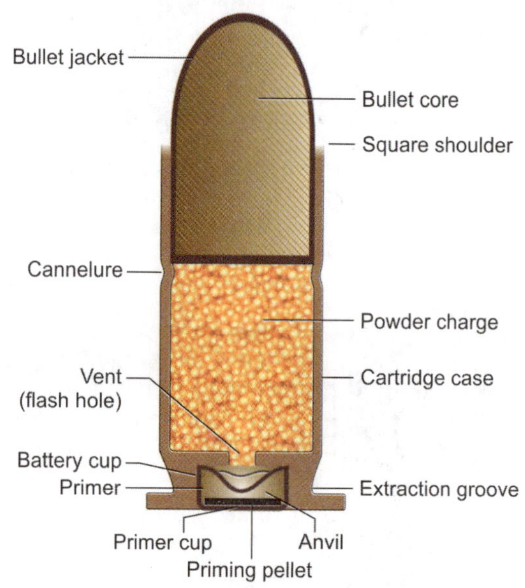

Fig. (8–64). Cartridge for rifled weapons.

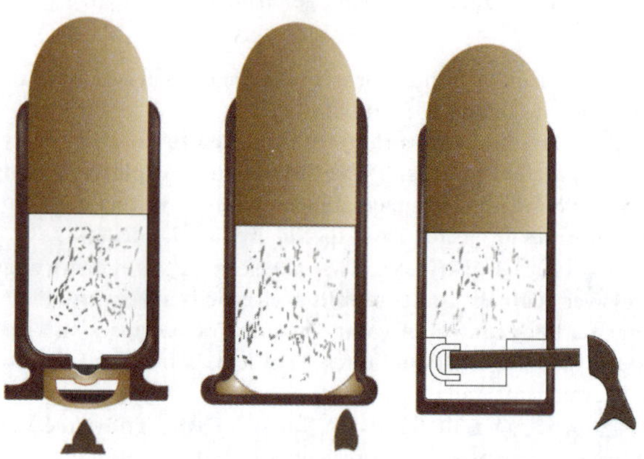

Fig. (8–65). Three types of cartridges. (1) Centrefire. (2) Rimfire. (3) Pinfire.

and burns it, which then flashes through the flash hole (fire holes or vents) in the centrefire case head, and ignites the powder charge. The primer used in shotgun cartridge is called a primer battery cup. This consists of a battery cup into which a primer cup fits. The battery cup supports the anvil and provides a flash hole. It is also held in place by friction. The primers which are used nowadays contain compounds of lead, antimony sulphide and barium, instead of mercury fulminate or lead azide. These minute particles can travel up to 7.5 to 15 cm. In rimfire cartridges no percussion cap is provided. The priming mixture is contained within the hollow rim of the cartridge and ignited when it is crushed between the rim walls of the cartridge head by the impact of the firing pin.

POWDERS: (1) BLACK POWDER: It consists of potassium nitrate 75%; sulphur 10%; and charcoal 15%. It is designated as FG, FFG, FFFG, etc., depending on the size of the grains. The more number of F's, the finer are the grains and the faster in burning. The powder grains are black, coarse or fine, without any particular shape. It burns with production of much heat, flame and smoke. Fine grains travel 60 to 90 cm. or more. One gram of powder produces 3,000 c.c. of gas. The gas consists of CO, CO_2, nitrogen, hydrogen sulphide, hydrogen, methane, etc., all at a very high temperature. It has largely been replaced by smokeless powder.

(2) SMOKELESS POWDER: It consists of nitrocellulose (gun cotton), (single-base), or nitroglycerine and nitrocellulose (double-base) or nitrocellulose, nitroglycerine and nitroguanidine (triple base). Triple based powder is commonly used. They produce much less flame and smoke and are more completely burnt than black powder. One gram produces 12,000 to 13,000 c.c. of gases. The colour varies from bright orange to bluish-black, and in shape from minute globules, flakes, square, rectangular, irregular discs, cylinders to longer threads. SEMI-SMOKELESS POWDER is a mixture of 80% of black and 20% of the smokeless type (DIMAIO, 1985 ⇒ 1000 lb/in²).

BULLETS (projectiles, missiles) Fig. (8–64, 8–65 and 8–67): The traditional bullet is made of soft metal and has a rounded nose. The metal is lead with varying amounts of antimony added to provide hardness. This is known as the round-nose soft bullet, and is usually used in rifles and revolvers. The tip of the bullet is called nose. The caliber of a bullet is its cross-sectional diameter. In revolver and pistol, the bullet is short and the point usually round or ogival. In rifle, the bullet is elongated with pointed end. Variations are: (1) Square-nosed, soft metal bullet, known as "wad-cutter", and used primarily for target shooting. (2) Hollow-point variety has a depression in the nose of the soft metal. This bullet is designed to expand or "mushroom" upon impact.

Mushroom bullets produce more serious wounds. Other types of bullets are: (1) Short flat-point. (2) Medium flat-point. (3) Medium round-nose. (4) Long round-nose. (5) Medium long sharp-point. (6) Medium sharp-point. (7) Flat base. (8) Sharp-point boat-tailed. (9) Pencil-point. (10) Streamlined with sabot.

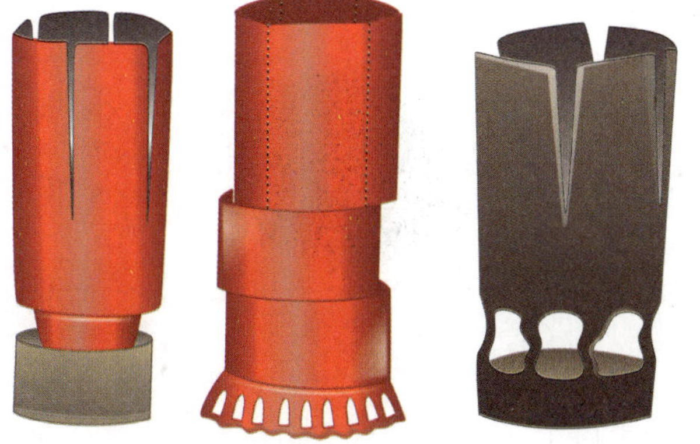

Fig. (8–66). Typical wads which may be recovered from the body at autopsy.

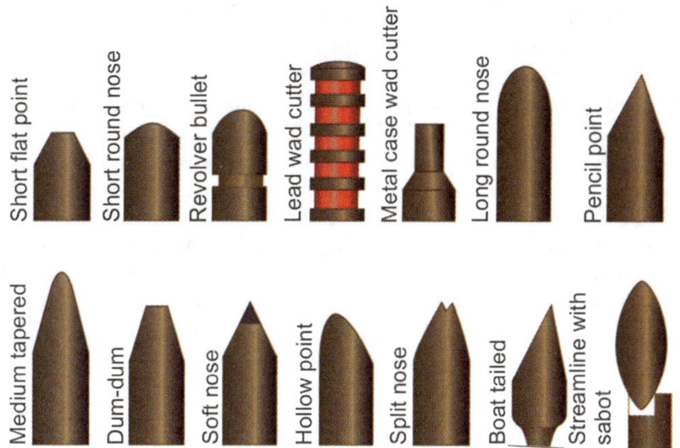

Fig. (8–67). Types of bullets.

Jacketed bullets are of two types: (1) The full metal jacket bullet in which a tough, heavy jacket covers all but the base, where the soft metal interior is exposed. The tough jacket may be made of steel, copper, nickel and zinc. (2) The semi-jacketed bullet is provided with a relatively thin but tough jacket, which covers the base and the cylindrical portion of the bullet, leaving the nose partly or fully exposed. This type is designed to expand or "mushroom" like the soft metal, hollow-point type. The combination of the above two is also available.

Bullets that distort at the nose such as soft-point or hollow-point bullets, creating a "mushroom" effect of deformation, cause greater damage than pointed-nose bullets. Larger bullets cause greater damage because of greater mass and kinetic energy. Jacketed bullets have greater penetrating power.

A Dumdum bullet is one which fragments extensively upon striking. They are not in use. Frangible bullets completely disintegrate. A bullet with a hole in the point is called hollow-point or 'express' bullet. Incendiary bullets contain phosphorus, so that it catches fire on hitting the target. Frangible bullet is made of iron which fragments on impact.

EXPLOSIVE BULLETS: Incendiary bullets contain explosive at the front end and cause fire in the target. They are banned. If explosive bullets are present in the body, ultrasound or microwave diagnostic techniques must be avoided, as they can cause the projectiles to detonate. The exploding bullet is of various types. The wound produced is larger than the usual. If the missile explodes, there is greater fragmentation of the bullet and increased destruction of the tissues. The surgeon and pathologist should wear goggles and use long-handled instruments to manipulate the missile during surgical operation or autopsy, as they are vulnerable to detonations of explosive missiles. The removed bullet should be handled with long rubber-covered forceps and kept in a padded container to protect it from excess impact, vibration and heat.

TRACER BULLET: The bullet contains a mixture of barium nitrate and powdered magnesium with strontium nitrate which burns during the flight of a bullet shedding red sparks. It leaves a visible mark or "trace' while in flight, due to which the gunner can observe the strike of the shot.

PLASTIC BULLETS: Baton round (plastic bullet) is a solid cylinder of polyvinylchloride (PVC), 38 mm. in diameter, 10 cm. long, weighing 135 g. It is fired from a smooth-bore weapon and is effective up to 50 to 70 metres. They are used for riot control. It should not be fired at a person under 20 metres range. It causes bruising and pain. Many injuries and some deaths have been reported. Police are instructed to fire at the lower half of the body to avoid serious injuries. Fracture of the skull, eye damage, fracture of ribs, limb bones, and contusions of liver, lung and spleen have been reported.

MECHANISM OF DISCHARGE OF PROJECTILE: A firearm is fired when the trigger is pulled, which is usually situated below, or below and behind the breech. The trigger releases a pin or hammer,

whose tip strikes the central recess at the base of the cartridge, above which is percussion cap, which contains explosive mixture known as priming, which explodes by heat created by the strike of the firing pin and sends a flash through a tiny hole into the main body of the powder-filled case, which sets fire to the powder charge or propellent, producing instantaneously a large amount of gas which is under high pressure. The cartridge case swells outwards, due to which the hold on the bullet (missile, projectile) is released, and forces the bullet into the barrel and passes out. The confined gas behind it gives recoil thrust to the gun. Noise of gun firing is caused by muzzle blast, or due to the suddenly released gases disturbing the air. If the velocity of the bullet is more than the speed of sound, then there is also a crack from that. The bullet reaches its maximum velocity as it comes out at the open end of the barrel and this is called muzzle velocity. The bullet is followed by a blast of highly compressed hot gas, particles of partially burnt and unburnt powder, smoke, flame and fragments of metal, cartridge and detonator, grease and wad or disc matter. The gases after leaving the muzzle expand at once to atmospheric pressure. High pressure and temperature exists just outside the muzzle, but this rapidly expands and cools. The blast has the shape of a cone whose apex is located at the muzzle. All these things produce some effect on the body at short ranges.

MECHANICS OF BULLET WOUND PRODUCTION: (1) BULLET VELOCITY: A bullet's ability to wound is directly related to its kinetic energy ($E = mv^2/2$) at the moment of impact. Because kinetic energy increases in direct proportion to weight (mass) of the missile and the square of its velocity, a bullet travelling at twice the speed of a second bullet of equal weight and similar shape, possesses four times much energy or wounding power. Tissue damage produced by high velocity bullets is disproportionately greater than that produced by bullet of ordinary muzzle velocity. A wound produced by a bullet, whose impact speed equals its muzzle velocity is more severe, than that produced by the same bullet, discharged from the same gun, whose speed has been reduced due to travelling a long distance before it strikes its target. High velocity bullets produce a clean circular entry wound and may perforate the body without showing any deviation in its path. Low velocity bullets may cause contusion or laceration of the margin and may be deflected within the body.

(2) TISSUE DENSITY: The greater the tissue density, the greater is the amount of energy discharged by the bullet's passing through it. A bullet may cause slight damage to the soft tissues, but the same bullet, at the same speed can produce extensive comminution of the bone.

(3) HYDROSTATIC FORCES: Hydrostatic forces cause excessive degree of destruction. When a bullet passes through a fluid-distended hollow organ, e.g., food-filled stomach, urine-filled bladder, CSF-filled ventricles of the brain, or a heart chamber distended with blood in diastole, produces extensive lacerations due to the explosive displacement of the liquid in all directions.

FIREARM WOUNDS

They are usually recognised without difficulty. Wounds produced by rifled weapons may simulate wounds inflicted by a red-hot poker or a burning pointed stick. Glancing wounds may simulate incised or lacerated wounds. A bullet that passes through glass or some other object, and then strikes the body may produce a wound resembling a laceration. **Firearm wounds cause crushing of the tissues and produce an actual hole. A stab wound causes a slit-like opening which tends to seal after the knife is withdrawn.**

WOUNDS FROM SHOTGUNS

Shotgun discharge contains lead pellets, soot in the form of smoke and debris, unburnt and burning propellant flakes or grains, flame and hot gases under pressure, detonator constituents and fragments of cartridge case. **The smoke extends up to 30 cm., flame up to 15 cm., and unburnt and partially burnt powder grains up to 60 to 90 cm.** The larger the caliber, the greater the distance to which the powder is discharged. **The cards travel for two metres, and wad for 2 to 5 metres. Marked variations occur between different weapons, different barrels of the same weapon, and different ammunitions fired from the same weapon. Ammunition plays a great role in the size and pattern of wounding.**

The character of a wound depends on. **(I) The Distance From which the Weapon is Discharged:** The discharge produces a long, shallow cone with its apex close to the muzzle of the shotgun. **A compact mass of shot emerges from the muzzle and begins to spread**, the divergence increasing progressively as the distance lengthens. Flame and hot gases follow the shot. High pressure and temperature exists just outside muzzle, which rapidly expands and cool.

(1) Contact and near contact wounds: They are single, usually round, equal to the bore in size, often ragged because of individual shot and tearing due to gases resembling exit wound, if present. In tight contact wound, soiling and burning are minimal or absent Fig. (8–68). As the gases are blasted within the wounds, the subcutaneous and deeper tissues show severe disruption. The rapid entry of gases causes a momentary vacuum immediately below the skin, which may cause extrusion of the soft tissues, e.g., fat through the wound. Particles of unburnt powder are driven to some distance through the wound and some of them are found embedded in the wound. These particles cause haemorrhage in deeper tissues and form aggregates of haemorrhages in the margins of the wound. Thus, **the margins of the wound will be contused. If the contact is tight (hard contact), muzzle impression (copy or recoil abrasion) is seen** due to firm mechanical pressure of impact of the metal rim against the skin, and also due to the subcutaneous expansion of gases lifting the skin forcibly up against the muzzle. The **muzzle imprint** may be an incomplete, indistinct bruise or rarely may be a perfect imprint of the end of the weapon. **Bruising can occur around the muzzle imprint. Muzzle imprint may be lost within the explosive damage associated with the discharge.** But, in a double-barrelled shotgun, the

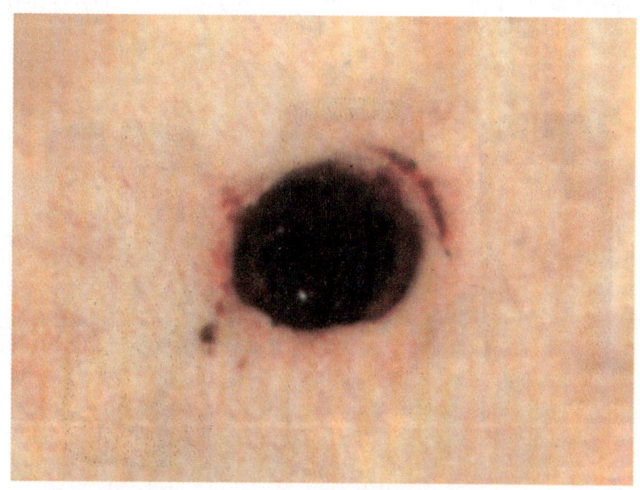

Fig. (8–68). Tight-contact shotgun wound of chest. Muzzle imprint is seen on the upper right side.

unused barrel often leaves a characteristic patterned abrasion. In many cases, muzzle impression is not produced due to rapid removal of the weapon by recoil. **The recoil, which takes the muzzle away from the skin, may loosen contact and if the muzzle is not pressed firmly, flame, gas and soot may escape sideways and cause singeing and blackening of the surrounding skin.** When a firearm is fired the shooter gets a jerk on the shoulder or wrist due to recoil movement of firearm. **In contact shot, the muzzle blast and the negative pressure in the barrel following discharge may suck blood, hair, fragments of tissues and cloth fibres several cm. back inside the barrel called "back spatter".** CO in the gases combines with haemoglobin and myoglobin due to which the wound of entry and the wound track appear pink. This decreases gradually, but may be seen very rarely at an exit wound. **Burning, blackening and tattooing of the tissue also take place in the depths of the wound.** The outer shots are deformed by their passage through the bore and choke. **Plastic wads retain their shape and diameter within the body, but felt and cardboard wads suck up blood and body fluids and swell.**

Contact shot over a bony area: Cruciate, stellate or ragged lacerations are seen especially if there is a thick bone immediately under the skin, such as skull due to the extreme force of the blowback phenomenon, as gases expand beneath the skin and lacerate the margins of the wound, as they exit through the original entry wound. **The internal damage is diffuse, but there is no cavitation. Contact wounds on the head produce greater disruption of the margins, and often show subsidiary linear tears in the skin extending from the margins of the main wound. A large irregular hole is produced in the skull, with fissured fractures running from its margins. The bone may show burning, blackening and tattooing in the margins. The entire contour of the face and head may be** destroyed, and the actual point of the muzzle impact of entry wound may be difficult to locate. Extreme mutilation is caused due to the explosive effect, because the gases have restricted space for expansion. **Comminution of the vault of the skull is usually accompanied by extensive fissured fractures,** or 'crazy-paving' fracture of the base of the skull, and the roofs of the orbits, and middle ears. **A large exit wound may be produced with disruption of the cranium and projection of brain tissue for some distance.** An eye may be blown out of its socket **(burst head)**.

An entrance wound in the mouth or nose may or may not be accompanied by an exit wound. Resistance by the hard palate reduces the power of the shot, and the shot lie mostly in the space between the skull and scalp, at the back or side of the head. Abrasions or bruising of one or both lips with or without laceration is seen. **Splitting of the angle of mouth may occur** due to blast. In the neck region a large exit wound or complete destruction may occur. On the chest, the skin and subcutaneous tissues may be peeled away from the rib cage to form a pocket which then collapses. **In contact or near contact wounds on the abdomen, coils of small intestine may lie outside the abdomen due to entry of gas into the peritoneal cavity.**

Loose contact: In loose contact or near contact shot, **some of the gases escape with the resulting scattering of the muzzle blast and an unusual arrangement of soot is seen on the skin known as corona,** similar to that as seen in rifled weapon wound. In loose contact with skin, the blast effect is less as compared to tight contact, and splitting of the wound margins usually does not occur.

Clothes: If the part is clothed, smoke will escape sideways and may be found in each layer of clothing and on the skin. The cloth may be singed at the edge of the hole, and there may be a ring of burning around the skin wound.

(2) Close Range (up to one metre): Within a distance of about 30 cm., tissues surrounding the wound are singed by flame, and blackened by smoke, and tattooed by unburnt or partially burnt powder granules. If the powder is smokeless, there may be greyish or white deposit on the skin round the wound. **The deposit of smoke is known as smudging, fouling or blackening.** This spreads more widely than powder tattooing. The blackening can be removed by a wet cloth. **Unburnt particles of the powder are embedded in the skin producing tattooing (stippling or peppering) Fig. (8–69).** The particles sticking to the epidermis or lodging in the epidermis superficially can be removed with pressure wiping, showing punctate wounds. **The hairs of the trunk and limbs may be completely burnt around the wound Fig. (8–70).** If the distance is greater, the keratin of the hair may melt with the flame, and then solidify on cooling, producing clubbed appearance of the hairs because of rounded bulges at the tips. **Soot soiling diminishes as the distance increases.** There may be a wide flare or narrow rim of hyperaemia or even blistering from the flame. **If the gun is fired at right angle to the body, the burnt area is circular, and if fired at an angle it is oval, the direction of the firing being indicated by the nearness of the wound to one or other end of burnt area. The end nearer the wound is the direction towards which the shot travelled.** Primer residues are easily removed from the skin by wiping, rubbing or washing. **The use of silencers to muffle the sound of discharge, reduce the amount of smoke and powder significantly and cause misinterpretation of the distance from which gun was fired. The burnt area darkens and parchmentises on drying after death.** Blackening and tattooing can be readily demonstrated by infrared photography on both skin and clothing. As range becomes greater, the intensity

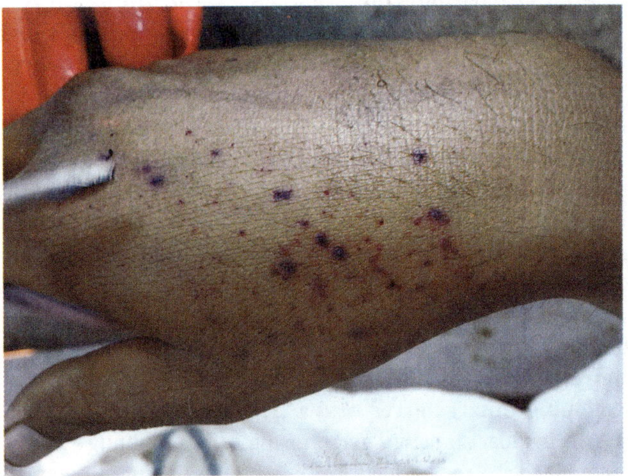

Fig. (8–69). Suicidal shotgun effect of tattooing on the back of the hand due to escape of gases from breech end of barrel.

***Courtesy*: Professor Manoj Kumar, BHU, Varanasi.**

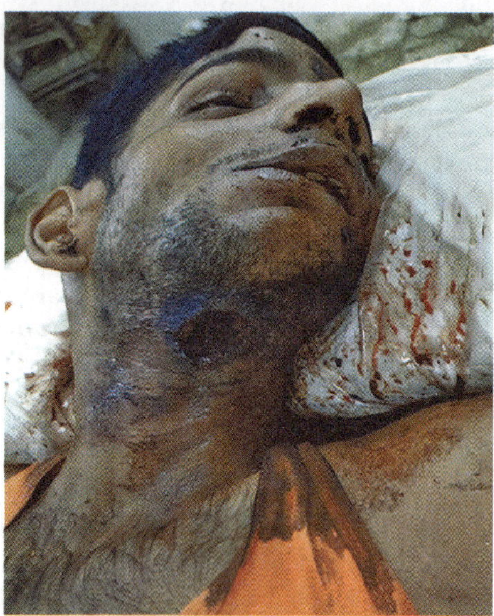

Fig. (8–70). Shotgun contract entrance wound on the floor of the mouth in suicide case.

Courtesy: **Professor Manoj Kumar, BHU, Varanasi.**

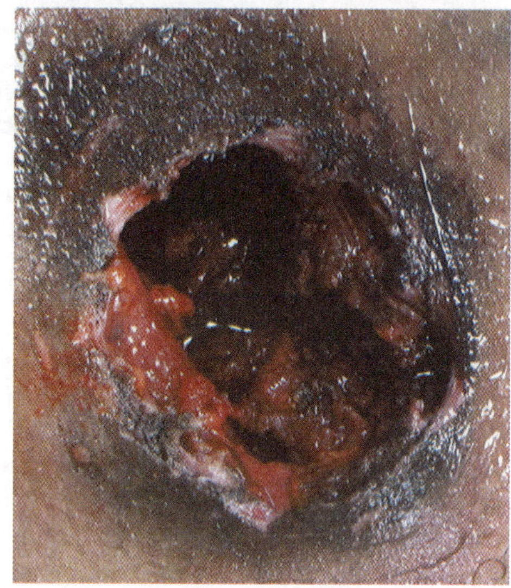

Fig. (8–71). Shotgun entry wound. Rat hole appearance.

of blackening and tattooing decrease and the spread increases in a fairly regular manner.

Between 30 cm to one metre: The wound is single, circular or oval, similar to contact wounds, though the blackening and tattooing are more extensive. The margins of the skin wound may be clean-cut or slightly ragged. There may be annular bruising around the wound due to tissue damage from the entry of gases. **Felt wads or plastic cups from the cartridge will be found in the depths of the wound.** The deeper tissues show marked disruption. In some cartridges, plastic granules may be used as a filler between the lead pellets, and this coloured material may be found within the wound or on the skin up to 2 to 3 metres and produces very fine, punctate abrasions around the pellet holes. **The plastic cup type wad opens up between 30 to 60 cm. so that four petals stick out, and a circular entrance wound is produced to form a square edged star or capital 'X' shape (Maltese cross) producing a characteristic bruise or abrasion of a similar shape encircling it. By 90 cm. air resistance folds back the petals and a single hole of entrance will be produced.** In the 0.410 ammunition, the plastic sleeve expands into only three petals and produces three abrasions.

At a distance of 60 to 90 cm: The tissues up to 30 cm. along the track, and around the wound may be cherry-red due to absorption of CO. **The small shot produce a single circular aperture, 2.5 to 4 cm. in diameter, with irregular and lacerated edges. There is no burning or blackening. Some amount of tattooing is usually seen.** The tissues within and around the wound are not cherry-red. **Between 30 cm to one metre, the rim of the wound is irregular and shows some scalloping, often referred to as a "rat-hole"** Fig. (8–71). There may be annular abrasions and bruising or "rat nibbling" from its resemblance to rodent teeth marks. **At close ranges, when the shots are bunched, they strike one another upon hitting the skin/clothing and are scattered after entering the body and cause much damage to the internal tissues.** In the skull, there is less disruption than that at contact range; bursting open of the skull and scattering of its contents is not seen. The column of pellets has a cutting action which produce a clean hole. When buck shot is fired from close range, the dispersal of the shot through the body may be minimal. **Shotgun wounds at contact and close range cause much more destruction of tissues than rifled weapons,** due to the greater amount of gas produced, because of larger amount of gunpowder.

(3) Short range (1 to 2 metres): A single circular aperture 4 to 5 cm. in diameter, with irregular and lacerated edges is produced. There is no burning, blackening or tattooing. The shot mass enters the body in one mass, producing a round hole, four to five cm. in diameter for all gauges and all chokes. **Wads may be found deep inside the wound up to two metres. Collect and preserve plastic sleeve, wadding and cardboard.** Annular or linear abrasions are caused by the impact of the clothing against the stretched skin during the penetration of the shot *en masse*.

(4) Intermediate Range (2 to 4 metres): The **minimal distance at which shot mass begins to spread is extremely variable. It may be one metre with sawed-off shotgun but is usually about two metres with cylinder bore guns and four metres with full choke guns. At a distance of two metres, the shot mass begins to spread and individual pellet holes may be detected, which are usually round and show a rim of abrasion at their margins. The wound of entry is irregular. Beyond two metres the wads often strike the body below the shotgun wound.** It may penetrate the skin or it may only bruise the skin. The wads found within the wounds are useful to determine bore of the gun.

At a distance of three metres: The central aperture is surrounded by separate openings in an area of about 8 to 10 cm. in diameter. As muzzle-target distance increases, the main entrance defect progressively becomes smaller, and individual pellet wounds increase in number. Occasionally, several individual pellet entrance wounds are in contact producing scalloped defects which are larger than the individual pellet holes.

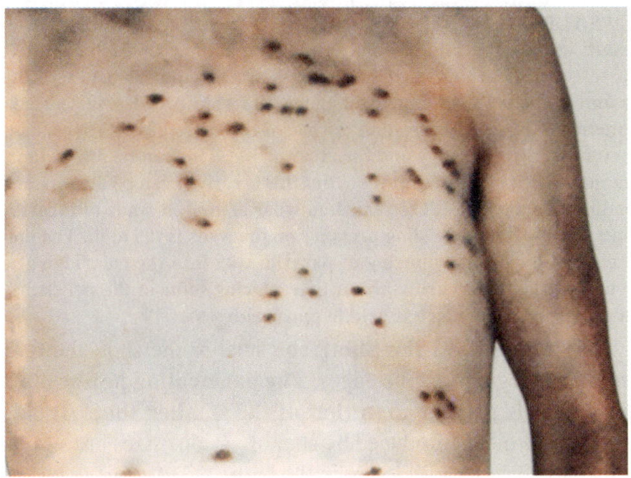

Fig. (8–72). Shotgun wounds from a distance of about 10 metres.

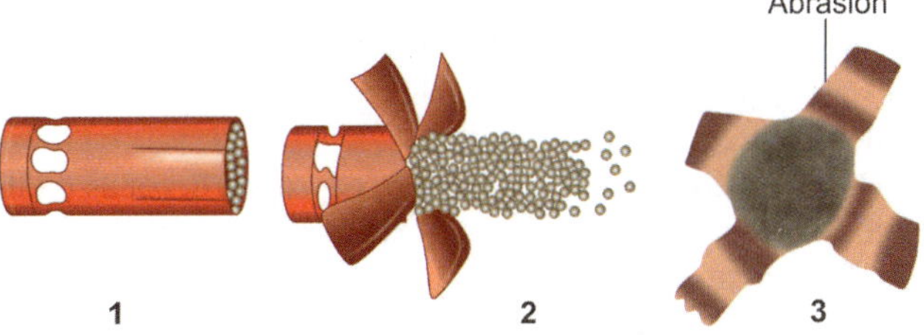

Fig. (8–73). Shotgun wad with enclosed lead shot in plastic cup. (1) Cup is not opened. (2) Between 30 to 60 cm. the sleeves of cup open and are forced backward. (3) Cross-like pattern of abrasion around the entry wound.

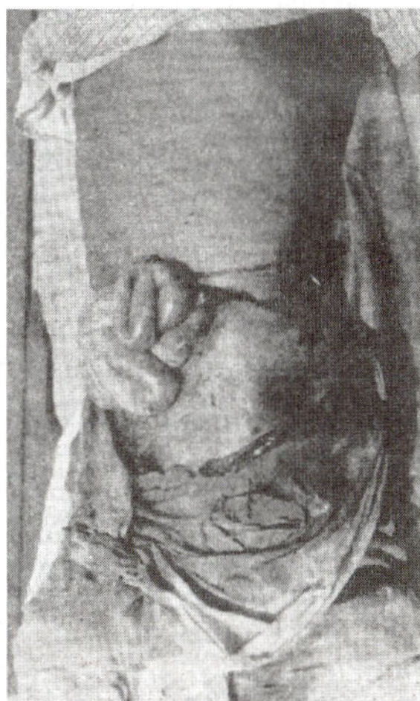

Fig. (8–74). Herniation of intestines through the entry wound of shotgun.

As lead is soft, pellets deform easily due to friction as they rub against the inside of the barrel. The heat can cause melting and fusion of pellets.

(5) Long or Distant range (above 4 metres): Distant wounds are those in which all shots penetrate separately. **At a distance of 4 metres, the shots spread widely and enter the body as individual pellets producing separate openings in an area of 10 to 15 cm. in diameter Fig. (8–72 and 8–74).** Each individual pellet reproduces its own track. In the skull, the energy of the shots is greatly reduced perforating the skin and bone, so that they usually do not travel the entire brain substance. Cavitation is usually minimal or does not occur, and distant contusions are rare. Laceration of blood vessels by pellets or bone fragments may produce infarcts. In shotgun discharge, there is no temporary cavitation. The spread of pellets from a fully choked barrel is:

10 metres	...	25 cm.
15 metres	...	35 cm.
20 metres	...	45 cm.
30 metres	...	75 cm.

The spread is almost double from an unchoked barrel Tables (8–10 and 8–11). **At about 30 metres, the pellets only penetrate the skin or muscle.** Death beyond a range of 30 metres is rare. It is possible for a single pellet or shot to cause death. The diameter of the wound is measured from the outermost of the individual pellet holes in centimetres. **For cylindrical barrels about one-third of the spread of shot in cm. roughly equals the range in metres which is very inaccurate. The estimation of range is difficult when replaceable or variable extensions called 'chokes' are used at the end of the muzzle of shotguns.** Some chokes and even the barrels themselves are replaceable. **Passage of shotgun pellets through any target before they strike the body, cause the pellets to spread, e.g., window glass, screen, layers of clothing or leather jacket. If a hand is held over the muzzle when discharge occurs, the pattern may be 7–8 cm across as it leaves the hand.**

Shotgun slugs usually produce large, gaping circular to oval defects with irregular margins. The internal injury is highly destructive and similar to that caused by high velocity rifles. **The wound caused by buckshot resembles bullet wound.**

Marked variations occur between different weapons and ammunition fired from the same gun.

COUNTRY-MADE FIREARMS: The injuries caused to the victim vary considerably depending upon the nature of projectiles. Metal scraps may produce small incised or incised-looking wounds; punctured wounds may be produced by nails, and lacerations and contusions by stone pieces. The distance up to which the smoke, flame and carbon particles travel is approximately half of that from factory made firearms. The pellets begin

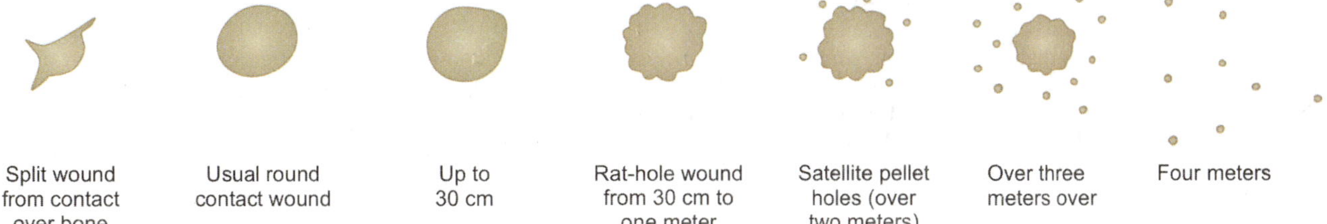

Fig. (8–75). Shotgun wounds at varying distances.

Table (8–10). Approximate spread of shot in centimetres at various distances

	5 metres	10 metres	15 metres	20 metres
Cylinder	20	50	65	75
Half-choke	13	30	40	50
Full-choke	8	25	35	45

Table (8–11). Percentage of shot falling within a 75 centimetres circle at various choke adjustments

Choke adjustment	Average percentage
Full choke	70
Three-quarter choke	65
Half-choke	60
Quarter-choke	55
Improved cylinder	50
No choke	30 to 40

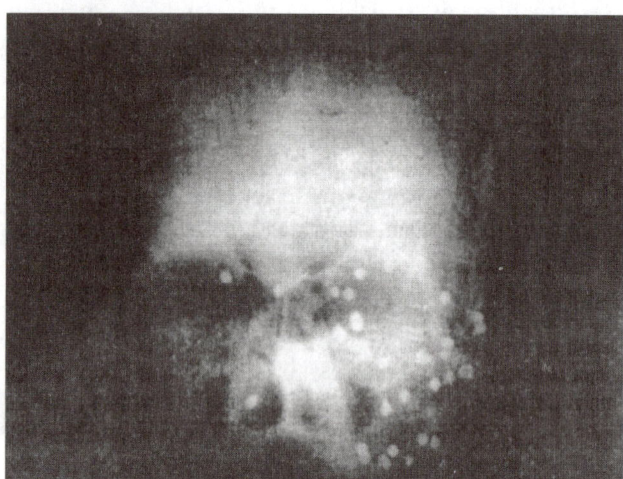

Fig. (8–76). X-ray of the skull showing multiple pellets underneath the subcutaneous tissues of the face over an area of 12 x 8 cm. A case of shotgun injury from a distance of 5 to 6 metres.

to disperse at a distance of 30 to 45 cm. The muzzle velocity is low and the barrel can accommodate a sub-caliber projectile or cartridge. As the characters of the firearms and components of the cartridge vary widely in country-made firearms, the data applicable to factory-made firearms to calculate the distance of firing cannot be applied. For estimating the distance of firing, the only ideal method is to carry out test firing with the suspected weapon.

BILLIARD BALL RICHOCHET EFFECT: At close range, while the shots are bunched, they strike one another upon impact on primary target, i.e., the skin or clothes, and spread out in a wide pattern as they pass through the body. This causes the shots to spread widely and may suggest a greater range of fire than actually occurred. Similar spread is seen if the shots strike any other intermediary object, e.g., door or window, before reaching the victim. The phenomenon is termed the billiard ball ricochet effect. The final shot spread as seen in X-ray Fig. (8–76) gives a true picture of the range of fire, only when the range of fire is great enough that the shots are spread out, before striking the target.

In decomposed and burned bodies where the skin pattern cannot be seen, the range of fire can be determined by X-rays.

BALLING OR WELDING OF SHOT: Balling of shotgun pellets results in the conversion of shot into a compact mass, which can travel for few metres in this form. In such cases, a circular or oval entrance wound of about 5 to 10 mm. in diameter, and widespread, small, circular punctures are seen, suggesting the use of two different weapons, one a shotgun at distant range and the other a rifle. This can be due to faulty manufacture or old ammunition, but this is rare. It can be due to hand-loading of cartridges, if too much powder is used, if wads of incorrect kind are inserted, or sealing pressure on the wads is too high. The most likely cause is due to pouring of paraffin wax into the cartridge after removing the outer cardboard or by replacing some of the pellets by a large ball-bearing which is held in place with wax.

(II) The Size of the Shot: The smaller the shot, the more minutely irregular are the edges. **The penetrating power of the large shot is greater than that of the smaller shot.** At close range, the wounds produced by shot of various sizes are similar, but small shots usually lodge in the body.

(III) The Nature of the Explosive: The extent of tattooing depends on bore of weapon, the type of powder used, the weapon and the range of blackening. **The greater the bore of weapon, the wider the area of blackening.** With smokeless powder, blackening and tattooing is less marked than with black powder at all ranges.

(IV) The Gun itself: The pattern of wound depends on the length of the barrel, the bore, absence or degree of the choke present. **Shorter barrels usually produce greater deposits over larger areas.**

The **direction of the fire** may be determined from the passage of individual shots through the clothes and tissues, from the grouping of shot marks and the direction of glancing shots.

Exit Wounds: Usually shotgun pellets do not exit from the body except: (a) Contact wounds. (b) Tangential wounds where some of the pellets have a very short track through the body. (c) Thin part of the body, such as the neck or extremities. (d) Wounds caused by large caliber buckshot or rifled slugs. Usually, a bruise may be seen in the deep tissue of exit site and shot may be felt under the skin.

At contact or near range, greater disruption of tissues occur compared to the entrance wound. The margins are everted as the unsupported skin is struck from within, the tissues tend to burst outward, and the skin fragments, but there is no singeing, blackening or tattooing of the margins. There may be small, separate wounds made by individual pellets that have become separated from the mass.

WOUNDS FROM REVOLVERS AND AUTOMATIC PISTOLS

The flame extends up to 8 cm; smoke up to 15 cm. and unburnt and partially burnt powder grains and small metallic particles up to 40 to 50 cm. with handguns Figs. (8–79 to 8–82) and up to 60 to 100 cm. in case of rifle. In case of pistol, distance from which powder residues can reach is about twice the length of barrel. The amount of smoke, flame and powder grains and the distances to which they will be carried will vary depending upon the type of gun powder used, the amount of powder load, the size and weight of the projectile, barrel length, caliber, the tightness of fit between the projectile and gun barrel and the type of firearm. Silencers will filter out a great proportion of soot and powder particles due to which the range appears greater than it actually was.

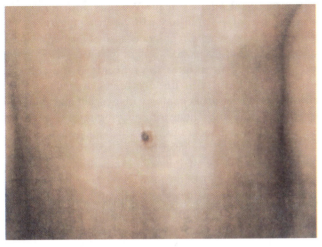

Fig. (8–77). Distant shotgun wound caused by a rifle slug.

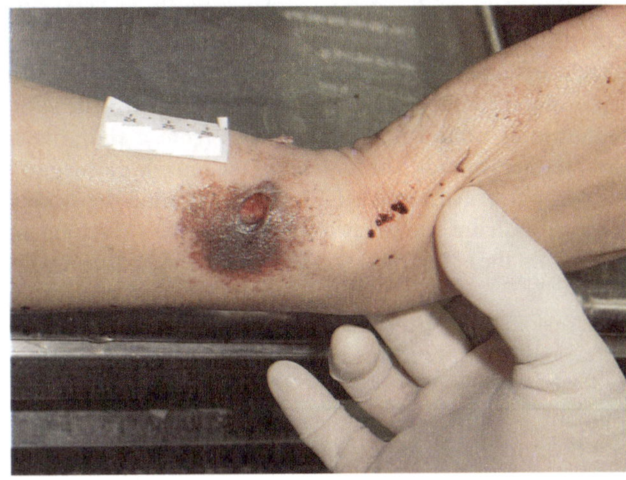

Fig. (8–80). Bullet wound of close range with powder effect around it.

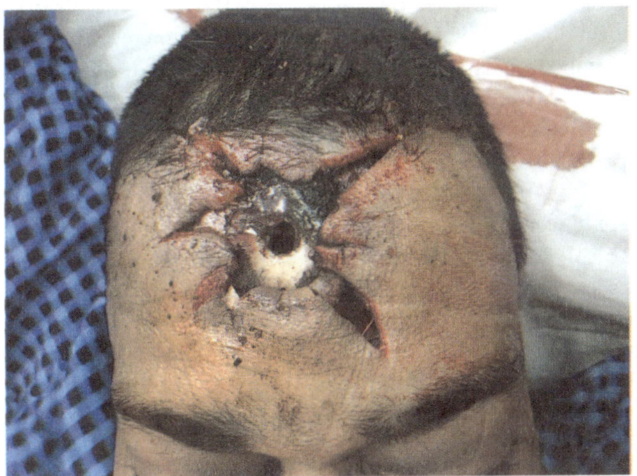

Fig. (8–78). Contact pistol stellate-shaped with blackening and burning around margins of wound.

Courtesy: Professor Manoj Kumar, HOD, AIIMS, Patna.

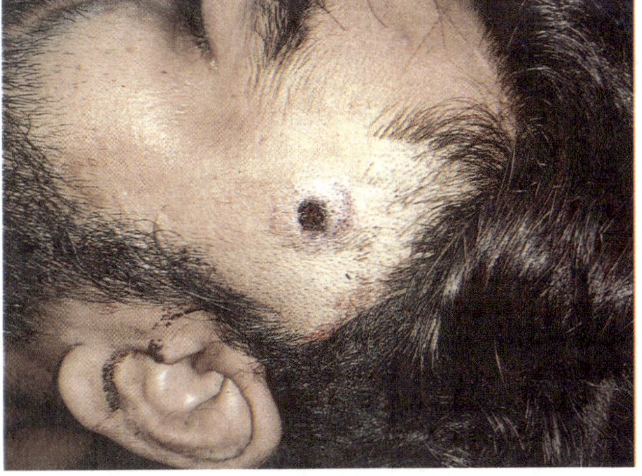

Fig. (8–81). Entry wound from a revolver showing abrasion collar.

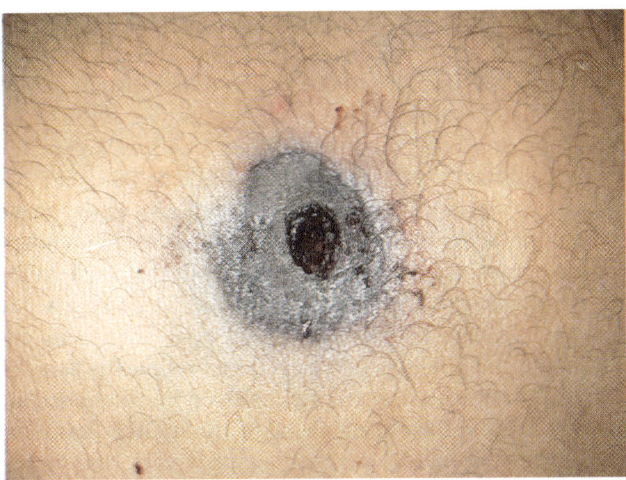

Fig. (8–79). From a revolver in the temple, muzzle mark is visible as a ring.

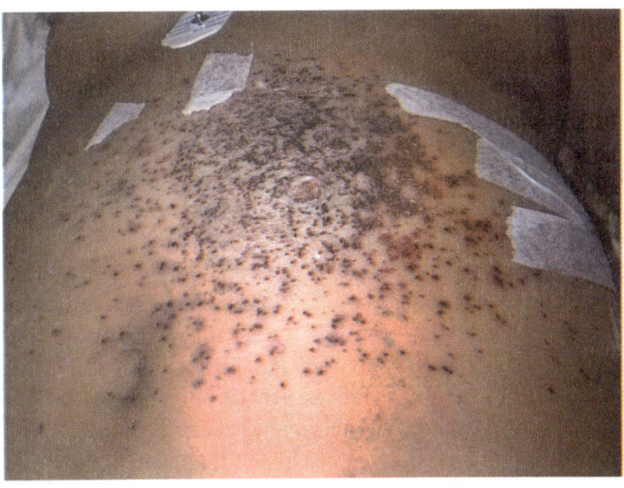

Fig. (8–82). Rifle entry wound showing tattooing, near shot.

Courtesy: Professor Manoj Kumar, BHU, Varanasi.

Entrace Wound (in-shot wounds): They may be classified on the distance of the muzzle of a firearm from the body; contact shot, close shot, near shot and distant shot. **(1) Contact Shot: In firm or hard contact (muzzle pushed hard against the skin), the resulting wound is similar to that from a shotgun. In some contact wounds, the imprint of the muzzle of the gun is found as patterned abrasion on the skin around the wound. This results from the great distension of the subcutaneous tissues from the entry of gases which forces the surface against the muzzle.** The mark may be an incomplete, indistinct bruise and occasionally a perfect imprint of the muzzle. Many muzzle impressions are not recorded due to the rapid removal of the weapon by recoil. When a firearm is fired, the shooter gets a jerk on the wrist due to recoil movement of firearm. **The discharge from the muzzle,** i.e. gases, flame, powder, smoke and metallic particles **are blown into the track taken by the bullet through the body. The wound is large and triangular, stellate, cruciate or elliptic, shows cavitation due to the expansion of the liberated gases in the skin and tissues, which show laceration. The margins are hyperaemic, contused and everted** due to gases coming out of the entering wound under pressure. Singeing of the hair may be present due to the escape of hot gases by the sides of the muzzle end. **The area immediately around the perforation is abraded,** and this thin rim of abrasion is usually **covered with powder residue.** In firm contact with the skin where the bone is not shallowly situated, the ever expanding gas continues to penetrate deeper, to be scattered in the soft tissues of the body. The wound is not eruptive or explosive in appearance. **Contact and close range discharges may cause pieces of skin, hair and adipose tissue fragments to enter the muzzle for several centimetres due to a momentary suction effect after pressure of gas blast subsides due to negative pressure in the barrel and possibly due to rapid relative cooling of the barrel called "back spatter".** Back spatter is more common with shotgun. Sometimes, blood may soil the hand of the person firing the gun.

Loose contact or near contact: In loose contact or near contact shot, some of the gases escape with the resulting scattering of the muzzle blast and an unusual arrangement of soot is seen on the skin known as corona. The **corona consists of a circular zone of soot deposit surrounding the bullet defect, but separated from it by a band of skin without a deposit of soot. This is due to the gases expanding about the muzzle, first at a velocity too high to allow for the settling out of soot, with a subsequent loss in velocity at a short distance from the muzzle, allowing the soot to finally deposit on the skin.** Wound has clear margin, everted, abraded and surrounded by soot. The blast effect is not as marked as in tight contact, and splitting of the wound edges does not occur. Evidence of burning is noted on microscopic examination in the edges of the contact and near-contact bullet wounds due to the flame of muzzle blast. Singeing of the hair may also be seen. **Tattooing begins when the muzzle to target distance exceeds one cm.** The powder residue is usually grossly visible in the subcutaneous and deeper areas. The entrance track is blackened by powder and smoke and seared and charred by flame. In loose contact, gas and soot escape from the side of the barrel, causing an eccentric area of burning and blackening.

Contact shot against head: Wounds appear, as very large explosive type of injury with bursting fractures. The skin wound is large and irregular because of the expansion of gases between the scalp and the skull which causes **eversion and splitting of the skin at the margins of the entrance wound. This results in undermined, ragged, stellate, triradiate or cruciform opening with everted margins from which tears radiate.** The tearing may be severe, as the gas raises a large dome under the skin which then ruptures. Such wounds are usually produced by large calibered pistols. A subcutaneous pocket containing blood mixed with gunpowder is formed by separation of the tissues. When a small calibered pistol is used, the wound may be small and regular. **Soot may be deposited on the bone surrounding the bullet hole.** This should not be mistaken for lead rubbed off on the bone during the passage of the bullet, which is seen only in a localised area. Frequently, soot passes deeper into the wound track and a faint gray or black discolouration may be seen on the inner surfaces of the skull around the bullet hole and on the dura mater. **Fissured fractures often radiate from the circular defect** due to the considerable sudden expansion resulting from the muzzle blast. **Fractures of the orbital roofs occur** due to the same mechanism, but the dura over the orbits is usually not damaged. In near contact shot, splitting of wound edges usually does not occur. Fractures of skull radiating from bullet hole are rare. **A bullet travelling the cranial cavity destroys the structures in its pathway and produces an expansile or explosive effect. A bullet fired from a short distance may produce an explosive effect sufficient to burst the scalp, shatter the skull and dislodge the brain. In less severe type of injury, a cone of damaged cerebral tissue is seen surrounding the wound track.** When a bullet moves through the body, it transfers kinetic energy to the surrounding tissue, which is thrown forcefully away from the bullet's path in a radial manner, and a **temporary cavity is formed in its path.** The margins of the wound of entry, subcutaneous tissues and muscles around the track of the bullet may be bright pink due to the presence of CO. **Abdominal wounds show cavitation because of the blast effect.**

When the part is clothed, the bullet hole in the cloth touching the muzzle is sometimes surrounded by a flat ring corresponding to the outline of the muzzle. **The loose fibres of the cloth in the centre of the bullet hole are often turned outward** due to the expanding gases returning through the defect. These fibres are usually blackened by smoke. In synthetic fabrics, melting of the ends of these fibres may be observed sometimes. **Varying amounts of soot is deposited on the edges of the bullet hole.** If the clothes are bloodstained, deposits of soot may not be recognised, but the inside of the garment may show large deposit of smoke. This is due to the spreading of smoke by the muzzle blast between the skin and the clothing and is seen commonly **if the shot passes through several layers of material. Each layer is blackened on both sides of the fabric, but the skin wound does not show blackening or tattooing.** If there is no intervening clothing, the smoke passes into the wound but a small amount is deposited on the wound edges, especially if contact with the muzzle was loose. Fine granules of powder and deposits of soot can

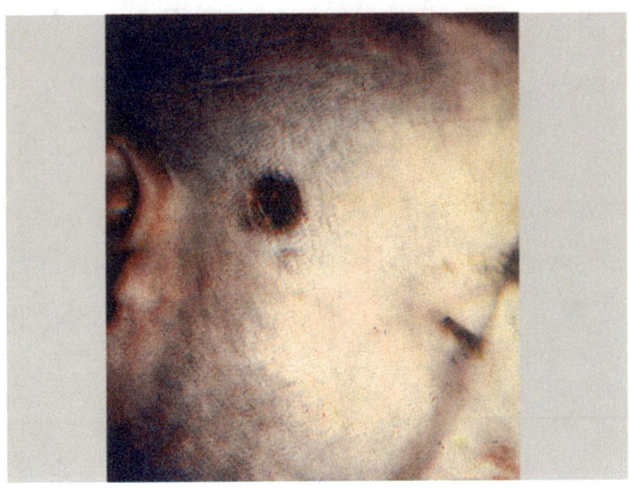

Fig. (8–83). Suicidal contact wound by revolver in the temple.

be demonstrated in the depth of the wound by a layer-wise dissection of the injury.

(2) Close Shot: This term is applied when the victim is within the range of the flame, i.e., 5 to 8 cm Figs. (8–79, 8–80 and 8–83). The term 'point blank' is used when the range is very close to or in contact with the surface of the skin. The entrance wound is circular with inverted edges, but the rebounding gases may level up or even evert the margins. A circular wound is produced only when the cone is at 90 degrees to the plane. In all other positions an ellipse wound is seen, its elongation increasing as the angle decreases. This pattern also applies to soot deposition. **The skin surrounding the wound is hyperaemic and shows some bruising, burning, blackening and tattooing.** Minute flakes of unburnt explosive are found on the skin. **The area should be swabbed with a water damped plain swab or preferably the skin can be cut around the wound and preserved unfixed and refrigerated.** The palms and soles are very resistant to powder tattooing. The blackening can be wiped off the skin by a wet cloth, but the tattooing cannot be wiped off. **Carboxyhaemoglobin** will be present in the wound track in diminishing concentrations **up to 30 cm** as the range increases. The length of the barrel of a firearm has considerable effect on the spread of smoke produced on the target, e.g., **a gun with a 5 cm. barrel will spread the smoke over a much larger area than a weapon having a 15 cm. barrel, fired from the same distance and using the same type of ammunition. Usually, as the distance between the muzzle and the target increases, the pattern of soot or powder on the target increases in diameter and the density of particle deposition decreases.** In handguns, up to 15 cm. from the muzzle, abundant gunpowder and diminishing amount of soot are deposited on the target. Powder tattooing consists of numerous reddish-brown or orange-red punctate abrasions surrounding the wound of entrance, which become more noticeable after a day or two and usually heal completely if the victim survives. Hair in the surrounding area may be clubbed, swollen at intervals by heat, or burnt. **Abraded collar and grease or dirt collar are present.** The internal injuries are almost same as in the case of contact shot.

(3) Near Shot: This term is applied when the victim is within the range of powder deposition Figs. (8–80 and 8–81), and outside the range of flame, and smoke, i.e., up to 50 cm. If the discharge occurs at a distance of about 15 cm., the lacerating and burning effects of gases are usually lost due to the dispersion cooling of the gases before they reach the skin. **The entrance wound is seen as a round hole, slightly smaller than the diameter of the bullet, due to elasticity of the skin, with a bruised and inverted margin and a zone of blackening and tattooing.** The individual tattoos are caused by the individual unburned powder grains being blown into skin. A small magenta-coloured zone, an actual micro-contusion is seen surrounding each tattoo point, which is caused by the trauma of the high speed impaction of the powder grain with rupture of small blood vessels and resulting minute haemorrhage. **If the bullet strikes the body at an angle, blackening and tattooing has a pear-shaped area, with the larger area on the side nearer the barrel.** Abundant gunpowder and diminishing amount of soot are deposited on the target. **As the distance increases, the intensity decreases and blackening and tattooing is spread out over a large area, and there is no singeing of the hair and skin. Between 30 cm. to 50 cm. there is no burning and blackening, but some amount of tattooing is usually seen.** Abrasion and grease collar are present. Occasionally, when the range of fire is short, small fragments of metal derived from the interior of the barrel of the gun or the bullet itself, are embedded in the skin in the vicinity of the entrance wound.

(4) Distant Shot **(Above 50 cm.) The entrance wound is smaller than the missile due to the elasticity of the skin, circular, and margins are inverted Fig. (8–84).** Distant entrance wounds of the palms and soles are irregular, often having a stellate appearance, without an abrasion ring, and look like exit wounds. **Burning, blackening and tattooing are not seen. The skin adjacent to the hole shows two zones, the inner of grease collar and the outer of abraded collar. In case of semi-jacketed bullet, the jacket separates as it goes through the body, and the core mushrooms into small pieces. X-ray gives a picture of "lead snowstorm".** The projectile need not strike the bone for this to occur. **If a semi-jacketed bullet passes through an intermediary target, the jacket may separate from the core, and both missiles may penetrate the body. When a bullet passes through an intermediary target, such as glass, may**

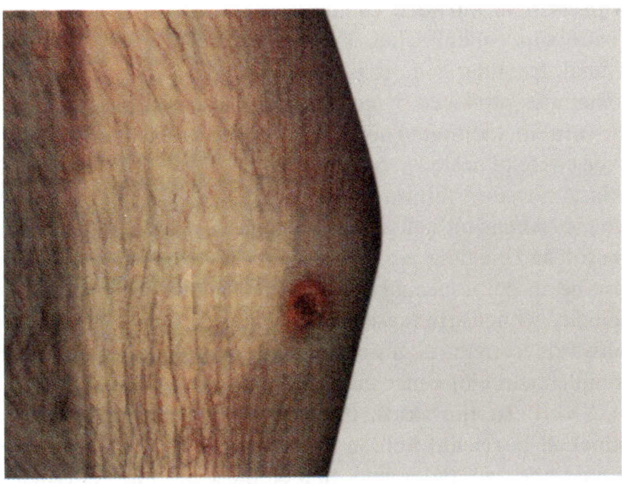

Fig. (8–84). Entry wound by a bullet fired from a distance.

cause superficial lacerations around the entry wound and these are referred to as pseudo-tattooing, which are larger and more irregular than that caused by powder. Intermediate targets, such as clothing, jewelery, items in pockets, furniture, doors, windows, walls, etc. modify the appearance of entrance wounds. The caliber of a bullet cannot be determined, if it strikes the skin surface obliquely.

Stretching and cavitation and dissipation of kinetic energy are the major causes of the lethal effects of a bullet, together with deformation and fragmentation.

Silencers reduce sound of firing and discharge of smoke and power significantly. The range of fire will be miscalculated.

THE ABRASION COLLAR (marginal abrasion): As the bullet strikes the skin, it first indents and then stretches the skin surface, so that perforation takes place through a tense area. After the bullet has perforated the skin, the elasticity of the skin causes the skin defect to contract. **The skin is abraded (abrasion collar) around the hole due to rubbing of the gyrating body of the bullet against the inverted epidermis and heat of the bullet. There is often a slightly wider circle of peeled keratin, where stratum corneum of skin is raised to form a slightly frayed edge around entry wound. A black coloured ring "grease or dirt collar" (bullet wipe soiling) is seen as a narrow ring of skin, lining the defect, and is sharply outlined.** This is caused from the removal of substances from the bullet as it passes through the skin, i.e., bullet lubrication, gun oil from the interior of the barrel, lead from the surface of the bullet, dirt carried on the surface of the bullet, as it travels through the atmosphere, barrel debris, etc. It is more marked in a distant shot. **Fouling refers to tiny lesions around the entry wound caused by fragments of metal** (from surface of missiles or interior of the barrel) **expelled by the discharge.** Friction between bullet and rifling may remove piece of lead jacket or barrel steel. They cannot be wiped off. **Infrared photography clearly indicates the presence of black ring around the bullet hole. Dirt collar is less common if the bullet is jacketed and may be absent when it has passed through clothing.** By contrast, **soot is dark in the centre and fades towards the periphery. The abrasion collar surrounds the dirt collar. The abraded collar is reddish at first, but becomes reddish-brown and then brownish-black as it dries. Some contusion is present in abraded collar, and as such, it is also called "contusion collar".** These two features are proof of an entrance wound. Irregular and occasionally patterned abrasion collar is sometimes produced by coarse article of clothing scraping on the skin. In addition to abrasion collar, there is often a slightly wide circle of peeled keratin, where the stratum corneum of the skin is raised to form a slightly frayed edge around the entry wound. **Abrasion collar may be absent** (1) When the tissues are soft and yielding, e.g., in the abdomen or buttocks. (2) It may also be absent, especially where skin is taut, and in some high velocity wounds. In these cases, small splits or tears radiating outwards from the edges of the perforation involving a part or complete circumference may be seen.

Skull: In the skull, the wound of entrance shows a punched-in (clean) hole in the outer table. The inner table is unsupported and a cone-shaped piece of bone is detached forming a crater that is larger than the hole on the outer table, and shows bevelling (sloping surface) Figs. (8–88 and 8–89). Fissured fractures often radiate from the defect. As the bone fragments have to pass through the dura before entering the **brain, lacerations are usually irregular and involve leptomeninges.** Pieces of bone from wound of entrance are often driven into the cranial cavity and may establish the bullet track. **Pieces of bone may produce short accessory wound tracks. At the point of exit, a punched-out opening is produced in the inner table and bevelled opening on the outer table. The**

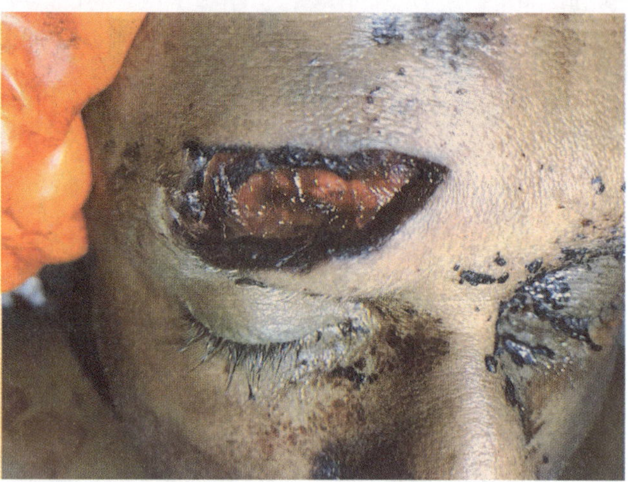

Fig. (8–85). Tangential shaped revolver wound with burning at the margins, resembling split laceration.

Courtesy: **Professor Manoj Kumar, HOD, AIIMS, Patna.**

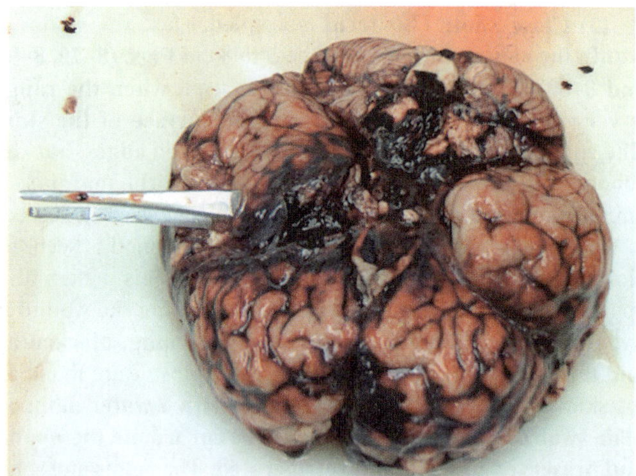

Fig. (8–86). Track and cavity caused by bullet passing through the brain.

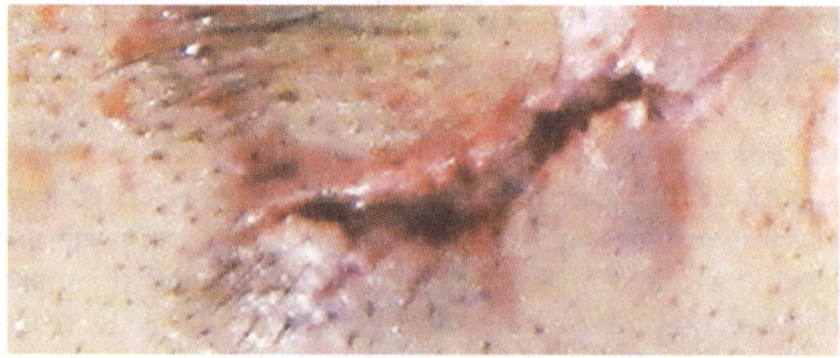

Fig. (8–87). Exit wound of revolver bullet.

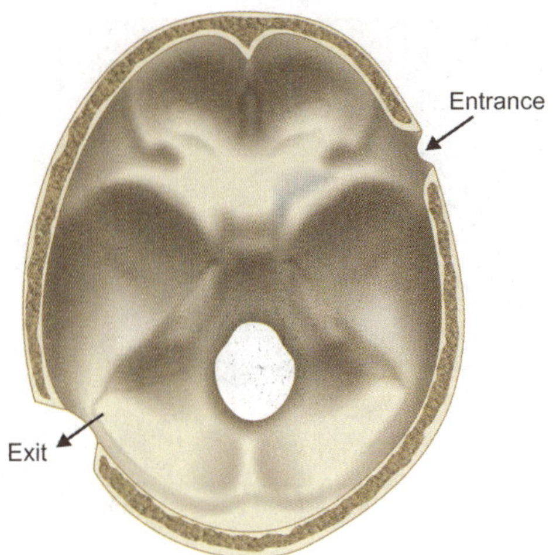

Fig. (8–88). **Shooting appearance of entrance and exit wounds in skull.**

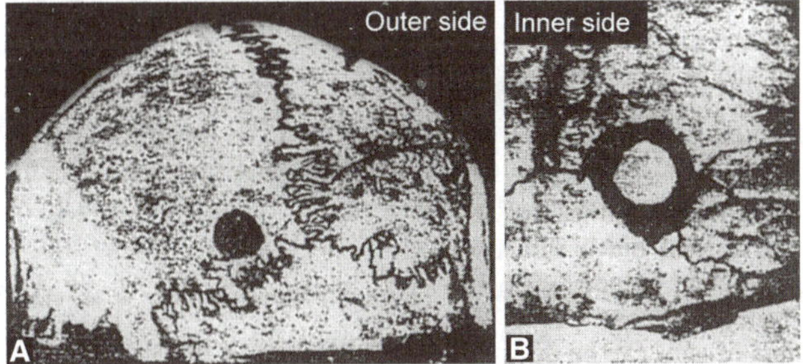

Fig. (8–89). **(A) Skull cap showing the entrance hole of a revolver bullet with clean-cut margins. (B) The inner side of the same bone showing bevelling of edges.**

wound is funnel-shaped, with the funnel opening up in the direction in which the bullet is travelling both in entrance and exit wound. Bevelling is produced when the unsupported diploe everts and fragments on the side where the bullet leaves, this in contrast to the approach side where the rim of the defect is supported by the underlying bone. **The exit wound is larger due to the deformity and tumbling of the bullet after entering the skull.** There are often fissured, sometimes comminuted fractures radiating from the central hole. **Asymmetry of the bevelling is useful in assessing the angle of fire.**

The same appearance is seen in sternum, pelvis, ribs, dentures and thumbnails.

Puppe's Rule: It can determine the sequence of shots, when several bullets have struck the cranium. This rule is applicable to any multiple blunt force, causing skull fractures. This rule has been developed by Madea in relation to bullet injuries. The test depends on the observations of the fracture lines either when they intersect each other, or when they intersect a cratered lesion, so that one can determine which crack or defect must have been formed first Fig. (8–90).

Direction: If the bullet strikes the body at right angle, the abrasion collar is circular and uniform because the scraping by the bullet is equal on all sides of the wound Fig. (8–91). **If the bullet strikes the body at an angle, the wound itself is round, but the marginal abrasion is oval or elliptical,** due to increased width on the side from which the bullet comes, due to

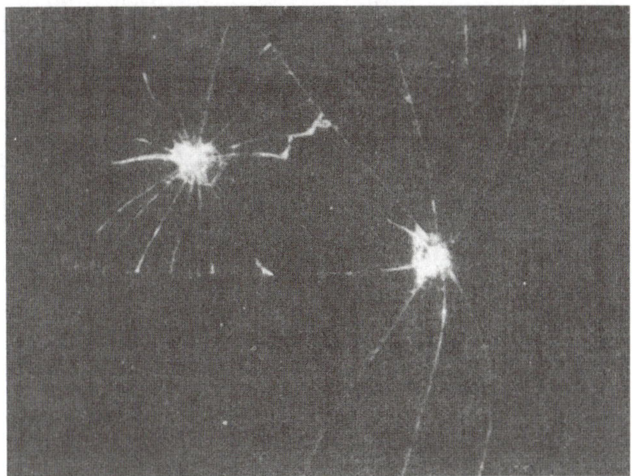

Fig. (8–90). **Piece of glass showing two impacts, each with radiating cracks, indicating that the blow on the right was made first. The cracks radiating from blow on left are arrested by those already present due to first blow on the right.**

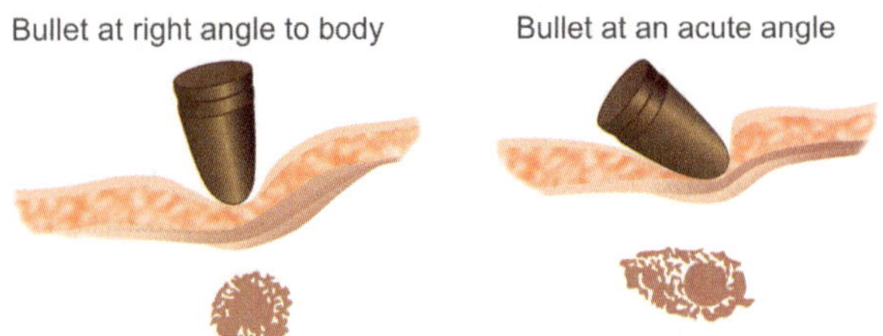

Fig. (8–91). **Abrasion collar of an entrance bullet wound.**

the bullet moving across a wider surface of the skin on that side. **The direction of the bullet is from the wide to the narrow side. Oblique angle will cause an elliptical mark,** the length of which increases as the angle decreases. When the bullet enters the body from an oblique angle, one edge of the wound is shelved or undercut below the margin distal to origin of discharge, which indicates the direction from which the bullet entered. Shelving is usually seen in the deeper layers of the skin rather than in the tissues below.

THE WOUNDING POWER OF BULLETS: The size and velocity of the bullet are the two most important factors. The wounding power of a bullet is proportional to its mass, multiplied by the square of its velocity. Another factor is the density of the tissue, e.g., destruction is greater in dense tissue such as bone than in soft tissues. The tissues show considerable damage due to the wobbling of a bullet within the body. A bullet travelling at high velocity produces a clean, circular punched-out aperture or slit and usually perforates the body. It is not deviated from its path by striking a bone, but may cause its comminution or splintering. A bullet of low velocity causes contusion and laceration of the margins. It is easily deviated and deformed by striking some hard object, and often lodges in the body. Large bullets cause greater damage than small ones. Round bullets produce larger wounds than conical ones. A bullet of smaller size than the calibre of the weapon may cause only bruising.

Clothes: If the shot is through a clothed surface, examination of clothing only can indicate its range. In a contact shot, the clothing usually shows a cross-shaped perforation and may be singed at the edge of the hole. **The inner surface of the garment may show abundant deposit of smoke, even if none is seen on the outside.** This results from spreading of smoke between skin and clothing by muzzle blast and is especially seen if the shot

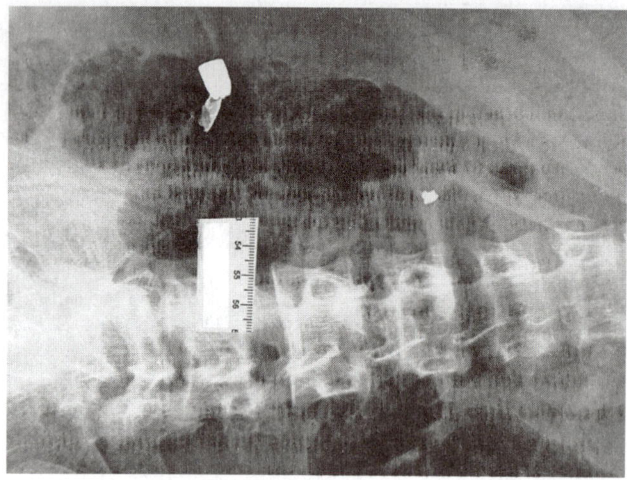

Fig. (8–92). X-ray photograph showing a fired bullet in.

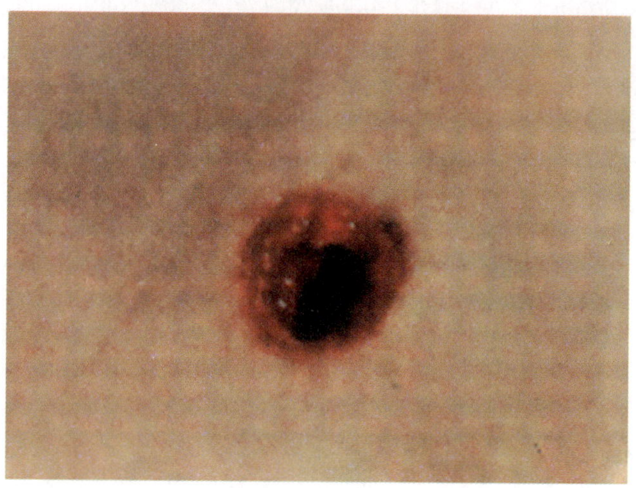

Fig. (8–93). Shored exit wound.

passed through several layers of fabric. **Each layer is blackened on both sides, while skin and wound may not show soot.** Cotton and polyester shirts allow gunpowder particles to pass freely, causing small holes in the fabric. In close shots, the clothing may absorb or filter out all of the products of discharge except the bullet. **An entrance hole in clothing, if made by a lead or full metal-jacketed bullet, may produce a grey to black rim known as "bullet wipe"** (grease, soot or debris from the barrel of the gun). Sometimes, pieces of cloth are carried into the wound of entrance.

Exit (outshot) Wounds: If the bullet fragments on impact, an exit wound may not occur. The bullet may be reduced to granules, and there may be difficulty to remove them from the body, even when identified by X-ray **Fig. (8–92)**. **Full metal-jacketed bullets usually exit undeformed. Exit wounds may vary considerably in size and shape Figs. (8–90 and 8–93). They may be round, stellate, cruciate, elliptical, crescent-shaped. An exit wound produced by a low velocity bullet or a tumbling bullet or a bullet passing sideways through the tissues may be elongated or slit-like resembling a stab, incised or lacerated wound.** The same appearance may be seen in a part of the body in which the skin folds or changes direction, e.g., in the buttock crease, under the arm, or in the groin or umbilical area. **Exit wounds of the head are usually star-shaped resembling contact entrance wounds. In some cases, the entrance and exit wounds may look alike. The exit wound is of help in determining:** (1) the direction of fire, (2) posture of the victim at the time of the shooting, and (3) the number of bullets in the body. **When the weapon has been fired in contact with the bone or at very close range, the exit wound is usually smaller than the wound of entrance. With increased range, the exit wound is larger than the wound of entrance. With high velocity bullet, the two wounds may be of the same size.** The edges of the exit wound may be puckered or torn and everted and pieces of contused, haemorrhagic subcutaneous fat may protrude through the defect. The edges are free from signs of burning, blackening or tattooing and there is no contusion or abrasion collar Table (8–12).

Shored exit wounds: If the skin at the exit wound is firmly supported, the exit wound appears as a circular or nearly

Table (8–12). Difference between wounds of entrance and exit of a bullet wound

	Trait	Entrance wound	Exit wound
(1)	Size :	Smaller than the diameter of the bullet. In close discharge, skin is torn.	Bigger than the bullet.
(2)	Edges :	Inverted.	Everted, puckered or torn.
(3)	Bruising, abrasion and grease collar:	Present.	Absent.
(4)	Burning, blackening, tattooing:	May be seen around the wound.	Absent.
(5)	Bleeding:	Less.	More.
(6)	Fat:	No protrusion except in contact shot.	May protrude.
(7)	Tissues within and around the wound:	May be cherry-red due to CO of explosive gases.	No colour change.
(8)	Approximation of edges:	Retains a small central defect.	Re-establishes skin's integrity.
(9)	Fibers of clothing:	Turned in and may be carried into the wound.	Turned out.
(10)	Lead ring or metal ring:	May be seen around the wound by radiological examination.	Absent.
(11)	Spectrography:	More metal is found around entrance wound, if bullet has only passed through soft tissues.	The exit wound may contain more metal if a bone is struck nearer to it.

circular defect surrounded by a margin of abrasion (usually broader than that of entry wound), resembling a wound of entrance (shored or supported exit wound). The shored type of exit wound caused by a bullet fired at long range or through clothing, or when the firearm is of small caliber and discharged in contact with the skin at a point where bone is not immediately below the skin surface, resembles wound of entry. Many shored exit wounds are caused if a firm object, e.g., a belt, the waist band of trousers, etc., brassiere, collar and tie, is pressed against the body at the site of exit wound, or if the body is leaning against a hard surface such as a wall, back of a chair or the floor, door, car seat, mattress, bedding, or if the person was lying down. In such cases the skin, crushed by the exiting bullet, produces an irregular, lopsided and large abrasion around or adjacent to the wound ("shored" exit wound). **In a fatty person, the edges of both the wounds of entrance and exit may be everted due to protrusion of fat. They may also be everted in decomposed bodies.**

Variations in exit wounds: The variation in the shape and large size of exit wound are due to: (1) The bullet tumbles in the body and fails to exit nose-end first. (2) The bullet is deformed. (3) The bullet breaks up in the tissues and exits as several pieces. (4) Fragments of the bone may be blown out of the body with the bullet. (5) The unsupported skin at the exit tends to tear and break into pieces. (6) Composition and velocity of missile. Rarely, slit-like exit wounds are seen probably due to the deformity of the bullet, caused by impact of the bullet on bone during its passage through the body. Such wounds are mostly seen on the head and over the shoulders. Occasionally, a bullet may be found protruding from an exit wound. In incomplete exit wound, bullet lacerates the skin, but is trapped and lodged within skin wound.

Sometimes an exit wound may be caused by a fragment of bone being expelled through the skin, but the bullet may remain in the body, or the jacket may separate and remain in the body and the bullet causing exit wound.

Large entry wounds: Entry wound may be larger than exit due to: (1) tearing of soft tissues by inrushing gases, (2) tumbling or yawning of bullet, (3) breaking of bullet with only a portion of it exiting, (4) tangential entry with focal avulsion of tissues, (5) bullet entering through folded or creased skin.

Revolvers and automatic pistols cause similar wounds, but penetrating power of bullets of pistols is much greater because of the greater velocity and because of their being coated with hard metal.

WOUNDS FROM RIFLE: The wounds inflicted on the body are similar to pistol wounds but produce more damage. They vary considerably and produce most unexpected results. The flame may extend up to 15 to 20 cm. Unburnt powder grains and small metallic particles are not found beyond one metre. Smoke is absent beyond 30 cm. from the muzzle.

In contact wounds, the burning and tattooing is not much. The blast effects are also much less and the splitting of the clothes or tissues is the same as that with the revolvers. The entrance and exit wounds may be of the same size and shape, if the bullet passes through the body without touching the bone; but even when no resistant structure is touched, there may be explosive effects and severe lacerated exit wounds. The entrance wound is usually smaller than the diameter of the bullet and looks like a wound made by forcing lead pencil into skin. Abrasion collar may not be present but the edges are depressed, may have microtears 1 to 2 mm in length, radiating from complete circumference of wound, and surrounded by a reddish zone which becomes brown on drying. Bruising of the deeper tissues around the track of the bullet is seen. If the bullet strikes at an angle, the skin may split or be turned up. If it strikes a bone, extensive shattering and comminution of bone takes place. In such cases, the wound of exit is usually a lacerated hole, varying from about 2.5 cm. to the size of the palm of the hand. Frequently, several small holes will be found around the large exit caused by fragments of bone being driven out. Bullet fragmentation is much more common in rifle injuries than those due to handguns. In wounds of the head within 300 metres, the brain is frequently pulped and a great part of the cranium slashed into fragments.

A bullet leaving the muzzle of service rifle rotates or spins round its long axis at the rate of about 2,500 revolutions per second, and for the first 200 to 300 metres, the base of the projectile has also a circular motion round the axis of flight, gradually losing this motion and continuing to spin in the true axis. If a resistant body is struck within a range of 200 to 300 metres, the effect produced by the spin of the bullet together with the intense liberation of energy is similar to that of an explosion, the tissues themselves exploding, not the bullet. This explains the shattering of bones such as pelvis, femur, skull, etc. It also explains the severe laceration seen even when a rifle bullet fired at short range passes through soft tissues only. At these ranges, the bullet commonly disintegrates, and causes effects which give the impression that more than one shot has been fired. Between 300 to 1,000 metres, the spin of the bullet becomes regular, and it passes easily through the tissues and cuts a clean hole through the bones. Beyond this, it behaves like a low-velocity bullet.

ALTERATION OF GUNSHOT WOUNDS: The appearance of a gunshot wound can be altered by the following conditions: (1) Drying of margins of the wound opening. (2) Decomposition of the body. (3) Healing of the wound itself. (4) Interference by emergency care personnel. (5) Surgical operation. (6) Interference by non-professional personnel at scene of death. (7) Washing or cleaning of the wound after death.

Airgun injuries: The missile is single and fired through a rifled barrel. 0.177 and 0.22 inch calibers are common. The pellet can enter skull and traverse whole width of brain but never produce an exit wound. They entry wound is small, but may show abrasion collar. There is no burning, blackening or tattooing.

X-RAY EXAMINATION OF GUNSHOT WOUND VICTIMS: It helps to (1) locate the bullet or pellets Fig. (8–75), (2) locate bullet fragments or jackets, (3) show the track of the bullet. Internal ricochet within the skull may be demonstrated, which helps to determine the direction of the fire, (4) determine the break up pattern of the bullet. This may also indicate the type of ammunition used, (5) determine defects in bone, (6) bullet embolism, (7) locate air embolism accompanying large vessel damage by the missile

ATYPICAL ENTRANCE WOUNDS: (1) (a) For a few microseconds after the bullet leaves the muzzle (up to about 50 metres for a pistol or 150 metres for a rifle), there may be a "TAIL WOBBLE' OR "TAIL WAG". This is partly responsible for the great tissue damage and the large atypical entrance wound at short range.

(b) The gyroscopic effect of the bullet diminishes as it reaches the end of its flight, until it begins to wobble, and then to tumble. In wobble, yaw or tumble, the impact of the bullet may be sideways or even backwards with an irregular lateral motion, due to which an irregular lacerated wound is produced. A bullet travelling in an irregular fashion instead of travelling nose-on is called a YAWNING BULLET, and a bullet that rotates end-on-end during its motion is called a TUMBLING BULLET. The amount of tissue crush might be three times greater when the bullet yaws to 90°.

(c) The tattooing seen on the skin may be altered by the use of 'silencers'. Muzzle-brakes and flash-hiders may produce peculiar blackening and tattooing patterns by allowing gases to pass in specific

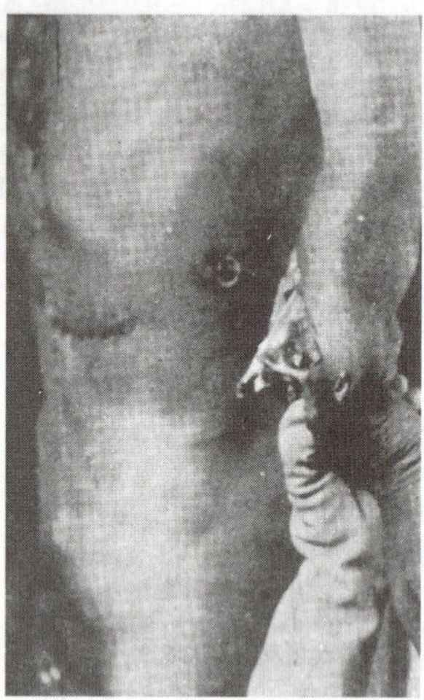

Fig. (8–94). Rifle bullet passing through the forearm and abdomen.

direction. Bullets fired through a shortened or sawn-off barrel, may be deformed or squeezed.

(d) In revolvers, weapon defects, such as cylinder misalignment will cause deformities of the missile, with breaking off of the metal fragments from the bullet occurring when the misalignment is great. Lesser defects of this type may cause tumbling.

RICOCHET BULLET: A ricochet bullet is one which before striking the object aimed at, strikes some intervening object first, and then after recocheting and rebounding (glancing) from these, hits the object. They are rare, as most bullets on striking a hard surface break up or penetrate the surface. The deflection of the bullet is partly due to the obliquity with which it strikes and partly due to rotating motion on its axis. **The critical angle of impact for ricochet for hard surfaces varies from 10 to 30º.** The bullet ricochets off at an angle smaller than the impact angle. The bullet may ricochet before or after striking the body and may produce a non-penetrating or a penetrating injury. **Ricocheting of a bullet may occur with inferior firearms and low velocity bullets. The bullet may be deformed and flattened before striking the skin Fig. (8–95). The degree of deformity varies depending on the texture of the bullet. This produces a large irregularly oval, triangular or cruciate entrance wound with irregular abraded margins. As the bullet loses gyrating movements, abrasion collar is absent. Burning, blackening and tattooing are also not seen.** Sometimes, a bullet may strike an object and tumble, and hit the body side on, producing an elongated wound of entrance like a keyhole. **The path of a ricochet is completely unexpected.** Particles of the substance against which the bullet is deflected or has struck, e.g., soil, fibres, paints, etc. may be found adhering to the bullet. The nose of the bullet may be found facing the entrance wound due to deflection in the body. **When the velocity is lost, the bullet only produces an abrasion or contusion.** Jacketed bullets have a greater ricochet potential than unjacketed bullets.

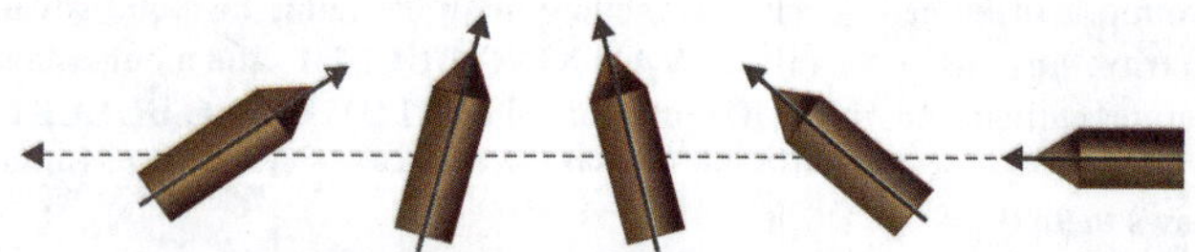

Fig. (8–95). Schematic depiction of "tumble' associated with missiles of very high velocities.

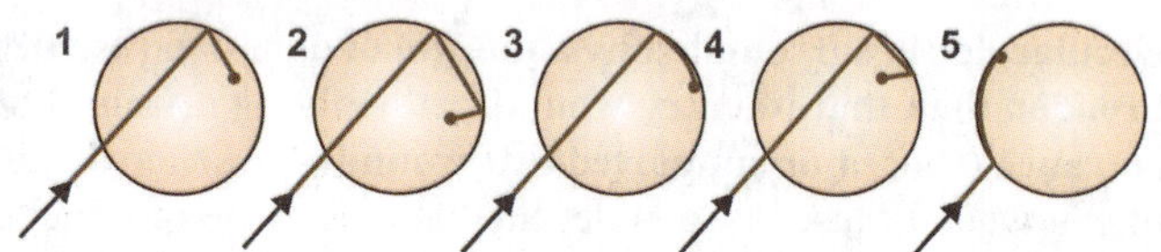

Fig. (8–96). Internal ricochet. (1) Single ricochet. (2) Double ricochet. (3) Inner tangential at contralateral side. (4) Inner tangential at contralateral side and ricochet. (5) Inner tangential at entrance side.

Internal ricochet: Sometimes, after passing through the brain, there is not enough energy left in the bullet to penetrate the skull. **It may rebound (ricochet) from the inner table of the skull like a billiard ball, producing a second track. If it ricochets for a second time, a third wound track is produced.** If the bullet enters the skull at an acute angle towards the inner table, it may move along the dura tearing the leptomeninges and blood vessels and produce a shallow wound track along the surface of the brain. The inner divergent course of the bullet may be combined with internal ricochet Fig. (8–96). **A bullet striking at a small angle with the surface may follow the curvature of the skull or a rib and emerge some distance away after having made a track in the subcutaneous tissues.**

(f) The bullet may strike the surface producing a contusion and fall to the ground. This is seen with relatively soft non-jacketed bullet fired from a firearm that has an eroded or worn barrel; and also when the ammunition used is of smaller size than the barrel of the gun.

(g) BULLET GRAZE OR SLAP: If a bullet strikes skin at so acute an angle that it does not perforate the skin, a grazing or slap wound is produced. It usually appears as reddish-brown, elongated, elliptical or triangular furrow or abrasion. The underlying dermis may or may not be involved, but the adjacent intact skin may be ecchymosed.

(h) The bullet strikes the sternum at just the right angle and is deflected, so that it continues around the rib cage, between the bone and the skin. It may come out at the back of the body after causing only a superficial injury; or it may lodge between the skin and the backbone.

Bullets that strike in unusual location may cause injury and death, but the wound of entry may be difficult to locate, e.g., ear, nostril, mouth, axilla, vagina and rectum.

(2) SINGLE ENTRANCE AND MULTIPLE EXITS: If the bullet splits up within the body and divides itself into 3 or 4 pieces, there will be only one entry hole, but several exits. The bullet striking a bone may break the bone into fragments, which act as secondary missiles producing multiple exits. Sometimes, the jacket of a bullet may separate from the inner part upon impact on a firm object, such as a button, a coin, a key in the pocket or on bone. In such cases, the jacket and the core each produce separate tracks. With the semi-jacketed bullet, lead core usually exits, and the jacket remains in the body. Sometimes, a fragment of metal separates from the bullet during its passage through the skull. The separated fragment proceeds under the skin until it exits at a distance of 3 to 5 cm. or remains lodged between the skull and the skin. The major part of the bullet will enter the skull and may exit in a different position. In such a case, a single bullet will produce two exit wounds. In bullet wounds of the head, many lead fragments may be found scattered throughout the brain and on X-ray may closely resemble a shotgun injury.

(3) BULLET STRIKING THE SKULL BUT NOT ENTERING IT: Bullets may graze or rub the top and sides of the cranium without entering it. In such cases, entry and exit wounds are found on the scalp about two to three cm. apart, while the skull between the two wounds shows an oval or elongated gutter-like depression (gutter wound; key-hole defect). When the bullet strikes the skull at an angle, it may rarely deviate from its path by impact on the bone, to produce a continuous

wound track under the skin without penetration of the skull. The track may proceed for considerable distance, the bullet following the curvature of the skull.

(4) MULTIPLE WOUNDS OF ENTRANCE AND EXIT FROM A SINGLE SHOT: A bullet may pass through an arm and the chest so that four wounds result. A bullet passing through the chest or abdomen and thigh and lower leg, produces six wounds. This occurs when the person is running or sitting in an unusual position. When the body surface is irregular, such as the breast or buttocks, several re-entries and exits can take place. In such cases, examination of clothing and detection of nitrites and nitrates and microscopic examination of the sections of the wound is useful. The features of re-entry wound resemble those of wounds caused by long range fire.

(5) ENTRANCE WOUND IS PRESENT BUT BULLET IS NOT FOUND IN THE BODY: This occurs when (a) the bullet entering the stomach may be vomited, (b) entering the windpipe may be coughed up, (c) entering the mouth may be spit out, (d) entering the gastrointestinal tract may be passed out in the faeces, and (e) when it is so deviated or turned on coming in contact with the bone, that it passes out by the same wound as it entered.

(6) UNEXPLAINED BULLETS IN THE BODY: **Occasionally, more bullets are found than there are entrance wounds.** This **occurs, due to defect in the weapon, or due to faulty ammunition, or with loaded firearm unused for several years** due to prolonged exposure to high environmental temperature or humidity. **When such a weapon is fired, the bullet travels a little distance within the barrel and may fail to come out from the muzzle. When it is fired again, the second bullet may go off carrying the lodged bullet with it, and both the bullets may enter the body through the same entrance wound.** This is called a **tandem bullet or piggyback bullet** (tandem=one behind the other) Fig. (8–97). The bullets may separate within the body, or before they hit the target. **The features caused by flame, smoke and gunpowder may be diminished or absent** and the wound may appear as if caused by long-range fire. This is because the pushing force of the second bullet is directed backwards due to obstruction caused by first bullet impacted in the barrel.

Souvenir Bullets: **If a bullet is present for a long time in the body, there will be no fresh bleeding in the surrounding area. A dense fibrous tissue capsule usually surrounds it.** A small scar indicates the original entrance wound. Lead poisoning may occur due to absorption of lead from lead bullets remaining in a body. Synovial fluid is capable of dissolving lead.

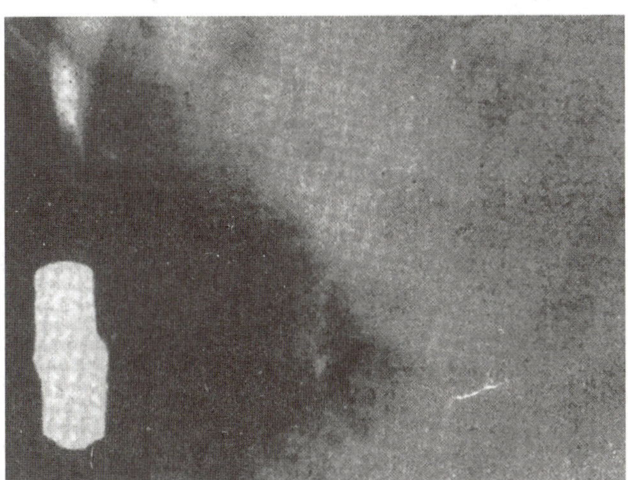

Fig. (8–97). Tandem bullet in the chest.

(7) FATALITIES WITH BLANK CARTRIDGES: A blank cartridge is one containing primer, gunpowder and wadding, but without a bullet or pellets. It contains ultrafast burning powder that explodes rather than burns. Wounds can be caused from the gases or from the closing part in the end of the cartridge. Wadding or gunpowder may cause laceration and may produce death from shock by pressure on nerves or by damaging main vessels, when blank cartridge is discharged close to the body. Distant shots with blank cartridge are harmless.

(8) FIREARM GOING OFF BY ITSELF: The firearm can go off by itself without any one touching the trigger due to some defect in its mechanism. Country-made guns and old worn guns may discharge on being pushed or thrown, or by the butt being dropped against the ground.

(9) FRANGIBLE BULLETS: They are designed to fragment upon impact, often to the point of disintegration. They are made mostly by lead or iron. Recovery and matching with a test bullet is difficult. If bone is penetrated, they are usually recovered in an eroded state. They do not ricochet.

(10) In some bullets, the component parts tend to separate on impact. Such bullets are partially jacketed at the base, with the tip remaining an uncovered lead core. The components separate on striking the body and create their own tracks.

(11) DUPLEX OR TANDEM CARTRIDGE: This is used in military rifles, and contains two bullets which enter the target at different points, separated by as much as 30 cm. The base of the forward bullet is notched, into which the second bullet fits closely. The base of the 'follow' bullet is not quite at right angle to its long axis, due to which there is a difference in line of movement of both the bullets.

(12) ARTEFACTS: (A) Surgical alteration or suturing of gunshot wounds create problems. The evaluation of the wound, whether it was an entrance or an exit wound becomes difficult (Kennedy phenomenon).

(13) BULLET EMBOLISM: Bullets entering an artery embolise into the femoral and popliteal arteries. With less frequent venous embolism, bullets enter veins of the lower limb or heart.

CONCEALED FIREARM WOUNDS: If the body is covered with blood, the blood clots may obscure the injury. A wound in the mouth, nostril, ear, eye, or in any of the body orifices, e.g., rectum or vagina may not be detected, if due care is not taken.

SCENE OF CRIME: Photographs: Before any items of evidence are moved, photographs must be taken from different angles to show respective positions of various items of evidence, including the victim. Photographs should also be taken after various objects are moved, for cartridge cases or bullets may be found under the victim's body, or they may be hidden by pieces of furniture, etc. Bullet holes in the walls, floor, ceiling or in the furniture should be photographed. Before undressing, the body should be photographed. After the clothes are removed, entrance and exit bullet holes should be photographed with identifying labels and rulers. The bullets, pellets, and wadding found in the body should be photographed. All areas likely to bear suspect's fingerprints, such as door knobs, glassware and the weapon should be examined for fingerprints.

EVIDENCE FROM SCENE: Collect: (1) The gun. (2) Fired bullets. (3) Empty cartridge cases, shells and wads. (4) Hairs, fibres and bloodstains. (5) Objects struck by or containing spent bullets, e.g., wood, cement, etc. (6) Glass shattered by bullets. (7) Areas showing fingerprints and footprints.

EVIDENCE FROM SUSPECT: Collect: (1) Clothes with trace evidence. (2) Victim's hair, clothing, fibres and blood. (3) Gunpowder and other evidence on the hands. (4) If there is a firearm at the scene, note (a) Exactly where found (b) Type of weapon (shotgun, rifle, revolver, pistol, etc.). (c) Mark initials on the butt or frame of the weapon. (d) Roll the weapon in a paper and send to the laboratory. (5) Unspent ammunition and empty cartridges or shells.

AUTOPSY: (A) CLOTHING: Clothes should be examined in situ and in relation to the injuries in the body. Take photographs. Cover the tears on clothes with cellophane sheets to prevent loss of residues.

Remove clothing layer by layer. List them all, and note their condition and the extent of blood-staining. Record the number and location of bullet holes. It is sufficient to describe the number of bullet holes in the outer garment and adding that bullet holes in the remaining clothes correspond in location to the outer garment. The location of bullet holes in clothes should be described in relation to the distance from collar, seams, pockets, heel level, etc. A single bullet may produce several holes due to the presence of folds in the garment, and simulate more than one shot. The holes in the clothing should be connected to those in the body to determine the direction of fire. The clothes should be dried. If damp clothes are packed, shrinkage may occur and position of the hole of the entry of the missile altered. Examination of the clothes help: (1) to establish the range at which the firearm was discharged, from the deposition of soot or powder tattooing, (2) to establish which defects are wound of entry or exit, (3) to locate the bullet. If no exit wound is present, either the clothing did not cover the area of the exit, or the bullet may be in clothing or fell away. The size of the bullet hole and the extent of soot and powder distribution should be measured and the density of tattooing noted. Note whether the fibres of the clothing are turned inwards or outwards. Clothing may be forced into the tissues in shotgun wounds. Probes, fingers, etc. should not be introduced through the defects in the clothing, as the direction or distribution of fibres will be changed and cause confusion in deciding the entrance and exit of a bullet.

Cover the tears on clothes with cellophane sheets to prevent loss of residues. The clothes should be preserved carefully in clean brown paper or plastic bags and sent to Forensic Science Laboratory for testing. The powder grains adherent to clothing should be carefully removed with forceps and preserved in a glass vial, as they may be lost from the clothes due to rough handling. Clothes should be folded in such a way, that the area of bullet holes and gunpowder soiling are not disturbed or contaminated. Infrared photography can be used to find out soot deposit on dark coloured or black fabrics. Ordinary X-ray can be used to search for larger metallic fragments for elemental content.

Number the entrance and exit wounds. In the case of multiple wounds, it is advisable to give a number to each wound, disregarding whether it was caused by entry or exit of a bullet.

Radiography of the relevant part of the body should be done to locate missiles, fractures, preumothorax and pneumoperitoneum.

(B) BULLET WOUNDS: If there are multiple wounds, they should be numbered. On the body diagrams, the wounds should be drawn as they appear on the body including burning, blackening, tattooing, abrasion collar, etc. Photographs of the wounds should be taken. Bullet wounds must be described with care: (a) the exact location of each wound should be noted in relation to its distance from the top of the head or the sole of the foot, (b) midline of the body, (c) a fixed anatomical landmark, e.g., "in the chest, 50 cm. below the top of the head, 8 cm. to the left of the midline and 2 cm. above the nipple". The size and the exact appearance of the wound is not preserved after excision due to the cutting of the elastic fibres.

(C) EXTERNAL WOUND: (1) (a) The character of the perforation, its shape (stellate, round, slit-like or irregular), and size should be noted. The hole in the skin should be carefully measured first, and then the abrasion collar and the powder pattern surrounding the borders of the entrance wound. Difference in the width of the abrasion collar at different points should be noted as they indicate the angle at which the bullet struck the skin. A circular wound requires only one diameter of measurements, e.g., the skin perforation is round and measured 8 mm. in width. It is surrounded by a uniform rim abrasion 2 mm. in width. An elliptical wound is measured across its widest and narrowest diameters and variations in width of abrasion recorded, e.g., the skin perforation measured 8 mm. by 3 mm. with the larger diameter running horizontally. A rim abrasion measuring from 0.5 mm. to 2 mm. surrounds the skin perforation with the wider area located at its lateral side. (b) The presence or absence of blackening and tattooing should be specifically noted, e.g., blackening and tattooing are absent, or the skin perforation is surrounded by an area of blackening and tattooing measuring 8 cm. by 5 cm. with the larger diameter running vertically. (c) Skin splits, contiguous and non-contiguous. (d) Muzzle imprint. (e) Soot deposit, including the corona. (f) Metal deposition. It is advisable to record the wound in the skin and the wound track through the body in one section. If the entrance wound is soiled with blood, it should be sponged carefully so that any tattooing of the skin may not be disturbed. After the wound has been examined, the skin around the entrance and exit wounds should be cut out including at least 2.5 cm. of the skin around and 5 mm. beneath the wound. They should be packed separately in rectified spirit, labelled and sent to the Forensic Science Laboratory.

ALTERATION BY MEDICAL CARE PERSONNEL: If surgical wounds are made on a shotgun or stabbing victim, the surgeon should make adequate documentation of their location and nature in his records or on the hospital chart, so as to prevent confusion, if the patient dies and an autopsy is performed. A scaled photograph or a diagram showing the numbered wounds is useful.

(D) TRACK TAKEN BY THE BULLET THROUGH THE BODY: Bullet tracks should be numbered and described individually. Probes should not be introduced through the track. The path taken by the bullet through the body should be carefully traced by dissection with the organs in situ. When multiple wounds are present, do not match up cutaneous entrance wounds with cutaneous exit wounds without verifying their pathways through the body. All the projectile paths in the torso should be followed through the body cavities. It is useful to measure the height of both entrance and exit wounds from the undersurface of the heel. This shows the direction of the track, and also the height above the ground at which the bullet entered and left the body, if the person was in standing position when struck. The bullet track should be described in relation to the planes of the body: (1) from front to back or from back to front, (2) from left to right or from right to left, (3) from above downwards (caudad), or from below upwards (cephalad). Angular estimates, i.e., vertical, horizontal and sagittal planes of the body are also useful to complete the description. To release the bullet from the bone without actually handling it, the segment of bone containing the bullet should be excised, or sawed, followed by manual bending. Frequently, the track of the bullet is unpredictable due to its deflection by bone, and the bullet may be found in a most unexpected situation. This point is very important when the question arises in the case of two wounds being found on the body not corresponding to the likely line of the track, as to whether they have been produced by one or two bullets. The bullet may take a straight path through the body, and in this case the relative positions of the entrance and exit wounds will indicate the direction of fire. When a cavity has been penetrated and blood has collected, the bullet should be searched in the effused blood. A high velocity bullet is rarely deflected. **To avoid prolonged search for the bullet in the body, X-ray examination should be done before autopsy.** Rib borders or the border of other bones must be examined for roughening or fracture, which may explain the deflection of bullet. If there are multiple tracks, each should be followed from the point of entrance to termination. The track made by the bullet widens as it goes deeper. If a bullet grazes a bone, it may produce a gutter with or without fracturing it. If a bullet passes through the bone, a track of tiny radio-opaque metallic particles removed from the surface of the bullet will be seen in X-ray. The size of pellets is difficult to measure after the shot is fired as it becomes deformed. All bullets and recognisable parts of bullets in the victim must be recovered, and described as to where it was found, whether it is intact, deformed or fragmented, whether the bullet is lead or jacketed, etc. Next to bone, the skin offers the greatest resistance to the penetration of a bullet. A bullet passing through the body may come to rest just underneath the skin on the opposite side. The type of missile and the point of recovery should be noted. The location and character of exit wounds should be noted. All wadding in the body should be recovered to know gauge of the shotgun and the type of ammunition.

When a rapidly travelling object is slowed by passing from a thin to a dense medium, there is a release of kinetic energy which may be so violent as to fracture bones in the immediate vicinity of the track although the bones are not actually struck. Shock waves will also pass through the tissues causing injury to organs, remote from the actual wound. When a high velocity missile passes through soft tissue, it is followed by cavitation due to the released energy. This primary cavity then collapses, and is followed by lesser secondary cavitation, which creates a negative pressure and debris is sucked into the track. When a high velocity missile strikes a relatively solid internal organ, such as the heart, this organ may disintegrate as if an explosive charge has been detonated in its substance.

BULLET TRACK IN THE BRAIN: Part of the energy of the bullet is spent by the tip to break the resistance of the tissues, and another part to push the tissues aside. This radial displacement producing transient cavitation is important with regard to the severity of tissue damage. If almost all the energy of the bullet is lost during penetration of the scalp, bone and dura, it passes through the brain without producing cavitation until it comes to rest. If the bullet passes through the brain with great velocity, the wound track expands immediately after the bullet has passed through. This expansion develops in few microseconds, during which time brain is suddenly pressed against the inner table of the skull and other firm structures, and momentarily bulges out of entrance and exit wounds and collapses equally fast. The track of damage may be 4 to 5 times the diameter of the bullet, as seen by a track of haemorrhagic pulped brain tissue. Prior to cavitation of brain, skull fractures result. **If the fractures extend beyond the area of entrance and exit and the cavitation is very severe, the skull may burst by the pressure of the brain. A large portion of the brain may be thrown out of the bursting skull and found relatively intact. This is known as KRONLEIN SHOT.** In such case, the entrance and exit wounds cannot be determined with certainty. If such explosion does not occur but cavitation is severe, the sudden pressure on the tissues surrounding the wound track causes immediate necrosis due to shearing forces acting on submicroscopic structures of cells. A ring of tissue haemorrhage is found outside the necrotic tissue. Contusions are also produced at a distance from the wound track due to displacement of portions of the brain due to the sudden space-occupying entrance of the bullet into the brain and by the associated cavitation. They occur independently of the location. **There may be herniation contusions of the parahippocampal gyri and cerebral tonsils, caused as the brain tissues are violently thrust against the edge of the tentorium and foramen magnum respectively.** Orbital plates may be fractured. Small caliber, low velocity bullets produce cavitation but fail to perforate the head on the opposite side. Sometimes, the entire track or one segment of it is found several times larger than the bullet. This occurs when the bullet passes sideways through the tissues or when it tumbles.

EXPLODED BULLETS: Bullets may be found in or on bodies either due to being fired from a gun or having been discharged from the cartridge as a result of heat-induced explosion. **An exploded bullet does not show land-and-groove markings and the cartridge case is devoid of firing-pin impression. Intense fire causes melting of ammunition and leaves a pool of molten lead which may stick to the body as tiny droplets.** X-ray shows "birdshot" pattern in films.

DESCRIPTION OF A FIREARM WOUND: There is a gunshot wound of entrance in the left anterior thoracic wall. This is just above and immediately medial to the left nipple and is situated 40 cm. below the top of the head and 10 cm. to the left of the midline. The wound is circular in shape, 0.8 cm. in diameter, and is made up of a 0.2 cm. radial dimensional abrasion ring concentrically placed about a 0.4 cm. diameter defect. There is no soot deposit or powder tattooing. A small amount of blood comes out from the defect upon manipulation of the body. A track is established from the gunshot wound of entrance on the left anterior thoracic wall, passes through the third interspace, through the lingua of the left lung, through seventh thoracic vertebra. Here, embedded in the bone, is recovered a full metal jacketed bullet of 0.25 caliber. This is marked 'X' and retained. A left haemothorax of 1200 ml. of fluid and clotted blood is present.

PRESERVATION, MARKING AND PACKING OF EXHIBITS: All bullets recovered from the body must be preserved with correct labelling of the relationship of each bullet to the corresponding wound. This is important in case of dacoity or rioting, to know which of the several weapons may have fired the fatal shot. It is important to state from which portion of the body, or from which internal organ it was removed. When more than one bullet or other foreign object has been removed from the body of a victim, or found in or about his clothing, each one should be labelled and placed in separate envelope. Care must be taken in removing a bullet from the body so that marks due to artefact, such as, scratches are not produced on the bullet. Such markings may make difficult subsequent identification of the bullet. **It is preferable to remove the bullets with bare fingers. A forceps protected with rubber tubing may be used.** The appearance of the bullet should be described accurately, e.g., intact, deformed, fragmented, lead or jacketed and the caliber if known. The bullet should be weighed, and if its base is not deformed, the diameter of the base should be measured. The recovered bullet should be dried and not washed, because washing removes the powder residue. **In shotgun injury, the doctor need not recover every pellet present. A few pellets should be recovered for the ballistic expert to determine the shot size and possibly type of ammunition. All buckshot pellets must be collected because they appear similar to bullets on X-ray examination.**

(1) FIREARMS: Identifying initials should be scratched on to gun's frame, receiver, or slide and on the gun barrel.

(2) FIRED CARTRIDGE CASES: The identification mark should be scratched on the inside of the open end. They may be wrapped in cotton and packed in cardboard boxes.

(3) FIRED BULLETS: The identification marks should be scratched on the base, or just above the riflings on the ogive but not on the end of the nose, for the nose may pick up trace evidence, e.g., the pattern of the weave of fabric through which it has passed. It is wrapped in cotton and packed in cardboard box. Each bullet should be packed separately.

(4) PELLETS, SLUGS, WADS, etc: They may be packed in cardboard box with cotton after drying and the container labelled.

(5) CLOTHES: The area of the powder tattooing should be preserved by fastening a cellophane paper over it, and packed in a box.

MEDICOLEGAL QUESTIONS

(1) IS THE INJURY CAUSED BY DISCHARGE OF FIREARM?

Firearm wounds are recognised by the appearance of clothing and examination of entrance and exit wounds, the track of the bullet, and the presence of bullet or pellets and residual matter in the clothing or around entrance wound and in the tissues.

(2) WHAT KIND OF WEAPON FIRED THE SHOT?

The kind of firearm can be determined by the size, shape and composition of the bullet, and examination of cartridge, shots and wad left in the body or found at the scene of the crime and the appearances of wounds. With the shotgun, the appearances of the wound are characteristic. In muzzle-loading gun, the wad consists of plug of paper or cloth; in breech-loading gun of circular discs of felt or cardboard, from which the bore of the gun can be determined. Stains on the clothes or skin may show whether black or smokeless powder was used, and microscopic and chemical examination of the stain is helpful in finding out the particular brand of powder. Evidence of recent fire can be made out for a few days, by examination of the weapon for mercury vapour. Spent cartridge contains residues of primer and detonator.

In firearm examination, the primary principles of identification are (1) determination of caliber and type; (2) number of rifling grooves; (3) width of rifling grooves; (4) direction (left twist or right twist) of rifling grooves; (5) pitch (angle of the spiral) of rifling. These are used to determine whether a bullet could have been fired in a type or model of a gun or specific weapon. The bullets expand into the grooves in the rifling, sealing the barrel and prevent excess escape of gases ahead of the bullet. **The firearms leave their signature on the cartridge case and on the bullet. With all rifled firearms, the bullet is slightly larger than the barrel, and as it passes through the barrel, its sides are marked by the rifling of the barrel (primary markings; class characteristics)** and cause the bullet to rotate. Class characteristics (bar codes) are determined before manufacture of the gun and result from manufacturing specifications, design and dimensions. The class characteristics in fired bullet identifications would be (1) caliber, (2) number of lands and grooves, (3) direction of twist of the rifling, (4) rate of the twist of the rifling, and (5) width of the lands and grooves. **They are most useful in identifying the make and model of gun involved. The surface of the bullet is also grooved by irregularities on the inner surface of the barrel itself (secondary markings; individual or accidental characteristics), which are specific for that particular weapon. These irregularities are produced by the sticking of the particles of the bullet to the bore when shots are fired and is known as 'metallic fouling'. Individual characteristics also result accidentally during manufacturing process, are usually microscopic in nature, and have random distribution.** These marks are more pronounced on lead bullets where the grooves score the bullet. For jacketed bullets, the land markings are more pronounced. **They are useful to identify one specific gun to the exclusion of all others ("bullet fingerprinting").** Sometimes, lead bullets may carry weave pattern of cloth. The bullet found in the body known as **crime bullet or exhibit bullet** is compared under a comparison microscope, with one fired from the suspected weapon known as **test bullet.** The suspected weapon is fired, using the same brand and type of ammunition into a box filled with cotton waste (bullet traps), a bag of rags, a sand bag, oiled saw-dust, blocks of ice, water tanks (bullet recovery tank) or against white blotting paper. Fresh pork skins, cleanly shaven are ideal for comparison with patterns on human skin.

From the fired cartridge case, the caliber and type of cartridge and its manufacturer can be determined, from the shape and size of the case and the stampings on the case head. Fired cartridge cases also may be identified with the firearm from which they were discharged by a study of the marks left on them by the weapon. They are: (1) The firing pin imparts its general shape, size and tooling imperfections, striking the primer in centrefire cartridges, or case rim in rimfire cartridge. (2) The internal pressure of firing, forces the soft brass head of the cartridge case against the breech face, which produces markings. (3) The extractor usually marks the rim of a cartridge case while withdrawing the cartridge from the chamber, but may also make marks as it slips over and engages the cartridge rim or at the time of disengaging the rim. The end of the extractor hook may produce markings against the case wall next to the head. (4) The ejector strikes the rim or head of cartridge sharply during ejection and usually leaves a mark. (5) The magazine or clip may leave both class and individual markings. Lips of a magazine usually mark the rim edges of cartridges as they are stripped from it and chambered. (6) Imperfections at the edge or mouth of the chamber will also mark the cartridge case as it is moved into and out of the chamber in loading and extraction.

(3) FROM WHAT DISTANCE AND DIRECTION WAS THE SHOT FIRED? The range of fire is determined by the presence or absence of the marks of smoke, flame, tattooing, etc., on or in the body of the victim. When the range is greater, it can be determined only approximately and with difficulty, from the nature of wounds and penetration. Test fire with suspect weapon using the same ammunition at varying distances until a similar spread of pellet markings and other findings is achieved on the target, is useful in estimating the range.

The direction of the track depends upon the posture of the body at the time of impact. The direction of fire may be determined from the position of entrance and exit wounds and the track, bearing in mind the possibility of deflection of bullet and the different relationships of the parts of the body during movement.

Sections of the skin and subcutaneous tissues taken from transcutaneous portions of bullet wound may provide evidence as to direction and range of fire. Carbonisation, desiccation or recognition of particles of debris embedded in epidermis near the bullet hole may indicate close range of fire and may distinguish entrance and exit sites. The findings of debris along the track and in laceration adjacent to it, suggest fire at contact range. The range from which the weapon was fired can be estimated by lead deposits around the entry wound. Swelling and homogenisation of dermal collagen caused by heat of bullet, is more marked at the entrance than the exit site.

(4) IF MULTIPLE WOUNDS OF ENTRANCE AND EXIT ARE PRESENT, COULD THEY HAVE BEEN PRODUCED BY A SINGLE BULLET? This has been already described.

(5) IF MULTIPLE WOUNDS ARE PRESENT, WERE THEY PRODUCED FROM THE SAME OR DIFFERENT WEAPONS? This is determined by examination of the wound and of the bullet, cartridge, shots, wad, etc.

(6) WHEN WAS THE FIREARM DISCHARGED? Tissue reaction to firearm injury is similar as for other types of injury. If black powder has been used, hydrogen sulphide may persist in the barrel for a few hours if breech is closed. The washing from barrels having discharged gunpowder are alkaline, contain nitrite, sulphate and thiosulphate. Smokeless powder leaves a dark grey deposit in the barrel of a recently discharged firearm. It forms a neutral solution with distilled water and contains nitrites and nitrates, but no sulphides. The mixture of gases of explosion has a peculiar smell, which can be noticed prominently up to 4 to 6 hours. After 24 hours no smell is experienced after the discharge of a gun. Due to backward escape of gases from a fired weapon, the hand of the person that fired the gun sometimes will receive gases and particles of unburnt powder on index finger, thumb and connecting web area. Rarely smoke deposit is found on both hands.

TESTS: (i) PARAFFIN TEST OR DERMAL NITRATE TEST: It detects gun powder residue (nitrates and nitrites). Melted paraffin is brushed on the surface of the hand. The wax is removed and inner surface of wax cast is treated with diphenylamine or diphenylbenzidine reagent. A blue colour develops where residue is present. It is obsolete.

(ii) HARRISON AND GILROY TEST: This test is not specific for firearm discharge residues, but only for certain elements or compounds to be found in such residues. This detects the presence of antimony, barium and lead. A cotton swab moistened with molar hydrochloric acid is used.

(iii) ATOMIC ABSORPTION SPECTROSCOPY (AAS) AND FLAMELESS ATOMIC ABSORPTION SPECTROSCOPY (FAAS): It detects antimony, barium and lead from primer and copper vapourised from cartridge case or the bullet jacket. Palms and backs of hands (four surfaces) are swabbed with four cotton swabs moistened with hydrochloric acid. A fifth swab is moistened with acid and used as control. This analytical system utilises high temperatures to vapourise the metallic elements of the primer residues and to detect and quantitate them. Typically the residue is deposited on the back of the firing hand of the suspect who fired the gun. Detection of primer residue in the palm suggest defense gesture rather than firing of a gun. In suicide with handgun, primer residue on the palm may be due to cradling the gun with this hand at the time of firing. With rifles and shotguns, residue is often detected on the non-firing hand that has been used to steady the muzzle against the body. If the person survives, loss of residue may occur due to washing of hand or rubbing them against different

materials. NAA and AAS can aid in (1) identifying holes in clothing, tissues, wood, etc. as bullet holes, from the presence of lead, antimony, barium and copper, (2) determining range of fire from concentration pattern of antimony around the bullet hole, (3) determining common origin of bullet fragments of shotgun pellets found at different places, from the concentrations of lead, antimony, arsenic, copper and silver in these alloys, and (4) determining from the presence of lead, antimony and barium on hands whether or not a person has fired a gun.

(iv) SCANNING ELECTRON MICROSCOPE-ENERGY DISPERSIVE X-RAY ANALYSIS (SEM-EDXA): It is the most sophisticated tool which can detect most minute traces of gunshot residue (GSR) found on the body of suspect. As a gun is fired, the GSR comprising chemical substances that burn and produce gases providing the velocity for the bullet, and metals such as antimony, barium, copper, etc. are also sprayed out and get deposited on the hands, clothes and even on the face of the person. In this gunshot residues are removed from the body using adhesive lifts. The material removed is scanned with SEM for the gunshot residues particles. The X-ray analysis capability is used to identify the chemical elements in each of the particles. The test is positive up to 12 hours after firing. The investigator can conclusively prove if the weapon was used by the suspect with a negligible margin of error.

(7) HOW LONG DID THE VICTIM SURVIVE? It depends on the cause of death, i.e., whether from shock and haemorrhage, injury to a vital organ or septic complications.

(8) HOW MUCH ACTIVITY COULD THE VICTIM PERFORM FOLLOWING THE INJURY? This varies considerably depending on the site of injury and the organ involved. If the bullet destroys motor area, brain stem or cervical cord or if a gaping laceration of the heart or aorta is produced, the victim becomes immediately incapacitated. Death is instantaneous if medulla is involved. Sometimes, through-and -through bullet wounds of the brain or heart do not cause immediate disability and the person may be able to carry out voluntary acts. In transection of a major coronary artery, prolonged survival is unlikely. Wounds of the auricles are most rapidly fatal; wounds of the right ventricle come next and the wounds of the left ventricle are the least rapidly fatal. The amount and rapidity of blood loss will also help to form an opinion about the extent of physical activity that would be possible. In any injury to other parts of the body, the victim may be able to walk about.

(9) IS IT A CASE OF HOMICIDE, SUICIDE OR ACCIDENT? In deciding the status of a particular case, all the available information should be obtained, including autopsy findings, the investigation of scene of death and the circumstances of the shooting. Each case will present its own problems Table (8–13).

(A) THE POSITION AND DIRECTION OF THE WOUND: These are very important. For suicide the sites of election are: (1) temple (about 60%), (2) centre of forehead, (3) roof of mouth, (4) midline behind the chin, and (5) left side or front of chest.

A SUICIDE using a revolver or pistol, usually shoots himself in the right temple region, (right handed person), the bullet passing almost horizontally or upwards and backwards through the head, and making its exit in the left parietal region. If the individual is left-handed, left temporal region is selected. Occasionally, a right-handed person holds the weapon with the butt projecting backwards and the thumb on the trigger, in which case the direction may be different. Sometimes, the gun is put into the mouth, nose, ear or on the face or undersurface of the chin, and fired upward into the brain. In some cases, the suicide interposes his hand between the pistol and his head, shooting himself through the palm of the hand. Suicidal wounds of the chest and abdomen are less common. On the chest, the gun is fired into the cardiac region in a backward direction with a slight deviation upwards or downwards either to the right or left. On the abdomen, the gun is fired into the epigastric region and produces perforations and lacerations of the upper abdominal viscera.

In rifle and shotgun, the butt is usually supported by ground and the weapon is fired by hand into the head, or the butt is supported against a wall and fired into the chest or abdomen. The person may attach some string or cord to the trigger and tie the loose end to his foot, lie down and discharge the weapon through the roof of his mouth. He may tie the cord to some firm structure and pull the barrel towards him, thus firing the weapon or he may press the trigger with a stick or some similar object. The presence of blood splashes on the hand which held the gun or the presence of an impression of the trigger or trigger guard on one or more fingers indicates suicide.

In **HOMICIDE**, a great variety of wounds can occur depending upon the circumstances. If there is a scuffle, some of the wounds may be from close range and the bullets may strike the body in various places and at different angles. If the victim runs, most of the entrance wounds will be on the back. If victim rushes at the assailant, the entrance wounds are on front of the body. If the assailant is in a panic or under strong emotion, a number of shots may miss the target or graze the skin. Wounds about the sides and limbs are suggestive of murder, if accident is excluded, and wounds about the back, and back of head are strongly suggestive of murder. Premeditated, calculated homicide by shooting can occur in a variety of ways. In gang feuds, the victim may be surprised and shot by enemies at close range into the back of the head and neck, with the bullet tracks parallel or only slightly deviating.

(B) THE NATURE OF THE ENTRANCE WOUNDS: This is very important. A contact wound is possibly suicidal, unless found on a part of the body which is not easily reached by the deceased, e.g., back of the chest or neck. Suicides usually pull the clothes aside to expose the skin before shooting themselves. Bullets vertically entering fatal parts like heart or head, indicate suicide. Several methods (combined suicides) or several attempts of committing suicide e.g., hanging and shooting indicate suicide. A close or distant shot is rarely suicidal.

(C) THE NUMBER OF WOUNDS: Multiple wounds are usually homicidal especially if they occur on the back or sides of the body or involve different regions of the body or are non-contact shots. Occasionally, multiple suicidal wounds are seen involving a single region like the temple, chest or abdomen or a combination of two different regions. When multiple suicidal wounds are fired serially, the injuries by the first shot do not incapacitate the victim immediately, enabling him to fire other bullets into his body. A bullet passing through the brain, causes

Table (8–13). Difference between suicidal, accidental and homicidal firearm wounds

	Trait	Suicide	Accident	Homicide
(1)	Site of entrance wound:	Head or heart.	Any area.	Any area.
(2)	Shot distance:	Contact or very close range.	Close or very close range.	Any range.
(3)	Direction:	Upward or backward.	Any direction.	Usually upward.
(4)	Number of wounds:	Usually one.	One.	One to many.
(5)	Hand pressing trigger:	Powder residue present.	Powder residue present.	Powder residue absent.
(6)	Position of the weapon:	Found at the scene.	Found at the scene.	Not found at the scene.
(7)	Scene:	Usually in his own house.	In his house or while hunting, etc.	Any place.
(8)	Sex:	Usually males.	Usually males.	Any sex.
(9)	Motive:	Insanity, incurable illness, financial loss, etc.	Nil.	Gang feuds, robbery, revenge, etc.

immediate unconsciousness, but if bone is involved without injury to the brain or a large vessel, the person may retain consciousness and power of motion. A bullet passing through the chest or abdominal viscera, in some cases does not incapacitate the victim and he may be able to shoot himself again.

(D) THE POSITION OF THE WEAPON: In suicide and accident, the weapon is usually found at the scene of the crime; the gun may bear the victim's fingerprints. The hand that fired the shot may show evidence of gunsmoke, powder deposits and traces of metals. With handguns, the effects of the components of a shot are commonly seen on the thumb, index finger and the area between them. Blood splashes may soil the gun and the hand, if the hand pulling the trigger is close to the wound. In cases of murder, weapon is usually not found near the victim. If the weapon is strongly grasped in the hand of the victim due to instantaneous rigor, it is a strong presumptive evidence of suicide.

In some cases of homicide, the scene may be altered to simulate suicide in order to conceal the crime. The assailant after producing a contact wound on the anterior surface of the body or an accessible part of head, may place the weapon in the hand of the deceased. In such cases, the thumb is usually found under and not around the gun handle, and the weapon is not tightly grasped. If the gun has been tampered with after shooting, e.g., removing of empty cartridge and substituting of unexploded cartridge, causes confusion. The absence of weapon is not conclusive of murder, for it may be removed by a person passing the place or in some fatal cases, the deceased is able to walk considerable distance, leaving the weapon behind.

(E) MOTIVE: When a person commits suicide, he usually has a motive, and he may leave a note or make preparations to kill himself.

(F) THE SCENE: Photographs of the scene, the body and the gun should be taken. Fingerprints on the weapon, doors, etc., are useful. If the gun is present at the scene, its position in relation to the body, its make, model, caliber, type of action and description of the ammunition should be noted. Any loose bullets found should be collected. If they are embedded in the walls, ceiling or furniture, they should be extracted and retained. The place in which the body is found, e.g., in a room in his own house, the state of the room, whether showing signs of struggle or not, the condition of the doors and windows whether locked or not, should be noted. If the body is found in the open, a search for footmarks and marks of struggle must be made.

(G) SEX: It is very rare for females to commit suicide by shooting, and rare for persons who are not used to firearms.

(H) DISPOSAL OF THE BODY: If the body is removed from the place of shooting or if an attempt is made to dispose off the body, commission of crime becomes obvious.

ACCIDENTAL WOUNDS: They are comparatively rare, and usually single. Most of the accidents are caused by carelessness or misuse. The technical reasons for accident are: (a) the construction of the weapon, (b) the absence of safety device, (c) the poor quality of the material used. Accidents occur when loaded weapons are handled carelessly or carried without safety catch, or when the victim slips while examining, loading or cleaning the weapon. The wounds are found on the front of the body, and frequently directed upwards. Sometimes, the victim is shot unintentionally by a person who is ignorant of firearms or careless in their use. Occasionally, when the police shoot on law breakers, an innocent bystander is struck by bullets Table (8–13).

Hunting accidents may result from (a) swinging the weapon through the line of hunters, (b) ricochetting bullets or pellets, (c) failing to unload the weapon when jumping over ditches, climbing fences or crawling through them, (d) failing to unload or uncock the weapon when it is carried or laid down. In case of a discharge caused by falling weapon, (a) the weapon or its muzzle will be some distance away from the body, and there cannot be a direct contact shot, (b) the weapon will show signs of force to allow a discharge, (c) marks will be found on the ground where the weapon dropped.

FAKED FIREARM WOUNDS: Firearm wounds are very rarely voluntarily inflicted for the purpose of attributing murder. They involve non-vital parts and are near wounds.

Concealed entrance wounds may be seen in mouth, ears, nostrils, axilla, vagina, anus and perineum.

IDENTIFICATION OF PERSON BY FLASH: It is possible to distinguish features with the help of a discharge from a gun or pistol up to a distance of about 8 metres, but the details of features of clothing cannot be made out. Thus, if the assailant is well-known to the victim, identification is possible.

BOMB EXPLOSION WOUNDS

A bomb is a container filled with an explosive mixture and missiles, which is fired either by detonator or a fuse. Terrorist bombs often involve only 2 to 10 kg. of explosives. When an explosion occurs, the explosive material produces a large volume of gas, and releases a large amount of energy. Pressure of up to 1,000 tons per sq. inch. can be generated. **A minimum pressure of about 700 kilopascals (100 lb/sq inch) is necessary for tissue damage in humans.** A person can be injured by an explosion in a number of ways.

(1) Disruptive Effects: If the victim is almost in contact with a large bomb he may be blown to pieces, e.g., when the victim is carrying it. The pieces can be scattered over an area of 200 metres radius. Many parts of the body are never found, having been disrupted into tiny fragments and mixed with the masonry and other debris of the bomb site. A bomb exploding on the ground may cause severe damage or traumatic amputation of the lower legs. A bomb which explodes when the victim is bending over it, may cause severe damage to arms, face and front of the chest. When the victim is a few metres away or with smaller explosion, disruption is usually limited to mutilation of a localised area Fig. (8–98).

(2) Burns: The temperature of the explosive gases can exceed 2000°C., and the radiated heat can cause flash burns. It burns nearby objects and clothing. The **flame causes extensive burns, which involve irregular area of skin to a different degree.** Tight clothing protects, so that beneath collars, bras, waist bands, socks and shoes, the skin may be quite normal.

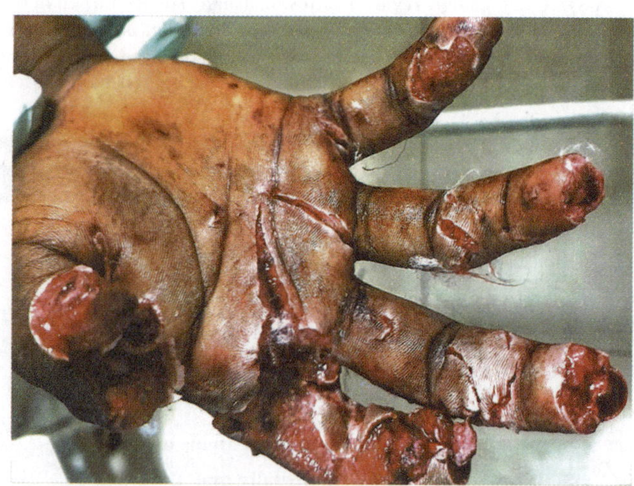

Fig. (8–98). Fire cracker explosion in the hand.

Courtesy: Dr Satish Phalkho, BHU, Varanasi, UP.

(3) Air Blast: An explosion produces a 'shock wave' which spreads concentrically from the site of explosion at about the speed of sound (1120 ft/sec). This wave of very high pressure is followed by a weak wave of negative pressure (below atmosphere), a suction which lasts about five times as long. A shock wave exceeding 700 kilopascals (100 lb/sq. inch) pressure is necessary to cause serious damage to the body. **The shock wave can throw the victim against a wall or toss him through the air causing blunt force injuries. The clothes may be blown off by the blast. The clothing should be retained for chemical analysis.** The shock wave passes through the body. **The homogeneous tissues like liver and muscle are not damaged. Blast injury of lungs is seen if the victim is within a few metres of explosion,** and at such range, the victim usually dies from other injuries. Lungs show subpleural patchy haemorrhages, scattered at random, often in the line of ribs. Sectioning of lungs shows more discrete scattered areas of haemorrhage, often with a tendency to be more central than periphery. Microscopically, alveolar ruptures, thinning of alveolar septae, enlargement of alveolar spaces and circumscribed subpleural, intra-alveolar and perivascular haemorrhages are the main findings. Desquamated alveolar and bronchial epithelium is seen lying free. **This causes reactive pulmonary oedema and blood-stained froth is found in the air-passages, and later bronchopneumonia. This specific pulmonary injury of air blast is called 'blast lung'.** The tympanic membrane most commonly ruptures with haemorrhage in the ear. Damage to cochlea is more frequent. Subperitoneal haemorrhage and haemorrhages in mesentery and omentum vary in size, and laceration of abdominal organs may occur. Intracranial haemorrhage, contusion of the brain, injuries of heart and aorta, pneumothorax, ruptured stomach and bowel may occur. **Death may occur from systemic air embolism,** from air which enters the pulmonary veins after blast damage to the lungs.

When the explosion is in the water, the pressure changes are called underwater blast. The physical changes are similar to those of explosion in air. Injuries occur mostly in gastrointestinal tract and less commonly in lungs. Most of the lung injury is due to pressure transmitted from abdomen through the diaphragm. Solid blast refers to a wave of energy that spreads through a rigid structure when an explosive is detonated near it and people in contact with its structure can be injured. Steel construction of tanks and warships conduct shock wave well and cause solid blast injury. The injuries are mostly skeletal. The fractures depend on the position of the person. Fractures of legs and vertebral column are more common. Gastrointestinal damage is more common than lung damage. In some cases, death may occur without any external injury.

(4) Flying Missiles: The blast may drive multiple fragments of bomb or pieces of nearby objects, e.g., gravel, glass, wood, brick, plaster, etc. through the air into the skin and **cause bruises, abrasions and puncture lacerations intimately mixed on the skin. This triad of injury (Marshall's triad) is diagnostic**

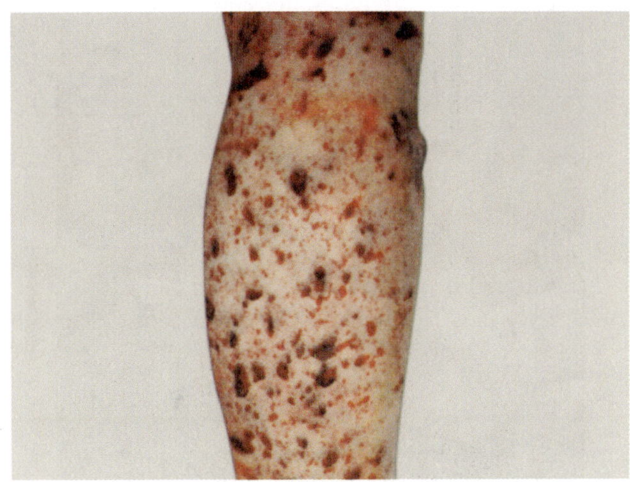

Fig. (8–99). Bomb explosion injuries showing bruises, abrasions and puncture lacerations.

Fig. (8–99). Most of the bruises and abrasions are less than one cm. in diameter, although they tend to unite. The puncture-lacerations are also usually of this size. They are ragged, sometimes with soiled margins, and may contain foreign material, such as scraps of clothing, wood or metal. The skin can be darkened by an explosion which drives dust into the skin and causes fairly uniform tattooing.

The force of the bomb explosion is extremely directional and the pattern of injury might indicate that the person was carrying the bomb or bending over it or sitting to one side of it.

(5) Falling Masonry: When a building is destroyed by a bomb blast, the persons inside sustain multiple injuries and die of traumatic asphyxia.

(6) Fumes: If a bomb explodes in a confined space, enough CO is produced to cause asphyxia. In a victim of bomb death, X-rays of tissues should be taken, as pieces of metal especially the detonating mechanism may be seen.

Incendiary bombs, e.g., napalm bombs primarily cause burns. A temperature of about 1000° C is produced. In incendiary bombs, usually phosphorus and magnesium are added. The **Molotov cocktail** is an incendiary bomb which is thrown by the hand. In a crude type of this bomb, a bottle is filled with gasoline and a rag to serve as a wick. The wick is lighted and thrown at the target. Various acids and chemicals are sometimes added to increase the destructive effects.

Autopsy: A complete body X-ray of the victim should be taken to identify fragments of explosive itself or metallic fragments within the body. Photographs or bodies and their fragments should be taken. All clothing should be retained for chemical examination. Splinters of wood, dust, glass or the explosive may be found deep within the wounds. Body may be shattered. Limbs may be blown off. Decapitation may occur. All types of injuries will be found in internal organs. Causes of death are mainly haemorrhage, shock, burns due to fire, radiation burns and burial in collapsed buildings.

DOMESTIC GAS EXPLOSIONS: They occur due to leaks in the gas supply. Natural gas explodes at concentrations in air between 5 to 15 percent. Ignition is usually caused by matches or candles, fires, sparking electric switches. The explosion is accompanied by a momentary flame

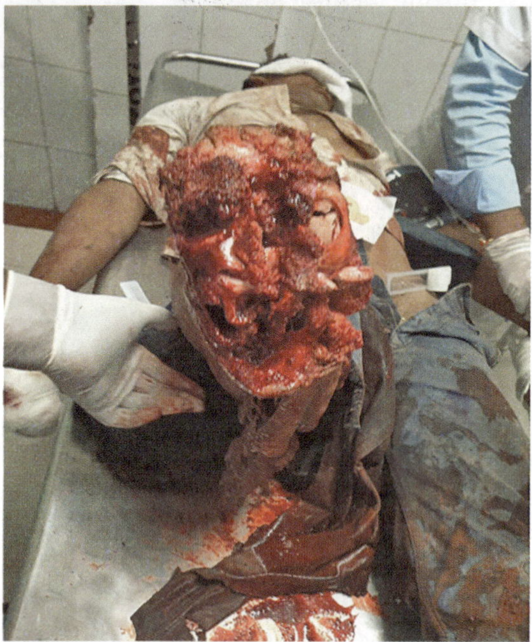

Fig. (8–100). **Cylinder blast victim with blown off right lower limb and torn garments due to blast.**

Courtesy: **Dr Satish Phalkho, BHU, Varanasi, UP.**

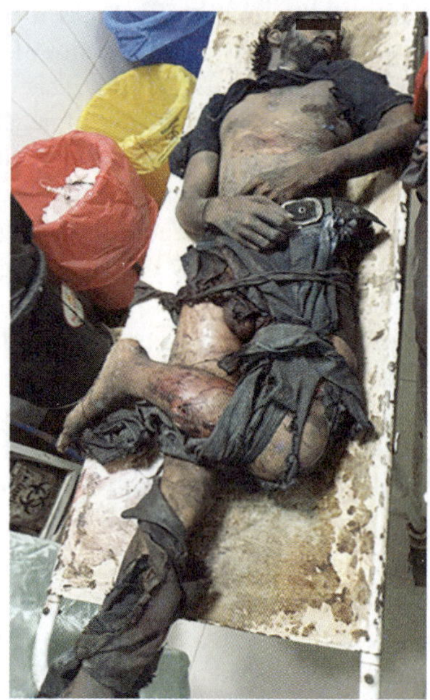

Fig. (8–101). **Deceased also died in balloon cylinder blast with torn clothing due to blast, chest and abdomen had severe damage to organs and tissues.**

Courtesy: **Dr Satish Phalkho, BHU, Varanasi, UP.**

that sets fire to furnishings. The air pressure usually rises to less than 10 psi, due to escape through broken windows and doors. Deaths are rare. The person can be thrown off their feet and injured. The damage is haphazard or diffuse. The flame singes hair and causes localised superficial burns of exposed surfaces. Most deaths occur when the building collapses and the victims are buried in the debris.

BALLOON GAS CYLINDER BLAST

In one unfortunate incident in a busy market one balloon filling gas cylinder blasted. Three persons were fatally injured and are shown in **Figs. (8–100 to 8–102)**, rest two were also critically injured but survived. Three fatally injured showed blown off lower limb, torn clothing, second showed blast effect and had severe injuries in chest and abdominal organs; third victim was hit by a piece of blasted-cylinder which torn her upper chest and damaged lungs and heart inside.

MECHANICAL EXPLOSION: Mechanical explosion occurs when a steam boiler bursts due to increased pressure. Heat and large volumes of gas are produced. The effects are similar to those of chemical explosion.

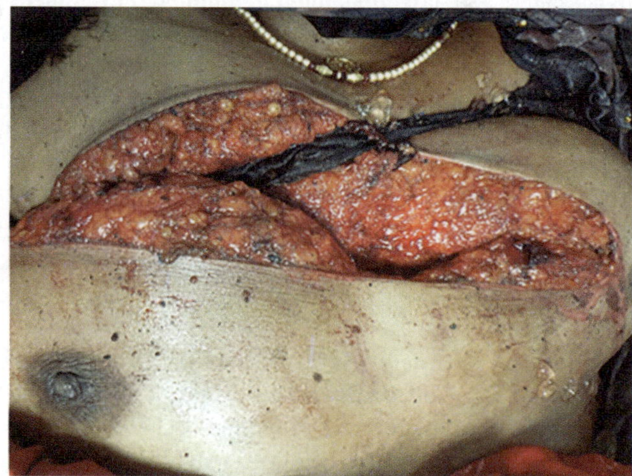

Fig. (8–102). **Oxygen cylinder blast victim where a piece of blasted cylinder made a deep cut wound of upper front of chest and damages chest wall, ruptured heart and lung inside.**

Courtesy: **Dr Satish Phalkho, BHU, Varanasi, UP.**

CHAPTER

9

REGIONAL INJURIES

FM 3.11: Regional injuries: Describe and discuss regional injuries to head (scalp wounds, fracture skull, intracranial haemorrhages, coup and contrecoup injuries), neck, chest, abdomen, limbs, genital organs, spinal cord and skeleton.
FM 3.12: Regional injuries: Describe and discuss injuries related to fall from height and vehicular injuries—primary and secondary impact, secondary injuries, crush syndrome, railway spine.

HEAD INJURIES

HEAD INJURY is a morbid state, resulting from gross or subtle structural changes in the scalp, skull, and/or the contents of the skull, produced by mechanical forces. The application of blunt force to the head may result in injury to the contents of the skull, either alone or with a fracture of the skull. The extent and degree of an injury to the skull and its contents is not necessarily proportional to the amount of force applied to the head. **Any type of craniocerebral injury can be caused by any kind of blow or any sort of head.**

SCALP: The thickness of the scalp in the adult is variable, ranging from a few mm to about 15 mm. Most wounds are caused by blunt force to the head, e.g., from falls or blows, and such wounds are contusions or lacerations.

CONTUSIONS: Contusions may occur in the superficial fascia, in the temporalis muscles, or in the loose areolar tissue between the galea aponeurotica and the pericranium. **Subgaleal haematoma does not show any colour change.** Contusions in the superficial fascia appear as localised swellings and are limited in size because of the dense fibro-fatty tissue of the fascia. A haematoma of the scalp may be very extensive and spread beneath the galea over most of the skull. (subgaleal haemorrhage). Deeper bruising in relation to the fibrous galea beneath the skin becomes visible when the scalp has been dissected and reflected. **A temporal bruise may later appear behind the ear, suggesting primary neck injury.** When the vault of the skull is fractured, blood may extravasate into the scalp tissues from the ruptured diploic veins. Bruises of the scalp are associated with prominent oedema. The veins of the scalp and face are connected with the parasagittal, lateral and cavernous sinuses through emissary veins which pass through the foramina in the skull. Infected wounds of the scalp and face may be complicated by thrombophlebitis, which may extend to the intracranial sinuses. **Bruising of the scalp is better felt than seen. Multiple contusions of the scalp may join together and become confluent which makes the interpretation of exact number of blows difficult. Its firm edge often feels like the edge of a depressed fracture of the skull. Lacerations of the scalp resemble incised wounds.** An oblique blow usually causes a large wound and direct blow a small wound.

LACERATIONS: If the scalp is lacerated by a blow, blood will be driven out of the vessels due to compression, and considerable bleeding will occur subsequently, but it will not be projected around the scene. If further blows are struck, blood will be projected about the scene under considerable pressure from the already lacerated vessels, and blood and tissue may adhere to the weapon and thrown in the direction of the uplift of the weapon. With repeated blows, blood will be splattered over the assailant, which will indicate the relative positions of the victim and assailant, and also whether they were inflicted with the right or left hand. Fall on to a flat surface, a blow from a wide, flat object will cause a ragged split which may be linear, stellate or irregular. Falls backwards against a ridge, such as a wall or a pavement kerb may cause a transverse laceration. **Temporal arteries spurt freely, as they are firmly bound and unable to contract,** and a fatal blood loss can occur from an extensive scalp laceration. Avulsion of a large area of scalp can occur in traffic accident, or if hair becomes entangled in machinery. Even after death, scalp injuries may bleed profusely, especially if the head is in a dependent position.

In case of homicide with head trauma, always retain a sample of victim's head hair, pulled from an area adjacent to the area of trauma.

FACE: EYES: Bleeding is more in facial wounds. A blow on the eye with a blunt weapon may cause a permanent injury to the cornea, iris, lens, or vitreous haemorrhage or detachment or rupture of the retina and traumatic cataract. The eyes may be gouged out with the fingers.

BLACK EYE (PERIORBITAL BRUISING) (Fig. (9–1), It is caused by (1) direct blow or kick in the front of the orbit, bruising lids, (2) injury to the forehead, the blood tracking down under the scalp, (3) fracture base of the skull in the anterior fossa, the blood leaking through cracked orbital plates. Roof of orbit may fracture due to fall on back of head. Fracture of medial wall and/or of orbital floor causes herniation of periorbital fat and inferior rectus muscle into maxillary sinus. X-ray shows a "tear drop" or polypoid mass in the roof of maxillary antrum (Racoon's sign).

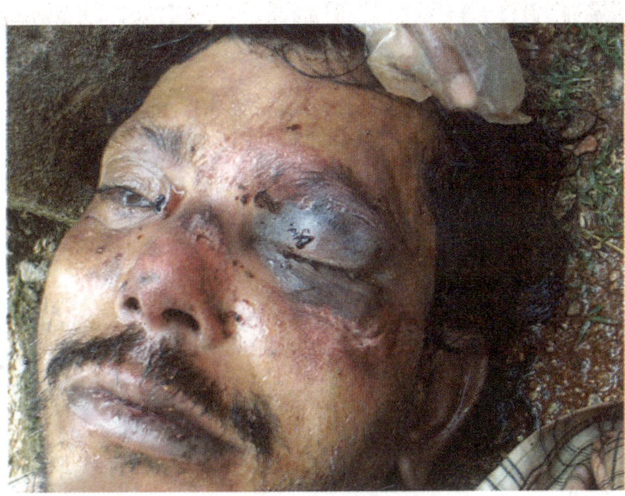

Fig. (9–1). Black eye.

NOSE: The nose may be bitten or cut off due to sexual jealousy or enemity. A blow on the head may cause nose bleeding due to partial detachment of mucous membrane without any injury to the nose.

EARS: A blow over the ears may produce rupture of the tympanum and deafness. The labyrinth may also be injured.

FACIAL BONES: A blow with a blunt weapon or fist, often fractures the nasal bones, and also ethmoid bone with radiating fractures into the supraorbital plates, if the force is severe. A blow with a blunt weapon may cause fracture of the maxilla and malar bones. Pulping of the face may result from striking with a heavy stone. The mandible is fractured by a blow from a fist, stick or by a fall from a height. A heavy blow on the jaw drives the condyles against the base of the skull, producing a fissured fracture. Very rarely, the condyles may be driven through the base of the skull.

TEETH: A fall or a blow with a blunt weapon may cause fracture or dislocation of teeth, with contusions or lacerations on the lips or gums and bleeding from the socket. X-ray of the jaw may show fracture of the alveolar margin at the site of dental injury.

SKULL

Never open the skull in a suspected cranial injury case until the circulation has been decompressed by opening the heart.

The outer table is twice the thickness of inner. In young males, the thickness of frontal and parietal bones is 6 to 10 mm and occipital bone 15 mm. The temporal bone is thinnest, 4 mm. Skull is thicker in the midfrontal, midoccipital, parietosphenoid, and parietopetrous buttresses.

FRACTURES: The force required to cause fractures of the skull varies greatly depending upon the area of the skull struck, thickness of skull, scalp and hair, direction of impact and other factors. Fractures may be caused by direct or indirect violence. **Direct injuries** may be caused by: (1) Compression as by midwifery forceps or crushing of the head under the wheel of a vehicle. (2) An object in motion striking the head, e.g., bullets, bricks, masonry, machinery, dagger, etc. (3) Head in motion striking an object, as in falls and traffic injuries. **Indirect injury** of the skull occurs from a fall on the feet or buttocks. Fractures of the vault occur from direct violence.

Under experimental conditions, a force of 400 to 600 pounds per square inch is required to fracture a cadaver skull covered by an intact, hair-bearing scalp, but 25 inch-pounds energy is sufficient to fracture empty human skulls lacking normal soft tissue coverings. The fracture may be simple or compound, i.e., associated with the injury to the scalp or nasal sinuses. There is no relation between the damage to the brain and linear fractures of the skull. Skull fractures can occur without any significant or detectable brain injury or any impairment of consciousness. Conversely, severe or fatal brain injury may occur without fracture of skull. A thin skull with a fracture may produce less brain damage than a thick skull without it.

MECHANISM OF FRACTURE OF SKULL

(1) FRACTURES DUE TO LOCAL DEFORMATION: If a small mass travelling at sufficiently great speed strikes the head squarely, it will drive inwards a piece of bone, shaped as cone-like indentation. At the apex of such a cone, the inner table will be stretched, but the outer table will be compressed, due to which the inner table fractures first. If the force continues to act, fracture of the outer table follows, and the completed fracture line runs from the central point radially. At the periphery of the indentation, the bone is bent in the opposite direction, and as the convexity of the bend is outwards, the outer table fractures first. The fracture lines tend to run circularly to enclose the base of the indentation. If the injuring force is not lost, a piece of bone fragmented by the radial fracture lines will be loosened and then depressed to form a comminuted fracture.

(2) FRACTURES DUE TO GENERAL DEFORMATION: Whenever the skull is compressed, e.g., laterally, there is a shortening in the line of pressure, while the vertical and longitudinal diameters are increased, due to which parts of the skull distant from the side of application of the injuring force are bulged and may fracture by bending.

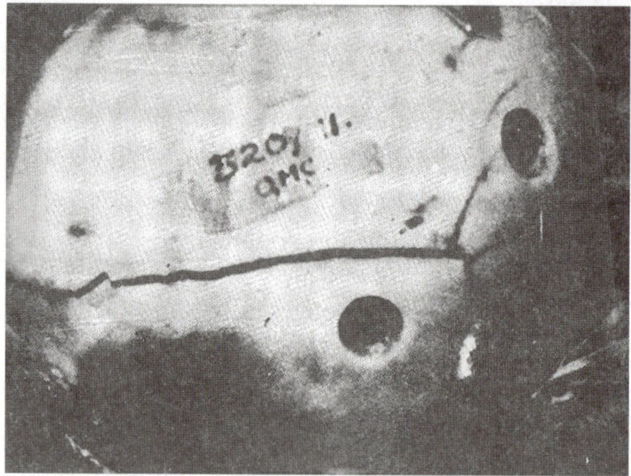

Fig. (9–2). Fissured fracture in the left parietal and occipital bones and two burr holes.

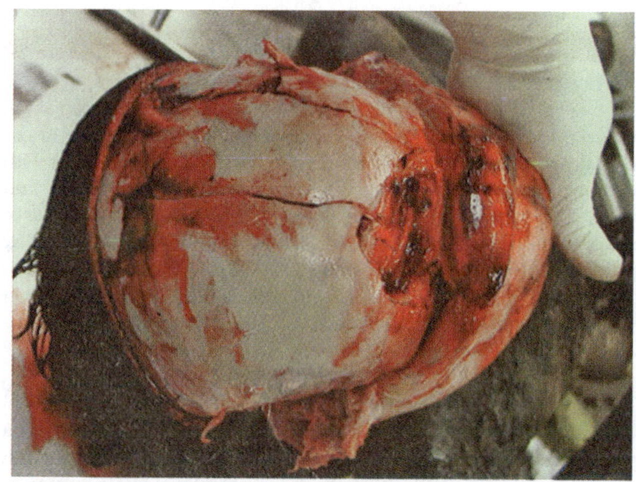

Fig. (9–3). Fissured fracture of vault of skull.

The head may be compressed: (1) Between two external objects, such as the ground and a wheel of a car. (2) Between an external object and spinal column. The latter method is common and is seen in motor car accidents, when an occupant thrown from his seat, strikes the head against resistant surface. It is also seen when the body is at rest, and a heavy object falls on the top of the head, driving the skull downwards on to the condyles of the atlas.

Fractures due to local deformation are commonly associated with those due to general deformation.

Types of Fracture Skull: (1) Fissured Fractures: They are produced by general deformation of the skull. **These are linear fractures involving the whole thickness of the bone or inner or outer table only Figs. (9–2 and 9–3). About 70% of skull fractures are linear. The outer table is capable of rebounding to its normal shape, while the more brittle inner table fractures.** It may be present alone or associated with other types. **They are likely to be caused by forcible contact with a broad resisting surface like the ground, blows with an agent having a relatively broad striking surface, or from a fall on the feet or buttocks. When a blow is struck on the side and the head is free to move, the fracture starts at the point of impact and runs parallel to the direction of the force. If the head is supported when struck, the fracture may start**

at the counter-pressure, e.g., in bilateral compression, the fracture often starts at the vertex or more commonly at the base. In both cases, the line of the fracture runs parallel with the axis of compression. A fall on the flat surface may show one or several fracture lines radiating from the point of impact, but the depression of bone fragments is not seen. **An extensive haematoma of the scalp will indicate the site of impact. In general, an injury of the head sustained by a fall is mostly situated in the level of the margin of the hat, while an injury due to a blow is commonly situated above this level.**

A fracture line tends to follow an irregular course and is usually no more than hair's breadth. Sometimes, a fracture line reaches a suture and follows its course for a while, and then starts again on its own way. **The fracture line is often red, but usually there is no haemorrhage.** At autopsy, blood can be allowed to run over the suspected fracture which is then washed. Blood will then mark out a fine fracture, which might otherwise be missed. Linear fractures do not tend to cross bony buttresses, such as glabella, frontal and parietal eminence, petrous temporal bone, and occipital protuberance. They tend to cross points of weakness, such as frontal sinuses, orbital roof, parietal and occipital squama. From the site and direction of the blow on the scalp, one can predict the likely fracture line. A blow over the glabella may cause shattering of the ethmoid sinuses and roof of the nose.

Multiple blows on the head: In persons having abnormally thin skull, minor violence may cause a fatal fracture. Fracture lines stop when the energy dissipates or when they meet a foramen, a suture or a preexisting fracture. **About 20% of linear fractures are not found on X-ray. In the case of the blow and subsequent fall, the fracture lines produced from a fall are arrested by those produced by the blow. If two blows are struck, the same results are seen and it may be possible to determine which of the blow was first struck.** The first blow to the skull will weaken the structure and subsequent blows may cause a degree of damage out of proportion to the force used, e.g. a second blow on an area of skull already fractured, may cause widespread collapse of the skull in that area, and the fragments of bone and the weapon itself may be driven far into the brain.

Anterior blows to the skull produce linear fractures of the orbit, often bilateral and the fractures cross the middle through the cribriform plate, and pass posteriorly through the pituitary fossa into the basal portion of the occipital bone. Blows to the anterior parietal bone produce fracture of the anterior temporal area, and with severe violence, linear fractures running towards the vertex and the anterior and middle fossae. Interparietal blows produce linear fractures running towards the base, involving the lesser wing of the sphenoid and pituitary fossa. The pituitary and hypothalamus may be damaged (micro-haemorrhages, ischaemic necrosis, avulsion) by blows to the side of the head causing fracture of the middle fossa. With posterior parietal blows, the fracture lines often cross the petrous temporal bone and extend towards the inner ends of the middle fossa into the posterior fossa. Blows on the occipital region produce fractures which extend towards the foramen magnum and often tend to run forwards to the lateral side of the occipital buttress and the foramen itself and may cross the petrous temporal bone and middle fossa. There may be fragmentation of one or both of the orbital plates. Blows high on the vertex tend to produce fractures which cross the midline, sometimes following suture lines.

The human adult head weighs about 4.5 kg. A linear fracture of skull may be produced when the head is hit on the side by a stone weighing 90 to 120 g. and when a weight of 2.25 kg is dropped through a distance of one foot.

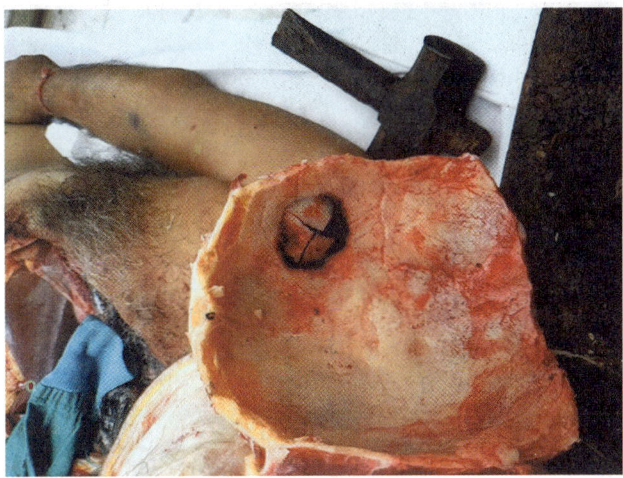

Fig. (9–4). Depressed (signature) fracture of the skull caused by hammer is shown in photograph.

Courtesy: **Professor Mukta Rani, LHMC, Delhi.**

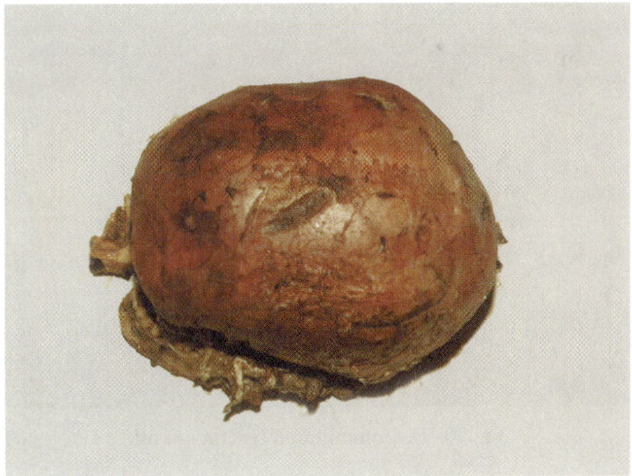

Fig. (9–5). Gutter fracture of skull.

(2) Depressed Fractures: They are produced with an object having relatively large amount of kinetic energy but small surface area, or when an object with a large amount of kinetic energy impacts only a small area of the skull Fig. (9–4). They are produced by local deformation of the skull. **In this, fractured bone is driven inwards into the skull cavity. The outer table is driven into the diploe, the inner table is fractured irregularly and to a greater extent and may be comminuted** Figs. (9–4 to 9–6). They are also called **"fractures a la signature" (signature fractures),** as their pattern often resembles the weapon or agent which caused it. **Localised depressed fractures are caused by blows from heavy weapon with a small striking surface, e.g., stone, stick, axe, chopper, hammer, etc.** Depth varies according to the velocity with which the impact is delivered. Rarely only the inner table may be fractured under the site of impact, leaving intact the outer table. **Sometimes, the depressed fracture may involve the outer table only.** A violent blow with the full face of a weapon completely detaches almost the same diameter of the bone, which is driven

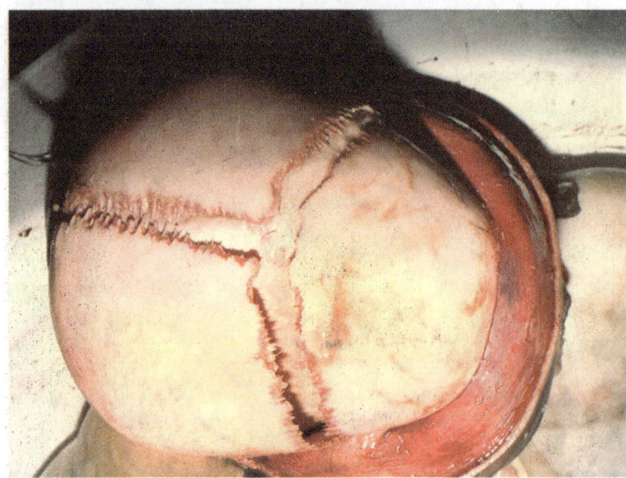

Fig. (9–6). Diastatic fractures of skull.

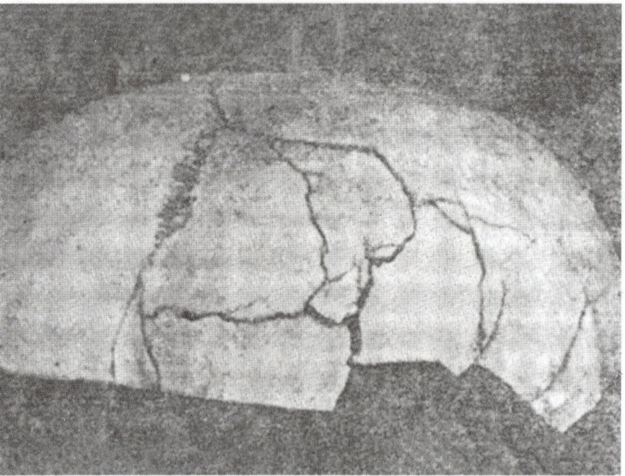

Fig. (9–7). Comminuted fracture skull.

inwards. A less violent blow, or an oblique blow, may produce a localised fracture with only partial depression of the bone. When a hammer is used, the fracture is circular or an arc of a circle, having the same diameter as the striking surface, and usually there are no radiating linear fractures. **The part of the skull which is first struck shows maximum depression.** When the butt of a firearm strikes the skull full faced, the fracture is rectangular, but if only the corner of the butt strikes, the fracture is triangular. Depressed fracture caused by a stone may be irregular or roughly triangular. **Linear fracture may radiate from the depressed fracture, indicating the direction of force.** Antemortem fractures in case of homicide often appear as localised depression of the skull. They show a shelving inward of the outer table of the bone along the edges of the fracture.

(3) Elevated Fracture: One end of fractured fragment is elevated over the surface of skull and the other end is depressed into cranial cavity. It is caused by a blow from heavy sharp weapon which elevated the fragment by lateral pull of the weapon while retrieving it.

(4) Comminuted Fractures: In a comminuted fracture there are two or more intersecting lines of fracture which divide the bone into three or more fragments Figs. (9–7 and 9–8). They are caused by a significant force striking over a

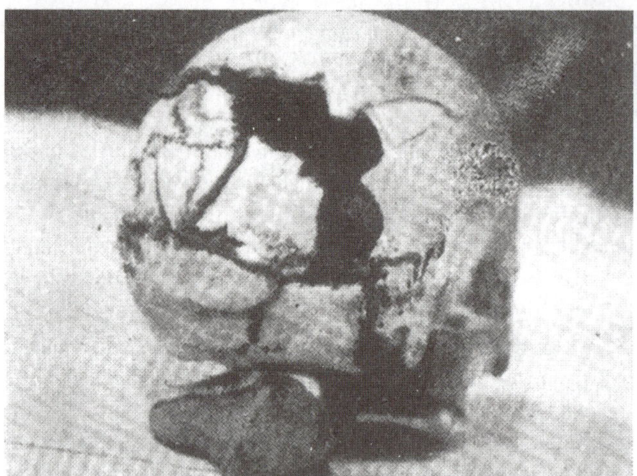

Fig. (9–8). Extensive comminuted fracture of the skull.

broad area, such as crushing head injuries, vehicle accidents, fall from a height on a hard surface, and from repeated blows by weapons with a large striking surface, e.g., heavy iron bar or poker, an axe, thick stick, etc. They may also result from a kick by an animal or by a bullet. It is often a complication of fissured or depressed fracture. **When there is no displacement of the fragment, it resembles a spider's web or mosaic. Fissured fractures may radiate for varying distances from the area of comminution (fragmentation).** When the force is great, the broken pieces of bone are displaced and some may enter the brain and others may be lost.

(5) Pond or Indented Fractures: This is a simple dent of the skull, which results from an obstetric forceps blade, a blow from a blunt object or forcible impact against some protruding object Fig. (9–9). They occur only in skulls of infants. **Fissured fractures may occur around the periphery of the dent.** The dura mater is not torn and usually the brain is not damaged. In an infant a blow often produces only a dent, like that seen in a Ping-Pong ball.

(6) Gutter Fractures: They are formed when part of the thickness of the bone is removed so as to form a gutter, e.g., in oblique bullet wounds Fig. (9–5). They are usually accompanied

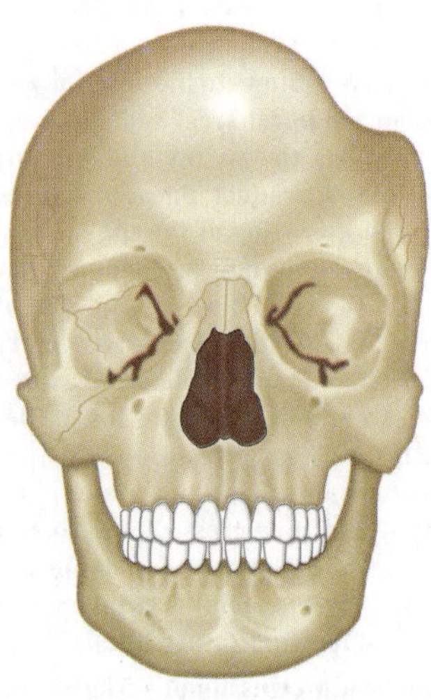

Fig. (9–9). Pond fracture.

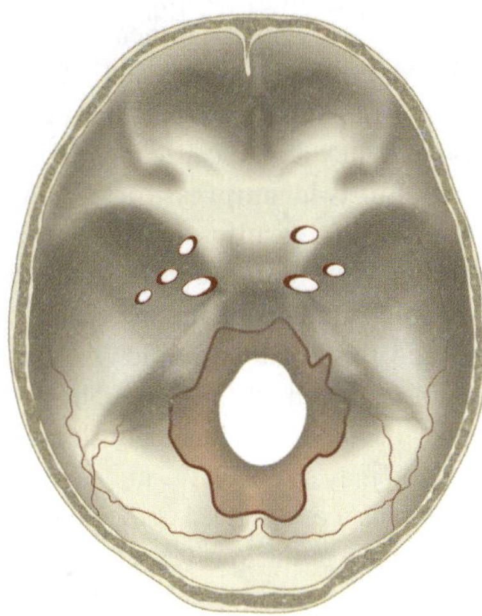

Fig. (9–10). **Ring fracture.**

by irregular, depressed fracture of the inner table of the skull. The dura mater and brain may be torn.

(7) Ring or Foramen Fractures Fig. (9–10): **It is fissured fracture which encircles the skull in such a manner that the anterior third is separated at its junction with the middle and posterior third. But usually the term is applied to a fracture, which runs at about 3 to 5 cm. outside the foramen magnum at the back and sides of the skull, and passes forwards through the middle ears and roof of the nose, due to which the skull is separated from the spine.** (1) **They are rare and occur after falls from a height on to the feet or buttocks.** In very severe cases, the spine may be driven into the skull cavity, and the vault of the skull may burst open (explosive type), giving the impression of an original massive fracture. **(2) A severe blow to the vertex may also cause a ring fracture,** but in this case the fracture of the vault will be depressed. **(3) A forceful blow on the chin in traffic accident may produce ring fracture.** There may be laceration of skin, but mandible is not fractured in most cases. They are thought to be produced from forces transmitted into the back of the skull through the mandibular joints. **(4) They are also caused by a sudden violent turn of the head on the spine,** shearing the vault from the base.

(8) Perforating Fractures: **These are caused by firearms and pointed sharp weapons like daggers or knives and axe.** The weapon passes through both tables of the skull leaving more or less a clean-cut opening, the size and shape of which corresponds to the cross-section of the weapon used.

(9) Blow-out Fracture: Blunt trauma to the eye in which the forces are transmitted via the globe to the bony orbit causing **fractures of medial wall and floor of orbit.**

(10) Diastatic or Sutural Fractures: **Separation of the sutures occur only in young persons, due to a blow on head with blunt weapon** Fig. (9–6). It may occur alone but often is associated with fracture. **It is usually seen in the sagittal suture.** They are particularly common in traffic accidents. They also occur secondary to increased intracranial pressure with resulting splitting of sutures.

(11) Expressed Fractures: **These occur as massive fragmentation/shattering of skull, where some pieces may be found outside the head.** They occur due to massive trauma often involving contact or close range firearm injuries or due to bomb blasts.

Sometimes in the skull, small portions of brim ossify from irregular independent centres and remain for variable periods of time as small bone known as Ossa Triquetra. The aperture left by separation of one of these bones may be mistaken for a fracture produced by a weapon.

FRACTURE BASE OF SKULL: **Basal fractures may be produced by: (1) Force applied directly at the level of the base. (2) General deformation of the skull wherever the forces are applied. (3) Extension from the vault. (4) Force applied to the base through the spinal column or face. In the base, fracture patterns are strongly influenced by the petrous buttress. Fracture lines which approach it from the middle or posterior fossa are turned either towards its apex or base, according to the angle at which they strike it. The middle of the body of the petrous bone is fractured only when the force is very great. Most basal fractures tend to meet at and overrun the pituitary fossa. Isolated fracture of the base is often due to transmitted force, either from the point of the chin or through the spine, except following blows in the temporal region. Fracture lines usually open into the basal foramina. The sphenoidal fissure is most commonly affected. The foramen magnum is not spared inspite of its thickened margins.**

Blows on the chin occasionally fracture the glenoid fossa. The force of a blow on the mandible, e.g., an upper cut in boxing, may be transmitted through the maxilla and its internal angular processes to the base of the skull and cause a fracture of the cribriform plate of the ethmoid. An oblique blow of great force applied to one side of the back of the head, will start a fracture in the underlying posterior fossa, which crosses the middle line to enter the middle fossa of the opposite side, and may end in the anterior fossa. Longitudinally or transversely directed forces always produce fractures in the corresponding axis. A fall on the back of the head or blow on the top of the head usually produces fractures of the roof of the orbits, especially in old people. These fractures may be comminuted and sometimes depressed. These fractures are supposed to be produced from the contrecoup of the orbital lobes of the brain on these paper-thin orbital plates. Sudden violent increase in internal pressure also produces fractures of roofs of orbit, especially in suicidal gunshot wounds of the skull. Fractures of the base of the skull may be: (1) Longitudinal, which divide the base into two halves. This may result from a blunt impact on the face and forehead, on the back of the head, or in front-to-back or back-to-front compression of the head, e.g., run over by a vehicle. (2) Transverse, which divide the base into a front and back half. This may result from an impact on either side of the head or side-to-side compression of the head as when run over by a vehicle. (3) Ring fractures.

Anterior fossa fractures are usually due to direct impact or a heavy blow on the chin. Blood and CSF may escape from the nose. Roof of orbit is fractured due to fall on back of head. Middle fossa fractures usually occur due to direct impact behind the ear. Posterior fossa fracture usually occur from direct impact on the back of the head. Basal fractures are usually associated with cranial nerve damage.

COMPLICATIONS: **(1) Fractures of anterior cranial fossa may involve the frontal, ethmoidal or sphenoidal air sinuses, with loss of blood from nose and mouth. (2) In fracture of cribriform plate if the dura and nasal mucosa are torn, CSF and even brain tissue can leak into the nose. (3) Leptomeningitis may result due to bacteria passing upwards from the nose. (4) Fractures involving paranasal sinuses may cause cranial pneumatocele. (5) Fractures of the middle fossa passing through the basiocciput or sphenoid bone may communicate with mouth, from which blood will run. (6) A direct communication between the cavity and the airway via the sphenoid sinus is produced in fracture of base of the skull involving the sella turcica. Blood may pass into the bronchial tree. Foci of inhaled blood are commonly seen in the lungs which indicate that death was not instantaneous. (7) A fracture of the petrous temporal bone may involve the middle ear, which allows blood and CSF to escape from the ear. The blood may pass into the mouth through the Eustachian tube, and may be swallowed. Tear of the posterior branch of the middle meningeal**

artery as it crosses a fracture of the temporal bone produces severe bleeding from the ear. (8) In posterior fossa fractures, extravasation of blood is seen behind the mastoid process or a large haematoma in the soft tissues of the back of the neck. (9) If the fracture reaches foramen magnum, cerebellar contusions may result, and the subsequent oedema may herniate the cerebellar tonsils fatally through the foramen. Cranial nerves may be injured by stretching or bruising but they are usually not severed. (10) Damage to surrounding structures. (11) Shock. (12) Portal of entry for bacteria. (13) Fat and bone marrow embolism. (14) Depressed fractures of the skull pressing the brain may cause severe dysfunction, coma and death.

THE CIRCUMSTANCES OF FRACTURE OF THE SKULL: Most of the fractures are due to an accident, e.g., a fall, or an injury by a motor vehicle. Multiple, localised and depressed fractures suggest homicide. Suicide by head injury is rare, because it is painful and cannot be produced easily. The victim is usually insane. It may be attempted by hitting the head against a wall or by driving a nail, etc., into the skull. Suicidal blunt impact injuries are grouped close to midline and directed to the top of the head.

AGE OF SKULL INJURY: Healing occurs without the formation of visible callus. The periosteal blood vessels are damaged, delaying the development of external callus. The edges of fissured fracture stick together within a week. The edges are slightly eroded and the inner surface of the skull may show pitting or deposition of lime salts in 14 days. The edges become slightly smooth and bands of osseous tissue run across the fissure in 3 to 5 weeks. When the edges are not in apposition, they become quite smooth in three months, or partially healed if close together. If there is much loss of bone, the gap is filled only with fibrous tissue.

INJURIES OF BRAIN AND MENINGES: The intracerebral lesions are divided according to the state of dura. If the dura is lacerated, e.g., by a bullet or any other object, such as fragment of bone, it is called open injury because it is open to infection. The brain is also lacerated. If the dura remains intact, it is called a closed injury, whether the skull is fractured or not. Blunt force to the head with a non-penetrating object or from a fall, or the head striking a flat surface or a firm object produce closed injuries. The mechanical force which produces a brain injury, usually produces injury of the scalp, fractures of skull and intracranial injuries. However, a fatal brain injury may be caused without any damage to the scalp or skull. Contusions are produced in the brain.

THE OCCURRENCE OF BRAIN INJURY: Brain injuries may be caused by: (1) Penetration by a foreign object, such as knife, bullet, etc. or fragments of skull in a depressed fracture. (2) By distortion of the skull. When a localised segment of the skull undergoes deformation, shear strains may develop in the brain tissue underlying the indentation, and a contusion may be produced in the surface layers of the brain tissue. If a fracture occurs, pieces of bone may penetrate the dura and lacerate the brain.

Contrecoup fractures: Fracture of the skull occurring opposite to the site of force is known as contrecoup fracture. This usually occurs when the head is not supported. This is explained by the sudden disturbance in the fluid brain content which transmits the force received to the opposite side, where the thrust of violent motion impacts against the cranial wall, which is unable to absorb this degree of disturbance.

MECHANISM OF CEREBRAL INJURY

Severe brain damage may be caused without actual blow or fall on the head, e.g. by shaking the infant as in child abuse, may cause subdural haemorrhage. A blow to the head will cause linear change in velocity or a rotational change in velocity about same axis. The forces involved are linear acceleration (or deceleration) forces due to the change in linear velocity and centrifugal and rotational velocity. Linear acceleration forces, tend to produce compressional or rarefactional (sound waves) forces which start from this point and travel back and forth through the brain, but they do not cause any damage. **The brain is easily distorted, but is incompressible. Change in velocity, either acceleration or deceleration, with a rotational element causes brain damage.** In either deceleration or acceleration of the head, the initial sudden change in velocity would set the head in rotation and this rotation would be transmitted to the brain which would glide within the dura. The area of the skull beneath an impact becomes momentarily depressed even if it does not fracture, and may strike on the underlying brain causing compression, and typical cone-shaped contusions are produced on the cortex, with the base at the surface. Other areas of the skull bulge outward simultaneously to accommodate the deformation. Gliding or shear strains are produced by the angular rotation of the head, which move adjacent strata of tissue laterally. The sudden arrest of the moving skull causes the deceleration of the skull first, but the momentum of the brain will cause it to continue in motion. In either deceleration or acceleration, the skull and brain cannot change their velocities simultaneously, and the brain will slow down or speed up only due to the restraint by the falx and tentorium, causing damage to the base of the cerebrum, corpus callosum and brainstem. Impact against the wide wall of the skull may cause diffuse contusion of the cortex. The shearing is more severe where the gliding is prevented by bony prominences, especially those of the anterior and middle fossae. As the cerebellum is smaller and lighter than the cerebral hemispheres, it is less liable to damage from rotatory movements of the head.

A blow to the side of the head may damage the medial surface of cerebral hemisphere on that side, especially in the region of the cingulate gyrus, because the soft brain is pushed violently against the free edge of the falx. Shearing strains caused by unequal rotational gliding and twisting of hemisphere may produce multiple haemorrhages and much direct damage to the fibres of the corpus collosum. **Holbourn postulates that brain tissue is injured when its constituent particles are pulled so far apart that they do not join up again properly when the blow is over. In the brain, the amount of this pulling apart is proportional to the shear strains.**

CONTUSIONS OF THE BRAIN: Contusion and laceration of the brain are two degrees of the same process. When a localised segment of the skull undergoes deformation at the moment of impact, shear strains may develop in the brain tissue underlying the indentation, and a zone of contusion may be produced in the surface layers of the brain. **When the head is rotated by an impact, the layers of brain tissue slide over each other at different depths in the cortex, which cause damage to the blood vessels. Contusion may occur on surface of cortex or deeper down.** There is no actual tearing of the tissues. They may occur without injury to the skull, but often there is a fracture of the skull. The period of unconsciousness varies, but it usually lasts from 30 minutes to several days. Pia-arachnoid is intact over surface contusions, and is torn in lacerations.

Cerebral contusions are circumscribed areas of brain tissue destruction, which are accompanied by extravasation of blood into the affected tissues. They are usually multiple and vary in size. They are produced by blunt force and are found in gray and white matter due

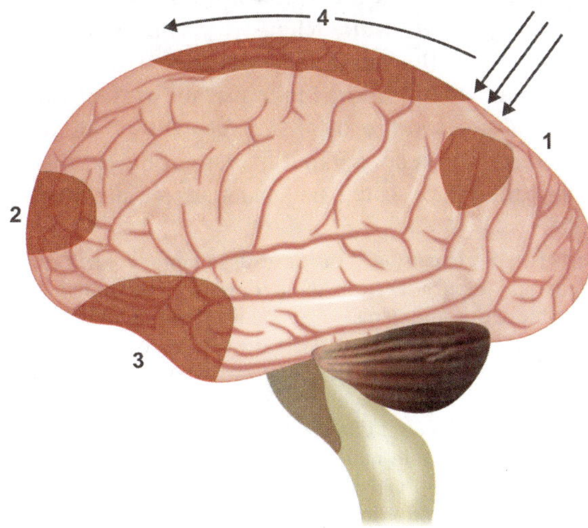

Fig. (9–11). Contusion and laceration of the brain. (1) Coup injury. (2) Contrecoup injury. (3) Dashboard injury in the region of the sphenoidal ridge. (4) Avulsion injury along the superior border of the hemisphere (the rotary vein).

to injury of blood vessels by mechanical stress. They present as streaks or groups of punctate haemorrhages. Contusions are most often found in the frontal and temporal lobes of the brain, and less commonly on the lateral and ventral surfaces of the cerebral hemispheres Figs. (9–11 to 9–13). If the haemorrhage is close to the surface of the cortex, there may be overlying focal subarachnoid haemorrhage. Deeper structures, e.g., basal ganglia, midbrain and brainstem are contused especially from impacts to forehead and vertex. The medulla may be contused in association with fractures which extend into the foramen magnum or involve the atlas and axis. Most haemorrhages occur at the crest of convolutions facing the dura of falx and tentorium. The haemorrhages are densely arranged and often elongated, radially pointing towards the white matter. Haemorrhage is first seen in the perivascular spaces along the shrivelled and collapsed blood vessels. It spreads along the sulcus and often involves several convolutions. Rarely, contusion haemorrhages occur in the cortex facing a sulcus. Traumatic contusion haemorrhages at the crest are recognised by their columnar arrangement perpendicular to the surface of the convolution. A larger haematoma may be formed by their union especially in persons with hypertension or in alcoholics. Many contusions are only seen on section of brain.

BLOWS: Blows to the back of head, usually due to falling backwards result in little or no occipital contusion, although there may be posterior cerebellar contusion or subarachnoid haemorrhage. They usually produce subfrontal and temporal lobe contusion. Blows to the top of the head produce minimal coup contusion but prominent contrecoup subtemporal or uncal contusion and less commonly subcerebellar contusion or laceration, which even result in posterior fossa subdural haemorrhage. In serious impacts, corpus callosum is lacerated. Blows to the side of the head produce a lateral coup lesion and more prominent contrecoup contusion, or laceration of the lateral aspect of the opposite hemisphere. There may be contrecoup contusion in the deep cortex or sylvian fissure. Blows to the front of the head usually do not produce cerebral contusion or laceration. There may be only diffuse subarachnoid haemorrhage, and contrecoup injuries to the occipital lobes are rare. In severe frontal injury, frontal coup laceration occurs. Contusions excite cerebral oedema in the adjacent brain and cause a rise in intracranial pressure. Old contusions appear as shrunken yellowish-brown areas known as "plaque jaures".

CONTUSION NECROSES: They are found at the crest of convolutions and form small clefts, irregularly-shaped holes, or trenches with sharply outlined walls, and usually brown in colour. They communicate with subarachnoid space, and do not contain any blood vessels. On section they are triangular or wedge-shaped, the wedge pointing into the white matter. The margins are straight. The area of necrosis is usually delineated by haemorrhage. If the necrosis is purely ischaemic, without haemorrhage, the gross lesion is seen in 10 to 12 hours after the injury as an area of swollen gelatinous parenchyma. The age of the lesion can be made out by the cellular reaction in the marginal areas. The first layer of cortex is always destroyed over contusion necroses, except for short stumps Figs. (9–12 and 9–13).

The combination of extensive contusion and an associated subdural haematoma is referred to as a 'burst' lobe, usually seen in frontal or temporal lobe and less commonly in a cerebellar hemisphere.

TYPES: Lindenberg and Freytag introduced new names for the contusions in the brain which do not fit into coup or contrecoup. Contusions found in deeper structures of the brain, such as white matter, basal ganglia, corpus callosum and brainstem along the line of impact, i.e., between the coup and contrecoup points, are called INTERMEDIARY COUP CONTUSIONS. Contusions caused by fracture of the skull are called FRACTURE CONTUSIONS. Contusions in the cortex and white matter of the frontal and central convolutions near the upper margin of the hemispheres show no relationship to the area and direction of impact. They are called GLIDING CONTUSIONS and are caused by stretching and shearing forces occurring in the region of arachnoid granulations, during to and fro gliding of the brain within the skull in moderately

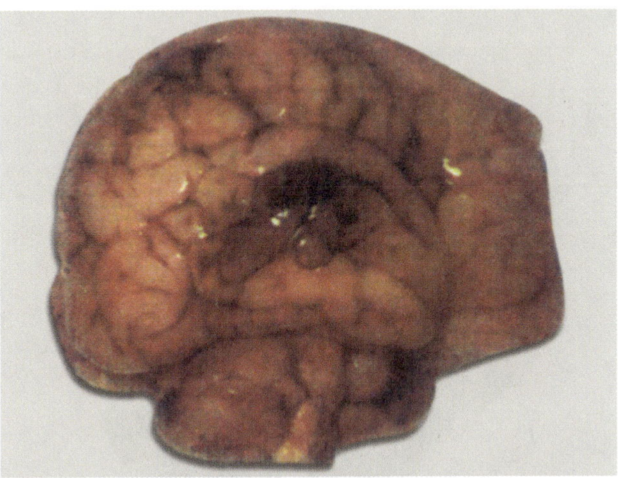

Fig. (9–12). Contusion of the right lateral side of the brain with subarachnoid haemorrhage.

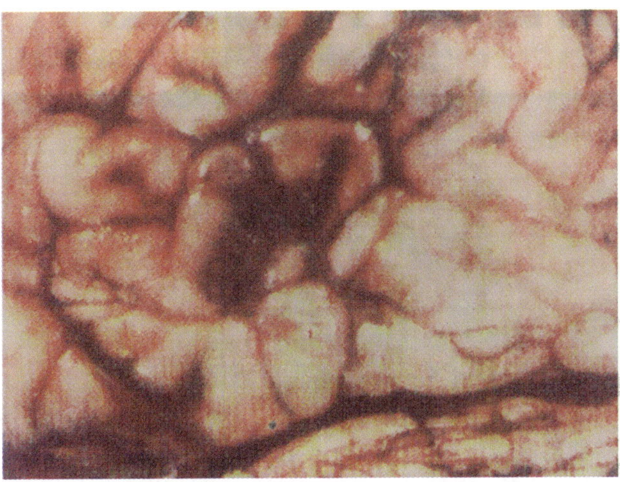

Fig. (9–13). Contusion of the brain.

severe impact. They are seen in falls and motor vehicle accidents. Contusions in the cerebellar tonsils and the medulla oblongata produced by momentary shifting of the brain toward the foramen magnum are called HERNIATION CONTUSIONS.

AGE OF CONTUSIONS: Ischaemic changes occur in neurons in an hour. Capillary proliferation begins in 5 days and is maximum at 10 to 12 days. Macrophages containing fat are present in small number during the first two weeks. Astrocytic proliferation occurs in few weeks, and a scar is left in about two months, which may have pale or golden yellow colour and are depressed.

LACERATIONS: Cerebral lacerations are traumatic lesions in which there is loss of continuity (tearing) of the substance of brain Figs. (9–14 and 9–15). **Surface lacerations are accompanied by ruptures of the pia mater and subarachnoid haemorrhages. They are usually surrounded by groups of contusions. When the parenchyma is completely disorganised, it is termed pulpefaction.** These tears are caused by stretching and shearing forces within the tissues produced by blunt force. In infants up to five months of age they are common, as the skull is easily deformed and the brain very soft. Lacerations are usually seen underneath skull fractures. In depressed fractures, the bone fragments tear the brain surface and may be driven into it. All penetrating injuries produce lacerations of brain. **Lacerations may also be produced without fracture of skull, when they are usually found in regions where the brain is in contact with projecting buttresses and ridges on the inner surface of the skull, e.g., the temporal poles and orbital surface of the frontal lobes.** Blunt trauma to the head, without fracture of the skull lacerate the corpus callosum or septum pallucidum, especially in younger individuals.

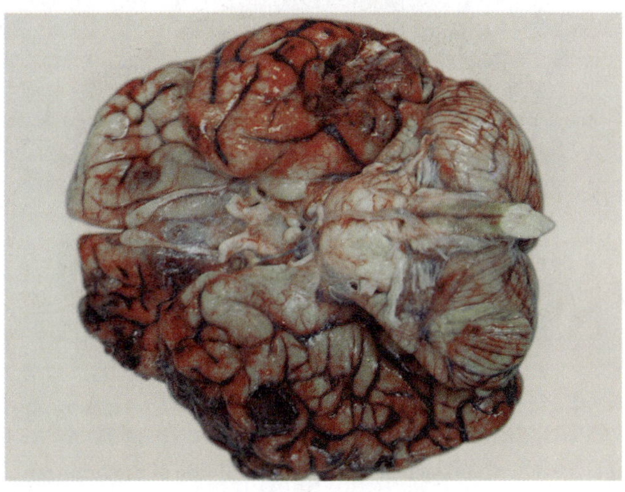

Fig. (9–14). Contusion of the lower surface of the brain.

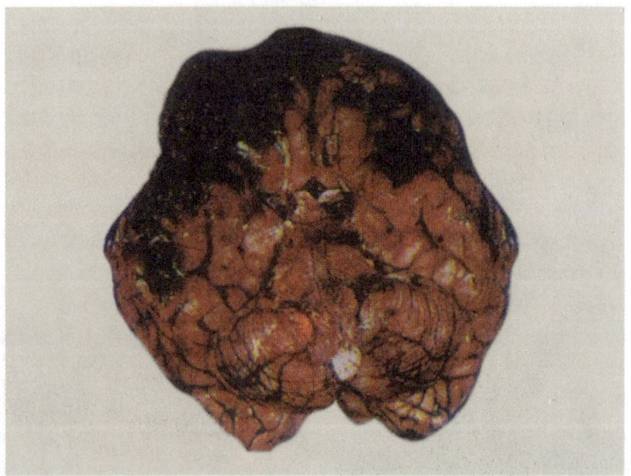

Fig. (9–15). Contusion and lacerations of base of the brain.

In severe hyperextension of the head, as in motor vehicle accidents, lacerations may be produced in the pyramids at the junction of the medulla oblongata and pons or avulsion of the brainstem at the pontomedullary junction. These lesions are usually associated with fractures of the base of the skull and of the upper cervical vertebrae. These slit-like, sometimes irregularly shaped lacerations often contain very little blood and may be mistaken for artefacts. Adhesions may develop between the brain and dura mater due to healing of surface lacerations, which may cause secondary epilepsy. Healing of deep lacerations involving ventricles may produce large glial cysts filled with CSF (traumatic porencephalic cysts.

CONTRECOUP LESIONS: Coup (blow; impact) means that the injury is located beneath the area of impact, and results directly by the impacting force. Contrecoup means that the lesion is present in an area opposite the side of impact Figs. (9–11, 9–14 and 9–16). Holbourn (Oxford physicist) in 1943, demonstrated that contrecoup lesions are chiefly due to local distortion of the skull, and sudden rotation of the head resulting from blow, which cause shear strains due to the pulling apart of the constituent particles of the brain. Holbourn defines **shear strain** as **"a strain produced by applied forces which cause or tend to cause adjoining parts of the body to slide relatively to each other in a direction parallel to their planes of contact".** A certain amount of shear may occur below the point of impact, particularly if the skull is fractured, which accounts for the coup, Fig. (9–16). **A much greater shear strain develops as a result of the rotation of the skull, and because the changes in the rotational velocity are usually greater at the pole opposite to the point of impact, contrecoup injuries are more extensive.** A line drawn between the centres of coup and contrecoup indicates the direction of impact relative to the head. In some cases, there may be no coup damage at all, only contrecoup. Fracture of the

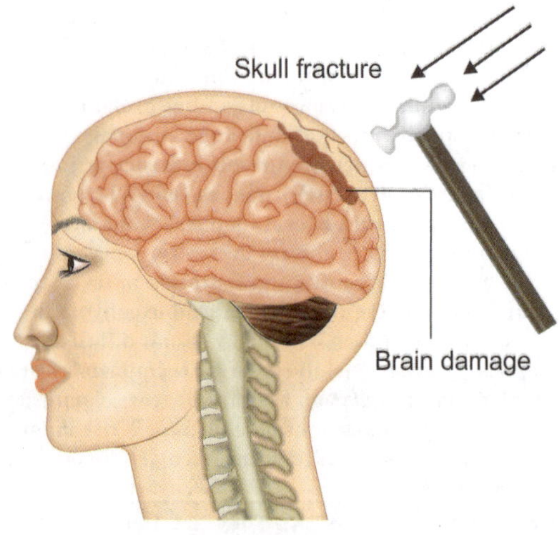

Fig. (9–16). Mechanism of coup injuries of the brain.

skull may not occur, even in the presence of severe coup and cortrecoup injuries. **Contrecoup injuries can also occur when a blow is struck on a fixed head Figs. (9–16 to 9–18).** If a person is lying on the ground or against some other unyielding surface, a heavy blow on the upper temporal or parietal area, may cause typical contrecoup injuries either in the contralateral temporal or parietal cortex, or against the falx on the inner side of the ipisilateral lobe. There is often coup injury also.

Mechanism: Contrecoup injury is caused when the moving head is suddenly decelerated by hitting a firm surface, e.g., striking the head on the ground during a fall, usually seen in traffic accidents. Subdural or subarachnoid haemorrhage may be caused as a contrecoup lesion. The sudden arrest of the head results in the brain which is still in motion, striking the arrested skull. A blow to the head causes the skull to move forward, but the brain lags behind for a brief period and the skull strikes the brain (acceleration injury). Another factor responsible for contrecoup injury is formation of a cavity or vacuum in the cranial cavity on the opposite side of impact, as the brain lags behind the moving skull. The vacuum exerts a suction effect which damages the brain Fig. (9–17).

Brain Injuries: Occipital injuries produce severe and extensive contrecoup lesions in the frontal region. The irregular bony prominences, particularly of the orbital and cribriform plates, and the lesser wings of the sphenoid, contuse or lacerate the base and produce blood-filled cavitation in the deep cortex and underlying white matter of the frontal lobes and the tips of the temporal lobes, sometimes with fracture of orbital plates. A blow at the front of the head may very rarely damage the inner and lower parts of the back of the brain by contact with the edges of the tentorium. This can also injure the brainstem and produce pontine haemorrhage. **Some authors are of the opinion that a fall on the frontal region will not produce occipital contrecoup injuries** due to the relatively smooth internal surface of the posterior cranial fossa. A fall on to the side of the head may cause a fracture of that side and contusion of the opposite side of the brain. **In temporal or parietal impacts, contrecoup injuries are likely to be diametrically opposite on the contralateral surface of the brain. A fall on the top of the head may produce contusion of the ventral surface of the cerebral hemisphere.** Rarely, a contrecoup lesion may be seen on the opposite side of the same hemisphere, e.g., a blow on the left parietal area may cause contrecoup lesion on the medial side of the left cerebral hemisphere against the falx.

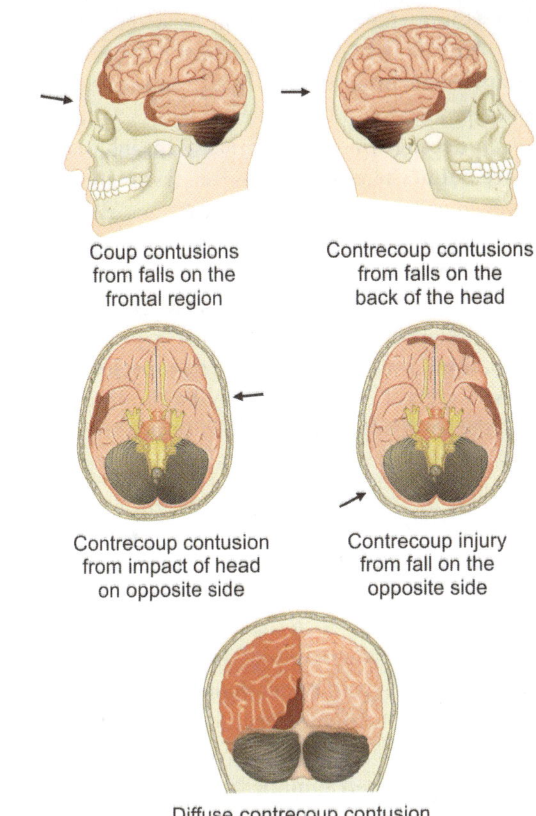

Fig. (9–18). Mechanism of coup and contrecoup injuries of the brain.

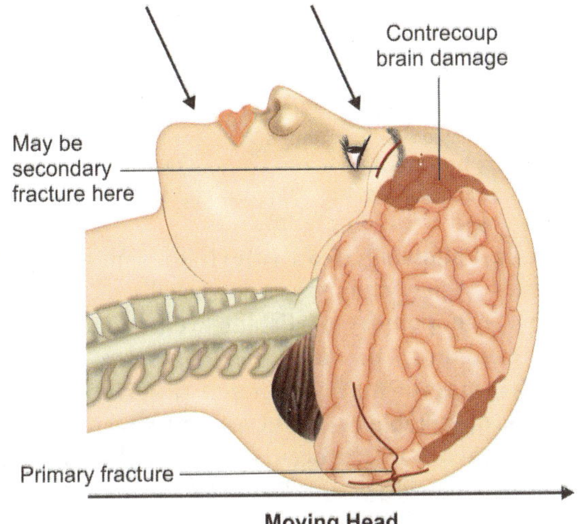

Fig. (9–17). Mechanism of contrecoup injuries of the brain.

M.L. Importance: A blow to the head produces coup contusions, while contrecoup contusions are either small or absent. A fall on the head produces contrecoup contusions while coup contusions are small or absent. Contrecoup injuries are rare before the age of three years. **Contrecoup injury is seen in skull, brain, liver, heart and lungs.**

CONCUSSION OF THE BRAIN

Concussion is a state of temporary unconsciousness (due to partial or complete paralysis of cerebral function), due to head injury, comes on immediately after injury, is always followed by amnesia, and tends to spontaneous recovery. True concussion may last for seconds or minutes. Loss of consciousness is believed to be a transient electrophysiologic dysfunction of the reticular activation system in the upper midbrain caused by rotation of the cerebral hemispheres on the relatively fixed brainstem.

Mechanism: Cerebral concussion occurs due to acceleration/deceleration of the head (the head freely

movable at some stage). The violent head movement causes shearing or stretching of the nerve fibres and axonal damage. **Severe injuries occur in coronal head motion only.** Sagittal head motion produces mild or moderate injury. **At low levels of acceleration/deceleration, anatomical damage of the axons does not occur, but there is physiological dysfunction.** The axon may recover completely or undergo degeneration. **With increased physical force, there is immediate structural damage of axons, with immediate stoppage of all activities.** In mild concussion, consciousness is not lost, and there is no confusion or disorientation, and amnesia may or may not be present. **In severe concussion, there is amnesia and loss of consciousness.**

Causes: Cerebral concussion may be produced by direct violence to the head, or by indirect violence as a result of violent fall upon the feet or buttocks, or by an unexpected fall on the ground in traffic or industrial accidents.

Features: During established concussion, the muscles are flaccid, pupils are dilated and unreacting, pulse is weak and slow, respiration is shallow. **As consciousness finally returns, there is a period during which the person appears to be lucid and in touch with his surroundings, but in fact he is not. He behaves automatically and not rationally or responsibly. The patient has no recollection of accident or injury, although he can usually recall events up to or within a few minutes of the occurrence. A post-traumatic amnesia may range from minutes to days, and its duration is usually proportional to the severity of the injury.** In some cases, amnesia after head injury may be permanent. If unconsciousness is prolonged, it is certainly due to obvious brain injury. **Concussion can be ruled out if unconsciousness does not occur immediately after a blow,** and if coma develops later, it is due to other pathology. **Blows to the neck or cervicocranial junction produce brainstem concussion.** With severe movement of the head, shearing stresses occur in the brain, which produce numerous small or punctate haemorrhages throughout the brain, "Commotio cerebri".

Theories: There are many theories as to the cause of concussion: vasomotor disturbances, impaction of the brain into the foramen magnum or tentorial opening, but the most acceptable hypothesis is **"diffuse neuronal injury",** a functional abnormality of the nerve cells and of their connections. Certainly, cerebral shift within the skull seems necessary to its production. Experimental evidence suggests that in concussion, direct damage occurs to the brainstem reticular formation. The nature of the interference with reticular formation function may cause damage to any part of the neurone; the cell body, axons or synapses and damage to synaptic junction between neurones. This damage may result from raised intracranial tension, brainstem deformation or shearing strain, but it commonly occurs with acceleration, or deceleration injuries than with injuries to the movable head. Death may occur without the patient regaining consciousness, or he may recover partially and then die suddenly, from concussion of vital cerebral centres. In cases of recovery, **post-concussion syndrome** may follow with headache, dizziness, nausea, vomiting, insomnia and mental irritability. **The victim may exhibit automatism. He may commit some violent or criminal act. Complete recovery takes place in less than ten days.** Diffuse axonal injury occurs when head acceleration occurs over a long time period, as in traffic accidents and falls from a considerable height.

Features of diffuse axonal injury are: (1) A focal lesion in the corpus callosum and other midline structures involving the parasagittal white matter, the interventricular septum and the wall of the third ventricle with some intraventricular haemorrhage. (2) A focal lesion in one or both dorsolateral sectors of the rostral brainstem. (3) Microscopic evidence of numerous axonal swellings and axonal bulbs. In fatal head injury greater or lesser axonal injury is almost always found.

Diffuse axonal injury (DAI) is a clinical condition, in which there is diffuse injury of the axons with immediate loss of consciousness and coma of more than six hours. In mild DAI, there is coma for 6 to 24 hours. In moderate DAI, there is coma for more than 24 hours, but there are no clinical signs of brainstem dysfunction. In severe DAI, there is coma of more than 24 hours with brainstem signs. It occurs due to vehicle accidents in about 90% of cases, and due to falls and assaults in about 10% of cases.

AUTOPSY: Autopsy may not show any change, but in some cases petechial haemorrhages may be found in the cortex, at the junction of the grey and white matter, in the roof of the fourth ventricle and under the pia mater of the upper segments of the cervical cord. Oedema, foci of myelin degeneration, etc., may be found. In mild DAI, some axons may be damaged. In severe DAI, there is shearing of axons in the white matter of the cerebral hemispheres, corpus callosum and upper brainstem, with focal haemorrhages in the corpus callosum and dorsolateral rostral brainstem. Microscopic examination does not show axonal injuries up to 12 hours after injury. After 12 hours, the axons first appear dilated, then club-shaped and finally appear as round balls known as "retraction balls", which indicates transected axons. The number of retraction balls begins to decrease 2 to 3 weeks after injury, and clusters of microglial cells appear, followed by astrocytosis and demyelinisation.

The interrogation of persons who have sustained head injuries: If a person becomes unconscious after head injury, he is likely to be mentally confused. **He usually suffers from amnesia to a varying degree and may not have recollection of sustaining an injury. A person involved in a traffic accident can walk around and talk to rescuers but may not, or only partially recollect the event.** The police may have to interrogate such persons in regard to events preceding and following the injury. **During interrogation the person should not be asked leading questions and no answer should be suggested. If such questions are asked, incorrect information may be obtained and the suggestions may become impressed on the mind of the person and he may have false memory in relation to the events. As such, the police should be advised to delay interrogating an accused person or a complainant who has sustained a head injury, until he completely recovers from his initial confusion.**

If the patient survives for about one hour BAPP (beta apoprotein precursor) may be identified in the axons of the damaged nerves by immunohistological techniques. At later stages, retraction balls may be identified by silver staining techniques.

Amnesia Following Head Injuries: Amnesia following head injuries is quite common and is usually associated with concussion. **The memory of distant events tends to return before the memory of more recent events. Permanent retrograde amnesia may vary from a period of seconds up to seven days** Table (9–1). **In a person recovering from concussion, events which occurred just before the injury are sometimes remembered indistinctly during the period of confusion, but there will be complete amnesia for these events after the return of complete consciousness.** As such, the patient

Table (9–1). Difference between drunkenness and concussion

	Trait	Drunk	Concussed
(1)	Face:	Suffused; flushed, warm.	Pale, clammy.
(2)	Pulse:	Fast, bounding.	Slow, feeble.
(3)	Pupils:	Contracted in coma, dilate on external stimuli and contract again. Reaction to light sluggish.	Contracted or unequal.
(4)	Breathing:	Sighs, puffs, eructates.	Shallow, irregular, slow.
(5)	Memory:	Confused.	Retrograde amnesia unrelieved by time.
(6)	Behaviour:	Un-cooperative, abusive, unresponsive, insolent, talkative.	Co-operative, quiet.

may make false accusations. Retrograde amnesia may also occur in injuries in which there is no loss of consciousness.

Post-traumatic Automatism: **Automatism refers to the behaviour that occurs when a person is unconscious and unaware that the act is taking place.** It is intimately associated with amnesia. After an accident, the patient may speak and act in purposive manner, but does not remember them afterwards.

Anterograde amnesia is characteristically seen in post-traumatic head injury.

Admission to hospital after head injury: A person who has sustained head injury, should be admitted in hospital for observation for at least 24 to 36 hours.

Head injury and acute alcoholic intoxication: **A person may be confused and disorientated after a head injury which may simulate acute alcoholic intoxication. If an intoxicated person sustains a head injury, it may not be possible to assess to what degree his condition is due to head injury or to alcoholic intoxication** Table (9–1). **Such person should not be kept in police custody but should be admitted in a hospital for observation.**

CASE: A slow moving car swerved into an intersection and over the curb onto the sidewalk. The right front door flew open, the driver was found sprawled across the seat in a pool of vomitus. The odour of alcohol was present and the driver was observed to be ataxic and incontinent, mumbling an incoherent story. A cursory examination resulted in a diagnosis of 'drunk', and he was sent to jail, where he was found dead the next morning. Autopsy revealed a cerebral haemorrhage, and no alcohol was present in the blood and only a mere trace in his urine. A chemical test of his breath or blood at the time he was examined would have indicated a low ethanol content, and other diagnoses might then have been considered.

OEDEMA OF BRAIN AND SWELLING: In brain swelling, oedema is mainly intracellular. The organ is enlarged and firm, but has a relatively dry cut surface. In oedema of brain, the fluid collection is interstitial. The organ is enlarged and soft and has a very watery cut surface. Swelling of the brain may occur following significant head injury, which may be focal, adjacent to an area of brain injury, diffuse involving both cerebral hemispheres, or involve one hemisphere only. Massive cerebral swelling can occur within 20 minutes following head injury. Swelling of one cerebral hemisphere is commonly seen in association with ipsilateral acute subdural haematoma Fig. (9–19). Increase in intravascular cerebral blood volume secondary to vasodilatation (congestive brain swelling) or an absolute increase in the water content of the brain tissue causes brain swelling. Cerebral oedema occurs due to increase in the water content of the brain. If brain swelling due to an increase in the intravascular cerebral blood volume is continued for some time, cerebral oedema will be produced due to increased vascular permeability. The brain weight may be increased by more than 100 g.

Brain swelling may not occur immediately after an injury, but may develop minutes to hours later. Delayed brain swelling of a significant degree is rare, which is usually diffuse and is seen in less severe forms of brain injury. With severe brain injury, diffuse brain swelling of a severe degree may occur immediately without the person regaining consciousness. It is asymmetrical if caused due to a mass in one side of the brain or subdural space, e.g. subdural haematoma or intracerebral haemorrhage.

Severe oedema presses down cerebral hemispheres upon the tentorium and herniate through the midbrain opening. The hippocampal gyrus may impact in the opening, lesser degrees causing grooving of the unci. Both these effects may lead to haemorrhage and necrosis at the sites of pressure. The rise in intracranial pressure impairs the venous return from the intracranial sinuses, but the arterial flow is not impaired, so further congestion and swelling occurs. Cerebral oedema can be caused or worsened by hypoxia.

AUTOPSY: The dura is stretched and tense and the brain is bulging with increase in weight. The gyri are pale and flattened with thinning of grey matter. The sulci are filled and cerebral surface is smooth. The cut surface is pale. Cerebral hemispheres and uncus may herniate. The ventricles may be reduced to slits due to swelling of adjacent white matter. The cerebellar tonsils may be impacted or coned into the foramen magnum Fig. (9–19). The normal anatomical grooving that often exists around the cerebellar tonsils should not be mistaken for "coning". True tonsillar herniation will show discolouration or even necrosis of the ischaemic, trapped tissue. Death is caused by compression of vital centres in brainstem.

Increased Intracranial Pressure: The causes are extradural and subdural haemorrhage, cerebral haemorrhage,

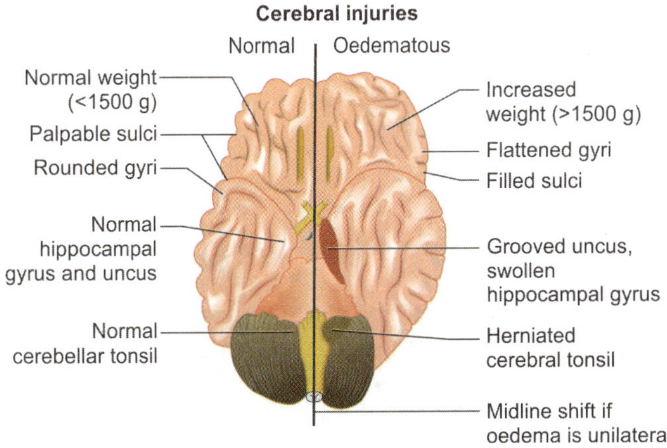

Fig. (9–19). Oedema of brain.

infarction of brain, tumour or abscesses of the brain or its coverings, dural sinus thrombosis, leptomeningitis, diffuse cerebral oedema, etc.

CEREBRAL COMPRESSION: Any increase in the size of the brain, e.g., generalised swelling or space-occupying lesions within the cranial cavity, result in compression of the brain. As the brain is incompressible, the compression will diminish the amount of CSF in the subarachnoid space and in the ventricles. A continued rise in intracranial pressure leads to a progressive interference with the blood supply of the brain. If there is increase in intracranial pressure above the tentorium, the adjacent uncus or inner margin of the temporal lobe is squeezed down through the hiatus along the midbrain, either on one or both sides, due to which the midbrain is squeezed from side to side and lengthens anteroposteriorly. This stretches the paramedian and nigral vessels which rupture to produce haemorrhages in the midline and along the substantia nigra, which is fatal. Sometimes, there is haemorrhagic infarction of the medial cortex of one occipital lobe, due to the twisting of posterior cerebral artery around the edge of the tentorium by herniation. A rise of pressure below the tentorium forces portions of the cerebellar lobes and tonsils of the cerebrum through the foramen magnum, and the medulla oblongata is compressed, which causes progressive failure of respiration. DURET HAEMORRHAGES are secondary herniation haemorrhages of the midbrain and pons, ranging from small streaks to massive confluent haemorrhage in the midline. They commonly occur with asymmetrical herniation of the brainstem. Uncal grooving and foraminal indentation of the cerebellar tonsils are common postmortem findings and must not be misinterpreted as evidence of uncinate herniation and cerebellar coning.

The suggestive evidence of cerebral compression are: flattening of the gyri, narrowing of the sulci, apparent decrease of CSF; deep grooved marking around the uncus of a temporal lobe and cerebellar pressure cone.

When severe brain swelling (or a space-occupying lesion) causes raised intracranial pressure above the tentorium, compression of the midbrain against the free edge of the tentorium may occur. This may be unilateral causing grooving of a cerebral peduncle (Kernohan's notch). When symmetrical the oedema forces the undersurface of the cerebrum against the tentorium so that the hippocampal gyrus is squeezed into the opening.

BRAINSTEM: It may be injured by (1) Stretching of peduncles when the hemispheres shift. (2) Deceleration against basisphenoid and dorsum sellae. (3) Lateral shift of peduncle against tentorial margin. (4) Stretch or avulsion from it of cranial nerves. (5) Traction on its vascular supply.

PONS: Spontaneous pontine haemorrhage is usually single, occupying from one-third to half of substance of pons. Traumatic haemorrhage occurs in a number of separate foci in the pons, which may unite if the victim survives for a sufficient time. Both types can rupture into the fourth ventricle. Pinpoint pupils not reacting to light in case of head injury indicates pontine haemorrhage. Primary haemorrhages in the brainstem are usually small and are seen in relation to the walls of the third and fourth ventricles and of the aqueduct. Haemorrhages in the restral brainstem are usually more numerous and severe than those into the medulla in rapidly fatal injuries. In most persons who die after prolonged unconsciousness, brainstem injuries are seen.

Respirator Brain: Autolytic processes proceed throughout the cerebral tissues and in the upper cervical spinal cord. Initially brain appears normal with areas of softening or duskiness. If the patient is kept on ventilator for days or weeks, cerebral sinuses are thrombosed and spinal cord frequently autolysed, and the brain will progressively become more gray, dusky, soft, and attains a near liquid state.

INTRACRANIAL HAEMORRHAGE

If the bleeding is small and thin-layered, it is called haemorrhage. If it is large and space- occupying, it is called haematoma. The application of a moderate force to the head may cause a severe intracranial haemorrhage, while a greater force may not produce haemorrhage. Injuries to the meninges may cause extradural, subdural or subarachnoid haemorrhage.

(1) EXTRADURAL HAEMORRHAGE

Anatomy: The dura is a strong and grey-bluish connective tissue membrane, the outer layer of which is firmly attached to the skull and the inner layer merges with the arachnoid **Figs. (9–20 and 9–21)**. It closely follows the contour of the brain but does not dip like pia mater. It forms the sinuses which are the drainage channel for the venous blood of brain, dura and bone. Extracranial veins also interconnect with the sinuses via emissary veins.

Causes: Extradural haemorrhage is caused almost exclusively due to trauma. At the moment of impact, the skull moves relative to the dura beneath it, and the dura is stripped from the bone. This produces an empty extradural space at the site of trauma. A blood vessel may be injured at the same time. The vessel injured depends upon the site of trauma. (1) **A blow over the lateral convexity of the head may fracture squamous temporal bone and injure the middle meningeal artery,** (usually posterior branch), especially in its posterior course as

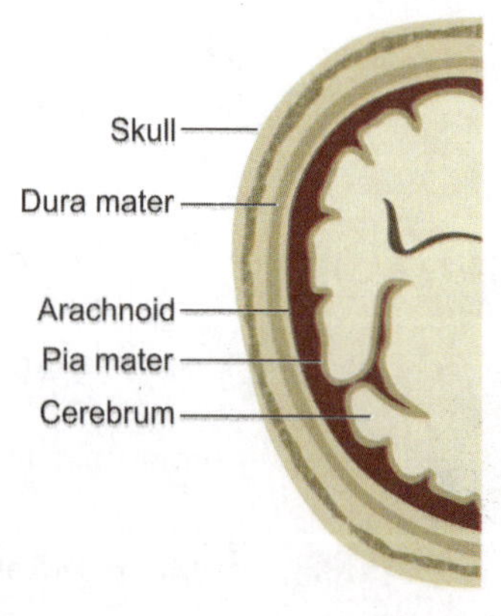

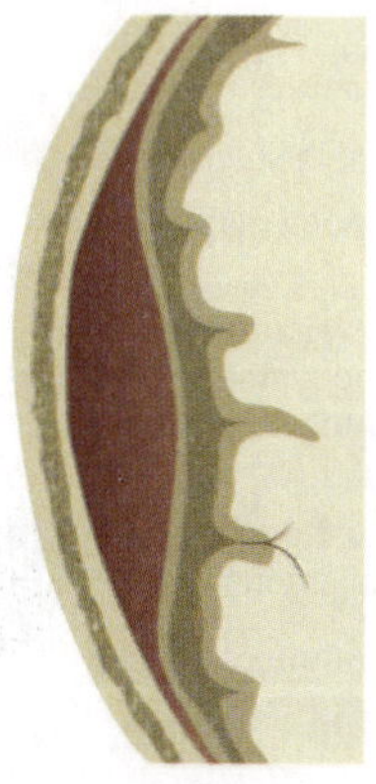

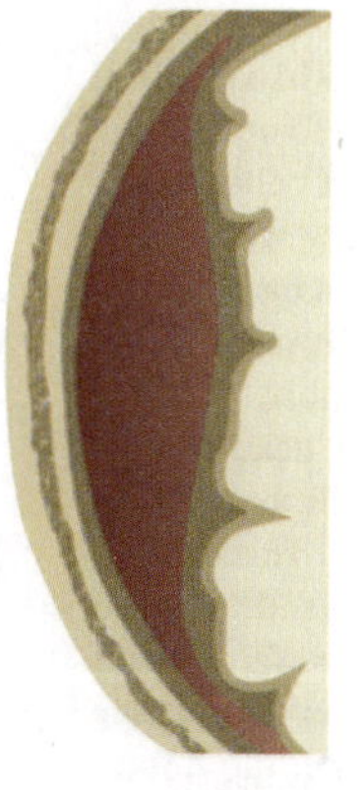

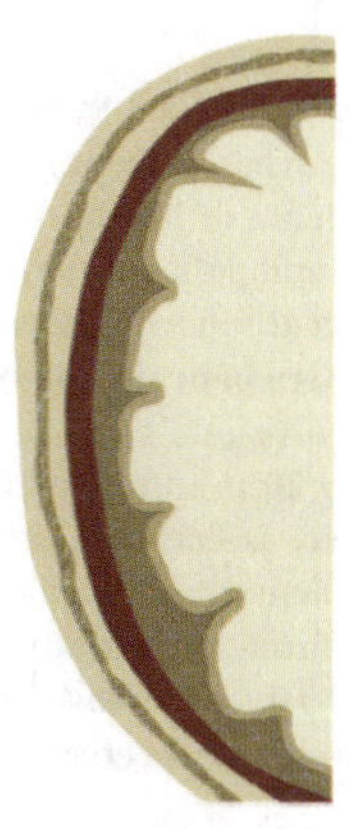

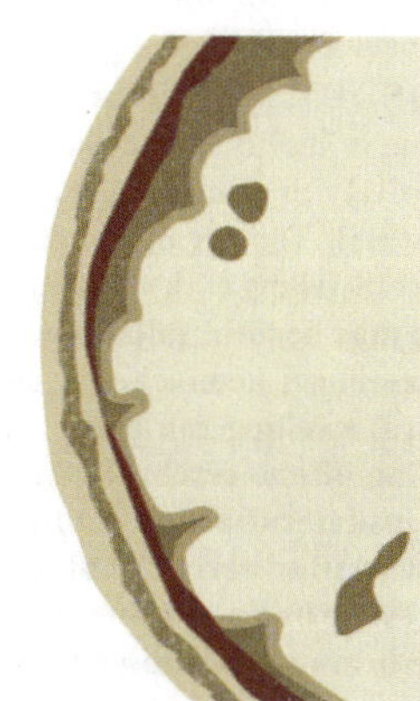

Fig. (9–20). Types of intracranial haemorrhage.

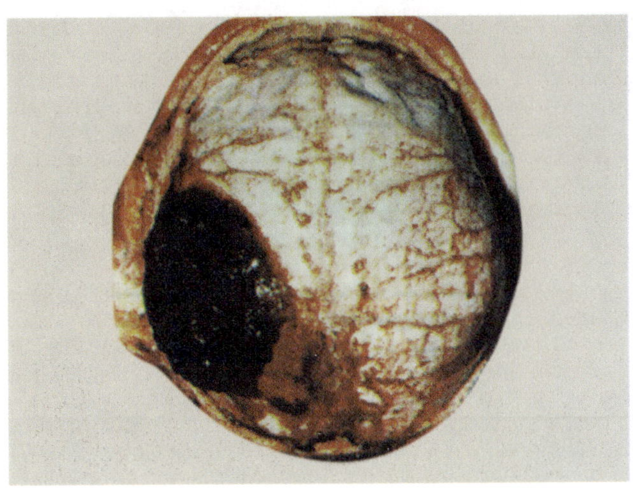

Fig. (9–21). **Extradural haemorrhage.**

it passes upwards and backwards across the temporoparietal region. Middle meningeal artery is a direct branch of internal maxillary artery. **Sometimes, the thin-walled meningeal veins which groove the bone are involved.** Venous bleeding will not produce sufficient pressure to strip dura from bone. **Less commonly, the posterior meningeal artery** near the foramen magnum (parieto-occipital haematoma) **or anterior meningeal artery** near cribriform plate are injured (fronto-temporal). (2) A blow over forehead involves the anterior ethmoidal artery. (3) A blow over the occiput, or low behind the ear, may tear the transverse sigmoid sinus and produce posterior fossa haematoma. (4) A blow on the vertex may cause haemorrhage from sagittal sinus. (5) Venous extradural haemorrhage accompanies fracture of skull (usually occipital), and is due to bleeding from the diploic veins. The haematoma is small, as the pressure is insufficient to tear back much of the dura. **In some cases the bleeding is both arterial and venous.**

It is the least common type of meningeal bleeding and is **seen in one to three percent of cases of head injury.** These haemorrhages are rare in the first two years of life due to the greater adherence of the dura to the skull, and the absence of a bony canal for the artery, but are common in adults between 20 to 40 years. **Haemorrhage may occur due to fall from a small height, or on being hit by a moving object, or after a minor accident.** Bleeding may continue for many hours or even a day after the injury. **In 90% cases, the fracture is of fissured type, but sometimes is depressed.** Rarely, the haemorrhage is found without any fracture of the skull or any external injury to the head. In almost all cases, **the haematoma is directly under the site of surface injury.** Bleeding from the main anterior branch of middle meningeal artery covers the motor area of the brain, and tends to run into the middle fossa.

Blood Clot: The clot has typical limitation due to the dural attachments at the suture lines. **The clot is sharply defined, presses the dura inward and causes a localised concavity of the external surface of the brain. The clot is oval or circular, rubbery consistency, reddish-purple, about 10 to 20 cm. in diameter, 2 to 6 cm. thick, weighs 30 to 300 g. and is adherent to the dura mater.** The clot is usually in the temporoparietal area or in the fronto-temporal or parieto-occipital region. Occasionally, it is frontal or seen in the posterior fossa. The haematoma cannot be contrecoup unless the skull has been grossly deformed. If it is bilateral, then trauma has been bilateral or a middle structure, such as the sagittal sinus has been injured. **Usually, 100 ml. is the minimum associated with fatalities.**

The accumulation of blood is most rapid when coming from a torn vein, and intermediate when both arterial and venous. About 50 percent of cases have a second haemorrhage; subdural, subarachnoid or intracerebral. Extradural haemorrhage at the base of the skull is rare. Extradural haematoma may occasionally spontaneously become smaller due to escape of the blood through a fracture into the subcutaneous tissues, and form a haematoma of the scalp. Small haematoma may undergo slow resorption by phagocytes derived from the perivascular cells of the dura.

CLINICAL FEATURES: In a typical case, there is a history of head injury which starts the bleeding, and will usually cause temporary unconsciousness. In about 25% of cases, there is no unconsciousness in the beginning. This is followed by a period of normal consciousness, the "LUCID INTERVAL" of few hours (2 to 4) to a week. Lucid interval is seen only in 30 to 40% cases. Lucid interval is not seen if the injury to the brain is sufficiently great, because of the overlapping of unconsciousness due to the brain injury and due to the pressure of extradural haemorrhage. As the pressure on the brain increases, the patient first becomes confused and may appear to be drunk. With increasing pressure, sleep and coma occur. Increasing weakness occurs in the face or arms on the side opposite to the haemorrhage and spreads to the leg. Pupil is dilated and not reactive to light, usually on the side of haemorrhage. Later there is bilateral dilatation and fixation of the pupils, decerebrate rigidity and death. The usual cause of death is respiratory failure due to compression of the brainstem.

AUTOPSY: There may be cerebral oedema and secondary haemorrhages in the pons. Tentorial herniation occurs largely from the pressure of the blood clot, and also due to the brain swelling beneath the haematoma. 20 to 50% cases are fatal. At autopsy, gentle removal of blood may show the break in the vessels and fissured fracture of the nearby skull, sometimes confined to inner table.

CHRONIC TYPE: Chronic extradural haematomas are rare and may or may not be associated with fractures of the skull. They are commonly seen in older children and young adults. In these cases symptoms are noted 2 to 3 days after injury. Sudden death may occur after several days.

(2) SUBDURAL HAEMORRHAGE: Anatomy: The arachnoid is a thin, vascular meshwork and is intimately applied to the inner surface of the dura. Subdural space is very narrow and contains a small amount of fluid permitting the thin and tough arachnoid to move relative to the dura Figs. (9–20, 9–22 and 9–23). The cerebral veins (bridging veins) cross this space to reach the sinuses. The arachnoid is attached to the dura by venous sinuses and arachnoidal granulations.

Causes: Subdural haemorrhage is commoner than extradural haemorrhage. It is common in childhood or old age. This occurs in the subdural space between the dura mater and the arachnoid due to: (1) Most cases are due to rupture of parasagittal bridging or communicating veins near sagittal sinus. (2) Rupture of inferior cerebral veins entering the sinuses at the base of the skull. (3) Rupture of dural venous sinuses. (4) Injury to cortical veins which are torn by sliding motion of the brain after the head has been arrested. (5) Lacerations or contusions of the brain and dura. (6) Rupture of an aneurysm or a superficial blood vessel malformation in the brain through the arachnoid into the subdural space. (7) Secondary to disease, e.g., cerebral tumour, cerebral aneurysms, or blood disorders. (8) Drugs such

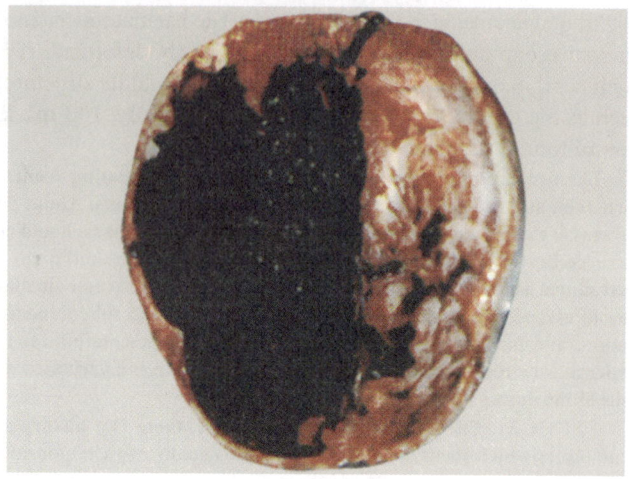

Fig. (9–22). **Subdural haemorrhage on base of the skull.**

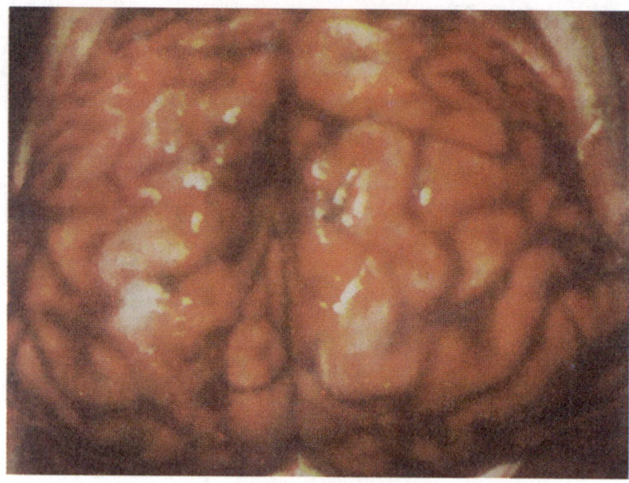

Fig. (9–24). **Subarachnoid haemorrhage.**

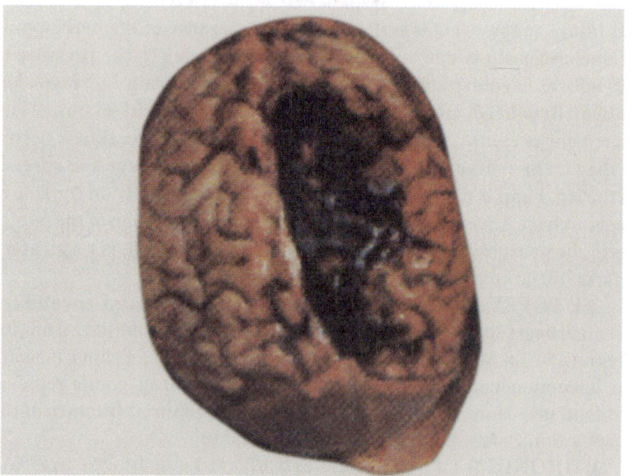

Fig. (9–23). **Subdural haemorrhage.**

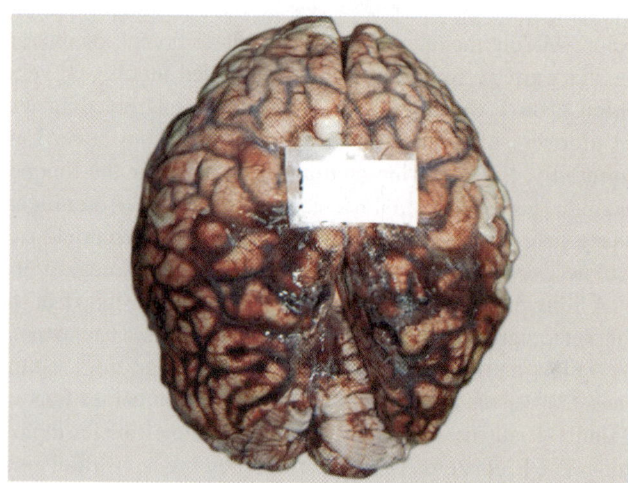

Fig. (9–25). **Subarachnoid haemorrhage.**

as dicoumarol, warfarin and heparin can produce subdural haematoma usually, but sometimes without a history of trauma.

In subdural haemorrhage due to head injury, if the person lives for some days, alcohol found in subdural hematoma at autopsy roughly corresponds to the blood level of the deceased at the time of head injury.

Mechanism: Subdural haemorrhage **arises from shear stresses in the upper layers of cerebrum** which moves communicating veins laterally sufficiently to rupture their junctions at either cortical veins or dural sinus surfaces. **It is caused due to change in velocity of head, either acceleration or deceleration,** almost always in a rotational component. When blunt impact strikes the skull, bleeding need not be situated directly under the area of impact.

Occurrence: Subdural haemorrhage may occur from relatively slight trauma, often insufficient to cause unconsciousness and usually not producing fractures of the skull, and may be associated with contrecoup contusions. About 70% occur due to falls and assaults and 25% due to vehicle accidents, and are especially likely to be found in alcoholics, old persons owing to atrophy or shrinkage of the brain and in children. It may occur in the absence of fracture of the skull or cerebral contusions or other visible brain injury. It occurs after the head impacts a hard surface and the brain is accelerated, which causes tearing of the parasagittal bridging veins.

Types: It is divided into three types according to the time of onset of symptoms after the injury. (1) In the acute type, haemorrhage occurs immediately and very rapidly after the trauma. (2) In the subacute type, the symptoms develop from several days to 2 to 3 weeks after injury, due to the pressure of the haematoma. The clot contains some dark fluid with formation of a thin peripheral membrane. (3) Chronic type results from slight trauma in which symptoms appear some weeks or months later.

(1) ACUTE SUBDURAL HAEMORRHAGE: It arises mostly from rupture of large bridging veins, rupture of one of the cortical arteries, or cerebral lacerations. Features: Rapid development of a subdural haematoma will cause compression of the brainstem and secondary brain haemorrhage. The cerebral convolutions retain their normal contours, because the blood presses both the crests and depths of the gyri. The haematoma causes displacement of the cerebral hemispheres with flattening of the convolutions of the opposite hemisphere as they are pressed against the dura and bone. **It is commonly seen over the upper lateral surface**

of the cerebral hemispheres but it may occur anywhere and may cover the entire side of the brain or even be bilateral. It is most commonly supratentorial. It usually appears as thick layers of blood over the superior surface of the brain, which drain down under gravity and cover the whole hemisphere, with a large accumulation in the middle and anterior fossae. The haemorrhage may remain fluid or may clot into a firm mass. **It is essentially venous or capillary and not arterial. The volume of the blood varies from a few drops or a thin-layered effusion to 150 ml. or more.** Fatal subdural haemorrhages are usually associated with contusions or lacerations of the brain and fractures of the skull. Often they accumulate gradually. With slow bleeding, a considerably large subdural haematoma can be tolerated without symptoms or serious side-effects. Usually, the vessels torn are so small that no main bleeding point can be discovered, either at operation or postmortem. **Small amounts of subdural haemorrhage are usually spontaneously absorbed.** Death may occur, if the haemorrhage is about 100 to 150 ml. Tears of sinuses produce clots in unusual positions, such as the posterior fossa over the occipital lobes or between the hemispheres over the corpus callosum. The sinuses are usually torn by penetrating wounds or depressed fractures.

In the acute type, the clinical picture closely resembles extradural haemorrhage, but the symptoms are delayed for 24 to 48 hours, instead of 2 to 4 hours. When there is a lucid interval, this may be longer than the average 4 hours of extradural haemorrhage. Subdural haemorrhage is almost always of traumatic origin. In the early period after the formation of haematoma, cerebral compression is not produced, but secondary changes in the haematoma may increase the size considerably. Death is very common due to secondary pressure upon the brainstem. Subdural haematoma produces some degree of cerebral shift and herniation, notably transtentorial.

Infarction: If infarction is due to subdural haematoma, it will be underneath it and is of more recent origin than the oldest portion of the haematoma. If infarction is due to stroke, there will be proximal disease of the cerebral arteries, such as severe atheroma in cervical carotid arteries, coronary atheroma, scarring of the heart muscle or disease of the valve. The infarction does not necessarily underlie the haematoma and will be as old as the oldest portion of the haematoma.

(B) SUBACUTE TYPE: This occurs when the bleeding is from smaller bridging veins. In this, the brain may or may not be damaged. The blood may be thin, watery due to haemolysis or dilution with CSF, but it may appear like that of the chronic type.

(C) CHRONIC TYPE: They are usually seen over the parietal lobe and near the midline and may be bilateral, often spread over the temporal or frontal lobe, and may extend to the base. It may be fairly localised and deep, or it may occur as a widespread surface film. It presents usually 3 to 6 weeks after the injury. The fluid in the haematoma is at first reddish-brown, often with fibrin clots. Later it has a darker colour, and after several weeks changes to mildly brownish colour. Sometimes, the interior may be much firmer and variegated in colour due to bleeds of different age. A small haematoma may be replaced by fibrous tissue. The original haemorrhage gets rapidly sealed off. As the original clot becomes absorbed, chemical changes which occur in it may cause a further haemorrhage to occur in it spontaneously. Further trauma also causes haemorrhage. This second haemorrhage then becomes sealed off. Successive haemorrhages perhaps from new blood vessels that penetrate the mass as part of healing process increase the volume and cause unconsciousness or death. Loculation is common with different coloured fluids or ooze in each lobule. This type of haemorrhage known as pachymeningitis haemorrhagica is usually seen in old persons. The brain atrophies in old age, and more space is produced in the skull for blood to accumulate. Many subdural haematomas are small, but some may measure 100 to 150 ml., which may be asymptomatic, but some may produce neurological symptoms. The haematoma will become gradually encapsulated by cells from the dura. The capsule is attached to the dura as the arachnoid does not take part in this encapsulation. This sac of blood will press on the gyri, flattening them and deforming the underlying surface of the brain. There is no shifting of the hemisphere toward the other side Fig. (9–26).

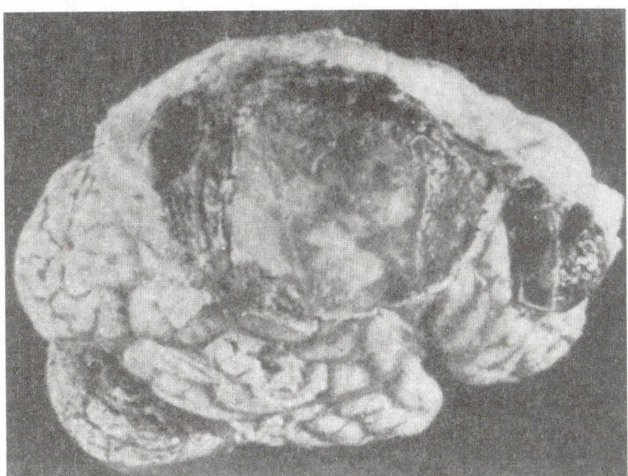

Fig. (9–26). Chronic subdural haematoma.

DATING OF SUBDURAL HAEMORRHAGE: A layer of fibrin is deposited on the dura beneath the haematoma after 24 hours. Fibroblastic activity at the junction of the clot and the dura by 36 hours, and a 2 to 5 cells thick layer of fibroblasts is seen after 4 to 5 days. and only fibrin is seen on the arachnoid side. After 4 days, red cells begin to lose their shape. The blood may begin to appear brownish after five days, but this is not reliable. Haematoma is invaded by capillaries and fibroblasts in 5 to 10 days. Haemosiderin-laden macrophages are seen. A membrane 12 to 14 cells thick is present by 8 days. In about 14 days, the membrane enclosing the arachnoid surface of the haematoma begins to form, and the dural membrane attains one-third to one-half the thickness of the dura. In 3 to 4 weeks, the haematoma is covered by a fibrous membrane that grows inward from the edges of the clot. In 4 to 5 weeks, the arachnoid membrane has half the thickness of the dura. The clot is liquefied completely and haemosiderin-laden macrophages are present in the membranes. The membrane is hyalinised on both its inner and outer sides in one to three months, with large capillaries invading the clot. This continues till complete resorption, leaving a gold-coloured membrane adherent to the dura.

SUBDURAL HYGROMA: When the arachnoid is torn, CSF may pass from the subarachnoid space into the subdural space. A large collection of fluid may accumulate and cause cerebral compression. This is called cerebral hygroma.

Persons suffering from subdural haematoma may be involved in arguments or fights, during which they collapse and die shortly.

(3) SUBARACHNOID HAEMORRHAGE: Anatomy: Pia mater is not a true membrane but is a surface feltwork of glial fibres, which are inseparable from the underlying brain. The space between the arachnoid and the very thin pia is genuine, and is called subarachnoid space. It contains the blood vessels of the brain, portions of its cranial nerves and a network of connective tissue fibres. It is filled with cerebrospinal fluid produced by the choroid plexuses of the lateral and fourth ventricles. The pia follows the surface of the convolutions along the sulci.

Causes: (1) Rupture of bridging veins near the sagittal sinus. Focal haemorrhages result from force applied to the head, usually accompanied by shaking of the brain and its coverings within the skull **Fig. (9–27)**. (2) Lacerations and contusions of the brain and

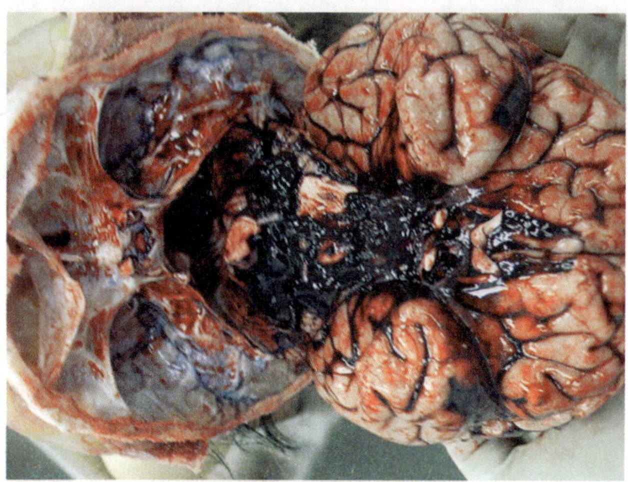

Fig. (9–27). Subarachnoid haemorrhage caused by rupture of berry aneurysms.

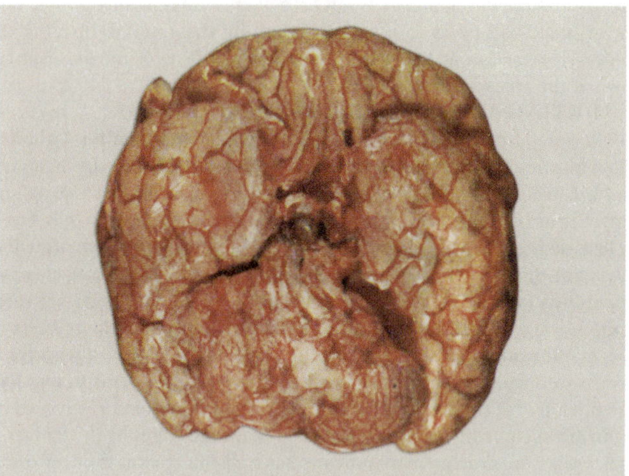

Fig. (9–28). Large berry aneurysm of posterior communicating artery.

the pia-arachnoid. (3) Rupture of a saccular Berry aneurysm, which account for 95% of aneurysms that rupture. In 20 to 30 % of cases multiple Berry aneurysms rupture **Fig. (9–28)**.

BERRY ANEURYSMS: Berry aneurysms develop over the years from developmental defects of the media of arterial wall. Size of aneurysms varies from few mm. to several cm. (usual 3 to 8 mm) Fig. (9–28). They are rare in children, and increase in frequency with age. Blood accumulates rapidly on the undersurface of the brain. With continued bleeding, blood passes along the fissures into the major cisterns and into the fourth ventricle. It may occur due to sudden rise of blood pressure due to emotional stress, such as assault, sudden exercise, sexual intercourse, etc. A second possibility is that a person with an already spontaneously leaking aneurysm may have a rapidly developing neurological or even behavioural abnormality that leads him into conflict with another person or a fall or a traffic accident. Alcohol also results in aggressive behaviour and a fight and fall, resulting in ruptured aneurysm. Spontaneous hypertensive subarachnoid haemorrhages occur due to rupture of microaneurysms called Charcot-Bouchard aneurysms that form at the bifurcations of small intraparenchymal arteries. They are seen in increasing number in the arteries of the brain with age and length of hypertension. The major sites of hypertensive haemorrhages are the putamen (55%), lobar white matter (15%), thalamus (10%), pons (10%) and cerebellar cortex (10%). These tend to be large, explosive lesions that greatly swell the pons and disrupt the central part of brainstem, usually with a ragged rim of white matter around the periphery. When an aneurysm ruptures, the victim seldom falls to strike his head. In most cases, the aneurysmal rupture is probably due to or consequent upon the fall and resultant head injury. The aneurysm should be examined at autopsy before fixation in formalin. To demonstrate the aneurysms, a constant stream of water should be poured over the base of the brain, while blunt dissection is made with the handle of a forceps or scalpel. Sometimes, the aneurysm is embedded in the brain surface. Intracranial aneurysms cause more than 50% cases of spontaneous subarachnoid haemorrhage. Berry aneurysms are most often found (about 90%) at the bifurcation of the middle cerebral, anterior cerebral (more common) and posterior communicating arteries. They are least common in vertebral artery. Rarely they can rupture into the subdural space or into cerebral hemispheres, with extension into the lateral ventricles, simulating an hypertensive intracerebral haemorrhage.

The victim of a spontaneous rupture of a berry aneurysm suffers a severe headache (thunderclap headache), neck stiffness and vomiting which may resolve or progress over hours or days to coma and death.

During assault the victim is physically and emotionally active, due to which the levels of catecholamines increase, and the high blood pressure may cause rupture of a weak aneurysm. A hard blow to the head may rupture a Berry aneurysm. A leaking aneurysm may cause behavioural abnormality leading to conflict with another person, an accident or a fall, and rupture of aneurysm. (4) Angiomas and arteriovenous malformations cause spontaneous subarachnoid bleeding. (5) Asphyxia. (6) Blood dyscrasias, leukaemias, etc. Minimal trauma may precipitate haemorrhage. (7) Tears of the ventricular ependyma. (8) Rupture of an intracerebral haemorrhage of non-traumatic origin (apoplectic haemorrhage or stroke) into the subarachnoid space. (9) A kick or a heavy blow on the side of the neck especially beneath the ear, can cause bleeding from the vertebrobasilar vessels in the posterior cranial fossa. (10) Sickle cell disease is a rare cause.

Traumatic subarachnoid haemorrhage over the base of the brain can be caused by lacerations of the internal carotid, vertebral, or basal arteries. These injuries can be immediately fatal if the haemorrhage is more than 30 ml. The most common causes of vertebral artery trauma are blows to the neck, motor vehicle accidents, falls, and cervical spine manipulation.

Vertebral Artery: The vertebral artery is injured due to overstretching of atlanto-occipital membrane and impact on muscles overlying the transverse process of upper cervical vertebrae. The damage may occur (1) in the canal of first cervical vertebra, (2) just below the axis, (3) just below the foramen magnum, (4) within the subarachnoid space above the foramen magnum. The blood tracks along the vessels and bursts into the spinal canal where pressure may be negative in the erect position. The violence causing the rupture may not cause any visible external injury, or the external injury may be so superficial as to escape notice. The lesion can be demonstrated by angiography and also by deep dissection of the upper cervical spine. The vertebral artery may rupture from sudden stretching due to partial dislocation of the upper cervical spine or atloido-occipital joint, or a fracture of the tip of the transverse process of the atlas. Mechanical forces, especially of a tilting and rotational nature, a blow to side of neck may cause dissection of the wall within the foramina of upper cervical spine. This causes blood to track upwards and medially to penetrate dura and enter inside the subarachnoid space of the posterior cranial fossa. A partial dislocation and vertebral artery injury commonly occurs, when the normal neuromuscular control of the neck muscle is lowered, leading to a slow and inadequate response to the blow. Surprise, disease, old age, arthritis and hypnotic drugs are some of the factors likely to influence this response.

Trauma: **In acute alcoholism, traumatic subarachnoid haemorrhage is more common due to loss of muscular coordination, resulting in excessive rotational forces within the head,** and also possibly due to increased bleeding from congested vessels which do not contract down, and the bounding pulse of the drunken man. The mechanism of haemorrhage is same as that for subdural haemorrhage.

This is the most common form of traumatic intracranial haemorrhage. In all cases of significant brain injury, some degree of subarachnoid haemorrhage is found. It may be the only complication of head injury but is often seen in association with other intracranial haemorrhages, with brain injuries and with skull fractures. This may be immediate or delayed until initial contraction and retraction of vessels has subsided. The latter is a reactionary haemorrhage (delayed post-traumatic subarachnoid haemorrhage). **Subarachnoid blood can be distinguished from subdural blood, because subdural blood will wash away under gently running water, whereas subarachnoid blood imparts a red colour to the brain that does not wash off.**

Autopsy: **It is mostly venous.** In the mild form, the subarachnoid haemorrhage is present as splashes of haemorrhage over the areas of contusion. In most cases it is diffuse overlying the cerebral haemispheres Fig. (9–26). Rarely, it causes scarring within the subarachnoid space, especially over the brainstem and in the basal cisterns. It can be unilateral or bilateral, localised or diffuse. It is usually found over the orbital surface of the frontal lobes, parietal lobes, and the anterior third of the temporal lobes. In most severe head injuries, it is present over the greater part of both hemispheres and is often accompanied by subdural bleeding. It spreads into the basal cisterns. The blood mixes with C.S.F. and may be distributed over the whole of the brain. A slightly yellow discolouration of the leptomeninges is seen as the subarachnoid haemorrhage becomes older.

Artefact: Subarachnoid haemorrhage may be produced as an artefact at autopsy during removal of the brain due to damage to the cerebral veins, and the arachnoid. It may also be produced postmortem due to decomposition with lysis of blood cells, loss of vascular integrity, and leakage of blood into the subarachnoid space.

If the victim survives for few hours, typical appearances of raised intracranial pressure may be seen at autopsy which may be contributed by progressive cerebral oedema. In most rapid deaths brainstem and cranial nerve roots are covered by a thick layer of blood clot which causes a widespread vascular spasm which may have an effect on vital centres in the brainstem. Rapid cardiorespiratory failure causes sudden collapse and death.

(4) INTRACEREBRAL HAEMORRHAGE: This may be found on the surface or in the substance of the brain. Haemorrhage into the brain due to trauma usually occurs near the surface. Relatively large, deep-seated traumatic haemorrhages are usually accompanied by other types of brain injury, e.g., cortical contusions **Figs. (9–29 and 9–30).**

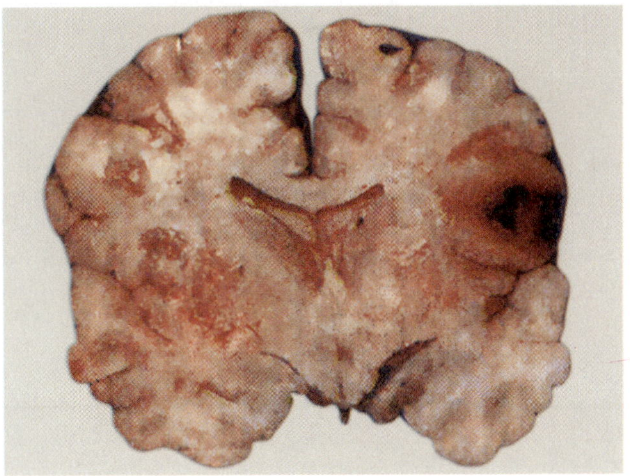

Fig. (9–29). Intracerebral haemorrhage.

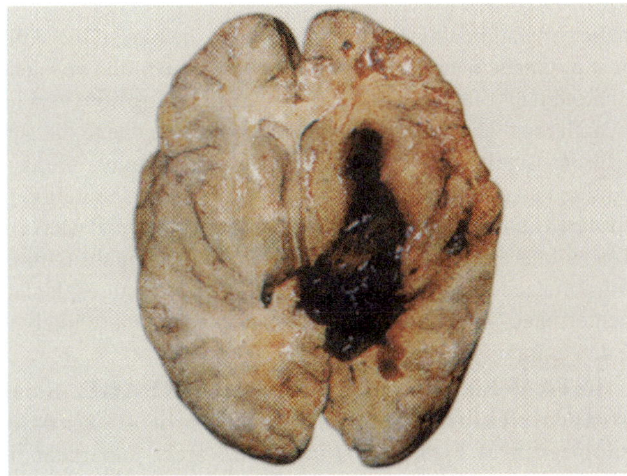

Fig. (9–30). Haemorrhage in the internal capsule, with extending into both lateral ventricles.

Causes: (1) Capillary haemorrhages are found in softening due to anoxia or arterial thrombosis or sinus thrombosis, in blood dyscrasias, in fat embolism and in asphyxial states. (2) Spontaneous haemorrhages in the region of the basal ganglia by rupture of lenticulostriate artery is common in middle-aged and elderly persons. (3) Angioma or malignant tumour of the brain. (4) Hypertensive cerebral vascular disease. Haemorrhage occurs in the thalamus, external capsule, pons and cerebellum **Figs. (9–30 to 9–32).** (5) Laceration of the brain. (6) Blow on the head, with or without fracture of the skull. They result from coup-contrecoup mechanism. (7) Intraventricular haemorrhages occasionally occur in the case of puerperal toxaemia in which there have been no fits.

Traumatic intracerebral haemorrhage results from coup-contrecoup mechanism. It is mostly seen in the fronto-temporal region and is often associated with fracture of skull. Acute massive traumatic intracerebral haemorrhage is associated with extensive and widespread injury to the brain. The patient becomes deeply unconscious from the moment of injury. Large haemorrhage may occur in the inferior part of the head of the caudate nucleus and pallidum from tears of small branches of the anterior choroid artery. They usually occur due to severe blows

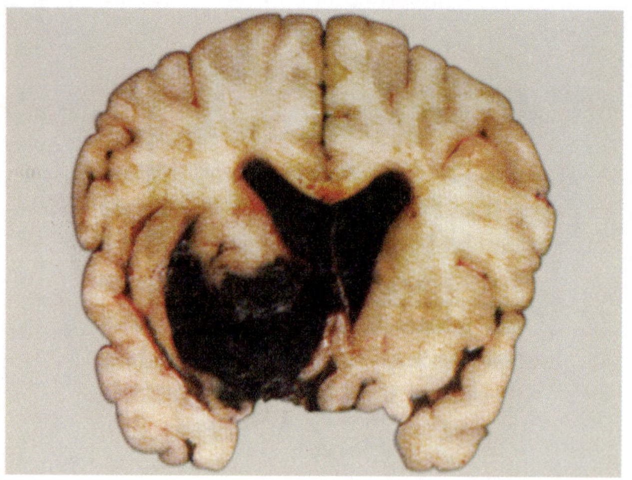

Fig. (9–31). Haemorrhage in basal ganglia on the left side extension into the ventricles.

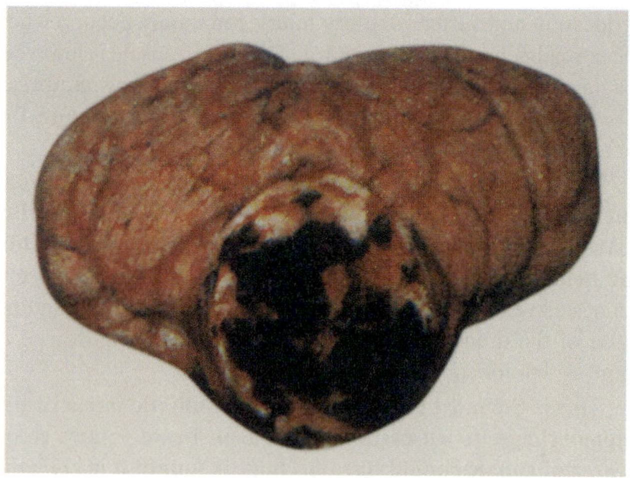

Fig. (9–32). Massive pontine haemorrhage.

on the vertex thrusting the brain down on to the base of the skull. Most traumatic haemorrhages occur at the time of the accident, but bleeding is often slow and in the nature of oozing from venules or capillaries. The continued slow oozing may be due to damage to further small vessels in the expanding haematoma. Clinical signs and symptoms may appear many hours after the injury. In rare cases, intracerebral haemorrhage may occur several weeks or even months after trauma, due to softening following the trauma, with damage to a blood vessel which ultimately ruptures. Isolate haemorrhages in the frontal or occipital lobes are more likely to be due to trauma.

INTRAVENTRICULAR HAEMORRHAGE: Small intraventricular haemorrhages occur in all kinds of craniocerebral Figs. (9–31) injuries. Rarely, subarachnoid haemorrhage enters the ventricles through the foramen of Magendi. **True traumatic ventricular haemorrhage as a sole finding occurs due to the head striking a firm object, e.g., a fall or a fall-like injury.** The bleeding may be from the choroid plexuses or from one of the veins of septum pallucidum. It may also be caused by rupture of an arteriovenous fistula. Intraventricular haemorrhages usually arise from the extension of non-traumatic intracerebral haemorrhage through the ventricle. Death may be rapid or delayed for several days.

Nontraumatic Intracerebral Haemorrhage: When disease is present, sudden rise of blood pressure due to physical exercise or excitement, e.g., alcohol, scuffle, assault, etc., may rupture vessels and produce haemorrhage. The commonly found diseases are cerebral aneurysm, degeneration of cerebral arteries, syphilis, and cerebral tumours, especially angiomata, and evidence of hypertension. If such person falls, and sustains a scalp wound before death, the haemorrhage may appear to be due to trauma. In such case, the age of the person, the site and extent of the haemorrhage, the presence of vascular lesions in the cerebral vessels and signs of cardiac hypertrophy and generalised arteriosclerosis are helpful in differentiating from traumatic haemorrhages Table (9–2). **The usual source of haemorrhage is rupture of a lenticulostriate branch of the middle cerebral artery, with bleeding into the basal ganglia and adjacent structures. Rarely, bleeding occurs in the pons or cerebellum.** At autopsy, the scalp and skull should be carefully examined for the presence of injuries and the entire cerebral vascular system must be examined for evidence of disease. **A single deep-seated haemorrhage in the brain is usually due to some disease.** Subarachnoid haemorrhage often occurs spontaneously from rupture of congenital aneurysms of blood vessels in the circle of Willis.

Table (9–2). Difference between post-traumatic intracerebral haemorrhage and apoplexy

	Trait	Post-traumatic haemorrhage	Apoplexy
(1)	Cause:	Head injury.	Hypertension, atherosclerosis, aneurysm.
(2)	Age:	Young individuals.	Adults past middle age.
(3)	Onset:	Distinct interval (few minutes to several hours) between violence and symptoms.	Sudden.
(4)	Position of head:	In motion.	Any position.
(5)	Region:	White matter of temporo-occipital or frontal region.	Ganglionic region.
(6)	Contrecoup haemorrhage:	May be present.	Not present.
(7)	Concussion:	May be seen; may become conscious before clinical effects appear.	Not present.
(8)	Coma:	Spontaneous variation.	Deep unconsciousness.

Intracranial haemorrhage due to violence can occur without any fracture of the skull or wound of the scalp. Extradural haemorrhage is always caused by mechanical violence. Subdural haemorrhage is almost always traumatic in origin, but may be caused by local inflammation. Traumatic haemorrhage in the brainstem is often well-circumscribed, sometimes rounded, typically lies between the aqueduct and the outer end of the substantia nigra.

AGE OF EFFUSION OF BLOOD: Recent effusion is bright red in colour, which becomes chocolate or brown after some days, and pale brownish-yellow in 12 to 25 days. As the time progresses, the coagulum becomes firmer and laminated. Microscopy is useful in forming an opinion on the relationship.

Comminution of the skull or extensive laceration of the brain usually produce immediate unconsciousness. Extradural and cerebral haemorrhage may not produce unconsciousness for several hours. Injury to the frontal lobes is less likely to cause rapid death than injuries to other parts of the brain. Skull fractures themselves are harmless. In about 20% of fatal head injuries, there is no skull fracture.

Cause of Death in Head Injuries: (1) Most deaths are due to damage to vital cerebral areas, located around the posterior hypothalamus, midbrain and medulla. Usually respiratory failure or paralysis is followed by permanent cardiac arrest. Vital centres may be compressed or concussed directly or they may be injured by secondary changes. (2) Raised intracranial pressure due to haematoma, contusions, lacerations, infarction or swelling is the common cause of death. (3) DAI. (4) Ischaemic brain damage. (5) Fat embolism. (6) Other causes of death are infections. In case of homicide with head trauma, always retain a sample of the victim's head hair, pulled from an area adjacent to the area of trauma.

NECK: Fractures of the hyoid bone or thyroid cartilage may occur due to falls injuring the neck, or when the neck comes in forcible contact with the handlebar of a cycle or the dashboard of a motor car. They can also occur in a fall against the side of a brick wall. A blow on the front of the neck may cause unconsciousness or even death due to vagal inhibition or by fracture of the larynx, usually involving the thyroid and cricoid cartilages and resultant suffocation from haemorrhage or oedema of the larynx. The mucous membrane of the trachea or larynx may be torn producing surgical emphysema and cause death by asphyxia. Non-penetrating laryngeal and cervical tracheal injuries can be produced by kicks with shod foot, judo, karate, and chop blows with the heel of the hand and by vehicular accidents due to striking the dashboard. Injury to atlanto-occipital junction is usually found in traffic accident victims.

Suicidal incised wounds are more common than homicidal, but punctured wounds are usually homicidal. In wounds of the trachea and of the larynx below the vocal cords, speech is not possible. Wounds of the larynx and trachea are not fatal, if the large blood vessels are not damaged. Wounds of the sympathetic and vagus nerves may be fatal, and those of the recurrent laryngeal nerves cause aphonia. An incision of the trachea may give rise to surgical emphysema in the cervical tissues.

Homicidal stab wounds may occur in any region of the neck, but are often found in the lower part. The wound is usually directed backwards, medially and downwards. It may injure the subclavian vessels or may extend through the apical pleura and penetrate the lung. Air may be aspirated into a cut cervical vein and produce pulmonary air embolism. The trachea or oesophagus may be cut, when the stab wound is directed medially. If large blood vessels, such as carotid arteries or jugular veins are cut, death occurs almost immediately.

VERTEBRAL COLUMN: High cervical injuries are best demonstrated by the posterior approach. The thoracic spine is better examined by the interior approach.

CAUSES: Fractures of the spine are caused by: (1) direct violence, and (2) indirect violence, as by forcible bending of the body or by a fall on buttocks or feet. Hyperextension is the most common mechanism of fracture of spine. Falling from a height, diving and being thrown from automobile are the common causes. The common sites of fracture are upper and lower cervical regions and junction of thoracic and lumbar segments. Fracture-dislocations and fracture of the laminae can damage the spinal cord.

FRACTURE OF TRANSVERSE PROCESSES: They are common in the regions of the lumbar spine, where the quadratus lumborum muscle is attached. Any extreme unguarded, sudden muscular contraction will produce a direct pull on the transverse process and may fracture one or more of these. Attempts to resist falling to one side may also cause strong contraction and fracture of one or more transverse processes. Rarely, if a person falls backward and strikes a projecting object, transverse process may be fractured.

FRACTURES OF SPINOUS PROCESSES: Spinous processes may be fractured by direct trauma, e.g., an object falling from a height and striking the fixed spine of a person, or from indirect violence by muscular pull, when the last cervical or first thoracic vertebra is usually fractured.

FRACTURE OF LAMINAE: They are usually caused by direct trauma, e.g.,a person falling against an object or receiving a blow usually in the neck region.

FRACTURE OF PEDICLES AND ARTICULAR PROCESSES: They result from a direct blow or severe fall upon the edge of some object. Articular processes may also fracture due to severe strain of the lumbar spine.

FRACTURE OF VERTEBRAL BODIES: Compression type (wedging) of the vertebral body occurs commonly in the lower dorsal and upper lumbar zone, particularly T12 and L1. It may occur in a fall from a height. A person falling from a height and landing on his feet may fracture one or both calcaneum(s) and the force may be secondarily transmitted to the spine, flexing it so violently that one or more vertebral bodies are crushed. If the flexion force is a general one, gradual compression occurs and the spongy bone of the vertebral body is compressed between the superior and inferior plates. If the fall is accompanied by tilts or torsion, pedicles or laminae may be fractured. If a heavy weight falls upon the flexed back or neck, wedge-compression lesions of the vertebral bodies occur with fracture-dislocation of the articular parts of the vertebrae. This may cause compression, laceration or crushing of the cord and paralysis of the body below the seat of injury. Firearm injury to the spine often breaks one or two vertebrae into several pieces.

Hyperextension fractures of the lumbar or dorsolumbar junction are rare. Hyperextension may cause crushing of the posterior portions of the vertebral bodies and the vertebral arches. Hyperflexion may cause comminution of one or more vertebral bodies with crushing of their anterior portions. In both types of injury spinal cord and meninges may be injured due to the displacement of portions of vertebral bodies or arches into the spinal canal. Hyperflexion can produce rupture of the posterior and hyperextension rupture of the anterior longitudinal spinal ligaments without fracture, which produce instability of the spinal column. Fracture-dislocation of vertebra results from a violent force, e.g., when a passenger is thrown out of the car in an accident. Such injuries are of two types. In the first type, there may be pure anterior dislocation of one vertebra upon the one below. In the second type, the pedicle is fractured with forward or backward displacement of the body of this vertebra upon the one beneath. Injury to the cord or cauda equina may be present.

Injuries to the atlas and axis are more serious than similar lesions in the lower cervical vertebrae, because of the possible paralysis of the respiratory centre. Forward dislocation of the odontoid process is usually fatal due to crushing of the cord.

SPINAL CORD: Spinal cord is injury during injury to the neck caused by sudden hyperextension of the neck followed by hyperflexion or vice-versa. Hyperextension is much more

dangerous in causing spinal damage. In hyperextension and hyperflexion, bleeding into the surrounding muscles, rupture of the anterior longitudinal ligament and tearing of intervertebral discs and of the annulus fibrosus may occur. Nerve roots may be torn or compressed and the spinal canal may be narrowed, distorted or even almost obliterated by fracture-dislocation of the vertebrae. Compression, ischaemia, haemorrhage and even pulping of the spinal cord may occur. **Upper two cervical vertebrae are commonly injured, especially dislocation of atlanto-occipital joint.** Fracture or dislocation of atlas frequently occurs when the vertex of the lowered head violently strikes the windshield of a decelerating vehicle.

Whiplash injuries: Fractures of the spine need not injure the cord, but the cord is rarely injured without associated fractures of vertebral column. "Whiplash injury" is an exception to this general rule. This is the injury sustained commonly by the occupants of the front seat. When the vehicle comes to a sudden stop, the forward thrust produces a state of acute hyperflexion, but this is converted into acute hyperextension as the forehead strikes the windscreen which causes injury to the cervical column. In such cases, and also due to a **sharp blow against the spinous process of an upper cervical vertebra (rabbit punch), fatal contusion or laceration of the spinal cord may occur without fracture of spine.**

Injuries: Spinal cord can be injured by penetrating wounds, by fracture and fracture-dislocation of vertebrae. **The spinal respiratory centre (origin of phrenic nerve) is mostly composed of C4 segment of spinal cord, with smaller contribution from C3 and C5 segments. Injury to brainstem and spinal cord above C4 can be rapidly fatal from disruption of cardiorespiratory regulation centres.** Injury to mid to lower cervical spine can cause death from compromise of respiratory function and/or spinal shock. **A puncture wound between first to third cervical vertebrae (pithing) may cause instantaneous death due to injury to the medullary centres or upper part of spinal cord.** Even a light blade may enter the cord between the laminae, as when the victim is bending when struck or the blade directed from below upwards. In the cervical region, the laminae are narrower and a horizontal thrust can penetrate the cord. **Quadriplegia occurs due to injury to the cord above the level of emergence of roots serving the brachial plexus (fourth cervical). Paraplegia occurs due to injury to cord at the level of the first or second thoracic segment.** The common sites of injury to the cord in order of frequency are: the lower cervical region, the thoracolumbar junction and the upper cervical region. Falls on the buttocks, and the lifting of heavy weights may cause protrusion of an intervertebral disc, and may compress adjacent spinal nerve root.

CONTUSIONS: Contusions of the spinal cord may result from a direct blow on the spine, indirect violence or penetrating wounds. Spinal contusions may occur without any fracture or dislocation of the vertebrae. The haemorrhages usually extend in the axis of the cord. Bleeding may occur either into the spinal meninges (HAEMATORRHACHIS) or into the substance of the spinal cord (HAEMATOMYELIA) Fig. (9–33). In some cases, bleeding occurs in the central grey matter of the cervical region, and may extend upwards and downwards. If the patient survives long enough, the haemorrhagic tissue breaks down to form a long fusiform cystic cavity filled with yellow fluid and surrounded by breaking down cord tissue.

Laceration of the cord with rupture of pia mater occurs with severe injuries. In rare cases, the entire cord may be completely severed.

COMPRESSION of spinal cord rarely occurs from effusion of blood from a fall. The cord is rarely penetrated in its upper part by sharp-pointed instruments. Firearm wounds may cause cord injury, even when missile has not entered the cord.

Concussion of the Spinal Cord: It may be caused due to some momentary collision of the cord against the wall of the canal or a transient deformity in the profile of the canal due to violent acceleration/deceleration or rotational strains. This commonly occurs in railway and motor car collision, and is known as **'railway spine'**. It also occurs from severe blows to the back, compression from dislocation or fracture of the vertebrae, damage by effusion of blood, fall from a height or a bullet injury. **It produces temporary paralysis, affecting the arms and hands or bladder, rectum, or lower extremities.** The symptoms may appear immediately or after some hours. These are headache, giddiness, restlessness, sleeplessness, neurasthenia, weakness in the limbs, amnesia, loss of sexual power and derangement of the special senses. **The paralysis is temporary and recovery occurs in about 48 hours.**

Momentary dislocation of the spine may occur especially in the cervical region, causing crushing of the cord, followed

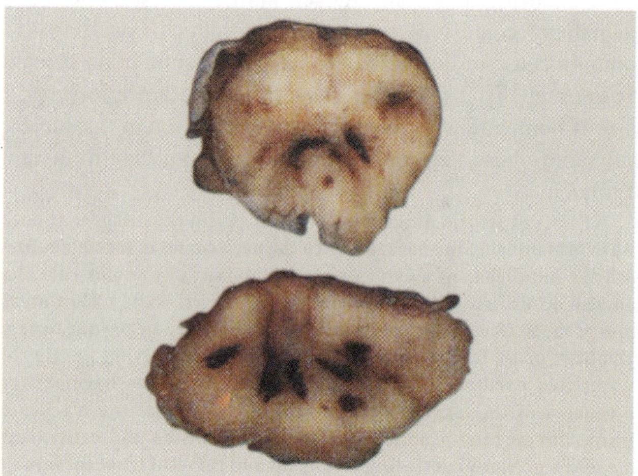

Fig. (9–33). Haematomyelia.

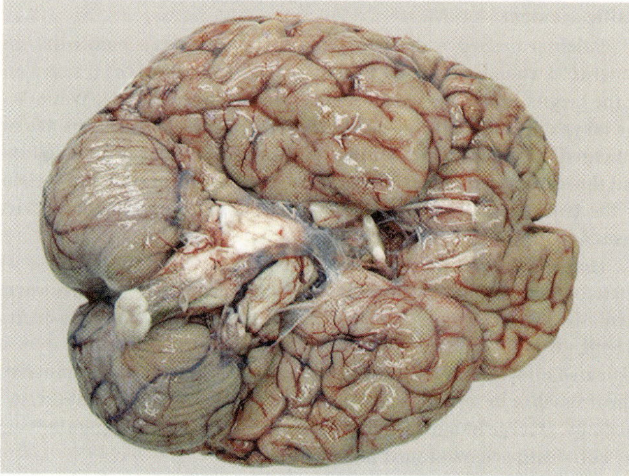

Fig. (9–34). Oedema of brain showing mushrooming of medulla oblongata and herniation of tonsils.

by self-reduction. Autopsy may show areas of haemorrhagic discolouration on the surface or in the substance of the cord, or there may be subthecal effusions of blood. Blows on the spine without fracture or dislocation, may be followed by oedema, venous thrombosis and softening of the cord.

CHEST: Injuries of the chest may be: (1) non-penetrating or 'closed', i.e., they do not open up any part of the thoracic cavity, and (2) penetrating or 'open'. Most closed chest injuries are caused by blunt force. Blunt force applied to the chest may cause abrasions and contusions of chest wall and injuries to the lungs, heart, large blood vessels or the oesophagus which may or may not be accompanied by external wounds of the chest wall or fracture of the ribs or the sternum. Severe blows on the chest wall may produce concussion of the chest, shock and death even when the viscera are not injured. Traumatic rupture of intrathoracic trachea and bronchus usually occurs due to compressive injury of the chest. The most frequent site is within 2.5 cm. of the carina, especially in the main bronchi.

A stab wound through the heart may pass down into the liver. Stab wounds through the lower part of the pleura may cross the costophrenic space without touching the lung and pass into the stomach producing pneumothorax and entry of stomach contents into the chest.

A penetrating injury of the chest, which damages only the parietal pleura may produce an open pneumothorax, communicating directly with the external air. The jagged end of a broken rib mass also causes this. This may be followed by an irritative pleural effusion and empyema. If visceral pleura is also damaged, air enters from the lung, even after the chest wound is closed. In this type, large volumes of air may accumulate under positive pressure. The other complications are: interstitial emphysema of the chest wall, lung, and mediastinum, haemothorax or haemopneumothorax.

RIBS: If compression is front to back, lateral rib fractures may occur, and if back to front, the ribs tend to fracture near the spine. If compression is from side to side, the ribs may fracture near the spine and sternum. The middle ribs from 4th to 8th are usually fractured. In fractures due to direct violence, the fragments are often driven inwards and lacerate the underlying structures. In a fall from a height, or when run over by a motor car or bullock cart, or compression of the chest by the knees or elbows, the ribs are fractured symmetrically on both sides, in front near the costal cartilages and at the back near the angles. Fracture of the ribs from muscular contraction during violent coughing, sneezing, etc., is very rare. In falls on to the side, rib fractures are often seen in the anterior or posterior axillary lines. Fractures of first three ribs usually produce severe injuries to the tracheobronchial airway and great vessels of the upper anterior chest. Fractures of 10 to 12 ribs can cause injury to the diaphragm, liver and spleen. Multiple unilateral or bilateral rib fractures give rise to a 'flail' or 'stove-in' chest, with consequent paradoxical respiration and interferes with respiratory exchange and also with blood return to the right atrium. In an adult, blood loss in multiple rib fractures may be one to two litres, due to injury to intercostal vessels which arise directly from the aorta.

STERNUM: Fractures of the sternum are not common. They may be caused by direct violence and usually occur transversely or by indirect violence as a result of forcible flexion or extension of the body. In artificial respiration, sternal fractures may occur at the level of third or fourth intercostal space.

LUNGS: Compression of the chest or blows from a blunt weapon produce contusions or lacerations. Pulmonary damage from compression may be gross or microscopic, focal or diffuse, and located centrally, peripherally or both. If the impact is severe, there may be internal laceration of the tissue either as multiple small areas of damage, or there may be a large irregular cavity, 'traumatic cavitation'. Lobes or parts of a lobe may be detached. The hilum may tear. Vessels in the hilum, especially veins may be torn. Extensive parenchymal lacerations can occur beneath an intact pleura. Lacerations are usually produced by the penetration of the lung tissue by fractured rib ends.

The presence of blood in pulmonary alveoli is not pathognomonic of haemorrhage by rhexis. In many types of anoxic death (natural and traumatic), alveolar capillary permeability is so increased by endothelial hypoxia that profuse haemorrhage occurs by diapedesis. Pulmonary parenchymal haemorrhage may also occur in severe passive pulmonary congestion, probably due to diapedesis and capillary rupture. Blood in airpassages and alveoli may be due to aspiration of blood from nasal and oral injuries.

Rapid accumulation of blood and air in thoracic cavity due to perforation of a lung or large bronchus can result in lethal mediastinal shift to the contralateral side. Minimal bleeding into thoracic cavity with tension pneumothorax can cause death several hours after injury. Sudden death following minor pulmonary injury can result from cardiac inhibition due to mechanical injury to the pleura. A wound of the lung causes frothiness of blood, which issues from the mouth and nose or in coughing. High explosive blast produces numerous haemorrhages into the lung tissue, intense capillary congestion, distension and rupture of vesicles. Contusions caused by direct violence occur on the surface of the lung or deep to the site of impact, and appear as single or multiple irregular haemorrhagic zones, or as horizontal bruises corresponding to the rib markings on the lateral surface of the lungs. Sudden compression of the chest may produce CONTRECOUP CONTUSIONS due to violent displacement of air in the lungs to the posterior surfaces near the angles of the ribs. They may extend laterally or forwards into the substance of the lungs. A pure pulmonary contusion heals rapidly and completely without residual scarring. Thin-walled blebs on the surfaces of the lungs indicate rupture of alveolar sacs from pressure on the chest. Pincer forces operating in V-shaped spaces in the chest produce wedge-shaped phrenico-costal contusion of the lungs. Stab wounds of the lungs are usually not fatal, unless a major pulmonary blood vessel has been severed. Pneumothorax is common. Spontaneous pneumothorax may occur following rupture of an emphysematous bulla. Iatrogenic pneumothorax may occur by external cardiac massage, percutaneously introduced subclavian catheters and continuous ventilatory support. In decompression multiple thin-walled, small emphysematous bullae appear on the surface of the lung.

DYSBARISM AND BAROTRAUMA

Dysbarism includes all adverse effects of pressure. Barotrauma is mechanical tissue damage caused by failure of a gas filled body cavity to equalize its internal pressure with changes in ambient pressure. It occurs most frequently under water.

When air is supplied at increased pressure, the contained nitrogen will progressively dissolve in the plasma and tissue fluids, which can produce narcosis, a state resembling drunkenness. This can occur at the depths greater than 30 m. If a diver with appreciable nitrogen dissolved in his tissues returns too quickly to normal atmospheric pressure, the dissolved gas will come out of solution and gas bubbles appear in the circulation, tissues and joint cavities, and can cause decompression sickness. Bubbles in the circulation can cause gas emboli which block small vessels and cause infarction, especially in central nervous system (CNS). The bubbles can interfere with coagulation system, causing platelet aggregation and disseminated intravascular coagulation. Subcutaneous emphysema can appear. This can also occur due to decrease from normal to low pressure, such as depressurization of an aircraft at high altitudes.

Physical damage: When sudden, or too rapid decompression occurs, physical damage may occur from volume changes. The gas in body cavities expands markedly as the diver rises and pressure effects from the contained gas will develop in paranasal sinuses, pulp cavities of teeth and middle ear. In the lung, the alveolar walls may rupture leading to interstitial emphysema. Bullae may appear on the pleural surface and, If these rupture, a pneumothorax is formed. Air may reach the mediastinum and track up the tissues to appear in the neck. Air can enter into the lung capillaries and veins. In most cases, smaller volumes of air enter into the systemic arterial circulation and impact in the arterioles and capillaries of target organs, especially the myocardium, spinal cord and brain, causing micro infarcts, hemorrhagic necrosis and loss of function of vital tissues. This pulmonary barotrauma may occur in only 2 or 3 m. of water.

Autopsy: Lungs may show oedema, patchy haemorrhages torn alveoli, focal emphysema and subpleural bullae. Pneumothorax and subcutaneous, mediastina, retroperitoneal and subpleural emphysema may be seen. Fat embolism may occur, both in post-descent shock and in decompression in both water and high altitude. Petechial hemorrhages may be seen in any part of CNS and spinal cord. Early infarcts may be seen if the victim survives for a day or more. Microscopically, ring-shaped hemorrhages around vessels may be seen in the white matter of brain. Adipose tissues and adrenal cortex may show micro-bubbles with a foamy appearance. Myocardium may show small foci of necrosis.

HEART: Contusions and lacerations of the heart may be caused by direct violence on the chest or by compression of thorax, or when a driver is forcibly thrown against the steering wheel. This may or may not be associated with external injury or fracture of the ribs or sternum. Cardiac contusions are usually seen on the anterior surface of either ventricle or the interventricular septum. Recent cardiac contusions are dark-red, haemorrhagic areas which are usually subepicardial. Cardiac contusions may simulate myocardial infarction, but are usually haemorrhagic, and transition from normal to haemorrhagic tissue is more abrupt upon microscopic examination. Antemortem contusions show localised interstitial haemorrhage and rupture of myocardial fibres. They usually heal completely, but rarely may undergo necrosis with rupture into pericardial sac. Large ones may be transmural. The commonest pincer lesion is a contusion of the right atrium at the entrance of the inferior vena cava. This is seen in compression injuries. It is produced by an impact between the liver and the heart across the right pericardio-phrenic angle. Some injury to the related part of the liver is common. It may cause sudden death several days after the injury. CONTRECOUP CONTUSIONS of the heart are seen over the posterior wall of the left ventricle. They are seen in traffic accidents in which the driver is thrown forward against the steering wheel and the heart is compressed against the vertebrae. Contusions may cause sudden death from ventricular fibrillation, or they may cause progressive circulatory failure and death after few hours or days. Foreign bodies, e.g., bullet, may remain embedded in the myocardium for years without producing any symptoms.

CARDIAC CONCUSSION: Cardiac concussion can occur after a sudden forceful impact directed at the mid-anterior chest wall in the region of the heart, i.e. COMMOTIO CORDIS. Death occurs due to ventricular fibrillation or asystole. The functional disturbance may be caused by reflex coronary vasoconstriction and myocardial ischaemia or by abnormal autonomic responses.

Lacerations of the pericardium and the heart may be caused by fracture of the ribs or the sternum. If the wound is small and oblique, the victim may live for some hours or days. Death may occur from shock and haemorrhage, haemothorax or cardiac tamponade. In falls from heights and in traffic accidents where the wheels of the vehicle passed over the trunk, sudden displacement of blood occurs into the thorax from the abdomen and the lower limbs leading to a rapid increase in intracardiac pressure. This may be sufficiently powerful to rupture the heart. Myocardial lacerations occur more frequently if the heart is filled with blood at the moment of impact, due to bursting force within the chambers. The heart is commonly torn due to compression, because the blood which it contains is incompressible. Auricular wounds are more dangerous than the ventricular. The heart may be ruptured by compression or from a blow or a fall, usually on its right side and towards its base. It may or may not be accompanied by marks of external violence or fracture. The common sites of traumatic cardiac rupture in order of diminishing frequency are: right auricle, right ventricle, left auricle, ventricular septum and valves. The only natural cause of rupture of the heart is softening or thinning by infarction, which invariably occurs in the left ventricle. Rupture of unhealthy muscle can be precipitated by any conditions associated with increased blood pressure and extra strain. Lacerations of valve cusps, leaflets, chordae tendinae or papillary muscles usually cause rapid cardiac failure.

Stab wounds of the heart are dangerous. If the left ventricle is pierced, the thickness of the muscle wall may restrict the bleeding, allowing time for surgical treatment. A stab of the right ventricle is more rapidly fatal, blood escaping through the wound to cause haemopericardium and cardiac tamponade. Blood accumulates faster in the sac than it can escape, either because bleeding rate exceeds drainage or exit hole becomes blocked by blood clot. 200 to 300 ml. of blood can cause death by increasing intrapericardial pressure and producing progressive external compression of the heart, with subsequent inadequate filling of chambers and interference with ventricular contractility. The right ventricle is more likely to be wounded, as it exposes its widest areas on the front of the chest.

In gross crushing injuries, if coronary artery is bruised, it may cause a traumatic coronary thrombosis within a few hours. Direct injury to the coronary arteries usually does not cause death. Separation of the heart from its attachments is possible due to traction force on the organs away from the neck.

Rarely, left anterior descending branch is injured due to blunt trauma to the anterior chest-wall. Atherosclerotic vessels are more susceptible to trauma. Diffuse inflammatory changes in heart muscle, i.e., traumatic myocarditis, is seen in head injuries resulting in death after a few days in a coma, or injuries affecting respiration with resulting hypoxia.

DIAPHRAGM: Wounds of the diaphragm may result from bullets or weapons which penetrate the cavity of the chest or abdomen, or by a severe blunt trauma to the anterior chest, severe, sudden blunt abdominal trauma with increased intra-abdominal pressure and upward displacement of abdominal viscera, or a fall from a height or from compression of the trunk. Rarely, an upward stab from the abdomen may puncture diaphragm. Lacerations may be unilateral or bilateral, anterior or posterior. It usually occurs near the central tendon on the left side and may be associated with visceral injury. It is frequently associated with fractures of the ribs and thoracoabdominal injuries. Death due to herniation of the abdominal contents into the chest (usually stomach, spleen, intestines and omentum in lacerations of left side), may be delayed for months or even years.

OESOPHAGUS: It is rarely ruptured near the lower end due to severe violence or vomiting. The ruptures are usually single, longitudinal splits on the lateral or posterior wall. Laceration can involve only mucosa or complete wall with perforation. Perforation of the oesophagus can result from the passage of instruments. A punctured wound of the oesophagus may produce mediastinal and cervical surgical emphysema and fatal mediastinitis.

COMPLICATIONS OF CHEST INJURIES: (1) Pneumothorax. (2) Haemothorax. (3) Chylothorax. (4) Interstitial emphysema. (5) Arterial air embolism. (6) Cardiac tamponade. (7) Air embolism. (8) Intraparenchymal haemorrhage. (9) Infection.

ABDOMEN: Injuries of the abdomen like those of the chest may be (1) non-penetrating or closed, and (2) penetrating or open. "Closed" abdominal injuries are caused by blunt force and occur in falls, in traffic accidents and in assault by blunt weapons. Abrasions, contusions and lacerations of the abdominal muscles occur due to blunt force. Profuse subcutaneous or deep-seated bleeding of the abdominal wall may track along the muscular and fascial plane to become more diffuse, and may cover a large area of abdominal wall, especially in the lower segment. Blood may track down the inguinal canal and appear in the scrotum or labia. Apparently trivial injuries may rupture abdominal viscera. In order of frequency, the structures most likely to be damaged in blunt abdominal trauma are: liver, spleen, kidney, intestine, abdominal wall, mesentery, pancreas and diaphragm. Injury to the stomach is caused by

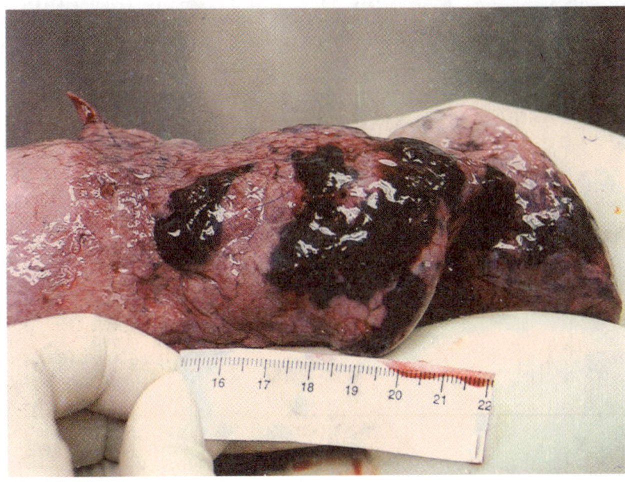

Fig. (9–35). Contusions in lungs.

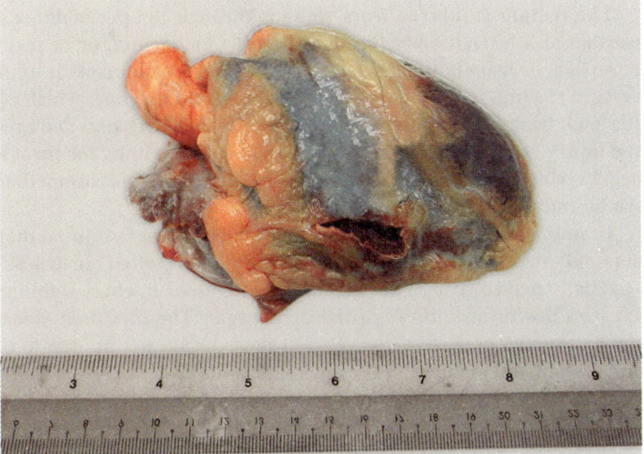

Fig. (9–36). Stab wound of heart.

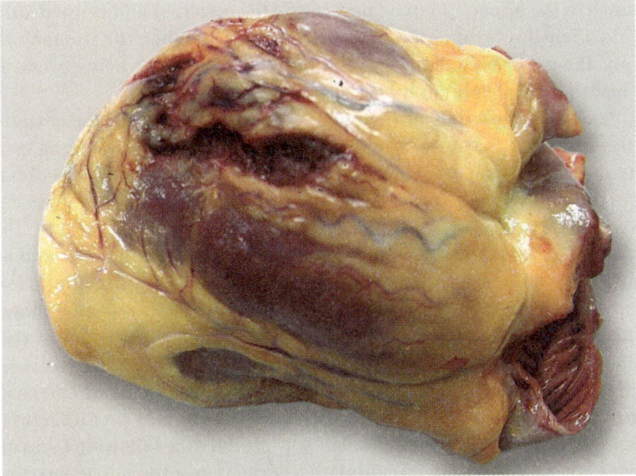

Fig. (9–37). Rupture of myocardial infarct.

localised blunt force applied to the epigastric or left upper quadrant, e.g. kick or a blow with a fist. This crushes the stomach between the anterior abdominal wall and vertebral column. There is usually a circular defect with ragged ecchymotic edges. Severe or fatal internal haemorrhage may occur without any sign of injury on the abdominal wall, especially if clothing overlies the area, probably due to compressive, absorbable nature of abdominal wall. If the victim anticipates the blow and tightens the abdominal muscles, this will disperse the force of impact and reduce the probability of internal injuries, e.g. in boxers. Sometimes, the skin of the abdomen and chest is not damaged, but the underlying muscles are torn by kicks, blunt weapons or street accidents causing protrusion of a portion of a viscus behind the skin. The firmer and denser a viscus, the greater is its friability. Solid organs are more readily lacerated by blows than hollow organs Figs. (9–38 and 9–39). Readily movable or displaceable organs have considerable capacity to absorb the force of blow without serious injury, because of their ability to "ride with the punch". The more sudden and forceful a blow to the abdomen, the more likely is the trauma to be serious and to involve solid viscera.

Penetrating wounds may be produced by a cutting or stabbing instrument, by a firearm, by the horns or claws of an animal or by a fall on a sharp projecting point. A single wound may result in injuries to more than one organ. Penetrating wounds of the lower chest may extend through the diaphragm and injure liver, spleen, stomach or intestines. When these wounds heal, the viscera protrude in the scar. A ventral hernia may take place. Penetrating wounds of the liver are relatively common than the spleen. The abdominal muscles may be torn by violent muscular action, e.g., convulsions of tetanus or in trying to escape a blow.

STOMACH AND INTESTINES: The jejunal portion of small intestine mostly occupies the umbilical and left iliac region; the ileum chiefly occupies the umbilical, hypogastric, right iliac, and pelvic regions. Injuries of the stomach and intestines may be caused by (1) forces of compression or 'crushing' forces, (2) traction or 'tearing forces', and (3) forces of disruption or 'bursting' forces. Compression forces produce

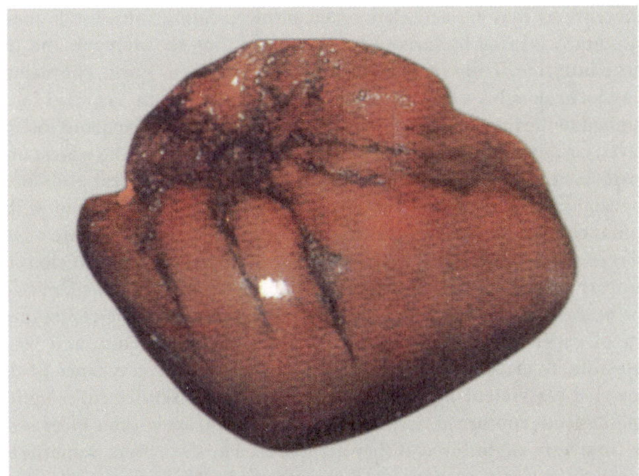

Fig. (9–38). Multiple lacerations of the liver.

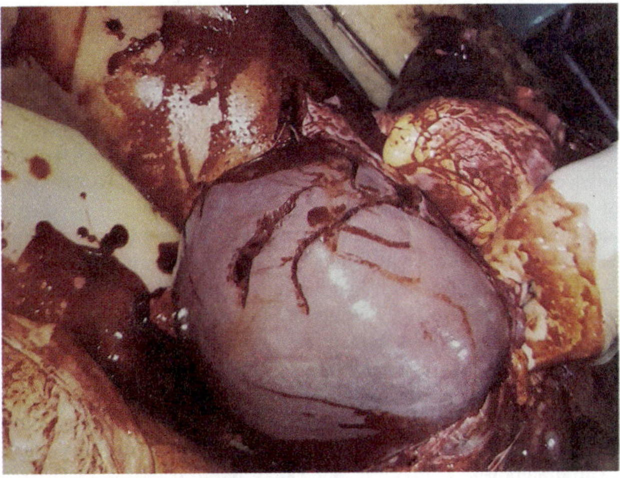

Fig. (9–39). Multiple lacerations of liver.

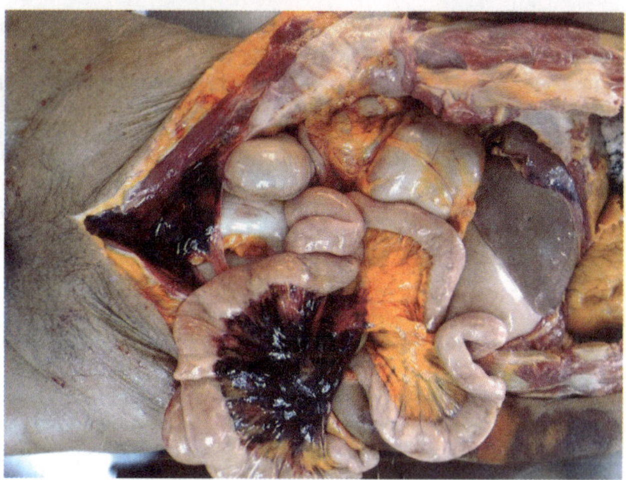

Fig. (9–40). Mesenteric contusions due to blunt trauma to the abdomen.

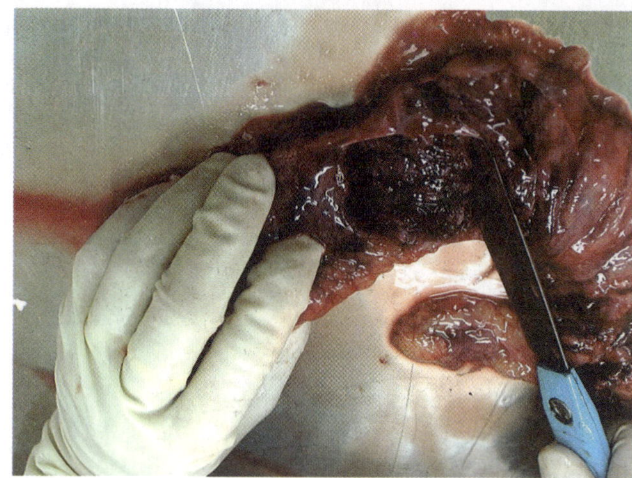

Fig. (9–41). Haemorrhagic pancreatitis.

contusions or lacerations. Contusion may occur in any of the layers of the bowel wall. Large contusion may form sloughs. Mesenteric blood vessels may be damaged and thrombosis in these vessels may produce infarcts of the intestine Fig. (9–40). Traction forces cause displacement of the stomach and intestines, but may stretch and rupture the attachment of the stomach or intestines, e.g., the mesentery may be torn near its intestinal attachment as a result of displacement of the small intestine. Lacerations may be complete or incomplete. Small intestine is more commonly injured by forces of compression than the stomach and the large intestine. Transverse colon is usually involved. Large contusions may form sloughs, which can cause delayed perforation. Traction force applied to the intestine may rupture the junction of the fixed and mobile parts, e.g., at the duodenojejunal junction. Duodenum is the widest and most fixed portion of small intestine. A blow to the central abdomen, especially in children may crush the duodenum against the front of the spinal column, sometimes transecting it clearly so as to simulate a cut. Forces of disruption, e.g., a blow over the abdomen cause contusions or ruptures. The ruptures are often multiple and occur along the length of the antimesenteric border of the bowel. The jejunum is the commonest site of rupture, followed by the ilium, duodenum, caecum, and large intestine. In crushing injuries there may be complete severance of the bowel. Less violent injuries produce a series of semicircular splits. Spontaneous rupture of the intestines may occur from chronic ulceration or from very slight force, if they are diseased or distended. Sometimes, paralytic ileus may occur due to injury. Thrombosis or haemorrhage may follow if the mesentery is contused or torn. The intestines and mesentery may be injured through the uterus by perforating instruments during a criminal abortion. Blast injuries may produce lacerations.

Compression may result in partial rupture of the stomach wall, with longitudinal mucosal tears, parallel to the lesser curvature. Similar injuries may be seen after forcible vomiting, e.g., in poisoning. More severe injury may cause laceration of the full thickness of the wall and rarely the stomach may be completely transected. The stomach distended with food or diseased from ulcer or cancer is easily ruptured by blunt violence, usually at the pyloric end and the lesser curvature. Traumatic rupture of the stomach may occur due to overdistention, as when an anaesthetic tube enters the gullet by mistake. Spontaneous rupture of the stomach may occur when there is an ulcer or even in the absence of disease. The stomach or small intestine may rupture due to an unexpected forceful blow, due to the relaxed abdominal wall musculature. The abdominal skin and the abdominal wall usually do not show any injury. Damage to the mesentery or mesenteric attachment of the intestine may be fatal because of the haemorrhage rather than inflammation.

Laceration of a single large mesenteric artery can cause death due to massive intraperitoneal haemorrhage. Colonic injuries are not common but midportion of transverse colon may be injured due to crushing between anterior abdominal wall and vertebral column.

The rectum is injured from wounds through the perineum, e.g., insertion of a foreign body through the anus for torture, or in sexual perversion, or from falling on a projecting point. A column of air under pressure rushing from the nozzle of a compressed air pipe, which is a little away from the anus may enter the bowel through the anus and cause fatal injury. Rupture of rectum or pelvic colon can occur by the tip of an enema syringe or a sigmoidoscope. The rectum of infants is sometimes torn by end of a thermometer.

In stab wounds of the abdomen, the small intestine is injured more commonly than the large intestine, and the stomach often escapes as it is partially protected by ribs, but may be involved in chest stabbings that pass downwards through the diaphragm. The intestinal wound may be situated at some distance from the external wound due to the compression and mobility of the intestines, and the depth of the wound is greater than the length of the penetrating object.

PANCREAS: It is located retroperitoneally. The tail crosses the upper pole of the left kidney. Wounds of the pancreas are very rare. The pancreas may be injured by compression forces, usually where the neck and body overly the second lumbar vertebra, when the viscera are crushed against the spinal column when the stomach is empty. A kick or a punch in the upper abdomen may injure the pancreas and cause death within a few days from inflammation Fig. (9–41). When the stomach is empty, the pancreas alone may be ruptured vertically by being pressed against the spinal column by the object struck.

Penetrating wounds of the pancreas are not common. Laceration of the pancreas may produce profuse intraperitoneal haemorrhage. Retroperitoneal fat necrosis, mesenteric fat necrosis or chemical peritonitis may result from the escape of pancreatic juice. Trauma to the pancreas can result in residual pseudocysts.

LIVER: It is the most frequently damaged abdominal organ and is second only to the brain in overall visceral susceptibility. Most injuries occur on convex surfaces. The liver is commonly ruptured by a blow, kick, crushing motor accidents, fall or by a sudden contraction of the abdominal muscles. They usually occur in association with other injuries, such as fracture of ribs, rupture of diaphragm, etc. Signs of external injury may or may not be present. Liver contusions may be difficult to recognise. Blunt force to the abdomen may produce the following types of hepatic lacerations: (1) Transcapsular lacerations over the convex surface of the liver under the site of impact. The lacerations are often shallow splits, branching out in a cobweb-like pattern across the surface of the organ. (2) Subcapsular lacerations over the convex surface of the liver under the site of impact. (3) Non-communicating or central lacerations in the substance of the liver. (4) Coronal lacerations over the superior surface due to distortion. (5) Lacerations of the inferior surface due to distortion. (6) CONTRECOUP LACERATION involving the posterior surface of the right lobe, at the point where it rests against the vertebral column.

If the force impacting the front of the liver is directed upward, it may lacerate the undersurface of the liver. If the force is directed downward and backward, superior surface is lacerated. If the force is directed straight at the liver along its anterior margin, lacerations occur both in the concave and convex surfaces. Transcapsular lacerations may cause rapid death from haemorrhage and shock. A subcapsular haematoma may rupture several hours or days after the injury and cause fatal delayed intraperitoneal haemorrhage. The right lobe is five times more commonly affected than the left. They usually involve the convex surface and inferior border but may only involve the deep substance of the organ, consisting of blood fissures. They are usually directed anteroposteriorly or obliquely. An impact on the right upper part of the abdomen may cause tearing of the liver close to its ligaments. Tangential or glancing blunt force to the right upper quadrant of the abdomen may separate the liver capsule from the underlying tissue with subcapsular haemorrhage. Rarely one lobe of the liver may be detached.

Mild degree of external violence may rupture the liver if it is diseased, e.g., fatty metamorphosis, abscess formation, malaria, bilharziasis. In newborn child, there may be a laceration in the liver or a large subcapsular haematoma which may not rupture for several days. This results from sudden pressure to the chest during delivery. In some cases, liver tissue emboli may produce fatal pulmonary embolism. In cases of central or subcapsular rupture, blood may pass through the bile duct into gastrointestinal tract. Penetrating wounds of the liver are relatively more common and may cause death by haemorrhage and shock.

Injuries of the GALLBLADDER and the extrahepatic bile ducts are rare, and are associated with injuries to other abdominal viscera. A gallbladder distended with stones may rupture spontaneously. The extravasation of bile into the peritoneal sac may cause peritoneal irritation and infection.

SPLEEN: The spleen lies in the left upper quadrant of the abdomen extending to the epigastric region, largely protected by the lower ribs. Penetrating wounds of the spleen are less common than those of liver, but bleeding is more profuse. The spleen may be injured by forces of compression or traction forces. Compression forces produce lacerations. Traction forces may tear the spleen from its pedicle. The spleen is ruptured usually in its concave surface, and is usually associated with injuries to other organs and rib fractures. Lacerations are usually transcapsular and may occur at the hilar or convex surfaces. They are often multiple and may simulate the alphabetical figures, Y, H, or L. Death from rupture of spleen is usually rapid, due to profuse haemorrhage. A relatively mild trauma or even the contraction of the abdominal muscle may predispose the spleen to rupture when it is diseased and enlarged, e.g., malaria, Kala Azar, and leukaemia. Spontaneous rupture of the spleen can occur in malaria, typhoid fever, haemophilia, leukaemia and infectious mononucleosis. A single blow may produce more than one rupture. Sometimes, the splenic substance may rupture without damage to the capsule. In such a case, death may be delayed for some days, as the capsule limits the rupture or prevents severe bleeding. Delayed splenic rupture following trauma usually occurs within two weeks. The effused blood under the capsule clots, presses on the rupture and prevents further bleeding. The clot may be disturbed due to sudden muscular excitement, with further bleeding and death.

COMPLICATIONS OF ABDOMINAL INJURIES: Laceration of the spleen produces rapid and copious haemorrhage. Laceration of the liver produces slow bleeding due to the relatively low pressure in the hepatic sinusoids but considerable bleeding occurs over a period of time. Peritonitis is more common in ruptures of the large intestine than ruptures of the small intestine due to the presence of pathogenic organisms in the colon. Chemical peritonitis is caused by leakage of gastric contents or pancreatic juice into the peritoneal cavity. Multiple contusions of the intestines may produce paralytic ileus.

UROGENITAL TRACT: KIDNEY: Injuries to the kidneys are not common as they are situated in relatively well-protected part of the body. Contusions and lacerations usually result from blunt force applied directly to the posterior or lateral aspect of the kidneys as from blows to loins. When the kidney is diseased, it may be injured from slight external violence. Contusions may be localised, or generalised and may appear as horizontal bruises corresponding to the rib markings over the posterior surface. Contusion about the upper pole of the right kidney is caused by its crushing against the lower ribs by force transmitted through liver.

Lacerations of the kidneys may be transcapsular, subcapsular and transrenal (tear extending from the capsule to the renal pelvis). In transcapsular and transrenal lacerations of the kidney, the capsule ruptures at multiple points often along lines which radiate from the hilum towards the convex border. These may cause haemorrhage into the perinephric fat and form a large perirenal haematoma. An extensive retroperitoneal haemorrhage usually occurs due to some secondary trauma, e.g., lacerations of the liver or the kidney, but it may occur as a primary traumatic lesion and cause death from shock. The kidneys may be ruptured when a person is run over by a vehicle, or falls from a height or is crushed. In transrenal lacerations, haemorrhage may occur as a primary traumatic lesion and cause death from shock. Blunt force applied to the loin may cause contusion or laceration of the renal pedicle. If the renal artery is torn, death may occur rapidly from haemorrhage. A partial tear of the artery may be followed by thrombosis and renal infarction. Contusion of pedicle may produce renal spasm and infarction. In falls from height, renal artery may be torn. Injuries of the ureters are rare.

The kidney is encapsulated and filled with blood and urine due to which a severe blow initiates forces which act according to PASCAL'S LAW, which states that the "force exerted upon any part of enclosed fluid is transmitted equally in all directions". Violent blows to a kidney can cause bursting injuries with fragmentation or multiple bisections.

Penetrating wounds are produced by bullets or pointed weapons usually through the loin, and other viscera are also injured, with retroperitoneal haemorrhage. Infarction of the kidney occurs due to direct injury to the renal artery, or a large intrarenal vessel. The complications may be sepsis, and the extravasation of urine into the surrounding tissues with the development of urinary fistula.

ADRENALS: The adrenal gland may be injured by the same force which damages the kidney and may be lacerated or crushed. Haemorrhage (adrenal apoplexy) may be rarely seen associated with other injuries.

BLADDER: In children, the anterior surface of the bladder is in contact with the lower part of the abdominal wall. Beginning at puberty, it slowly begins to descend in the pelvis. The bladder may be lacerated from a fall, a kick or a blow on the abdomen. When the bladder is distended, the peritoneum over the upper surface is stretched and tears, which often extends through the bladder wall and urine is extravasated into the peritoneal cavity. When the bladder is only partially distended, blunt force to the lower abdomen may cause an extraperitoneal rupture. Rupture of the bladder usually occurs in association with fracture of the pelvis. In extraperitoneal ruptures, the urine may extravasate upwards to the level of the kidneys or downwards along the spermatic cord into the scrotum, which may produce cellulitis and death. Spontaneous rupture of the normal bladder is rare, but may occur when it is ulcerated or diseased (tuberculosis, carcinoma, cystitis, etc.), when there is obstruction in the urethra. During parturition, the bladder may rupture due to the pressure of the child's head. It may rupture by a cystoscope, catheter or other body introduced through the urethra.

Stab wounds of the lower abdomen may penetrate bladder and may cause rapid death from haemorrhage. There may be extraperitoneal extravasation of urine. A high velocity bullet penetrating the distended bladder causes an explosive effect on the urine, which may produce extensive laceration of the bladder.

The male urethra may be ruptured usually under the pubic arch by a kick in the perineum, by a fall on a projecting substance, by fracture of pubic bone or by a foreign body. Forcible catheterisation or cystoscopy, especially in the presence of some obstruction can cause rupture of urethra from within. The tear in the urethra may be complete or partial, and the wound may communicate with the skin. Usually damage occurs in the bulbous or membranous urethra. Violent displacement of a full bladder, as in crushing injuries of the pelvis may rupture the posterior urethra. The female urethra may be ruptured by an act of rape.

FEMALE GENITAL ORGANS: Contusions and lacerations of the vulva and vagina may be due to kicks during assaults, or falls on a projecting substance. Wounds of vulva caused by a blunt weapon may resemble incised wounds. Lacerated wounds of the vulva may bleed profusely. The vaginal wall may be lacerated during delivery, which may extend into the bladder or rectum.

The uterus, ovaries or the Fallopian tubes may be contused or lacerated in severe compression injuries of the pelvis. The non-gravid uterus is not usually injured. The gravid uterus may be ruptured by a blow, kick, trampling on the abdominal wall, or by instrumental criminal abortion, or in obstructed labour. Placenta may separate from uterus and cause death of foetus. Penetrating wounds are not common.

MALE GENITAL ORGANS: The penis may be injured by a squeeze or crush, and the engorged erected penis may be completely avulsed from the pubes by forceful pull. Self-inflicted injuries may be seen in insane persons. Accidental injuries are rare, but they may be injured or amputated from motives of revenge. Penile strangulation may occur due to placement of a constricting apparatus around the penis. Oedema developing in the distal portion prevents removal of the device Fig. (9–42). The testicles are contused from blows, kicks and squeezes. **Compression or crushing of the testis may cause sudden death from cardiac inhibition.**

LIMBS: Abrasions, contusions and deep lacerated wounds involving the muscles and extending up to the bone are common in traffic and industrial accidents. Deep-seated limb injuries affecting the muscles, vessels, nerves or bone may occur without any external evidence of injury.

FALLS: When a person becomes unconscious while standing or walking he will fall forward. When a person is pushed from the front, he may fall on his back. An alcoholic may stagger for some time and fall forwards or to one side. In epileptic convulsions, the person falls backwards due to spasm of the muscles of the back. In cases of brain stroke, the person may fall on to the side of hemiplegia.

AORTA: Rupture of the thoracic aorta may occur in traffic accidents; the driver's chest striking the steering wheel, or the front seat passenger's chest striking the dashboard, or impact of the occupant's chest against the pavement following ejection, or pedestrian sustaining a violent impact to the chest or been run over. Falls from height and crushing chest injuries also cause rupture of aorta. A transverse tear of the aorta immediately above the cusps of the aortic valve may occur when a violent force compresses the heart and intrapericardial portion of the ascending aorta. This is associated with fractures of sternum and upper ribs. Lacerations are usually transverse and may be associated with rib and/or vertebral fractures. Most common site is in the descending thoracic aorta, just distal to the origin of the left subclavian artery. Rarely, a periaortic haematoma due to laceration of aorta may produce a false aneurysm. Traumatic rupture of abdominal aorta may occur in automobile accidents. Spontaneous rupture of the aorta may occur from local disease.

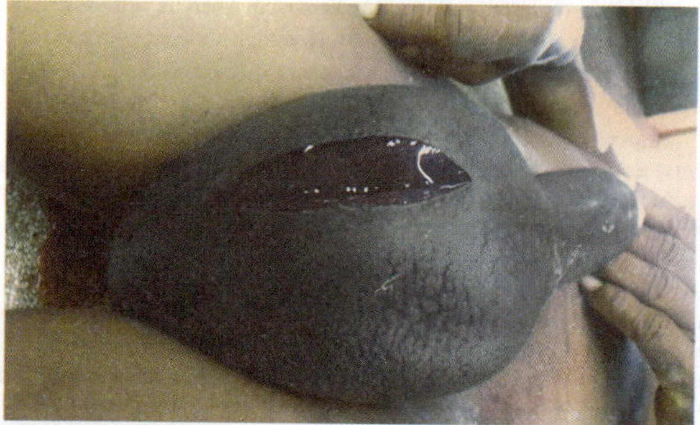

Fig. (9–42). Bruising of scrotum and penis.

Courtesy: Dr. Tamil Mani, Associate Professor; Pudukottai, Chennai, Tamil Nadu, India.

INJURIES OF ARTERIES: A direct injury of a large artery of the limb, e.g., the brachial or femoral artery, may produce contusion or partial or complete rupture of the arterial wall which can cause immediate localised arterial spasm (traumatic segmentary arteriospasm). Arteriospasm is commonly seen in fracture of the limb bone, and occurs when the bone ends or fragments contuse or lacerate an artery.

Contusions of the arteries are usually found in the intima, and are usually associated with tears of the intima and thrombus formation. Arterial contusions are common in crush injuries of the limbs. When an artery is lacerated or punctured, e.g., by a bone fragment or by a bullet, a perivascular haematoma may form in the surrounding tissues. The blood at the periphery of the haematoma may coagulate and organise, and if the central portion of the haematoma remains fluid, a direct communication may be maintained between the artery and the haematoma forming a false aneurysm. This aneurysm may gradually increase in size and rupture resulting in profuse haemorrhage and death. True traumatic aneurysms are rare. It may occur when outer coat of a large artery is injured, e.g., a tangential bullet injury of a vessel.

A penetrating wound of a limb, e.g., from a bullet or a stab may extend through an artery and the accompanying vein, and produce an arteriovenous fistula. In a large arteriovenous fistula situated in proximal part of a large limb artery, considerable amount of blood may leak into the related vein. Muscle necrosis and gangrene may occur due to impairment in the blood supply to the limb. Progressive cardiac decompensation and death may occur due to fall in arterial pressure and the rise in venous pressure.

Arterial thrombosis and embolism, traumatic segmentary arteriospasm, true and false traumatic aneurysms and arteriovenous fistulas may impair the circulation in a limb. Sensory and motor nerve endings are highly susceptible to ischaemia. Muscle tissue becomes necrosed. Ischaemia persists for six to 8 hours, and skin becomes necrosed in 24 hours. Fibrosis of necrosed muscles cause shortening of the muscles and produce deformities and contractures (Volkman's ischaemic contracture). Most commonly occlusion of the brachial artery results in deformities and contractures of the forearm and hand.

VEINS: Minor injuries may damage the veins. Contusion of the wall or tearing of the intima may occur in trauma. A thrombus may form at the site of damage to the intima which may become dislodged and give rise to pulmonary embolism. Pulmonary air embolism may occur in laceration of a large vein in an open wound to a limb. Fat embolism may result from laceration of vein in regions of extensive damage to adipose tissue. The inferior vena cava may be torn transversely by severe trauma.

PERIPHERAL NERVES: Incised or puncture wounds may divide peripheral nerves. They may be lacerated in certain types of fractures, e.g., the musculospiral nerve may be lacerated in fractures of the shaft of the humerus. Compression or crushing injuries may cause contusion or concussion of nerves. Traction forces may injure the nerves, e.g., the ulnar nerve may be stretched in fracture-dislocations of the elbow joint. Ischaemia of limb due to arterial injury may result in paralysis and anaesthesia, even when the nerves are not directly injured.

BONES: Fractures of the Extremities: (I) DIRECT FORCE: (1) Penetrating fractures. (2) Focal fractures occur when a small force is applied to a small area resulting in a transverse fracture. Overlying soft tissue injury is relatively minor. **(3) Crush fractures** occur when a large force is applied over a large area. Overlying soft tissue is extensively injured, and often the fracture is comminuted. In severe impact injuries of the legs, the fracture may be transverse, oblique, spiral, segmental, comminuted, longitudinal split, tension-wedge or compression-wedge type.

(II) INDIRECT FORCE: (1) **Traction fracture:** In this the bone is pulled apart by traction, e.g. transverse fracture of patella due to violent contraction of the quadriceps muscle. (2) **Rotational fracture:** The bone is twisted and a spiral fracture is produced. It occurs only when the bone is subjected to torsional force. (3) **Vertical compression fractures** produce an oblique fracture of the body of long bones with the hard shaft driven into the cancellous end. (4) **In angulation and compression fractures,** the fracture line is curved. (5) **Angulation, rotation and compression** fractures are oblique.

Contusion of bone and of its periosteum occurs due to a blow or a fall. Fractures may occur from falls, blows or the action of the muscles. In direct violence, fracture occurs at the site of impact, and some injury to the overlying soft tissue is always present. They may be compound or comminuted. If the violence is indirect, a simple fracture occurs in a region distant from the site of impact of the force, e.g., a fracture of the head of the radius or of the lower end of the humerus caused by a fall on the extended palm. In a simple or closed fracture, there is no communication between the bone and the air. A fall on the outstretched hand will cause Colles' fracture (fracture of the distal end of radius). A compound fracture from indirect violence may occur when a fragment of bone pierces the skin from the inside. The sharp ends of the fractured bone produce injuries of the soft tissues. In a compound or open fracture, there is a communication between the bone and the air through a wound. Clavicle is commonly fractured at the junction of middle and lateral one-third. The sudden contraction of the muscle during an unexpected movement may fracture a bone, e.g., the olecranon or the patella may be fractured by the sudden contraction of the triceps or the quadriceps muscles respectively. Most spontaneous fractures occur due to disease, e.g., osteoporosis, osteomalacia, Paget's disease, etc. Green-stick fracture is an incomplete fracture involving only part of the distance across a bone shaft, with bending or crushing of the bone. It occurs in young children. In childhood, slipping of an epiphysis is common, e.g., in distal end of the radius, internal epicondyle of the humerus, capitulum, and distal end of the tibia.

When a car dashes against a tree or a wall, injury to spine and fractures of the limbs may result from indirect violence. In an accident, fracture occurs at the weakest part of the bone, is usually spiral or oblique without a bruise or wound. Fractures of metacarpal bones occur usually by striking the closed hand (fist) against a firm surface (Boxer fractures).

AUTOPSY: At autopsy a fracture may be suspected when there is extensive swelling and discolouration of the skin, or when there is abnormal mobility, or crepitus is found. The tissues surrounding suspect fracture should be dissected to determine injuries to the soft parts. In adults blood loss in compound fracture of femur may be 1 to 3 litres, closed fracture of femur 1 to 2 litres, humerus 200 to 500 ml, pelvis 2 litres, closed fracture of lower leg 0.5 to 1 litre and fracture dislocation of ankle 0.5 to one litre. Different types of fracture of long bones are given in Fig. (9–43).

DISTINCTION BETWEEN ANTEMORTEM AND POSTMORTEM FRACTURES: Fractures caused some hours before death show signs of effusion of blood, laceration of muscles and oedema, which are not seen in a fracture produced after death.

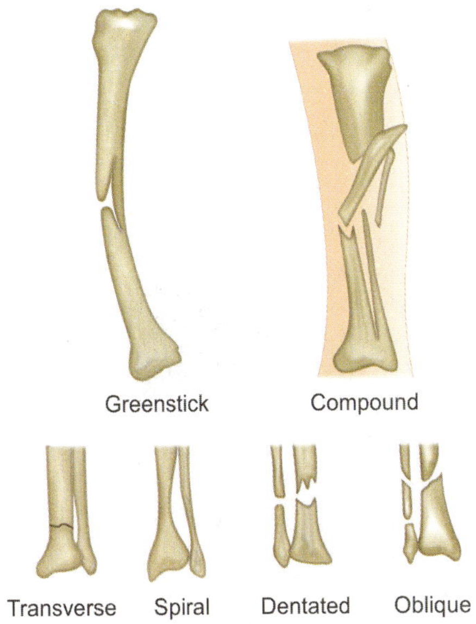

Greenstick   Compound

Transverse   Spiral   Dentated   Oblique

Fig. (9–43). Various types of fractures.

A fracture produced shortly before, or shortly after death has same characters, except that in the former there may be more effused blood, which penetrates further into the adjacent tissues.

AGE OF FRACTURE: Haemorrhage occurs at the time of injury, and the haematoma formed around the fracture is usually clotted within 12 to 24 hours. A fibrin network is formed within hours. Histologically, some necrosis of the bone is seen in two days. Acute inflammatory changes are seen within hours of injury and last for several days. After partial organisation of blood clot, the fracture gap may be filled with condensed highly eosinophilic fibrin. Within one to two days, there may be migration of polymorphs into the necrotic tissue and later macrophages. Osteogenic granulation tissue is formed accompanied by hyperaemia and oedema in four days. New vessels are formed and numerous fibroblasts are seen in seven days. Small areas of bone are laid down around blood vessels in an irregular interwoven manner within a week. This woven bone is formed equally by periosteal, endosteal, and marrow reticulum cells. The fibroblasts lay down reticulin and then collagen, which is usually well marked by ten days. A haematoma, resulting from a fracture usually gets absorbed in 10 to 14 days. Cellular elements give rise to osteoblasts and chondroblasts which produce a matrix of collagen and polysaccharides impregnated with calcium, called callus in two weeks. Much of the damaged marrow is invaded by vascular fibrocellular tissue by 15 to 20 days. By X-ray examination, callus is not readily visible for three weeks. The periosteal callus gap is usually obliterated by 30 days. Callus is formed into hard bone in about two months, although the bone still undergoes reconstructive modelling. After healing is complete, an approximate estimation of the age can be given from the extent of remodelling, the smoothness of edges, and the form of trabeculae passing through the line of fracture. The last thing to occur in fracture healing is regaining of full joint motion.

If a fracture is inadequately immobilised, repeated movements of the limb cause tearing of the granulation tissue with recurring hyperaemia, continued resorption of bone and delayed union.

JOINTS: Injuries may be caused by blows or fall or by dislocations. Any injury to the synovial membrane, the intra-articular cartilages, the ligaments, or the capsule of a joint may be accompanied by a transudation of serous fluid into the joint cavity. Laceration of the synovial membrane or the joint cartilages, or fracture-dislocations cause haemorrhage into joint cavity. Serous effusions are absorbed, but blood is organised with intra-articular adhesions. Dislocations may occur due to direct violence like falls, blows, or muscular action, or spontaneously when the joints are diseased. They are not dangerous unless they occur between the vertebrae, or are compound. Punctured or incised wounds of the joints are likely to become infected. To determine the range of movement at a joint, graduated protractor is used.

The estimation of age of dislocation can be made by the colour change if bruise is present. In older cases, the amount of new fibrous tissue or the formation of false joints may give some idea of the age of the injury.

FALLS FROM HEIGHT: Factors influencing the pattern of injury: (1) Height. (2) Orientation of body at point of impact: In majority of falls, vertical landing with feet first is common and next common being with head first. (3) Surface impact: The surface on to which a body falls determines the pattern of deceleration and energy exchange. (4) Deceleration: Quicker the body is brought to rest, greater will be forces acting on it.

In a typical case of primary impact with the feet (about 60%), the bones of the feet (calcaneum and other tarsal and metatarsal bones) are fractured (usually comminuted and often open) and the tibias may be driven through the soles of the feet; fracture-dislocation of the ankles; comminuted or oblique fractures of the tibiae and fibulae; fractures of the femurs (shafts, condyles or neck); pelvic fractures; fractures and dislocations of the vertebral column associated with lacerations or transection of spinal cord; ring or comminuted fractures of the base of the skull and injuries to the brainstem and inferior surface of the brain. Fractures in the lower limbs could be unilateral or bilateral. There may

be lacerations of the liver and spleen. The aorta usually ruptures at the junction of the aortic arch with the descending thoracic aorta. Intimal tears are often seen along the thoracic or abdominal aorta. Ruptures or lacerations of the pulmonary trunk, arteries and veins and of the superior and inferior vena cavae are less common. This full range of injuries does not occur in every case.

In primary head impact open comminuted or depressed skull fractures with brain lacerations and partial or complete extrusion of the brain may occur (about 10%). This may also be seen with primary impact of the feet and subsequent secondary head impact.

Imprint abrasions and contusions are common when the body lands on hard patterned surfaces. Bruising of the palms and fingers may be seen if the victim clings into the edge of the building or parapet before releasing the grip. Perineal bruising due to relative movement of the pubic-perineal region against the clothing may be seen in vertical feet-first impacts, which may be misinterpreted as resulting from sexual assault. All sorts of lacerations may be sustained. Bodies may be transected or decapitated as they hit other objects. Usually, the greater the height of the fall, the more severe are the injuries. In most cases, the posture or orientation on impact determines the regional preponderance of injuries. The body can bounce off the surface as it impacts and then fall some short distance away.

The severity of injuries is not directly related to the distance of the fall of the person. Some persons may die after falling from a standing position on to the back of the head, but some may survive a fall of many metres. In old people, falls can cause fracture of the neck of the femur, ribs, arms, and pelvis. When a person falls or jumps from a height, the trajectory is downwards and outwards, and the distance the body strikes the ground is variable. Much depends on whether the victim fell passively from near the wall or projected himself outwards at the top. The body turns and twists in an unpredictable manner during fall. A person falling 15 metres attains a speed of 17m/s. When falling from a high building, the displaced air tends to act as a cushion which drives the body from the wall. A simple fall can result in a body impact some distance from the foot of the building, which is not an evidence of a push or of a deliberate jump. The site of primary impact shows most severe injury. Sometimes, two areas may strike the ground simultaneously, e.g. head and shoulder, or the person may bounce and two or more major impacts occur. If the person falls on to the head, both vault and base can fracture, with extrusion of brain. When the person falls to the side of the body, fractures of multiple ribs, shoulder girdle, arms, and contusions and lacerations of back, buttocks or limbs, and severe abdominal and thoracic injuries can occur. The lungs are most sensitive to deceleration; pulmonary haemorrhages and haemothorax are common. The liver is most commonly injured followed by heart and aorta. The aorta tears usually either at its origin or at the end of the thoracic arch.

Occasionally, extensive and severe internal visceral and skeletal injuries may occur in the absence of any significant external injury, if the body lands upon a relatively soft surface, such as a grass patch.

TRAFFIC ACCIDENTS

A large variety of injuries are sustained by persons involved in traffic accidents.

INJURIES TO PEDESTRIANS: Patterns of injury: (1) Primary impact injuries (the first part struck). (2) Secondary impact injuries (further injuries caused by the vehicle). (3) Secondary injuries, sometimes called tertiary injuries, (injuries caused by the victim's striking objects, such as the ground). Diagrams indicating the location, nature and extent of injuries are of value to establish injury patterns.

In **primary impact injuries, the part of the body involved depends upon the position of the person in relation to the vehicle when struck,** i.e., whether crossing the road from one side to the other or walking with or against the traffic. The injuries also depend upon the relative heights of various parts of the vehicle, i.e., bumper, fender, radiator, door handles, etc.

Bumper injuries: In the typical case, the victim is struck by the front of the vehicle, and sustains so-called bumper injuries on legs. These injuries may be severe with **fractures of tibia and fibula often compound and extensive soft tissue damage.** They may also be minimal or absent externally. Usually the tibia is fractured, with forward displacement of the bone fragment which was struck. The fracture is usually spiral or wedge-shaped. **The base of the triangular fragment of bone indicates the site of impact, and the apex points in the direction in which the vehicle was travelling** Fig. (9–44). If the leg is lifted, the fracture is often transverse. If the vehicle was braking violently at the moment of impact, the front end of the vehicle dips down and the legs are injured at a lower level. Frequently, bumper injuries are at different levels on the two legs or absent on one leg, which suggest that the victim was walking or running when struck. The fracture is at a higher level in the leg that was in contact with the ground. If the individual was oriented sideways to the impacting vehicle, bumper fracture will be seen in one leg only. In children, the bumper usually produces fracture of the femur.

Secondary impact injuries: If the foot is fixed, a fracture results, and the buttocks and back will come in contact with the car and then pushed forward Fig. (9–45). **He may sustain a fracture-dislocation of the lumbar or thoracic spine, sometimes associated with the fractures of adjacent ribs.** The detached portion of the vertebral column may move forward transecting the cord and thoracic aorta. If the feet slide forward, the whole body will fall backward with a secondary impact of the head against the windshield, or he may be thrown into the air, or to one side and strike the ground. If the person falls on the hood, the tangential force directed by the hood to the buttock and thigh may cause separation of the skin and subcutaneous tissues from the muscle, producing a pocket in the upper thigh and buttock. Large amount of blood may collect in this pocket, which is often not seen externally.

Secondary injuries: When he is thrown clear of the vehicle soon after the impact, he may sustain secondary injuries which vary greatly in severity. They may be abrasions, contusions, fractures of various bones including the skull.

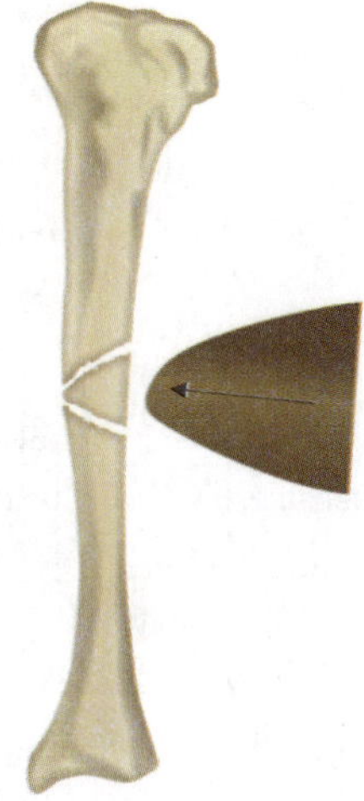

Fig. (9–44). Wedge-shaped fracture of tibia in a pedestrian with bumper injuries.

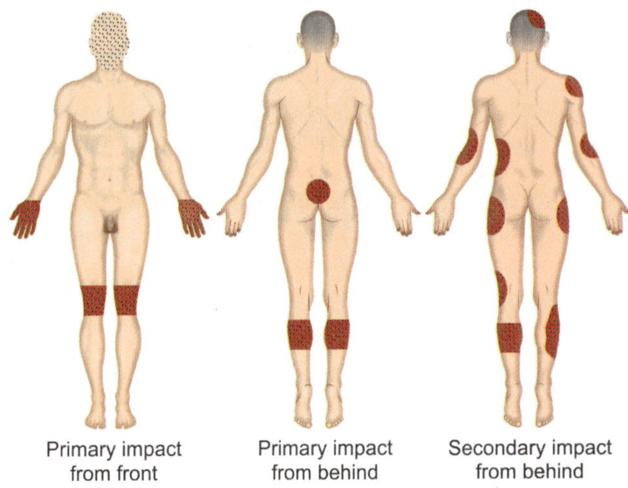

Fig. (9–45). Impact injuries; primary (cross-hatched); secondary (dotted).

Front Impact: If the person is facing the vehicle, he may sustain intra-abdominal injuries, and injuries to the chest wall and the thoracic contents. Direct impact to the thorax may cause rupture of the aorta below the arch at the level of the ligamentum arteriosum, due to the sudden increase of intravascular pressure. There may be bruising of the right atrium and sometimes laceration or rupture of the heart. Splenic lacerations cause slow oozing. Injury to the intestinal tract is less common.

Rear Impact: **If the victim is struck from behind, a characteristic series of superficial, parallel linear and irregular linear tears of the abdomen or the inguinal regions are seen due to overstretching of the skin which appear dry, yellow and bloodless** Fig. (9–46). If the vehicle travels at high speed, deep lacerations may be produced due to the same mechanism. If the victim is run over by the vehicle, similar injuries may be produced due to overstretching of the skin by the passing wheel, and the crushing weight of the vehicle on the body Fig. (9–46). An impact against a mudguard or headlamp may result in fracture of the pelvis or fracture-dislocations of the sacroiliac joints. They leave patterned imprints on the skin. The pubic ramus opposite to the buttock or hip involved is usually fractured. **The margins of the lacerations show contusions in primary impact injuries, and abrasions in secondary impact injuries.** A rear impact of a pedestrian is often associated with fracture of cervical spine, and often dislocated at the base of skull due to whiplash. The thoracic and lumbar areas may be crushed by impact of the hood. **Many impacts are on front corner of the car** and pedestrian may be knocked diagonally out of the path of the car. If thrown into the centre of the roadway the person can be run over by another vehicle.

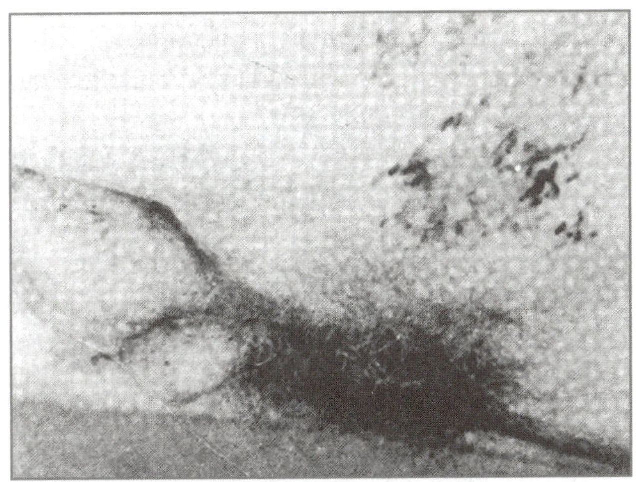

Fig. (9–46). Linear superficial tears of the inguinal region and lower abdomen in a pedestrian struck from the automobile from behind.

Side impact: When a pedestrian walks into the side of a vehicle, pressure abrasions or tears on the side or front of the face are produced which are sometimes patterned. A hand, forearm or elbow may intervene between vehicle and either the face or trunk. The chest or loin may be injured sometimes with fractured ribs and rupture of lungs, diaphragm, spleen or liver. Tearing wounds may be caused by protruding objects, such as door handles, or with cuts from broken glass. If the person falls and is run over by the back wheels, crushing injuries of the head, trunk and limbs are seen.

Injuries depending on the speed of vehicle: At a speed of 20 kmph, the person can be thrown away. At a speed of 40 to 50 kmph., if the vehicle strikes a person below the centre of gravity of his body, (below waist line, just below brim of pelvis), he is thrown upward and slides on to the hood(bonnet) of the vehicle (scooping-up) and may sustain superficial abrasions of his elbows, shoulders and head, or severe injuries from striking the bonnet or protruding objects and especially the windscreen or windscreen pillars at either side. Impact with the windscreen and secondary injuries cause fractures of ribs, arms, pelvis and injuries to the abdomen. Often the injuries are found more on one side, usually on the opposite side to the point of primary impact. Subsequently, the person slides sideways off the hood and sustains a final impact with the road's surface, usually by the head and occasionally with the buttocks. Fractures of the sacroiliac joints and fractures and dislocations of cervical spine due to sudden unexpected hyperextension of the neck following initial impact are common. Atlanto-occipital dislocation and partial disruption of intervertebral disc are common. When the vehicle travels at a greater speed (80 to 100 kmph), the pedestrian may be thrown higher and falls on the vehicle roof sometimes somersaulting so that the head strikes the roof. He can then slide or thrown over the back of the car on the road behind the vehicle. In general, the higher the speed more severe the injuries.

Injuries caused due to straight and high-front vehicle: If a fast moving bus, truck or van having a straight and high front end hits an adult, the impact is naturally much higher, at hip or even shoulder level and may cause primary damage to pelvis, abdomen, shoulder-girdle, arm or head. Even low speeds can cause severe injuries. If the body is hit at hip level, the victim will be pushed directly forwards in front of the vehicle. If the body is hit high up, the upper part of the body will be pushed down, or he may be carried on the radiator grille for some distance and fall in front of the vehicle as it slows down or comes to a halt, and the victim may be run over. If clothing or part of the body becomes engaged under the bumper or in the wheel arches during the initial impact, the person will be dragged underneath, instead of being thrown upwards. Protruding objects may cause serious injuries. In children, impact with the front of a vehicle is above the centre of gravity. The victim is pushed down and run over.

It is always not possible to associate injuries sustained by pedestrians with specific features of external automobile design, especially when the victims are children or the accident is of the low speed type.

The most extensive fractures are produced by the head striking a flat surface. In pedestrians, the head is injured by direct impact with the vehicle and by striking the road. Both impacts produce fractures involving almost all parts of the skull, especially the base. Fractures may extend transversely across the base of the skull through the middle fossa to the lower parietal bone on each side. Extensive injuries of the brain are caused under such distortion and with added severe acceleration or deceleration. Extensive surface laceration with much subarachnoid and often subdural bleeding may occur. Haemorrhage into the basal ganglia and severe laceration of the corpus callosum may occur. Bleeding into the uncus and brainstem are rare.

Rolling Injuries: Rolling injuries are produced when a vehicle with a low chassis, "rolled" the victim along the roadway as it passed over him. They are usually located on two or more body surfaces and run circumferentially. **They are mostly abrasions, grease soiling and burns from the exhaust system.** There may be fractures of the skull, neck, shoulder, shoulder-girdle, ribs, vertebrae or pelvis. Patterned imprints may be present caused by parts on the undersurface of the chassis. The elasticity of skin and tissues tends to keep the body in one piece, though broken. At very high speeds (130 kmph), impacts result in hemisection of the victim.

Injuries due to run over: If the person is run over, there may be: (1) Tyre marks, often spread a little due to yielding and flattening of the body from pressure. A body may be dragged and turned over due to being run over. In this case, tyre marks or grease from the undercarriage of the vehicle may sometimes be seen on surface of body in contact with road, while the opposite side of the body shows brush burns. (2) Grazes. (3) Avulsion. The rotatory effect against a fixed limb may strip off almost all tissues down to the bone. The avulsed wound may be segmental or circumferential, the latter completely encircling arm or leg. If scrotum or abdominal wall are injured, testes or intestines are extruded. Avulsion of an ear occurs if a tyre passes over the head of the victim. The tear is behind the ear if the vehicle rolls from back to front in relation to the victim, and in front of the ear, if vehicle travels in opposite direction. (4) If the brakes of the vehicle are applied, the wheels will lock and long lacerations are produced due to the shearing action of tangential force. Complete amputation of a limb or decapitation may occur. (5) Burning of the skin due to the heat produced by sliding of the body and discharge of hot exhaust. (6) Deep crushing of the internal organs and flattening deformities of the head, chest, or pelvis. (7) Decapitation or complete amputation of an extremity may occur. (8) When a child is run over by a vehicle, fractures may not be produced, because of the elasticity of partly cartilaginous skeleton.

OCCUPANTS OF THE VEHICLES: Injuries to driver: Most of the vehicular accidents are frontal (two vehicles colloiding head-on or vehicle striking a fixed object occurs in about 80% of all vehicular accidents) causing violent deceleration. If the impact is gross, the engine or front wheel assembly may be forced back into the seating area intruding upon driver. Similarly, the roof or front corner pillar may cave in on top of the driver. The occupants of the vehicle will continue to move forwards, at the same speed the car was travelling, even though the vehicle has stopped. The unrestrained driver first slides forwards so that his legs strike the fascia parcel shelf area, knees hit the bottom of the dashboard causing fractures of patella or distal femur, and his abdomen or lower chest strikes the lower edge of the steering wheel. Dislocation at the hip-joint or fracture of neck of femur may occur. This is called **"secondary accident".** Then the body flexes across the steering wheel and begins to rise. The heavy head goes forward and there is flexion of cervical and thoracic spines. The head strikes the windscreen, the upper windscreen rim or the side pillar. The windscreen may break and the driver may be ejected through the broken glass on the bonnet or on the road.

The driver may be thrown forward and strike the chest on the steering-wheel or the upper abdomen on wheel-rim **Fig. (9–47).** The horn boss may strike the sternum and produce a transverse fracture usually at third intercostal space, and crush the heart or split the aorta. The wheel-rim may crush the liver, spleen or kidneys. In some cases, lungs are contused or lacerated, due to fractured ribs penetrating the lung tissue. Pneumothorax may be present. Liver may be lacerated near its attachment or impact sites anywhere in right or left lobe. Central tearing of upper surface is common, which may even transect the organ. Spleen shows shallow tears, often around the hilum. Rarely it may be avulsed from the pedicle. Mesentery and omentum often show bruising and rarely laceration. Transection of the aorta usually occurs immediately distal to the origin of the left subclavian artery. There may be transverse lacerations of the intima of the aorta (ladder tears). The heart may show contusions, laceration of the pericardial sac, rupture of right and left atrium, right ventricle and interatrial septum. In high speed impacts, heart may be completely avulsed from its base and found lying loose in the chest. The throat may be crushed across the horn-ring or the top of the steering-wheel. These are often known as **'the steering-wheel impact type of injury Fig. (9–47).** Modern design has reduced the danger of injuries by steering column by making the column

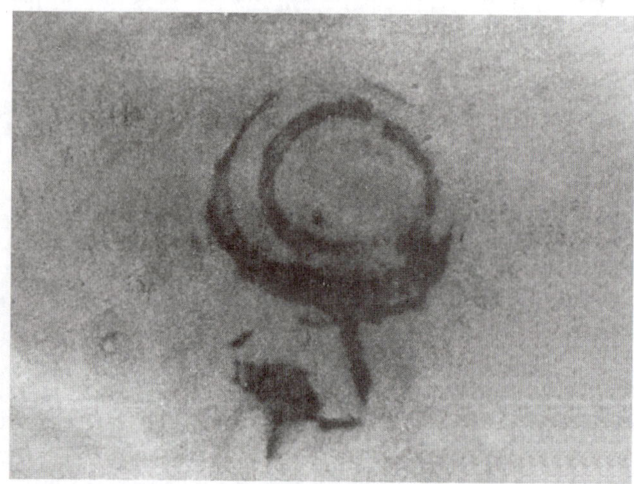

Fig. (9–47). Steering wheel impact injury.

telescope, hinged or collapsible. Facial lacerations and fractures of facial skeleton, especially nose and maxilla may occur.

If the driver appreciates that the accident is unavoidable, he may put some of the force on his hands on the steering-wheel and avoid full impact of his chest against it, or severe impact of the head against the windscreen, and may sustain injuries to the wrists or forearms. Transmitted fracture of the femur or pelvis occurs if attempt is made to apply the brakes. The driver and front passengers may split the head or face on a shattering windscreen frame, or may sustain a fracture-dislocation of the cervical spine due to hyperflexion of the head or being thrown up as well as forward. Dislocation of atlanto-occipital joint is found in about one third of all fatal motor vehicle accidents.

Whiplash injury: It is caused due to a violent acceleration or deceleration force applied to the passenger, usually front seat occupant. When the vehicle comes to a sudden stop due to head-on obstruction, the heavy head continues to move forward (acute hyperflexion). When the body comes to rest, or the head strikes an obstruction in front, there is then a reactionary hyperextension as the head is thrown backwards, this **double movement being known as the 'whiplash'.** If a vehicle is hit violently from behind by another vehicle, then the head is thrown violently backwards into hyperextension and then comes forwards after body stops movement. In either case, this violent extension-flexion movement can cause atlanto-occipital dislocation in 20 to 30% cases, or less commonly a fracture-dislocation in the lower part of the spine at about C 5 and 6. Laceration of tendons and joint capsules, intra-articular haemorrhages and tears with separation of cartilaginous lining of articular surfaces may occur. Fatal contusion or laceration of the spinal cord may occur without fracture of spine. Fracture or dislocation can also occur in the upper dorsal spine, often around T 5 to 7. **Head restraints (head rests) prevent hyperextension of the neck to certain degree.**

Head injuries: The head strikes the upper part of the window glass, frame and adjacent roof; upper limbs and thorax strike the window-sill and adjacent door structures; and hip and abdomen strike the arm-rest area. Head injuries are caused mainly by contact with portions of the vehicle interior located at head level, e.g., upper part of the side door and window-frame and glass, windshield, sun visor and its hinges and rear vision mirror. When the forehead strikes the windshield, shallow penetration produces U-shaped, L-shaped, right angle or linear cuts or abrasions, and deeper penetrations lacerations. Multiple, short linear, angular, rectangular and square, punctate lacerations of the face are produced due to the shattering of the windscreen glass into multiple small rectangular, square or cubical fragments with relatively blunt edges **("sparrow foot" marks;** dicing injuries). They are relatively superficial. Thin pieces of windscreen glass may be embedded in the wounds or may be found loose in the clothing. There may be partial avulsion of the skin. The windshield of some modern vehicles consists of two panes of glass that are laminated to either side of a relatively flexible plastic sheet. Occupants who impact the windshield may break the outer glass layers, deform the plastic layer and sustain minor vertically grouped incised wounds on the forehead. But if the windshield is penetrated, deep incised wounds will be caused on the head and neck. These wounds may bleed profusely. Impaction of the head with the windscreen can cause fracture of the base of the skull, closed head injury and fractures of the cervical vertebrae. Basal fractures tend to run along the petrous ridges through the sella turcica **(Hinge Fractures)**.

Front seat passengers: The pattern of injuries are almost similar to that of the driver, except steering wheel injuries. In a head-on crash, the front passengers move forward in a seated position, the knee striking the rigid metal lower panel, chest and abdomen striking the upper portion of the panel and the head is thrown against the windshield. Abrasions and lacerations are produced on the shins and knees, or one or both patellae are fractured, or knee joint is crushed. Abrasions and lacerations on the dorsum of the foot and on the toes, may be caused by hyperflexion of the toe at the time of impact. The femur or the pelvis may be fractured by being thrown against the dashboard or shelf-edge. In forward crashes, the floor of the vehicle frequently bends inward, twisting the foot on the ankle and causing fracture-dislocations. Sometimes, the foot may be trapped and the shaft of the tibia or fibula fractured, as the occupant's body moves forward.

Front-to-side collisions: Injuries to the face due to shattering of the glass can be seen on either or both sides of a driver. In these, doors on the side opposite to impact are opened. If the impact is from the right side, the driver will sustain external injuries mostly on the right side of the body. Injuries are usually more severe than those sustained in frontal collision and usually involve the chest and abdomen. The right arm or leg may be fractured. Rib fractures occur mostly on the right side. Heart may rupture. Liver and right kidney may be lacerated. Fractures of the base of the skull and neck may occur. If the impact is from the left side, the injuries tend to be more severe on the left side.

Back seat occupants: During violent deceleration, unrestrained back seat occupants are projected forwards and strike the back of the front seats including head rests and suffer from fewer facial, neck, pelvic and arm injuries but more abdominal trauma. They may be thrown over the seats and fall on the front seat passengers or sometimes ejected through the windscreen.

Thoracic injuries: Aorta is usually ruptured with deceleration. It may be associated with a severe whiplash effect on the thoracic spine. The aortic rupture is circular and clean-cut, and appears as sharp as if it has been transected with a knife. Sometimes multiple transverse intimal tears are seen adjacent to the main rupture, the so-called "ladder tears". Contusion of the pericardium and myocardium may be seen even without fractures of ribs. The posterior surface of the heart may be damaged from impact against the spine. In high speed impacts, the heart may be completely avulsed from its base and may be found lying loose in the chest cavity. The auricles and ventricles may be lacerated. The heart may be lacerated directly from fractured ribs, sternum or external objects. Blunt impact often produces a line of bruising down the posterior part of the lung where it lies in the paravertebral gutter. Air bullae or blood blisters may be seen under the pleura overlying the bruised areas. Haemothorax or pneumothorax may be present. The interior of the lung may be pulped due to transmitted force or large variations in intrathoracic pressure during the impact.

Abdominal injuries: The liver may rupture in any part. Usually there is central laceration of the upper surface, which may extend deeply and may transect the organ. There may be shallow, multiple, parallel tears in the upper surface of the right lobe. In subcapsular tears a haematoma is formed which can rupture later. Sometimes there is gross pulping and disruption or internal laceration without surface injuries. Shallow tears are produced in the spleen usually around the hilum. Rarely the spleen may be avulsed from the pedicle. There is often contusions of mesentery and omentum.

Sometimes, the door may spring open and the person may fall out **(occupant ejection)**. Occupants thrown out of the car can sustain injuries to any area of the body, and multiple injuries to the chest and abdomen are common with multiple limb fractures. When the **car overturns,** the occupants may be pinned and crushed, showing classical traumatic asphyxia, or the chest and abdomen may be crushed with serious injury to the heart, lungs, liver, spleen or kidneys. Depending on the circumstances of the accident, the occupants are burned, asphyxiated or drowned while trapped in the interior of a car.

Roll-over crash: If the passenger compartment remains intact, the belted occupants frequently survive the crash, as the vehicle does not stop suddenly and impact is spread over a period of time. Non-belted occupants tumble around inside the vehicle. Fractures and subluxation of cervical spine may occur.

Seat Belt Injuries: Seat belts are of the lap strap and shoulder diagonal type, which are of the "inertia-reel" type, which allow slow movement but jam at a sudden tug. They are less effective than three point belts consisting of both diagonal and strap. A seat-belt acts in the following ways: (1) It restrains the body against severe deceleration, keeping it away from windscreen, steering wheel and other obstructions. (2) It spreads the deceleration force over a considerable area of broad strap against the body surface. (3) The strap stretches during deceleration and reduces G-forces by slightly extending the time of deceleration. (4) It prevents ejection from the vehicle into the road. It reduces risk of death by about 40%. Small intestine avulsions, intestinal, omental and mesenteric lacerations and intestinal contusions and perforations occur, known as "seat belt syndrome", due to acute flexion over a lap strap. Rupture of the spleen, liver, pancreas, caecum and bladder occur due to compression between belt and vertebrae. Abrasions, contusions and haematomas of the lower abdomen and chest wall can occur as a direct result of seat belt trauma. The abdominal aorta can be crushed. Transverse fractures of lumbar vertebrae, usually at the second or third segment of interspace can occur due to acute trunk hyperflexion over the belt fulcrum. The posterior arch, pedicle or transverse processes may be fractured. Bruising of skin and underlying muscles and fracture of clavicle and sternum occur where the belt crosses them.

Air bags: It consists of a large fabric bag, which is normally folded into steering wheel hub in the case of driver's position and into fascia in front of front-seat passenger. In this sodium azide is converted into nitrogen gas in milliseconds. Deflation is also rapid. They are intended to provide protection in frontal crashes. They protect chest from impact on steering wheel and column and prevent whiplash motion of the head by providing a more gradual deceleration of head and neck and also protect the face. At least one airbag related injury occurs in 43% of airbag deployments. Adults of short stature and children are particularly liable. About 95% of injuries are minor. Fatal lesions are caused by impact of chest against airbag. Fatal injuries include cervical spine dislocations or fractures, basal skull fractures and injuries to thoracic and abdominal viscera. Facial bruising and fractures of arms are seen. Eye injuries are common, such as mild corneal abrasions, chemical burns, globe rupture or perforation. Air bags alone reduce fatalities by about 14% in drivers compared with 45% of lap-shoulder belts used alone. If both are used fatalities are reduced by 50%.

Tail-gating occasionally occurs with cars driving into the back of large trucks. In such case, the windscreen and front of the passenger compartment are smashed with severe injuries to the head and shoulders and in some cases decapitation of the occupants of the front seat.

Delayed deaths: Delayed deaths can be caused by continuing bleeding, secondary haemorrhage, renal failure from hypertension and/or extensive muscle damage, fat embolism, local or systemic infections, myocardial or cerebral infarction.

Triage is the sorting out and classification of casualties of war or other disaster, to determine priority of need and proper place of treatment.

(2) CYCLISTS AND MOTOR CYCLISTS: This includes motor cycles, motor scooters, mopeds and pedal cycles. Accidents to cyclists and motor cyclists are commonly caused by turning in front of a vehicle from one side or the other. The cycle is hit, and the person is thrown violently to the ground or into some other object or on to the car. In being thrown, they may injure the groins or legs by protruding objects, such as handlebars or projection levers or mirrors, long tears being common. The handlebar may tear the liver or the spleen and cause massive internal bleeding. The head or shoulder may hit some object first, or they may be thrown beneath a vehicle and crushed like any pedestrian. Primary impact injuries may be to the leg or to the chest if the victim runs into a stationary vehicle, often causing a ruptured heart or aorta. Injuries to legs may occur in relatively low speed accidents due to the machine falling heavily on them. Falling from the vehicle, especially at speed can cause visceral damage, especially rupture of the liver and spleen. **Pillion riders** falling off the backs of motor cycles have a laceration of the back of the head, a fracture of the posterior fossa, contrecoup contusions of the frontal lobes and abrasions of the back and elbows.

Crash helmet: Crash helmet reduces friction of the head against the ground, and makes deceleration less drastic by allowing the protected head to skid across the ground. Helmets reduce the risk of head injury by about 30%, and fatalities by about 40%. When a crash helmet is worn, the crown may be protected, but the whole head may be "eggshell" on to the base or cervical spine with fracture of the spine. Occasionally, when the helmet is pinned or crushed, the chin strap may be drawn upwards and cause strangulation. Although helmets do decrease fatalities, their greatest value is protection at lower speed or tangential impacts. Severe brain damage may occur even when a helmet is worn. A helmet which shows only glancing linear abrasions indicates the likelihood of a less severe brain injury than

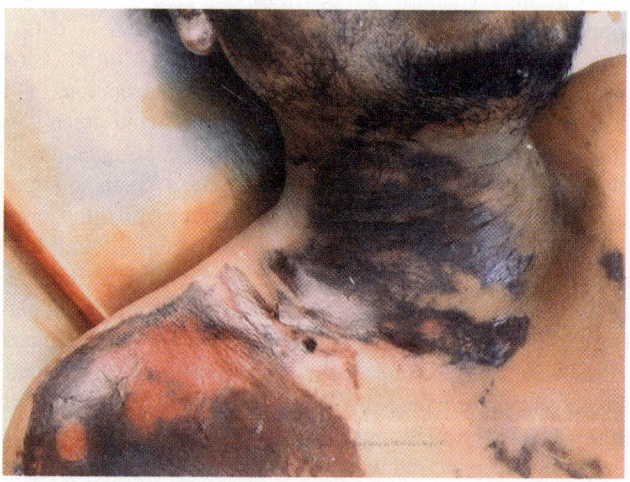

Fig. (9–48). Abraded contusions of front on of neck and chest in road traffic accident.

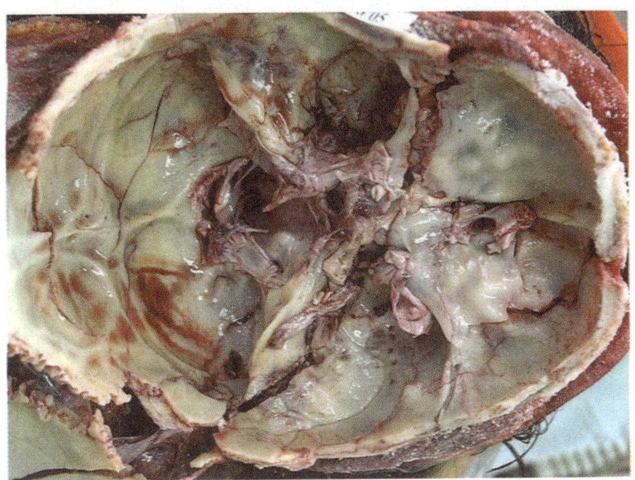

Fig. (9–49). **Hinge fracture of the skull (motor-cyclists) fracture.**

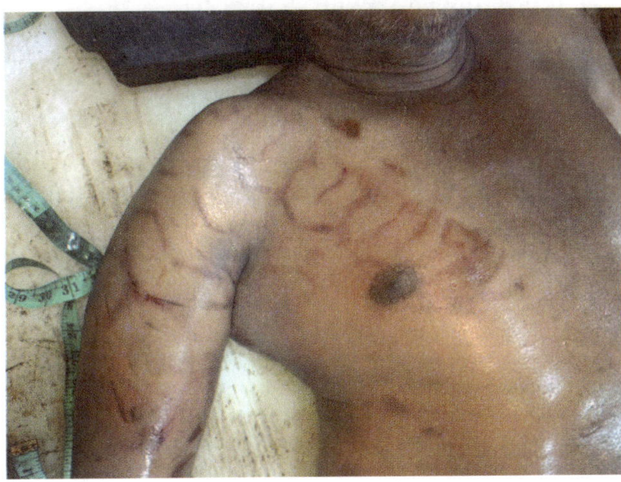

Fig. (9–50). **Tyre tread marks on back due to run over by a vehicle.**

one in which there is direct impact imprint. Cortical contusions and lacerations are common. Brain tissue may extrude through compound fractures of the skull.

Head injuries: About 50% of helmetless motor cyclists sustain head injury. The person falls head-on into some hard surface, or slides and tears the unprotected brow, face or ears with flattened or depressed fracture of the skull Fig. (9–49). The brain is crushed or torn and bleeds from multiple sites. Impact on the crown of the head may produce ring fracture around the foramen magnum. Sudden deceleration often causes whiplash injury of neck. Instantaneous death may occur due to injury of medulla associated with fractures and/or dislocations of the atlanto-occipital and atlanto-axial areas. The classical fatal injury in both motor cyclists and pillion passengers is fracture of the skull, usually from secondary impact with ground. Temporoparietal fractures are common often with contrecoup brain injury. In many types of road accidents or due to a very heavy impact on one side of the head, a fracture is produced across the floor of each middle fossa passing through the pituitary fossa, often associated with fissured fractures passing upwards to the temporal bones. At autopsy, **the base of the skull is seen divided into two halves, each moving independently of each other like a hinge, the so-called motor cyclists fracture.** Hinge fractures are usually associated with injuries of the brainstem, particularly ponto-medullar tears.

Bicycle spoke injury: It occurs when a rider or passenger on a bicycle slips from the seat and the foot or leg passes through the spokes of the wheel. In this soft tissue is crushed, with internal avulsion or damage.

Tail gating: The motor cyclist may drive into the back of a large vehicle, e.g., truck, known as "under-running" or "tail-gating". This may occur due to the sudden and unexpected stoppage of the truck or when the motor cyclist is at high speed in darkness. In such cases, the motor cyclist's head and shoulders are smashed against the tail-board. In extreme cases decapitation may occur.

INVESTIGATION OF AUTOMOBILE ACCIDENTS: Investigation of traffic accident should include: (1) study of the accident scene, (2) mechanical and engineering examination of the involved vehicles and of each component whose failure could affect safety in

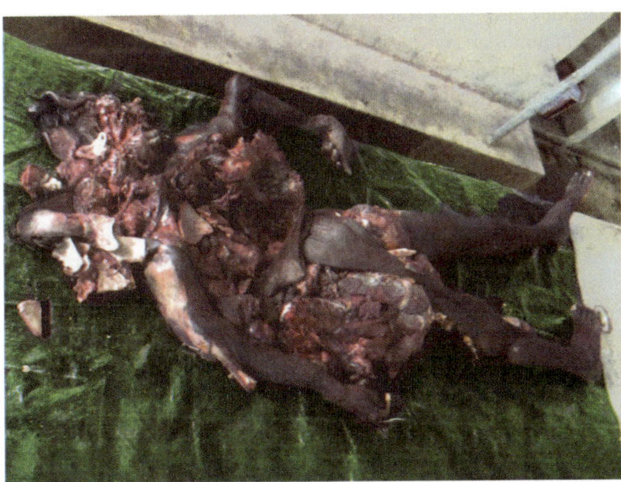

Fig. (9–51). **Crushed and multilated body in road traffic accident.**

Courtesy: **Dr Tamil Mani, Associate Professor, Pudukottai, Tamil Nadu, India.**

motion, (3) complete autopsy of all dead victims, (4) physical and psychiatric examination of surviving drivers, (5) personal and social histories of surviving persons.

EXAMINATION OF THE SCENE: The investigation of the scene of accident consists of a search for traces left by the vehicle, and traces left by the victim of the accident, who may have been struck by the vehicle or thrown from it.

(A) TRACES LEFT BY VEHICLES: (1) SKID MARKS: The location, direction and length of skid marks are a reliable guide as to the speed of the vehicle at the time the brakes were applied. They are important for the reconstruction of an accident and evaluation of the statements made by the driver. Skid marks should be measured and sketched. Their shape and location should be recorded by photographs.

(2) DIRT FROM THE UNDERSURFACE OF THE VEHICLE: The location of such dirt dropped on the highway due to impact of a vehicle with some resisting substance may be of value in accident reconstruction. It may provide evidence as to which vehicle was violating traffic rules.

(3) TYRE MARKS: Tracks leading to and from the scene indicate direction of travel, speed and attempts to stop or avoid collision. Tyre marks are usually caused by the skin being forced into the grooves of the tyre tread, the edge of the raised rubber tracing out the pattern. They are helpful in the identity of the vehicle as each tyre has individual character caused by skid, cuts by glass, nails, sharp stones, etc.

(4) MATERIAL FROM THE VEHICLES: This may consist of glass from broken headlight, windshield or window mirrors, parking lights, metal parts from the grille, door handles, etc., fragments of paint or enamel from the vehicle. Puddles of oil, water or antifreeze may give evidence of damage to the vehicle if the vehicle was driven away or removed after the accident. These can be matched with the suspect's car found later.

(B) TRACES LEFT BY VICTIM: Blood, fragments of tissue, hair, and fragments of clothes may be found at the scene due to injury to the victim. The location of such evidence should be sketched and the material preserved and sent to the laboratory for examination.

THE CASE VEHICLE: The vehicles involved in accidents are photographed from various angles to record the type and amount of damage. Measurements of the vehicles are made to determine the amount of deformation and collapse of various structures. Photographs of the interior of the vehicle should be taken, especially areas of deformation and of impact points, i.e., steering wheel, the instrument panel, bent knobs, broken windshields, interior of the doors, etc. The investigators should look for items of evidential and correlative value, such as human tissue, blood, hair, cloth fibres, etc. at the possible points of impact. The undersurface of the chassis should be examined for blood, hair and fibres from clothes. The location of vehicles, the type of road and its surface in the vicinity of the accident, the location and position of victims on the road, distance and direction of the victims from the impact, and size and direction of blood on road should be noted, photographed and drawings made showing various details of the accident.

THE ACCIDENT VICTIMS: In a fatal accident, when the victim is still at the scene, photographs of the victim should be taken to show his position relative to vehicle if he was ejected.

THE AUTOPSY: The main objects are: (1) To construct the accident to determine its cause. (2) To find out the cause of death. (3) To find out the manner of death. (4) To establish identity of the victims. (5) To identify the driver and reconstruct the position of the victims prior to the accident. (6) To differentiate injuries caused by being hit from those caused by being run over. (7) To identify the automobile in cases of hit-and-run. (8) To determine the significance of previous injuries in case of delayed death.

(A) CLOTHES: The clothes should be examined while still on body to determine any evidence to indicate what part of the vehicle struck the victim. Paint, smudge marks, grease and oil marks and dirt on the garment must be noted. The clothes may sometimes show clear imprints of tyre. Pieces of glass or metals may be found in or on clothing. All of these may assist in reconstructing the accident and in identifying the unkown vehicle in a hit-and-run accident.

(B) THE BODY: Complete autopsy must be carried out, including for the presence of any natural disease which might have contributed for the accident. All types of trace evidence either in the clothing, hair, on the skin or in the wounds must be retained, especially in a hit and run case. Patterned injuries must be photographed with a scale in view. Blood should be collected for grouping and DNA fingerprinting in a hit and run case to identify a vehicle if found with blood or tissue traces upon it. Blood analysis for alcohol in a driver or screening for drugs of dependence and common medicines that might have caused drowsiness should be carried out. The description of nature, size, extent and location of the injuries may identify some wounds on the body with some object or part of the vehicle in question. Primary impact injuries vary in extent and severity in different cases depending on the position of the pedestrian, and on the speed of the vehicle, and the part of the vehicle hitting the person, etc. The distance of wounds from feet should be recorded, because the position of these wounds will indicate which part of the vehicle struck the person, and will serve to corroborate or contradict the evidence of witnesses. The secondary impact injuries should also be described. Drag marks may indicate that the victim had crawled from the vehicle and was not ejected. They show typical brush burning without significant haemorrhage in the skin and subcutaneous tissues. Valuable information may be obtained from the victim's injuries, regarding the mechanism of the accident. **Every injury cannot be interpreted and the patterned injuries should be primarily considered.** It is useful to make a diagrammatic representation of injuries on a body outline.

CAUSE OF DEATH: When a person is found in a crashed vehicle, it should be determined whether he died from injuries sustained in the accident or due to a natural cause.

(A) DISEASE AND ACCIDENTS: In the causation of accidents, diseases do not contribute very much. Natural disease can cause accident and death of driver, the commonest cause being coronary artery disease. A person suffering a heart attack while driving, usually slows down or stops the vehicle in time to avoid collision, and no major injuries are sustained by the occupants or the pedestrian hit. Diabetics who take insulin, rarely experience hypoglycaemic attacks while driving, which may cause an accident. An attack of angina, valvular heart disease cerebrovascular accidents, and migrainous headaches may cause an accident. Minor vision defects, colour blindness, and defective hearing do not contribute much for an accident. Epilepsy is a well known risk. **Physical fatigue usually does not affect the accident, but mental or psychological fatigue, 'tiredness' may affect. Driver falling asleep is a major cause of accidents.**

(B) DRUGS AND ACCIDENTS: **Drunken driving** is a major cause of accidents. A serious lack of control is produced by an overdose or a normal dose of insulin not covered by sufficient intake of food. Drowsiness and accidents may be caused by morphine, pethidine, cannabis, cocaine, benzodiazipines, tranquilisers, amphetamine, antihistamines and some hypotensive drugs.

(C) PSYCHOLOGY AND ACCIDENT: Disorganisation of skilled reactions may occur in persons who are emotionally upset or suffer from anxieties.

CAUSE OF DEATH: Severe blunt force injuries alone or in combination with minor natural disease will point to a traumatic cause of death. The pattern of injuries and their circumstances of death will indicate whether death is accidental, suicidal or homicidal. Severe natural disease alone or in combination with insignificant trauma will point to a natural manner of death. Minor trauma may be sufficient to cause death either by affecting diseased organs or by affecting vital areas, e.g. nervous centres of the brain or the conduction system of the heart.

Deep injuries of the back of the neck, such as:(1) haemorrhage in the atlanto-occipital joints, (2) fractures of atlanto-occipital joints, (3) extensive muscular haemorrhages, (4) extradural or subdural spinal cord haemorrhages , (5) contusions and lacerations of upper cervical cord, may be caused due to vehicular accident. These may be missed in the usual autopsy and cause of death may be given as natural. **Car exhaust gas may seep into the vehicle and precipitate a fatal accident or an apparent natural death.**

In the case of pedestrians, cardiovascular or cerebrovascular disease and reduced mobility may lead to accident. Defects in sight and hearing may have contributed to accident, though this is almost never detectable at autopsy. A dead body lying in a street may be run over by a vehicle. In such case, large amount of blood may be found in the body cavities and also some degree of haemorrhagic infiltration of tissues at the site of gross traumatic lesions.

Death may occur a long time after the person sustains injuries in a traffic accident. A continuous chain of symptoms from the accident to death (bridging symptoms) and morphologic proof that the changes of natural disease complicating the trauma can be traced to the time of the accident, will prove causal relationship in delayed traffic deaths.

Wrong determination of the cause of death may result from (1) faulty reconstruction of accident, (2) incomplete gross and microscopic autopsy, (3) misinterpretation of pattern of injury, (4) improper ageing of injuries, (5) incomplete toxicologic examination.

MURDER BY MOTOR VEHICLE: A crime may be committed with the help of an automobile in the following ways. (1) **Premeditated murder** of a pedestrian with an automobile.

(2) HIT AND RUN: The driver of the vehicle kills or injures a person accidentally and leaves the scene to avoid blame. The vehicle and driver will have to be identified. Examination of the scene, of the body, and collection of gross and trace evidence, e.g., tearing of the clothes, grease marks, oil, road dust, broken lamp or windscreen glass, metallic or paint fragments from the vehicle, blood, urine, hair, etc., on the clothes and on the body is helpful. The clothes may show a tyre tread pattern. Matching studies of blood type, hair, dirt, grease, paint, oil, rust, etc. found on the victim and the vehicle in question can lead to the identification of the vehicle involved. Measurement of the leg fractures from the heels of the feet, and the height of other body injuries sustained from the protruding parts of the vehicle, may aid in the identification of the suspect vehicle. The pattern of injuries and other findings may help to determine the position of the victim at the time of first vehicle contact.

RUN OVER INJURIES: If a person is run over by a vehicle and dragged, impact injuries may not be found, but the clothes are torn and avulsion of skin and compression injuries of internal organs are present. The body or clothing of the victim may show oil and rust from the low parts of the vehicle and the vehicle may show fibres of clothing, hair, and blood from the victim on some of its low parts. Tyre tread patterns on the clothes or skin is valuable evidence.

(3) ACCIDENT FAKED TO CONCEAL CRIME: Rarely, a person may be killed by other means, and the body placed in a vehicle is pushed off the road to make the scene look like an accident. In such a case, careful evaluation of all the injuries is necessary. Sometimes, a murder victim is burnt in a vehicle to conceal the crime. Sometimes, putrefaction indicates the body to have been dead prior to the fire.

SUICIDE BY MOTOR VEHICLE: Some vehicular accidents are suicidal. Suspicion may arise from the circumstances preceding the accident, e.g. family quarrel, financial crises, threats of suicide, previous suicide attempts, history of depression, suicide note, etc. The characteristic of a suicidal death by a driver is a head-on collision with a roadside object, pole or bridge-support at a high rate of speed, without evidence of an effort to apply the brakes or to evade striking the object. The accelerator pedal imprint is an additional evidence of the deliberate nature of the crash. Rarely, premeditated homicide may be disguised as an accident. Suspicion should arise when the accident cannot be reconstructed.

IDENTIFICATION OF DRIVER: The driver can be identified by: (1) The presence of steering-wheel impact type of injuries. (2) Finding of paint or glass from the door on the driver's side on the victim's body or clothes. (3) Finding of cloth fibres, hair and tissue from the suspected driver on the driver panel, door or glass on the driver's side or on the steering wheel and columns. (4) The brake or accelerator pedal design is imprinted on the sole of the driver's shoe. (5) Matching of the blood group of the driver with that of blood of the driver panel, driver door and steering assembly.

SENSING DIAGNOSTIC MODULES (Black boxes): If the vehicle is equipped with black box, it will continually monitor a number of vehicle functions, such as speed, throttle position, engine RPM, brake use, impact velocity, seat belt use, air bag deployment, etc. On impact, the device stores all the recorded data collected over the last five seconds or so.

AIRCRAFT INJURIES: Most of the aircraft accidents occur on landing (35%), or take-off (35%). The sudden deceleration on crashing causes breakup of the aircraft and injuries to the occupants.

CRASH ACCIDENT: Both on landing and take- off the passengers are usually secured to their seats with lap type safety belts, which are fixed to the back of the base of the seats, and pass over the hips to tie across the abdomen just above the symphysis pubis. Many types of injuries are seen, in the relatively intact bodies. Fracture spine, especially thoracic spine are very common. These are usually hyperflexion injuries due to rapid deceleration when the aircraft strikes the ground. The forward momentum throws the head, on to the back of the front seat causing facial injuries. There may be fracture of the base of the skull, especially ring fracture. Fracture of the lower legs due to seat displacement is typical of the landing time accident, while fracture of the femur and internal injuries due to vertical deceleration, indicate a deep stall type of accident. Intrathoracic injuries occur due to squeezing of the chest by pressure against the sternum, which may rupture or detach the heart. Ruptures of the liver, spleen, kidneys and abdominal aorta occur. Death may be due to burning or CO poisoning. The seats may break loose due to which almost any type of injury may result. In about 20% of fatal crashes fire occurs.

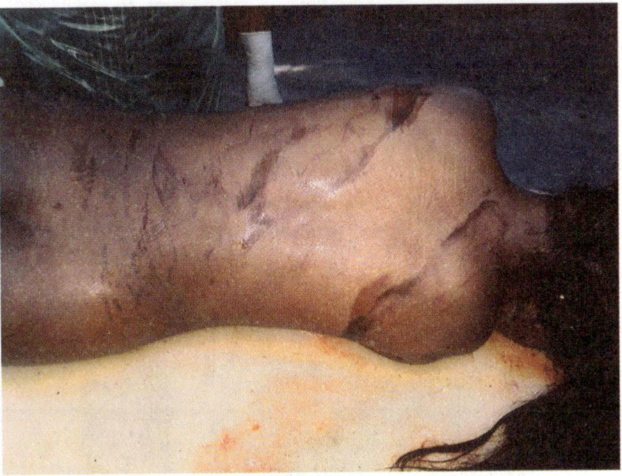

Fig. (9–52). Run over a vehicle showing patterned tyre mark.

Courtesy: Dr Tamil Mani, Associate Professor, Pudukottai, Tamil Nadu, India.

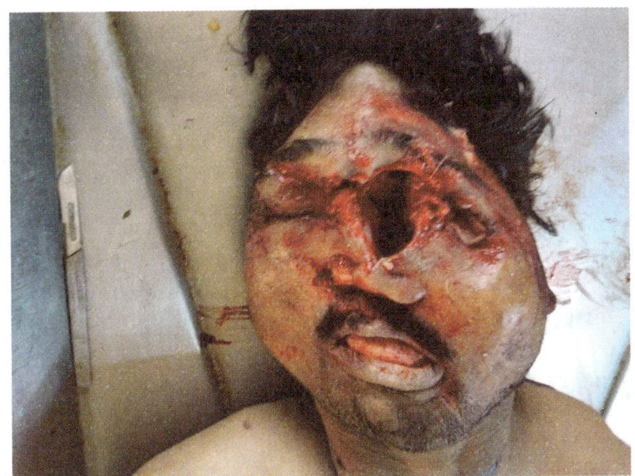

Fig. (9–53). Crush injury of face due to heavy brunt object.

FLIGHT ACCIDENTS: The cabins are pressurised to prevent anoxia while in flight. If a door or window breaks, cabin pressure falls and anoxia may produce death. The rush of air out of the cabin is sufficient to blow a standing or even seated man out with it. The injuries vary from total disintegration of the body to relatively minor injuries. When a plane breaks up at a relatively high altitude, fragmented bodies may be distributed over wide area.

AUTOPSY: (1) Identification and autopsy of the pilots for natural disease and toxicological analysis. (2) Examination of clothing of all fatal casualties. (3) Determination of cause of death of all casualties. (4) Preservation of blood specimens from all casualties for COHb and alcohol estimation and lactic acid estimation. Brain lactic acid levels exceeding 200 mg% indicate hypoxia. (5) Collection of urine, bile and viscera for detection of any poison. (6) Collection of specimens of lung from all casualties for assessment of agonal period.

BOXING INJURIES: A wide range of injuries are produced, but the head is frequently injured. Fracture of skull is rare, but **subdural haemorrhage,** usually within one of the middle cranial fossae, due to tearing of dural emissary veins, **is the most common cause of death** due to prolonged repetitive punching, occurs in about one-third of fatal cases.

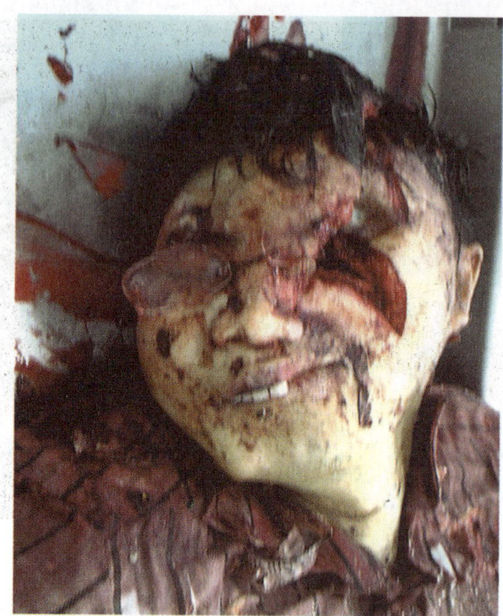

Fig. (9–54). **Crush injury of face due to fall of construction material from height.**

Some victims may show pontine haemorrhage, the so-called **"boxers haemorrhage".** Retinal detachment, choroidal tears and vitreous haemorrhages may occur. Fifth metacarpal bone may be fractured (Boxer's fracture). Deterioration in speed and coordination is the chief symptom of the onset of punchdrunk (traumatic encephalopathy or dementia pugilistica) condition, which may arise years after the last injury. **Punchdrunk syndrome in its final form is recognised by slurred speech, defective memory, slow thought process, stiff limbs, ataxia, broad-based gait, outbursts of violence,** Parkinsonian-like facial appearance and dementia. The intracranial findings in boxers are: subdural, subarachnoid and intracerebral haemorrhage, diffuse axonal injury, focal ischaemic lesions, dissecting aneurysms, cortical atrophy, slight hydrocephalus, thinning or tears of corpus collosum, scars or patches of gliosis, loss of neurones from the cerebellum and substantia nigra, and contusions of the brain. **The changes are broadly similar to that in Alzheimers disease.** These injuries can cause cerebral oedema, herniation of the brain, secondary brainstem injuries, and hypoxic injuries of the brain. The mechanism is not known, but probably repeated blows to the head produce small haemorrhages and degenerative changes in brain, especially in the region of corpus striatum, thalamus, deep temporal gray matter, septal regions and on certain neurons along the cerebellar pathways. There is enlargement of the ventricles due to loss of white matter and a perforation of the septum pallucidum.

RAILWAY INJURIES: ACCIDENTAL INJURIES: When the person walks on the track, primary injuries are seen on the front or the back, due to contact with the protruding parts of the engine. Secondary injuries are produced due to being thrown or run over which are soiled with oil and dust. When the person is crossing the line, primary injuries are seen on the side of the head and shoulders. If the person is bending down, the primary injuries are seen on the back and the buttocks, and secondary injuries on the face and front of the body. When the person walks at the side of the line, the shoulder or head may be hit by some protruding part of the train. When a person falls from the train, multiple injuries are produced. When a person leans out of the window, head injuries are produced due to railway fixtures, bridge abutments or tunnel sides, etc., and the person may be found in the carriage or on the side of the track. A person trying to board a fast moving train may be thrown off or may get crushed between train and the platform. A shunter may be squeezed between the buffers during uncoupling rolling stock. When a person is run over by a train, very severe mutilation of the body may occur and the body may be severed into many pieces and soiled by axle grease and dirt from the wheels and track. Wheel marks, dirt and grease contamination may be seen on the body. In collisions, and derailment, fractures of the legs and spine are produced. Head injuries, contusions, cuts and burns are also produced. Most injuries are produced due to crushing and trapping within distorted carriages Figs. (9–55 to 9–59).

SUICIDAL INJURIES: The injuries are extensive and due to primary impact. If a person lies down on the track, extrusion of organs, traumatic amputations of the limbs or trunk or decapitation may occur. Wheel marks and dirt and grease contamination may be found on the body.

Sometimes, a person is killed and the body placed on the railway track to simulate suicide or accident. Examination of the scene of the crime and the body for marks of violence will often solve the problem.

MASS DISASTERS

Disaster means a catastrophe, mishap calamity or grave occurrence in any area, arising from natural or man made causes or by accident or negligence which results in substantial loss of life, or human suffering or damage to, and destruction of property, or damage to, or degradation of, environment, and is of such a nature or magnitude as to be beyond the coping capacity of community of the affected area.

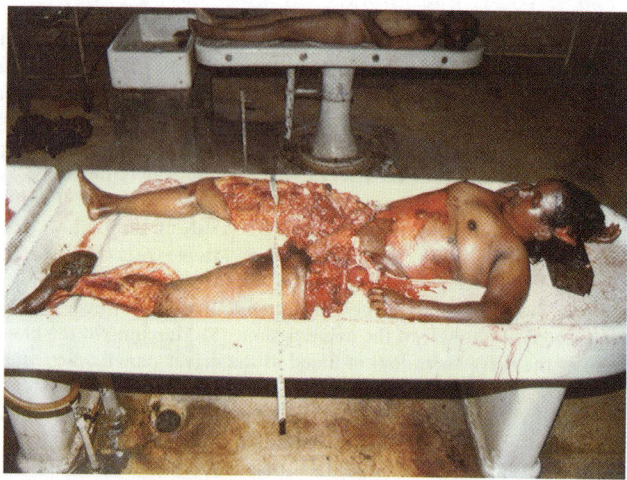

Fig. (9–55). **Multiple injuries caused by run over of a train.**

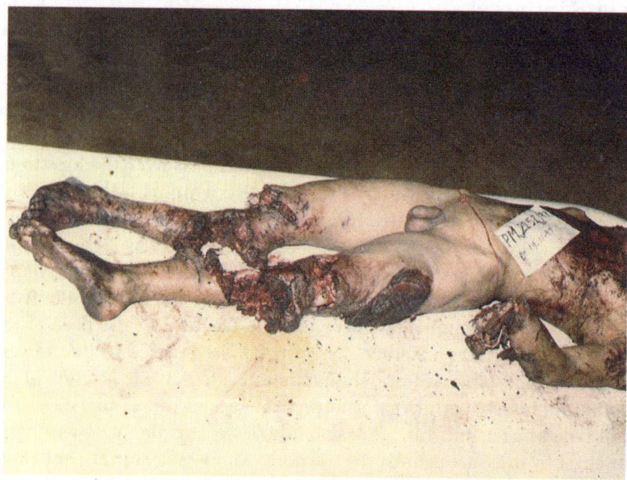

Fig. (9–56). **Multiple injuries caused by runover of a train .**

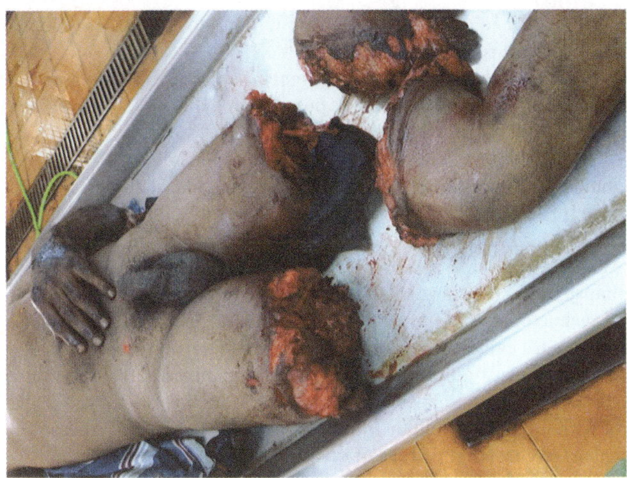

Fig. (9–57). Traumatic amputation of both thighs and forearm due to run over by a train.

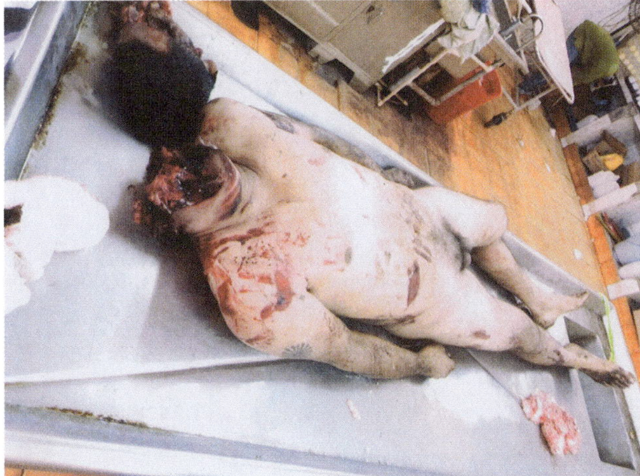

Fig. (9–58). Decapitation due to run over by a train.

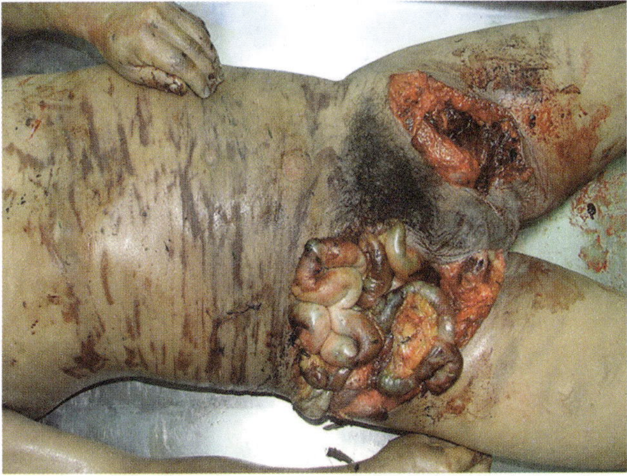

Fig. (9–59). Injuries caused due to run over by train.

CLASSIFICATION OF DISASTERS: (A) NATURAL: (1) Non-biological—earth quake, cyclone, flood, drought, heat wave, volcanic eruption, landslide. (2) Biological—disease epidemic, mass poisoning (food/liquor).

(B) MAN MADE: (1) Accidental transportation (road, rail, sea, river, and air), building collapse, mining accidents, dam-bursts, food poisoning, fires. (2) Industrial—fires, explosions, leakage of toxic substances/gases. (3) Civil disturbances—riots and demonstrations. (4) Warfare—conventional (bombardment, exchange of fire, shelling), and non-conventional (nuclear, biological and chemical warfare, terrorism).

OBJECTS OF PATHOLOGICAL INVESTIGATION: (1) To retrieve and reconstruct bodies and fragmented bodies decently. (2) To establish personal identity. (3) To conduct autopsies on some or all of these bodies. (4) To establish the cause of death in same or all, especially air-crew and drivers and to assist in constructing the cause of disaster. (5) To obtain material for toxicological analysis (especially alcohol and CO) where appropriate. (6) To seek evidence of the cause of the disaster from autopsy examination, such as bomb or detonator fragments that may be embedded in the bodies.

FIRST STATGE (AT THE ACCIDENT SITE): (1) Isolation, demarcation and protection of the site by a security cordon. (2) In case of survivors establishing a system of triage to determine priority for transport to the hospital. (3) Identification of precise site of occurrence and preparation of a detailed sketch of the disaster site showing main pieces of wreckage and position of bodies. (4) Photographs: (a) Long view: showing general location and conditions, which are taken from eye level if the area is large, several photos are required. (b) Intermediate views: They should cover the general area surrounding the deceased, showing conditions in general and relating the overall scene to specific items and places. The deceased should be photographed from different angles. (c) Close-up views: To record injuries on the deceased and particular items of evidence at the locus. Injury photographs should be taken at right angles to the body using a scale. (5) Maintain the relationship between clothing and personal effects found at the scene and the respective remains. (6) Locate bodies and label them with a serial number and photograph them in situ. Mutilated bodies and fragments (prosthesis, a portion of a jaw, fingers, skin containing tattoos) should also be numbered and labelled. (7) Record each body and place it in a suitable container for transfer to mortuary. Make sure that things belonging to one body are not assigned to another. (8) Everything must carry the same number which has come from the body including clothing, wallets, rings, teeth, jewellery, etc. (9) Providing information regarding the victims to the press and relatives. (10) Counselling the relatives of the victims. (11) Transport bodies to mortuary as soon as possible.

SECOND STAGE—IN THE MORTUARY

AUTOPSY: (A) EXTERNAL: (1) Note state of body—entire, mutilated or fragmentary remains. (2) For each unknown remains, as well as for multiple remains, prepare photographs, diagrams and tables for comparison between the unknown and known features. (3) Note presence or absence of P.M. changes. (4) Note injuries—size, site, number, nature, age, and special features, if any. (5) Examine for comparison with medical records, eyeglasses, including frames and lenses. (6) Look for contact lenses. (7) Review reports of missing persons, statements of witnesses and relatives in mass disaster situations and content of passenger manifests provided by representatives of airlines, bus, train, etc. following aircraft accidents. (8) Examine, describe, record, and photograph the clothing and other physical evidence. Describe the size, colour, condition, and type of each garment. Record descriptions of laundry marks, labels, and name tags. (9) Examine personal effects, such as rings, watches, belt buckles, and bracelets for engraved markings. Determine if keys found on the remains provide access to the home or vehicle of the missing person. (10) Obtain fingerprints for comparison. (11) Remove and examine dentures if present. Examine teeth for comparison with antemortem dental records and X-rays. Age can be determined by examination of ground sections of teeth. Examine denture for name and identification number. (12) Examine skeletal remains to determine race, sex, age, evidence of prior disease or injury, etc. (13) Occupation marks, moles, tattoos, operation scars, congenital defects, pre-existing disease, old injuries and fractures. (14) Radiological examination of entire body for foreign bodies, which is particularly useful in mutilated bodies. (15) Compare hair with known hair. (16) Confirm gross pathological findings by microscopic examination. Determine the age of antemortem injuries. (17) Establish and maintain a chain of custody for physical evidence.

(B) INTERNAL: The following points need special attention. (1) Stage of putrefaction of internal organs. (2) Surgical removal of any organ carried out in life. (3) Evidence of pre-existing disease, nails, plates, etc. due to surgery. (4) Nature, extent and degree of organ injury. (5) Evidence of organic disease causing sudden death such as coronary occlusion, cerebro-vascular accident, etc. (6) Evidence of poisoning. (7) Presence of foreign bodies.

SPECIMENS TO BE COLLECTED AND PRESERVED. The exact specimen required to be collected would depend on the nature of the disaster. They could be: (1) Clothes if charred or blood stained. (2) Foreign bodies. (3) Viscera, blood and urine for chemical analysis. (4) Obtain blood for grouping, Rh typing, sex chromatin, karyotyping and DNA fingerprinting. (5) Retain tablets or capsules found in stomach. Preserve blood for alcohol, drugs, CO, etc. (6) Internal organs for histopathological examination.

THIRD STAGE—COMPARISON OF RECORDS: (1) Compare all evidence collected with information made available by relatives and establish the identity of the deceased. (2) A minimum of seven to eight points of comparison must tally to confirm identity. (3) It is essential that record of all medical and dental examination including X-ray films be filed for future reference.

Last task to be performed in the mortuary is the examination of any fragments of bodies, with, so far as possible, matching of those fragments with the bodies from which they originated.

Not only many clues to identity be found in separated fragmented remains, but occasionally important evidence about the cause of the accident can be ascertained.

CAUSE OF DISASTER: (1) Evidence of organic diseases like coronary occlusion, cerebrovascular accident, etc., can produce sudden collapse in the pilot or driver. (2) Evidence of poisoning due to alcohol or psychotropic drugs affecting higher mental faculties. (3) Explosion injuries with evidence of retained explosive material suggest sabotage.

The autopsy findings relating to the driver, pilot and flight crew must be reviewed in close cooperation with all the other investigating agencies, and with all other available information as to the circumstances of the incident to construct picture of the incident.

Reception of bereaved relatives: Interview for description of missing persons including clothing, jewellery, dentures, teeth, any peculiarities, etc., and comparing with the remains. Coordination and cooperation with press and media.

CHAPTER

10

MEDICOLEGAL ASPECTS OF WOUNDS

FM 2.15: Describe special protocols for conduction of medicolegal autopsies in cases of death in custody or following violation of human rights as per National Human Rights Commission Guidelines.
FM 3.4: Mechanical injuries and wounds: Define injury, assault and hurt. Describe IPC pertaining to injuries.
FM 3.5: Mechanical injuries and wounds: Describe accidental, suicidal and homicidal injuries. Describe simple, grievous and dangerous injuries. Describe antemortem and postmortem injuries.
FM 3.7: Describe factors influencing infliction of injuries and healing, examination and certification of wounds and wound as a cause of death: Primary and Secondary.
FM 3.8: Mechanical injuries and wounds: Describe and discuss different types of weapons including dangerous weapons and their examination
FM 3.30: Describe and discuss issues relating to torture, identification of injuries caused by torture and its sequalae, management of torture survivors.
FM 3.31: Torture and human rights: Describe and discuss guidelines and Protocols of National Human Rights Commission regarding torture.

Offences against human body are described under sections 299 to 377, 394, 396, 397, 459, 497 and 498A of I.P.C. together with punishments.

HOMICIDE: Homicide is **killing of a human being by another human being.**

Types: (1) Murder (S.300, I.P.C.). (2) Culpable homicide. (a) amounting to murder (S.299, I.P.C.), (b) not amounting to murder (S.304, I.P.C.). (3) Rash or negligent homicide (S. 304 A, I.P.C.).

Justifiable Homicide: This is the homicide which is justified in the circumstances which led to the killing of a person. This may occur (1) in the administration of justice, like execution of sentence of death, (2) the maintenance of justice, e.g., in suppressing riots, or executing arrest, or killing in course of violent crime, e.g., a woman who kills a person who attempts to rape her.

Excusable Homicide: This is the homicide caused unintentionally by an act done in good faith. This includes (1) killing in self-defence when attacked, provided there is no other means of defence, (2) causing death by accident or misadventure, (3) death following a lawful operation, (4) homicide committed by an insane person.

The terms justifiable and excusable homicide are not used in Indian law.

INJURY: Any harm whatever illegally caused to any person in body, mind, reputation or property (S. 44, I.P.C.).

CULPABLE HOMICIDE: Culpable homicide is causing death by doing an act (1) with the intention of causing death, or (2) with the intention of causing such bodily injury as is likely to cause death, or (3) **with the knowledge that such act is likely to cause death** (Sec. 299, I.P.C.).

Explanations: (1) A person who causes bodily injury to another who is suffering from a disorder, disease or bodily infirmity which accelerates the death of the person, shall be deemed to have caused his death. (2) Where death is caused by bodily injury, the person who caused such bodily injury shall be deemed to have caused death, although by skilful treatment, the death might have been prevented. (3) The causing of the death of a child in the mother's womb is not homicide. But it may amount to culpable homicide to cause the death of a living child, if any part of that child has been brought forth, though the child may not have breathed or been completely born.

MURDER: Culpable homicide is murder (1) if the act by which the death is caused is done with the intention of causing death, or (2) if it is done with the intention of causing such bodily injury as the offender knows to be likely to cause death, or (3) if it is done with the intention of causing bodily injury which is sufficient in the ordinary course of nature to cause death, or (4) if the person committing the act knows that it is so immediately dangerous, that it must in all probability cause death, or such bodily injury as is likely to cause death and commits such act without any excuse (S.300. I.P.C.).

Exceptions: Culpable homicide does not amount to murder, if the act by which death is caused is done: (1) under grave and sudden provocation, (2) in good faith of the right of private defence of person or property (S.96 to 106, I.P.C.), (3) for the advancement of public justice, (4) without premeditation, and (5) when the person above the age of 18 years takes the risk of death with his own consent.

COMMENT: During a quarrel, death may occur from rupture of the heart, the bursting of an aneurysm, cerebral or subarachnoid haemorrhage, hypertension or any other natural disease. If it can be proved from autopsy that death resulted from a natural cause, and that the infliction of the injury did not operate in any way either immediately or remotely, the assailant will not be responsible for the death of his victim. In these cases, death might have taken place about the same time and in the same circumstances whether there was a quarrel or not.

Death may occur from a slight injury inflicted on a previously diseased organ, e.g., miliary aneurysms, fatty degeneration of the heart, duodenal ulcer, ulcerative colitis, enlarged spleen especially due to malaria, amoebic abscess, hydatid cyst, tuberculosis, disseminated sclerosis, Parkinsonism, etc. Dissemination of a neoplasm might be accelerated by direct injury. Acceleration of the progress of an already fatal illness may also occur following injury. In law, a causal relation is established if trauma aggravates, hastens or precipitates a disease condition. It is not necessary that the trauma be an aetiologic cause. In such cases, if injury accelerates the process of dying or precipitates death, the assailant is not guilty of culpable homicide, but he can be charged of simple or grievous hurt, if it can be proved: (1) that he had no intention to kill his victim, (2) that he could not have possibly known the existence of that disease, and (3) that the same injury would not have caused death when inflicted on a healthy person. A person can be convicted of culpable homicide, if he causes bodily injury to another who is suffering from disease, disorder or physical weakness and thereby accelerates the death of the other person, if he had intention to kill or had the knowledge that such injury is sufficient or likely to cause death.

To substantiate a charge of murder or culpable homicide, it is necessary to prove that the injury inflicted on the deceased was actually the cause of death, and the act was committed with the intention of causing such bodily injury as the offender knew that it was likely, or sufficient in the ordinary course of nature to cause death. If these conditions are not satisfied, the assailant may be convicted under the offence of culpable homicide not amounting to murder, or grievous or simple hurt, according to the circumstances of the case, including the kind of weapons and the site of the violence.

A BODILY INJURY WHICH IS LIKELY TO CAUSE DEATH is one in which death is not merely possible but is likely. It constitutes a grave danger to the life of the affected person due to its severity or of the structures involved. It applies in special cases where person injured is in such a condition or state of health, that his or her death is likely to be caused by an injury which would not ordinarily cause the death of a person in sound health, and where the person inflicting the injury knows that owing to such condition or state of health, it is likely to cause the death of the person injured.

A BODILY INJURY WHICH IS SUFFICIENT IN THE ORDINARY COURSE OF NATURE TO CAUSE DEATH is one as a result of which death is very probable. Death must be the result of the direct effects of the injury. If there was a lesser probability of death resulting from the act committed, the finding will be that accused intended to cause injury likely to cause death. An injury sufficient in the ordinary course of nature to cause death, need not cause death inevitably and in all circumstances. The sufficiency is the high probability of death in the ordinary way of nature. It is not always easy to decide whether or not an injury is one that is sufficient in the ordinary course of nature to cause death. Some examples are: stab injuries or rupture of the heart; injury to the large blood vessels; stab on the abdomen, chest or other parts of the body injuring an internal organ or a large blood vessel; hurt causing rupture of spleen, liver or an internal organ; severe injuries of the brain and spinal cord; incised wound on the neck; compound fracture of the skull; squeezing of the testicles; penetrating wounds or rupture of the gastrointestinal canal; extensive burns and scalds; hanging or strangulating a person; smothering or gagging; drowning; failure to tie the cord after it is cut in a newborn; administering large dose of poison, etc. A number of injuries, none of which is sufficient in itself to cause death may together by their cumulative effect be sufficient to cause death.

The offence is culpable homicide, if the body injury intended to be inflicted is likely to cause death. It is murder, if such injury is sufficient in the ordinary course of nature to cause death. The distinction is fine but appreciable. The nature of the weapon has to be considered. A blow from the fist or a stick on a vital part may be likely to cause death; a wound from a knife in a vital part is sufficient in the ordinary course of nature to cause death.

S. 302, I.P.C.: Punishment for murder: Death, or imprisonment for life, and also fine.

S.303, I.P.C.: Punishment for murder by life convict (death).

S. 304, I.P.C.: Punishment for culpable homicide not amounting to murder: Imprisonment for life, or up to 10 years and also fine. **"Provided that if death is caused to a girl or a woman, the accused committing such homicide shall be punished with imprisonment for whole life and shall also be liable for fine which may extend to two lakh rupees."**

S. 304-A, I.P.C. Causing death by negligence: "Whoever causes the death of any person, by doing any rash or negligent act not amounting to culpable homicide shall be punished with imprisonment for a term which may extend to two years or with fine, or with both.

S.305, I.P.C.: Abetment of suicide of child or insane prson (ten years imprisonment).

S. 306, I.P.C.: Abetment of suicide: Suicide is the act of taking one's own life voluntarily. If any person commits suicide, whoever abets the commission of such suicide, shall be punished with imprisonment for a term which may extend to ten years, and shall also be liable to fine. There must be instigation, cooperation or intentional assistance given to the would be suicide.

Dyadic death: A person killing someone and then committing suicide.

S.307, I.P.C.: Attempt to murder is punishable with ten years imprisonment.

S.308, I.P.C.: Attempt to commit culpable homicide is punishable with imprisonment up to seven years or with fine or both.

S.309, I.P.C.: Attempt to Commit Suicide: Whoever attempts to commit suicide and does any act towards the commission of such offence, shall be punished with simple imprisonment for a term which may extend to one year, or with fine, or with both.

Shooting, hanging and stabbing are a 'hard' way of committing suicide and typically a male choice; poisoning and drowning are 'soft' ways of committing suicide.

S. 319, I.P.C.: HURT: Hurt means bodily pain, disease or infirmity caused to any person. It does not include mental pain. S. 312 to 328 of **I.P.C.** deal with causing hurt and their punishments.

Infirmity is any inability of an organ to perform usual function, which may be temporary or permanent. A temporary mental impairment or terror would constitute infirmity.

S.320, I.P.C.: GRIEVOUS HURT: Any of the following injuries are grievous. (1) Emasculation. (2) Permanent privation of sight of either eye. (3) Permanent privation of hearing of either ear. (4) Privation of any member or joint. (5) Destruction or permanent impairing of the power of any member or joint. (6) Permanent disfiguration of the head or face. (7) Fracture or dislocation of a bone or tooth. (8) Any hurt which endangers life, or which causes the victim to be in severe bodily pain, or unable to follow his ordinary pursuits for a period of twenty days.

COMMENT: Grievous hurt is hurt of a more serious nature. It is very difficult to draw a line between those bodily hurts which are serious and those which are slight. To make out the offence of voluntarily causing grievous hurt, there must be some specific hurt, voluntarily inflicted, and coming within any of the eight kinds enumerated in this section.

(1) Emasculation: It means depriving a male of masculine vigour. Amputation of penis, injuries to the genitals or head, fracture pelvis with injury to parasympathetics, fracture spine at the level of lumbar 4 and 5 with injury to sacral segments of spinal cord (erigentes nerve, genital branch of genito-urinary nerve) can result in impotence. **If the testes are removed before puberty, impotence is the rule, but if they are removed after puberty potency is retained.**

(2) Permanent privation (loss) of sight of either eye: The gravity of such injury lies in its permanency because it deprives a person of the use of the organ of sight and also disfigures him. It can be caused by gouging out of eyes, poking eyes, chemicals, etc. Permanent loss does not mean that it should be incurable, e.g., loss of sight occurring due to corneal opacity resulting from injury to the cornea may be curable by corneoplasty. It constitutes grievous injury.

(3) Permanent privation of the hearing of either ear: It deprives a man of his sense of hearing. Such injuries may be caused by a blow on the head or the ear, or by blows which injure the tympanum or auditory nerves or by thrusting something or pouring hot liquid into the ear or by a blast which causes deafness.

(4) Privation of any member or joint: The term **'member' means an organ or a limb being part of man capable of performing a distinct function.** It includes eyes, ears, nose, mouth, hands, feet, etc. If the joint becomes permanently stiff, so that normal function is not possible, it is grievous injury.

(5) Destruction or permanent impairing of the powers of any member or joint: In ordinary course of life, the use of limbs and joints of the body are very essential to the discharge of the normal functions of the body. Their deprivation causes lifelong crippling and makes the person defenceless and miserable. It causes great hardship to human body by its retention without normal function which is like amputation. Stricture due to burns, corrosives or any other injury, damage to tendons due to blunt or sharp force injury, leading to permanent impairment of powers of joints, muscles constitute grievous injury.

(6) Permanent disfiguration of the head or face: The word 'disfigure' in this section means **to cause some external injuries which detracts from his personal appearance, but does not weaken him,** e.g., cutting off a man's nose or ears. Branding a girl's cheeks which leaves permanent scars amounts to disfigurement.

"A cut on the bridge of the nose of a girl caused by a sharp weapon like razor or knife has been held to be permanent disfigurement even though the internal wall separating the nostrils was intact".

(7) Fracture or dislocation of a bone or tooth Fig. (10–1): Fracture of either outer or inner table of the skull is considered a fracture. If a cut resulted only in a scratch or cut, and did not go deep to any length into the bone, it will not be fracture, otherwise it should be deemed to be one. It is not necessary that a bone should be cut through and through, or that there should be any displacement of any fragments of the bone. **If there is a break by cutting or splintering of the bone, or there is a rupture or fissure in it, it would amount to a fracture. Dislocation means displacement Fig. (10–1). Mere looseness of teeth will not amount to dislocation.** It has to be proved that the tooth was originally not loose, and that there was fracture or dislocation by the injury. Fracture or dislocation of a bone or tooth causes great pain and suffering to the injured person and is considered grievous hurt.

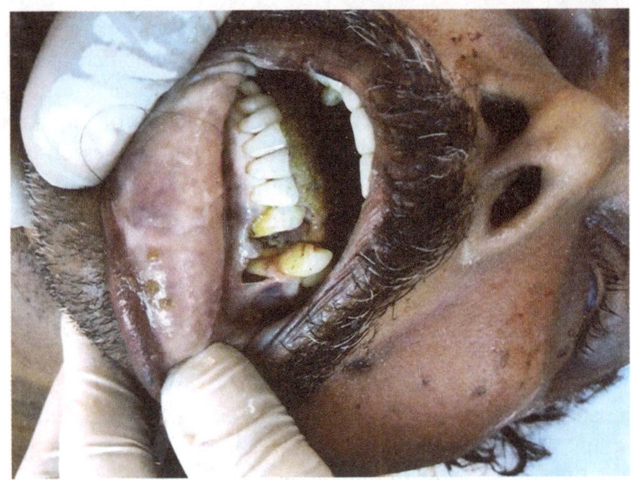

Fig. (10–1). Disarticulation of canine teeth. A case of grievous injury.

(8) Any hurt which endangers life, or which causes the victim to be in severe bodily pain, or unable to follow his ordinary pursuits for a period of 20 days: Some hurts which are not like those kinds of hurts which are mentioned in the first seven clauses, may be most serious. A wound may cause intense pain, prolonged disease, or lasting injury, but does not fall within any of seven clauses. A beating may not mutilate the sufferer or fracture his bones, but may be so cruel as to bring him to the point of death. The eighth clause provides for such hurts. Under this, three different clauses of hurt are included. They are: (1) any hurt which endangers life, (2) any hurt which causes the victim to be in severe bodily pain for a period of 20 days, and (3) any hurt which prevents the victim from following his ordinary pursuits for a period of 20 days. The three clauses are independent of each other, and a hurt of any of the three clauses would be a grievous hurt.

Any hurt which endangers life: An injury can be said to endanger life, if it is itself such that it may put the life of the injured in danger. An injury caused on a vital part of the body cannot be called grievous hurt, unless the nature and dimensions of the injury or its effects are such that the doctor is of the opinion that it actually endangers the life of the victim. Administration of harmful drug to a person to make him unconscious is not grievous hurt, even though in some cases death may be caused if the drug is given in large dose. If the life of the person is not endangered, it is not a case of grievous hurt. **To designate an injury as grievous hurt, danger to life should be imminent.**

Dangerous injuries are those which cause imminent danger to life, either by involvement of important organs or structures, or extensive area of the body. If no surgical aid is available, such injuries may prove fatal. The concept of injury dangerous to life is not very precise. As such, it is not enough if the medical witness makes simple statement that the injury in a particular part is dangerous to human life. He should place all relevant data, namely the nature and extent of injury, the kind of weapon used, the part of the body struck, whether the injury caused haemorrhage or shock, affected important structures or organs, or was very extensive, or otherwise caused imminent danger, and should also state the various grounds on which he considers the injury to be a dangerous one. Some examples of injuries which endanger life are: stab on the abdomen or head or vital part, hurt causing rupture of spleen, squeezing testicles, incised wound on the neck, compound fracture of the skull, rupture of an internal organ, injury of a large blood vessel.

Any hurt which causes the victim to be in severe bodily pain, or unable to follow his ordinary pursuits for a period of 20 days: The length of time during which a sufferer is in pain, disease or incapacitated from pursuing his ordinary occupation is a defective criterion of the severity of a hurt. It is employed not only in cases where violence has been used, but also in cases where hurt has been caused without any assault, e.g., by the administration of drugs, the setting of traps, the digging of pitfalls, the placing of ropes across a road, etc. **The extent of hurt and the intention of the offender are considered for giving punishment.** It is difficult to prove that an injured person was in severe bodily pain for 20 days, but it is easier to prove that he was unable to follow his ordinary pursuits due to the hurt. The opinion of the doctor attending on the patient is important, on the point of his disability. **A mere stay of 20 days in the hospital does not make injury grievous,** unless the injured person was in severe bodily pain, or unable to follow his ordinary pursuits for a period of 20 days. **Ordinary pursuits include acts of daily routine of a person, such as eating food, taking bath, going to the toilet, etc. but do not refer to the duties that constitute the job of a person.** An injury which endangers life may cause severe bodily pain for 20 days, but an injury which causes such pain may not be dangerous to life, but it is still a grievous hurt under this clause.

The possibility of correction of any of the above through surgery should not be a factor while assessing such injury.

The line between culpable homicide not amounting to murder and grievous hurt is very thin. In the former, the injuries must be such as are likely to cause death, in the latter the injuries must be such as to endanger life. The likelihood of death resulting from an injury will depend upon severity of injury, the structures involved, age of the individual, and the state of health of the injured. Where there is no intention to cause death, or no knowledge that death is likely to be caused from the harm inflicted and death is caused, the accused would be guilty of grievous hurt if the injury caused was of serious nature, but not of culpable homicide.

In case of hurt, the duty of the medical witness is only to describe the facts. It is the Court that must decide whether it is simple or grievous. The entry made in the wound certificate as simple or grievous is only meant to guide the investigating officer.

ILLUSTRATIONS: (1) "A woman was confined to a hospital for 17 days due to certain injuries inflicted on her, but her life was in danger for three days only. It was held that the injuries were grievous".

(2) "The thrusting of a lathi into the anus of a man has been held to be the causing of grievous hurt which endangers life".

(3) 'During an altercation, the victim was stabbed on the left forearm with a knife, due to which the radial artery was injured and the victim died soon after due to haemorrhage. It was held that the offence is neither murder, nor culpable homicide not amounting to murder, as the forearm is not a vital part. The accused was held to be guilty of voluntarily causing grievous hurt with a deadly weapon".

(4) "In case of injury to the abdomen, where intestines had come out of the wound, it was held to be grievous hurt".

"A deep injury which may be deep to the bone, but without a cut in the bone or fracture is not grievous hurt".

"Where death is caused as the result of an injury which is not intended to cause death, and was not in normal conditions likely to cause death, it is neither grievous hurt nor culpable homicide not amounting to murder".

Coma for 20 days due to head injury constitutes grievous injury.

SIMPLE INJURY: Simple injury is one which is neither extensive nor serious and which heals rapidly.

S.321, I.P.C.: Voluntarily causing hurt.

S.322, I.P.C.: Voluntarily causing grievous hurt.

S.323, I.P.C.: Punishment for voluntarily causing hurt: Imprisonment up to one year, or with fine up to one thousand rupees or both.

S.324, I.P.C.: Voluntarily causing hurt by dangerous weapons or means (3 years imprisonment) or with fine or both.

S.325, I.P.C.: Punishment for voluntarily causing grievous hurt: Imprisonment for a term extending to seven years and also fine.

S.326, I.P.C.: Voluntarily causing grievous hurt by dangerous weapons or means: Imprisonment for life or up to ten years and also fine.

Dangerous weapons or means include any instrument for shooting, stabbing or cutting or any instrument, which used as a weapon of offence, is likely to cause death; fire or any heated substance; poison or any corrosive substance; explosive substance or any substance which is harmful to the human body to inhale, to swallow, or to receive into the blood or by means of any animal.

S.328, I.P.C: Administering stupefying drug with intention to cause hurt, etc.

S.340, I.P.C.: Wrongful confinement (imprisonment up to one year or fine or both, S.342, I.P.C.)

S. 351, I.P.C.: An assault is an offer or threat or attempt to apply force to body of another in a hostile manner. It may be a common assault or with an intent to murder. S.352 to 358 I.P.C. deal with punishments for various types of assaults.

S.352. I.P.C.: Assault or use of criminal force (imprison up to 3 months or fine)

S. 362,I.P.C.: ABDUCTION: Whoever by force compels, or by any deceitful means induces, any person to go from any place, is said to abduct that person. Abduction may take place against any person of any age. For abducting a person force, compulsion or deceitful means are used. Free and voluntary consent of the person abducted condones abduction. Intention of the abductor is an important factor in determining guilt of the accused. It is not a substantive offence and is punishable only when done with some other intent under S.364 to 369 I.P.C. The offence continues as long as the abducted person is removed from one place to another.

DOWRY DEATHS

The Dowry Prohibition Act of 1961, defines 'dowry' to mean any property or valuable security given to or agreed to be given either directly or indirectly: (a) by one party to marriage to the other party to the marriage, or (b) by the parents of either party to marriage or by any other person to either party to the marriage in connection with the marriage of the said parties, but does not include *dower or mahr* in the case of persons whom the Muslim Personal Law applies to. It excludes presents in the form of clothes, ornaments, etc. which are customary at marriages, provided the value thereof does not exclude ₹ 2000/-.

S.3 of the Act provides for penalty for giving or taking dowry and S.4 penalty for demanding dowry.

In some cases newly married girls are abused, harassed, cruelly treated and tortured by the husband, inlaws and their relatives for or in connection with any demand for dowry. In extreme cases, the woman is killed by burning or some other method.

Legal Aspects: S.304–B., I.P.C. (Dowry Death): (1) **Where the death of a woman is caused by any burn or bodily injury or occurs otherwise than under normal circumstances within seven years of her marriage** and it is shown that soon before her death she was **subjected to cruelty or harassment by her husband or any relative of her husband** for, or in connection with, any demand for dowry, such death shall be called "dowry death", and such husband or relative shall be deemed to have caused her death. (2) Whoever commits dowry death shall be punished with imprisonment of not less than seven years, but which may extend to life imprisonment.

S.498–A, I.P.C.: Whoever being the husband or the relatives of the husband of the woman, subjects such woman to cruelty shall be punished with imprisonment for a term which may extend to three years and shall also be liable to fine.

Cruelty has been defined as any wilful conduct which drives the woman to commit suicide or grave mental or physical injury to her or harassment of the woman with a view to coerce her for dowry.

S.113A and 113B, I.E.A., deal with presumption as to abetment of suicide by a married woman, and presumption as to dowry death.

S.174 (3) Cr.P.C.: Procedure in dowry death (suicide, suspected murder, request by a relative; doubt of cause of death, police consider necessary). Police has to enquire and report.

Dowry deaths occur either by murder of a married woman or she herself committing suicide being unable to bear harassment or cruelty for not fulfilling the promises by her parents or her relatives or of those interested in her marriage. Ovarian steroidogenic activity in women reaches peak during luteal and premenstrual period, which causes physical and psychological tension in women. Suicidal tendency is more in some females in luteal and premenstrual phase. Look for signs of neglect, malnutrition, physical injuries, poisoning, infertility, pregnancy and menstrual phase. Such murders are invariably committed secretly either in the house or at a place where outsiders may not witness it. The bride may be burnt or killed by various methods. The usual defence in all dowry death cases is that either the woman committed suicide, or death occurred accidentally due to burns while cooking food.

In premenstrual and menstrual phase, due to hormonal imbalance many females become oversensitive and depressive even on trival issue and may commit sucide. Hypothyroidism is associated with paranoid and depressive behaviour due to which she may commit suicide.

The doctor should make a record of the history of the injuries and the persons responsible for it, when the victim is brought to the hospital, noting the time and the name of the person who gave the history. The condition of the victim should be recorded at frequent intervals. Care should be taken that no person has discussion with the victim before doctor records the statement of the victim to avoid any undue influence being exerted on her. A Magistrate may be called to record the dying declaration. Visit to the scene of crime by the doctor and other forensic scientists is very helpful in determining the manner of death.

Inquest should be conducted by a Magistrate or police officer not below the rank of deputy superintendent of police, and autopsy should be carried out by two doctors in case of dowry death.

WOUND CERTIFICATE: The casualty medical officer or any other medical officer may be called upon to examine injured person. Medicolegal injury cases should be examined without delay at any time of day or night. All details of examination of injured person, whether admitted into hospital or treated as outpatients have to be entered in an **Accident Register,** maintained in all Government hospitals. **This register is a confidential record and should be in safe custody of the medical officer.** It has to be produced in a Court of law if asked for. A detailed and accurate record should be made by the doctor at the time of the examination. The doctor is required to fill in a printed form of injury or wound certificate, one copy of which is sent to the investigating police officer in a sealed cover, and the other is retained for future reference.

If an injured person is brought to hospital, and labelled as M.L.C. the doctor should inform the local police station over telephone or by a letter of intimation.

Preliminary particulars: The following particulars should be noted. (1) Serial number. (2) Name, age and sex of the injured person and address. (3) Father's or guardian's name. (4) Date, time and place of examination. (5) Name and number of the accompanying police constable and the police station to which he belongs. (6) Names of the persons who had accompanied the injured person with their address. (7) A brief statement of the injured person about the exact nature of incident, where the incident took place, time and date of incident, details of physical force used in assault. This is to be recorded **as "alleged by the patient".** (8) Two identification marks. (9) The size of the victim, i.e., stature, body weight and development. (10) The consent of the person for examination should be taken. If the condition of the patient is serious, dying declaration should be recorded.

The following are the various entries in the wound certificate.

(1) Nature of each injury: All injuries observed, however insignificant they may appear should be noted. The nature of each injury, i.e., abrasion, contusion, incised wound, lacerated wound, stab wound, burns, fracture, dislocation, etc., should be noted. It may be convenient to deal with multiple injuries by grouping them according to their kind and severity. Alternatively, it may be better to **group them anatomically, e.g., injuries of the head, of the trunk or of a limb. A lens should be used** to get an accurate idea of the nature of the edges, ends and floor of a wound. Note whether the edges are smooth, ragged, abraded, contused, inverted or everted, and the ends sharp, blunt, square, split or show tailing. **The presence of any foreign material in the wound,** e.g., metal, glass, splinter of wood, broken point of a knife, pellet, bullet or wad of a firearm, hair, dirt, etc., should be noted, preserved and handed over to police. Photographs are useful. The position of injuries can also be shown on body sketch.

(2) Size, shape and direction of each injury: All injuries should be measured with a tape and never guessed, and the amount of blood extravasated should be measured and **photographs or sketches, showing the position and size of the wounds is desirable.** The shape of the wound, e.g., circular, oval, triangular, elliptical, etc., should be noted and also the bevelling of the edges. The direction of the wound, i.e., horizontal, vertical, oblique, etc. should be noted with regard to the anatomical position of the body. In case of stab and firearm wounds, direction of the wound should be noted. The pattern of the wound if any should be noted.

(3) On what part of body inflicted: The exact situation of wound with reference to some anatomical landmark, e.g., the middle line, a bony structure, a joint, the navel or the nipple should be mentioned. Technical terms should be avoided as far as possible. Photographs are useful. The position of injuries can also be shown on body sketch.

(4) Simple, grievous or dangerous injury: Against each injury, it should be noted whether it is simple, grievous or dangerous. **The injured person must be kept under observation, if the nature of a particular injury cannot be made out at the time of examination,** e.g., in head injury where the symptoms are obscure or abdominal injuries with vague symptoms. In all injuries, **when a fracture of a bone is suspected, an X-ray examination should be done** for confirmation. In such cases, the report should not be given hastily, if there is pressure from the police.

(5) By what weapon inflicted: In many cases, the examination of the wound and clothes give a fairly definite information about kind of weapon. With stabs and incised wounds there is not much difficulty; wounds caused by broken glass may simulate either, but irregularity of the edges will be found in some parts of the wound, and if glass pieces are found it clears all doubts. Wounds made by blunt instruments, blows or kicks over bony prominences may simulate incised wounds, but an examination with hand lens helps the diagnosis. **If medical officer is shown a weapon and asked, "Were the wounds caused by this weapon?" he should never answer in the direct affirmative, but should state that wounds could be caused by that weapon or were caused by similar weapon.**

Any weapon sent by the police, which is alleged to have been used in producing injuries should be examined for marks of blood stains, hair, pieces of cloth, etc., adherent to it and should be returned to the police after it is sealed. A foreign body found in a wound, e.g., a piece of glass, a splinter of wood, the broken off point of a knife or the bullet, shots, or wadding of a firearm, may indicate the manner in which the wound was inflicted, and may even help to identify the weapon with which the injury was caused, e.g., the broken point of a knife with a missing point which it is alleged was the weapon used; or if the knife produced has a perfect point, it will be clear that it could not have been the weapon employed. A stabbing instrument is likely to break when it passes through the sternum or skull or enters a vertebra. The broken part remains within the body. **Any foreign body found in the wound should be preserved.** Presence of dust, coal or grease should be noted as they give a clue to the nature of injury.

The clothes should be examined for the presence of cuts, tears or burns, and it should be seen if these injuries correspond to the injuries on the body. If the clothing was very loose and was disarranged during the struggle or folded on itself, these may not coincide with the wounds.

(6) Whether the weapon was dangerous or not? A dangerous weapon is any instrument for shooting, stabbing or cutting or any instrument which used as a weapon of offence is likely to cause death.

(7) Remarks: The general condition of the patient should be noted under this column, such as conscious or unconscious, bleeding from the ears, nostrils, mouth, etc., paralysis, state of shock, B.P., pulse, respiration, temperature, etc. The age of the injury should also be noted. It is only possible to give an approximate time. **The age of the injury is very important for its appearance may or may not correspond to the time when it is alleged to have been inflicted, and all the injuries found on a person may not have been produced on the same day.**

A proper examination and documentation of a wound may reveal the nature of the wounding object, the direction of force, the approximate age of the wound, the character and manner of injury, etc. A careful search should be made for wounds in the concealed parts, e.g., axilla, nape of the neck, rectum, vagina, inner canthus of eye, etc.

Laboratory investigations recommended and treatment prescribed should be noted.

When a victim of suicide, homicide or accident dies in the hospital, the medical officer should report the matter to the police immediately. In civil cases, when a party wishes to have medical evidence given on their behalf, the medical officer is entitled to charge reasonable fee. In criminal cases, permission of the Government is required to give evidence for the defence. **When a dead body is brought to the hospital, do not examine the injuries.**

TORTURE

The World Medical Association (Declaration of Tokyo, 1975) defined torture in relation to detention and imprisonment as **"The deliberate, systematic or wanton infliction of physical or mental suffering by one or more persons** acting alone or on the orders of any authority, to force another person to yield information, to make a confession or for any other reason".

S. 330, I.P.C.: Voluntarily causing hurt to extort confession, or to compel restoration of property is punishable with imprisonment up to 7 years.

S. 331, I.P.C.: Voluntarily causing grievous hurt to extract confession or to compel restoration of property is punishable with imprisonment up to ten years.

S. 339, I.P.C.: Wrongful restraint. Imprisonment up to one month (S.341, I.P.C).

The ethical aspects concerning the doctors with regard to torture are dealt in: (1) Declaration of Geneva, 1948, states that no one shall be subject to torture or to cruel, inhuman or degrading treatment or punishment. (2) Declaration of Tokyo, 1975. (3) Principles of medical ethics relevant to the role of health personnel, particularly physicians in the protection of prisoners and detainees against torture and other cruel, inhuman or degrading treatment of punishment (U.N. 1984). (4) World conference on human rights, 1993. Freedom from torture is a right which must be protected under all circumstances, including in times of internal or international disturbance or armed conflicts.

Torture may be carried out by (1) Criminal and terrorist groups, and (2) By the police or other security force personnel during the detention and interrogation of prisoners and suspects.

Objects: (1) To obtain information if a person is suspected to have committed a crime against person or property or indulged in antinational or terrorist activities. (2) To sign a document confessing a crime. (3) To take revenge against a person or his family members by rape, kidnapping, etc. (4) To obtain testimony incriminating others. (5) To spread terror in the community by militant groups or by dictators ruling the country. (6) To destroy the personality of individuals who raise their voices against dictatorial rule, or oppression in the society.

METHODS: The methods of torture are wide and varying. **(I) PHYSICAL ABUSE:** (1) **Beating** is the commonest form. Fist, foot or an instrument, such as *lathi,* metal or wooden bars, whips, belts, cycle chains, etc., are used. The usual target is the back, but injuries may be seen on almost any part of the body. Abrasions, contusions, lacerations and fractures may be found. Bruises in abdominal wall and rupture of internal organs may be seen. Poking with stick, baton, rod, etc. is common. (2) **Falanga** (falaka, bastinado): In this canes or rods are used to beat on the soles of the feet, or rarely to the palms of the hands or hips, which is very painful and debilitating. Contusions are found deep in the tissues. Faint red lines may be seen, and often hyperpigmentation along the lines of injury. Aseptic necrosis may occur. (3) **Telefono:** It consists of repeated slapping of the sides of the head (over ears) by the open palms of the assailant. This may cause rupture of ear drums and injury to the inner ear. (4) **Beating on the abdomen** while lying on a table with the upper half of the body unsupported. In this bruises and rupture of viscera may be seen. (5) **Beating the head** may produce contusions and lacerations of the brain, intracranial haemorrhages and skull fractures, cerebral cortical atrophy, etc. (6) Fingers are twisted or pencils, etc., are kept between two fingers and squeezed hard. **Fingernails are pulled out** using pliers. Pins and pointed objects are introduced underneath finger and toe nails. (7) Making the victim **chew hard on pieces of metals,** stones, etc., or pulling teeth by clips, pliers or forceps and drilling the teeth to expose pulp cavity. (8) **Mutilation:** Chopping of ears, nose, fingers, etc. (9) **Disfiguration by** throwing corrosives on face or other parts of body. (10) Use of continuous **high-pitched sound.** (11) **Forced immersion** of head often contaminated with urine or faeces, until the stage of suffocation **(wet submarino, latina).** Foreign material or debris is found in upper respiratory and upper GI tract. (12) Tying of a **plastic bag** over the head up to the point of suffocation (dry submarino). Asphyxial signs will be present. (13) **Suspension of body by the wrists.** Bruises or scars about the wrists and joint injuries are seen. (14) **Suspension of body by the arms or neck:** Bruises or scars at the site of binding. Prominent lividity in the lower limbs. (15) **Suspension by the ankles:** Bruises or scars about the ankles. Joint injuries. (16) Head down from a horizontal pole placed under the knees with the wrists bound to the ankle **(Parrot's perch, jack).** Bruises or scars on the anterior forearms and backs of the knees. Marks on the wrists and ankles. (17) The victim is asked to **stand in hot sun on one leg** for prolonged periods. Dependent oedema may be seen. (18) Forced straddling of a bar **(saw horse):** Perineal or scrotal haematoma. (19) **Burns** caused by cigarette butts is common. Other methods are application of heated solid body, molten rubber dripped on skin, kerosene soaked rags wrapped around limbs and set fire, hot iron, throwing boiling water or acid, etc. (20) **Cold:** Victim is made to lie on a cold and damp floor or on an ice slab without clothing. (21) **Electric shock (cattle prod):** A magneto delivering high voltage may be used in which burns may not be found on the skin, but it causes severe pain. Sometimes, main voltage of 110 or 240 volts is used, which produces burns, and can cause death in some cases. The genitals especially the penis and scrotum are the targets, and in females nipples, but the current may be applied anywhere. (22) Heated metal skewer inserted into the anus **(black slave):** Perianal or rectal burns. (23) **Dehydration:** Vitreous humour electrolyte abnormalities. (24) **Exposure to dogs or other wild animals** to produce bites. (25) **Disfigure or maim the victim** by inflicting incised wounds on the face, nose, ear lobes, fingers, trunk, etc. (26) **Shooting** through the knee or lower limbs **(knee-capping).** (27) **Disallowing sleep.** (28) **Chepuwa;** The legs and thighs are tied very tightly with bamboo sticks, etc., to induce severe pain. (29) Hair may be plucked or the person may be dragged by the hair. (30) Scratching with knife and sprinkling lime juice or **chilli powder.** (31) **Application of irritant substances** to cause itching or pain. (32) **Ghotna** involves rolling a wooden log or iron rod up and down the thighs, while the log is weighted by one or two policemen standing on it. This causes rupture of muscle fibres and blood vessels. severe pain and often unconsciousness and the victim is unable to walk for several weeks. The ghotna may also be applied by placing it behind the knees and then forcibly flexing the legs over it.

(II) MENTAL TORTURE: (1) **Solitary confinement** in a dark place. (2) **Blindfolding** for a long time, or frequent transfer from one place to another blindfolded. (3) **Starving** the victim. (4) Causing **mental anguish** by giving false information to victim regarding tragedy involving wife and children. (5) **Enforced use of psychotropic drugs.**

(III) SEXUAL TORTURE: (1) Infliction of **injuries to private parts** or introducing foreign bodies into the rectum or vagina, or mutilation of breasts or genitals. (2) **Raping the victim or undressing before others,** or sexually tortured by trained animals, etc. (3) Suspension of weights on the penis and scrotum. (4) **Forced sex with convicts.** (5) Application of **chilli powder** or other irritants to genitalia.

(IV) PHARMACOLOGICAL TORTURE: Various drugs, such as drugs to induce self-disclosure, muscle relaxants, pain—inducing drugs, or psycho-pharmacological drugs, etc.

SEQUELAE: Infection, disfiguration of face, impairment of hearing and sight, psychic disturbances, such as anxiety, depression, phobias, sleep disturbances, suicidal tendencies, etc., and social stigma. Death may occur rarely.

EXAMINATION: ISTANBUL PROTOCOL (V.N. 1999) is the first set of international guidelines for documentation of torture and its consequences. The doctor should obtain complete history from the patient about methods of torture. Symptoms and disabilities following torture are to be recorded. Details of acute and chronic symptoms should be noted. The injuries should be recorded in detail and marked on body diagrams. Photographs of injuries should be taken with a scale placed near the injuries. All the systems of the body should be examined completely. X-rays should be taken and CT scan done to detect minute fractures and soft tissue injuries.

TREATMENT: The principles of treatment are: (1) Developing a good rapport with the victim. (2) Empathising with the victim and his family. (3) Avoiding situation or objects that remind the victim of the torture event. (4) Psychotherapy. (5) Rehabilitation, counselling and re-assurance should be provided.

In India, **National Human Rights Commission (NHRC), State Human Rights Commission (SHRC)** and Human Rights Courts have been constituted for better protection of human rights and connected and incidental matters thereto.

Human Rights and Forensic Medicine: Human rights are based on the United Nations (UN) Universal Declaration of Human Rights (1948). It states 'Everyone has the right to life, liberty and security of person' (Article 3) and 'No one shall be subjected to torture or to cruel, inhuman or degrading treatment or punishment' (Article 5). Forensic expert has humanitarian as well as legal role in context of Human rights and its violation. It is based on different activities: exhumation and examinations of bodies in singular or mass graves, autopsies on fresh bodies, examination of living torture victims, studies of documents like medical records, police reports and autopsy reports, court appearances in human rights courts and publication of reports, scientific articles, text books and conducting training courses.

DEATH IN CUSTODY

Custody death refers to death of a person when under state, either for interrogation, prevention, trial, or in prison jail or detention jail, in police station or prison officers attempting to detain a criminal or a person escaping or attempting to escape from police custody or prison. Person may die during (1) process of arrest, (2) during interrogation, (3) in cell, (4) during third degree torture.

(A) DURING ARREST: (1) Traumatic asphyxia may occur if the offender resists arrest, and a number of policemen fall upon him to overpower him. If there is a struggle, blunt injuries sustained by the offender by the use of fist, arm or leg, riot stick, etc., by the police or from head injury from falls against ground, wall, etc., may cause death.

(2) HOG-TYING (total appendage restraint procedure) is a type of physical restraint in which the person is placed in prone position with

his wrists and ankles bound behind his back and secured by a cord. The person may have difficulty in breathing or may become unresponsive. Rarely, death may occur due to varying degress of asphyxia with heart disease, sympathomimetic drug abuse, and the body's physiologic response to stress and exertion. Death often occurs not during physical restraint but soon following the restraint.

(3) CHOKE OR CAROTID HOLDS: A choke (bar arm control) or a carotid sleeper hold, do not involve the use of a mechanical implement.

(I) IN CHOKE (BAR ARM) HOLDS forearm is placed straight across the front of the neck. The free hand grips the wrist and pulls it back, which causes obstruction of the airway and carotid arteries and immediate unconsciousness. The hypopharynx is also occluded by displacement of the tongue Fig. (10–2). Fracture of the hyoid bone or larynx may occur if great force is used. Rarely death may occur due to hypoxia and release of catecholamines due to struggle, resulting in fatal cardiac arrhythmia, especially if the deceased consumed cocaine or similar drug. Pressure on the carotid bodies can cause death by sudden cardiac arrest.

(II) In the CAROTID SLEEPER HOLD (lateral vascular neck restraint), standing behind a person the arm is placed about the neck with the antecubital fossa centered at the midline of the neck. The free hand grips the wrist and the arm is pulled backwards, which compresses the carotid arteries and jugular veins but not vertebral arteries and the trachea Fig. (10–3). Consciousness is lost in 10 to 15 seconds. If pressure is released the victim regains consciousness in 10 to 20 seconds. The neck structures are not damaged. Rarely death may occur due to hypoxia and release of catecholamines.

Most deaths occur immediately after an arrest in which there is a violent struggle. Hypoxia may exacerbate pre-existing ischaemic heart disease, resulting in myocardial infarction or cardiac dysrhythmias.

Death in custody can be due to: **(1) Natural Disease:** The emotional upset may precipitate an acute cardiac crisis in the presence of severe pre-existing disease. A large number of custody deaths are natural, triggered by stressful event. Following diseases must be specifically looked for: diabetes, epilepsy, asthma, coronary artery disease, tuberculosis and pancreatitis. **(2) Death immediately after struggle:** hypertensive bleeding or dysrhythmias. **(3) During Lockup:** (A) If the offender was severely intoxicated, he may die of acute alcoholic poisoning, or he may aspirate the vomit and die of choking. (B) The drunken offender may fall on a hard surface on the occiput. If on autopsy contrecoup injuries are found, it indicates deceleration injury rather than an assault with a weapon. (C) Physical injuries may also occur from falls in drug addicts used to amphetamine, cocaine or hallucinogens. **(4)** A person with illicit drugs in his possession may swallow the drugs to avoid detection on being caught and may die suddenly while in custody. **(5) Drug related death:** Overdose, deprivation, drug carrier through body. **(6)** A person may have injuries that were sustained before he was arrested or sustained during arrest may die in custody. **(7) Torture by various methods:** By kicking and stomping, or a backward blow from the point of an elbow on the face, neck, or abdomen, fist blows, etc., inflicted with sufficient force can cause severe damage and death. Some methods of physical abuse may not leave any apparent marks of violence, such as hair-pulling, face slapping and blows to the side of the eardrum. Blows to the abdomen may not cause any apparent mark. Pinching, squeezing and blows to the testes may produce bruising of the skin and swelling and tenderness of testes. The soles may be stuck with a baton, ruler, etc. In many custody or restraint related deaths, physiologic processes have a prominent role in death, which are not identifiable at autopsy.

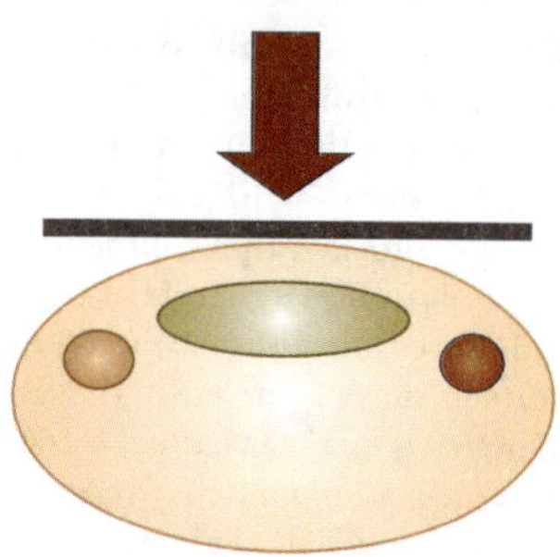

Fig. (10–2). Carotid hold. Force applied across the front of neck compressing the airway.

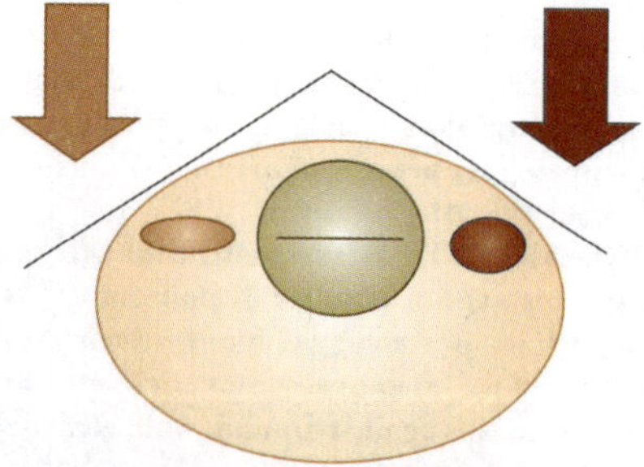

Fig. (10–3). Carotid sleeper. Direction of force on neck aimed at compressing the carotid arteries.

The most common physical sign found in cases of custodial torture are: (1) Scars in soles of feet, (2) Muscle and joint disorders, (3) Scars in parts of body, (4) Scars of burns, (5) Chronic pain due to faulty healing of fracture, (6) Broken or missing nails, (7) Broken or missing teeth, (8) Peripheral nerve damage, (9) Loss of hearing, (10) Enlarged feet, (11) Habitual subluxation of the shoulder or knee, (12) Deviation of nasal septum.

Suicide in custody: Suicides in custody are quite common. Any object may be used to commit suicide. The common method is hanging. Sometimes, a poison may be consumed, or he may jump from a height, or cut his throat or a large blood vessel, blunt force injuries.

Investigation is done by a magistrate and postmortem is conducted by a team of doctors.

ASSAULT: In the adrenaline response of "fight or flight", the shock element of pain is greatly suppressed. The usual shock effect may be damped down considerably in an assault and only the sheer physical and haemodynamic sequelae of the injury will eventually lead to a slowing down, then collapse and death.

Autopsy in Custodial Death: National Human Right Commission (NHRC) has laid down protocol to be followed in cases of deaths in police action, custodial deaths and death in prison.

The NHRC directed to promptly report all deaths in police and judicial custody within 24 hours of the occurrence, to the Commission. While conducting postmortem examination of the deceased, photographs of the deceased should be taken and the postmortem examination of the deceased should be video filmed.

The aim of video-filming and photography of postmortem examination should be: (i) to record the detailed findings of the postmortem examination, especially pertaining to marks of injury and violence which may suggest custodial torture, (ii) to supplement the findings of postmortem examination (recorded in the postmortem report) by video graphic evidence so as to rule out any undue influence or suppression of material information (iii) to facilitate an independent review of the postmortem examination report at a later stage if required. However, in cases of deaths in jail, the requirement of videography in postmortem examination can be relaxed to some extent.

Protocol for video-filming and photography of postmortem examination: (i) At the time of video-filming of the postmortem examination the voice of the doctor conducting the postmortem should be recorded. The doctor should narrate his prima-facie observations while conducting the postmortem examination. (ii) A total of 20-25 coloured photographs covering the whole body should be taken. Some photographs of the body should be taken without removing the clothes. The photographs should include the following: (a) Profile photo-face (front, right lateral and left lateral views), back of head. (b) Front of body (up to torso-chest and abdomen)—and back. (c) Upper extremity—front and back. (d) Lower extremity—front and back. (e) Focusing on

each injury/lesion-zoomed in after properly numbering the injuries. (f) Internal examination findings. (2 photos of soles and palms each, after making incision to show absence/evidence of any old/deep seated injury). In firearm injuries while describing, the distance from heel as well as midline must be taken in respect of each injury which will help later in reconstruction of events. (iii) Photographs should be taken after incorporating postmortem number, date of examination and a scale for dimensions in the frame of photographs itself. (iv) While taking photographs the camera should be held at right - angle to the object being photographed. (v) Video-filming and photography of the postmortem examination should be done by a person trained in forensic photography and videography. A good quality digital camera with 10X optical zoom and minimum 10 mega pixels should be used.

Other precautions to be taken before conducting postmortem examination include: (i) Both hands of the deceased need to be wrapped in white paper bags before transportation. The dead body afterwards should be covered in special body bags having zip pouches for proper transportation. (ii) Clothing on the body of the deceased should not be removed by the police or any other person. It should be collected, examined as well as preserved and sealed by the doctor conducting the autopsy, and should be sent for further examination at the concerned forensic science laboratory. A detailed note regarding examination of the clothing should be incorporated in the postmortem examination report by the doctor conducting the autopsy. (iii) In case of alleged firearms deaths, the dead body should be subjected to radiological examination (X-rays/ CT scan) prior to autopsy.

The postmortem report has to be prepared in the new proforma. The postmortem report along with the recorded video film and photographs should be sent to the Commission within 2 months of the incident. In some cases of custodial death, after postmortem the viscera is sent for examination and viscera report is called for. In such cases, the postmortem report and other documents should be sent to the commission without waiting for the viscera report. The viscera report should be sent subsequently as soon as it is received.

SUDDEN DEATH DURING OR IMMEDIATELY AFTER A VIOLENT STRUGGLE OR DURING EXERCISE

Sympathetic stimulation causes an increase in heart rate, force of myocardial contraction and blood pressure. During exercise, there is a progressive rise in systolic pressure, with little change in diastolic pressure. There is progressive increase of heart rate with exercise (maximum rate is about 180 to 200 beats per minute), before reaching a plateau. Systolic pressure increases to 160 to 210 mm Hg, due to which there is a decrease in peripheral resistance. **During exercise, serum potassium levels increase. Sudden death occurs not only during exercise, but often during first few minutes after cessation of strenuous exercise.** Highest levels of catecholamines occur during the first 3 minutes after cessation of exercise. Norepinephrine levels increase 7 to 10 times over baseline values and epinephrine 3 to 8 times. Potassium concentration falls rapidly, reaching hypokalaemic levels within 1 to 2 minutes post-exercise. Norepinephrine interacts with alpha-1 receptors and causes vasoconstriction of coronary arteries, due to which the supply of oxygenated blood to the myocardium is decreased. **The combination of rising catecholamines and falling potassium during first few minutes after exercise may make the person susceptible to post-exercise arrhythmias (post-exercise peril). Sudden death occurring after exercise is probably caused by this mechanism, with ischaemia sensitizing the heart to arrhythmogenic properties of catecholamines and hypokalaemia. If the person suffers from heart disease, a focal area of myocardial ischaemia develops, with fatal cardiac arrhythmia.**

Occasionally, an individual becomes unresponsive and dies either during or shortly following a physically intense struggle with police and/or other individuals. The struggle often arises when an agitated, excited, psychotic or otherwise hyperactive person resists arrest. Commonly, these effects are due to the toxic effects of cocaine and/or amphetamine abuse.

During high intensity exercise, e.g., a struggle, and sometimes physical upset of being arrested and confined may have affected the blood pressure and heart rate sufficiently by an adrenaline response to have precipitated an acute cardiac crisis in the presence of severe pre-existing disease.

In some cases, sudden death during or following struggle can be caused by natural disease that is not diagnosable anatomically, such as Wolff-Parkinson White syndrome, the prolonged Q-T syndrome, etc.

Sudden cardiac death can also occur due to psychological stress, due to fatal or potentially fatal cardiac arrhythmias with and without underlying heart disease. This is caused by stress-induced sympathetic stimulation.

Emotional stress such as anger, anxiety and fear have an effect on the heart and increase sympathetic output and may precipitate fatal dysrhythmia, particularly in those with significant heart disease, such as severe coronary artery atherosclerosis or cardiac hypertrophy. The heart and CNS are neurally linked. Both parasympathetic and sympathetic nerves innervate the heart with a complex interaction of impulses contributing to the cardiac plexus and influencing the arrhythmogenicity of the myocardium. Cardiac-neural interactions may help explain the deaths of individuals collapsing following a severely stressful, fearful, life-threatening, emotionally charged event and also sudden deaths of some persons with seizure disorders of subarachnoid haemorrhage. **The stress associated with assault or simply fear of severe injury may precipitate catecholamine release and stress the myocardium into fatal dysrhythmia.** However, the emotional response may be complicated by additional factors, such as physiological stress or exertion and minor or sublethal physical injuries sustained during an altercation, which would enhance the argument supporting the link between the crime and death of the victim. **If the person suffers from heart disease, a focal area of myocardial ischaemia develops with fatal cardiac arrhythmia.**

Emotional deaths: In charged emotional atmospheres, some persons collapse suddenly due to stress as in football and cricket play grounds, where spectators are unable to bear emotional pressures. Similar charged situations are also seen in interpersonal conflicts, fights, agitation, hysterical behaviour, physical fights bearing minor injuries. Cardiac-neural interactions cause cardiac inhibitions or arrhythmias. These become more immediate and prominent in persons having underlying cardiac hypertrophy and ischaemic disease. Emotional response period varies in each person but usually within 1 to 2 hours.

Alcohol and sudden death: Sudden death of a person with a history of alcohol abuse may occur during a struggle. Chronic alcoholics may have prolonged QT-interval, which is associated with sudden death and also have increased levels of norepinephrine. Arrhythmias can be aggravated by catecholamines released during a violent struggle. **If the heart is predisposed to fatal arrhythmias by the action of alcohol, then the released catecholamines during a violent struggle can produce a fatal arrhythmia.**

Autopsy: A complete history should be obtained including medical records of the deceased. **Autopsy is negative.** A complete autopsy should be performed and microscopic examination of all organs especially the heart and complete toxicological examination should be done. Diseases that can cause sudden and unexpected death, such as cardiovascular diseases, epilepsy, asthma, diabetes etc., should be sought for. Blood should be examined for alcohol in cases where the offender has consumed alcohol.

HOMICIDE BY HEART ATTACK: Davis (1978) has published guidelines for certifying homicides by heart attack which require that (1) The crime be of such a nature, that if physical injury has occurred, a homicide charge would be supported. (2) The victim realises an implicit threat to his safety. (3) The circumstances be of an obvious emotional nature. (4) Cardiac arrhythmia and collapse occur during criminal act or in the ensuing emotional response period. (5) Chronic heart disease be demonstrable.

EXCITED DELIRIUM: Agitated or excited delirium (acute psychotic episode) is an acute confusional state marked by intense paranoia, hallucinations, hyperactivity, incoherent shouting, aggression and demonstration of excessive strength and violence towards objects and people. It may also occur in the absence of stimulant drugs in persons with endogenous mental disease, such as schizophrenia, schizoaffective disorders, delusional disorders and drug or alcohol intoxication. **The most common causes are toxicity from stimulant drugs especially cocaine, methamphetamine and psychotropic patients who stop taking their medication. Sudden cardiac death associated with a severe metabolic (lactic) acidosis may occur.** A violent struggle occurs in an attempt to restrain the persons from injuring themselves or others. **Immediately after the struggle ends, the levels of catecholamines continue to increase for about three minutes, while the level of potassium drops considerably. These two factors predispose to the development of an arrhythmia.** The individual becomes unresponsive and dies without responding to resuscitation. **Cocaine has a double effect. It causes increased release of catecholamines from the adrenals and inhibits norepinephrine reuptake due to which coronary arteries contract, reducing myocardial perfusion. In such cases,** the **cause of death** can be given as **"cardio-pulmonary arrest during violent struggle" in individual under influence of cocaine, alcohol, etc.**

CAUSES OF DEATH FROM WOUNDS

The causes of death from the wounds are: (1) Immediate or direct. (2) Remote, delayed or indirect.

IMMEDIATE CAUSES: (1) HAEMORRHAGE: Haemorrhage means escape of blood from the cardiovascular system.

Types: Haemorrhage is classified as capillary, venous, arterial or cardiac, depending upon its origin. Haemorrhage may be external or internal. When bleeding occurs due to various types of wounds, it is called traumatic haemorrhage. Bleeding occurring in the absence of trauma is called spontaneous haemorrhage. Petechiae are minute haemorrhagic spots, usually of capillary or venular origin. Ecchymoses are larger areas (1 to 2 mm) of extravasated blood. A haematoma is localised collection of blood, usually clotted, forming a tumour-like swelling in a tissue. **Apoplexy is large effusion of blood into an organ, but the term is commonly used for cerebral haemorrhage.**

The loss of blood from the circulation may be due to wounds of the heart, or of the larger blood vessels, or to a severe laceration of an organ or structure, which is very vascular. The haemorrhage may occur at the time of injury (primary haemorrhage). Secondary haemorrhage (reactionary haemorrhage) occurs from the same site as primary haemorrhage but is usually delayed for several hours (up to 24 hours or more) after the injury. It may occur due to a rise in blood pressure (which accompanies the recovery from shock), and muscular movements, which loosen the blood clot, and the erosion of vessel walls which occur in infection.

(a) EXTERNAL HAEMORRHAGE: It may produce syncope and death either rapidly, if a large vessel has been injured, or slowly if a number of small vessels have been damaged. In partial transection of an artery, retraction does not occur and bleeding is more. The sudden loss of blood is more dangerous than the same quantity lost slowly. When leakage is slow, body can compensate for loss of a greater volume, both by adjustment of vascular bed and by restoration of blood volume by transfer from other aqueous compartments. A minor injury may produce death from haemorrhage in persons with haemorrhagic diathesis or haemophilia. An approximate idea of loss of blood may be had from the soaking of clothes, and the surroundings of the victim, and from the anaemic state of the viscera.

(b) INTERNAL HAEMORRHAGE: It may occur in penetrating wounds, gunshot wounds, and due to rupture of organs or vessels. The blood escapes from the divided vessels, either internally or externally as it remains fluid even after death. Blood in the pleural cavity does not clot, because of rapid defibrination due to movements of the lung.

Wounds can continue to bleed copiously after death due to passive leakage, especially if the injured part of the body is dependent, i.e., lower than the rest of the body. Blood can also accumulate in large quantity within the pleural and peritoneal cavities after death.

MECHANISM OF DEATH: (1) The rapid loss of one-third of the blood of the body causes death due to irreversible hypovolaemic shock. Due to severe fall in blood pressure, cerebral ischaemia and death from cerebral anoxia occurs. Children, women and old people die from the loss of much smaller quantity. (2) Haemorrhage can kill rapidly creating increased pressure in or on a vital organ which interferes with its vital function, e.g., an effusion of 300 to 400 ml. of blood into the pericardial sac interferes with the heart's action (cardiac tamponade); a small haemorrhage into the medulla will fatally interrupt the functions of the vital centres there; an intracranial haemorrhage may cause death from cerebral compression. (3) Bleeding into the trachea or bronchi can cause rapid death from asphyxia due to the blood acting as a mechanical barrier to respiratory efforts, which cause asphyxia. The victim literally drowns in his own blood.

AUTOPSY: The pathologic findings in death from haemorrhage are pallor of the skin and mucous membranes, and of all viscera (especially renal cortex), and a small amount of blood in the blood vessels. In the typical case, the heart is contracted and shows streaky minute subendocardial haemorrhages on the left side of ventricular septum, and papillary muscle.

(2) REFLEX VAGAL INHIBITION: In this, there may not be visible external injury.

(3) SHOCK: Shock is a circulatory disturbance characterised by hypoperfusion of cells and tissues due to reduction in the volume of blood or cardiac output, or redistribution of blood resulting in a decrease of effective circulating volume.

Primary Shock: **Primary or neurogenic shock (vaso-vagal shock or reflex cardiac arrest) results from a sudden reduction of venous return to the heart due to neurogenic vasodilation with pooling of blood in the peripheral vascular bed,** especially in the splanchnic area. There is yawning, sighing respirations, nausea and vomiting followed by unconsciousness, but the attack rarely lasts for more than a few minutes. There is pallor, coldness of the extremities, weak rapid pulse and low blood pressure. **The cardiac output is unchanged. It may follow any form of stress. Psychological factors, such as fear, grief, anxiety, emotion and pain due to various causes also play a large part.** It may occur when a few ml. of blood are withdrawn, or from the sight of blood or an anticipation of injection.

ACUTE NEUROGENIC CARDIOVASCULAR FAILURE: The sympathetico-adrenal division stimulates the cardiovascular system to meet the demands of the body in physical and emotional stress, especially in an emergency. The parasympathetic division has a tonic and inhibitory control on the cardiovascular system. These two divisions act together and provide a balanced control to meet the varying needs of the body. There is much individual variation and in some persons constitutional imbalance of the autonomic system seems to be present, with increased sympathetic or parasympathetic tone.

Sympathetico-adrenal stimulation occurs in emotional disturbances, such as fear, especially when accompanied by painful sensations. The peripheral nerves convey both pressor and depressor afferent fibres. Stimulation of the pressor fibres causes generalised vasoconstriction with a rise in blood pressure. Stimulation of the depressor fibres cause generalised vasodilation with a fall in blood pressure. Weak stimuli of afferent nerve fibres cause depressor effects and stronger stimuli cause pressor effects. Painful stimuli are associated with pressor effects. Strong and painful stimuli excite pressor afferent fibres of peripheral nerve. The sympathetico-adrenal division is stimulated by physical exertion, cerebral anaemia, hypoglycaemia, low oxygen tension or a high CO_2 tension in the blood. The stimulation is caused both by direct action on the medullary centres and by reflex action through the chemoreceptors of the aortic and carotid bodies. Sympathetico-adrenal stimulation results in rapid pulse, increase in myocardial contractility and irritability, extrasystoles and generalised vasoconstriction with a rise in blood pressure, and may lead to sudden, fatal circulatory failure from ventricular fibrillation, Hypotension resulting from pain or fear, from loss of effective circulating blood volume, drugs or reflex action will cause hypoxia. Hypoxia from a low cardiac output or respiratory inadequacy will render the ventricular cells more sensitive to catecholamine release and lead to ventricular fibrillation. Circulatory failure due to ventricular fibrillation usually occurs after several minutes.

PATHOLOGY: There may be some pre-existing cardiac disease, such as coronary artery sclerosis, cardiac hypertrophy or fibrosis, fatty myocardium, chronic valvular disease (esp. aortic valves), or syphilitic atresia of the coronary orifices. Signs of earlier chronic congestive failure, i.e., chronic passive congestion of organs and dependent oedema may be present. Pulmonary congestion and oedema are present and may be marked. Pleurae show petechial haemorrhages, which may be very numerous.

DIAGNOSIS: The possibility of the neurogenic cardiovascular failure should be considered when a healthy person dies suddenly without any adequate cause. The cause of death as ventricular fibrillation precipitated by reflex sympathetico-adrenal stimulation may be inferred, if some pre-existing cardiac lesion is found at autopsy, if the fatal symptoms were those of a hyperacute congestive cardiac failure (with acute dyspnoea and cyanosis), and if acute congestive visceral changes are present.

Secondary Shock: **It is more serious and may be fatal. There is progressive circulatory failure and damage to the tissues.** It is called secondary or delayed shock, because the circulatory disturbance usually develops gradually or after a latent period following the injury. Apart from haemodynamic alterations, there are disturbances in the molecules of cells due to diminished perfusion of the tissues. Intracellular metabolism is disturbed with anaerobic glucose metabolism and increased production of lactic and other acids, which may cause disruption of lysosome, release of their lytic enzymes and death of cells. The production of adenosinetriphosphate is decreased, which results in a reduction of protein synthesis, and disturbance in the transport mechanism and cell membrane permeability. Associated with this is a reduction in oxygen consumption, interference with enzyme system, metabolic acidosis, water and electrolyte disturbance and renal insufficiency.

PATHOGENESIS: Reduction of blood flow with poor cellular perfusion (anoxia) is the essential feature of shock. Three basic pathophysiologic derangements are: (1) reduction of actual circulating blood volume, (2) decreased cardiac output, and (3) widespread vasodilation of the capacitance vessels (capillaries and veins).

Stages of Shock: **(1) Nonprogressive phase:** In this reflex compensatory mechanisms are activated and perfusion of vital organs is not affected. **(2) Progressive state:** In this tissue perfusion is reduced with increasing circulatory and metabolic imbalances. **(3) Irreversible stage:** This occurs after severe injury to the cells and tissues.

MECHANISM: During early shock a number of neurohumoral mechanisms, such as baroreceptor reflexes, catecholamines, antidiuretic hormone, activation of renin-angiotensin axis, and generalised sympathetic stimulation maintain cardiac output and blood pressure. There is tachycardia, peripheral vasoconstriction and conservation of fluid by the kidneys. During the progressive phase, vital organs suffer from significant hypoxia. Hypoxia causes impairment of intracellular aerobic respiration, followed by anaerobic glycolysis and excessive production of lactate, which causes metabolic lactic acidosis. Due to lowering of pH in the tissues, arterioles dilate and blood begins to pool in the capillaries. This causes diminished cardiac output, and anoxic injury to endothelial cells, leading to disseminated intravascular coagulation. When the tissue hypoxia is widespread, the function of vital organs deteriorates. The patient is confused and the urinary output begins to fall.

Types: Shock can be classified on the basis of the stressful circumstances under which it occurs. **(1) Haemorrhagic shock (hypovolaemic shock):** This occurs when the blood loss is sufficient to impair peripheral perfusion, which produces a sufficient degree of systemic anoxia. Loss of 10 to 40 per cent of the total blood volume produces shock. **(2) Traumatic or wound shock:** This is the most common type of shock. The blood volume may be reduced due to haemorrhage from ruptured vessels, an excessive loss of plasma from damaged capillaries or venules at the site of injury, or a combination of both factors. In some cases, blood loss is not significant and the shock may be due to neurogenic mechanisms. It has also been suggested that the major factor is absorption of products of tissue autolysis from the area of injury, which causes a generalised increased vascular permeability. Infection of the wound and bacterial endotoxins may also play a part. **(3) Burn shock:** It results from loss of plasma, resorption of necrotic tissue and bacterial sepsis following extensive burns. **(4) Surgical shock:** It occurs either during or immediately after surgical procedures. It may be due to a combination of causes; anaesthesia, loss of blood and plasma, emotional reactions, infections and probably liberation of substances from severely traumatised tissues that may influence the circulation. **(5) Cardiac or cardiogenic shock:** It results from

Table (10–1). Classification of shock

Types of shock	Clinical examples	Principal mechanisms
Cardiogenic:	Myocardial infarction, rupture of heart, arrhythmias, cardiac tamponade, pulmonary embolism.	Failure of myocardial pump due to intrinsic myocardial damage or extrinsic pressure or obstruction to outflow.
Hypovolaemic:	Haemorrhage, fluid loss (e.g., vomiting, diarrhoea, burns).	Inadequate blood or plasma volume.
Septic:	Overwhelming bacterial infections: Gram-negative septicaemia ("endotoxic shock") or Gram-positive septicaemia.	Peripheral vasodilatation and pooling of blood; cell membrane injury, endothelial cell injury with DIC.
Neurogenic:	Anaesthesia, spinal cord injury.	Peripheral vasodilatation with pooling of blood.

the decreased cardiac output, reduced blood flow and deficient delivery of oxygen to the tissues following injury to the pumping mechanism. **(6) Septic shock:** It develops in the presence of severe infection. Loss of fluid from the circulation (generalised increased vascular permeability), or pooling of the blood in the peripheral vascular bed (vasodilation) cause circulatory failure. **(7) Endotoxic shock:** This is closely related if not identical to septic shock. It is seen in patients having Gram-negative infections. Bacterial endotoxins induce intravascular coagulation prior to endothelial damage Table (10–1).

Surgical shock does not occur in head injury unless it is extremely severe, or there has been excessive blood loss from scalp wound, other injury to trunk or limbs.

Postmortem Appearances: The findings in secondary shock are circulatory changes, and degeneration and necrosis in various organs. The circulatory changes include congestion of all the internal organs, petechial haemorrhages in the serous cavities and oedema of the viscera.

Brain: The brain may develop ischaemic encephalopathy. The changes occur if the person survives for 12 to 24 hours. At first there is swelling or shrinkage of neurons. Later the nucleus becomes pyknotic. Later, nerve cells die and are replaced by fibrillary gliosis.

Kidneys: The renal changes are those of acute tubular necrosis. The renal changes begin within 24 hours, and become marked in another 7 to 10 days. The kidneys are normal in size, but in some cases they may be slightly enlarged. If extensive muscle injury or i.v. haemolysis are also associated, peculiar brown tubular casts are seen.

Lungs: They are not affected in hypovolaemic shock. When vascular collapse is caused by bacterial sepsis or trauma **"shock lung"** is seen. **The lungs resemble liver, are dark red, firm, airless and heavy. There is capillary congestion, interstitial and intra-alveolar oedema and haemorrhage, interstitial lymphocytic infiltration, alveolar hyaline membrane, thickening and fibrosis of alveolar septa and necrosis of alveolar epithelial cells.** The capillaries contain an accumulation of leucocytes, clumps of platelets and often microthrombi. In some cases, secondary or terminal pneumonia may be superimposed.

Heart: Fatty change occurs in about 20% cases after 18 hours and becomes well-marked in 3 to 4 days. **Subendocardial haemorrhages and necrosis sometimes appear in all forms of shock.**

Gastrointestinal tract: The lesions are multifocal and widely distributed throughout the bowel. Patchy mucosal haemorrhages and necroses ("haemorrhagic enteropathy") may be seen. The mucosa of the gastrointestinal tract is often congested and oedematous, and may show haemorrhage, erosions or ulcerations in 2 to 3 days especially in those who are on mechanical ventilator for more than 2 days. The intestinal tract may contain blood-stained fluid. The blood is fluid and dark–red.

Liver: Gross appearance of the liver is not altered. Fatty changes develop after 18 hours, which may extend from the central areas to lobules. Central necrosis occurs with severe perfusion deficits.

Spleen: In septicaemia, there may be enlargement and softening of the spleen and non-specific toxic signs in other organs such as the heart and liver.

Adrenal: Focal lipid depletion of the cortex occurs after 24 hours and is well marked by third or fourth day.

Foci of necrosis may be present in the lymph nodes, spleen and pancreas.

Mental (nervous) shock: It is the mental state resulting from an unpleasant experience, which may be physical or psychic.

(4) MECHANICAL INJURY TO A VITAL ORGAN: Severe injury to a vital organ, such as crushing of brain, heart, etc. is rapidly fatal.

Death may occur from a slight injury inflicted on a previously diseased organ, e.g., rupture of enlarged spleen, perforation of a chronic intestinal ulcer; bursting of an aneurysm, etc. In such cases, the assailant cannot be charged with culpable homicide but is convicted of simple or grievous hurt, if it is proved that his intention was not to kill his victim, that he could not possibly have known the existence of disease, and that the same injury could not have proved fatal when inflicted on normal healthy individual.

REMOTE CAUSES: Though the injury does not directly cause death, the victim may die after a varying period from remote causes. **Even when the victim dies of complications, an assailant is responsible, provided death can be traced to likely result of the injury.** In a charge of murder, death should be clearly connected with the injury. **The assailant is responsible even if the victim was in a bad state of health when attacked, and if the injury inflicted by the accused accelerated or precipitated the death.**

(1) Infection: Wound infection may be caused by: (1) Organisms normally present on the body surfaces, e.g., Streptococci, Staphylococci, B.pyocyaneus, Coliform bacilli, Freidlander's bacilli, and Cl.welchii. (2) Organisms invading the tissues from the environment, e.g., Streptococci, Staphylococci, C. diphtheriae, Coliform organisms, Cl.welchii and Cl.tetani. **Primary wound infection** is caused by organisms, which are carried into the wounds at the time of the injury, e.g., from the skin, clothing, dirt, etc. **Secondary wound infection** is caused by organisms which invade the wound after injury, e.g., by airborne droplet infection, contaminated dressings, etc.

(a) DIRECT INFECTION: Infection at the site of an open wound, such as a stab wound, or a gunshot wound, and fracture of anterior cranial fossa communicating with an air sinus may cause meningitis. (b) REMOTE INFECTION: Uterine infection following upon criminal abortion may cause meningitis. (c) TRAUMA: At the site of infection, such as bruising of a pre-existing staphylococcal lesion of the bone may produce septicaemia or pyaemia. (d) Infection may be due to an indirect result of injury which creates a local area of lessened resistance, e.g., abscess may form around simple fractures of bone, contusion, or in traumatic infarcts of liver, kidneys and spleen. Dead tissue and extravasated blood provide favourable environment to bacterial growth. (e) If the general vitality is depressed, hypostatic pneumonia, pyelonephritis, cystitis, decubital ulcers, etc. may develop.

Pyogenic cocci may produce a localised abscess (usually in staphylococcal infections) or a diffuse spreading cellulitis (usually in streptococcal infection). B.proteus, B.pyocyaneus and B.coli produce suppurative lesions in association with pyogenic cocci. In clostridium cellulitis, the infection is confined to the connective tissues which produce gas, but the muscles are affected. In gas gangrene there is a massive and rapid necrosis of muscle tissue which causes severe toxaemia.

Septicaemia is the presence of rapidly multiplying highly pathogenic bacteria in the blood. In this, there may be enlargement and softening of the spleen, and non-specific toxic signs in other organs, such as the heart and liver. Pyaemia is the dissemination of small septic thrombi in the blood which cause their effects at the site where they are lodged. Bacteraemia is the presence of small number of bacteria in the blood which do not multiply significantly. Chronic inflammation is a prolonged. process in which tissue destruction and inflammation occur at the same time.

(2) Gangrene or Necrosis: Gangrene is death of a part accompanied by putrefaction. It results from severe crushing of part and tearing of blood vessels **Fig. (10–4).**

(3) Renal failure following trauma: (acute tubular necrosis; crush syndrome): The cause is obscure, but may involve the juxtaglomerular apparatus and the renin angiotensin system, and disseminated intravascular coagulation effects on the glomeruli. It may occur in cases of trauma to the limbs in which necrosis of the muscles occur, which may be due to ischaemia

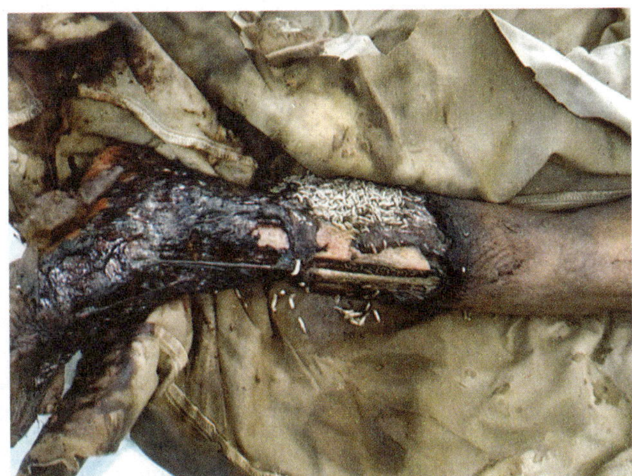

Fig. (10–4). Gangrene of foot and leg.

***Courtesy:* Professor Mukta Rani, Lady Hardinge Medical College, New Delhi.**

of direct compression. **It results from severe crushing of the muscles, especially those that involve the lower limbs,** e.g., under fallen masonry, industrial and vehicular accident, torture by rolling a rod over thighs, etc. In traffic accidents, necrosis of muscle may occur without any prolonged crushing injury. Death usually occurs in one to two weeks after the injury. It is also seen in extensive burns and certain poisons, e.g., mercuric salts or carbontetrachloride. The effects are similar to those associated with incompatible blood transfusion. **There are no specific gross changes in the kidney.** Microscopic examination reveals degeneration and necrosis of focal portions of distal part of Henle's loop and the distal convoluted tubules. **Cellular infiltration is seen in the interstitial tissues around the degenerated and necrosed tubules.** The distal tubular segments and the collecting **tubules contain casts of haeme compound.** The casts may be due to reduced filtration rather than tubular damage. The glomeruli and proximal convoluted tubules appear normal.

(4) Neglect of Injured Person: Death may occur from complications arising from a simple injury due to improper treatment, or negligence on the part of the doctor, or to negligence or wilful disobedience on the part of the patient.

(5) Surgical Operation: The assaulted person is not bound to submit himself for operation. If death occurs due to this omission, the assailant becomes responsible. If death follows a surgical operation performed for the treatment of an injury, the assailant is responsible for the result, if it is proved that the victim would have died even without the operation, and that the operation was thought necessary and was performed by a competent surgeon with reasonable care and skill. A doctor cannot swear that an operation would have saved the life of the victim. He can only affirm that it might have provided the victim a better prospect of recovery. When anaesthesia is given to an injured person before operation, and if the person dies during its administration, and if it is agreed that the patient would not have died but for its administration, the person causing injury is liable to be punished for culpable homicide. If hurt or wound is not fatal, and if it is clearly proved that death of the victim is caused by application of harmful medicines by himself or those about him, this cannot be regarded as murder. **An operation on an assaulted person should not be undertaken unless it is clearly indicated. Consultation with another surgeon is advisable.**

(6) Natural Disease: Some natural disease may be present which was the actual cause of death, but in which death was accelerated by assault, e.g., persons suffering from miliary aneurysms, fatty degeneration of the heart, amoebic liver abscess, hydatid cyst, enlarged spleen, etc. may die due to slight violence, **which may be a precipitating cause.**

(7) Supervention of Disease from a Traumatic Lesion: Fibrous scar tissue formed due to healing may contract and produce complications, e.g., fibrous scar in a hollow muscular organ may produce stricture and obstruction. If a fibrous scar is under continuous tension, it may stretch and produce complication, e.g., a fibrous scar in the wall of an artery may bulge into a traumatic aneurysm. Damage of an artery by a bullet may produce false aneurysm, which may rupture later. Direct injury to the coronary artery by thoracic trauma may be followed by coronary thrombosis. Meningitis, encephalitis, brain abscess may follow head injury. A wound of the abdominal wall after healing may be followed by strangulated hernia with fatal result. An injury affecting lower portion of spinal column or cord may cause paraplegia which may cause death from septic cystitis or bed sores and general exhaustion.

(8) Thrombosis and Embolism: The most common sites of thrombosis are in deep femoral, the popliteal and posterior tibial veins, and occurs usually in traumatic lesions of lower extremity, especially fractures of long bones. **Leg vein thrombosis may occur after any period of stagnation or pressure on the legs and has been reported in long-distance air passengers called Economy Class Syndrome. About 10 to 20% of fatal pulmonary emboli occur in the absence of trauma. Other veins, such as the venous sinuses of dura mater or subclavian or axillary veins, external and internal iliac veins, prostatic plexus, uterine and ovarian veins, occasionally develop bland thrombi after traumatic injury. Arterial thrombosis and embolism is rare. Pelvic vessels are rarely involved in pregnancy and abortion. Bullet wounds and stab wounds of the carotid arteries may injure the intima and a thrombus may develop at the site of the injury followed by embolism of middle cerebral arteries.**

The thrombus usually develops in 10 to 20 days and is detached in part or whole and travels to pulmonary artery. A large embolus in the pulmonary trunk often produces a noticeable fullness before the vessel is opened. The embolus which blocks the pulmonary trunk causes death in few minutes due to vagal inhibition, acute asphyxia or right-sided heart failure, and no infarction is found in the lungs. Infarction of lung is seen when the artery to a bronchopulmonary segment or smaller vessel is blocked. Pulmonary emboli should be differentiated from postmortem clots. In all cases of pulmonary embolism, examine the legs for presence of thrombi.

Pulmonary emboli are cylindrical in shape firm, brittle with a dull, matt, striated surface from fibrin lamination, often branch and frequently curled. Older thrombus tends to be greyish-red and varies in colour from place to place. Side branches may be seen that do not correspond to the branches of the pulmonary artery in which they lie. **Postmortem emboli are dark-red, soft and jelly-like with a shining, glistening surface.** When pulled out of the vessel it forms a cast of the branches and does not pour out of the cut small vessels.

OBSTRUCTION BY EMBOLI: When a large embolus obstructs the bifurcation of the pulmonary artery or one of its main branches, an immediate acute dilatation and failure of the right side of the heart occurs (acute cor pulmonale). When smaller branches of the pulmonary arteries are obstructed, generalised vasospasm occurs and causes sudden sharp increase in blood pressure in the lesser circuit with marked dilation and over-distension of the right ventricle. Systemic shock occurs with peripheral hypotension and interferes with coronary flow. The entire complex causes immediate stoppage of vital functions.

For examination of deep leg veins incise the midline of the calf, expose and reflect the gastrocnemius muscle and then cross-section and squeeze it to see if thrombi can be expressed from the veins at this level.

UNUSUAL TYPES OF EMBOLI: Unusual types of pulmonary embolism are sometimes produced by trauma. Fragments of bone marrow may be found as emboli in smaller branches of the pulmonary artery, usually following fracture of bones containing marrow. Fragments of liver parenchyma may enter torn hepatic veins after blunt force injury to liver and may be carried as emboli. Laceration of brain accompanied by tearing of venous sinuses may lead to pulmonary embolus. Foreign bodies may enter veins or arteries and are transported as emboli, e.g., bullets and pellets.

(9) Fat Embolism: Causes: (1) Fracture of a long bone; the incidence is up to 2%, and 10% in multiple fractures, especially with pelvic injuries, (2) an injury to adipose tissue which forces liquid fat into the damaged blood vessels, (3) injecting oil into circulation, e.g., in criminal abortion, (4) occasionally due to natural disease without trauma as in sickle cell anaemia. Certain non-traumatic conditions, e.g., diabetes, following blood transfusion, fatty change in the liver as seen in chronic alcoholics, septicaemia, steroid therapy, acute pancreatitis,osteomyelitis, lipo-suction, decompression sickness (Caisson's disease), in too rapid ascent to high altitudes without a functional pressurised cabin or under simulated flight conditions in decompression chambers, (5) in cases of severe antemortem burns. In every injury involving bone or subcutaneous tissue, fat embolism occurs to some degree, especially crushing of buttocks or breasts. **Pulmonary fat embolism unless it is gross enough to cause ventilatory embarrassment by widespread plugging of capillaries has no significance.**

The presence of fat droplets in the blood stream indicates that the injury was produced during life, except in case of burning and advanced putrefaction. Charring after death may produce a picture similar to fat embolism. Large amounts of liquefied fat are derived from fat cells in the tissue in putrefied body. When cardiac massage is done, fat enters the blood vessels even if the circulation has stopped. If during resuscitation, the sternum or ribs are fractured, bone marrow embolism is seen in the lungs.

CLINICAL FEATURES: The emboli enter the pulmonary vessels and obstruct the flow of blood through the lungs. Cyanosis, precordial pain, rapid pulse and respiration, hyperpyrexia and petechial haemorrhages caused by impaction of fat droplets in small venules on any part of the body, typically seen in the conjunctivae, on the chest and axillae may develop in 8 to 20 hours. There may be fever, thrombocytopaenia, fat globules in the urine, and sputum and renal failure. Death may occur with severe dyspnoea about 30 hours after the trauma. In such cases, fat globules are probably transported to the lungs in moderate quantities at intermittent intervals until the circulation is obstructed.

Tests: A piece of lung tissue in 20% caustic potash is compressed by a coverslip and examined under the microscope as a rapid method of identification. After a few minutes, red cells disappear and fat is seen lying as plugs in the pulmonary capillaries. They appear highly refractile and show a narrow dark edge. The diagnosis is made by microscopic examination of frozen section of the lungs, stained for fat with Sudan III (orange colour), Scharlach R or osmic acid (black).

AUTOPSY: Fatal pulmonary embolism can be diagnosed after injury to a limb, when an embolus is found in the pulmonary artery or one of its branches, and when a part of a thrombus or the site of thrombus can be demonstrated in one of the veins of the limbs. Pulmonary emboli are cylindrical in shape with parallel contours, often branched, frequently curled and show no relationship in shape to the vessel in which they are found. Death usually occurs about the tenth day, but may be delayed up to three weeks. The pulmonary vessels, arterioles and capillaries are seen filled with globular fat emboli. The lungs show congestion, oedema and slight hypostatic pneumonia. The brain, heart and kidneys may show few scattered emboli. Bone marrow fat is scanty in children, due to which fat embolism is rare. **20 to 100 ml. of free fat causes embolic death.**

Cerebral fat embolism: Cerebral fat embolism develops when the fat emboli are forced through the pulmonary capillaries into the systemic circulation in sufficient quantity to affect the brain. About 14 to 18 hours after injury, clusters of petechial haemorrhages are seen in any part of the body, but especially over front of chest, shoulders, neck due to impaction of fat globules in capillaries and death occurs in one to two days. The brain, kidneys and myocardium are most vulnerable target organs. At autopsy, petechial haemorrhages are seen in the white matter of cerebral and cerebellar hemispheres and brainstem, and appear as a ring of red blood cells around a necrotic zone of brain tissue in the centre of which lies a small arteriole plugged by a fat embolus. Death from fat embolism of the brain occurs when vital centres are affected.

Brain embolism: Trauma to the head accompanied by disruption of the brain can result in small amounts of brain entering the dural venous sinuses, if the patient survives long enough and cause embolism.

(10) AIR EMBOLISM: Causes: (1) Incised wounds of the lower cervical or clavicular regions involving the jugular or subclavian veins. Penetration by bullet does not usually produce air embolism. (2) A wound of the sagittal sinus inside the skull. (3) Faulty technique in giving intravenous injection with the gravity or similar apparatus. (4) Crush injuries of chest. (5) Positive pressure ventilation in newborn infant. (6) Injection of air or fluid mixed with air or soap water into the pregnant uterus for procuring abortion. (7) Caesarean section, version or manual extraction of the placenta may introduce air into uterus. (8) Oral-genital sex in a pregnant woman. (9) Injection of air under pressure in Fallopian tube to test its patency. (10) Subclavian vein catheterisation. (11) Air encephalography. (12) Artificial pneumothorax and pneumoperitoneum. (13) Caisson's disease.

PULMONARY AIR EMBOLISM: Air entering the venous system is carried to the heart and pulmonary arteries, which causes mechanical obstruction of the pulmonary arterial vasculature. This causes churning of the blood and air producing froth. The churning can result in the development of complexes of air bubbles, fibrin, platelet aggregates, erythrocytes and fat globules thus further occluding the vasculature, which causes death. Large volume of air causes obstruction in the pulmonary vasculature and also in the right ventricle. **About 100 ml. of air introduced under pressure is necessary to produce fatal pulmonary air embolism.** Paradoxical air embolism, i.e. air crossing from the venous to the arterial circulation, usually occurs due to a septal defect or a probe patent foramen ovale.

Two factors favour pulmonary air embolism. (1) Fixation of walls of veins, e.g., in the clavicular and pelvic regions, the upper dorsal spine and the dural membranes. When these veins are cut, they do not collapse and haemorrhage occurs, followed by negative pressure in the vessel. (2) The suction effect of the respiratory movements and heart's action on such veins as the jugular, subclavian and vertebral has a tendency to create a negative pressure in the vessels during the phase of inspiration. **Pulmonary air embolism is rarely seen following injury to peripheral veins. Air injected into a limb artery is not harmful, as most of the gas is absorbed rapidly.** If there has been a considerable delay between death and autopsy, the air can dissipate, presumably dissolving into the tissues.

Systemic air embolism: It occurs when air in sufficient quantity enters a vein of the pulmonary system and is carried through the left side of the heart to block arterioles and capillaries in different parts of the body, especially in the brain and the heart. Platelets are also consumed, adhering to fibrin thrombi. Fibrinolysis is activated. Air entering carotid artery passes into cerebral circulation. **Penetrating wounds of the chest are the common cause,** e.g., puncture wound in a lung which does not collapse may penetrate a vein and a bronchiole and allow air to enter the vein. **Crushing injuries of the chest and major or minor surgical procedures upon the thorax also produce air embolism. Arterial air embolism may occur in dysbarism.** Surgical emphysema may occur in upper thorax and neck region due to leakage of gas from lung damage or pneumothorax or both. **1 to 2 ml. of air may be enough to produce death, because the air travels directly from lungs to the left side of the heart, from which it can be forced into the coronary or the cerebral arteries.** Air bubbles in the cerebral veins can be due to artefact produced by removing the skull. **Death from air embolism commonly occurs within a few minutes and usually not delayed beyond 45 minutes.**

Oxygen in the heart indicates air embolism, because it is not present in appreciable quantity if the gases were those of decomposition. Frothy blood resembling air embolism can be found especially in the right ventricle (1) due to handling the heart before it is opened at autopsy, (2) putrefaction, (3) postmortem event, and (4) artificial respiration in the dying or recently dead. The source from which air was derived should be established, e.g., if source is regarded as pregnant uterus, air bubbles should be found in the veins draining the large pelvic veins and the inferior vena cava.

DIAGNOSIS OF AIR EMBOLSM: For the diagnosis of systemic air embolism, the internal carotid and the basilar arteries are ligated before the brain is removed. The skull vault should be removed, without puncturing the meninges. Examine the meningeal vessels for visible air bubbles. In acute cases, gas bubbles will be visible within the cerebral arteries, but not in the cortical veins. The presence of bubbles in the pial veins is an artefact. Then submerge the brain in water, release the ligatures, cut the vessels and slightly compress them and watch for air bubbles. An airtight, water-filled glass syringe with a needle can be used to collect gas from blood vessels, heart or cavities. **In artificial respiration in a dying person right ventricle may contain frothy blood.**

X-ray examination of the whole body may detect large quantities of air. Air bubbles in the retinal arteries can be demonstrated with an ophthalmoscope. The gas is collected from the heart and brought into contact with an alkaline pyrogallol solution, which turns brown in the presence of free oxygen and indicates antemortem air embolism.

AUTOPSY: The head should be dissected first, to look for air in cerebral arteries. The sternoclavicular joint should not be opened in cases of air embolism, as pulling back the sternum may suck air into the veins. The lower part of the sternum is cut at the manubrium. Clamping of ascending aorta and vena cavae prevent the escape of air into these vessels. The chest cavity is filled with water. The coronary arteries are incised and massaged and the escape of gas bubbles is observed. The epicardial veins usually have a beaded appearance, with numerous air bubbles along the length. Air in the coronary arteries indicate systemic embolism. **In air embolism, right ventricle is distended with air under pressure and bright-red frothy blood is found in the right side of the heart, vena cavae, pulmonary arteries and coronary veins.** The blood is fluid throughout the body, the viscera are congested, and petechiae are present in the serous surfaces and in the white matter of the brain. Make a small incision on the pulmonary artery and each chamber of the heart and look for the air bubbles rising to the surface of the water. The pericardial sac should be filled with water. A 50 ml syringe is filled with water and a large-bore needle attached. The right ventricle should be punctured. If air is present it will be seen to bubble up through the water in the syringe. Aspirometer will measure the amount of air which can be analysed by gas chromatography. In embolised air CO_2 is less than 15%, nitrogen is higher than 70% and oxygen is reduced to 8 to 15% place air from heart into a bottle containing 2% alkaline pyrogallol solution. Oxygen containing air stains the solution brown. Gases of decomposition have no effect.

(11) ADULT RESPIRATORY DISTRESS SYNDROME (ARDS): It occurs due to heavy impacts on the thorax, blast injuries to the chest, pulmonary infections, toxins, systemic shock, irritant gases, aspiration of gastric contents, near drowning, etc., in which there may be "diffuse alveolar damage". The victim may suffer from severe dyspnoea and progressive respiratory failure due to poor exchange of gases. The lungs are dark-red, congested, become stiff and oedematous, and retain their shape after removal, and may be double in weight. Histologically, intraalveolar exudates, hyaline membrane, alveolar and interstitial oedema, and patchy alveolar haemorrhages are seen in the lungs. Later, cellular proliferation is seen and in 50% of persons who survive, lungs become fibrotic.

RESPIRATORY LUNG: It is similar to ARDS. It is seen within a few days, but usually after many days or weeks in a patient who dies after being on mechanical ventilation. The lungs are stiff, rigid, heavy, but not obviously oedematous. Areas of collapse and haemorrhage with formation of hyaline membrane is seen. Microscopically, proteinaceous fluid and a mixture of proliferative cells may be seen in the alveoli.

(12) DISSEMINATED INTRAVASCULAR COAGULATION (DIC): It occurs due to trauma, infection, shock, burns, sepsis, malignancy, severe non-specific stress, etc. and other acute events. It is a consumption coagulopathy associated with blood clotting mechanism. There is an abnormal activation of the coagulation process within the blood vessels. Damaged tissue from trauma and burns can trigger thromboplastin-initiated coagulation; entry of tissue cell elements, especially from red cells, brain and placenta are particularly potent. Particulate matter, such as bacteria, micro-emboli of all types including fat and air emboli, can precipitate coagulation via factor XII. Vascular endothelial damage and stasis of blood flow have similar effect.

Fibrin is consumed and precipitated in vessels causing both vascular obstructive effects and a haemorrhagic diathesis from depletion of the coagulative system. There can be postmortem fibrinolysis, and as such it may be difficult to demonstrate fibrin histologically. Lungs, liver, kidney and adrenals should be examined for fibrin. The complications are microvascular obstruction leading to infarction and bleeding in skin and internal organs.

AUTOPSY: DIC is confirmed at autopsy by the unusual amount and distribution of bleeding in the body and by the finding of fibrin clots and the signs of ischaemia, of infarction of many organs on microscopy.

(13) SUPRARENAL HAEMORRHAGE: Suprarenal haemorrhage is rarely a terminal event, usually after some trauma to the body not related to direct injury to the suprarenal vessels, but appears to be neurologically mediated via the sympathetic nervous system. The sudden collapse and rapid death usually occurs a few days after the trauma varying from 2 to 21 days. At autopsy one or both adrenals are swollen (3 to 5 cm) due to bleeding in the medulla, the cortex being tightly stretched. The causes are: (1) Trauma of all types. (2) Breech births or foetal anoxia. (3) Meningococcal septicaemia (Waterhouse Friedrichsen Syndrome) and disseminated intravascular coagulation. (4) Infective and postoperative septicaemia (often Gram-negative). (5) Haemorrhage into a secondary deposit. (6) Thrombosis of central vein with adrenal infarction. (7) Hypertension and chronic renal failure.

MEDICOLEGAL QUESTIONS ON TRAUMA

(1) Can postmortem injuries be distinguished from antemortem injuries?

Severe bleeding from a wound indicates that it is antemortem. Injuries which usually result in active bleeding may produce little or no bleeding if they were sustained during severe shock resulting in hypotension and peripheral vascular collapse. **Injuries caused soon after death which lacerate vessels distended with fluid blood can cause haemorrhagic infiltration of tissues. Injuries inflicted shortly before death cannot be distinguished from those inflicted shortly after death.** Wounds produced shortly before death are not always associated with thrombosis or fibrin deposition. Absence of swelling does not exclude antemortem injury. White blood cells are capable of movement for few hours after cardiac arrest. This makes a "vital reaction" to injury of doubtful reliability. **The physical components of vital reaction are: swelling, effusion of lymph, leucocytic infiltration, pus formation or evidence of repair** Table (10–2).

HISTOPATHOLOGY: In injury after somatic death, margination and a limited emigration of leucocytes may occur. Marked cellular exudation and reactive changes in the tissue cells are seen in antemortem wounds only. However, the absence of tissue reaction does not necessarily indicate postmortem origin of wounds due to (1) if the victim dies soon after infliction of injury, (2) in small wounds the degree of cellular injury may not be sufficient to cause emigration of leucocytes, or there may be resolution of the reaction, (3) the circulatory failure occurring in severe injuries may interfere with normal reaction.

The intensity of the local reaction to an injury depends upon: (1) the severity of the injury, (2) the vascularity of the injured tissue, and (3) the presence or absence of infection or foreign bodies due to which the age of an antemortem wound cannot be determined within narrow limits.

HISTOCHEMICAL CHANGES IN INJURED TISSUES: The histochemical demonstration of an enzyme depends upon its action on the substance upon which the enzyme acts. The reaction product resulting from enzyme activity forms an insoluble deposit at the site of enzyme action. If this deposit is not coloured, it is made visible by use of suitable chemicals. The intensity of final dye indicates the relative intensity of the enzyme activity. In trauma to the living tissue, two zones are seen around the wound: (1) close to the edge of the wound, there is a zone 0.2 to 0.5 mm. wide, which becomes necrotic with decreased enzyme activity (negative vital reaction). (2) Immediately beyond this layer, there is a 0.1 to 0.3 mm. zone of reaction, where a number of enzymes become increased in concentration during the reparative process (positive vital reaction), compared to the normal level in the areas outside the wound. In postmortem wounds, positive vital reaction zone does not develop. In the positive zone esterases and adenosine triphosphatase increase within an hour after injury. At around two hours, aminopeptidase, at four hours, acid phosphatase, and at five hours, alkaline phosphatase activity increases. These changes can be demonstrated for a few days after death, if autolysis is prevented by refrigeration. The wound sample is excised with a rim about 1–2 cm, surrounding the wound. It is divided into 2 parts. One specimen is fixed in 10% formalin, automatically processed and cut in the form of 5 to 6 micron paraffin sections and stained by HandE for histological study. The other specimen is freshly frozen on a block of solid carbon dioxide for enzyme histochemical study. The freezing is completed by setting another block of dry ice on the tissue specimen.

BIOCHEMICAL TIMING OF WOUNDS: Tissue cathepsins increase almost immediately if the stroma is damaged, and can be demonstrated within 5 to 10 minutes. Serotonin appears in maximum concentration in about 10 minutes and histamine in 20 to 30 minutes after wounding. To establish the antemortem nature of the wound, the level of histamine should be at least 50% greater and that of serotonin, at least twice the concentration of the control skin. Serotonin and histamine contents are measured spectroflurometrically. Postmortem wounds do not show these reactions Fig. (10–5).

Enzyme reactions in a wound are specific indicators of its vital origin. They take place quicker than any other reliable change yet known. The reactions in wounds inflicted on different parts of the body are similar. The presence or absence of reactions is not affected by any period of delay between death and examination. The reactions are not affected by therapeutic measures, such as the application of antiseptic agents Fig. (10–5).

Senility, severe illness and cachexia and widespread multiple injuries may distort the usual pattern by reducing the ability to produce these reparative enzymes. In contused wounds the reactions are less useful as the damage is more diffuse and there are no definite zones. For the tests about 2 gm of skin freed from subcutaneous fat are required.

(2) Can the time of infliction of the wound be determined?

WOUND HEALING: The changes vary according to the size of a wound, the type of wound, the tissue, and the age and health of the victim.

Table (10–2). Difference between antemortem and postmortem wounds

Trait		Antemortem wounds	Postmortem wounds
(1)	Edges:	The edges are swollen, everted, retracted, and wound gapes.	Edges do not gape, but are closely approximated.
(2)	Haemorrhage:	Abundant and usually arterial.	Slight or more and venous.
(3)	Spurting:	Signs of spurting of arterial blood on the body, clothing or in its vicinity present.	No spurting of blood.
(4)	Extravasation:	Staining of the edges of the wound and extravasation in neighbouring subcutaneous and interstitial tissues which cannot be removed by washing.	Edges and cellular tissues are not deeply stained. The stain can be removed by washing.
(5)	Coagulation:	Firmly coagulated blood in wounds and tissues present.	No clotting or soft, friable clot.
(6)	Vital reaction:	Signs of vital reaction present, i.e., inflammation and repair.	No signs of vital reaction.
(7)	Enzyme histochemistry:	Increased activity of esterases, adenosine triphosphate, aminopeptidase, acid and alkaline phosphatase.	Diminished or no enzyme activity.

Only an approximate time can be determined. Healing by first intention means union in a clean incised wound with good apposition of the edges. In healing by secondary intention, granulation tissue is formed.

Enzyme histochemistry contributes to the timing of wounds inflicted 1 to 8 hours before death. The biochemical methods are most useful for the timing of wounds, inflicted during the last hour before death.

HISTOPATHOLOGY: Vasoconstriction begins within few seconds. Dilatation of capillaries occurs within few minutes, accompanied by increased permeability to plasma protein. Fibrin appears in the wound within a few minutes, but can also appear in postmortem injuries. Migration of polymorphs may be seen in dilated small vessels in half to 4 hours but is not a reliable sign of antemortem injury. Basophilic mast cells lose their granules within 4 hours. In 4 to 12 hours, leucocytic infiltration is marked. At about 4 hours some extravascular emigration may begin. After 12 hours, a scanty mixture of lymphocytes and monocytes appear. Tissue oedema and swelling of vascular endothelium occurs. In 12 to 24 hours, leucocytes form a marginal palisade. Macrophages and mononuclear cells increase. Removal of necrosed tissue begins. In about 15 hours, mitoses are seen in fibroblasts. Epidermis begins to spread across and down the surface of the scab and down the sides of a cut into the wound. At about 48 hours, leucocytic infiltration is at its peak. Repair begins with many fibroblasts appearing, and elastic fibres are scarce. In about 72 hours, new capillaries begin to bud from vessels, and granulation tissue forms. In 3 to 6 days, collagen begins to form, and giant cells appear around necrotic debris. Haemosiderin appears from the third day. In 3 to 6 days, epithelium grows actively on the surface. In 10 to 14 days, vascularity decreases, and cellular reaction subsides. Fibroblasts are very active, and collagen is laid. Epidermis becomes thin and flat. Elastic fibres are less compared to adjacent undamaged tissue. Regression of cellular activity occurs by 12 days in both epidermal and dermal tissue. After two weeks, collagen and elastin increase, and vascular scar is formed, which gradually becomes more dense and avascular. Contraction starts about 5 to 7 days after wounding and stops at 6 weeks. Histochemical wound changes are shown in Fig. (10–5).

(3) Can a lethal degree of internal trauma be present without any external indication of trauma? Yes. A wedging type of blow to the lower chest and upper abdomen may tear the aorta, as in traffic accidents. The weight of the individual who applies his knee to the upper abdomen of another may cause a rupture of the liver and death. Manual strangulation and smothering may not leave external signs of trauma. Fractures of ribs, vertebrae or pelvis with accompanying lethal visceral injuries can occur without external indications of serious violence.

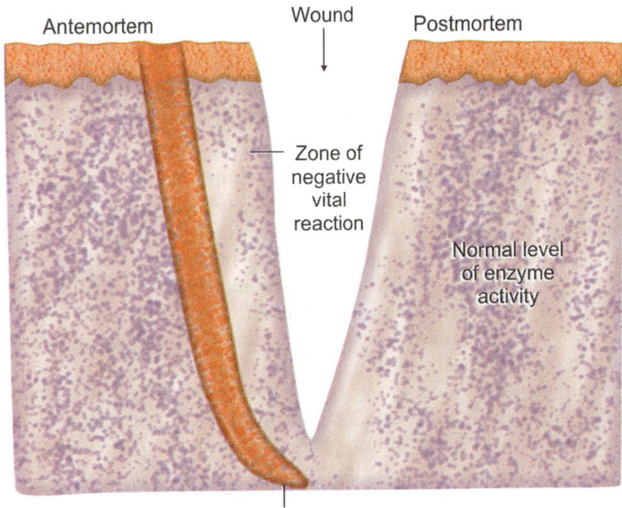

Fig. (10-5). Histochemical wound changes.

(4) Can resuscitative efforts produce injuries which cannot be differentiated from the injuries already present?

Yes. In perimortem injuries (that occur during the act of dying), haemorrhage may be seen involving the soft tissues. Contusion-abrasion of chest wall, fractures of ribs, fractures of the sternum, contusions of the heart, contusions and lacerations of the liver and spleen, rupture of the heart and duodenum usually occur during resuscitation.

(5) Can there be much delay in death following the infliction of trauma?

Yes. The victim may die after a varying period from remote causes. The rupture of liver, spleen, aorta and other organs may be delayed by hours, days and sometimes weeks after the organ was weakened by the traumatic lesion.

(6) Which of the several injuries caused death?

The actual cause of death must be found out, and **when there is more than one wound, it may be necessary to determine which one of them caused death, since the wounds may not have been made by the same assailant, nor at the same time.** This may be done by examining the wounds individually and noting which of them involved injury to some vital organ or large blood vessel, or led to secondary results causing death.

(7) Would the victim have survived had he been given more prompt medical assistance?

A very guarded reply should be given, depending on the nature and extent of injuries, because there is much individual variation.

(8) Can the wounds be altered from their original appearance?

The wounds may be altered in many ways. In the living, the wound may be altered by healing and treatment. In the dead person, the wound might have been altered by resuscitative measures applied and by insects, animals and decomposition.

(9) Are there situations where more than one type of weapon was employed with any frequency?

Such situations are not rare. In gang feuds, the victim may be suddenly attacked by a number of persons with different types of weapons. The victim may be waylaid and a number of different types of injuries inflicted. Sometimes, a suicide uses different types of weapons, as some methods fail to produce death.

Death need not occur very soon after the assault, if it can be established that assault could have precipitated an infarct in a myocardim already compromised by coronary stenosis. The blow may never actually be struck or it may fail to hit the body, yet the threatened person may suffer a transient hypertension or tachycardia that may precipitate a subintimal haemorrhage that leads to death.

(10) How long did the victim live, and could he have carried out voluntary acts after receiving a fatal injury?

In cases where the injuries are presumed to have caused rapid death, a medical witness may be asked to state whether a person is capable of speaking, walking or performing any other voluntary act, which would involve bodily and mental power for some time after receiving the injury. The length of time the deceased could have lived after infliction of injury will depend upon multiple factors, including blood vessels and tissues injured, age and health of the person, the degree of associated shock and the rate of bleeding. A very guarded reply should be given, because individuals vary in their reaction to injuries. Victims of severe frontal lobe wounds may have prolonged survival periods. If the brain stem is destroyed by a penetrating injury or in wounds of basal ganglia, or aortic arch is completely transected, immediate incapacity occurs. Most other injuries do not cause sudden death or rapid loss of function. In severe injuries of the brain, sometimes a person survives, although the damage done might have been expected to have caused instant death. A person may remain conscious for several minutes before dying from a severe intracranial injury. Sometimes, a person may die from a blow which produces no obvious naked-eye changes in the brain. A single stab wound of the skull and brain are not immediately fatal, and the victim may walk or run. Stab wounds of the heart are dangerous, but often rapidly disabling or fatal. Immediate death is likely when the auricles are extensively torn or punctured, but in less severe wounds, powers of voluntary acts and walking are retained for some time. In slanting ventricular perforation, at first there may not be bleeding but later there may be mild oozing which may cause death. Perforations of the right ventricle bleed more rapidly than those of the left, as it is relatively thin-walled. The victim may be able to run 100 to 200 metres before collapsing. Small perforations of the left ventricle may seal themselves with minimal blood loss. With an extremely lacerated heart or severed large artery an individual can retain consciousness at least for 10 to 15 seconds. If a major coronary artery is completely cut, prolonged survival is not possible. In the adrenal response of "fight or flight," the shock element of pain is greatly suppressed. Thus, in an assault only the sheer physical and haemodynamic sequelae of the injury will lead to a slowing down, then collapse and death. In the interval, the injured victim may be able to perform normal physical activity. In fatal electrocution in which the heart stops functioning, the person can walk and talk for 20 to 30 seconds before dropping dead. Muscular powers are retained in ruptures of liver, spleen or kidneys, unless there is marked immediate blood loss. When the windpipe is divided, the voice is usually lost. Stab wounds of back of neck are not immediately incapacitating unless they sever the spinal cord or medulla oblongata and the victim may be capable of movement for some time. It is not possible to say from an examination of wounds in a dead body, as to how long the person might have lived, or how much voluntary activity he might have performed before death, after infliction of the injury. It is safer to say what is ordinarily expected.

CASE: (1) Glaister reported a case in which the man shot himself with a 0.45 caliber pistol beneath the chin. The bullet entered the cranium and pulped the frontal and temporal lobes of the brain and exited through a 4 cm. defect in the skull. Following this injury the man walked from a garden shelter (where the shooting had occurred and where later pieces of skull and brain were found on the ceiling), walked around in the garden for at least 165 metres, returned to the shelter for some time, then walked home to his house, where he arrived at least one hour after the shooting. He spoke in normal fashion to the maid who admitted him, hung up his overcoat and umbrella, and walked upstairs to his room. Death did not take place until at least 4 hours after the shooting.

(2) A 28-year-old man was shot at from a range of 3 metres in the anterior chest with a 12 bore sawed-off shotgun. He ran about 16 metres before he collapsed and died. At autopsy anterior wall of right ventricle showed a ragged 3 cm. opening. Multiple pellet perforations were present in the right lung. The right pleural cavity contained 2500 ml of blood and pericardial sac 400 ml of blood. Wad was found in both main pulmonary arteries at the lung hila, carried to these sites as emboli from the right ventricle.

(3) A 37-year-old man was stabbed in the chest with a butcher's knife. Following the injury, he got into his car and drove four city blocks; lost control of the vehicle and crashed into a parked car. He proceeded to the hospital and died in the emergency room about 20 minutes after the injury. At autopsy there was a 6 mm slit-like cut in the right ventricle of the heart, and 1400 ml. of blood in the left pleural cavity and in the pericardial sac.

(4) A 23-year-old man who was stabbed with a kitchen knife, walked and staggered a distance of 110 metres and died at the hospital a few minutes after arrival there. At autopsy, there was a 6 mm. cut in the left ventricle of the heart and the aorta and 1900 ml. internal bleeding.

(11) Can the degree of trauma be quantitated?

There is much individual variation in the reaction to trauma. At best the amount of degree of injury can only be roughly estimated as mild, moderate, severe, or extreme.

(12) What is the relationship of trauma and natural disease?

TRAUMA AND MALIGNANCY: There is strong evidence that trauma does not induce neoplasia, and that the co-existence of the two processes is purely co-incidental. Often, trauma merely calls attention to a pre-existing tumour that had not previously been noted. Since trauma disrupts tissue, it might activate a pre-existing tumour to grow and spread more rapidly. In rare cases there is apparent relationship, between tumour and some preceding trauma to the part. Often, trauma merely calls attention to a pre-existing tumour that had not previously been noted. Repeated minor trauma is called chronic irritation. With repeated minor trauma and disruption of tissue, the cellular proliferations of regeneration and repair become continual. In few cases, cancer develops after many years, e.g., cancer of the skin adjacent to a chronic osteomyelitic sinus that has drained for a number of years. Skin cancers developing in burn scars have been well recognised. Since trauma disrupts tissue, it might activate a pre-existing tumour to grow and spread more rapidly.

EWING'S POSTULATES should be satisfied before accepting a relationship between trauma and new growth. They are: (1) There must be evidence of previous integrity of the injured part. (2) Undeniable and adequate trauma must be proved. (3) There must be proof of reasonable time interval between injury and appearance of tumour. (4) The disease must develop at exact site of the injury. (5) The nature of the tumour must be proved.

The role of direct trauma in rupturing an aneurysm is not certain. A large, fragile aneurysm on the circle of Willis might be damaged by a substantial head injury.

TRAUMA AND MYOCARDIAL INFARCTION: A blow or some physical trauma may precipitate a myocardial infarct or arrhythmia. The emotional upset that accompanies injury, or even the threat of fear of an injury, can cause death due to transient hypertension or tachycardia that may precipitate a subintimal haemorrhage, arrhythmias, or cerebral or subarachnoid haemorrhage. Physical effort which can damage a diseased heart in some cases can be traced to unusual job or to the performance of unfamiliar or unaccustomed work, to accidents or other trauma, and to the extra physical demands while working with a defective equipment.

Acute coronary occlusion may be due to a dissecting aneurysm of an atheromatous coronary artery and follow direct trauma. Direct injury to the coronary artery causing death is unusual. Traumatic coronary thrombosis rarely occurs when the walls of the artery are injured.

Sudden release of epinephrine following extreme terror in a person with a normal heart can cause ventricular tachycardia, which can progress to ventricular fibrillation and death, severe injury and the associated anxiety, pain, anger, fear, apprehension associated with it may impose on extra load in person with organic heart disease, may precipitate a cardiac infarction or sudden collapse and death during exertion.

A heart attack my occur while at work, either incidentally by normal progression of a chronic disease process or due to unusual physical or mental strain. The risk is greater in those who were otherwise sedentary and that long-term moderate exercise is associated with a reduced risk. Some cardiologists feel that a heart attack never occurs after physical effort, while others believe it can occur. If the attack occurs within seconds or minutes after unusual effort, the causal connection can be established with certainty only in direct trauma to the heart occurring during work. Attacks occurring few days later may be due to haemorrhage in an atherosclerotic plaque in the coronary artery which initially narrows the lumen, but later causes occlusion.

Acute bacterial endocarditis may occur following an injury. The vegetations can be detached forming septic thromboemboli and can lodge in the brain, kidneys, etc. causing septic infarcts, increased intravascular pressure due to strenuous physical effort may cause a vessel to rupture, e.g., Aortic aneurysm, varicose veins.

Mechanical forces responsible for heart injury are: (1) Penetrating foreign objects, e.g., missiles and stab wounds. (2) Migrating foreign objects, e.g., needles, bullets, metal fragments, etc. (3) Non-penetrating mechanical forces transmitted to the heart, e.g., (a) Compression forces from direct blows to chest, from crushing chest injuries or transmitted from injury to the abdomen or legs. (b) Contusive forces and jarring forces from direct blow to the chest or transmitted from decelerative accidents. (c) Bursting forces from increase of intracardiac blood pressure due to direct compression of heart from chest injuries or transmitted from compression of the abdomen, and (d) Tearing, disruptive forces transmitted from decelerative accidents. (4) Intracardiac-introduced instruments, e.g., cardiac catheterisation and implantation of pacemakers.

TRAUMA AND CORONARY THROMBOSIS: Evidence of injury to the chest wall, such as contusion of the chest wall, fracture of the sternual or of sternal ends of left third and fourth ribs and mechanical injury to heart especially in the region or directly to the thrombosed vessel will establish traumatic origin of coronary thrombus.

TRAUMA AND SUBARACHNOID HAEMORRHAGE: An assault is rapidly followed by the signs of subarachnoid bleeding and subsequent death. A heavy blow to the head, jaw or neck can rupture, split or weaken the fragile wall of a large, thin-walled aneurysm. In fights, the victim is physically and emotionally active, so that adrenal response is likely to be present. Muscle tone, heart rate and blood pressure are increased by catecholamines, and it is likely that raised internal blood pressure in a weak aneurysm is a far more potent reason for rupture than a blow on the head. Another possibility is that a person with an already spontaneously leaking aneurysm may have a rapidly developing neurological or even behavioural abnormality that causes a fight, or into a dangerous physical position, such as a fall or a traffic accident. Rupture can occur in young to middle aged persons during innocent activities, such as jogging, intercourse, and sporting exertion, probably because of a transient rise in blood pressure and pulse rate.

TRAUMA AND NERVOUS SYSTEM: It is difficult to refute completely the direct cause and effect relationship between: (1) Head injury and meningitis. (2) Head injury and epilepsy. (3) Head injury and psychosis. (4) Head injury including occupational stress and rupture of a congenital cerebral aneurysm.

The following conditions should be satisfied before accepting a relationship between injury and post-traumatic psychosis. (1) Prior to injury the patient had been a mentally well adjusted person. (2) The injury had produced organic damage to the central nervous system. (3) The injury was severe enough so as to threaten the life. (4) The nature of injury was such as to affect the structure or function of certain parts of the body to which emotional importance is attached, e.g., genitals, eyes, face, hands, breasts. (5) The victim was obsessed about the outcome from the time of injury. (6) The psychosis developed within a reasonable time after the injury was sustained. (7) The psychotic thoughts had a positive relationship to the assault or accident that was responsible for injury.

Traumatic Neurosis: It is a specific disease entity characterised by increased irritability or startle reaction, repetitive dreams of again being in the situation where the trauma occurred, a phobic fear of returning to the accident scene, marked anxiety and withdrawal from previously enjoyed or tolerated social and sexual activity. Pure form is rarely seen, but psychiatric sequelae, such as conversion hysteria, anxiety, and phobic or other neuroses or psychotic depression, or schizophrenia can occur.

As a general rule, settlement tends to cure compensation neurosis, whereas in anxiety neurosis, indemnification has no effect on the mental disturbance.

Trauma and alimentary system: A blow to the epigastric region may cause death by cardiac inhibition. Trauma may cause perforation of peptic ulcer and death. Fatty or diseased liver may rupture due to trauma. A kick or punch on upper abdomen may injure duodenum or pancreas and cause death.

CHAPTER

11

THERMAL DEATHS

FM 2.24: Thermal deaths: Describe the clinical features, postmortem finding and medicolegal aspects of injuries due to physical agents like heat [heat-hyper-pyrexia, heat stroke, sun stroke, heat exhaustion/prostration, heat cramps (Miner's cramp) or cold (systemic and localized hypothermia, frostbite, trench foot, immersion foot)].

FM 2.25: Describe types of injuries, clinical features, pathophysiology, postmortem findings and medicolegal aspects in cases of burns, scalds, lightening, electrocution and radiations.

Thermal deaths are those which **result from the effects of systemic and/or localised exposure to excessive heat and cold.**

COLD

Exposure to cold produces hypothermia which is defined as an oral or axillary temperature of less than 35°C. The body can tolerate dry cold much better than wet cold (immersion). Wetness increases heat loss considerably. The direct effects of cold are prominent in fatty tissue and myelinated nerve fibres. Indirect effects are mostly ischaemic, due to vascular damage. **The ability of the hypothalamus to regulate temperature is completely lost below 30°C.** Fat persons and women tolerate cold better, than lean persons and men.

LOCAL EFFECTS: (1) The cold produces first a blanching and paleness of the skin, due to vascular spasm. (2) It is followed by erythema, oedema and swelling due to the later vascular dilatation and paralysis and increased capillary permeability. (3) Blister formation is the third more advanced stage which can involve skin, subcutaneous tissues, muscles and nerves. Either the tissues become frozen stiff, hard and necrotic by direct effect of cold, or the necrosis follows vascular occlusion, thrombosis, obliterating endarteritis, secondary inflammation and infection of the damaged tissue.

The localised effects of cold are (1) Trench foot and immersion foot. Trench foot and immersion foot are the result of prolonged exposure to severe cold (5 to 8°C) and dampness, such as typically seen in soldiers during winter warfare, especially in trenches and in persons exposed to prolonged immersion or exposure at sea. The extremities are affected in those conditions. Blister formation with ulceration and localised dry gangrene occurs. (2) Frostbite is infarction of the peripheral digits with oedema, redness and later necrosis of the tissue beyond a line of inflammatory demarcation Figs. (11–1 to 11–3). It may affect only the skin or may extend deeply. It occurs due to exposure to greater extremes of cold (–2.5°C), develops more rapidly and in addition to the extremities, it frequently affects other parts, e.g., nose, ears and the face. In frostbite, necrosis with blister formation and gangrene occurs. Skin becomes hard and black in about two weeks.

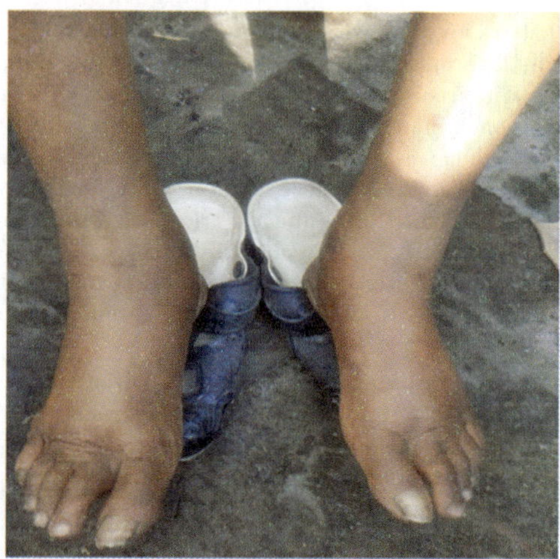

Fig. (11–1). Frostbite of first and second degree with bluish, swollen feet on both sides up to ankle areas in exposed area in a winter season.

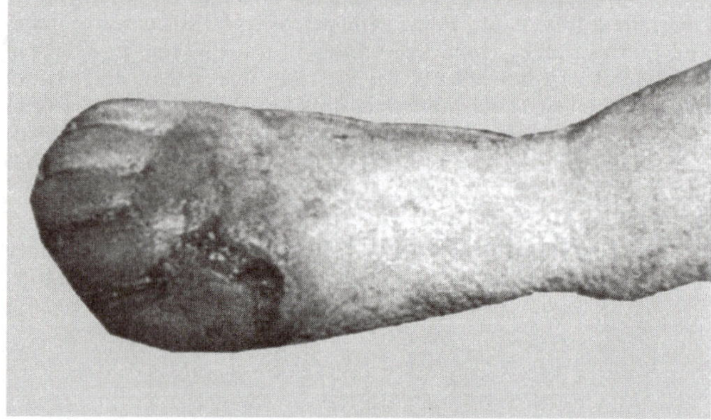

Fig. (11–2). Frostbite foot.

GENERAL EFFECTS: Ill-effects are manifested in three stages which merge imperceptibly, leading to death. In the first stage, the patient feels cold and shivers and the body temperature falls. In the second stage, shivering stops when the temperature is at or below 32°C. The victim is depressed, and with further cooling he becomes lethargic, drowsy and sleepy, which gradually passes into stupor and coma. The muscles stiffen and mobility is impaired. If he tries to walk, he may feel as if drunk. Respiration, circulation, metabolic and enzymatous processes and oxygenation of all cells are slowed down or blocked. In the third stage, the temperature is lowered to 27°C or even less, which if maintained for 24 hours or longer is fatal. Death results from the ultimate failure of the vital centres due to anoxia.

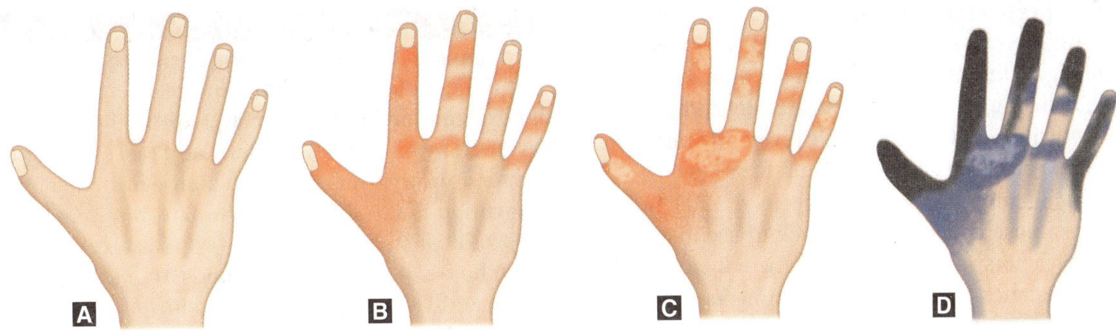

Fig. (11–3). **Frostbite stages: (A) Normal skin. (B) Frostnip: No permanent damage or change in temperature occurs. Skin shows a colour change along with a numb/irritant feeling. (C) Superficial frostbite: Skin feels warm and appears swollen and blistered. This is due to the osmotic forces resulting from formation of ice crystals inside the tissue. (D) Deep frostbite: Tissue starts turning blue-black and there is loss of function.**

POSTMORTEM APPEARANCES: EXTERNAL: **Pink or brown-pink areas with indistinct blurred margins, particularly over and around joints such as knees, elbows and hips is characteristic. There may be pink patches on cheeks, chin and nose. The extremities may be cyanosed. Oedema may be seen in the feet and lower legs. PM lividity is bright pink.**

INTERNAL: **The appearances are not characteristic. The subcutaneous tissues are relatively avascular. Ice crystals can be found in blood vessels, heart and interstitial tissue spaces. The blood is often of a bright red colour due to the retention of oxygen by haemoglobin at low temperatures. The stomach mucosa is studded with numerous brown-black acute erosions, ulcerations and haemorrhages similar to those seen in many types of pre-death stress. A variable degree of fat necrosis of the pancreas is seen in about 50% cases. Areas of stiff, yellow fat necrosis are seen in pancreas and adjacent areas of omentum and mesentery. Pulmonary oedema and micro-infarcts in many organs are common. Perivascular haemorrhages in the brain and small infarcts in the heart is seen. Internal organs are congested.**

Medicolegal Importance: Most deaths are the result of accidents, especially in drunkenness, mountaineering or persons lost in snow-drifts and those who have been immersed in ice cold waters. Infanticide and homicide in adults, where unconscious persons are left in freezing temperature are rare.

RECIPROCAL OR PARADOXICAL UNDRESSING: **This is a strange condition seen in accidental hypothermia, particularly in old persons. The cause of the condition is not known.** It may be due to long exposure to severe cold producing paralysis of the thermal regulatory mechanism. This results in **failure of vasoconstriction of arterioles of the skin which results in a flow of blood from the core of the body, thus giving an exaggerated sensation of warmth. Terminal hallucinations occur. Because of the great discomfort, the person may take off some or all of their clothing.** The person is found dead in extremely cold environment. In such case, there may be suspicion of sexual offence. Death may occur if the body temperature falls.

THE HIDE-AND-DIE SYNDROME (Terminal burrowing behaviour): In very rare cases of hypothermic death, the disoriented, dying, hypothermia victim, who while attempting to protect himself from the cold, may hide himself in corners, in cupboard or under piles of furniture or household goods. More commonly a naked or partly clothed old person is found amid a scene of utter confusion with furniture pulled over and drawers and cupboards emptied out, but the disturbance is at a low level and the tops of tables, etc. are not disturbed. This may lead to suspicion of homicide and robbery. Outdoors, he may attempt to burrow into snow, bush, or other constituent of environment. The signs of hypothermia are usually found. The problem arises as to whether the victim became hypothermic first which lead to mental confusion causing strange behaviour, or whether due to some mental aberration, the person began behaving abnormally. Terminal mental confusion, delirium and hallucinations occur.

NEONATAL COLD INJURY: **It results from a failure of the metabolism to prevent a fall in temperature in a body kept in an unsuitable cold environment. The symptoms appear usually in the first week of life. The rectal temperature is usually below 32°C. The children become increasingly lethargic and drowsy and refuse food. The outstanding feature is swelling of the extremities, with pitting oedema, particularly the hands and the feet, and the eyelids. Localised hardening of the skin and subcutaneous tissue overlying oedematous parts, starts in the distal part of the legs and spreads to involve the trunk. The face, hands and feet are red, which is a striking and constant finding. The heart rate is slow. Pulsation of peripheral arteries is absent. Respirations are shallow, slow and may be irregular. Infants lie still, though conscious. The skin is cold. The haemorrhagic tendency is manifested by gastrointestinal bleeding, petechial haemorrhages and oozing of blood from scratches and injection sites.**

DIAGNOSIS: **Massive pulmonary haemorrhage without evidence of infection, frothy blood-stained secretion in the nose or mouth, mild ascites and oedema and cyanosis of the extremities is suggestive. It may be mistaken for sclerema or haemorrhagic pneumonia.**

MEDICOLEGAL IMPORTANCE: **It is a method of killing illegitimate and unwanted infants.**

HEAT

Three clinical conditions may result from exposure to high environmental temperature: (1) heat cramps, (2) heat hyperpyrexia, and (3) heat prostration.

(1) HEAT CRAMPS **(miner's cramps, stoker's cramps or fireman's cramps): They are caused by a rapid dehydration of body through the loss of water and salt in the sweat. It is seen in workers in high temperature, when sweating has been profuse. The onset is usually sudden. Severe and painful paroxysmal cramps affecting the muscles of the arms, legs and abdomen occur. The face is flushed, the pupils dilated and the patient complains of dizziness, tinnitus, headache and vomiting. Intravenous injection of saline gives rapid relief.**

(2) HEAT PROSTRATION **(heat exhaustion, heat syncope, or heat collapse): Heat prostration is a condition of collapse without increase in body temperature, which follows exposure to excessive heat. It is precipitated by muscular work and unsuitable clothing. There is extreme exhaustion and peripheral vascular collapse. The patient feels suddenly weak, giddy and sick. He may stagger or fall. The face is pale, the skin cold, the temperature subnormal. The pupils are dilated, the pulse small and thready and the respiration sighing. The patient usually recovers if placed at rest, but death may take place from heart failure.**

(3) Heat Hyperpyrexia or Heat Stroke: A fever above 41.5°C is termed hyperpyrexia. Heat stroke is a condition characterised by rectal temperature greater than 41°C., and neurological disturbances, such as psychosis, delirium, stupor, coma and convulsions. The term **thermic fever** or **"sunstroke"** is used when there has been direct exposure to the sun.

Predisposing factors: High temperature, increased humidity, minor infections, muscular activity and lack of acclimatisation are the principal factors in the initiation. Where there is 100% humidity, a temperature of 32°C in the environment may lead to heat stroke. Other factors are old age, pre-existing disease, alcoholism, use of major tranquilisers, obesity, lack of air movement and unsuitable clothing. **Failure of cutaneous blood flow and sweating, the factors which control body temperature, leads to a breakdown of the heat regulating centre of the hypothalamus.**

Types: Heat stroke is of two types: (1) **Exertional heat stroke** most commonly occurs in athletes, military personnel or other persons working hard in a hot environment. A persisting sweating as a result of increased catecholamine production can be seen in about 50% of individuals. (2) In old persons usually over 60 years **during heat** waves. **In the classic form sweating is usually absent.**

CLINICAL FEATURES: The onset is usually sudden, with sudden collapse and loss of consciousness. In some cases, prodromal symptoms of headache, dizziness, nausea, vomiting, weakness, faintness, staggering gait, purposeless movements, mental confusion, muscle cramps, restlessness and excessive thirst occur. The temperature rises to 40°C to 43°C or more. The skin is dry, hot and flushed, with complete absence of sweating. The pupils are contracted. The pulse is rapid (usually more than 130 p.m.) and later becomes irregular. The breathing is rapid, (usually above 30 breaths p.m.) deep and of Kussmaul type. When temperature rises above 42°C. vasodilatation occurs with decrease in blood volume leading to circulatory collapse and cardiac failure. Blood pressure is low. Convulsions occur and the patient becomes delirious or comatose. The fatal period is five minutes to three days. Death results from centre paralysis of medullary heat regulating centre.

Postmortem Appearances: They are not specific. The temperature remains high after death. Rigor mortis (RM) sets in early and disappears early. Lividity is marked. **C.N.S:** The brain is congested and oedematous and petechial haemorrhages are seen in the white matter. Cerebral hemispheres are increased in weight and show flattening of the convolutions. **R.S.:** Trachea and bronchi contain frothy haemorrhagic fluid. The lungs show oedema, congestion and haemorrhages. **Heart**: Dilation of right auricle, flabbiness of muscle, petechial or confluent subepicardial and subendocardial haemorrhages and degeneration of myocardium. **Liver:** Congestion and centrilobular necrosis. **Kidneys:** Congestion, oedema and increase in weight. In case of longer survival, tubular necrosis and haemoglobinuric nephrosis is common. **Adrenals:** Pericapsular haemorrhages, engorgement of sinusoids and cortical degeneration. **General:** Petechial and confluent haemorrhages and disseminated intravascular coagulation are seen in most organs.

HYPERTHERMIC ANHYDROSIS OR DESERT SYNDROME: The features are like that of heat exhaustion. After profuse generalised sweating for several days, perspiration stops suddenly in all parts of the body below the neck region but persists in face and neck. There is hyperkeratotic plugging of sweat glands leading to functional failure of sweat apparatus. Papular rashes appear over face and neck. It was observed in U.S. soldiers having training in deserts.

BURNS

A burn is an injury which is caused by application of heat (by conduction or radiation) or chemical substances to the external or internal surfaces of the body, which causes destruction of tissues. Radiation causes damage through conversion of infrared frequencies into thermal heat on absorption at the skin interface. The minimum temperature for producing a burn is about 44°C for an exposure of about 5 to 6 hours. At 65°C, two seconds are sufficient to produce burns and full thickness destruction of skin occurs within seconds above 70°C.

Varieties of Burns: The external appearances of burns vary according to the nature of the substance used to produce them. (1) A highly **heated solid body** or a molten metal, when applied to the body for a very short time may produce only a blister and reddening corresponding in size and shape to the material used. **It will cause destruction, or even charring of the parts, when kept in contact for some time. The epidermis may be found blackened, dry and wrinkled.** The hair may be singed or distorted. **Hair singed by the flame becomes curled, twisted, blackish, breaks off or is totally destroyed** Fig. (11–4).

(2) Burns produced by **flame** may or may not produce vesication, but **singeing of the hair and blackening of the skin are always present.** Roasted patches of skin or deeper parts may be seen. Dry heat causes burns by direct conduction or radiation to the skin Fig. (11–5).

(3) Burns caused by **kerosene oil, petrol,** etc. are usually severe and produce **sooty blackening of the parts and have a characteristic odour** Fig. (11–6).

(4) Burns caused by **explosions** in coal mines or of gunpowder are usually very extensive and produce **blackening and tattooing** due to driving of the particles of the unexploded powder into the skin.

(5) Burns due to **X-ray and radium** vary from **redness of the skin to dermatitis,** with shedding of hair and epidermis and pigmentation of the surrounding skin. Severe exposure may produce burns with erythema, blistering or dermatitis, or ulceration with delayed healing and ill-formed scars. Fingernails may show degenerative changes and wart-like growths. Infra-red rays may cause necrosis of the skin.

(6) Burns caused by **ultraviolet rays** (the sun or mercury vapour lamp) and infrared rays produce **erythema or acute eczematous dermatitis.**

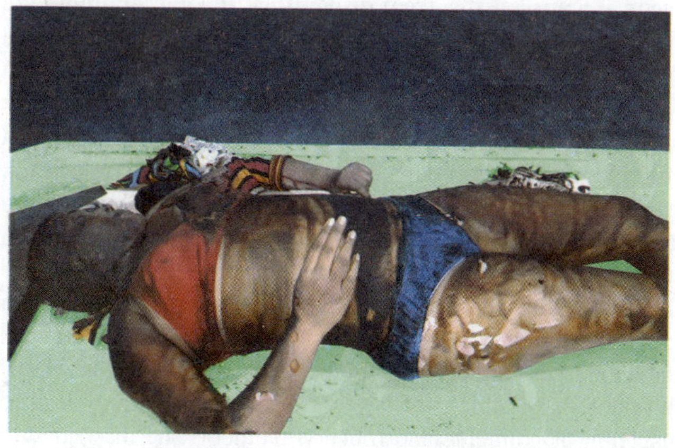

Fig. (11–4). Burns of first degree.

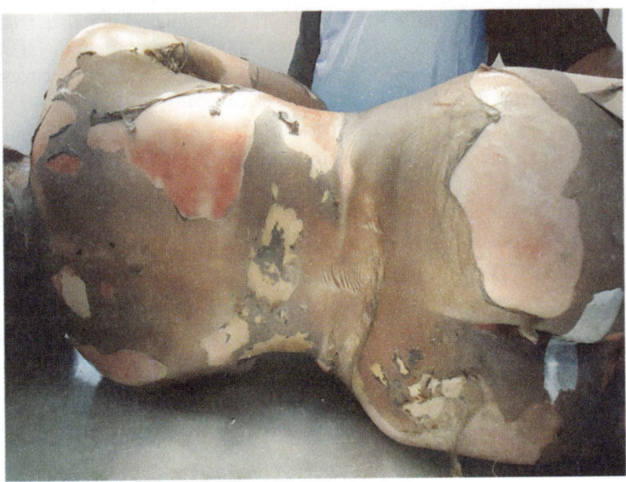

Fig. (11–5). Dermo-epidermal burns.

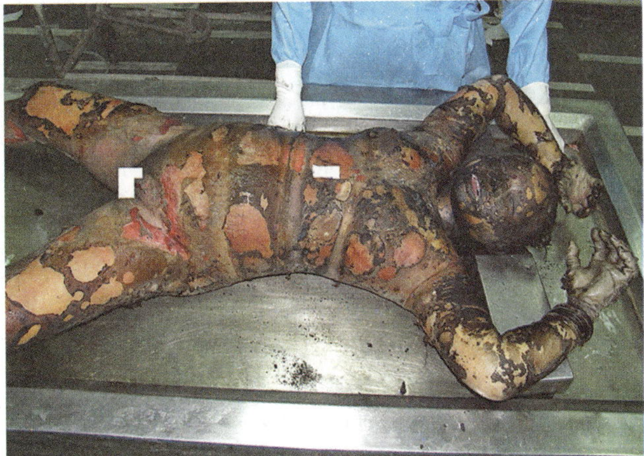

Fig. (11–6). Various degrees of burns.

(7) Radiant-heat burns **are caused by exposure to a heat source,** e.g. sun burn, a type of electromagnetic wave.

(8) Microwave burns **are well-demarcated, full thickness burns without charring.**

(9) Burns from corrosive substances **show ulcerated patches and are usually free from blisters; hair is not singed and the red line of demarcation is absent.** They show distinct colouration and are usually uniform in character. Strong acids produce dark leathery burns upon the skin. Strong alkalis cause the skin to slough and leave moist, slimy, greyish areas. Hydrofluoric acid and bromine cause necrosis of the skin and tissues.

(10) Electrical burns.

Degree of Burns: Dupuytren divided burns into six degrees, but they were merged into three degrees by Wilson. The precise depth of a burn can be measured by a high frequency ultrasound device.

(1) Epidermal: **The affected part is erythematous** (red). There is capillary dilatation and transudation of fluid into the tissues causing swelling. A split may occur in the epidermis or at the epidermal-dermal junction to **form a blister (vesicle or bulla), which is covered by white, avascular epidermis, bordered by red, hyperaemic skin usually 5 to 20 mm. across. The base is bright red when burst.** Singeing of the hair is present. The blister contains gas and fluid containing protein. When epidermis is lost, the dermis becomes reddened, inflamed and exudes plasma and tissue fluid. These burns are very painful. Repair is complete without scar formation.

(2) Dermo-epidermal (third and fourth degrees Dupuytren): **Whole thickness of skin is destroyed with destruction of dermal appendages.** The central zone of necrotic tissue is surrounded by first degree burns, or a zone of hyperaemia or both. **These burns appear as shrivelled, depressed areas of coagulated tissue, bordered by reddish blistered skin.** The lesions may be brown or black, due to charring and eschar formation. **The necrotic tissue separates usually within a week, and leaves an ulcer which heals with scar formation.** Contraction of the scar tissue may produce disfigurement or impaired function, according to the site and size of the burns. **Pain and shock are greater than in first degree burns.**

(3) Deep: In this, there is a **gross destruction not only of the skin and subcutaneous tissue, but also of muscle and even bone.** Nerve endings are also destroyed, and as such the **burns are relatively painless. The appearances are similar to those of the second degree, but in a more severe form. The burnt part is completely charred.**

Clinical classification (1) Superficial, when less than full thickness of skin is involved. (2) Deep.

Effects: The effects depend on: (1) The degree of heat: The effects are severe, if the heat applied is very great. The body of an adult does not burn completely in a burnt house, as the temperature usually does not exceed 650°C. **For purpose of cremation, a human body has to be incinerated for one-and-half hours at 1000°C. The ashes weigh two to three kg., and contain bone fragments which can be identified as human.** (2) The duration of exposure: The symptoms are more severe if the heat is applied for a long time. (3) The extent of the surface: The estimation of the surface area of the body involved is usually worked out by the "rule of nines" (Wallace), 9% for the head and neck (head 7%, neck 2%); 9% for each upper limb; (arm 4%, forearm 3%, hand 2%), 9% for the front of each lower limb; 9% for the back of each lower limb; (thigh 10%, leg 5%, foot 3% for each lower limb); 9% for the front of chest; 9% for the back of chest; 9% for the front of the abdomen; and 9% for the back of abdomen, 99% of the body Fig. (11–7A). In children surface area is estimated as given in Fig. (11–7B) and Table (11–1). The remaining one percent is for the external genitalia. **Palmar surface of patient's hand is about one percent of body surface area.** Involvement of 50 percent of the body surface will prove fatal even when the burns are only of the first degree. **Skin surface is about 4.6 sq. metres in an adult.** (4) The site: Burns of the head and neck, trunk or the anterior abdominal wall are more dangerous. (5) Age: Children are more susceptible, old people less. (6) Sex: Women are more susceptible.

Local effects of thermal injury include: vascular thrombosis and tissue necrosis, increase evaporation of water from burnt surface and local heat loss.

CAUSES OF DEATH: **(1) Primary (neurogenic) shock due to pain, etc. (2) More than half of deaths from burns occur within the first 48 hours usually from secondary shock, due to fluid loss from burned surface. Circulatory collapse may occur with 15% of burns of total body surface area. (3) In smoke inhalation apart from CO, the other factors which contribute to death are oxygen deprivation, cyanide, free radicals**

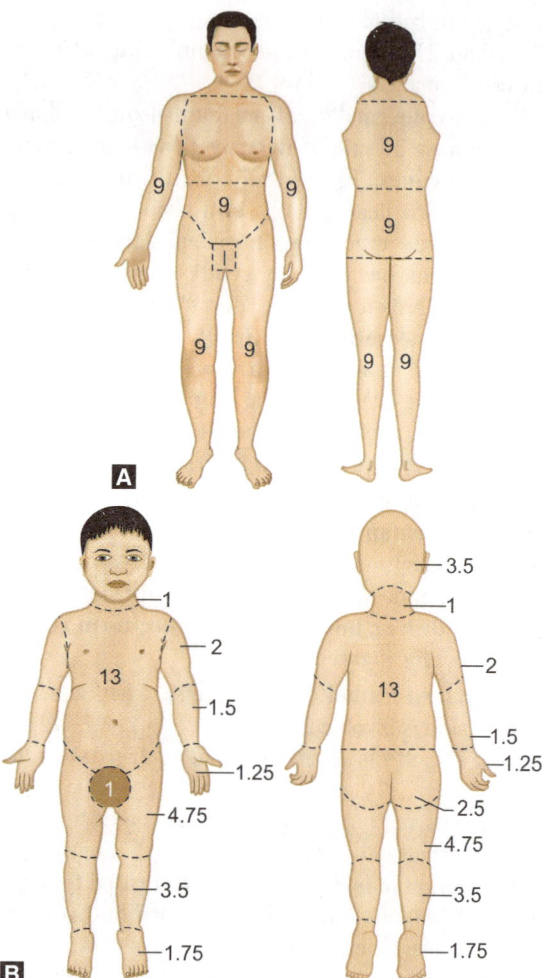

Fig. (11–7). (A) Estimation of the extent of surface burns. (B) Estimation of the extent of surface burns in children.

Table (11–1). Estimation of percentage of body surface area burned (Lund and Browder)

Area of Body	1 to 4	5 to 9	10 to 14	Adult
Head and neck	19	15	14	09
Front of trunk	16	16	16	18
Back of trunk	16	16	16	18
Upper limb	19	19	19	18
Lower limb	30	34	34	36
Genitalia	0		1	1

(inactivate surfactants, thus preventing oxygen from crossing the alveoli into the blood), and non-specific toxic substances. (4) Toxaemia, due to absorption of various metabolites from the burnt tissue persists up to 3 to 4 days. (5) Sepsis is the most important factor in deaths occurring four to five days or longer after burning. (6) Biochemical disturbances, secondary to the fluid loss and destruction of tissue, e.g., hypokalaemia. (7) Acute renal failure, due to lower nephron nephrosis occurs on the third or fourth day. (8) Gastrointestinal disturbances, such as acute peptic ulceration, dilation of the stomach, haemorrhage into intestines. (9) Oedema of glottis and pulmonary oedema due to inhalation of smoke containing CO and CO_2, if the person dies in a burnt house. (10) Accident occurring in an attempt to escape from a burning house or by injuries due to falling masonry, timber or other structures on the body. (11) Pyaemia, gangrene, tetanus, etc. (12) Fat embolism is rare. (13) Pulmonary embolism from thrombosis of veins of the leg due to tissue damage and immobility. (14) Often, multisystem failure. (15) Death may occur years after recovery from malignant transformation of a burn scar (Marjolin's ulcer).

In severe burns, respiratory distress may be due to oedema of upper air way, pulmonary oedema and inhibition of respiratory excursions by tight eschar. Delayed deaths in burns may occur from respiratory failure due to ARDS, or pulmonary embolism due to prolonged immobilisation.

Postmortem Appearances:

Clothes: If clothing is ignited, combination of flash and flame burns occur. Pure cotton fabrics transmit more thermal energy to skin than polyster-cotton blend fabrics. Cotton fabrics ignite easier and burn faster, producing a larger, deeper area of burn. As the fabric weight increases, the area burned decreases. Knit fabrics produce smaller areas of burn than woven fabrics. Nylon and polyester fabrics melt and stick to skin and may produce far more serious burns. Long loose garments catch fire easily and are more dangerous than close fitting garments. The clothes should be removed and examined for the presence of smell of kerosene, petrol, etc. For analysis of volatile substances, fragments of clothing should be placed in a glass container with a screw-top cap. If placed in a plastic bag, the volatile material may escape. Any container found should be examined for finger prints.

External: Heat rigor may be observed in the muscles. **It is difficult to determine the time of death as body temperature, postmortem hypostasis and rigor mortis cannot be assessed. Decomposition is accelerated with burns limited to the body surface, but greatly reduced in a severely burned body.** Hair is singed, or completely burnt. In lesser degrees of burns, ends are bulbous at intervals. **Portions of the body where clothing is tight, e.g., under the belt, shoes, brassier or buttoned collar are often comparatively unaffected. The use of flammable liquid, such as kerosene or petrol often results in patchy charring of various severity, i.e. while some areas are charred deeply, others areas are burned less severely.** Dry leather-like burnt skin may also reveal the presence of residual accelerants. Sometimes, skin and hair in the armpits and the gums are spared. The colour of light hair changes on exposure to heat. At about 120°C for 10 to 15 minutes, brown hair becomes slightly reddish. There is no change in the colour of the black hair. First degree burns usually disappear after death due to gravitation of blood to dependent parts, but capillaries of burnt area will contain clotted blood. **The face is swollen and distorted. The tongue protrudes** and may be burnt due to the contraction of the tissues of the neck and face. **Froth may appear at the mouth and nose due to pulmonary oedema** caused by heat irritation of the air-passages and lungs and heart failure due to asphyxiating effect of COHb. **It indicates that the deceased was breathing while the fire was in progress. In the hands, the skin detaches as glove,** due to deposition of fluid between the layers of the skin, including the fingernails. By removal of the superficial layers of the skin by wiping or rubbing, tattoo marks become visible. **The burnt areas will be found reddened and blistered or charred. Blisters** may be present either in the main burn or as islands beyond the periphery. The whole of the burned area may form one large blister or be a confluence of blisters. Blisters are due to increased permeability of superficial blood vessels due to heat. They contain serous fluid containing albumen and chlorides and red and white cells. The fluid coagulates on heating or on treatment with nitric acid.

The blisters of a second degree burns cannot be distinguished from blisters seen in CO poisoning, deep coma, antemortem and postmortem gasoline exposure and peeling of the skin seen in the early stages of putrefaction. **When these various types of blisters burst, they leave a pale, moist, raw surface which becomes yellow, tan and finally dark brown and leathery as it dries.** The degree of burning in each area should be assessed. Occasionally, anus is dilated and rectal wall protrudes through the opening.

Pugilistic Attitude (boxing, fencing or defence attitude): The posture of a body which has been exposed to great heat is often characteristic. **The legs are flexed at the hips and knees, the arms are flexed at elbows and wrists and held out in front of the body, head slightly extended, all fingers are hooked like claws. Contraction of paraspinal muscles often causes a marked opisthotonus, in an attitude commonly adopted by boxers Fig. (11–8).** Degree and severity of contractures depend on intensity of heat and duration for which heat was applied. Muscles are contracted, desiccated and carbonised on the surface. This stiffening is due to the coagulation of proteins of the muscles and dehydration which cause contraction. The flexor muscles being bulkier than extensors contract more due to which joints of all limbs are flexed. It occurs whether the person was alive or dead at the time of burning.

Heat Ruptures: In severe burning or charring **skin contracts markedly and heat ruptures occur, either before or after death. They are produced by splitting of the soft parts. These splits may be anywhere, but are usually seen over fleshy areas of the body,** like calves, thighs and extensor surfaces, joints and on the head. Splits of abdominal walls occur parallel to muscle fibres. **These ruptures or splits in the skin may be several centimetres in length,** and **superficially they may resemble lacerations or even incised wounds Figs. (11–9 and 11–10). They can be differentiated by:** (1) Absence of bleeding in the wound and surrounding tissues, since heat coagulates the blood in the vessels. (2) Intact vessels and nerves are seen in the floor. (3) Irregular margins. (4) Absence of bruising or other signs of vital reaction in the margins. **When the skin is completely burnt, the underlying muscle usually shows rupture due to heat.**

Sometimes, the charred skin cracks easily when an attempt is made to remove the body from a house destroyed by fire. These tears are commonly seen around joints, especially the elbows, shoulders and knees.

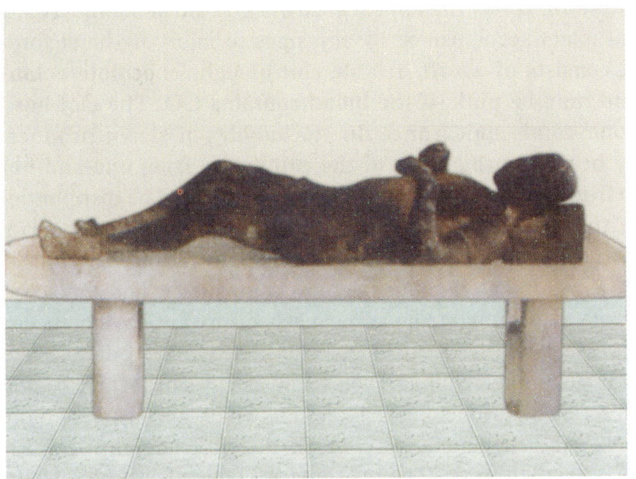

Fig. (11–8). Puglistic attitude in a case of burns.

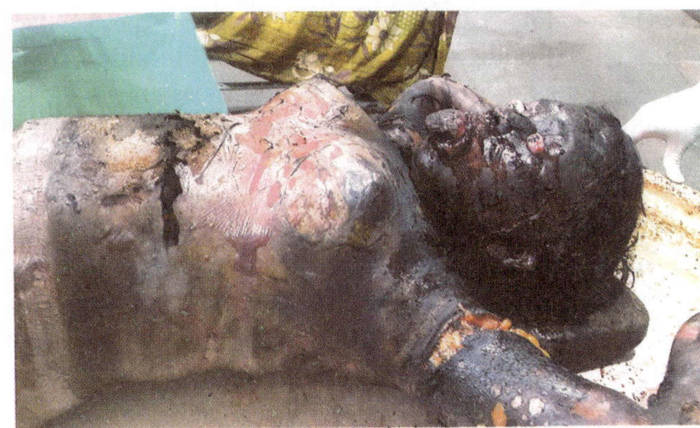

Fig. (11–9). Heat ruptures in left axilla in burning.

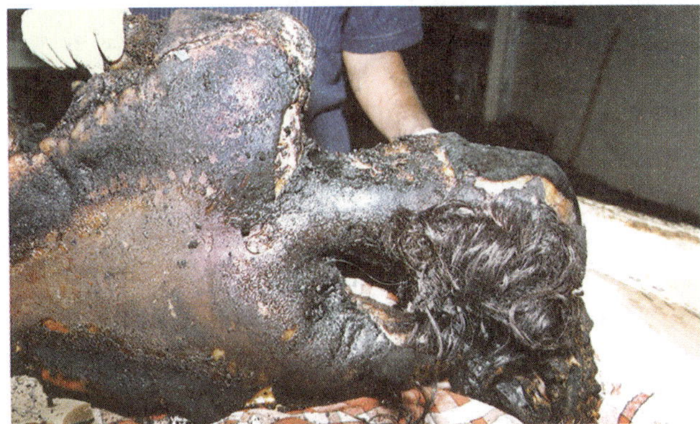

Fig. (11–10). Heat ruptures on scalp and left shoulder.

Flash burns: Flash burns are a variant of flame burns. **They occur due to sudden ignition or explosion of gases or fine particulate material, e.g. explosions, or ignition of highly inflammable liquids or gases, and produce a uniform first and second degree burns of all of the exposed areas of skin due to brief but intense exposure to heat.** If clothing is ignited, a combination of flash and flame burns occur.

Other effects: Obesity and clothes contribute to faster and more complete destruction of a body in a fire. If the adipose tissue is ignited, prolonged local smoldering may cause severe skeletal damage, including amputation. Human bodies burn readily, especially when the subcutaneous fatty tissues have ignited. **Often, some parts of the body are preserved, if they are protected from the flames. In sitting persons, the buttocks may be spared; if the head falls forward between the knees, the abdomen is spared. The hands and feet may drop off if the burning is sudden and intense,** and they may be preserved with slight damage because they fall away from the source of the fire. **Flexion of the limbs by heat may cause tumbling of a burnt body from a bed or chair to the floor, if the body was not well balanced. Partial burning of the abdominal wall associated with gas expansion within the intestines may produce rupture of the abdominal wall,** in the charred burnt victim. The intestines may protrude through this defect. **Flame burns usually have a patchy distribution and vary in size and shape.** Sometimes, the body may be covered with a black or brown layer of smoke which does not penetrate into skin creases. On straightening the flexed neck or limb, the paler skin in the crease is exposed which may mimic a ligature mark. **In severe burns, the skin may be stiffened, yellow-brown and leathery, muscles are shrivelled and desiccated even carbonised on the surface. Beneath that there is a zone of brownish pink cooked meat and under that normal red muscle. Drying after death of areas that were weeping serum leaves a stiff, parchment-like surface. At greater depths, more moist and normal working soft tissues are seen.** As the tissues are shrunken, stab, gunshot and other wounds may be shrunken to a small size. **Muscles under the burnt area are pale, brownish and part-cooked.** This occurs after death due to heated environment. **At greater depth, more moist and normal looking soft tissues are seen.** Black, brittle masses are found in the tissues merging into cooked dry muscle beneath. **Burnt bone has a gray-white colour,** often showing a fine superficial network of heat fractures on its cortical surface. The soft tissue of the face may be completely burnt exposing the skull. In a charred body, the corneas are white and translucent and lenses opaque and the front teeth may partially or completely disintegrated. When considerable destruction of body occurs, it is difficult to differentiate antemortem from postmortem burns. The outer tables of the exposed cranial vault may show a network of fine criss-crossing heat fractures. Rarely the body cavities may be opened by partial destruction of their walls and hollow organs like stomach and intestines may rupture. If the flame is unchecked, the body will be reduced to a shapeless, coal-like mass and finally to heap of grey and yellow ashes **Figs. (11–11 and 11–12)**.

Establishment of Identity: In a charred body the weight and stature are unreliable, as they are greatly altered due to drying of the tissues, skeletal fractures, and pulverisation of intervertebral discs due to the heat. **The stature may be less by several centimetres and weight loss may be up to sixty percent.** The features are changed due to contraction of the skin. Moles, scars and tattoo marks are usually destroyed. In a badly charred body cheeks act as insulation and protect posterior teeth for a considerable time, but anterior teeth may be charred and friable. **If a person is killed during the blaze, the teeth are extensively destroyed than when he was killed prior to fire, because the lips behave differently in the two cases. When a living person is burnt the teeth become loose in their sockets, whereas in a dead person the teeth are firmly attached. Teeth crack when exposed to heat. Enamel crowns are completely lost while roots remain intact but opaque.** Dental charts should be prepared and X-rays of the jaws taken, which can reveal metal pins, fillings, etc. which can be compared with previous charts of the suspected person. Postmortem X-rays can be compared with the previous X-ray of the suspected person. Complete X-rays of the body of the victim are useful to locate possible old fractures, bony abnormalities or foreign bodies. The finding of metal staples, steel wires, pins, plates, screws and artificial joints indicate surgical procedure. **Presence of some disease, absence of uterus, ovaries, appendix, one kidney,** etc., **presence of pacemaker, valve implant,** etc. may be helpful. In a badly charred or incinerated body, the sex can be determined by finding the uterus or prostate which resist fire to a marked degree, and by pelvic bones, and age by teeth and by observing centres of ossification in the bones and the condition of the epiphyses. If the whole body is destroyed, personal effects such as keys, jewellery, watch strap, shoes, buttons, belt-buckle, etc., may help in identity. **DNA extracted from blood** from cardiac chambers or from any human remains is analysed using PCR (DNA fingerprinting) and compared with the alleged biological parents.

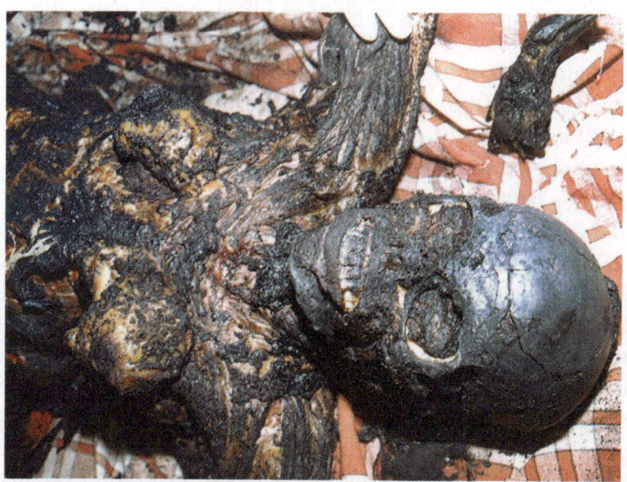

Fig. (11–11). Charring of the body due to burns.

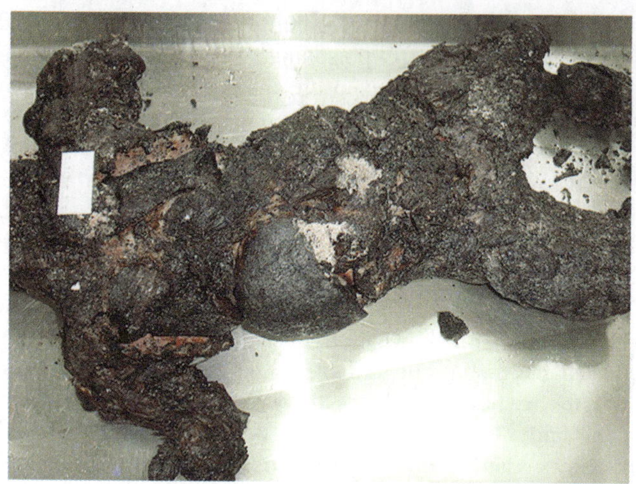

Fig. (11–12). Charred body recovered from a burnt house.

Internal: Heat haematoma occurs when the head has been exposed to intense heat, sufficient to cause charring of the skull. It has the appearance of extradural haemorrhage, but is not accompanied by any signs of injury by blunt force. **It consists of a soft, friable clot of light chocolate colour, and may be pink, if the blood contains CO. The clot has a honeycomb appearance due to bubbles of steam produced by heat. The thickness of the clot varies from one-and-half to fifteen mm., and the volume up to 120 ml. The distribution of the clot follows closely the distribution of the charring of the outer table of the skull Figs. (11–13 and 11–14).** The parietotemporal region is the most common site and sometimes frontal or occipital region. The mechanism of its development is obscure. It may be due to blood being boiled from the diploic layer of bone through emissary veins and venous sinus which rupture or shrinkage of meninges and brain, which may aspirate blood from the venous sinuses. **The carboxyhaemoglobin level in heat haematoma will be the same as in peripheral blood.** Heat haematoma will contain carboxyhaemoglobin, but **extradural**

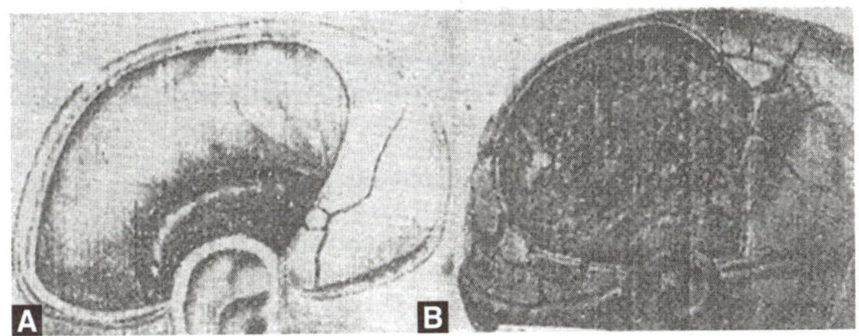

Fig. (11–13). (A) Extradural haemorrhage. (B) Heat haematoma with skull fractures.

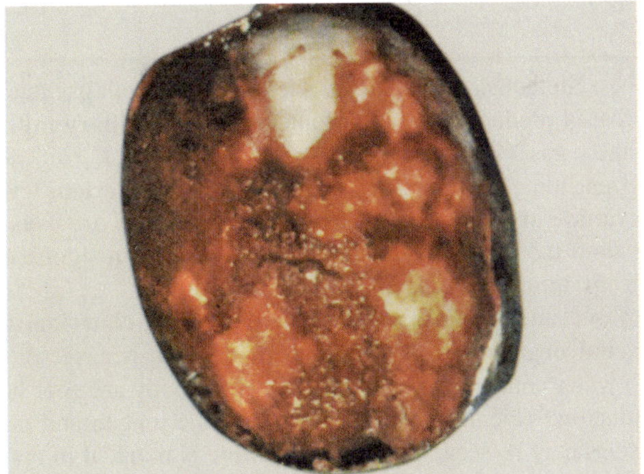

Fig. (11–14). Heat haematoma.

haemorrhage caused by injury before the fire began, will not show carboxyhaemoglobin. The dura underneath the haematoma is greatly shrunken which compresses the brain. The dura may split under tension and brain tissue may ooze out and form a mass of frothy paste. The adjacent brain shows hardening and discolouration from the heat. The basic difference between traumatic extradural haemorrhage and haematoma due to burns is given in **(Table 11–2)**.

Thermal fractures of the skull: The skull fractures occur most commonly in areas where the skull has been severely burned **Fig. (11–15)**. **There are two types of thermal fractures of the skull.** (1) Intracranial increase of steam pressure causes separation of ununited sutures or an intracranial explosion occurs, producing **fractures with gaping defects and widely separated bony margins.** (2) The fracture occurs due to rapid drying of the bone with contraction, and only involves the **outer table of the skull. In this type there is no displacement,** and the lines of fracture are frequently stellate. **Skull fractures are usually seen on either side of the skull above the temples. Sometimes they may be bilateral. They consist of several lines which radiate from a common centre and in some cases may fragment.** The skull is often friable with flaking of the outer table. Heat fractures usually do not involve the sutures of the skull even in young persons with un-united sutures. **Heat fracture may cross a suture line.** When the body is completely burnt, bones from the neurocranium are commonly found as pieces up to 10 cm in size, but not facial skeleton.

In fire victims, fractures of long bones are caused due to excessive shrinkage of the muscles, which exert unduly great pull on the tendons and bones. Peculiar, characteristically curved

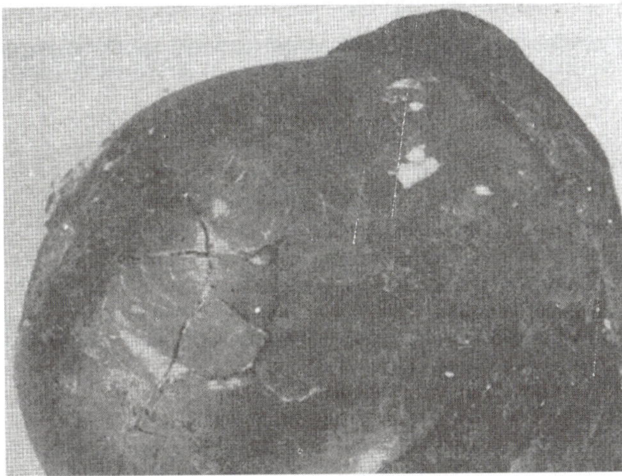

Fig. (11–15). Heat fractures in the skull due to burns.

fractures are often seen in bones of extremities exposed to very high temperatures. **Prolonged application of heat to the neck can make the hyoid bone so fragile that it breaks on gentle manipulation.** Burnt bone has a grey-white colour, usually showing fine superficial network of heat fractures on its cortical surface, which may crumble on handling.

CO levels: In death due to burns, the **CO levels in the blood will be more than ten percent and may reach 70 to 80%,** though children and old persons die at levels of 30 to 40%. In heart and lung disease, low levels of CO are found in deaths. **The blood is cherry-red, which may change to brownish due to heat.** The level of CO saturation of the blood is dependent on concentration of CO in the inhaled air, the duration of exposure, the rate and depth of respiration, the haemoglobin content of the blood and the activity of the victim.

Absence of CO: CO may be absent in blood due to various reasons, such as rapid death, convection air currents, low production of CO, flash fire (as in the conflagration of a chemical plant), inhalation of superheated air resulting in death by suffocation, in warfare, or in an explosion when death is instantaneous.

Death from suffocation: If death has occurred from suffocation, aspirated blackish coal particles are seen in the nose, mouth, larynx, trachea, bronchi, oesophagus and stomach and blood is cherry-red. Such particles are embedded in frothy mucus which covers the congested mucosa. **The presence of carbon particles in the terminal bronchioles on histological examination is absolute proof of life during the fire Fig. (11–16). Presence of carbon particles and an elevated CO saturation together are absolute proof that the victim was alive when the fire occurred.** The soot is better seen by spreading a thin film of mucus on a clean sheet of white paper. The amount of soot in the air-passages depends on the type of fire, the amount of smoke produced and the duration of survival in the smoke-contaminated atmosphere. Incision of trachea before evisceration should be done for the presence of soot. If the mouth is open, some passive percolation of soot may be found at the back of the pharynx, but it cannot be carried beyond the vocal cords, and also it is not found in the lower oesophagus and the stomach. In absence of CO in blood and soot in the airways, death may result possibly due to poisoning with CO_2 and/or O_2 deficiency.

Table (11–2). Difference between extradural haematoma due to burns and due to blunt force

	Trait	Epidural haematoma due to burns	Epidural haematoma due to blunt force
(1)	Cause:	Charring of the skull due to intense heat.	Blunt force to the head.
(2)	Situation:	Anywhere. Usually bilateral.	Usually adjacent to Sylvian fissure.
(3)	Distribution:	Diffuse.	Localised.
(4)	Characters:	Thin, granular, soft, friable clot of light chocolate colour, honeycomb appearance: evenly distributed or sickle-shaped.	Discoid shape; localised, more rubbery consistency, reddish–purple.
(5)	Skull:	May be fractured.	Associated fracture in temporal area.
(6)	CNS:	No injury.	Frequently injured.
(7)	Carboxyhaemoglobin:	Present.	Absent.

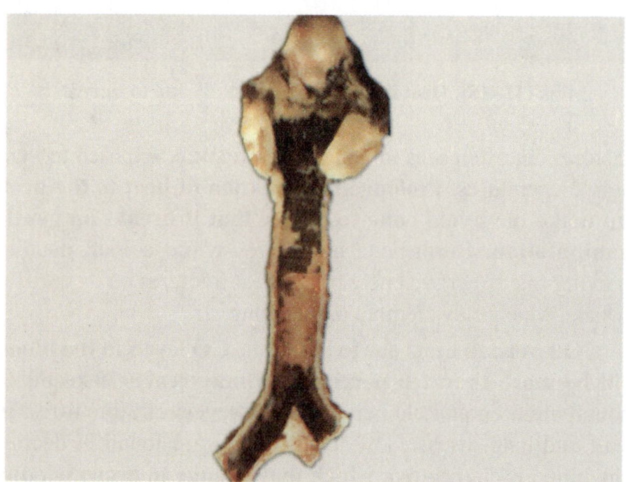

Fig. (11–16). Soot in the larynx and trachea in case of burns.

Inhalation of flame or superheated air: If flame or superheated air is inhaled, burns are seen in the interior of the mouth, tongue, fauces, nasal passages, larynx and air-passages with destruction of vocal cord epithelium and acute oedema of the larynx and lungs. Heat effects on the pharynx and epiglottis can occur postmortem, through passive percolation of hot gases through the open mouth. Dry heat burns are limited to the oropharynx and upper airway. Death may occur rapidly by shock or acute respiratory insufficiency. The interior of the larynx, trachea and main bronchi may be thickened and blanched, or reddened and the cells become swollen, pale and ballooned. If the temperature is too low, to burn the lining. The mucosa of the air passages is shed into the lumen of the viscus, and smaller peripheral air passages are choked by a mass of desquamated epithelial cells, mucus and carbon particles. **Sometimes, inhalation of smoke produces vomiting which may be inhaled and found in the smaller bronchi.** If the victim survives for a few days, inflammatory changes occur in the larynx, with sloughing of mucosa, ulceration and secondary infection.

Poisonous gases: Cyanides and oxides of nitrogen are produced due to burning of plastic and synthetic material. Burning of nitrogen containing substances, e.g. nitrocellulose film may liberate nitrogen oxide and nitrogen tetroxide. Burning of wool or silk liberate ammonia, hydrogen cyanide, hydrogen sulphide and oxides of sulphur. **The inhalation injuries of the lungs are chemical injuries caused by the byproducts of incomplete combustion.** These produce **pulmonary oedema** due to injury at the endothelial-epithelial interface, **alveolar collapse** due to decreased production of surfactant and **bronchociliary injury.** All these gases contribute to death.

Depending on the materials burning in the fire, **various levels of cyanide are found in the blood, but the levels are usually less than 0.3 mg.%. Cyanide can be produced in significant concentration by decomposition of the body.**

Viscera: Even in cases of severe external charring, the internal organs are usually well preserved, because of its high water content and as the tissues of the body are poor heat conductors. Haemorrhage in the root of the tongue and neck muscles may be seen. **Visceral congestion is marked in many cases. Petechial haemorrhages are usually found in the pleurae, pericardium and endocardium.** Haemoconcentration is present, and frequently there is some tissue oedema and excess of fluid in the serous cavities. **Sometimes, brain, liver, lung, etc. may be cooked,** i.e., hardened and discoloured. The brain is usually shrunken, firm and yellow to light-brown due to cooking. Flattening of the gyri and obliteration of sulci may occur due to thickening and contraction of the coagulating dura against the surface of the brain. The dura mater is leathery. **The dura may split and the brain tissue may ooze out,** forming a mass of frothy paste. The pleurae are congested or inflamed. The lungs are usually congested, and show marked oedema; they may be shrunken and rarely anaemic. The lungs are heavy, airless and consolidated. They may be hardened and discoloured. **The vessels of the lungs may contain a small amount of fat** due to a physico-chemical alteration of fat already present in the blood. Macrophages may contain pigment particles. Necrosis of the alveolar epithelium and necrotic debris is present as a membrane in cases of shock lung or adult respiratory distress syndrome. Signs of infection and inflammation may be present in delayed deaths. **Due to heat, sometimes blood is pressed out of the lung tissue into the alveoli, airway, mouth and nostrils.** This may simulate blood that was inhaled during life due to injury. A small amount of blood caked over the inner surface of chest cavity may also occur in the same way. The heart is usually filled with clotted blood and may show interstitial oedema and fragmentation of myocardial fibres. **There may be inflammation and ulceration of Peyer's patches and solitary glands in the intestines.** Occasionally, stress ulcers **(Curling ulcers) are produced in the duodenum commonly in the first part, in less than 10% cases, about the tenth day in extensive burns of the body.** Curling's ulcers are usually sharply punched-out mucosal defects, which may be superficial or deep. **Petechiae**

of stomach and duodenum, often with erosions, occasionally acute ulcers, is a more common finding. The gastric ulcers may occur within a day of burning.** There may be bacterial or fungal colonies in the floors of the ulcers. Erosion of large vessels occasionally produce fatal haemorrhage. The large bowel may also be involved. The spleen is enlarged and softened with oedema and necrosis of lymphoid germinal centres. The liver may show cloudy swelling or necrosis. **Jaundice may occur.** The kidneys may show cloudy swelling, capillary thrombosis and infarction. **Presence of heme casts in medullary tubules is common.** Renal obstruction leads to microcirculatory insufficiency and renal ischaemia. The adrenals may be enlarged and congested. **When more than 30% of the skin surface is burnt, haemoglobinuria occurs.**

Laryngeal Oedema: It may be caused by allergic anaphylactic reactions, infections, tumours, inhalation of flame or superheated air, inhalation of irritant gases, etc. **Inhalation of superheated steam causes laryngeal, tracheal and respiratory burns. The latter may progress to adult respiratory distress syndrome.** The amount of oedema will decrease with postmortem interval and only wrinkling of mucous membrane may be present. Microscopically, eosinophils may be seen.

Collection of blood: **Blood should be obtained from the heart or major vessels and placed in a tightly stoppered container.** It need not be collected or kept under oil. If blood is clotted, the clot should be preserved. **For CO analysis, if no blood can be obtained, use spleen, marrow, liver or muscle in that order.** Blood should be preserved by fluoride for analysis of cyanide.

Age of Burns: The ageing of the burns is very inaccurate and depends upon the agent, the extent, and their depth. Redness appears immediately, and vesication in about an hour. The exudate begins to dry in 12 to 24 hours and forms a dry, brown crust within 2 to 3 days. The red inflammatory zone disappears in 36 to 72 hours, and pus may form under sloughs. Superficial sloughs fall off in four to six days, and deeper sloughs within two weeks. After this, granulation tissue covers the surface and a scar is formed after several weeks Fig. (11–17).

HISTOPATHOLOGY: The blood vessels in the floor of the blister are dilated. Within 6 hours, inflammatory reaction with polymorphonuclear leucocyte infiltration occurs in the dermis, which is highest in 48 to 72 hours. In 12 to 24 hours, there is some necrosis and degeneration of epidermal cells in the central zone. The epidermis may be coagulated, thinned and deeply staining. The cells in the deeper layers of the epidermis become elongated and flattened with their long axes tending to be oriented more at right angles to the skin surface, closely resembling streaming of epithelial cells as in electric mark. In 48 to 72 hours, migration of epidermal cells is pronounced, and there is increased proliferation of epithelial and connective tissue cells. Small haemorrhages may be seen in the deepest layers of the skin. Vacuolisation in the epidermal and dermal layers is a characteristic feature.

Marjolin's ulcer: Untreated or non-healing wounds may lead to chronic ulceration which may undergo malignant transformation, so called Marjolin's ulcer (squamous cell carcinoma).

Antemortem and Postmortem Burns: In antemortem burns, a zone of hyperaemia (line of redness), which varies in width, but is usually five to twenty mm. is present at the edge of the burnt area except in cases of immediate death Figs. (11–18 and 11–19). It is due to oedema of tissues and capillary dilatation and merges with the edge of the burn which may show blistering or charring. **It involves whole thickness of true skin. It is permanent and persists after death.** Heat applied up to

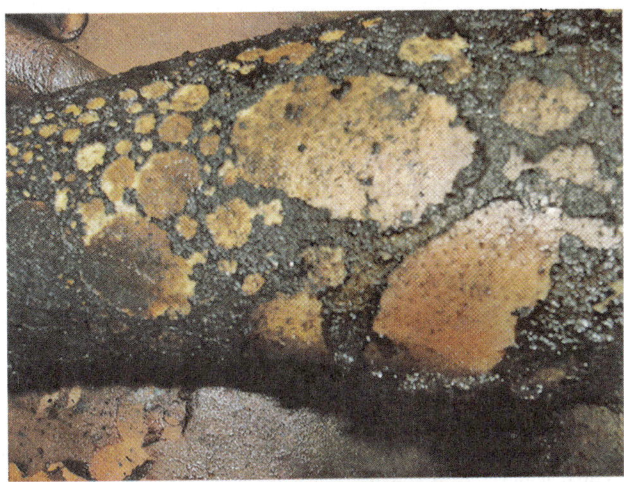

Fig. (11–18). Postmortem burns.

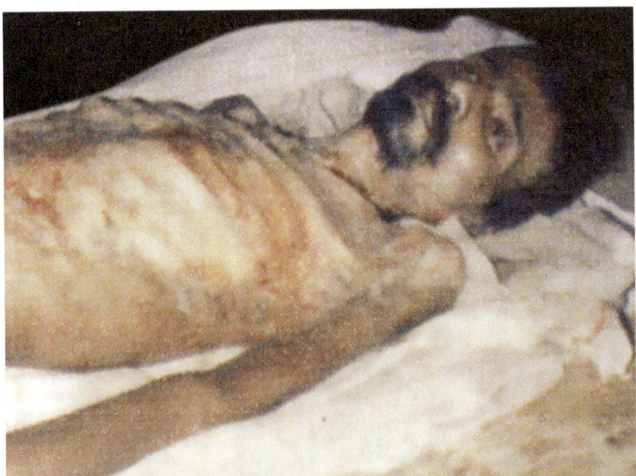

Fig. (11–17). Extensive burns showing unhealthy granulation tissue after 2 months of survival.

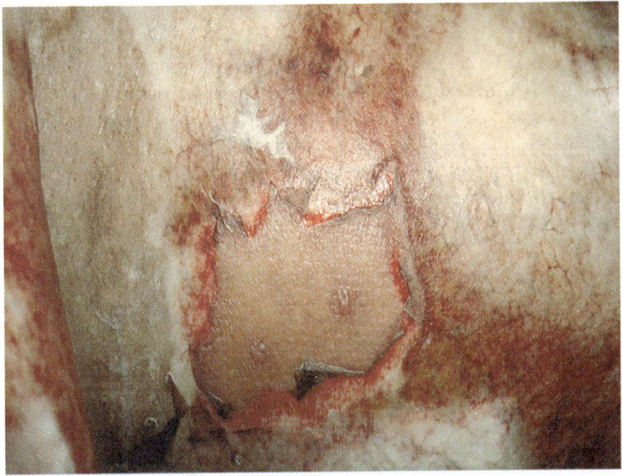

Fig. (11–19). Antemortem burns showing a zone of hyperaemia at the edge of the burnt area.

one hour after death can produce a red line of erythema. If the person is alive, the skin beyond this zone shows erythema, which tends to disappear after death. **If the whole body is burnt, line of redness will be absent.** The antemortem blister appears as a raised dome and contains gas or fluid. The base and periphery show reddening with swollen papillae. In antemortem burns, the skin adjacent to burnt area shows an increased reaction for SH groups in all layers, and increase in ATP and esterases in one to 2 hours, aminopeptidases in 2 to 4 hours, acid phosphatases in 4 to 6 hours and alkaline phosphatases in 8 to 12 hours. Acid mucopolysaccharides are present in the superficial zone of burnt area Table (11–3). **If a dead body is in contact with petrol or kerosene, skin is burnt which is similar to that seen in dry heat burns.**

Postmortem blisters are pale-yellow, and the contained fluid is thin and clear. **The base of the postmortem blister is dry, hard and yellow.** The protein content of serous fluid is not of much value to differentiate antemortem and postmortem burns. **Postmortem burns show dried scorching of the skin surface, like burnt paper.** Sometimes blisters with a red rim can be seen in postmortem burns, due to contraction of dermal capillaries forcing liquid blood to the periphery of the burn or blister. In some cases deep burns may not show inflammatory reaction, due to heat thrombosis of dermal vessels. Burns produced shortly before or after death cannot be distinguished either by naked eye or by microscopic examination.

CIRCUMSTANCES OF DEATH: The distribution of burns on the clothing may indicate the manner in which it was ignited, the posture of the victim at the time, the path taken by flames and to discover that unburnt cloth was saturated with some inflammable material. Splash patterns burnt into the floor and floor coverings, holes in the floor, particularly holes of the 'tongue and groove' type and the characteristic odour of petroleum fuels and solvents are all useful indicators of the use of inflammable material. Differentiation is mostly a matter for the police investigation. The inhalation of CO often causes severe muscular incoordination, weakness, and confusion due to which the victim is unable to escape and dies of asphyxia, the body being burnt after death.

ACCIDENT: Large number of deaths are accidental. Accidental burning deaths may occur inside the kitchen, in factories, house conflagrations, flaming of highly inflammable fuel, electrical short circuits, manufacture and playing with fireworks, dropping lighted matches, falling asleep while smoking a cigarette which drops on to the bed or chair, faulty heating appliances or electric wiring, leakage of cooking gas, etc. Infants, children, epileptics, intoxicated or drugged persons or helpless from other causes may fall into a fire. Lamps or stoves may explode and set fire to the clothes. Clothes of women may catch fire accidentally while cooking. In such cases, burns are usually found on the front of thighs, abdomen, chest and face. There may be severe burning of the hands due to the victim trying to extinguish the fire by beating out the flames. The feet and ankles are usually not burnt. Multiple deaths from burns may result from plane crashes or automobile accidents. In industry, burns may be caused by explosions from inflammable liquids and by flashes from furnaces. If the body is lying on a flat surface, the skin resting on the surface may be well preserved, even though the body as a whole may be severely charred.

SUICIDE: Occasionally, women commit suicide by pouring kerosene on their head and clothes before setting fire to themselves due to domestic worries, disappointment in love or acute or chronic disease. Extensive second and third degree burns, more concentrated on the front are seen over the whole of the body; only the skin folds, such as the axillae perineum and soles being spared. Sometimes, a person may keep a piece of cloth in her mouth to suppress her cries. Sometimes, suicidal burning is a mode of public protest. Self-immolation may be performed as an acute emotional reaction. Some of the victims have schizophrenia. In case kerosene, petrol, etc. is found on the body including head hair in high amounts, it is likely to be either suicide or homicide.

HOMICIDE: Murder by burning is rare. When blunt object injuries are inflicted, and then body is exposed to fire, blood from contusions will not show carboxyhaemoglobin, though this is present in circulating blood, indicating antemortem burns. If an inflammable fluid such as kerosene, petrol, etc., is poured on a person lying on his back and then burnt, there will be burning of the sides of the neck, sides of the trunk, between the thighs and other areas, especially if the clothing is absent in those areas, as the fluid runs downwards. Parts of the body which are in contact with ground do not show burning. Sometimes, fire, hot metals, boiling water and corrosive substances are used with criminal intent. A drunken man may push or throw his wife or child on the fire, and sometimes lighted lamps may be used as missiles. Burns may be inflicted on the pudenda of women as a punishment for adultery. Attempts may be made to burn a body after homicide with the object of concealing the crime. In such cases, the body should be examined for marks of violence, e.g., stab wounds, bullets, strangulation, etc. The usual signs of death by throttling, suffocation or blows may be completely destroyed. Examine internal organs for evidence of trauma or disease or poisoning. The possibility of postmortem injuries caused by firemen, fire-rescue members, or during transportation to mortuary must be considered. Examine internal organs for evidence of trauma or disease or poisoning. Blood should be preserved for alcohol CO and for other toxicological examinations. The possibility of postmortem injuries caused by foremen, fire-rescue members, or during transportation to mortuary must be considered.

Cigarette burns are circular, to oval, semilunar or lunar like areas of 0.3-0.5 cm with reddish yellow parchment-like area of first and second degree. If the cigarette has been stubbed out on the skin, a larger and irregular burn is produced contaminated with ash and debris **Figs. (11–20 and 11–21).**

SELF-INFLICTED BURNS: Burns are sometimes self-inflicted in order to support a false charge.

SCALDS

A scald is an injury which results from the application of liquid above 60°C or from steam. The destruction does not extend as deeply as in burns. **Water at 70°C can cause full thickness scalds of the skin in one second of contact.** It resembles a first degree dry burn, but the shape of scald tends

Table (11–3). **Difference between antemortem burns and postmortem burns**

	Trait	Antemortem burns	Postmortem burns
(1)	Line of redness:	Present.	Absent.
(2)	Blister:	Contains serous fluid with proteins and chlorides. Base is red and inflamed.	Contains air and thin clear fluid. Base is dry, hard and yellow.
(3)	Vital reaction:	Marked cellular exudation and reactive changes in the tissue cells present.	Absent.
(4)	Enzymes:	Peripheral zone of burn shows increase in enzyme reaction.	Peripheral zone does not show increase in enzyme reaction.

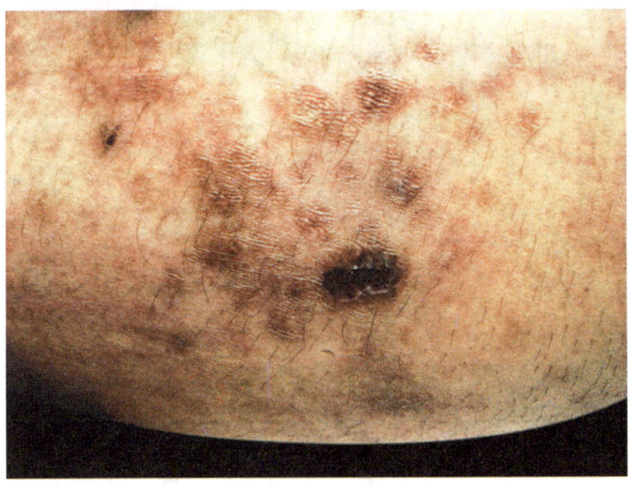

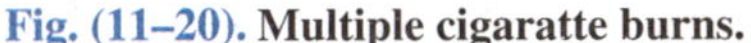

Fig. (11–20). **Multiple cigaratte burns.**

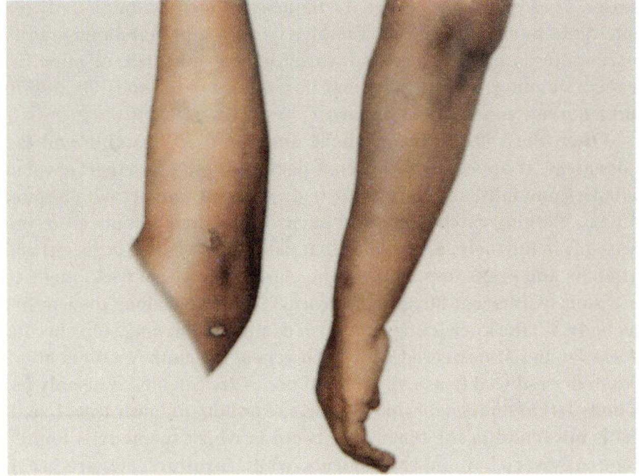

Fig. (11–21). **Cigarette burns on the upper extremity.**

Table (11–4). **Difference between burns from dry heat, moist heat and chemicals**

	Trait	Dry heat	Moist heat	Chemicals
(1)	Cause:	Flame, heated solid body, or X-rays.	Steam or liquid above 60°C.	Corrosive chemicals.
(2)	Site:	At and above the site of contact.	At and below the site of contact.	At and below the site of contact.
(3)	Splashing:	Absent.	Present.	Present.
(4)	Skin:	Dry and wrinkled, may be charred.	Sodden and bleached.	May be destroyed.
(5)	Vesicles:	At the circumference of burnt area.	Over the burnt area.	Very rare.
(6)	Red line:	Present.	Present.	Absent.
(7)	Colour:	Black.	Bleached.	Distinctive.
(8)	Charring:	Present.	Absent.	May be present.
(9)	Singeing:	Present.	Absent.	Absent.
(10)	Ulceration:	Absent.	Absent.	Present.
(11)	Scar:	Thick and contracted.	Thin and less contracted.	Thick and contracted.
(12)	Clothes:	Burnt.	Wet; not burnt.	May be burnt; show characteristic stains.

to be different. The severity of a scald depends on duration of contact with the skin and temperature of fluid. **Redness appears at once and blistering will take place within a few minutes.** The intensely red base of a severe scald is at first covered with wrinkled, macerated epidermis. **If blistered skin is removed, it will leave a pink raw surface and later the exposed dermis becomes brownish, hard and dry. Blisters have an hyperaemic zone around them. There is a reddening and swelling of the papillae in the floor of the blister. The blister fluid contains white and red cells.** A postmortem blister does not show hyperaemia in the surrounding area and the floor is not red. Scalds show soddening and bleaching but do not singe the hair, and do not blacken or char the skin Table (11–4). **Superheated steam** soddens the skin which becomes dirty-white colour.

Degrees of Scalds: (1) Erythema by vasoparalysis. (2) Blister formation due to increased permeability of the capillaries. (3) Necrosis of the dermis.

Features: The injury is limited to the area of contact and is more severe at the point of the initial contact. **Scalding can occur through clothing**. Clothes worsen the damage by prolonging contact with hot liquid and reducing the cooling effect of evaporation. Scalded areas are usually large, but may be small if caused by splashing. **Streaks of liquid run downwards from the main area causing lines of blisters. Sticky liquids, such as syrup, oils and tar cause more severe scalds than hot water.** There is usually a sharply demarcated edge, corresponding to the limits of contact of the fluid. The scalded skin may swell and exude serum. Scars of scalds are much thinner than those of deep burns and cause less contraction and disfigurement.

If inflammable fluids are used, signs of trickling of the burning fluid will be present on some parts of the body, e.g. if kerosene is splashed on a body lying on its back and then ignited, runs of burning liquid will be seen on the sides of the neck, sides of the trunk, between the thighs, etc. When scalds are extensive death usually occurs from shock, fluid and electrolyte disturbance and secondary infection.

Toxic epidermal necrolysis due to disease or drugs cause blistering and separation of superficial layers of skin with a raw weeping surface has a close similar appearance to a scald.

OCCURRENCE: Scalds are usually accidental due to bursting of hot water bottles, bursting of boilers, splashing of fluid from cooking utensils, or pulling over saucepans or kettles by children, etc. (splash burn). Occasionally, children suck the spouts of kettles, which causes severe steam scalds of the mouth and air-passages with oedema of the glottis. Suicide by scalding is rare. Boiling water may be thrown with intent to injure. Murder by scalding is rare. Steam burns are rare.

SPONTANEOUS HUMAN COMBUSTION (Preternatural combustion) :

This is very rare. During putrefaction, inflammable gases are produced in abdomen due to the action of microorganisms upon organic

matter. These gases are ignited if a flame is nearby. A human body may sometimes burn away almost completely, with minimal damage to the surrounding area. This occurs invariably near a hearth, or open fire-grate or chimney. The burning may be confined to the body, its clothing and a narrow zone of floor or carpet.

Often the victims are alcoholic and confused, instable and lack judgement. It appears that when a person usually an elderly woman collapses and falls, and part of the body comes in contact with a source of heat, clothing catches fire and burns the limited amount of oxygen available in the room, after which that part is ignited, and adjacent body fat melts and soaks into clothes. The clothing acts as a wick, melts the next zone of adjacent fat, and the process is repeated along the length of the body, till the knee joints are reached, and the burning stops because of less fat and also covered with less layers of the clothes. Often, all soft tissues are reduced to ash and most of bones are calcined. The only part of body left undamaged is likely to be one or both of lower legs. Usually CO is not found in the blood. The room in which the body is found is frequently very hot and the contents, walls, furniture, etc. are heavily soiled by soot, but there is no fire damage to any of the objects in the room.

ELECTRICAL INJURIES

PHYSICAL FACTORS: Voltage is the fundamental force or pressure that causes electricity to flow through a conductor and is measured in volts. Resistance is anything that impedes the flow of electricity through a conductor and is measured in ohms. Current is the flow of electrons from a source of voltage through a conductor and is measured in amperes. The injuries caused by contact with electrical conductors depend upon: (1) THE KIND OF CURRENT: Alternating current is 4 to 5 times as dangerous as an equal voltage of direct current. An alternating current is one that reverses its direction at regular intervals. In direct current, current flows in the same direction. (2) THE AMOUNT OF CURRENT: The amount of current that will flow through or over the body may be determined by the formula $A = V \div R$, where A is current in amperes, V is potential difference in volts and R is the resistance of the body in ohms. The flow of the current through the body is great, if the voltage is high (more than 1000 volts) or if the resistance is low. Electrocution is rare at less than 100 volts, and most deaths occur at more than 200 volts. In India, the voltage of domestic supply is usually 220 to 240 volts, alternating current with 50 cycles per second. Currents of 10mA cause pain and muscle contractions, over 60 mA are dangerous, and 100 mA is fatal. High voltages (more than thousand volts) may cause the victim to be thrown clear, while lower tensions, around 240, cause muscle contraction, due to which the victim holds on to the source of the current. (3) THE PATH OF THE CURRENT: Death is more likely to occur if the brain stem or heart are in the direct path of the current. (4) DURATION OF THE CURRENT FLOW: The severity is directly proportional to the duration of current flow. Electrocution is death caused by passage of electric current, Figs. (11–22 and 11–23).

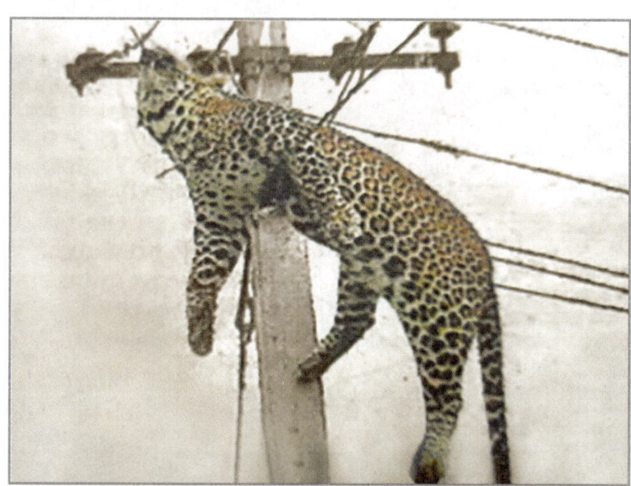

Fig. (11–22). The body of leopard dangling on an electric pole.

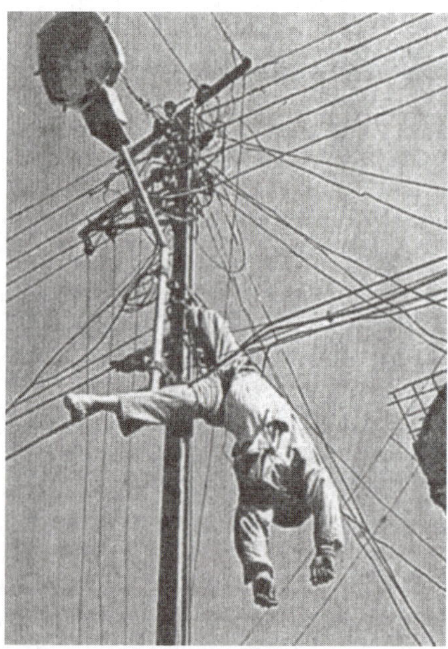

Fig. (11–23). Electrocution during working on a pole for repairs.

Electrical injuries consist of (1) Fatal electrocution, (2) electric shock, (3) burns. For an electric shock to occur there must be contact by the body with both a positive and negative pole, or alternatively, the 'earth'. The earth may be any object not insulated from the ground. When earthing of the body is poor, as with dry and rubber shoes, carpets, wooden floors and upstair premises, fatal electrocution is uncommon. The effects of electricity depends on the voltage and the resistance offered by the body. If the body is well insulated, it does not conduct the current and no harm results. Dry skin offers high resistance but the resistance is diminished when the skin is moist or covered with sweat. Blood has a low resistance, and as such within the body, electricity tends to be conducted along blood vessels. Predisposing factors are unexpectedness of shock, anxiety, fear and emotions, exhaustion, cardiovascular and other diseases.

Local Effects: The current passes through the skin producing heat, which causes boiling and electrolysis of tissue fluids. The skin explodes and rolls back from the surface. **A well-moistened skin may not show electrical burn, while a thick dry skin may show well-marked electrical burn.**

(1) The electric mark (Joule burn): It is specific and diagnostic of contact with electricity and is found at the point of entry of the current. It is seen in accidents with high tension currents Fig. (11–24). It is endogenous thermal burn due to the heat generated in the body from electricity. These marks are round or oval, shallow craters, one to three cm. in diameter, and have a ridge of skin of about one to three mm. high, around part or the whole of their circumference. The crater floor is lined by pale flattened skin Fig. (11–25). In some marks, the skin may break within or near the margin of the crater, resembling that of a broken blister. When contact is more prolonged, the skin in the mark becomes brown and with further contact, there may be charring. If the conductor contains copper, the electric mark can have a bright green colour. **Occasionally, the mark may have a distinctive pattern,** that of the shape of the conductor, especially where this is a linear wire or a shaped metal object. **A characteristic feature is the presence of an**

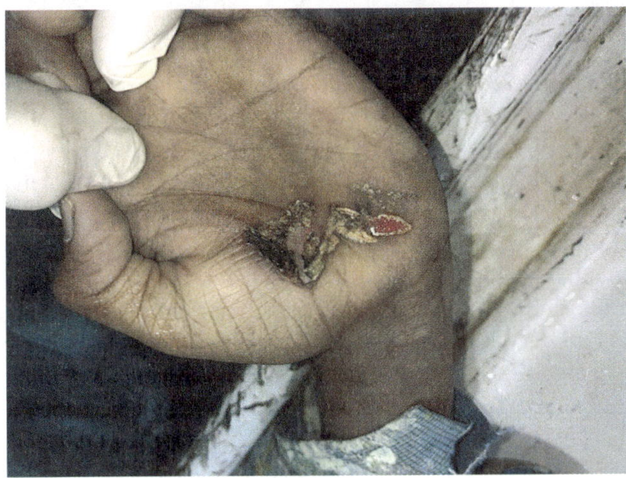

Fig. (11–24). **Entrance electric marks on the palm of the hand.**

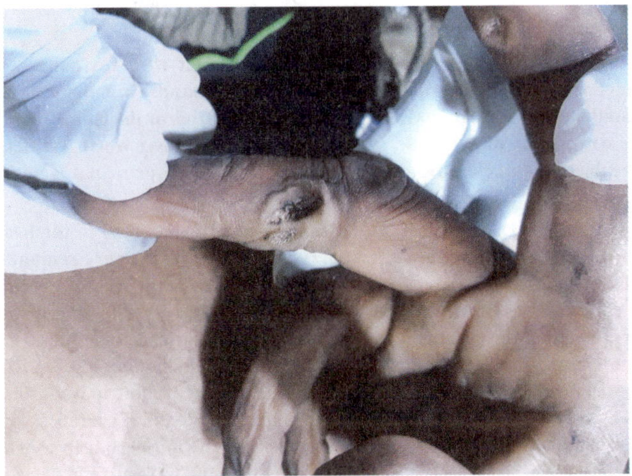

Fig. (11–25). **Joule burn on index finger.**

areola of blanched skin seen at the periphery of the electric mark, which survives death and is pathognomonic of electrical damage. Often there is hyperaemic border outside the blanching. Occasionally, an alternating spectrum of blister-reddening-pallor-reddening is seen. They are commonly found on exposed parts of the body, especially on the palmar aspect of the hands.

Histological examination of the electric mark usually shows coagulation of the dermis, with separation of the epidermis in some areas, and in other areas the cells become elongated and arranged in parallel rows at an acute angle, or almost at right angles to the dermis.

(2) Flash or Spark Burns: The intense heat which may result from flash-over produces burns, which resemble thermal burns (exogenous burns). In spark burn, there is an air gap between metal and skin. Here a central nodule of fused keratin, brown or yellow in colour is surrounded by the typical areola of pale skin. The burns may be as small as pinpoints, or deeply seated and contracted if contact is prolonged or very high voltage is applied.

High voltage burns may be very severe with charring of the body. High tension injuries are caused by flash, flame or the current itself. Multiple individual and confluent areas of third degree burns are seen. Soft tissue can be destroyed over a wide area. **1000 volts will jump several mm and 100 kilovolts about 35 cm.** Very high voltage currents **produce massive destruction of tissue with loss of extremities and rupture of organs.** When bone is involved, periosteum may be elevated or superficial layers of the bone may be destroyed or fracture may occur. Sometimes, multiple lesions are found in the region of flexures of a limb where the current has passed across the joints, instead of passing around it. High tension electrical currents may produce multiple, small, discrete, pitted burns due to arcing from the conductor to the body without direct contact. In high voltage contacts, the skin of wide area may be brown or greyish, partly from heat effects and partly from metallisation. **Multiple burnt or punched-out lesions are produced due to the arc dancing over the body surface over large areas which present 'crocodile flash burns' Fig. (11–26).** Flash-over often produce **'arc eye'.** High amperage has an explosive blast-like effect and may produce injuries resembling bullet, stab or incised wounds.

Absence of burns: (1) In low voltage electrocution, if the area of contact is relatively large, e.g. when a hot wire is grasped with a wet hand, or when a person is electrocuted in bath tub. (2) When the area of contact is small in low-voltage electrocutions. (3) Brief contact with a live wire, may not produce burns. In this case, the person may collapse from ventricular fibrillation and fall away from the wire.

(3) Electric burns or splits: When the electrical conductor is a wire, a linear burn may occur. **When burn is linear, such as that from a bare wire pressed against the skin, the areola has a pale zone parallel to central burn.** Where the tip of the wire or rod is at right angle to the skin, the mark may be present as a circular hole, penetrating skin, muscle and even bone, so as to simulate a bullet hole. When the current passes from a metal conductor into the body, metallic ions are embedded in the skin and even in subcutaneous tissues. If copper or brass conductors are involved, a bright green imprint may be seen, which persists for some weeks during life. **The splits are dry, hard, firm, charred, insensitive, with ragged edges, and their form is round, oval, linear, or of irregular shape.** The depth of the lesion is much greater than appears on the surface. Shedding of the superficial layers of the skin is common, and some of this may be found attached to the conductor. Wrinkling of the skin may

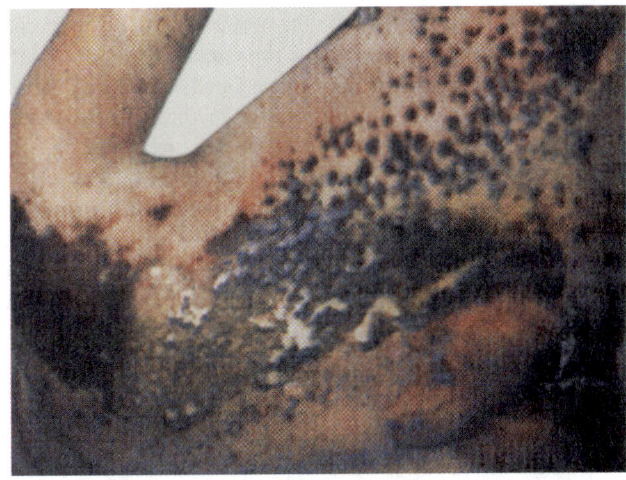

Fig. (11–26). **Crocodile skin appearance in high voltage electric shock.**

be found and occasionally localised oedema of a limb. Aseptic necrosis develops, which often extends beyond the burns in area and depth and may lead to sloughing.

HISTOPATHOLOGY: Microblisters develop within the squamous epithelium and in the external horny layer, due to the cooking effect on the tissues. They represent defects through which the steam exited. Larger vacuoles are produced within the epidermal cells, the nuclei of which are fusiform, hyperchromatic and show a peculiar distortion with stretching and narrowing of the contour and produce palisade-type appearance. This change is called streaming of the nuclei. These flattened cells usually stain darker than the normal cells with haemotoxylin and eosin. The nuclei of the vascular media tend to be twisted to resemble spirals, which may be seen at distant points from the site of contact with the electrode. There may be localised degeneration of the intima. Tearing of elastic fibres and the overlying intima is common and may cause secondary thrombosis.

Exit Marks: These are variable in appearance, but they have some of the features of entrance marks. There may be more damage of tissues, and they are often seen as splits in the skin at points where the skin has been raised into ridges by the passage of current; splitting of these ridges may be continuous or interrupted.

Postmortem Appearances: External: The examination of the scene may be much more important than the postmortem of the body. The clothing, including shoes, gloves and headgear should be examined for burns. **In cardiac arrhythmia, victim will be pale, and in respiratory paralysis cyanosed.** The eyes are congested and the pupils dilated. Rigor mortis appears early, and postmortem lividity is well developed. **In about 50 to 60% cases there are external marks of electric burning, and contusion or laceration at the point of entrance and exit of the body. In some cases, the lesions may extend through subcutaneous tissues and involve muscles and bone.** A number of greyish-white circular spots, which are firm to the touch and free from zone of inflammation may be found at the site of entrance and exit. Severe convulsions caused by electrical discharge may cause fractures of the spine or limbs. **Extensive ecchymosis may be found on the skin of the trunk.** In some cases, external lesions may be absent and frequently they are so slight as to require careful search. Occasionally, only the hair is singed. Arcing of the current may produce characteristic pit-like defects on the surface of the hair. Current marks may be hidden inside the oral cavity, from putting live wires into the mouth or from drinking at a water fountain in contact with electric current. They may be found in the urethra due to urination on a high tension wire. **In some cases, the entrance and exit marks cannot be determined grossly.** Occasionally, the site of entrance may be determined by histochemical methods or by electron microscopy from the deposition of metal particles on the skin. **Any metallic objects on the body will produce corresponding burns on the skin,** because it becomes heated by the passage of the current. This metallisation is due to the volatilisation of the metal, particles of which are driven into the skin. **Differentiation between antermortem and postmortem electrical burns is not possible.**

Extensive burning may occur, even beneath clothes when a person dies in front of an electric or gas fire.

Internal: The appearances are usually those of asphyxia. The lungs are congested and oedematous, and the brain, meninges and parenchymatous organs are congested. Petechial haemorrhages may be found along the line of the passage of the current, under the endocardium, pericardium, pleura, brain and the spinal cord. In some cases, irregular tears and fissures in the brain tissue and rupture of walls of arteries are seen. There may be necrosis of the intima, or of the complete wall of the blood vessels. Vascular thromboses may be seen in the vicinity of electrical burns. Skeletal muscle in the path of the current may show Zenker's degeneration. **High amperage has an explosive effect and may produce injuries resembling bullet, stab or cut wounds. Small balls of molten metal, derived from the metal of the contacting electrode, so-called current pearls, may be carried deep into the tissues. Heat generated by the current may melt the calcium phosphate, which is seen radiologically as typical round density foci (bone pearls or wax drippings).** There may be bone necrosis, and zigzag microfractures. A foetus may survive the electrocuted mother or a surviving mother may abort after electric injury. Occasionally, no lesions can be found either externally or internally. Death in these cases may be due to vagal stimulation.

TREATMENT: If the person is in contact with the source of electricity, he should not be pulled with bare hands, but the current should be switched off or the victim moved by a stick or the hands should be wrapped in dry cloth or newspaper, or rubber gloves worn. Artificial respiration and closed chest cardiac massage are the principal forms of treatment.

CAUSE OF DEATH: Circuits from any of the limbs to the head involve the brain stem and upper cervical cord. Arm-to-arm circuit may also involve the upper cervical cord. In these cases, death probably occurs from paralysis of medullary (respiratory) centres. Arm-to-arm or left arm to either leg circuits involve the heart and death occurs either from ventricular fibrillation or cardiac arrest without fibrillation, Fig. (11–30). Death need not be instantaneous. Individuals may be able to walk some distance and talk before the onset of collapse and death. If current is low, but contact time is great (minutes) death occurs by muscle paralysis with secondary asphyxia. Death in high voltage is due to respiratory arrest or electrodermal injuries. In non-fatal cases, hemiplegia or paraplegia, loss of sight, hearing and memory may occur or there may be no effect.

In delayed deaths, unconsciousness occurs, often accompanied by signs of circulatory and respiratory failure. Death may occur after a few days from infection, or from haemorrhage due to damage to blood vessels.

MEDICOLEGAL ASPECTS: Death by electric currents are usually accidental from defective electric appliances or negligence in the use of equipment, flying kites and short-circuit. Erection of electrified wires to protect property or to attach a live wire to door knobs, gates, railings, etc. against thieves may cause death of intruder. In industry, deaths may result from contact with live overhead cables or from handling of charged lamps, tools or switch gears. Rarely, death may occur during convulsive therapy to mental patients (iatrogenic) but cases of suicide, and even homicide have occurred. The viscera should be analysed to know whether the victim was impaired at the time of the accident. Suicide is rare. A person usually winds wires round his fingers or wrists, which are then connected to the mains supply by means of a plug and the current is switched on.

Judicial Electrocution: Death penalty is carried out in the electric chair in some states in the U.S.A. The condemned man is strapped to a wooden chair and one cap-like electrode is put on the shaven scalp which is moistened with a conducting paste and the other on the right lower leg, and **a current of 2,000 volts and 7 amperes is passed for one minute through the body**. After tetanic spasm and loss of consciousness, **the same current is passed through the body a second time for one minute.** Third degree burns are produced at the site of contact between the electrodes and skin. The brain is heated up to 60°C. and vacuolation occurs around the vessels.

LIGHTNING STROKE

PHYSICAL FACTORS: A flash or bolt of lightning is due to an electrical discharge from a cloud to the earth. The electric current is direct with a potential of abut twenty-thousand amperes and about one hundred to thousand million volts or more. Along the track of the current much energy is liberated, most of which is converted into light. A single flash of lightning stroke lasts about 1/1000 of a second, due to which no burns or only minor burns and singeing of hair may be seen. It is attracted by the highest points. It passes normally along the outside of a conductor, and as such, persons in buildings are relatively safe from electrocution. Dry skin and dry clothes are bad conductors, whereas wet skin and wet clothes are good conductors. Lightning or atmospheric electricity differs from ordinary electric current only in degree. The effects are seen in an area about 30 metres in diameter. A lightning bolt may injure or kill a person by a direct strike, a side-flash, or conduction through another object. In a direct strike or a side-flash strike, the current can spread over the surface of the body, enter it or follow both routes. In a side-flash strike, the flash of lightning hits an object, e.g. a tree, and jumping from it, strikes the person. Rarely a person may be injured while indoors, while in the shower or bathtub, the current travelling along water pipes, or while using the telephone.

FACTORS INFLUENCING INJURIES: Four factors are involved: (1) Direct effect from electric discharge passing to earth. (2) Surface 'flash' burns from the discharge. (3) Mechanical effect due to force of displaced air around the flash by heat expansion, and (4) Compression effect due to air movement in its return wave.

Clothes: The clothes are usually burnt or torn at the point of entrance and exit. In some cases, the clothes may be stripped off the body and thrown to some distance. In exceptional cases, clothing is not damaged even though the person is killed by lightning. Conversely, clothing may be burnt without any injury to the person.

Study of pathology of lightening is called Keraunopathology.

Postmortem appearances: External: The expanded, displaced air causes disruptive or blast-like lesions, e.g., contusions, lacerations, fractures, ruptures of organs, wounds of almost any variety, burns, etc. Extensive ecchymoses may be seen on the skin of the trunk. **Internal:** Belts and boots may be ruptured. Rigor mortis may appear soon and pass off quickly. Intense oedema of the skin develops at points of entry of current in those who survive, probably due to paralysis of local capillary and lymphatic vessels. If the patient survives for some time internal vessels will show clots and thrombi and affected organs will show necrosis and gangrene.

Signs of asphyxia are present. Leptomeninges may be congested or lacerated. The brain may be congested or oedematous. Subarachnoid and intracerebral bleeding may occur. Patches of haemorrhages may be seen under the pleura and pericardium. Lungs are congested. Blood vessels may be thrombosed or ruptured. Rupture of ear drum and haemorrhage in middle ear may be seen.

The burns may be: (1) Linear: These vary from 3 to 30 cm. or more in length, and 0.3 to 2.5 cm. in width. They are often found in the moist creases and folds of the skin. Irregular, linear, first degree burns may follow skin creases, esp. if damp from sweating.

(2) Arborescent or Filigree Burns (Lichtenberg's flowers): **They are superficial, thin, irregular and tortuous markings on the skin. These markings have a general pattern resembling the branches of a tree. This fern-like pattern of erythema in the skin is usually found over the shoulders or the flanks Figs. (11–27 and 11–28).** It appears within few minutes to one hour of accident.

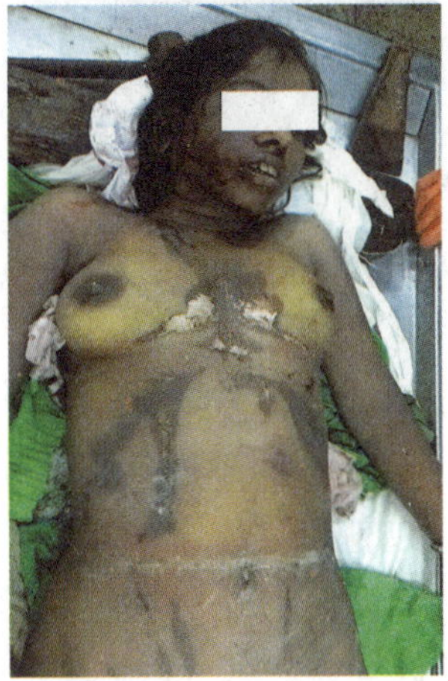

Fig. (11–27). Burns due to lightning.
Courtesy: **Dr Satish Kumar Khalkho, BHU, Varanasi**

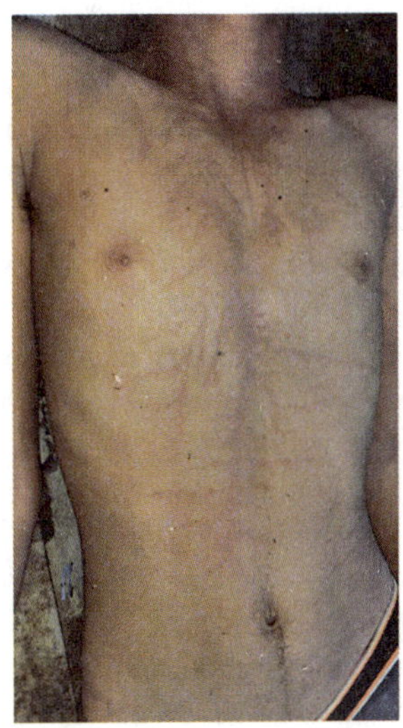

Fig. (11–28). Filgree or arborescent burn marks in a case of lightning.
Courtesy: **Dr Radhey Khetre, Associate Professor, GMC, Aurangabab MS.**

Mechanism: The mechanism by which this pattern occurs is not known. It may be caused due to the slight staining of the tissues by haemoglobin from lysed red blood cells along the path of the electric current or rupture of smaller blood vessels at several places giving rise to ecchymoses. They may be superficial burns producing mere erythema of skin which indicate the path taken by the current. They seem to be caused by electron showers induced by lightning, or from boiling of the intercellular fluid following the fascial planes Fig. (11–29). **They indicate the paths taken by the discharge, and disappear in one to two days if the person survivers Fig. (11–30). These marks are seen rarely. Red streaks following skin creases or sweat-damped tracks are more likely**

(3) Surface Burns: They are true burns and occur beneath metallic objects worn or carried by the person, which are fused by the flash.

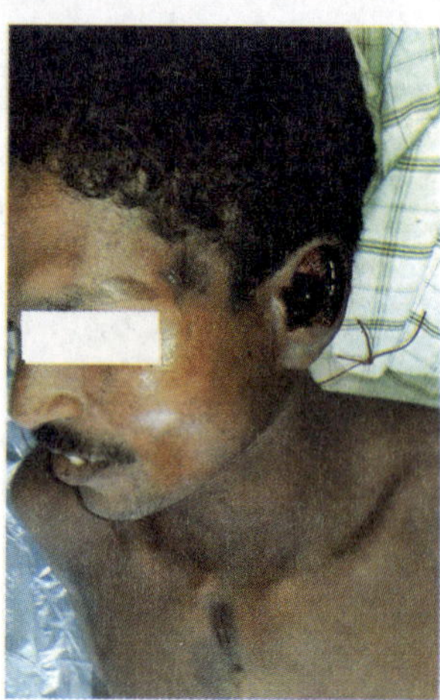

Fig. (11–29). **Bleeding due to rupture of tympanic membrane in lightning.**

Courtesy: **Dr Satish Kumar Khalkho, BHU, Varanasi**

Keraunoparalysis (Lightning paralysis), is a transient paralysis of lower limb and is associated with extreme vasoconstriction and sensory disturbances of one or more extremities.

Cause of Death: Involvement of the central nervous system with paralysis of the heart or of the respiratory centre or electrothermal injuries cause death.

Survived person may be unconscious or confused for several hours after the event and subsequently exhibit neurological signs, which usually resolve within a few days.

Medicolegal Importance: Most deaths occur in the open, e.g. persons sheltering under trees, open fields, especially if they are carrying or wearing something which may attract lightning. Persons seated in motor vehicles do not suffer harm due to insulation provided by tyres or due to not having a circuit within it. **Less than half of the persons struck by lightning are killed. Death is always due to accident. Sometimes, the appearances left on the human body closely resemble those produced by criminal violence. Thus a person may be found dead in an open field or on the highway and body may show contusions, lacerations and fractures.** In such cases, the diagnosis should be based on the history of a thunderstorm in the locality, evidence of effects of lightning in the vicinity of the body, and fusion or magnetisation of metallic substances.

RADIATION

The decomposition of atoms accompanied by emission of radiant energy such as alpha, beta, or gamma rays is known as radioactivity. Thorium, uranium, and cadmium emit radiant energy. Radiation causes damage through conservation of infrared frequencies into thermal heat on absorption at the skin surface. Man is exposed to ionising radiation from: (1) Industrial applications. (2) Medical applications (a) traces, (b) internal therapeutic agents, (c) external therapeutic techniques. Man is exposed to slight amount of radiation from cosmic rays, nuclear reactor accidents, television sets and nuclear weapon testing.

Radiation Syndrome: With doses of 200-250 rods illness with rising mortality is seen. More than 500 rods result in 100% mortality. With less severe but lethal dose, nausea and vomiting occur immediately followed by diarrhoea. About fifth day vomiting, dehydration, profound electrolyte imbalance, circulatory collapse and death occurs.

Delayed Effects: These are seen many months or years later. They are: (1) Malignant tumours and Leukaemia. (2) Dermatitis, ulceration and infection. (3) Gangrene. (4) Depression of all elements of bone marrow. (5) Increased permeability of blood vessels. (6) Cataract. (7) Sterility in both sexes. (8) Osteosarcoma. (9) Stillbirths, congenital malnutritions, mental defects.

Legal problems are: (1) Negligence of treating doctor. (2) Compensation where workers when they are exposed to radiation due to fault of establishments.

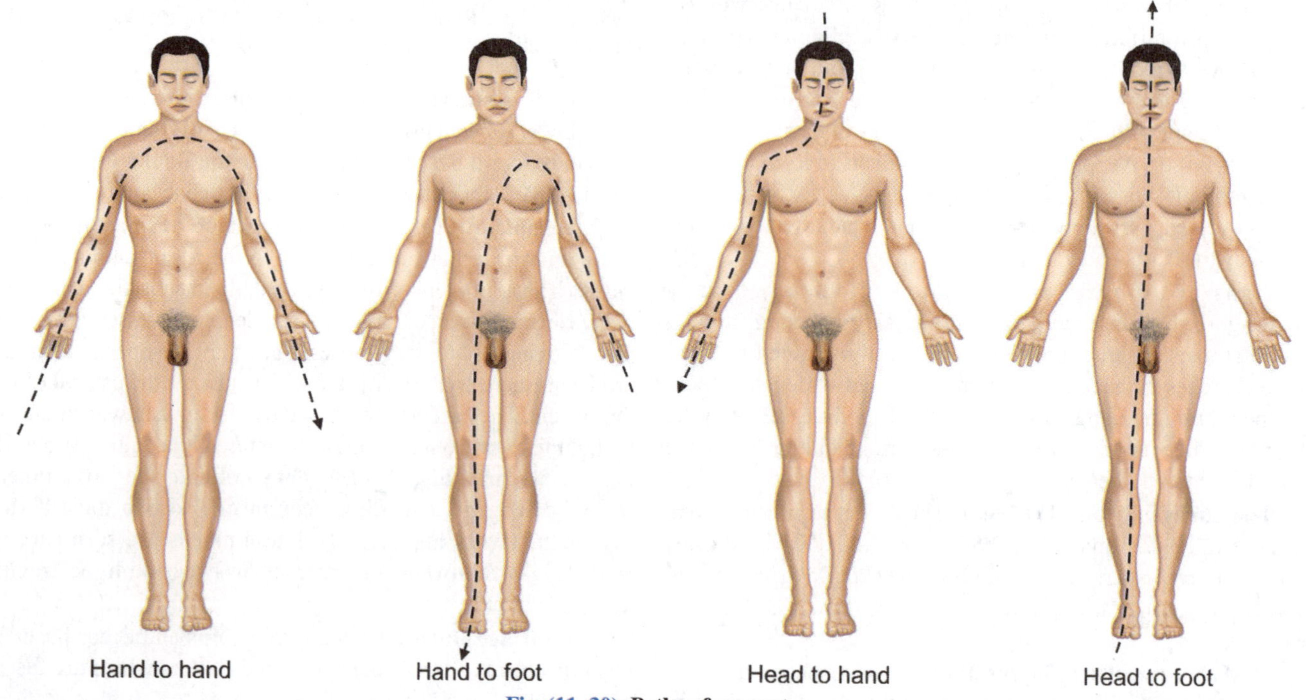

Fig. (11–30). **Paths of current.**

CHAPTER

12 STARVATION

FM 2.26: Describe and discuss clinical features, postmortem findings and medicolegal aspects of death due to starvation and neglect.

Starvation may occur from the actual withholding of food or from the administration of unsuitable food.

Types: (1) Acute and (2) Chronic.

Causes: Acute starvation results from sudden and complete stoppage of food. Chronic starvation results from gradual deficient supply of food. Starvation deaths may be due to (1) famine, (2) being trapped in pits, mines or landslides, (3) neglect on the part of the parents or guardians, (4) wilful withholding of food, and (5) wilful refusal to take food.

Symptoms: In acute starvation, there is a feeling of hunger for the first 30 to 48 hours, which is followed by pain in the epigastrium which is relieved by pressure. After four to five days of starvation, general emaciation and absorption of the subcutaneous fat begins to occur. The eyes are sunken and glistening, the pupils are dilated, the cheeks sink and the bony prominences become visible. **Bichat's buccal pad of fat is among the last subcutaneous adipose tissue to disappear.** The lips are dry and cracked, the tongue coated and dirty, and thirst is intolerable. The saliva is thick and scanty. The voice is weak and whispering. The skin is dry, rough, thin, inelastic, wrinkled and pigmented. Emaciation may be extreme, the abdomen concave from costal margins to iliac crests and limbs become thin and flaccid with loss of muscular power. **Muscular weakness is progressive and may be severe. Cardiovascular changes are those of progressive insufficiency.** The pulse is slow at rest, but on exertion paroxysmal tachycardia supervenes. The temperature is subnormal. Constipation is usual, but towards death diarrhoea and dysentery are common. The urine is scanty, turbid and highly concentrated, and shows evidence of acidosis. The loss of weight is most marked and constant. **In the last stage, the body is reduced to an extreme state of emaciation Fig. (12–1).** The ribs are prominent, with concavities in the intercostal spaces and sunken supraclavicular fossae. Before death the body has an offensive odour. **Death usually occurs when 40% of the original weight is reached.** The intellect remains clear till death, though in some cases delusions and hallucinations of sight and hearing occur.

MECHANISM: As starvation continues, at first rapid mobilisation of protein stores occur which are converted by the liver to glucose, which is mainly used to supply energy to the brain. After that, the main means of energy production is lipolysis. Adipose tissue releases free fatty acids. In the liver they are the substrate for synthesis of ketone bodies, which are used as fuels for skeletal and heart muscles and brain. As complete depletion of fat stores approaches, protein is again rapidly used as a source of energy.

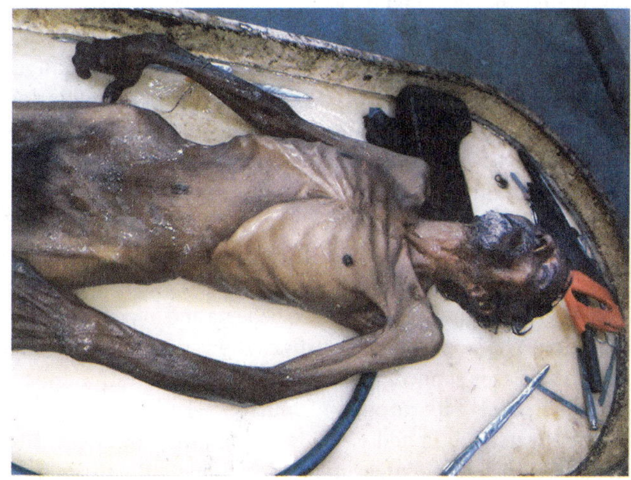

Fig. (12–1). **Starvation.**

CHRONIC STARVATION: The changes are constant and develop in a constant order. (1) Loss of well-being, hunger and hunger-pains. (2) Mental and physical lethargy and easy fatigue. (3) Progressive loss of weight which is rapid in the first six months. (4) Polyuria. (5) Increasing cachexia, the body weight is reduced by about 40% of the normal. Pigmentation and anaemia. (6) Hypothermia, peripheral vascular stasis in cold and hypotension. (7) Extreme lethargy, gross mental retardation and loss of self-respect. (8) Oedema, first in the feet and lower limbs. (9) Reduced resistance to infection causing diarrhoea, dysentery, tuberculosis, etc.

The blood sugar, proteins, chlorides and cholesterol are lowered. Non-protein nitrogen and urea, plasma free acids and ketone bodies are raised.

Cause of Death: Death occurs from exhaustion, circulatory failure due to brown atrophy of the heart, intercurrent infection or multiorgan failure with ventricular fibrillation. Dehydration and hypothermia contribute to death.

Fatal Period: If both water and food are completely withdrawn death occurs in 10 to 12 days. If food alone is withdrawn death occurs in 6 to 8 weeks or even more. **Death usually occurs when about 70 to 90% of body fat, and 20% of body protein are lost.** Newborns may survive for 7 to 10 days without food or water.

FACTORS INFLUENCING THE FATAL PERIOD: (1) Age: The very young and the old suffer the worst. (2) Sex: Females withstand starvation for a longer period. (3) Condition of the body: Fatty, healthy people stand starvation better. (4) Temperature: Exposure to cold or

excessive heat hastens death. (5) Physical exertion: Active physical exertion hastens death.

Postmortem Appearances: External: Rigor mortis sets in and disappears early. The face is pale, the skin inelastic and pigmented. Sometimes, follicular hyperkeratosis develops. Subcutaneous patches of oedema are seen around the ankles and inside the thighs. **In the wet type, there is marked oedema of face, trunk and limbs with ascites and pleural effusions.** Trophic skin changes and infections are common. Pressure sores on buttocks, heels and spine may occur. The hair is dry, lustreless and brittle, and nails are also brittle.

Internal: Fat is almost completely absent in the subcutaneous tissues and also in the omentum, mesentery and about the internal organs, which is never seen in wasting disease. The fat of the female breast and of the orbit is spared till late. Subepicardial fat becomes replaced by a watery gelatinous material. In children, the skeleton shows spinal curvature, rickets and dental defects. In adults progressive demineralisation and osteomalacia are seen. Stress fractures may occur. **All organs and tissues show changes similar to premature senility. There is extreme emaciation and general reduction in size and weight of all the organs except the brain,** which is sometimes pale and soft. Muscles are atrophied and darker due to increase in lipochrome. The fibres lose striations and become more uniform from granular degeneration. The heart is small from brown atrophy and the chambers are empty. The lungs are pale and collapsed, and exude very little blood when cut. Rarely, there may be oedema and hypostatic basal congestion. The stomach and intestines show atrophy of all coats and the mucosa is stained with bile. The walls of intestine appear like tissue paper with atrophy of mucosa. The bowel contains offensive watery fluid and gas. **There may be superficial but extensive non-specific ulceration of the bowel like those seen in ulcerative colitis.** The liver is atrophied and may show necrosis due to protein deficiency. Spleen is shrunken. The gall bladder is distended with bile. The kidneys show atrophy of the nephron. Blood volume is markedly reduced, and there is marked anaemia. The urinary bladder is empty. There may be evidence of some intercurrent disease.

Medicolegal Aspects: The exclusion of disease likely to cause loss of weight, e.g., malignant disease, progressive muscular atrophy, Addison's disease, diabetes mellitus, tuberculosis, pernicious anaemia, chronic diarrhoea is essential. Sometimes, it may be impossible to determine whether it was the cause or effect of malnutrition, e.g. tuberculosis. **If marked loss of weight and especially the absence of fat are found at autopsy, and there is no evidence of disease, a diagnosis of death due to starvation can be made.**

Right to life as guaranteed under article 21 of the Constitution of India, does not include the right to die, and as such **arrest and forcible feeding of persons going on hunger strike is lawful. Loss of weight and acidosis with ketone bodies in urine are the criteria to advise forced feeding.**

SUICIDE: Sometimes, persons fast voluntarily, for the purpose of exhibition. Lunatics and hysterical women may refuse food. Fasting may be undertaken by persons to attract public attention, e.g., fast unto death, for rectification of grievances.

HOMICIDE: The victim is usually an infant, or any other person, e.g., aged or feeble-minded are starved with evil intention. Illegitimate children are frequently starved to death. Children starved by their parents or guardians is known as "Baby-farmer".

ACCIDENT: Accidental starvation may occur during famine, being trapped in pits or mines, landslides, shipwreck, etc. It may be due to ignorance which leads to a failure to provide enough food or to provide food of the right kind. It may also occur in stricture or cancer of the oesophagus or ankylosis of jaw. Signs of neglect and emaciation may be seen in drug addicts, where the desire for the drug is more than the desire for food. Either due to psychiatric causes, usually of a paranoid schizophrenic nature or due to senile dementia, some persons, usually old, refuse to spend money on food, clothes, etc.

CHAPTER

13

MECHANICAL ASPHYXIA

FM 2.20: Mechanical asphyxia: Define, classify and describe asphyxia and medicolegal interpretation of postmortem findings in asphyxial deaths.
FM 2.21: Mechanical asphyxia: Describe and discuss different types of hanging and strangulation including clinical findings, causes of death, postmortem findings and medicolegal aspects of death due to hanging and strangulation including examination, preservation and dispatch of ligature material.
FM 2.22: Mechanical asphyxia: Describe and discuss pathophysiology, clinical features, postmortem findings and medicolegal aspects of traumatic asphyxia, obstruction of nose and mouth, suffocation and sexual asphyxia.
FM 2.23: Describe and discuss types, pathophysiology, clinical features, post mortem findings and medicolegal aspects of drowning, diatom test and, Gettler test.

Mechanical asphyxia is a broad term in which enough external pressure is applied to the neck, chest or other areas of the body, or the body is positioned in such a way that respiration is difficult or impossible Fig. (13–1).

HANGING

Hanging (self-suspension) is that form of asphyxia which is caused by suspension of the body by a ligature which encircles the neck, the constricting force being the weight of the body.

Classification: (I) Depending on degree of suspension: (a) Complete hanging: Body is completely suspended without any part of the body touching the ground. **(b) 'Partial hanging':** the body is partly suspended, the toes or feet touching the ground, or is in a sitting, kneeling, lying down, prone or any other posture, with only the head and chest off the ground. **The weight of the head (5 to 6 kg), chest and arms act as the constricting force. The whole weight of the body is not necessary, and only a comparatively slight force is enough to produce death. (II) Depending on position of the knot: (a) Typical hanging: The ligature runs from the midline above the thyroid cartilage symmetrically upward on both sides of the neck to the occipital region and the knot is over the central part of back of neck.** (b) **Atypical Hanging:** The knot is anywhere other than on the occiput, i.e. on the right or left side or front of the neck.

Ligature: A suicide will use any article readily available for the purpose, like a rope, cord, metallic chains and wires, leather strap, belt, bed sheet, scarf, *dhotie, saree, turban, sacred thread,* etc. **The doctor should note whether the mark on the neck corresponds with the material alleged to have been used in hanging, and if it is strong enough to bear the weight and the jerk of the body. He should also note its texture and length, to know whether it was sufficient to hang.** Before removing the ligature from the neck, it should be described as to the nature and composition, width, mode of application, location and type of knot, and take a photograph. Sometimes, the rope will break or become detached and the deceased will be found lying on the ground with a ligature around his neck.

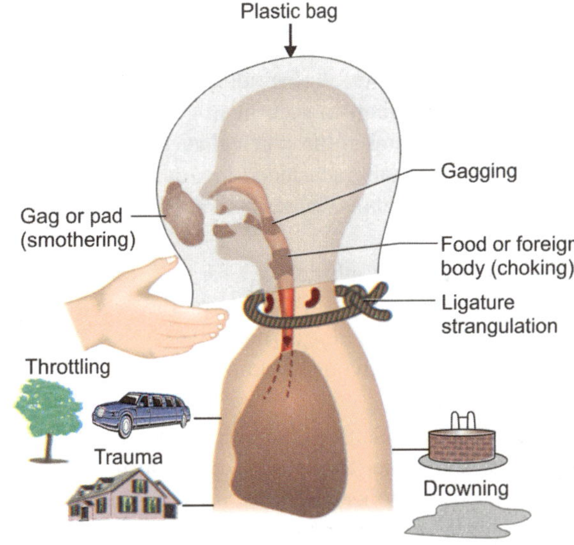

Fig. (13–1). Mechanical asphyxia.

SYMPTOMS: The first symptoms are loss of power and subjective sensations, such as flashes of light and ringing and hissing noises in the ears. There is intense mental confusion, all power of logical thought is lost; the individual can do nothing to help himself even if it were possible. These are followed by loss of consciousness (within 15 seconds when a thin rope is used), and as such it is regarded as a painless form of death. Then follows a stage of convulsions. The face is distorted and livid, eyes prominent, and there is violent struggling. Respiration stops before the heart, which may continue to beat for about 10 to 15 minutes.

Cause of Death: (1) **Asphyxia:** The constricting force of the ligature causes compressive narrowing of laryngeal and tracheal lumina, and forces up the root of the tongue against the posterior wall of the pharynx, and **folds the epiglottis over the entrance of the larynx to block the airway. Obstruction of the airway**

usually causes struggle, known as air hunger. If entry of air into the lungs is completely prevented, death occurs rapidly with marked asphyxial signs. A tension of 15 kg. on ligature blocks the trachea. (2) **Venous congestion:** If the knot is situated in the chin area, **venous flow is obstructed, but arterial flow may continue.** The jugular veins are blocked by the compression of the ligature which results in stoppage of the cerebral circulation, and a rapid rise in venous pressure in the head and unconsciousness. This occurs if ligature is made up of broad and soft material, which cannot sink into tissue to any depth. The jugular veins are closed by a tension in the rope of 2 kg. (3) **Combined asphyxia and venous congestion**: This is the commonest cause. (4) **Cerebral anaemia**: If the knot is situated in the region of nape of neck, **both arterial and venous blood flow are cut off** by pressure of the noose on both sides of neck. Pressure on the large arteries on the neck produces cerebral anaemia and immediate coma (10 to 15 seconds). If pressure is immediately released, consciousness is regained in 10 to 12 seconds. Death will be slow and asphyxial features are less marked. This occurs with ligature made of thin cord, which sinks deeply into tissues. **A tension of 4 to 5 kg. on ligature blocks carotid arteries, and 20 kg. the vertebral arteries. This is much less common than venous occlusion.** (5) **Reflex vagal inhibition from pressure on the vagal sheath or carotid bodies.** Fear, apprehension, struggling and possibly alcohol, may heighten the sensitivity of vagal mechanism. The release of catecholamines during such adrenal response may sensitise the myocardium to such neurogenic stimulation. (6) **Fracture or dislocation of the cervical vertebrae.** This occurs when there is a free fall and sudden jerk during hanging as in judicial hanging. The above causes may act independently or in concert.

Delayed Death: Death delayed for several days is rare. Delayed deaths occur due to (1) aspiration pneumonia, (2) infections, (3) oedema of lungs, (4) oedema of larynx, (5) hypoxic encephalopathy, (6) infarction of brain, (7) abscess of brain, (8) cerebral softening.

The secondary effects of hanging in persons who have recovered are sometimes hemiplegia, epileptiform convulsions, amnesia, dementia, cervical cellulitis, parotitis, retropharyngeal abscess, amnesia, and dementia.

Fatal Period: Death occurs immediately if the cervical vertebrae are fractured, or if the heart is inhibited; rapidly if cause is asphyxia, and least rapidly if coma is responsible. **The usual period is 3 to 5 minutes. Most hangings cause gradual, subtle and painless death.**

TREATMENT: After the ligature is cut to remove the constriction of the neck, artificial respiration and stimulants should be given.

Postmortem Appearances: External: Ligature mark on the neck: The ligature mark in the neck is the most important and specific sign of death from hanging. It depends on: **(1) Composition of ligature: The pattern and texture is produced upon the skin,** e.g., if thick rope is used, its texture may be impressed in the form of superficial abrasion. **(2) Width and multiplicity of ligature: When ligature is narrow, a deep groove is made** because much more force per sq. cm. of ligature is directed inwards. A broad ligature will produce only a superficial mark. If the ligature is passed twice round the neck, a double mark, one circular, and the other oblique may be seen. The ligature may have one, two, or more layers. There may be multiple congested areas, where the skin has been caught between the various layers. **(3) The weight of the body suspended and the degree of suspension:** Heavier the body and greater the proportion of the body suspended, the more marked is the ligature impression. **(4) The tightness of encircling ligature: The ligature impression is deeper opposite the point of suspension,** but it may tail off very rapidly if ligature consists of loop rather than a noose. If the noose tightens completely around the neck, the ligature mark will be seen completely encircling the neck. **(5) The length of time body has been suspended: Longer the suspension, deeper is the groove.** Even a soft, broad ligature can cause a clear-cut groove if suspended long. If the ligature is cut down within a short time and a soft broad ligature has been used, there may be no external mark. **(6) Position of the knot: The main force applied to the neck by ligature is opposite to the point of suspension.** If the point of suspension is in occipital region, front of the neck is involved. If in front, the depth of the groove is limited posteriorly by cervical spine. **(7) Slipping of ligature during suspension:** Frequently, only the portion adjacent to the knot moves. There is a tendency for the ligature to move upwards, this being limited by the jaws. The upward movement may produce double impression of ligature. The lower mark is usually very superficial and is connected by fine abrasions, caused by the slipping ligature, to the mark made by ligature in its final position. Record circumference of the neck.

Knot: (1) A **slip knot (running noose) Fig. (13–2)** is produced by attaching a rope to itself, creating a loop which can be tightened to produce a running noose. (2) A **binding knot** is a knot in which rope passes at least once around the neck, and is held in place by two ends of the rope being knotted together. This produces a **fixed noose**. (3) **Reef knot** is a flat knot used in tying reef-points consisting of two loops passing symmetrically through each other that will not slip. (4) **Granny knot** is knot like reef knot, but asymmetrical, apt to slip or jam. **Noose** is a loop with running knot which ties the firmer the closer it is drawn. It is frequently in the form of a simple slip-knot to produce a running noose or fixed by granny or reef-knot; occasionally a simple loop is used. **The knot is usually on the right or left side of the neck, ligature usually rising behind the ear to the point of suspension. Sometimes, the knot is in the occipital region and rarely under the chin.** After suspension in hanging, the knot is at higher level than the remainder of ligature, the movement of knot being due to the act of suspension. The involvement of

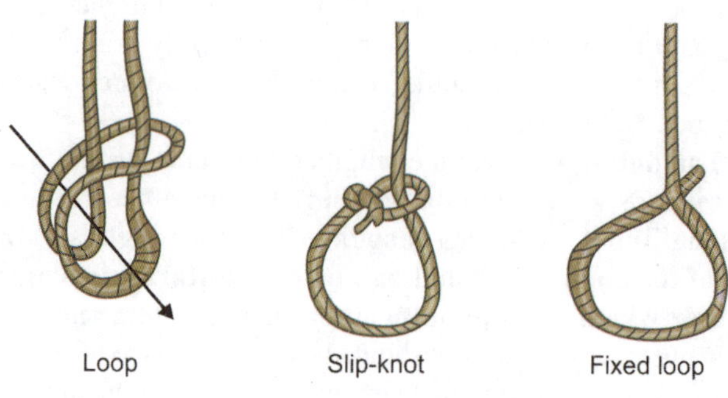

Fig. (13–2). Types of ligature.

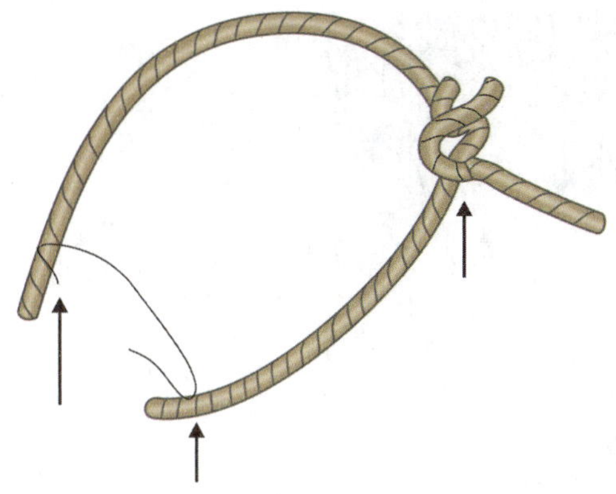

Fig. (13–3). **Method of preservation of noose in hanging and strangulation.**

another party may be suggested by certain types of knots and nooses. **In the majority of hangings, the ligature consists of a single loop. Removal of the noose from the neck is done by cutting the noose away from the knot and tying the cut ends with string or wire** Fig. (13–3).

Description of Ligature Mark: The description of the ligature mark should **include its direction, continuous or interrupted, colour, length, depth and width, ligature pattern if any, the areas of the neck involved, and its relation to local landmarks. The ligature produces a furrow or a groove in the tissue which is pale in colour, but it later becomes yellow-brown or dark-brown and hard like parchment (rope burns), due to the drying of the slightly abraded skin. The course of the groove depends on whether a fixed or running noose has been used. A fixed noose is one in which the rope is knotted (granny or reef knot). A running noose is one in which the end of rope is passed through the loop made from other end (slip knot).** (1) When the loop is arranged with a fixed knot, the course of the mark is deepest and nearly horizontal on the side opposite to knot, but as the arms of the ligature approach the knot, the mark turns upwards towards it. This produces an inverted 'V' at the site of the knot, the apex of the 'V' corresponding with the site of the knot **Fig. (13–4)**. An impression from a knot may be found if the ligature is tight on the skin, usually on one or other side of the back and occasionally beneath the chin. (2) In the case of a fixed loop with a single knot in the midline at the back of the head, the mark is seen on both sides of the neck and is directed obliquely upwards towards the position of the knot over the back of the neck. (3) In the case of a fixed loop with a single knot in the midline under the chin, the mark is seen on the back and both sides of the neck, and is directed obliquely forwards towards the position of the knot over the front of the neck. (4) In the case of a fixed loop with the knot in the region of one ear, the mark

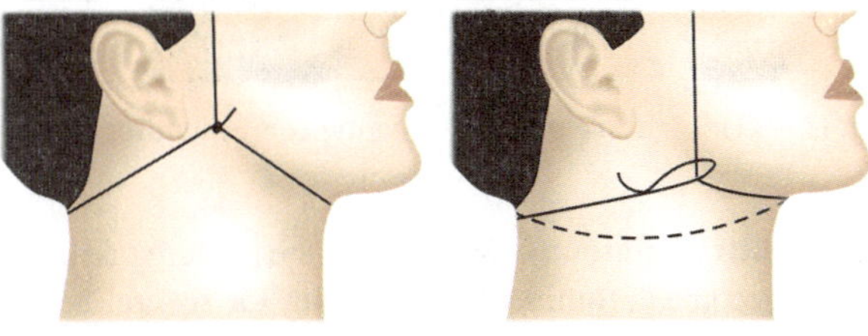

Fig. (13–4). **The position of the ligature mark on the neck.**

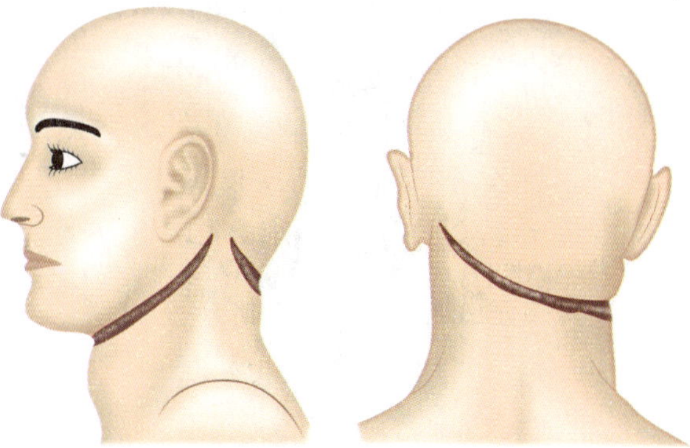

Fig. (13–5). **Ligature mark in hanging. Point of suspension is just posterior to the left ear, with the furrow crossing the anterior neck above the larynx, showing inverted V furrow.**

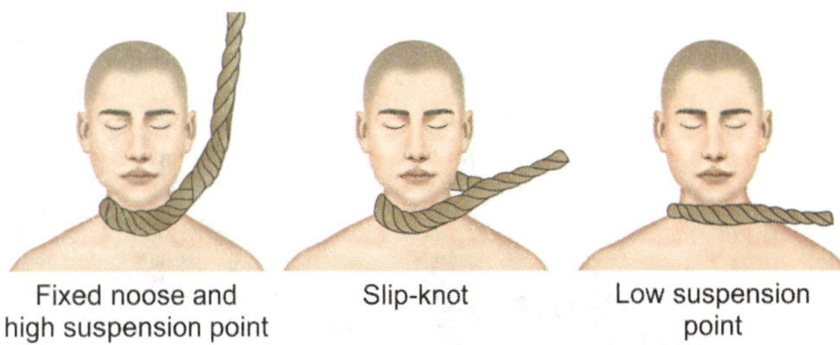

Fig. (13–6). **Types of suspension of the body in hanging.**

differs on each side of the neck **Fig. (13–5)**. On the side of the knot, the mark is directed obliquely upwards to the knot, and on the other side it is directed transversely. If the ligature is in the form of a loop, the mark will be most prominent on the part of the neck to which the head has inclined and less marked over the region of the open angle of the loop. (5) If a running noose fails to tighten, the mark may resemble one produced by a fixed loop. If the noose is a belt, a single ligature will produce two parallel ligature marks, as the upper and lower edges of the belt dig into the skin.

Horizontal ligature mark is seen Fig. (13–6): (1) When a running noose is applied, the weight of the body will cause the noose to tighten in a mainly horizontal position. The mark is seen on both sides of the neck, and is usually directed transversely across the front of the neck resembling that of a ligature mark in strangulation, except that it is likely to be seen above the level of thyroid cartilage. (2) In hanging from a low point of suspension, the groove produced by the ligature is less well marked, and may be at about the level of the upper border of the larynx and more horizontal. (3) In partial hanging when the body leans forward, a horizontal ligature mark may be seen.

The junction of the noose and the vertical part of the rope of the noose is pulled upwards and away from the skin and so no mark is left. The apex of the triangle formed in this way is called the suspension peak or point and indicates the position of the junction of the noose and vertical part of rope. This suspension peak is a distinguishing feature from ligature strangulation. The firmer muscular tissues at the back of the neck do not show clear and deep grooves, as are seen at the front or sides of the neck. **Along the edges of the depression, a narrow zone of congestion or haemorrhage will be seen above**

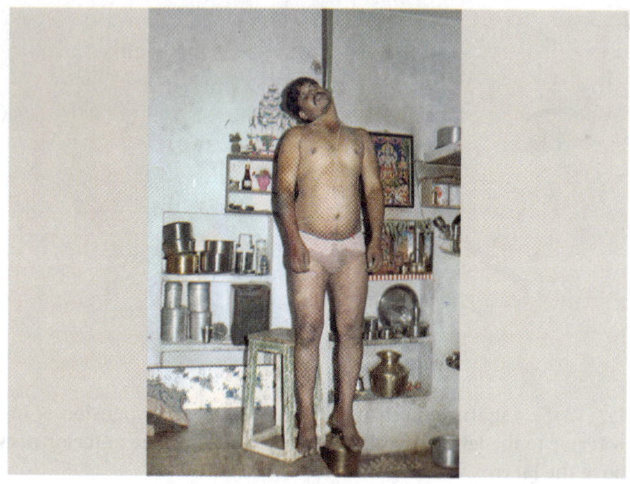

Fig. (13–7). **Suicidal hanging.**

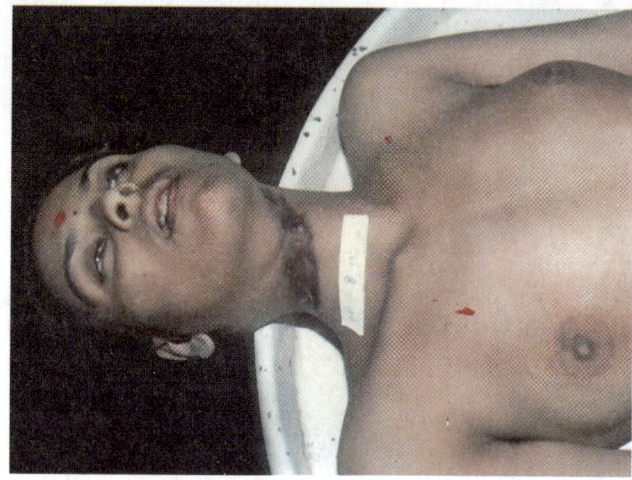

Fig. (13–9). **Ligature mark of hanging.**

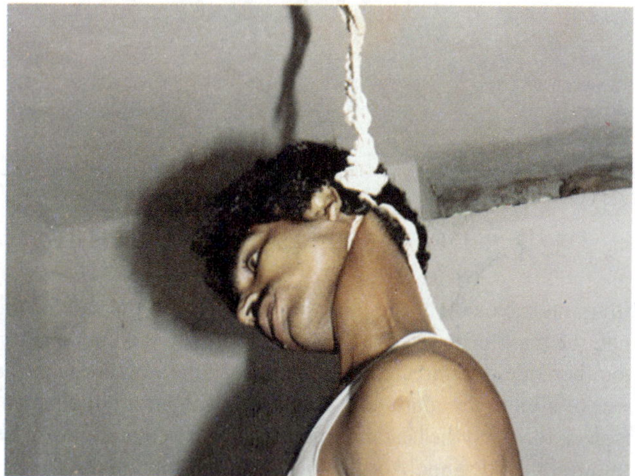

Fig. (13–8). **Suicidal hanging.**

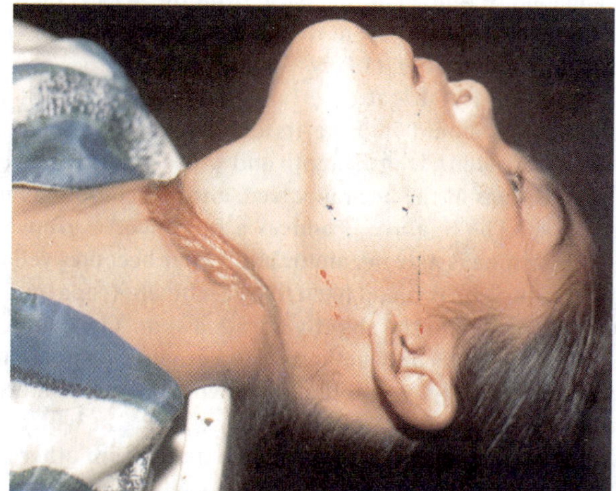

Fig. (13–10). **Ligature mark of hanging.**

and below the groove at some point, usually the deepest point, if not throughout its course. This is not an indication of vital reaction, but is due to displacement of blood laterally from under the zone of maximum pressure. In some cases, the lower margin of the groove is pale, and upper margin red due to postmortem dilatation and distension of vessels and small haemorrhages may be present. Blisters containing serum may result from friction of a tight noose. Ecchymoses and slight abrasions in the groove are rare. **Ecchymoses alone have no significance as to whether hanging was caused during life or not, but abrasions with haemorrhage are strongly suggestive of suspension taking place during life.**

Features Figs. (13–8 to 13–11): The mark is situated above the level of thyroid cartilage, between the larynx and the chin in 80% of cases. It may be at the level of the cartilage in about fifteen percent, and below the cartilage in about 5% cases, especially in partial suspension. **The width of the groove is about, or slightly less than the width of the ligature. Any well-defined pattern in the ligature is likely to be produced in the groove permitting a match of patterns.** Ligature pattern may be better appreciated by examining under oblique lighting and using a magnifying lens. **Rarely, a narrow wire may be used**

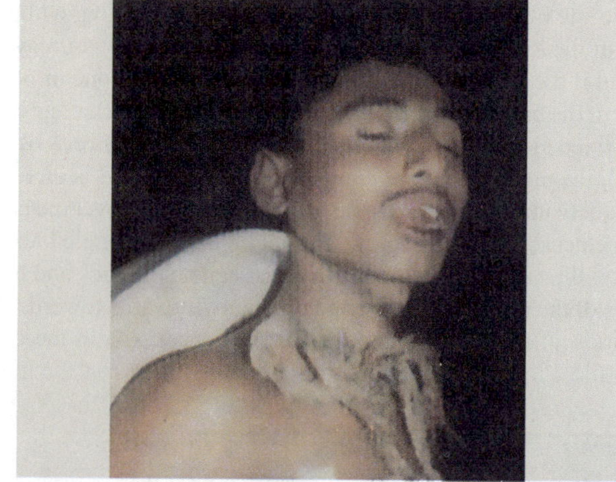

Fig. (13–11). **Ligature mark of hanging corresponding to the ligature used.**

("cheese-cutter" method). When fresh, the ligature mark is less clear, but becomes prominent after drying for several hours. A portion of skin and deeper tissue in relation to ligature should be examined microscopically for evidence of **tissue reaction, which**

if present indicates antemortem hanging. The absence of tissue reaction does not exclude antemortem hanging (Gordon, et al). Fabric ligature mark: When a folded cloth has been used, there may be great difference between the appearance of the neck mark and the size of the ligature. When fabric is pulled tight, certain parts of it become raised into ridges, which form the ligating surface, and only these may be reproduced on the skin. **When nylon, silk or terylene fabrics are used, they may leave a mark only 2 to 3 mm. wide. A loop made of soft material, e.g., towel, scarf, etc. may not produce a ligature mark, but the knot may produce an abrasion due to its firmness. If there is no ligature, the mark should be taped, as it may pick up some fibres by the ligature** and facilitate the identification of the material of which the ligature was made. The ligature mark of hanging may be reproduced by dragging a body along the ground with ligature passed round the neck soon after death. However, hanging may occur without visible marks on the victim's neck. If there is a beard, or if a portion of clothing is caught between the ligature and the skin, no ligature mark may be found under it. **The ligature mark may disappear after several hours following removal of the ligature. Decomposition obliterates the ligature mark.**

Pseudo-ligature mark: In obese persons or infants, skin folds on the neck may resemble a ligature mark, especially after refrigeration of the body has caused coagulation of the subcutaneous fat. When there is swelling of the neck tissues due to decomposition, marks may be produced by jewellery or clothing.

Partial Hanging: Hanging may occur simply by leaning against the noose secured to a chair or door knob, the leg of a table, a bedpost or rail, or the handrail of a staircase, which is slightly higher than the position of the head, the deceased being in a kneeling position, or fall back or forward and lie prone with only the face and chest off the ground. In these cases, only the weight of chest and arms can cause fatal pressure on the neck. In these cases, **the constricting force is less and congestive changes in the face are more marked, and petechiae are seen,** because carotid arteries and jugular veins are occluded, but vertebral arteries continue to supply blood to the head. **Bradycardia and fibrillation due to neural or neurohumoral mechanism may cause death when suspension point is very low. Hanging may occur when pressure is applied only at the front of the neck, e.g., by the arm of a chair, rung of a ladder, etc.** In such case, the marks on the neck may be indistinct or absent. **Decomposition sets in relatively early in the congested face of a partially suspended body.**

Signs of asphyxia: The petechial haemorrhages present in the skin and conjunctivae (25% of cases) remain, as they are extravascular. They occur more frequently in incomplete suspension. **The signs of asphyxia are most marked in cases in which the noose was placed high up on the throat. Obstruction of the jugular veins, while the arteries remain patent (incomplete suspension), leads to severe engorgement of the head and neck with numerous petechiae.** If asphyxial process is slow, face will be dusky-purple, congested and often swollen. Occasionally, the congestion drains away from the head, in spite of the ligature being still in position. This probably occurs through the vertebral venous plexus, which is not easily compressed as the jugular veins. The brain is often drained of blood in this way. **Slow asphyxia is the exception in hanging and is likely to occur only when the point of suspension is a low one, or ligature exerts pressure below the chin and does not encircle the neck. When suspension is complete or in the standing posture, asphyxial signs are slight, face is pale petechial haemorrhages are relatively uncommon** due to the complete obstruction of the arterial system (absence of pooling of blood in the head and no increased pressure), but are usually present when hanging has been from low point. In death due to vagal inhibition face will be pale. **Majority of victims of hanging are seen with pale faces.** When pressure is applied on the neck, the progression of pure asphyxial process may suddenly stop, by the superimposition of vagal inhibition, so that the intensity of congestive changes may be of any degree in any given death. **The neck is stretched and elongated and the head is always inclined to the side opposite to the knot. The face is usually pale,** due to cerebral ischaemia (occlusion of carotids and vertebral arteries and drainage by secondary vertebral venous system) or vagal inhibition, but is sometimes congested and swollen due to leakage of oedema fluid into the soft tissues (swelling often disappears when the body is cut down), if the veins were constricted before the arteries. **The eyes are frequently protruded and firmer than usual** due to congestion. The conjunctivae are usually congested. When knot is situated in front of one ear, conjunctival haemorrhages may be one-sided. The eyes are closed or partially open, and the pupils are usually dilated. If the ligature knot presses on cervical sympathetic, the eye on the same side may remain open and its pupil dilated **(le facie sympathique).** It indicates antemortem hanging.

Other signs: The tongue is usually swollen and blue especially at the base, and usually forced against the teeth when the jaw is shut, or the tip may be found projecting between the lips, due to the noose lifting the glossopharyngeal skeleton, causing protrusion the tongue. The protruding part of the tongue is usually dark-brown or even black due to drying. The lips, and the mucous membrane of the mouth are blue. **Saliva may be found dribbling from the angle of mouth, when the head is drooping forward.** This is due to the increased salivation before death due to the stimulation of the salivary glands by the ligature or congestive hypoxia. Salivation is increased by stimulation of pterygopalatine ganglion. **Slight haemorrhage or bloody froth is sometimes seen at the mouth and nostrils, and some blood may be found under the head.** This results from rupture of engorged blood vessels, and should not be mistaken for evidence of foul play. Occasionally, haemorrhage into the middle ears is seen due to excessive congestion. The hands are clenched, especially in violent hanging. Engorgement of the penis with blood occurs from hypostasis; it may be semierect, and semen may be found at the tip. Urine and faeces may escape due to relaxation of the sphincters. If the body has been suspended for some time, **postmortem hypostasis is seen in the legs, feet, hands and forearms,** while the upper part of the body will be pale. **Petechial haemorrhages may be found in the skin of the legs in two to four hours Fig. (13–12).** If the body is removed within four hours after death and is placed in supine position, postmortem hypostasis in the limbs will fade and new areas of lividity will appear along the back and buttocks.

Internal: The neck should be examined after removal of the brain and viscera from the chest and abdominal

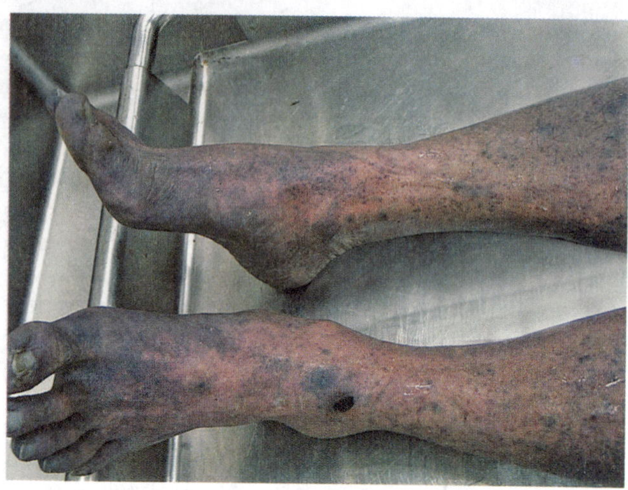

Fig. (13–12). **Petechial haemorrhages on legs and feet in complete hanging.**

cavities. Superficial incision of the groove may show small haemorrhages in the underlying layers of skin, caused by the direct pressure and indirect stretching of these structures produced by the ligature without tissue reaction. **The tissues under the mark are dry, white and glistening with occasional ecchymoses in the adjacent muscles. Haemorrhages in strap muscles are present in about 25%, and the platysma and sternomastoid are ruptured (5 to 10%), if violence has been considerable. In some cases (5 to 10%), the intima of the carotid arteries show transverse splits** (under the groove, usually around the region of sinuses) on ipsilateral side related to the location of ligature knot, which appear to be due to traction rather than direct pressure, with extravasation of blood in their wall due to stretching and crushing. It indicates that the victim was alive at the time of hanging. **Several horizontal intimal tears scattered along the carotid arteries at different levels are sometimes found in hanging associated with a long drop.** To demonstrate these tears, the carotid arteries should be opened to the level of mandible. The vertebral arteries show rupture, intimal tears, and subintimal haemorrhages in some cases. Injury to the trachea is unusual. **Petechial haemorrhages may be found on the epiglottis, in the larynx and trachea.** Bruising of the deep muscles at the base of tongue occurs from crushing of this area against hard palate by upward push of ligature. The lymph nodes above and below the ligature mark are congested. The trachea is usually congested. **The lungs are congested, oedematous and exude bloody serum on section in cases of constriction occurring at the end of expiration; but they are pale if constriction occurred at the end of inspiration. Subpleural ecchymoses may be found. The abdominal organs are usually congested.** The brain is usually normal, but may be pale or congested according to the mode of the death. **Subarachnoid effusions are common.** Bleeding into the outer layers of the intervertebral discs (red stripes in between the vertebral bodies) of lumbar vertebrae (Simon's haemorrhages) may be seen in bodies suspended for a long time.

Fractures of hyoid bone: Opinion varies regarding the frequency of fracture of the hyoid bone. Estimates range from 0 to 60%, but the average is 15 to 20%. Fractures are rare below 40 years because of the elasticity of the cartilage and mobility of the joints. **The fracture is common in persons above 40 years and involves the great horns, at the junction of inner two-thirds and outer one-third.** The fracture is usually a direct result of the ligature, but it can be a traction or **"tua"** fracture.

The fracture of superior horns of the thyroid cartilage depends on location of the knot, location of ligature, length of ligature and possible swing. It may also occur due to indirect force caused by stretching of thyrohyoid ligament and thyroid membrane. **It occurs in about 40% of cases above 40 years.** A jump from a tree may damage the vertebrae at atlanto-occipital joint.

DIAGNOSIS: (1) Ligature mark around the neck, (2) presence of abrasions, ecchymoses and redness about the ligature mark, (3) trickling of saliva from the mouth, (4) ecchymoses of the larynx or epiglottis, (5) rupture of the intima of the carotid, (6) congestion and haemorrhage in lymph nodes above and below ligature marks, (7) absence of any other cause of death and (8) postmortem signs of asphyxia.

THE CIRCUMSTANCES OF DEATH: Scene of Crime: Note the posture of the body, any signs of violence or disorder of furniture, etc., and the condition of the clothing of the deceased. The texture and length of ligature should be noted to know whether it was sufficient to hang. If the ligature had broken and the victim is found on the ground, free ends of the ligature should be compared to know whether they coincide and that a break had occurred. The accessibility of suspension point should be noted by measuring the height from ground to hanging point (suspension point), and height of support to reach the suspension point.

SUICIDAL HANGING: Hanging is a common method of committing suicide worldwide. A typical method of self-suspension is to attach a rope to a high point, such as a beam, window-casing, ceiling fan, branch of a tree, etc. The lower end is formed into either a fixed loop or a slip-knot which is placed around the neck. The accessibility of suspension point should be noted by measuring the height from ground to hanging point (suspension point) and height of support to reach the suspension point. The victim stands on a stool, chair or other platform and jumps off or kicks away the support, due to which the body is suspended. The body must be in a position compatible with self-suspension. It is important to examine the point of attachment and the surrounding area. If the point is high, then it is likely that there will be recent disturbance of dust caused while attaching the ligature. The deceased's hands and sometimes part of his clothing may also show the presence of corresponding dust marks. There may also be disturbance of dust from the attached cord or from an abraded area particularly if a beam has been used to attach the ligature. Complete suspension of the body in the absence of any platform is unusual in suicide. The hands and feet are sometimes tied by the victim before hanging himself, to prevent a change of mind. The position of the ligature with reference to the knot and the manner in which it is attached to the support must be compatible with self-suspension. Determination of purpose will often compensate bodily infirmity. Blindness or age is no bar to hanging. A person with tracheostomy can commit suicide by hanging as death occurs due to vagal inhibition. The victim might pull away the ligature to free himself from the constriction and if he had long nails, nail marks may be inflicted on the neck. Sometimes, the upward movement of the rope at the time of suspension may scratch the skin. In an attempted resuscitation, scratches or nail marks on the neck may be produced by another person. Superficial abrasions and sometimes small contusions overlying bony prominences of the limbs and trunk may be found in suicidal hangings due to contact of the body against nearby objects during voluntary or early involuntary movement. Sometimes, a person may hang himself after other forms of suicide, e.g., cutting the throat or wrists, stabs, firearm wounds, ingestion of poison, etc., have failed to produce death. Unusual positions, e.g., where the parts of the body touched the ground, kneeling or reclining, are almost diagnostic of suicide Fig. (13–13). Suicide pacts effected by hanging are rare.

The body should be photographed from various angles Figs. (13–14 to 13–16). Cellophane tape should be applied to the palms, fingers and

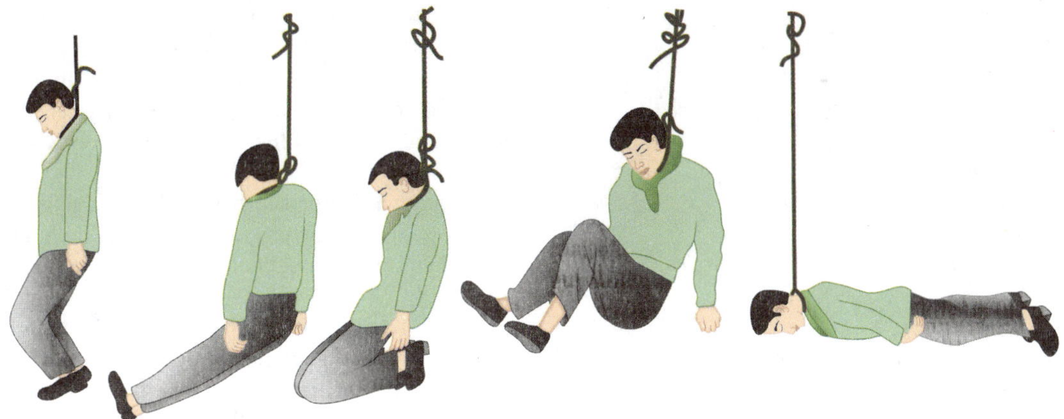

Fig. (13–13). **Partial hanging.**

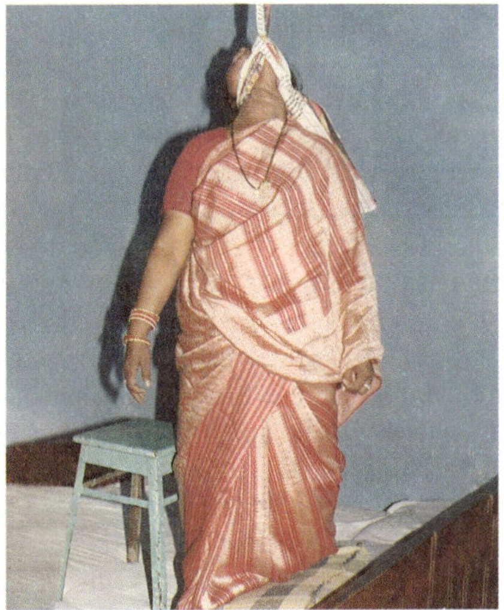

Fig. (13–14). **Ligature knot on front of neck in hanging.**

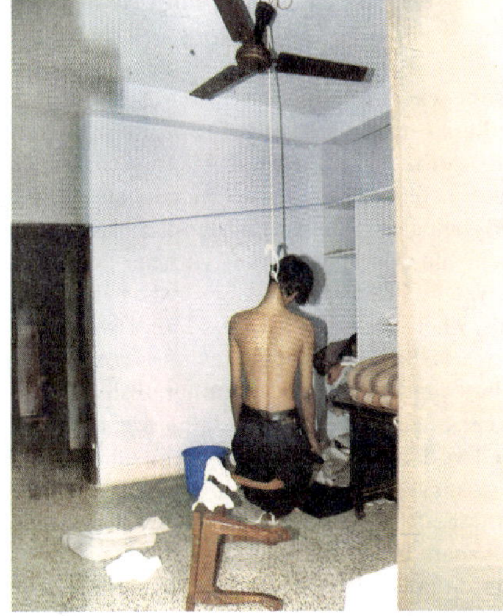

Fig. (13–16). **Partial hanging (sitting position).**

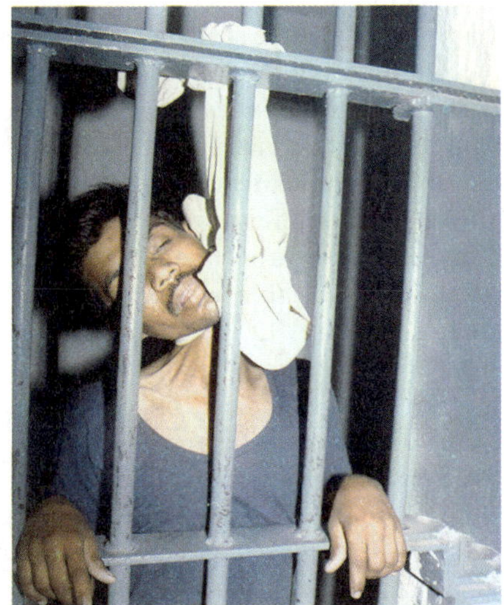

Fig. (13–15). **Partial hanging in police lockup.**

ligature mark, removed and folded inwards for detection of fibres from the ligature. Nail clippings can be examined for presence of fibres. Measure the distance from the ground to suspension point, ground to the feet, and height of stepping device if any. Measure the circumference of the neck.

If any external injuries are present, the doctor must decide, whether they are self-inflicted, occurred during convulsive phase preceding death, produced when the body was cut down or occurred when the swinging body contacted other objects or during attempted resuscitation or homicide.

Complex suicide: The person plans more than one method of suicide to make sure that death will occur.

Complicated suicide: When during the original suicidal method, unintentional trauma occurs which leads to death, e.g., a person hanging himself from a branch of tree, the branch breaks and the person dies due to complications of fall.

Suicide pact: Where more than one person decide to kill themselves **Fig. (13–17)**.

MULTIPLE METHODS OF SUICIDE: CASE: (1) A man was found hanging. The examination of the scene and information obtained by the police were consistent with suicide. However, the body had a bullet wound on the right side of face and another in the palm of the left hand; five cut wounds of the throat; cuts over the left wrist, dividing the muscle tendons but not blood vessels. Apparently he had attempted to shoot himself, to cut his throat, and the blood vessels in the wrist, all of which failed. In desperation, he hanged himself.

(2) A highly pessimistic person determined to commit suicide, decided to hang himself. He selected a tree with a stout branch overhanging a cliff, the sea being 16 metres below. He procured a dose of opium to prevent any pain in the process of hanging. To make certain that death occurs, he decided also to shoot himself. The noose adjusted, opium swallowed,

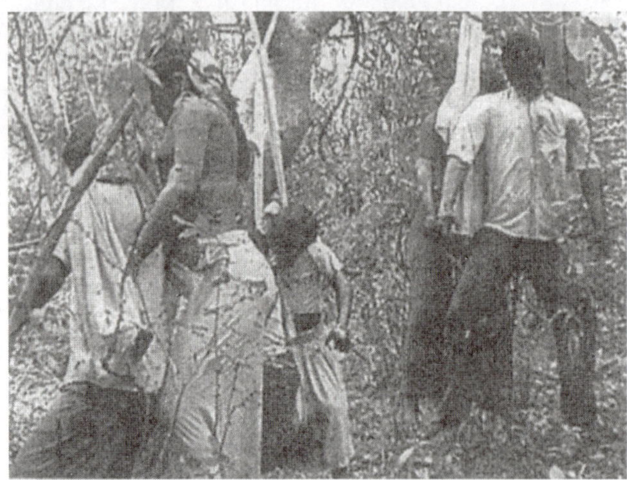

Fig. (13–17). Suicide pact by hanging of a family of five persons.

and the revolver cocked, he stepped over the cliff, and as he did so fired. His aim was altered by the jerk of the rope, and the bullet missed his head but partly cut through the rope. The rope broke due to the jerk of the body, and he fell into the sea 16 metres below. He swallowed sea water, vomited the poison, and swam ashore a wiser man.

(3) A 42-year-old woman was found with her head submerged in the blood-stained water of her bath tub. Her wrists, ankles and neck showed incised wounds. There was a star-shaped bullet wound on her forehead and at autopsy a 0.38 caliber bullet was recovered from the brain. In addition, she had consumed a large number of sleeping pills.

(4) A 40-year-unemployed male took poison, tried to hang himself, stabbed himself with a knife and finally jumped out of seventh-storey window only to survive and land up in a hospital and police custody. He made all these attempts after stabbing his girlfriend to death in a Bangkok hotel room in the morning, and writing on the wall with her blood. "If you think money is more important, we should die together".

ACCIDENTAL HANGING: (1) It is seen in children during play while imitating judicial hanging or in athletes who are in the habit of exhibiting hanging. Some padding between ligature and neck suggests accident. (2) Workmen in falling from scaffolding may be hanged by becoming entangled in ropes. (3) When boys climb trees or railings they may loose their foothold and in falling, some garment is caught by branch of tree or bar and is drawn tight round the neck. (4) Infants wearing restraining apparatus may wriggle partly out of it, and become asphyxiated by its tightening around their neck as they try to crawl away or fall over the side of the bed. (5) The ligature need not completely encircle the neck to cause death. It is sufficient if it is applied beneath the chin so as to compress the sides of the neck, e.g., suspension of the chin by the steering wheel of a motor car, the tailboard of a lorry or cart, the edge of a sofa or the arm of chair. (6) A person who slips when descending a ladder may be suspended by one of its rungs, or a slip on a staircase may result in suspension on the edge of one of the treads. (7) It may be associated with abnormal sexual behaviour.

HOMICIDAL HANGING: It is extremely rare. It is difficult for a single assailant to carry it out, unless the victim becomes unconscious by injury or by a drug, or is taken unawares, or is a child or a very weak person. Homicide should be suspected (1) where there are signs of violence or disorder of furniture or other objects, (2) where the clothing of the deceased is torn or disarranged, (3) where there are injuries, either offensive or defensive, (4) the knot is tied to the back of neck, (5) mouth is gagged, (6) limbs are tied, (7) evidence of stupefication by drink or drugs. In all doubtful cases, circumstantial evidence is important.

If an individual is suspended upside down for a long time, death can occur in a few hours to a day either from acute cardiac or respiratory failure or a combination of both.

LYNCHING: The name is derived from captain William Lynch, who used to order hanging on the spot publicly without trial in USA, where a black rapist was used to be lynched by angry white mob with a view to teaching others a lesson for committing offence. **It is homicidal hanging.** It may be killing by beating by mob to punish a person in cases of robbery, caste marriages, honour killing, thieves, vehicle drivers for causing death of persons, etc.

Honour Killing: Murder of daughters/sisters for defying parents wish and marrying a person of their choice out of caste/ religion due to the thought of bringing disrepute to the family and community.

Postmortem suspension of body (P.M. hanging): A person might be ligature strangled and then hanged. In this case the ligature marking will not have the classic inverted V configuration of hanging. **A ligature applied to the neck within two hours of death will produce a ligature mark.** Look for signs of dragging to the place of suspension. When a dead body is suspended, the rope is usually tied first around the neck, and then around the beam, branch of a tree, etc. **The beam shows evidence of the rope having moved from below upwards as the body has been pulled up. In true suicidal hanging, the rope moves from above downwards.** Further, fibres from the rope may be found on the hands of the victim in suicidal hanging, but not in case of postmortem hanging. The rope should be examined for presence or absence of any paint similar to one on the beam. In most cases, the internal signs are clearly not those of hanging, although in most cases ligature mark cannot be distinguished. Rarely, for motives of revenge, fraud or for some other reason, a victim arranges his suicide to appear to have been a murder.

JUDICIAL HANGING: In India, legal death sentence is carried out by hanging the criminal. The face of the person is covered with a dark mask, and **he is made to stand on a platform above trapdoors which open downwards when a bolt is drawn.** A rope to allow a drop of five to seven metres according to the weight, build and age of the person, is looped round the neck, with the knot under the angle of the right jaw. The placement of the knot beneath the chin, in the submental position is said to be more effective. **On drawing the bolt, the person drops to the length of the rope. The sudden stoppage of the moving body associated with the position of the knot causes the head to be jerked violently.** This causes **fracture-dislocation usually at the level of the second and third, or third and fourth cervical vertebrae. Bilateral fractures of either the pedicles or laminae of the arch of the second, third or fourth cervical vertebrae occur (hangman's fracture).** Less commonly, dislocation of the atlanto-occipital joint or odontoid process of the axis vertebra occurs causing pulping of the spinal cord and transection of the cervical cord causing the neck to be lengthened considerably. The upper cervical cord is stretched or torn across. With proper judicial hanging, there is a rupture of the brain stem between the pons and the medulla. This results in instantaneous and irreversible loss of consciousness (due to destruction of reticular formation) and in irreversible apnoea (due to destruction of the region of respiratory centre). **It results in immediate unconsciousness, but heart beats and respiratory movements may continue up to 10 to 15 minutes until hypoxia causes arrest, and spasmodic muscular jerking may occur for a considerable time.** The pharynx is usually injured and the carotid arteries may be torn transversely, either partly or completely. Asphyxial signs are not seen in properly performed judicial hangings.

STRANGULATION

Types: (1) Strangulation by a ligature, (2) Manual strangulation or throttling, (3) Garroting, (4) Mugging, (5) Bansdola.

LIGATURE STRANGULATION: Strangulation by ligature is that form of asphyxia which is caused from constriction of the neck by a ligature without suspending the body.

SYMPTOMS: Sudden and violent compression of the windpipe causes almost immediate insensibility and death. If the windpipe is partially closed, buzzing in ears, congestion and cyanosis in head, vertigo, tingling, muscle weakness, bleeding from the mouth, nose and ears, clenching of the hands and convulsions occur before death.

Cause of Death: Death may be due to: (1) **Asphyxia, due to elevation of the larynx and tongue, closing the airway at pharyngeal level. It is difficult to occlude the airway at laryngeal or tracheal level,** due to the rigidity of the strong cartilages except when extreme pressure is applied. (2) Cerebral anoxia or venous congestion. (3) Combined asphyxia and venous congestion. (4) Vagal inhibition, and (5) Fracture-dislocation of cervical vertebrae (rare).

Ligature: The ligature may consist of a wide variety of objects such as cords, wires, ropes, belts, scarves, ties, towels, stockings, bed linen, etc.

Postmortem Appearances Figs. (13–18 to 13–25): (A) **External: The ligature mark: The appearance of ligature mark on the neck varies considerably, depending upon nature of ligature, amount of resistance offered by the victim and amount of force used by the assailant. It is usually a well-defined and slightly depressed mark at any level on the neck, but usually about the middle or below the thyroid cartilage. The mark completely encircles the neck transversely** Table (13–1), but is more prominent at the front and sides than at the back. The skin of the front of the neck is more likely to be damaged by a ligature than the thicker, tougher skin at the back of the neck. **Sometimes, the ligature mark is seen only at the front.** The mark may be absent on the back due to the presence of clothing or long hair between the ligature and the skin. A ligature mark may be interrupted at the front by the presence of the clothing or by the victim's fingers in an attempt to pull the ligature away. **If a knot has been applied, there may be a wider area of bruising at the site of the knot. If the ligature has been tightened pulling on the crossed ends, the mark is likely to be more prominent at the site of cross-over, and the marks produced by the two ends will be at different levels.** The mark of cross-over may be at the front, back or side according to the position of the assailant. **The mark may be oblique as in hanging, if the victim has been dragged by a cord, after he has been strangled in a recumbent posture. Multiple turns produce a complex mark** in which it may be possible to trace the number of turns, but a complex ligature composed of several pieces knotted together may produce a mark which simulates multiple turns, though there was only one. **Occasionally, a ligature mark may be seen only across the front of the neck, if the assailant presses from the front, or pulls from the back, using a cord stretched between two hands.**

Twisted cords with a rough surface, if tied around the neck several times in parallel, may squeeze a skin fold and compress the capillaries inside leading to haemorrhage into the fold. Vesicles containing fluid may also form in these folds.

Rarely, a narrow wire may be used, the so-called "cheese-cutter" method. When narrow ligature, e.g., a cord, wire or thin

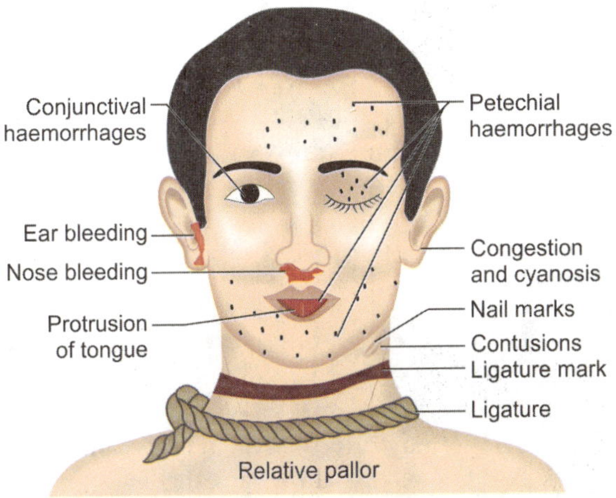

Fig. (13–18). **Signs of strangulation.**

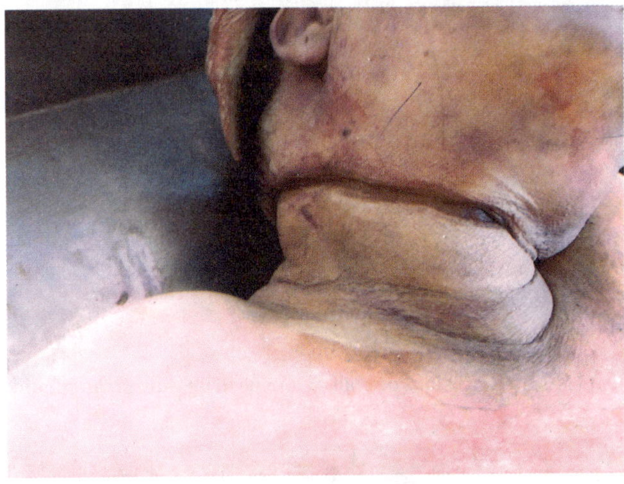

Fig. (13–19). **Transverse ligature mark on front and right side of neck in ligature strangulation.**

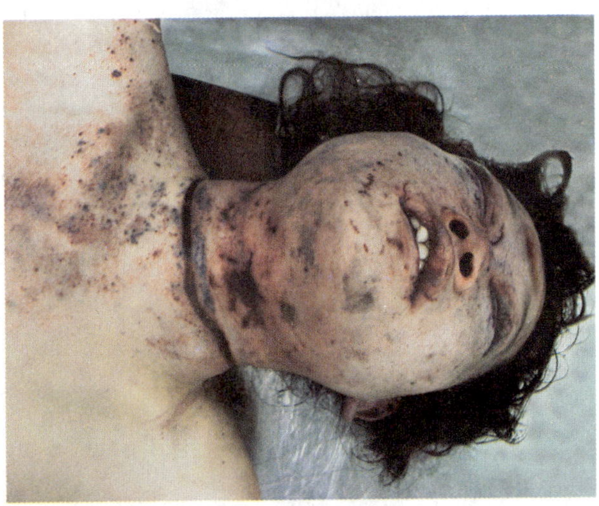

Fig. (13–20). **Strangulation by ligature with nail marks around lips and front of neck area above ligature.**

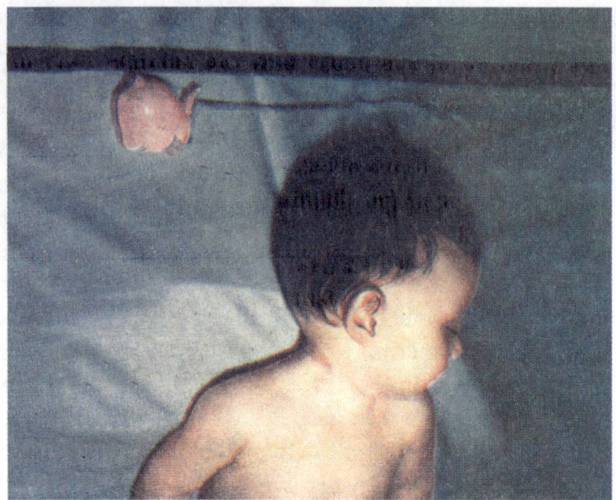

Fig. (13–21). Homicidal ligature strangulation. Ligature mark produced by the rubber tube of the toy (shown above head) looped around the neck.

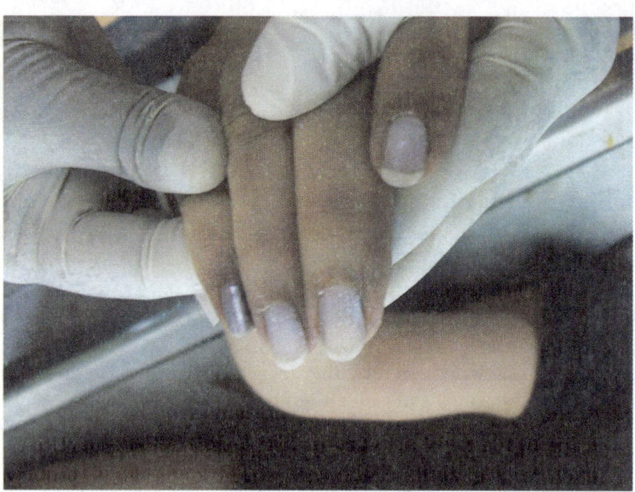

Fig. (13–22). Cyanosed finger nails in asphyxia.

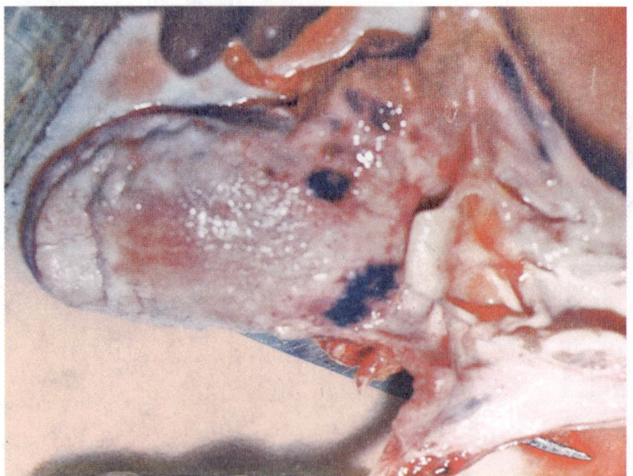

Fig. (13–23). Contusions on root of tongue in ligature strangulation.

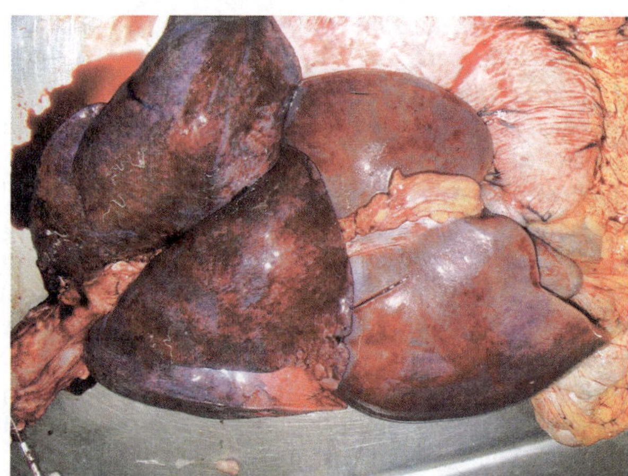

Fig. (13–24). Ligature strangulation. Intense congestions of viscera of chest and abdomen.

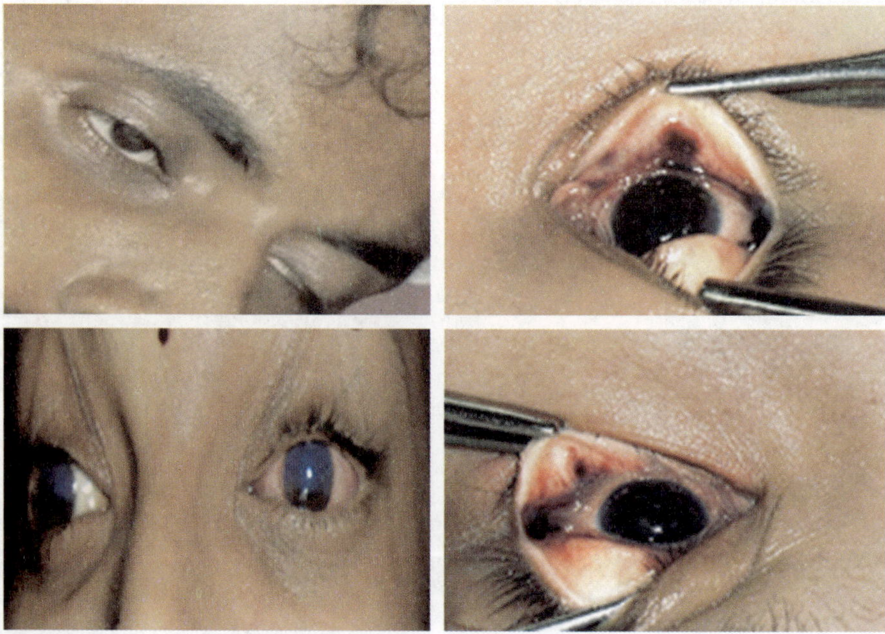

Fig. (13–25). Eyes in hanging and strangulation.

rope has been tightly forced into the skin, the skin may stretch and after the ligature is removed, the elastic recoil may make the ligature mark slightly narrower than the actual diameter of the ligature itself. **If the ligature is still in position when the body is examined, it may appear to be deeply embedded in the skin, and on removal a deep groove may be seen in the skin.** This embedding may be increased by oedema of the tissues, especially above the ligature, which initially may not have been applied so tightly. The swelling can continue to develop to some extent even after death, increasing the depth of the groove, possibly due to some passive transudation of tissue fluid even after stoppage of circulation.

Strong pressure may lacerate the skin or cut into the deeper tissues and cartilages. When a folded cloth has been used, there may be great difference between the appearance of the neck mark and the size of the ligature. **When nylon, silk or terylene fabrics are used, they may leave a sharply defined mark only two to three mm. wide, resembling a mark caused by a narrow cord or wire.** The reason for this is, that when a broad piece of cloth is tightly stretched by pulling, certain parts of it become raised into ridges which form the ligating surface and only these may be reproduced on the skin. **These marks are usually less well demarcated at the edges than a cord or rope. These marks may fade if the neck is not examined soon after death, and if there was no abrasion.** The neck should be examined under ultraviolet light to visualise a suspected mark made by soft material. **The base of the mark is usually red (may be pale), especially if the ligature was of soft material, but cords, ropes and wires tend to abrade the surface, which on drying becomes hard, yellow or brown and parchment-like.** There may be exudation of tissue fluid which later dries, forming a stiff film, which tends to become more prominent as the interval lengthens after death. **Petechial haemorrhages are usually found immediately adjacent to the ligature mark, which is a confirmation that the mark was made during life. A narrow zone of reddening, congestion or bruising is also common immediately above and below the groove,** due to lateral displacement of blood from the squeezed area. This does not necessarily indicate that the ligature was applied during life. **The skin is pale below ligature mark, and puffy, oedematous, congested, cyanotic and haemorrhagic above the ligature.** Scratches may be found on the skin of the neck near the ligature caused by the attempt of victim to pull away the ligature. They are usually vertical, but may be irregular or crescentic. The fingernails of the deceased should be examined for fragments of skin and blood. In cases of homicide also, fingernails should be clipped and examined. **A body which is wet, may not reveal fingernail marks until drying of the skin.** The pattern of the ligature may point to the agent, e.g, a woven belt, plaited electric wires, links of chains, spiral rope patterns, etc. **If a rough ligature, e.g., a rope is used, and if there is some movement of the rope on the skin during a struggle, the skin may show marked abrasions and haemorrhages, and the deep muscles of the neck are grossly bruised. The ligature mark of strangulation is not obliterated by putrefaction, but is better preserved than the skin beyond it,** because of compression of the underlying blood vessels, and preventing the access of bacteria. **Even if the mark is obscured, subcutaneous haemorrhages in relation to the mark may be found.** Pulling a U-shaped ligature against the front and sides of the neck while standing at the back can cause death.

Depth, width, direction, raised ridges of skin, zones of hyperaemia, presence of duplicate strangulation marks, dried excoriations due to slippage of the implement, marks due to textile weave pattern and structure, distribution of petechiae in the skin, bruising, scratch marks and blisters in the strangulation mark should be noted.

Pseudo-strangulation: (1) Occasionally marks are seen on the dead bodies of infants and children in whom the neck is short. These depressed marks are produced from folds in the skin due to bending of the head. (2) In the elderly, pale crease marks may be seen due to overlapping rolls of skin, especially when head has been propped up with a pillow. (3) It can also be seen in decomposing bodies with tight collars, buttoned shirt at the neck or other clothing round the neck. In these cases, a deep groove simulating ligature mark of strangulation is produced due to the swelling of the tissues around the tight-fitting garment, as the body decomposes.

EXAMINATION OF LIGATURE: If at autopsy, the ligature is still in place around the neck, it should be removed by dividing it away from the knot, so that the knot may be preserved. The knot should be secured by tying the component parts with strings so that they do not fall apart as the ligature is removed see Fig. (13–3). Photographs (at close range) should be taken before the ligature is removed. The ligature should always be examined for the presence of blood, fragments of epidermis, hair or other suspicious substances. Record circumference of the noose of the ligature material as well as that of the neck of the victim.

If the nature of ligature is in doubt, before disturbing the neck, a search should be made for fibres or other material from the ligature, on the skin and adjacent clothing. This can be done by sticking five cm. lengths of transparent adhesive tape to the suspected area and stripping them off. This is then transferred to microscope slides and examined. The pattern produced by the ligature can be made out by examining the neck with oblique light or by ultraviolet light.

Signs of struggle: If there has been a struggle, abrasions and contusions may be seen on the face and other parts of the body. If the assailant kneels on the chest or abdomen of the victim, fractures of the ribs and injuries to the internal organs may be present.

Signs of Asphyxia: A sudden compression of the windpipe often makes a person powerless to call for help, and causes almost immediate unconsciousness and death. If there is slight vagal effect and some venous obstruction, there will be slight congestion of head and neck and occasional petechial haemorrhages. **With moderate venous constriction and some respiratory obstruction, asphyxial signs are moderate. When constricting force is great, (respiratory and venous obstruction) asphyxial signs are marked. Intense congestion and deep cyanosis of the head and neck is seen,** because the vertebral arteries continue to supply blood to the head and venous drainage is very less. **The face is puffy, oedematous, congested and cyanotic.** The eyes are wide open, bulging and suffused, with confluent scleral haemorrhage; the pupils dilated, the tongue swollen and often bruised, dark-coloured and protruded. Petechial haemorrhages are common in the skin of the eyelids, conjunctivae, face, forehead, behind the ears and scalp. **Bloody froth may escape from the mouth and nostrils,** and there may be bleeding from the nose and ears. The hands are usually clenched. The genital organs may be congested and there may be discharge of urine, faeces and seminal fluid. These asphyxial signs may be absent if death occurs quickly from vagal inhibition, due to pressure on carotid sheath.

Internal: **The neck and its structures should be examined after removal of brain and chest organs,** to allow blood to drain from the neck blood vessels. **There may be superficial haemorrhage under the ligature mark, though this is often minimal. There is severe engorgement and haemorrhage into the tissues in and above the area compressed. The adjacent muscles of the neck are usually lacerated. The deep muscles of the neck show little or no bruising, if the ligature used is soft and yielding. In some cases, no external mark is seen on the surface of the neck, but extensive bruising of the deeper tissues may be found.** The extent of the bruising depends upon the degree of pressure used. **A ligature which is tightly applied on the neck until death occurs, may fail to produce any bruising.** Subcapsular and interstitial thyroid haemorrhages are common. The mucous membrane of the pharynx, pyriform sinuses, epiglottis and larynx usually show areas of haemorrhagic infiltration. Lymphoid follicles at the base of the tongue and the palatine tonsils are congested; the posterior lingual mucous membrane, submaxillary and parotid glands may be studded with petechiae. The intima of the carotid arteries are not usually damaged, but a deeply sunken narrow ligature applied with force may damage the carotid arteries.

Bruising of the root of tongue and floor of the mouth may occur. Haemorrhage may be seen under the mucosa of the larynx, especially beneath the vocal cords as a direct result of compression and due to stasis of blood rather than asphyxia. These haemorrhages are larger than petechial haemorrhages of asphyxia. **The larynx, trachea and bronchi are congested and contain frothy, often blood-stained mucus.** False haemorrhages may be present in the back of the oesophagus and on the anterior spinal ligaments. The carotid arteries are damaged, if a narrow ligature is applied with force. **The lungs are markedly congested and show ecchymoses and large subpleural haemorrhages. Silvery-looking spots under pleural surface due to rupture of the air cells which disappear on pricking, are seen in more than 50% cases.** Due to putrefactive gas formation bullae will slip under the fingers if it is smoothened being subpleural, while emphysematous bullae will not. Pulmonary oedema may be present. Microscopically, there is usually intense interalveolar congestion with haemorrhages of varying size, fluid in the alveoli, areas of collapse and intervening areas of ruptured alveoli. **The air-passages often contain large areas of desquamated respiratory type epithelium, red blood cells and fluid. The parenchymatous organs show intense venous congestion,** and in young persons' ecchymoses are usually seen on the heart and kidneys. The brain is congested and shows petechial haemorrhages.

Injury to the hyoid bone is not common, because the level of constriction is usually below the bone. **If ligature is wide, sometimes fracture may occur. In older persons, fracture can be caused by** (1) direct lateral compression from the sides of the neck, by pressure applied high up under the angles of the jaw. (2) indirect violence, in which the bone is drawn upwards and immobilised by the various muscles which are attached to its upper surface when the neck muscles are contracted, as in attempt to resist strangulation. **Fracture of the thyroid cartilage is more common, especially of one or both superior horns.** Fracture of thyroid laminae and cricoid cartilage is less common than in throttling and occurs only when considerable force is used, or if some solid object is included in the ligature and applied over the front of the neck. Trachea is rarely broken Table (13–1).

Table (13–1). Difference between hanging and strangulation

Trait	Hanging	Strangulation by ligature
(1) Ligature mark:	It is oblique, does not completely encircle the neck; usually seen high up in the neck between the chin and larynx. The base is pale, hard and parchment-like.	It is transverse, completely encircling the neck below the thyroid cartilage. The base is soft and reddish.
(2) Abrasions and ecchymoses:	About the edges of ligature mark not common.	About the edges of the ligature mark are common.
(3) Bruising:	Of the neck muscles less common.	Of the neck muscles more common.
(4) Neck:	Stretched and elongated.	Not stretched or elongated.
(5) Subcutaneous tissues:	White, hard and glistening under the mark.	Severe engorgement and haemorrhage into tissues in and above the area compressed.
(6) Hyoid bone:	Fracture may occur.	Fracture is uncommon.
(7) Thyroid cartilage:	Fracture is less common.	Fracture is more common.
(8) Larynx and trachea:	Fracture rare.	Fracture may be found.
(9) Emphysematous bullae:	Not present on the surface of the lungs.	Very common on the surface of the lungs.
(10) Carotid arteries:	Damage may be seen.	Damage is very rare.
(11) Face:	Usually pale and petechiae are not common.	Congested, livid and marked with petechiae.
(12) Signs of asphyxia:	External signs less marked.	External signs well-marked.
(13) Tongue:	Swelling and protrusion is less marked.	Swelling and protrusion is more marked.
(14) Saliva:	Often runs out of mouth.	Absent.
(15) Bleeding:	From the nose, mouth and ears not common.	From the nose, mouth and ears common.
(16) Involuntary discharge:	Of faeces and urine less common.	Of faeces and urine more common.
(17) Seminal fluid:	At glans is more common.	At glans is less common.

MEDICOLEGAL QUESTIONS: (1) WHETHER DEATH WAS CAUSED BY STRANGULATION? In death due to strangulation, the general features of asphyxial death are present. Their local distribution in the head and neck is strongly presumptive of strangulation. This is confirmed by the ligature mark on the neck. Evidence of violent compression or constriction of the neck during life is obtained from the presence of bruising or ecchymoses about the marks on the neck, haemorrhages in the strap muscles, under the skin, in the sides of the tissues around the trachea and larynx, in the larynx and in the laryngeal structures themselves. The ligature mark alone is not diagnostic, for it may be indistinct or absent, if a soft ligature material is used. The ligature mark may be produced by the application of a ligature to the neck even after death. Certain marks on the neck produced after death may simulate ligature mark.

The possibility of other causes of suboxic or asphyxial death should be excluded. In the absence of ligature mark in the neck or deeper injury, it will be difficult to form an opinion, except from circumstantial evidence. In cases of putrefaction, a medical opinion about strangulation can be given fairly, if there are signs of mechanical violence applied to the neck, e.g., fracture of the larynx or hyoid bone, bruising of the muscles and visible skin impressions. Indistinct marks on the neck, patches of discolouration or signs of asphyxia cannot be relied upon as evidence of strangulation in a putrefied body.

A medical opinion should be based on all the facts connected with the position of the body, the nature and direction of the ligature and the effects produced on the neck and structures below the skin. The mere presence of a cord or ligature around the neck of a dead body does not confirm the diagnosis, for it may be put around the neck for a malicious purpose. All marks of violence on the body of a supposedly strangled person should be carefully examined, to determine whether they could cause death, or whether they can be explained on other grounds. Strangulation by ligature has to be differentiated from hanging Table (13–1).

(2) WHETHER THE STRANGULATION WAS SUICIDAL, HOMICIDAL OR ACCIDENTAL?

SUICIDAL STRANGULATION: Suicide by strangulation is rare. Various methods of tightening the ligature are employed by the victims. The number of knots, tightness and method of knotting should be considered. (1) The ligature is tightened like a tourniquet, but the person can apply a single or double knot, before consciousness is lost. In most cases, some mechanical device is always made to keep the ligature tight after insensibility develops. (2) Several turns of rope are tied round the neck with a knot which is usually single and in front, or at the side or back of the neck. (3) A cord may be tied around the neck and twisted tightly by means of a stick or some other solid material inserted between the ligature and the skin, and twisted around several times. When consciousness is lost, although grip on stick is released, the ligature will not become loose as it gets arrested against the shoulder or chin (Spanish Windlass Technique). (4) A running noose is applied to the neck, and the free end of the rope to which a weight is attached, is thrown over the end of the bed on which the victim lies. (5) A person may strangle himself by leaning with the whole weight of his body on a cord passed round the neck and attached to a fixed point.

In suicidal strangulation, the signs of venous congestion are very well developed above the ligature, and are especially prominent at the root of the tongue. This severe congestion probably results by the slow tightening of the ligature, and also because it is usually so secured that it remains in place after death, preventing postmortem drainage of blood. Injuries are usually less marked because less force is used. In all cases of suicidal strangulation, the ligature should be found *in situ*, and the body should not show signs of violence or marks of struggle. If ligature is still present, the number of turns and type of the knots require detailed study. The application of ligature with several turns, whether closed with a half-knot or even a complete knot, is consistent with suicide. A single turn of a broad ligature of rough cloth, closed with a half-knot indicates suicide. A correct medical opinion may be usually formed from the course and direction of the tie, the way in which it was secured or fixed to produce effective pressure on the windpipe, and the amount of injury to the muscles and parts beneath.

ACCIDENTAL STRANGULATION: (1) Children may get entangled in ropes during play, or the neck may be caught in window cords, etc. (2) Infants are sometimes strangled in their cots when the neck is caught inside bars, in restrainers, braces, etc. (3) Occasionally, an infant is strangled with a string attached to a toy tied to the crib. (4) Persons under the influence of alcohol, epileptics, and imbeciles may be strangled either by a tight scarf or collar and neck tie. (5) It may occur if an intoxicated person rests the neck against a bar or other hard object. (6) It may occur when a string used in suspending a weight on back, slips from across the forehead and compresses the neck. (7) In industry, belts, ropes or parts of clothing may be caught in the rollers or other parts of the moving machinery and cause accidental strangulation. (8) Accidental strangling may occur in uterus when the movement of the foetus causes the umbilical cord to encircle the neck. In such case, there is relatively slight cervical tissue injury. Wharton's jelly is not damaged and lungs are usually incompletely expanded.

HOMICIDAL STRANGULATION: Strangulation is a common form of murder. Virtually all cases of strangulation are homicide. Many of the victims are adult women and frequently strangulation is then associated with sexual assault. Usually there is a single turn of ligature round the neck, with one or more knots (granny or reef knots) at the front or side of the neck. When there are two or more firm knots, each on separate turns of the ligature, homicide is almost certain. There may be more than one ligature mark, each of varying intensity and crossing each other, in parallel or at an angle to each other. Abrasions are usually seen due to movement of the ligature across the neck. Fingernail marks may be seen, either from the victim attempting to remove the ligature, or from the assailant attempting to secure the ligature, and/or restrain the neck from moving, or even attempting manual strangulation. The victim's clothing may sometimes be caught in the ligature during a struggle and produce marks, which require careful evaluation. The mark may either completely encircle the neck or may be seen only at the front, when the ligature is pulled tightly from behind. The mark may also be sloping if the ligature is pulled upwards from behind, and the position is high up at the level of the hyoid bone. Sometimes, a ligature is passed over the body, and then tied to the hands and feet to simulate suicide. In such cases, the manner of tying should be examined. The presence of a complex type of knotting in the cord, e.g., the presence of reef knot, suggests homicidal strangulation. Infanticide by strangulation may be caused by winding the umbilical cord round the infant's neck. In such cases, the cord will show appearances indicative of rough handling with displacement of Wharton's jelly, and other signs of violence are present on the body. Sometimes, homicidal strangulation is feigned by an individual to bring a false charge against his enemy. Hysterical women sometimes feign it without any obvious motive.

Evidences of struggle are usually found, but if the person is taken unawares, and the ligature is suddenly placed around the neck and pulled tightly, the person loses consciousness quickly and is unable to offer much resistance. If the person is weak and infirm, or made unconscious by blows on the head or by intoxicating drugs and in children, there may be few or no signs of struggle. If the clothing of the deceased is torn or disarranged, it indicates that a struggle has taken place. If there is a struggle, both assailant and victim may show abrasions and contusions. Entanglement of hair or clothing with the ligature should be regarded as suspicious of homicide.

Strangulation should be assumed to be homicidal until the contrary is shown. As a rule, the murderer uses far more force than is necessary, and as such, injuries to the deeper structures are well marked. If the ligature is around the neck with two or three knots at the back of the neck, it is presumptive of homicide. The ownership of the ligature may sometimes become an important clue, e.g., if the ligature found around the dead body may be proved to correspond with parts of the same material found in the possession of suspected assailant. Unusual ligatures

may narrow the search for the assailant, since they may be material of the kind used in a particular occupation. If the ligature is removed or lies loose, unless explained, are presumptive of homicide. If the ligature mark in the neck does not accurately correspond with the ligature found, it is presumptive of homicide. Sometimes, circumstantial evidence, such as time, place, locked doors and windows, motive, etc., is almost the only evidence for a suggestion either of suicide or homicide.

Ligature marks produced after death do not show bruising. Either a grooved impression is seen on the skin which is not injured, or yellow or brown abrasion without signs of vital reaction. There may be ligatures or other marks around the limbs especially wrists and ankles, which may be placed either before or after death.

In a charge of murder, it may be suggested that the deceased might have been accidentally strangled in a state of intoxication, either by a tight scarf or collar and tie. When there is pressure on the windpipe, the victim attempts to pull the ligature, and scratches may be found on the neck, which may arouse a suspicion of throttling. If the relations of the body to surrounding objects and the constricting agent have not been disturbed, cases of accidental strangulation present no difficulty. If the body has been removed from the place in which it was first discovered, or the ligature has been removed, the presumption of accident can only be established from the description given.

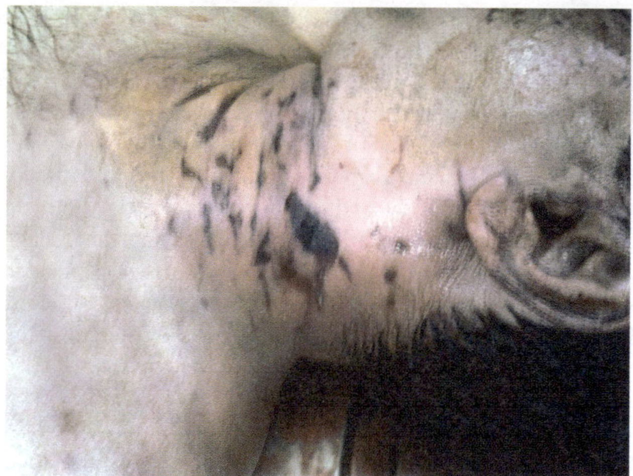

Fig. (13–26). Fingernail abrasions on front of neck in manual strangulation.

Courtesy: **Professor Mukta Rani, LHMC, Delhi**

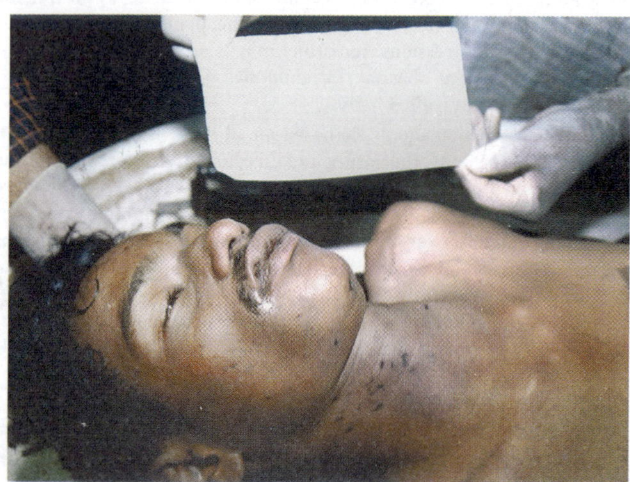

Fig. (13–27). Manual strangulation vertical finger nail marks on neck.

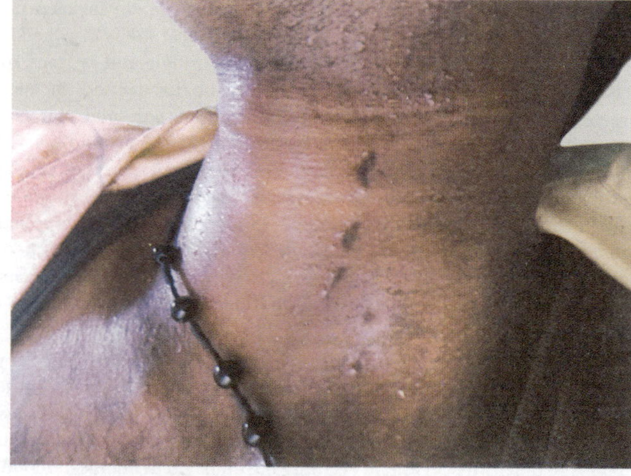

Fig. (13–28). Vertical nail marks on neck in manual strangulation.

THROTTLING OR MANUAL STRANGULATION

Asphyxia produced by compression of the neck by human hands is called throttling. Death occurs due to occlusion of carotid arteries or vagal inhibition which is much more common than in ligature strangulation, hanging excepted. Occlusion of airway plays minor role.

Postmortem Appearances: External: Bruises on the neck: The situation and extent of the bruised areas on the neck will depend upon the relative positions of the assailant and victim, the manner of grasping neck, and the degree of pressure exerted upon the throat. The bruises are produced by the tips or the pads of the fingers. Their shape may be oval or round and of the size of the digits (1.5 to 2 cm.), but continued bleeding into the contused area usually increases the size. If the fingers skid across the skin surface, longer, irregular marks may occur, along the jaw margins and chin. Usually, more force is used than is necessary to kill the victim. (1) A grip from right hand from the front produces a thumb impression on the right side of the victim's neck, which is usually under the lower jaw over the cornu of thyroid. Several finger marks are seen on the left side of the neck obliquely downwards and outwards and one below the other, but sometimes are grouped together and cannot be distinguished separately. (2) In a grip from behind the victim, the pressure is applied all around the neck, but some areas of bruising are more prominent due to the pressure of the fingertips. (3) When both hands are used to compress the throat, the thumb mark of one hand, and the finger marks of other hand, are usually found on either side of the throat. Sometimes, both thumb marks are found on one side, and several finger marks on the opposite side **Figs. (13–26 to 13–28)**. (4) A grip from both hands, one being applied to the front and the other to the back, produces bruises on the front and back of the neck. (5) In the case of children, or where the victim's neck is small, or the assailant's hand relatively large, the bruises may be towards the back. (6) Due to the shifting of the grip and sometimes the frank struggle of victim, bruises may be seen anywhere, even at the posterolateral sides of the neck and on the upper chest and collar bones.

Bruises may be seen over the prominence of the larynx and at the level of the cricoid. They may also be seen in the grooves on either side of the larynx. They may also be seen over the prominence of larynx and at the level of the cricoid. As such, it cannot be definitely determined which hand was applied from which side. In such cases, it is not possible to tell whether an assailant seized the victim from front or behind. Sometimes movement of fingers may cause large irregular bruises. **When fresh, the bruises are soft and red, but after several hours they appear brown, dry and parchment-like. If a soft material is kept between the hand and throat, bruising may not be seen. If the pressure upon the neck is maintained until after the death of the victim, bruising may be absent,** because there has been no blood flowing to extravasate from the damaged vessels. **Rarely, in throttling there are no external or internal injuries. This occurs if the victim is unconscious and amount of pressure to the neck is minimal.**

Fingernail abrasions: If the fingertips are pressed deeply, the pressure of the **nails produce crescentic marks on the skin.** They are more likely to be seen at the site of the thumb than the fingers, because when throat is gripped, the thumb exerts more localised pressure, and is less likely to move than the fingers during the struggle of the victim. Fingernail abrasions are of two types. (1) When the pressure is static, regularly curved, comma-like, dash-like or straight, up to 1.5 cm. in length and a few millimetres in width. (2) **When the nails skid down the skin, parallel, linear lines, several centimetres in length may be seen. Many scratches may be several millimetres wide and placed a centimetre or so apart, are produced by the victim herself, while trying to pull away the assailant's hand.** As most victims are females, the nails may be long and the scratches more severe than those caused by the assailant. These defence scratches are seen in parallel lines in a vertical direction in the long axis of the neck, but are often random. **Fingernail abrasions are much less common than bruises.** Victim's fingernail scrapings may contain fragments of skin, blood, hair and fibres. Irregularity of the nails of the assailant may leave signature on the victim's skin. **The alleged assailant should be examined to correlate any injuries that may have been inflicted on him by the fingernails of victim, and his fingernail scrapings should be taken.** If one hand only is used, there may be more extensive abrasions on the side of the neck to which the fingers were applied, the thumb making few scratches. If numerous scratches are found on the left side of the victim's neck, the inference will be that the throttling was by the right hand of the assailant and vice versa. Haemorrhage in the subcutaneous tissues and the muscles underlying nail marks is usually scanty when compared with external injuries. In some cases, linear impression is produced. **It is commonly assumed that the concavities of the crescentic abrasions follow the anatomical shape of the nail margin. But the results may be completely contrary.** According to Gordon and Shapiro, the shape of the fingernail, largely determines the result. **Nails with straight border give unpredictable results. As the nails become more pointed towards the centre of the free border, paradoxical results are more common.** Fixation of the skin at the centre occurs where the nail digs in with escape at the margins, so that when the traction releases, the mark appears inverted, with the convexity facing the finger pad. In some cases, the injuries are indefinite abrasions, which may not be noticed unless examined carefully. A wet body may not show fingernail marks until drying of the skin has occurred.

Signs of asphyxia: Face is usually congested and cyanotic above site of throttling with petechiae of conjunctivae and sclerae. Fine petechiae may be present on the face. The tongue may or may not be bitten, but is usually protruded. Congestive-asphyxial signs appear in 15 to 30 seconds of pressure on the neck, but if a change in grip occurs and fingers impinge on carotid structures reflex cardiac arrest occurs, so that the intensity of congestive changes may be of any degree in any given death.

Signs of struggle: Bruises and abrasions may be found on other parts of the body. In cases where the victim has been forced to the ground and has been held down, bruising may be found: (1) in the scalp tissues over the back of the head, (2) in the tissues overlying the spinous processes of the lower cervical and upper dorsal vertebrae, (3) in the tissues overlying the posterior surface of the scapulae, (4) over the muscles of the front of the chest and abdominal wall if the assailant kneels on the victim. If the force is considerable, fracture of ribs and contusions and lacerations of the abdominal organs may occur. Fingernail marks and fingertip bruising of the face are quite common. There may be an attempt to obstruct mouth, producing injuries of the lips.

DISSECTION OF THE NECK: The neck structures should be dissected *in situ* and in a bloodless field. The block removal of the neck structures (as in routine autopsies), may produce artefacts in the neck tissues which resemble bruises. When the tongue and neck structures are firmly grasped and pulled upon, the hyoid bone may be fractured. Bruising invariably occurs in throttling, and is very important in the absence of external marks and fracture of the neck structures. To obtain a bloodless field in the neck, the head should be opened, and the brain removed as in routine autopsy. The abdominal and thoracic organs should be removed as in routine autopsy. The head is then moved slowly up and down and allowed to drain of blood. Then an incision should be made from the chin to the manubrium sterni, or a V-shaped incision made on the neck extending from the mostoid process on either side to the manubrium sterni Fig. (13–29), and the platysma dissected laterally on both sides. If the veins are damaged, they should be ligated to prevent bleeding, as otherwise the blood will infiltrate into the tissues and may be mistaken for contusions. The sternomastoid muscles are cut from their attachments.

The common carotid artery is cut longitudinally, looking for any bruising around the bifurcation. Tears of the intima of the carotid

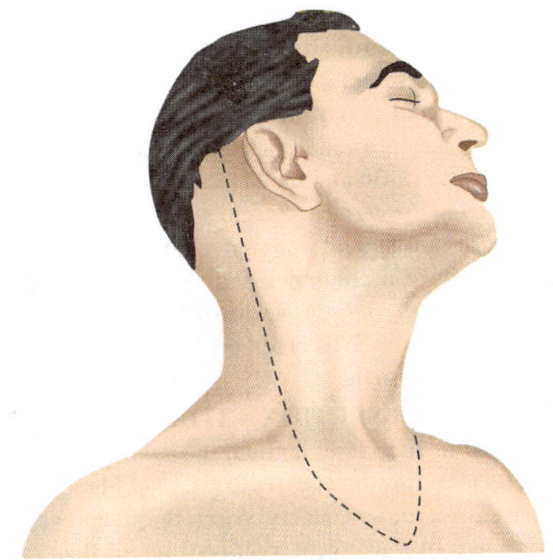

Fig. (13–29). V-shaped incision for dissection of neck.

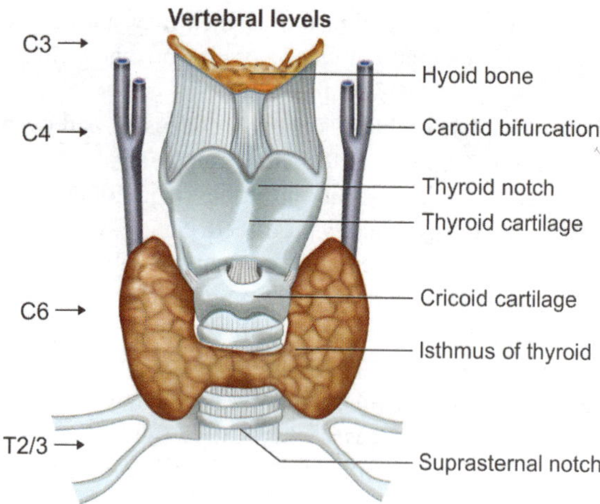

Fig. (13–30). Structures on the front of the neck.

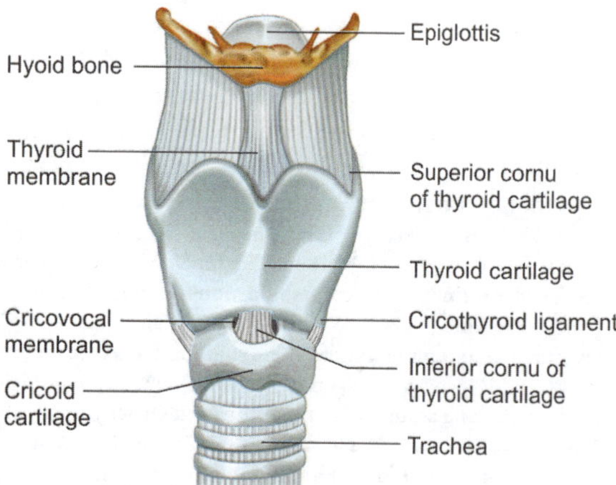

Fig. (13–31). Hyoid, larynx and trachea.

artery are usually seen half to one cm. below the bifurcation of the vessels. Toothed dissecting forceps should not be used as it may damage the intima which resembles a tear. The hyoid bone is identified and the suprahyoid and infrahyoid muscles are reflected, noting for any contusions. Sectioning of thyrohyoid ligaments between greater cornua of hyoid bone and superior cornua of thyroid cartilage permits manipulation of both structures independently for possible fractures. The hyoid bone is grasped at the body in one hand and each greater horn is tested with the other hand by bending it outwards and inwards to note the presence of a fracture. The hyoid bone is removed from the neck and any fracture if present is confirmed. The fracture appears as an irregular break in the continuity of the bone and is usually associated with haemorrhage at the site of fracture. The thyroid cartilage is exposed by dissecting the thyroid gland through the isthmus and the middle constrictor muscle. The larynx and trachea are examined for the presence of any fractures Figs. (13–30 and 13–31).

Usually injuries of the cervical vertebral column and spinal cord are missed. The neck organs should be removed, the anterior longitudinal ligament of the vertebral column is exposed and examined. Incise posterior side of the neck and dissect down to the spinous process and the ligaments surrounding the foramen magnum, and odontoid process is cut. Expose the spinal cord.

POSTMORTEM DISSECTION ARTEFACTS OF THE NECK: During routine postmortem examination, the holding of organs and the incision of vessels often produces extravasation of blood into the tissue spaces. These are dissection artefacts. When the structures of the neck are removed *en masse* by downward traction from the floor of the mouth, blood will extravasate in the deep connective tissues. If an autopsy is carried out within a few hours of death or if the head and neck are congested owing to the position of the body after death, haemorrhage may occur into the spaces between the muscles of the neck, when the structures are being dissected or removed. All the structures of the neck should be examined *in situ* to ensure that postmortem artefacts are not mistaken for antemortem bruises.

Internal: Bruising of neck structures: The soft tissues of the neck are compressed and forced upwards and backwards against the cervical vertebrae. **Bruises may be found in the dermis, in the superficial fascia, in the deep fascia, the muscles, in the substance of the thyroid gland, and sometimes under the capsules and in the substance of the submandibular glands. Bruises are usually separate. In some cases, bruising may be absent externally, although the deeper tissues may show fairly extensive bruising. Rarely, there are no external or internal injuries, if the victim is unconscious and amount of pressure to the neck is minimal. The mark on the surface of the neck may not exactly correspond with the internal bruising, because of the mobility of the skin** which may alter the relationship which normally exists between it and underlying structures. The extent of bruising depends upon the degree of pressure used. In some cases, a small area of bruising on either side of the midline and usually over the thyroid cartilage or the hyoid bone may be the only finding. **Sometimes, the bruising of the muscles is very slight,** and as such the muscles of the neck should be dissected individually *in situ.* Tissues at the back of the neck may show bruising when counterpressure has been exerted. The muscles surrounding the larynx, both anteriorly and posteriorly frequently show well marked bruising. **The sternomastoid and deeper strap muscles may show patches and bleeding or even frank haematoma and may be torn. The platysma muscle may be bruised.**

There may be deep haemorrhage in the neck tissues surrounding or adjacent to the bifurcation of the common carotid artery. **Carotid arteries show intimal tears in 10 to 15% of cases at or near the carotid sinus.** Haemorrhages may occur in pharynx, epiglottis, tonsils, base of the tongue, the larynx immediately below the vocal cords and also beneath the capsule of the thyroid, submaxillary and parotid glands and lymphatic glands of the anterior triangle of the neck. **Deep haemorrhages may be present in the base of tongue, usually at the sides.** Deep congestion is seen in central or whole posterior part of tongue. **The larynx is usually squeezed, as the pressure is bilateral.** To demonstrate the fractures of laryngeal cartilages, it is essential to strip the larynx of its attached muscles and ligaments. **Minor fractures of larynx may not be fatal. Bruises of the laryngeal mucous membrane is frequent,** sometimes accompanied by severe laryngeal swelling which may or may not be accompanied by fracture of the hyoid bone and laryngeal cartilages. **The surface of the epiglottis may show a shower of petechial haemorrhages or frank haemorrhage.** Deep haemorrhages may be present in the base of the tongue. The lungs show congestion and with subpleural petechial haemorrhages. **Pulmonary oedema** and subpleural blebs may be present. **A fine froth, often blood-stained is seen in the bronchi.** The air passages often contain desquamated epithelium. Microscopically, haemorrhages are seen in the interstices under the pleurae and through rupture of the alveolar walls. Some areas are overdistended with ruptured alveoli and other areas are collapsed. The brain is usually congested and may show petechial haemorrhages in the white

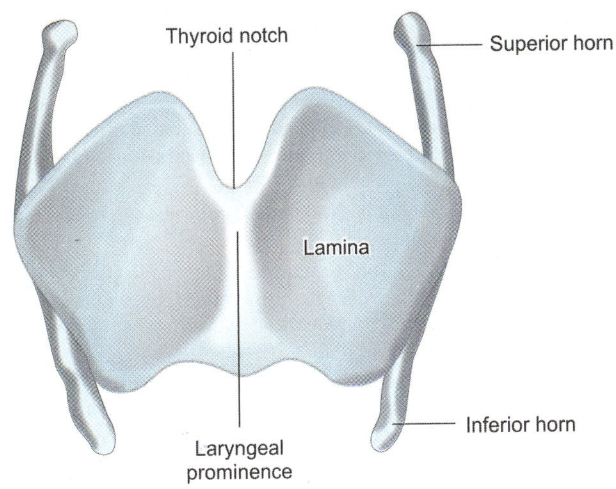

Fig. (13–32). **Thyroid cartilage.**

matter. Subarachnoid haemorrhages and rarely areas of small haemorrhages in the brain may be present. Haemorrhages may be found over the brain. Other internal features are similar to that of strangulation.

Artefacts: Spurious collections of blood are commonly found behind the pharynx, larynx and on the front of the cervical spine. In most cases it is an artefact produced by overdistension and rupture of the venous sinuses, forming the pharyngo-laryngeal plexus, which can occur in natural deaths and may be either peri- or early postmortem in origin. They can be mistaken for evidence of throttling. Similarly, there can be small collection of blood around the hyoid and thyroid cartilages which can be mistaken for strangulation. Banding of the oesophagus is another artefact, especially when the tissues are congested. These bands are pale areas in the mucosa caused by postmortem hypostasis being prevented from settling by the external pressure of larynx, trachea and aortic arch.

Thyroid cartilage Fig. (13–32): The superior horn of thyroid cartilage is much more fragile and fractures much more commonly than greater horn of hyoid bone. Fracture of the superior cornu of the thyroid cartilage at its base is common due to the local pressure, but the extent of damage varies. **Often only the right horn may be broken to which the thumb was applied.** It only indicates pressure applied to the neck, but is not a threat to life. Fracture of a horn even with slight bleeding can be produced after death by rough handling of the body, e.g., by hyperextension of the neck, and as such it is not proof of injury during life. **The sole finding of a fractured horn without injury to skin or deeper structures is of no value.** Fracture of the ala of the thyroid cartilage occurs often either in the midline or obliquely or spirally across the left or right lamina, if pressure is much greater. **Fractures of the thyroid cartilage are more serious than those of the hyoid bone.** This injury is more common in blows to the front of the neck, either by the fist or the edge of the hand, punching, kicking, arm-locks or fall on to a ridged object, such as gate or chair-back. They are usually vertical and near the junction of the laminae in the midline, and are the result of a direct blow upon the laryngeal prominence. The body of the thyroid cartilage can be broken by a **Karate blow** to the front of the neck or by contact with the handlebar of a bicycle or the edge of a chair or any projecting object. Sudden death may be caused through vagal inhibition of the heart or laryngospasm. In **"commando punch"**, the edge of the hand is brought forcibly across the side of the neck or the front of the larynx. Blows directly to the larynx, indirectly stimulate the sinus region, or the laryngeal sensory nerve endings and may trigger the cardio-inhibitory reflex.

Hyoid bone: Fractures of the hyoid bone with inward driving of its distal fragments occur in 30 to 50% of cases, either due to direct lateral compression or due to indirect violence. In direct violence, the hyoid is drawn up and held rigid by the powerful muscles attached to its upper and anterior surface. Violent downward or lateral movement of the thyroid cartilage or pressure between the hyoid bone and the thyroid cartilage will exert traction through the thyrohyoid ligament and produce fractures of the hyoid bone. **Fractures of the thyroid cartilage and hyoid bone are usually found in old people with calcified thyroid cartilages and rigidly ossified hyoid bones, but are very rare in young children.** Laceration of pharynx may occur following fracture of hyoid bone.

Fracture of the cricoid cartilage (shaped like a signet ring with the signet part at the back) anteriorly through the narrow bridge in a spiral or oblique fashion rather than at the wider posterior plate **occurs almost exclusively due to the anteroposterior compression against the spine,** e.g., by the thumbs or the forearm of the assailant. Rarely it may break either during transit, or from incorrect autopsy techniques. It can also occur by allowing neck to fall against a hard surface or sharp edge during removal from place of death or during handling in mortuary. Focal haemorrhage is always seen around fracture caused during life. **If bleeding is not seen by the naked eye, but histology of the fracture site shows some red cell extravasation, this can be accepted as antemortem in the presence of surface bruises, scratches, muscle bleeding, intralaryngeal and tongue haemorrhages.** Fractures of the cricoid cartilage is seen only in fatal cases of throttling. Severe injury to the internal cervical structures, e.g., bilateral comminuted fracture of the larynx, is usually caused by a blow to the neck or a fall on the neck rather than throttling. Larynx composed of nine cartilages is situated opposite to 3 to 6 cervical vertebrae in adult males and little higher in females. In these conditions, the fractured margins are driven inward.

CAUSE OF DEATH: Pure asphyxia from strangulation is rare, as considerable pressure is necessary to obstruct the trachea which will also block the jugular and carotid systems. Occlusion of the airway probably plays a minor role in causing death. The carotid arteries lie over the transverse processes of fourth, fifth and sixth cervical vertebrae and any anterolateral impact in this position can compress them against the underlying bone. The usual mechanism of death is occlusion of carotid arteries. A shifting grip may suddenly impinge upon the carotid vessels causing sudden death. Thus, there may be a period of partial asphyxia terminated suddenly by the onset of cardiac arrest. About half of the deaths are due to vagal inhibition, in which the amount of force need not produce any damage either to skin, deep tissues or the arteries. Rapid or instantaneous death can occur due to sudden cardiac arrest, when a pale face with no signs of asphyxia are seen. This is commonly seen in throttling, often in hanging and less often in ligature strangulation. If a victim of throttling survives, amnesia and neck pain are common.

PALMAR STRANGULATION: The palm of one hand is placed horizontally across the mouth and nostrils without using the fingertips, its pressure being reinforced by placing the other

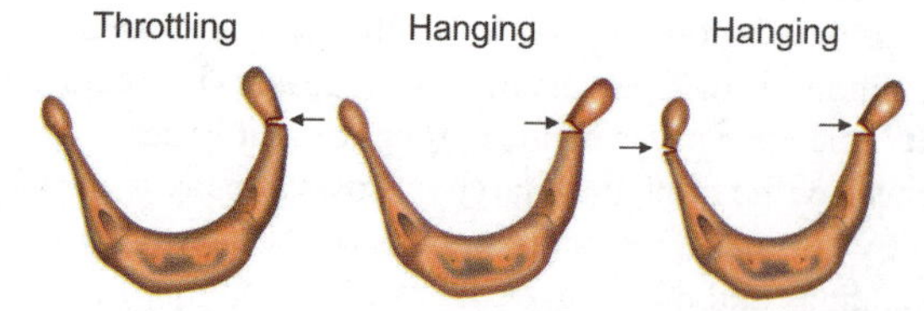

Fig. (13–33). Fracture hyoid bone in throttling and hanging.

palm on the top of it at right angles, the heel of the upper palm pressing upon the front of the neck. In such case, the face is congested with petechiae. Diffuse bruising with fracture of thyroid cartilage may be seen. In most cases the victim is intoxicated.

HYOID BONE FRACTURES: Classification: (1) Inward compression fractures. (2) Anteroposterior compression fractures. (3) Avulsion fractures.

Hyoid bone lies at the root of the tongue where the body is difficult to feel. The greater horn lies behind the front part of sternomastoid, 3 cm. below angle of mandible and 1.5 cm. from the midline.

Inward Compression Fractures: This is seen in case of throttling, where the main force is an inward compression acting on the hyoid bone. **The fingers of the grasping hand squeeze the greater horns towards each other, due to which the bone may be fractured within one cm. of the tip, and the posterior fragment is displaced inwards. The periosteum is torn on the outer side of the bone, but not on the inner side.** In such cases, if the body of the bone is grasped in one hand, and the distal fragment between the finger and thumb of the other hand, the distal fragment can be easily bent in an inward direction, but outward movement is limited to the normal position only Fig. (13–33). At the joint between the greater horn and body of hyoid, a similar fracture may be seen. In some cases, bilateral inward fractures may occur. In cases of putrefaction and maceration, if the soft tissues are not attached to the bone, it is difficult to say whether the small fragment was fractured inwards or outwards. The bone should be preserved with the soft tissues attached, if it has to be kept as an exhibit.

Anteroposterior Compression Fractures (Abduction fractures): In cases of hanging, the hyoid bone is forced directly backwards, due to which the divergence of greater horns is increased which may fracture with outward displacement of the posterior small fragment. In such case, the periosteum is torn on the inner side of the fracture only, due to which the fragment can be easily moved outwards, but inward movement is limited to the normal position only. **Like the inward compression fracture, anteroposterior compression fracture may occur either in the greater horn or at its junction with body, and it may be bilateral.** When compression is severe, the small fragment may be completely detached from the bone and may lie either medially or laterally to the rest of the bone. In such cases, *in situ* examination of the hyoid bone in the neck only will decide whether the fracture was inward or outward. **Outward fractures of the greater horn of hyoid bone are seen in ligature strangulations, run over motor vehicle accidents, blows on the front of the neck, etc.** In these cases, the hyoid bone is grossly fractured with outward displacement of the fragments and multiple fractures of other structures are also found.

In some cases of bilateral fracture of hyoid bone in hanging, one greater horn is fractured outwards and the other inwards Fig. (13–33). **This may be explained as follows: The hyoid bone is pressed backwards, as well as moves from side to side in hanging, due to which posterior end of the greater horn may be caught against a bony ridge or sides of the vertebrae. An inward fracture of the imprisoned greater horn occurs because of the continued side to side movement and counter-pressure. An outward fracture of the other greater horn occurs due to the further compression of the vertebral column.**

Inward compression or anteroposterior compression fractures are not of much practical value.

Avulsion (Tug or Traction) Fractures: Violent lateral or downward movements of the thyroid cartilage or the pressure between the cartilage and hyoid bone will produce traction through the thyrohyoid ligaments, leading to fracture of the hyoid bone.

Demonstration of Fractures: 1% aqueous solution of toluidine blue solution is applied to suspected areas of fracture and left for 15 seconds and then cleaned with water. By examination with stereomicroscope, fractured sites would appear bluish.

The cartilaginous separations between the greater horns and the body, and the joints between the lesser horns and the body, or the presence of incomplete bony union of the hyoid parts, should not be mistaken for fractures. Triticeous cartilages are little nodules embedded in the thyrohyoid ligament. These may be confused with a fracture of the superior horn of thyroid cartilage. They are a normal anatomic variant and can be palpated as nodules and easily moved in different directions. Improper dissection of the neck may produce postmortem fracture. The neck should be X-rayed in lateral oblique views to demonstrate fracture of the hyoid and cricoid.

MEDICOLEGAL QUESTIONS

(1) WHETHER DEATH WAS CAUSED BY THROTTLING?

The usual diagnostic signs of death due to manual strangulation are: (1) Cutaneous bruising and abrasions. (2) Extensive bruising with or without rupture of the neck muscles. (3) Engorgement of the tissues at and above the level of compression. (4) Fracture of the larynx, thyroid cartilage and hyoid bone. (5) Cricoid cartilage is almost exclusively fractured in throttling. (6) General signs of asphyxia.

When all the signs are present, the diagnosis is easy. In the absence of external signs , or when they are equivocal, care is necessary. The pressure must be applied for two minutes or more to cause death. Fingernail abrasions are often produced due to the victim trying to free himself from the throttling grip. The examination of the nails of the victim and assailant may indicate their origin. When a suspended body shows extensive injuries to the neck structures, there is a strong probability that the victim was first throttled and then suspended after death. In such case, signs of violence on the body, and sometimes of rape, if present are helpful. The discolourations produced in decomposing bruises are usually localised, but similar areas of decomposition may be found when decomposition affects localised antemortem intravascular collections of blood in the cervical tissues, or localised patches of postmortem lividity. Hyoid bone fracture is strongly suggestive of throttling.

When throttling has been attempted at about the moment of death, one cannot be certain whether the deceased was alive or dead at the time. Nail marks will appear much the same whether produced just before or just after death, but contusions are only produced during life.

(2) WHETHER THE THROTTLING WAS SUICIDAL, HOMICIDAL OR ACCIDENTAL?

SUICIDAL THROTTLING: Suicide by throttling is not possible, because the compression of the windpipe produces rapid unconsciousness and the fingers are relaxed. Sometimes, a person might try to strangle himself with his hand, and upon failure might use a ligature. In such case, the degree to which the impressions exist will usually clear the doubt.

HOMICIDAL THROTTLING: Throttling is a common mode of homicide because the hand is immediately available. It is a method of

choice in infants. The victims are usually infants, children or women. Adults can be throttled when under the influence of drugs or drink, or stunned or taken unawares. In an adult, signs of struggle are usually present, but if the throat is forcibly grasped and firmly compressed, the victim cannot struggle. The assailant may also sustain injury, especially scratches and bruising of the face and arms, or his hands and fingers may be bitten. The alleged assailant should be examined to correlate any injuries that may have been inflicted on him by the fingernails of the victim, such as scratches, which are found mostly on the back of the hand and face. The fingernail scrapings of the assailant should be taken to compare any debris found and the tissue types of the victim. Sometimes, it is preceded by rape or attempted rape. The victim may have been held down by the throat during intercourse or throttled to stop her cries. If contusions and fingernail abrasions are present on the neck, the presumption must be of homicide. The defence may allege that such marks have been produced due to fall by the deceased while his hand was passively applied to his neck, the marks being produced accidentally by the pressure of his own fingers. This is highly improbable.

ACCIDENTAL THROTTLING: A sudden application of one or both hands on other person's throat as a demonstration of affection, in joke, as a part of physiological experiment, etc., may cause death from cardiac inhibition. The victim cannot have died instantaneously if there is bruising, for bruising requires a beating heart.

(3) HOW MUCH FORCE COULD HAVE BEEN USED BY AN ASSAILANT ? If there is severe damage to neck structures, it indicates use of considerable force, and is indicative of intent to injure, if not to kill. If there is fracture of hyoid bone or larynx, it indicates the use of appreciable force and is homicidal in nature, for it cannot be an accidental touch or momentary grip. A brief and minor contact with the neck would be consistent with restraint, without intention of injuring and causing death. Minor damage or absence of damage to the neck structures is presumptive of innocence, but sometimes deliberate interference with the neck structures can kill without producing much damage, e.g., the karate blow. If only slight changes are seen in the neck structures, a guarded opinion should be given about the probable degree of force used.

BANSDOLA: One strong bamboo or stick is placed across the back of the neck and another across the front. Both the ends are tied with a rope and tightened due to which the victim is squeezed to death. Sometimes, a stick is placed across the front of the neck, and the assailant stands with a foot on each end of the stick. If a stick or foot is used, a bruise is seen in the centre of the neck across the windpipe corresponding in width to the substance used. If two sticks are used, a similar mark will be seen on the back of the neck. Sometimes, the chest may be squeezed forcibly between two sticks placed across the back and front of the upper part of the chest. This interferes with respiration and causes laceration of the muscles and fractures of the ribs.

GARROTTING: The victim is attacked from behind without warning. The throat may be grasped, or a ligature is thrown over the neck and quickly tightened, by twisting it with a lever (rod, stick, ruler, etc.), within the ligature. The assailant is then able to tie the ligature with one or more turns. In this way, a single assailant can kill a healthy adult male. This method is usually used in lonely places to kill travellers and to rob them. This method had a refinement in which the neck was forced against a sharp spike which penetrated the spinal cord, which results in sudden loss of consciousness and collapse. Garrotting as a mode of judicial execution was once employed in Spain. An iron collar around the neck was tightened by a screw for strangling (Spanish Windlass).

MUGGING: Strangulation is caused by holding the neck of the victim in the bend of the elbow. Pressure is exerted either on front of the larynx, or at one or both sides of the neck by the forearm and upper arm. The attack is usually made from behind. The postmortem appearances are those of ligature strangulation with a broad object, i.e. the signs are minimal. Sometimes, a diffuse abrasion may be seen along the margin of the jaw due to the friction of the forearm. Internally, there may be diffuse bruising, but this may be slight or absent. There may be bruising behind the larynx and in the strap muscles of the neck. Fracture of superior horn of thyroid or hyoid is rare. In some cases, the neck may be pressed by the foot or knee. When the neck is stamped on repeatedly, there will be crushing of the larynx and trachea, and bleeding in the soft tissues with swelling. Death may occur due to asphyxia or reflex cardiac arrest.

COMPRESSION OF THE NECK: This is a broad term used for non-specific causes of neck pressure which may be sudden. In hard compression, such as kicking or stamping or jumping on the neck, or karate chops, and flying kicks, soft tissues are grossly damaged. There may be vertical fracture of the laminae of thyroid cartilage, cricoid or upper tracheal rings. Hyoid bone and thyroid cartilage tend to be flattened and broken outwards. Death may be rapid with crush injury, and seepage of blood into the tissues, or it may be asphyxial due to swelling or obstruction of the airway. Surgical emphysema may be present. **Soft, prolonged neck compression occurs in wrestling, carotid sleeper hold and choke hold.**

SUFFOCATION

Suffocation **is a general term to indicate that form of asphyxia, where entry of air to the lungs is prevented by any means other than pressure on the neck or drowning.**

ENVIRONMENTAL SUFFOCATION: Death from hypoxic hypoxia may usually result from breathing in a vitiated atmosphere. A vitiated atmosphere is deficient in oxygen which is caused by displacement of oxygen from the atmosphere by inert gases or by gases generated in the atmosphere. CO, CO_2, methane, sulphuretted hydrogen, sulphur dioxide, nitrous oxide, chlorine and phosgene are commonly found in vitiated atmosphere. **CO displaces oxygen from the atmosphere, and sulphur dioxide prevents haemoglobin from combining with oxygen. Deaths are almost always accidental. The concentration of oxygen in air is about 21%, nitrogen 79%, and CO_2 is 0.033%. An oxygen concentration of 16% or less is dangerous, and with 5% concentration, consciousness is lost rapidly and death occurs within a few minutes.** (1) Suffocation occurs in airtight place or one in which ventilation is negligible. This may occur when children become locked in old disused refrigerators or when they lock themselves into large boxes or trunks during play. (2) Lack of oxygen in the atmosphere may occur in the vicinity of lime kilns and wells or excavations in chalk rock, where the oxygen is displaced by CO_2. (3) In a confined space, such as tanks, grain-bins, silos, deep tanks of a ship, fermenters, tanning vats, unused wells, sewers, etc., hazardous gases, vapour, dust or fumes may accumulate or the oxygen may be deficient. A person may be suffocated on entering such a confined space. (4) Inhalation of irrespirable gases, such as CO_2, CO, hydrogen sulphide or smoke from a burning house , or entering into disused wells produce suffocation. **CO_2 and methane are the most commonly encountered suffocating**

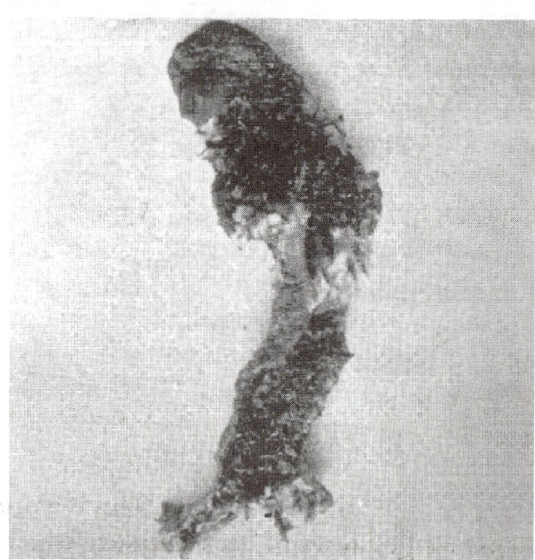

Fig. (13–34). Smothering. The victim fell into a heap of husk and inhaled the material into his air-passages.

gases. Death occurs due to lack of oxygen. (5) Reduction of atmospheric oxygen as in decompression, such as cabin failure of aircraft at high altitudes. (6) It also occurs in ship's tanks or other industrial metal chambers, in which oxygen is replaced by nitrogen. (7) In deaths associated with replacement of oxygen with an inert gas, such as helium, rapid death is common before hypoxia had any physiological effect. **In hypoxic death, petechial haemorrhages are absent. Congestion and cyanosis may or may not be present.**

SMOTHERING: This is a form of asphyxia which is caused by closing the external respiratory orifices either by the hand or by other means, or blocking up the cavities of the nose and mouth by the introduction of a foreign substance Fig. (13–34), such as mud, paper, cloth, etc. Smothering has been used synonymously with suffocation by some authors.

Suicide by Smothering: (1) **Suicidal smothering by the hand is impossible.** (2) Suicide is possible by burying the face in a mattress or lying against the bed clothing to obstruct the nose and the mouth. It is usually seen in the mental patients or prisoners. (3) Sometimes, in cut-throat wounds, the trachea may be completely cut and the soft parts may obstruct the trachea and the victim is smothered. (4) Suicidal smothering can be effected by tying a polythene or similar bag over the head.

Accidental Smothering: Most fatal smotherings are accidental. (1) Suffocation rarely occurs when an infant 3 months or less, turns on its face and buries it in soft pillow or mattress. The fabric that becomes stained with saliva, nasal mucus and vomit may form an impervious seal and prevents the passage of air. The weight of the head presses the nostrils and mouth against the fabric. **It is not necessary that the mouth and nostrils should be completely closed at the start, for as obstruction increases and congestion develops, saliva, mucus, oedema fluid and traces of blood will pour out into the mouth and cause obstruction to breathing.** Infants covered with heavy blankets or bedding will not die of smothering. (2) An epileptic or intoxicated person may smother himself accidentally by burying his face in a pillow that is impervious to air, or covering with bed clothes. (3) A person may accidentally fall into a large quantity of semisolid or finely divided material like mud, ashes, grain, sand, coal dust, etc., so that his mouth and nose are covered by the substance. The victim may struggle, inhale some of the material into his air-passages, and swallow some into his stomach in an effort to breathe. (4) Children may be suffocated accidentally while playing with plastic bags. Death may occur even if the open end of the bag is not tied around the neck due to cardiac inhibition due to CO_2 narcosis. Even a flat plastic sheet may adhere to the face in some way and block the nose and mouth which is exaggerated by attempts to breathe. **Face is pale. Signs of asphyxia are faint or lacking in case of plastic bag suffocation. Moisture usually collects in the bag.** (5) Smothering from plastic bags may occur due to the addictive habit of "glue-sniffing", in which the organic solvents of certain glues is used as an intoxicant, by putting some into a plastic bag and inserting the head to obtain a high concentration of vapour. In such cases, chemical analysis is essential. (6) Plastic bags may be applied to the head for experiment or auto-erotic exercise, as partial asphyxia is believed to increase sexual sensation. (7) It also occurs if the membranes remain round the head of the newborn after delivery.

Homicidal Smothering: Homicide is possible where the victim is incapacitated from drink or drugs, very weak, child or old person, in ill-health and when the victim is stunned by a blow. Usually, the mouth and nose are closed by a hand or cloth, or the face may be pressed into a pillow (gentle homicide). Smothering can be caused by pinching the nose of the child with one hand, while the other hand is used to push the jaw to close mouth **Fig. (13–35)**.

Autopsy: External: Obstruction by bed clothing, a pillow, a cushion, etc., applied with skill, may not leave any external signs of violence, especially in the young and the old. When the face is pressed into a pillow, the skin around the nose and mouth may appear pale or white due to pressure. Pressure marks on the face can rarely be distinguished from postural changes, where circumoral or circumnasal pallor is caused by passive pressure of the dependent head after death which prevents gravitational hypostasis from entering these areas. **Petechiae and congestion are rarely seen unless the victim struggles and fights for breath. Saliva, blood and tissue cells may be found on the pillow. If the orifices are closed by the hand, there may be scratches, distinct nail marks, or laceration of the soft parts of the victim's face.** The lips, gums and

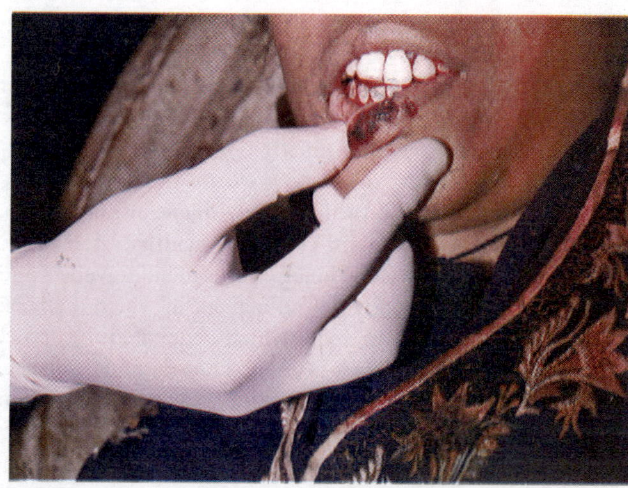

Fig. (13–35). Smothering. Contusion of inner side of lower lip.

tongue may show bruising or laceration. Slight bruising may be found in the mouth and nose, which should be confirmed by microscopy. **The asphyxial signs and symptoms are severe, because death usually results due to slow asphyxia and often the fatal period is three to five minutes. The head and face may show intense congestion and cyanosis with numerous petechial haemorrhages in the skin of the face and beneath the conjunctivae.** Blood may ooze out from the mouth and nose. The tongue may be protruded and may have been bitten. Often, the head and face enclosed in a plastic bag are pale, with few petechial haemorrhages in the eyelids and pericardium or there may be no asphyxial signs. Death is rapid due to reflex cardiac arrest, rather than a purely hypoxic process. Moisture inside the bag is not proof of breathing as evaporation from the skin, nose and mouth can produce moisture.

Internal: Mucus may be found at the back of the mouth. Air passages often contain eosinophilic fluid with red blood cells and varying amounts of desquamated respiratory epithelium. Slight acute emphysema and oedema of the lungs with scattered areas of atelectasis, petechiae and congestion are the major findings. The internal organs are deeply congested and sometimes show small haemorrhages. In the absence of localising signs at autopsy, the background to the death and the circumstances in which the body was found are of help. The finding of the material from the victim such as mucus, squamous epithelium on the smothering material is also of help. **If a person is buried alive, earth and sand will be found in the respiratory tract.**

Homicidal smothering is extremely difficult to detect. The autopsy may reveal asphyxia, but there may not be any corroborative medical evidence to prove foul play. The pathological changes must be interpreted keeping in view the medical history of the deceased, the scene of death, and the specific circumstances surrounding the death.

GAGGING: This is a form of asphyxia which results from forcing a cloth into the mouth, or the closure of mouth and nose by a cloth or similar material, which is tied around the head. A gag (such as rolled up cloth) pushed into the mouth sufficiently deep to block the pharynx will cause asphyxia. Initially, the airway may be patent through the nose; collections of saliva, excessive mucus with oedema of the pharynx and nasal mucosa, progressively causes complete obstruction. There may be congestion of the face and fine petechiae of the face, sclerae and conjunctivae. It is almost always homicidal and the victim is usually an infant. It is not possible for one person to gag and bind another. **Sudden death due to reflex vagal inhibition may occur. The gag should be examined for buccal epithelial cells.**

Gagging is usually resorted to prevent the victim's shouting for help, and death is usually not intended. The victim's hands are tied behind to prevent their removing the gag, and the legs are tied together to prevent walking or running for help. It should be noted, as to how the cloth piece is wrapped round the nose and mouth, how it is tied, and how far the mouth gag is stuffed inside the mouth.

OVERLAYING: Overlaying or compression suffocation results due to compression of the chest, so as to prevent breathing. It occurs when the mother or other person shares a bed with an infant. During sleep, the older person rolls on to or crushes the infant. The thoracic movements are limited and respiratory exchange is either reduced or completely prevented. In many such cases, the mother or older person goes to the bed under the influence of alcohol. It is very rare. Flattening of the nose and face (smothering) may or may not be seen. These parts are pale. The nostrils are often filled with froth, which may be blood-stained and this may stain the pillow or garment. The usual findings are those of asphyxia. Death may occur from neurogenic cardiac arrest.

Traumatic asphyxia and smothering: When a person is buried in loose earth or sand or in grain silos, he may die due to occlusion of the nose and mouth and immobilisation of the chest and abdomen by external pressure sufficient to prevent respiratory movement.

CHOKING

Choking is a form of asphyxia caused by an obstruction within the airpassages, usually between the pharynx and bifurcation of trachea. The individual develops a sore throat, hoarseness, respiratory difficulty and then suddenly collapses. Choking from objects being lodged in the posterior hypopharynx, blocking glottis and oesophagus is commonly seen in the very young, elderly, psychiatric patients or in the infirm, particularly where the ability to swallow or masticate is severely impaired. **It is commonly associated with alcohol intoxication, neurological injury or senility.**

Accidental Choking: Choking is almost always accidental. (1) Choking commonly occurs during a meal when food is accidentally inhaled, especially when the victim is laughing or crying. (2) Vomited matter may be inhaled by a person under the influence of drink or of an anaesthetic, during a fit of epilepsy, or while in a state of insensibility from other causes. (3) Infants usually regurgitate clotted milk after a meal, and this may fall into the larynx. (4) Choking may occur due to inhalation of blood from facial injuries, such as a broken nose, or dislodged teeth, and laceration of the lips and gums inflicted during fight, if the victim becomes unconscious and lies on his back. Sometimes, blood may be found as far as the smaller bronchioles. (5) Impaction of solid bodies, such as a large bolus of food, piece of meat, fruit stone, onion, potato, corn, button, coin, rag, rubber teat, seeds, live fish, mud, leaves, cotton, or a set of false teeth, extracted teeth in dentistry, blood and cloth after ENT operation, such as tonsillectomy may cause asphyxia. (6) Gauze packs inserted during an operation can be inhaled and cause death. (7) In adults, false dentures may impact in the throat sometimes during anaesthesia. (8) Children often place objects like marbles or coins in their mouths, which may pass into larynx or trachea during a sudden deep inspiration. (9) Objects like rubber balloons may be inhaled by children during play **Fig. (13–36)**. (10) Choking due to regurgitation of food may occur during rape or violent sexual intercourse **Fig. (13–37)**. (11) In head injury, irritation of the brain causes vomiting, which may be inhaled. (12) Food aspiration following suppression of the gag reflex by tranquilizing drugs is sometimes seen in lunatic asylums. The foreign body becomes arrested at, or just below the vocal cords **Figs. (13–36 and 13–37)** and may produce an inflammatory reaction with oedema. (13) Insect bites especially those of bees, wasps and hornets, and drug reaction from penicillin, etc., can

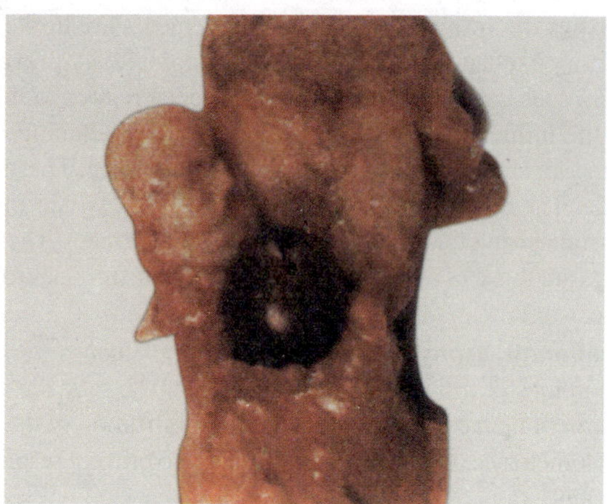

Fig. (13–36). Chocking from a grape.

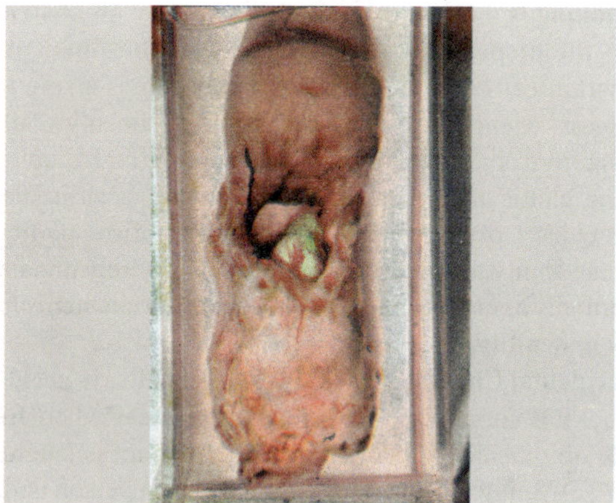

Fig. (13–37). Chocking due to a bolus of food.

cause swelling of the lining membranes of the larynx and death within a few minutes due to an allergic reaction. (14) A blow to the front of the neck may cause severe swelling of the mucosa of the airway due to oedema and haemorrhage. (15) In an epileptic, the tongue falling against posterior pharyngeal wall during an attack, may result in choking. Death may occur due to reflex vagal inhibition.

Very rarely pins, safety pins, small bone pieces may be lodged in the air passages for relatively long periods without causing serious trouble.

If there is struggle to breathe and attempts to remove the occluding object are unsuccessful, asphyxial changes are well marked. When a foreign body is inhaled, there is immediate acute respiratory distress, but once this has passed, the victim has little subsequent distress. Complications may develop after a latent interval.

Autopsy: Great thickening of epiglottis and epiglottic folds by jelly—like oedema and inflammatory tissue will be found occluding entrance to larynx. Mucus may be found at the back of mouth and throat in considerable quantity. Microscopically, lungs show intense interalveolar oedema and congestion, haemorrhages of varying sizes and collection of desquamated respiratory type epithelium.

Suffocation may occur from diseases, such as diphtheria, infectious mononucleosis, H. influenzae infection in children, rupture of aortic aneurysm in air passages, haemoptysis in pulmonary tuberculosis, a tuberculous gland eroding into a bronchus and prolapsing into its lumen, acute oedema of the larynx due to inhalation of steam or ingestion of irritant substances, pharyngeal abscess, epiglottitis, laryngeal and bronchial growths, haemorrhage into the trachea, etc., and from the effects of certain poisons.

Choking from external causes may occur from impaction of a relatively large foreign body, a bolus of food, or a denture in the oesophagus, compressing the trachea. This may rarely cause death by vagal stimulation.

Suicidal Choking: It is rare. The victims are usually mental patients (dementia or psychoses) or prisoners. For this a foreign body is thrust into the throat.

Homicidal Choking: Choking as a mode of infanticide may be caused by stuffing a wad of paper or cloth into the pharynx or larynx. It is very rare and is practicable only when the victim is suffering from disability or disease.

Cause of Death: (1) Cardiac inhibition is the common cause. (2) Asphyxia. (3) Laryngeal spasm. (4) Delayed death may result from pneumonia, lung abscess or bronchiectasis.

CAFE CORONARY: This is a condition in which a **healthy but grossly intoxicated person (restaurant patron), who begins a meal, suddenly turns blue, coughs violently, then collapses and dies, without much fuss. Death appears to be due to sudden heart attack. At autopsy, a large piece of poorly chewed food (bolus or a piece of meat) may be found obstructing the larynx. The clinical signs of choking are absent,** because of the high blood alcohol content which anaesthetises the gag reflex. Death is caused due to reflex vagal inhibition of heart.

TREATMENT: A blow on the back or on the sternum may cause coughing and expel the foreign body. If there is difficulty in breathing and cyanosis, first aid is given by application of pressure on the abdomen (Heimlich manoeuvre) till the patient recovers or loses consciousness. A person standing behind the patient and using hands with fingers interlinked exerts pressure in the region of the pit of the stomach may expel the object. If this is not successful, the foreign body should be removed from the hypopharynx with the middle and index fingers or with forceps.

Autopsy: The foreign body which caused the occlusion of air passages will be found in the mouth, larynx or trachea. **When food or vomited matter has been inhaled, particles of food material may be observed embedded in thick mucus in the trachea and bronchi, and particles may be drawn into the bronchioles which distinguishes the condition from those cases in which food is forced up the oesophagus and falls into the larynx after death.** Typical findings of asphyxia are absent. Toxicological examinations for alcohol and sedatives is essential.

TRAUMATIC ASPHYXIA: Mechanism: Traumatic asphyxia results from respiratory arrest due to mechanical fixation of the chest, by an unyielding substance or object, so that the normal movements of the chest wall are prevented. Fatal cases are only due to accident. Usually, there is a gross compression of the chest and usually abdomen by a powerful force, due to which chest expansion and diaphragmatic lowering are prevented.

Causes: (1) Multiple deaths are likely to occur when there is an outbreak of fire in a theater or whenever large crowds gather in an enclosed place. Some are crushed by the weight of the crowd, the chest being pressed violently, or may even get trampled on and crushed under feet **(riot crush or human pile deaths).** (2) Another common cause is crushing by falls of earth or stone usually in a coal mine or during tunnelling or in a building collapse even if head remains above the fallen soil. Similarly, burial in grain, sand, coal or mineral, may have the same effect. (3) Sometimes, the victim is pressed to the ground by some heavy weight as by a motor vehicle or other machinery. (4) A person repairing a car may be crushed when the jack slips and the vehicle falls on top of him. (5) It may occur in assault cases, where the victim is jumped or stamped upon and crushed by one or more assailants. (6) It occurs in industrial disasters, earthquakes and landslips. (7) Trapping between a vehicle and wall or between buffers of two railways trucks. (8) Occasionally, it results from indirect compression, when the body is subjected to force in such a manner that his thighs and the knees are driven against his chest, the so-called "jack-knife" position.

Postmortem Appearances: **An intense congestion, petechial and confluent haemorrhages and cyanosis of deep purple or purple-red colour of the head, neck, and upper chest above the level of compression is the prominent feature.** The purple-red colour is due to haemorrhage into the tissues around the dilated blood vessels. Below this level, the skin is pale or mildly cyanosed. **Areas of pallor seen at the level of the collar of the shirt, folds or creases in the garments, buttons, braces, etc., are another characteristic feature.** The face, lips and scalp may be swollen, congested and dotted with petechiae and ecchymoses Fig. (13–38). Fractures of the ribs, and other bones may occur. **If the patient recovers, the purple colour gradually disappears in ten to fourteen days, without the colour changes seen in bruises.** Heavy pressure on the chest primarily compresses the thinner right side of the heart, but left side continues to pump blood for some time. Retrograde displacement of blood from the superior vena cava into the subclavian veins and the veins of the head and neck results from sudden compression of the chest or abdomen. The spread of the hydrostatic force to the veins of the upper limbs is prevented by valves in the subclavian veins. The displacement of the blood into the valveless veins of the head and neck causes the rupture of distal venules and capillaries. These ruptures produce numerous petechial haemorrhages into the skin, eyelids, conjunctivae, mucous membrane of the mouth and usually bleeding from the nose and ears. **The conjunctivae and sclerae are grossly congested and haemorrhagic.** The bleeding in the eyes may form blood blisters which bulge through the eyelids and may occupy the whole of the sclera. Petechial haemorrhages may be seen over the surface of the cerebral hemispheres. The lungs are usually dark, heavy and have subpleural petechial haemorrhages. The right heart and all the veins above the aorta are markedly distended. Internal organs are congested.

BURKING: **Burking is a method of homicidal smothering and traumatic asphyxia**. William Burke and William Hare, made their living by digging up bodies from graveyards and supplying them to the medical schools for dissection. Later they killed 16 persons in Edinburgh, during the years 1927 and 1928, and sold their bodies to Dr. Robert Knox for use as specimens in his anatomy classes. A victim usually alone or away from the family, was invited to their house and given alcohol. Then the victim was thrown to the ground and Burke used to kneel or sit on the chest and close the nose and mouth with his hands, and Hare used to pull him round the room by the feet. Hare turned approver.

POSTURAL OR POSITIONAL ASPHYXIA: **It occurs when an individual acquires a certain body position in which his breathing is impaired, often because of neck twisting with kinking or compression of the trachea and/or elevation of the tongue into the posterior hypopharynx.** In addition, the normal venous return to the heart may be impaired. **Body is typically inverted (upside-down), and the weight of the abdominal contents press against the diaphragm pushing it upwards, thus compressing the thoracic organs which combined with decreased respiratory movements, leads to cardiorespiratory failure and death. It is always accidental.**

Causes: It occurs in a variety of situations. (1) It is most common in situations where a violent or physically aggressive person is physically or mechanically restrained on their stomach, face down or in a prone position. (2) When a person falls in a well and wedged between the walls. (3) **An intoxicated person may slide out of bed so that his head and chest, hang down from the edge and the remaining body rests at an upper level** Fig. (13–39). (4) From forcible flexion of the neck on the chest or

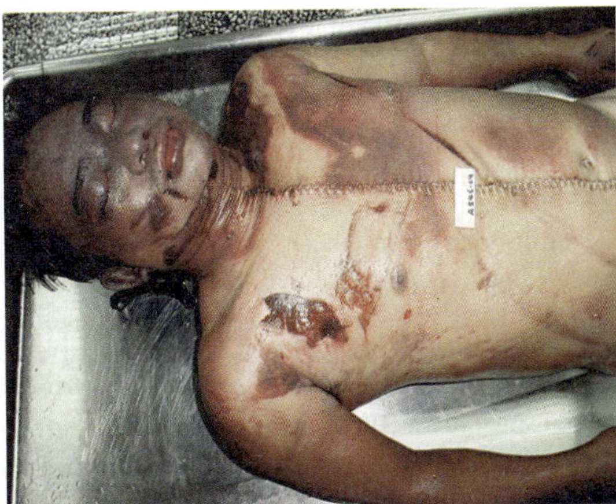

Fig. (13–38). Traumatic asphyxia caused by fall of a heavy object on the chest.

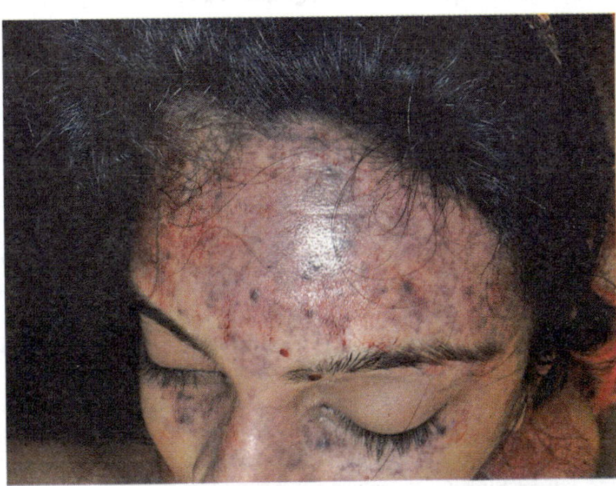

Fig. (13–39). Postural asphyxia. Marked congestion, cyanosis and petechiae are seen on the face.

when he collapses in a narrow space and neck is bent or twisted. (5) Occasionally, it results from indirect compression, when the body is subjected to force in such a manner that his thighs and the knees are driven against his chest, the so-called "jack-knife" position. **There is usually marked congestion, cyanosis and petechiae in the face and neck.**

The diagnosis is essentially based on (1) the body position must obstruct normal gas exchange, (2) it must not be possible to move to another position, (3) other causes of natural or violent death must be excluded.

DROWNING

Drowning is a form of asphyxia due to aspiration of fluid into air-passages, caused by submersion in water or other fluid. Complete submersion is not necessary, for submersion of the nose and mouth alone for a sufficient period can cause death from drowning. Death in shallow water can occur in the case of alcoholic stupor, epileptics or infants. About 150,000 person die from drowning each year around the world.

DURATION OF SUBMERSION IN FATAL CASES: When a person falls into water, he sinks partly due to the force of the fall, and partly to the specific gravity of the body which is 1.08. The specific gravity of fat is 0.92; bone 2.01, muscle 1.08, soft organs 1.05, and brain 1.04. Shortly afterwards, he rises to the surface due to the natural buoyancy of the body. In sudden immersion into cold water, the victim may take a deep inhalation of water due to reflex from stimulation of the skin. He may hold his breath for varying periods until the CO_2 in his blood and tissues reaches sufficient levels to stimulate the respiratory centre. At that time, an inevitable inhalation of water may occur. When he cries for help and struggles, he is likely to inhale water, which produces coughing and drives out large volume of air out of lungs, and leads to disturbance of the rhythm of the breathing. He may vomit and aspirate some gastric contents. His struggle increases and again he sinks. If this occurs during inspiration, he will inhale more water. The cerebral hypoxia will continue until it is irreversible and death occurs.

With warm water, cerebral anoxia becomes irreversible between three to ten minutes. Consciousness is usually lost within three minutes of submersion. The struggle for life with rising and sinking of the body goes on for a variable period, depending on the vitality of a person, until he remains submerged. Convulsive movements then occur, followed by coma or suspended animation and death. Immersion in cold water may be followed by immediate circulatory collapse, irregularity of heart beat and death. In freezing water death occurs in 5 to 10 minutes. At 6°C, incapacitation is likely to occur within 30 minutes and death in less than one hour. A body in fresh water usually sinks to the bottom, but in deep salt water, the body may not sink to the bottom but floats several metres under the surface, depending on salinity.

THE MECHANISM OF DROWNING: Brouardel carried out experiments with dogs as follows. The four limbs of the dog were fixed to a wooden board, and a weight of lead was fixed to the lower end. A cannula was introduced into the femoral artery to record the blood pressure and heart beats, and a pneumograph attached to the epigastrium for recording respiratory movements. The dog was then lowered into a tub filled with water. The dog's head was kept about 30 cm. below the surface throughout. The process was divided into five stages. (1) The stage of surprise lasting for 5 to 10 seconds. The animal inspired once or twice but inactive. (2) The first stage of respiratory arrest, lasting for about one minute. The dog was violently agitated, fighting against its bonds and obviously trying to reach the surface. The mouth was shut and respiration arrested. (3) The stage of deep respiration, lasting for about one minute. The dog made some deep inspirations and expelled white foam to the surface. The agitation stopped. The eyes and mouth were open. A few swallowing movements were noted. (4) The second stage of respiratory arrest, lasting for about one minute. Thoracic movements were not observed. The corneal reflex was lost and pupils were widely dilated. (5) The stage of terminal gasps, lasting for about 30 seconds. The dog made 3 or 4 respiratory movements. The lips and jaw muscles showed fibrillary contractions. The whole process of drowning of these dogs in fresh water took 3 to 4 minutes. Under identical conditions, sea water is approximately twice as lethal as fresh water. In man, probably the course is similar except rising to the surface once or more. Hypoxic convulsions may occur in the fourth stage.

Kylestra (1965) reported that mice submerged in suitably oxygenated physiological saline solution, could survive for 18 hours. If this medium was replaced by sea water or tap water, the mice succumbed in less than twelve minutes. The volume inhaled is also important. Modell (1966) showed that in dogs, if the volume inhaled exceeded 44 ml. per kg. body weight, the chance of survival was very small. The critical volume of sea water was twenty-two ml. per kg. In humans, it is believed, similar phenomenon occur in drowning.

Types: Drowning is of four types: (1) **Wet drowning**: In this, **water is inhaled into lungs and** the victim has severe chest pain. This is also known as **primary drowning (typical drowning),** in which **death occurs within minutes of submersion secondary to cardiac arrest or ventricular fibrillation.** Hyperkalaemia is only a relatively minor factor. (2) **Dry drowning: In this type, water does not enter the lungs, but death results from immediate sustained laryngeal spasm due to inrush of water into the nasopharynx or larynx. Thick mucus, foam and froth may develop, producing a plug. This is seen in 10 to 20%** cases of immersion and is commonly seen in children and adults under the influence of alcohol or sedative hypnotics. Resuscitated victims have panoramic views of past life and pleasant dreams without distress. (3) **Secondary drowning** (post-immersion syndrome or near drowning): **Near drowning refers to a submersion victim who is resuscitated and survives for 24 hours**. The person may or may not be conscious. These **persons may develop hypoxaemia resulting in brain damage, electrolyte disturbances, pulmonary oedema, haemoglobinuria, sepsis, metabolic acidosis, chemical pneumonitis, cerebral oedema, cardiac arrhythmias and myocardial anoxia.** Death may occur from half to several hours after resuscitation in about 20% of cases. In survivors, about 5 to 10% develop most serious neurologic damage. (4) **Immersion syndrome** (hydrocution or submersion inhibition): **Death results from cardiac arrest due to vagal inhibition** as a result of (a) cold water stimulating the nerve endings of the surface of the body, (b) water striking the epigastrium, (c) cold water entering ear drums, nasal passages, and the pharynx and larynx which cause stimulation of nerve endings of the mucosa. Falling or diving into the water, feet first, or "duck-diving" by the inexperienced, or diving involving horizontal entry into the water with a consequent blow on the abdomen cause such accident. Alcohol increases such effects, due to the general vasodilation of skin vessels, and possibly by some central effects on the vasomotor centre. This type of very rapid death on immersion is also said to occur in emotionally tense individuals, such as intending suicides, in whom the nervous reflex arcs seem more active. This is seen in one to two percent of cases of drowning. **Deprivation of oxygen caused by obstruction of alveolar spaces is a factor in all types of drowning, especially as the time of immersion lengthens.**

The Pathophysiology of Drowning: The pulmonary alveolar lining is semi-permeable. If water enters the alveoli, an exchange of water takes place through the alveolar lining. The extent and direction of this exchange depends on the

difference between the osmotic pressure of the blood and the water.

(1) Drowning in Fresh Water or Brackish Water: In drowning in fresh water (0.05% NaCl), **two-and-half litres or more of water may be inhaled and absorbed in three minutes; blood volume may increase by 50%** causing a great strain on the heart due to hypervolaemia. Haemodilution leads to haemolysis, relative anaemia, myocardial hypoxia, haemoglobinaemia, and haemoglobinuria, marked hyponatraemia and hyperkalaemia. Calcium levels may fall to two mEq/L. Fresh water alters or denatures the protective surfactant which lines the alveolar wall, while sea water dilutes or washes it away. The denaturing of surfactant can continue even after a person is successfully resuscitated. Loss or inactivation of pulmonary surfactant (lipoprotein) and alveolar collapse decrease lung compliance, resulting in severe ventilation perfusion mismatch, with up to 75% of the blood perfusing non-ventilated areas. The defective functioning of surfactant leads to pulmonary oedema with transudation of protein-rich fluid into the alveolar spaces, hypoxia and secondary metabolic acidosis. Acute respiratory distress syndrome (ARDS) may result from aspiration if the person survives. Severe hypotension may occur during and after the initial resuscitation period. When water is inhaled, debris plugging the patient's airway and release of inflammatory mediators cause increased peripheral airway resistance with pulmonary vasoconstriction, development of pulmonary hypertension, decreased lung compliance and fall of ventilation perfusion ratios. **The concentration of serum electrolytes (sodium and calcium) decreases considerably.** Proteins and haemoglobin are also reduced. The serum **potassium increases** (a powerful myocardial toxin). This increased load causes rapid overburdening of the heart and produces pulmonary oedema. The oedema fluid contains serum proteins. The heart is subjected to hypoxia, overfilling, sodium deficit and potassium excess. Cardiac arrhythmias leading to ventricular tachycardia and fibrillation occur, probably due to hypoxia and haemodilution. Hypoxaemia and hyperkalaemia may directly damage the myocardium, decreasing cardiac output. Metabolic acidosis may impair cardiac function.

(2) Drowning in Sea Water: Due to the high salinity of sea water (usually over three percent NaCl), **water is drawn from the blood into the lung tissue, and produces severe pulmonary oedema, and hypernatraemia.** This causes haemoconcentration. Simultaneously, in an attempt to re-establish osmotic balance, salts from the water in the lungs pass into the blood stream. A marked bradycardia occurs, probably due to the raised plasma sodium level. Heart failure may occur due to myocardial anoxia and increased viscosity of blood. **Slow death occurs from asphyxia.**

Haemodilution is far more dangerous than haemoconcentration. The red cells are crenated in sea water drowning and lysed in fresh water drowning, and potassium sodium ratio is greatly increased.

Causes of Death: (1) **Asphyxia:** Inhalation of fluid causes obstruction to the air-passages. Circulatory and respiratory failure occur simultaneously, due to anoxia of both the myocardium and the respiratory centre. (2) **Ventricular fibrillation:** In fresh water drowning death may occur in three to five minutes from a combination of anoxia, and a disturbed sodium-potasium ratio producing arrhythmias of the heart-beat, ventricular tachycardia and fibrillation. Severe hyperkalaemia is only a relatively minor factor. (3) **Laryngeal spasm** may result from inrush of water into the nasopharynx or larynx. (4) **Vagal inhibition** is due to icy cold water, drunkenness, high emotion or excitement (intending suicides) and unexpected immersion. (5) **Exhaustion.** (6) **Injuries:** Fracture of skull and fracture-dislocation of cervical vertebrae may occur due to the head striking forcibly against some solid object. Concussion may occur due to striking the head against some hard substance, or the water itself while falling from a height.

Fatal Period: Death usually occurs in **four to five minutes of complete submersion in fresh water and 8 to 10 minutes in sea water.**

TREATMENT: Artificial respiration and closed-chest cardiac compression should be started immediately. In fresh water drowning an external defibrillator should be applied to the chest and the electrolyte balance should be restored. In sea water drowning administration of oxygen and correction of haemoconcentration by infusion of hypotonic fluids should be carried out. The mouth and nostrils should be cleaned and air-passages kept clear by repeated suction. The body should be wrapped in warm blankets and stimulants given.

Direct mouth-to-mouth or direct mouth-to-nose breathing are the best methods of artificial respiration. The patient is made to lie on his back, and the head is hyperextended. The operator takes a deep breath and then breathes directly mouth-to-mouth or mouth-to-nose, or through a specially designed tube. The patient is allowed to exhale passively. This is repeated about fifteen to twenty times per minute. This should be continued for about an hour or till natural respirations are restored.

CLOSED-CHEST CARDIAC MASSAGE: The patient is made to lie on the back. The operator places his hands one on top of the other, on the lower end of the patient's sternum. Forcible rhythmic compressions are made 60 to 80 per minute to empty the blood from the ventricles. The force of compression must be sufficient to produce pulsation in the carotid and femoral arteries.

Postmortem Appearances: External: The postmortem signs are variable and none of them is pathognomonic. If the body is removed from the water shortly after death, the clothing is wet and the skin is wet, cold, moist and pale because of vascular contraction on the surface. Mud, silt, sand, sea weed, water weed, algae, small aquatic animal life, etc. may be present on or in the body, such as mouth, nostrils, ears, etc. **The postmortem lividity is light-pink in colour** (simulating the colour in CO poisoning) due to the presence of unreduced haemoglobin in the superficial blood vessels due to cold, whether antemortem or postmortem, but in some cases it is dusky and cyanotic, or it may be a mixture of the two. **Postmortem staining is usually found on the face, the upper part of the chest, hands, lower arms, feet and the calves, as the body usually floats face down, buttocks up, with legs and arms hanging down in front of the body.** The face may or may not be cyanotic, the conjunctivae are sometimes congested and few petechial haemorrhages are seen beneath the conjunctivae, especially in the lower eyelids. The pupils are dilated. The tongue may be swollen and protruded. Petechial haemorrhages are rarely seen in the skin. Rigor mortis appears early, especially when a violent struggle takes place before death. Vomiting, micturition, defecation and seminal emissions may occur agonally.

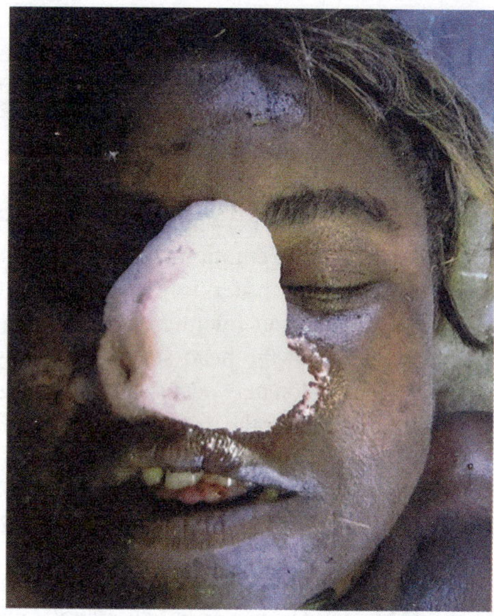

Fig. (13–40). Drowning. Copious froth from the nostrils.
Courtesy: Professor M. Reddy; Manmohan Reddy, Swaziland.

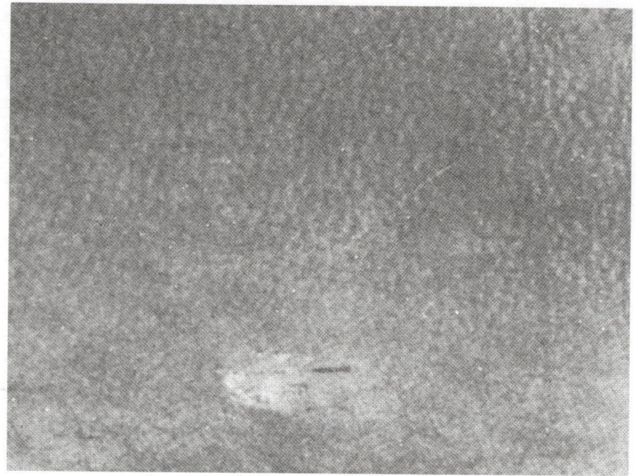

Fig. (13–41). Cutis anserina.

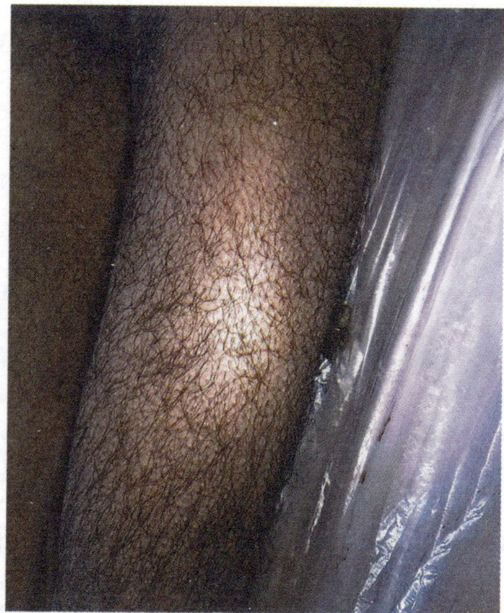

Fig. (13–42). Cutis ansetina.
Courtesy: Dr. Satish Phalkho, BHU, Varanasi.

Froth: A fine, white, lathery froth or foam is seen at the mouth and nostrils, which is one of the most characteristic external signs of drowning Fig. (13–40). The inhalation of water irritates the mucous membrane of the air-passages due to which the tracheal and bronchial glands secrete large quantities of tenacious mucus, and the alveolar lining cell irritation produces oedema fluid. Vigorous agitation of the seromucoid secretion and the surfactant with aspirated water and retained air, by the violent respiratory efforts, converts the mixture of endogenous secretions and drowning medium into froth. **The froth consists of protein and water and the fine bubbles do not readily collapse when touched with the point of a knife due to presence of surfactant. Froth is more common in drowning in sea water. Froth is usually white, but may be blood-stained,** because of slight admixture with blood from intrapulmonary bleeding. If wiped away, it gradually reappears, especially if pressure is applied on the chest. Froth is seen in death due to strangulation, acute pulmonary oedema, electrical shock, during an epileptic fit, in opium poisoning and putrefaction, but in all these cases it is not of such a large quantity as in drowning, and the bubbles are also much larger. Froth formation in respiratory tract suggests pulmonary oedema. Putrefaction converts froth into bubbly, reddish, foul-smelling fluid.

Cutis anserina or goose-skin or goose-flesh, in which the **skin has granular and puckered appearance may be seen on the anterior surfaces of the body particularly on the thighs. It is produced by the spasm of the erector pilae muscles,** attached to each hair follicle, and can occur in living when the skin comes in contact with cold water **Figs. (13–41 and 13–42).** It may occur on submersion of the body in cold water immediately after death, while the muscles were still warm and irritable. It is also produced by rigor mortis of the erector muscles. Agonal contraction of erector pilae is common. It is rarely seen in India, as the water is usually warm. Retraction of the scrotum and penis is due to the same cause, and has the same value. These changes have been designated **"reaction phenomenon".**

Cadaveric spasm: Weeds, gravel, grass, sticks, twigs, leaves, etc. present in the water may be firmly grasped in the hands due to cadaveric spasm. This strongly suggests that the person was alive when he drowned, because it indicates the struggle of the person for his life. This is seen rarely. The old adage about a **"drowning man clutching a straw"** contains a large amount of scientific truth. Damaged nails and abraded fingers showing sand, mud, or other materials under the nails due to struggle has the same significance.

Washer woman's hands: Soddening of the skin occurs due to absorption of water into its outer layer. It is first seen on the fingertips in two to four hours and spreads to the palm and the backs of the fingers, and the back of the hand, in that order in about twenty-four hours. **Wrinkling of the skin begins to appear shortly after immersion, bleaching of epidermis in four to eight hours, and the bleached, wrinkled and sodden appearance is seen in twenty hours. The skin becomes sodden, thickened, wrinkled, and white in colour, known as "washerwoman's hands" Figs. (13–43 and 13–44).** This is seen early in warm water. Area protected by clothing develop

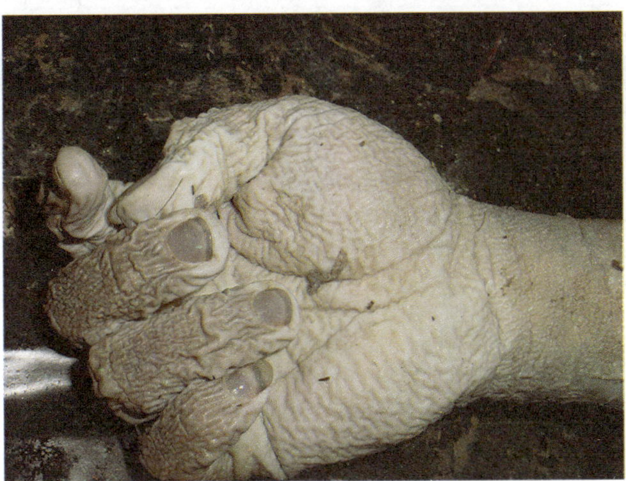

Fig. (13–43). Washerwoman hand in drowning.

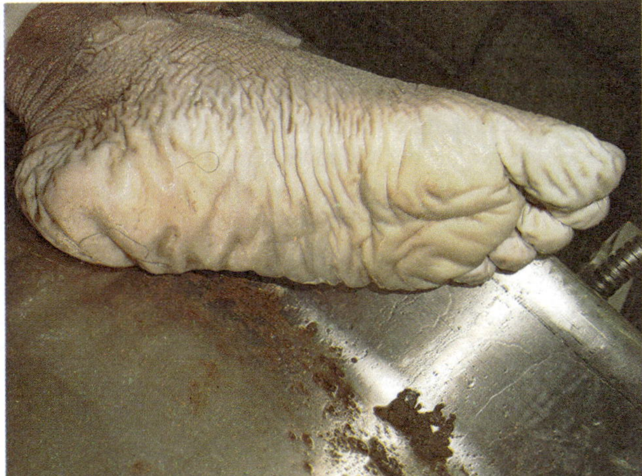

Fig. (13–44). Washerwoman feet in drowing.

these changes later. The accuracy of timing is not possible due to variations in environmental conditions. Similar progress and changes are seen in the skin of the foot, but when shoes are worn, it takes almost twice as long,

Contusions and abrasions produced during life may not be seen after removal from water, but are seen after the drying of the skin. In a few hours after removal from the water, the face may be bloated, either livid or black, later changing to a deep green. The discolouration is usually not found on surfaces which have been in close contact, as in the armpits and upper limbs, if they are in close contact with the body, and the lower limbs if they are close together. The stains are usually not seen on the parts which have been closely wrapped in clothing due to pressure which prevents accumulation of fluids.

Internal: Lungs: **The lungs are voluminous, may completely cover the pericardial sac, and bulge out of chest when the sternum is removed.** This is known as **ballooning** and is due to presence of fluid and air in the bronchi. The lungs are overdistended, and the alveolar walls are torn. Peripheral displacement of air by water distends the air spaces and the **medial aspects of each lung approach the midline.** The oedema fluid in the bronchi blocks the passive collapse that normally occurs at death, holding the lungs in the inspiratory position. In addition, there is often an element of over-distension caused by valvular action of bronchial obstruction. This produces **impression of ribs (grooves) on lateral surface of lungs, which is an important sign of drowning. On section, an oedematous condition due to the presence of watery, frothy, sometimes blood-stained fluid is seen. Drowning fluid actually penetrates alveolar walls to enter the tissues and the blood vessels. This has been described as emphysema aquosum. It is present in about 80% of cases and is presumptive evidence of death from drowning. If the victim is unconscious at the time of drowning, mere flooding of the lungs with water, but without formation of columns of froth occurs, which is known as oedema aquosum**. The foam acts as a "check valve". **The more powerful inspiratory efforts allow air entry to the lungs, but expiratory efforts are insufficient to expel air, water and foam. The lungs feel doughy and readily pit on pressure. The alveolar walls may rupture due to increased pressure during forced expirations, and produce small intrapulmonary haemorrhages, which when present subpleurally are called "Paltauf's haemorrhages". Paltauf's haemorrhages are shining, pale pink or bluish-red, and may be minute or 3 to 5 cm. in diameter.** They are usually present in about 50% of cases in the lower lobes of the lungs, but may be seen on the anterior surfaces of lungs, and the interlobar surfaces. **Red and grey patches may be seen on the surface, due to Paltauf's haemorrhages and patchy interstitial emphysema respectively.** The degree of ballooning is reduced in cases of pulmonary fibrosis and when extensive pleural adhesions are present. **Usually the lungs are congested moderately, but may be pale** due to the forcing out of blood from the lungs, and compressing of the vessels in the inter-alveolar septa by the air and water trapped in the alveoli. **Petechial haemorrhages on the surfaces of the lungs are absent (or very rare),** due to compression of the blood vessels in the interalveolar septa by the water. Few non-specific petechial haemorrhages can be found in the fissures and around the hilum, which are seen irrespective of cause of death.

Lungs in fresh water drowning: In fresh water drowning, the lungs are ballooned but light in weight (about double the normal weight). **They are pale-pink or pale grey** due to squeezing out of blood from compression of the vessels in interalveolar septa by the trapped air and water in the alveoli and appear uniformly emphysematous. **They retain their normal shape and do not collapse when they are removed from the chest.** A crepitus is heard on sectioning and each portion retains its normal shape. On compression, little froth is squeezed out, and there is no fluid in the tissue unless there is oedema.

Lungs in salt water drowning: In salt water drowning, the lungs are ballooned and heavy, weighing up to 2 kg. They are purplish or bluish in colour, sodden and jelly-like in consistency and pit on pressure. When removed and placed on a flat surface, they tend to flatten out. **On sectioning of the lung, crepitus is not heard.** Copious amounts of fluid pour out of the cut sections even without compression. The shape of the sectioned portion is not retained. When squeezed, the tissue is found to be filled with fluid in most parts of the lungs, i.e., they are wet and sodden Table (13–2). Occasionally, small intra-alveolar haemorrhages are seen in both fresh water and sea water drowning

Table (13–2). Difference in lungs between fresh water and sea water drowning

	Trait	Fresh water drowning	Sea water drowning
(1)	Size and weight:	Ballooned but light.	Ballooned and heavy.
(2)	Colour:	Pale pink.	Purplish or bluish.
(3)	Consistency:	Emphysematous.	Soft and jelly-like.
(4)	Shape after removal from the body:	Retained; do not collapse.	Not retained; tend to flatten out.
(5)	Sectioning:	Crepitus is heard. Little froth and no fluid.	No crepitus. Copious fluid and froth.

which causes the red staining of the foam in the respiratory tract. The pleurae may be discoloured by haemorrhages, but petechial haemorrhages of asphyxial type are not found. Petechial haemorrhages may be present in the subepicardial region of the heart posteriorly.

If the body remains in water for several hours, or if the postmortem is delayed for several hours after removal of the body from the water, these changes become less marked, and the difference in appearance between the fresh water and sea water drowning lungs are not clear. **If there has been delay between death and examination, froth in the lungs and air-passages and overdistension of the lungs is not seen in most cases of drowning.**

Dry lung drowning: In death due to laryngeal spasm, very little water may enter the lungs but asphyxial signs are present. In laryngeal spasm, there is no anatomic evidence. It is a diagnosis of inference and exclusion. In many cases of drowning, relatively dry lungs (dry lung drowning) are observed. This may occur if circulation continues for a short time after removal of the victim from the water or if resuscitative measures are carried out. In such cases, most of the water in the lungs is absorbed into the hypertonic plasma while the lungs remain distended. It has been suggested that this is likely to occur if laryngeal spasm supervenes to prevent further water entry, so that continued circulatory function can remove intra-alveolar fluid into the plasma.

Froth appears within two minutes of drowning, and its quantity varies depending on the length of the submersion, and the violent respiratory efforts. The mucosa of the air-passages is congested. Froth in the air passages varies from body to body. They may be completely filled by it, but **usually the froth is seen in secondary bronchi and beyond, if autopsy is delayed for several hours. This is one of the characteristic signs of drowning,** but if artificial respiration has been performed, especially by means of a respirator, the amount of froth and fluid in the air-passages may be greatly reduced.

The fluid in the respiratory passages is of the same nature as the medium in which the body was found and substances like fine silt, grit, sand, weeds, diatoms, or various forms of algae can be found. If the matter has penetrated deeply into the lung it is useful evidence, but its presence in the trachea may be due to passive entry after death.

In secondary drowning lungs are rigid, stiff and heavy and show features of adult respiratory distress syndrome.

Hydrostatic lung: If **a dead body is thrown into water, due to the hydrostatic pressure water passes into the lungs.** This **"hydrostatic lung"** will simulate the "drowning lung". According to Eisele, a "drowning lung" may be produced in a body remaining at the depth of 2 metres for 20 hours. **A drowning lung together with the frothy fluid is diagnostic.**

Inhalation of water causes obstruction of the pulmonary circulation. This results in dilation of the right side of the heart and the large veins, which contain dark fluid blood. **The blood is fluid due to the dilution by inhaled fluid and release of plasminogen activator** from the damaged endothelium of pulmonary capillaries. The intima of the aorta is stained red.

Stomach: The stomach contains water in 70% of cases. If the chemical and microscopic nature of the water is same as that of the medium of submersion, it is a valuable confirmatory evidence of drowning, but it is possible that the victim might have drunk the same water shortly before death. **When a disagreeable liquid which would not be swallowed voluntarily and which corresponds to the drowning medium, e.g., liquid manure, or muddy water containing debris is found in the stomach, it is a valuable indication of drowning.** The amount should be measured and examined for foreign substances. Water is not found in the stomach, if the person died from syncope or shock and in putrefaction. Gastric mucosa is often soft and heavy. Gastric mucosa shows micro-ruptures due to overstretching as a result of ingested fluid **(SEHRT's sign)**. If entire gastric content is allowed to stand in a beaker for an hour, it will segregate into 3 layers, i.e., solids at bottom, liquid in middle and foam on the top **(Wydler's sign). The small intestine may contain water in about 20% cases. This sign is regarded as positive evidence of death by drowning** as it depends on peristaltic movement which is a vital act.

The brain is congested, swollen with flattening of the gyri. The other organs are congested. When the struggle is violent, the victim may bruise or rupture muscles, especially those of the shoulder-girdle. **Violent respiratory efforts may force some water into the middle ear through the Eustachian tubes (UENO's sign) and is suggestive of antemortem drowning.**

Haemorrhages are found in the middle ear in about half the cases of drowning. **Haemorrhage in temporal bone or in the mastoid air cells, is seen in large number of cases.** Water may also be present in maxillary and sphenoid sinuses **(Sveshnikov's sign).** The increased pressure transmitted from the surrounding water to the body and tending to be uniformly distributed, more easily compresses air in closed cavities than the body tissues. The lining of these cavities absorbs fluid and swell up followed by vascular engorgement and haemorrhages into the chambers. **Temporal bone haemorrhages** are also seen in deaths due to hanging, head injury and CO poisoning.

Cutis anserina, washerwoman appearance of the palms and soles, pulmonary oedema, and haemorrhage into the

petrous and mastoid bones can be found in a victim of drug overdose thrown in water, and the victim of heart attack collapsing into water.

Occasionally, the individual vomits during the unconscious gasping phase of drowning, and stomach contents may be found in the air-passages.

Spleen may be small and anaemic due to vasoconstriction **(Sabinsky's sign).** Ratio of weight of both lungs and weight of spleen is more or equal to 14.1 in death due to drowning (Drowning index).

Microscopic examination of lungs from freshly drowned persons shows distension of alveoli, alveolar ducts and bronchioles, with extension, elongation and thinning of the septa and compression of the alveolar capillaries. Some alveolar walls may have been ruptured. Capillary congestion, intra-alveolar haemorrhages and protein-rich oedema fluid are often present. Intra-alveolar and intra-capillary red cells may not contain haemoglobin. Histological changes in lungs are inconstant and unreliable.

DIATOMS: They are microscopic unicellular or colonial algae. They have a complex structure of their cell-walls which are usually strongly impregnated with silica and contain chlorophyll and diatomin, a brown pigment. Diatoms belong to class Bacillariophyceae. Diatom secretes hard siliceous outer box-like skeleton called a frustule. **They resist heat and acid. There are about 25,000 species. They vary considerably in size from 2 microns to one mm. in length or diameter.** Most species are from 10 to 80 microns in length and if elongated, up to 10 microns in width. **Diatoms measuring up to 60 microns in diameter and parts of larger diatoms are said to enter the pulmonary circulation during drowning.** The diatom skeletons are readily recognisable as radially or axially symmetrical structures. **Their shape may be circular, triangular, oval, rectangular, linear, crescentic, boat-shaped, etc. Fig. (13–45). Their presence varies from place to place, and there are seasonal variations at the same place.** They occur in cultivated soils and on surface of moist rocks and in the atmosphere. **Large numbers of free floating diatoms are found in both fresh water and sea water.** Certain foods, notably shell fish contain large quantities of diatoms. They may be demonstrated in human organs by: (1) direct digestion of the material with nitric acid and sulphuric acid, (2) incineration in electrical oven and then dissolving the ashes with nitric acid, (3) direct microscopic examination of the lungs. Water is squeezed out from the lungs, centrifuged and sediment examined, (4) microscopic examination of tissue section, whereby optically empty sections are produced.

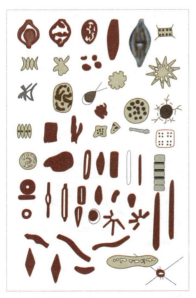

Fig. (13–45). Diatoms and planktons.

The drowning fluid and the particles in it, e.g., diatoms and planktons, pass from the ruptured alveolar wall into lymph channels and pulmonary veins and thus enter the left heart. Only a live body with a circulation could transport diatoms from the lungs to the brain, bone marrow, liver and other viscera, and skeletal muscle. They are also found in the bile and urine. The bone marrow is highly suitable and reliable. The bone marrow of long bones, such as the femur, tibia and humerus or sternum is examined for diatoms Fig. (13–47). The sternum is washed in distilled water. The periosteum is removed from the posterior surface. A piece of rectangular bone is removed with a sharp and clean knife and the marrow is curetted out from the gutter. Kidney, lung, liver or brain is also washed and 1x1 cm. pieces cut from the deeper tissue.

Technique: Five grams of bone marrow or liver, kidney, brain, etc. is put in separate test tubes and covered with five times the volume of concentrated nitric acid, and left at room temperature for one to two days to allow digestion. Alternatively, they can be heated in a water-bath overnight. This process chars, blackens, and destroys organic matter. Diatoms have silica shells and as such are not destroyed. The tube is centrifuged, the supernatant acid poured off and replaced with distilled water. This process is repeated 2 or 3 times to dilute the acid. The deposit is examined under phase-contrast or dark-ground illumination. The silica skeletons of diatoms are birefringent when viewed microscopically with polarised light. **The number of diatoms found in the tissues is relatively small.** Strong acid digestion markedly reduces the yield.

It is claimed by some Japanese workers that using detergent or enzyme digestion instead of destructive acid, even soft-bodied algae and protozoa can be recovered from the tissues in drowning.

Control samples of about 2 litres water should be obtained from the site of accident for comparison. About 15 ml. of iodine solution is added to this to kill microorganisms, and allowed to settle overnight. The bulk of the water is poured off and the remainder centrifuged to recover diatoms. **The finding of similar diatoms in the water and in the body tissues is in favour of drowning. Diatom test is often negative in undoubted cases of drowning in water full of diatoms.** Diatoms from the alimentary canal may enter the circulatory system and reach the various organs in the body, and occasionally may be found in cases other than drowning.

ALTERATIONS IN BLOOD (GETTLER TEST): Normally, the chloride content is almost equal in the right and left chambers of the heart, and is about 600 mg. per 100 ml. When drowning occurs in fresh water, water tends to pass from the lungs to the blood and the blood gets diluted by as much as 72% in 3 minutes, and the blood in the left side of the heart will show chloride content up to 50% lower than usual. In drowning in sea water, water is absorbed from the pulmonary circulation into the alveolar spaces which may be up to 42% and due to the haemoconcentration, the chloride content in the left side of the heart shows an increase up to 30 to 40%. A 25% difference in chloride is significant. The test is of doubtful value.

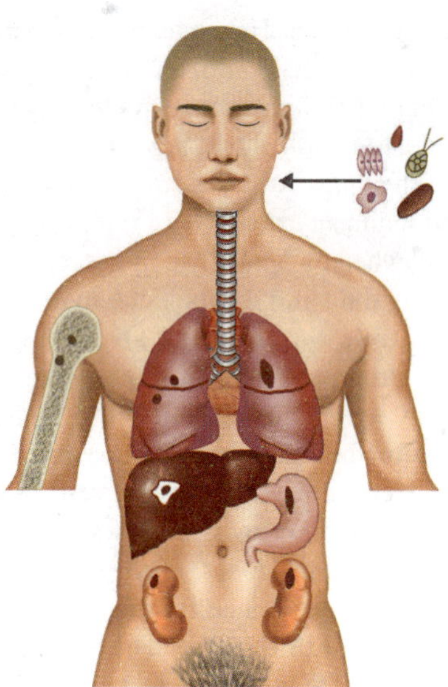

Fig (13–46). Diatoms in drowning.

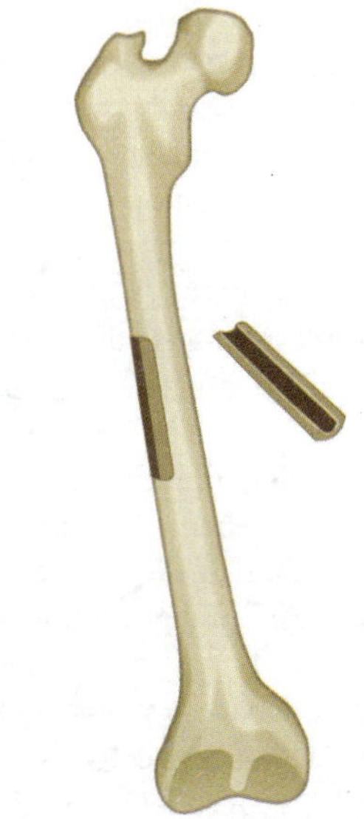

Fig. (13–47). Method of securing a specimen of bone marrow.

Plasma Specific Gravity: In drowning, the specific gravity of plasma from the left side of the heart is less than that of the plasma in the right side. In non-drowning cases the reverse is the case.

Magnesium: The magnesium content of the blood on the left side of heart is more than 1.25 mg/1000 ml than on the right side in salt water drowning.

SERUM STRONTIUM: Abdallah, et al (1985) reported raised serum strontium levels in deaths due to drowning, which was reciprocally related to the volume of the water aspirated. This will differentiate death due to drowning from postmortem immersion of a body. Differences in the strontium concentration of blood from left and right heart are always greater than 75 µg/1 in sea water drowning (Azparren,et al., 1994).

M.L. PROBLEMS: Dead bodies are commonly found immersed in water and other fluids in all manner of places and circumstances. Such cases prove the most difficult medicolegal problems. The circumstances surrounding each individual case are important. It should be remembered that drowning is not limited to deep water situations like sea, tanks, rivers, lakes, wells, etc., but persons under the influence of drugs or drink, infants, epileptics can fall face down in a puddle or ditch and die of immersion.

Diagnosis: All tests may be corroborated in early recovery but ultimately not dependable in later recoveries. The autopsy diagnosis of drowning can pose problems, because the findings are often minimal, obscure or completely absent. Drowning is one of the most difficult modes of death to prove at postmortem, especially when the body is not examined in a fresh condition. The diagnosis is basically one of exclusion based largely on the history and investigative reports of the case. **When the findings are negative, cause of death may be given as "consistent with drowning" or even to admit that the cause of death is "undetermined".** The reliable signs of drowning at autopsy are: (1) Fine, white froth at the mouth and nose. (2) The presence of weeds, sand, mud, etc., firmly grasped in the hands. (3) The presence of fine froth in the lungs and air-passages. (4) The voluminous water-logged lungs. (5) The presence of water in the stomach and intestines, and (6) Finding of diatoms in the tissues.

ABSENCE OF SIGNS OF DROWNING: The above signs will not be found, if death occurs due to vagal inhibition. In death from syncope, or when a person is in a state of helplessness from drink or other cause, or when a person receives an injury during fall into the water which prevents him from struggle, the signs will be slight. In dry drowning, the postmortem appearances are those of asphyxia. If the postmortem is delayed for a few hours, or if any appreciable delay has occurred before recovery of the body from water, the signs of drowning will not be found to a great extent.

DECOMPOSITION OF BODY: If the body remains in water, lividity appears in the head, neck and chest, and putrefaction begins in the same place and produces the appearance of diffuse scalp haemorrhage. The blood becomes more fluid and water is found in gradually increasing quantity in the pleural cavities. A body removed from water undergoes rapid decomposition. In moderately advanced putrefaction the diagnosis is difficult, the only evidence being the presence of water in the pleural cavities due to diffusion of water from the lungs, which finally collapse, and froth in bronchi. In advanced putrefaction the signs are completely absent. Algae get attached to exposed portions of drowned bodies, multiply and form a layer over the skin, which may be seen in 3 to 4 days in summer. Scraping of the algae will remove the superficial layers of the skin, due to which small abrasions may disappear.

THE CIRCUMSTANCES OF DROWNING: Bodies recovered from water may have died of: (1) natural disease before falling into the water, (2) natural disease while already in the water, (3) injuries before being thrown into water, (4) injuries while in water, (5) hypothermia in the water, (6) drowning. The manner of death cannot be interpreted from an autopsy alone. The findings have to be viewed together with the circumstances.

ACCIDENTAL DROWNING: (1) Occasionally, swimmers, fishermen and dock workers may be drowned accidentally, but it is common in non-swimmers. (2) It also occurs while bathing in tanks, rivers or sea. (3) Women may fall accidentally into a well while drawing water from it. (4) Children may fall in ponds or lakes while playing near their banks. (5) Usually, children die from drowning in shallow water, but adults usually epileptics, or under the influence of drink or drugs, or collapse due to coronary artery disease or dizziness due to hypertension may fall face down into shallow water and die. Drowning and near drowning are major causes of morbidity and mortality in children. (6) Accidental drowning in the swimming pool sometimes results from jumping off the diving board. Impact of the forehead on the floor of the pool may cause hyperextension of the head and loss of consciousness with subsequent inhalation of water. In such cases, haemorrhages are seen in the deep neck muscles in the region of C_1 and C_2 with or without vertebral fractures.

DEATH IN THE DOMESTIC BATH: A sudden collapse from coronary or cerebrovascular disease may cause loss of consciousness, leading to immersion of head and death. Similarly, epilepsy or a fall producing a disabling head injury may also cause death. Other causes include CO poisoning, alcohol or drug intoxication and electrocution. In such cases, it should be established whether the head was really in the water and if so, whether the water was inhaled. A sample of the bath and tap water should be collected. Bruising of the head is usually seen from falling or being struck. Grip marks (finger-tip bruises) on legs or arms indicate forcible immersion. Natural disease should be excluded at autopsy and the viscera preserved for chemical analysis.

CASE: BRIDES OF THE BATH: John Lloyd took an insurance policy in the name of his wife. A few days later, she was found dead in the bathtub. At inquest, a verdict of accidental death was recorded. Lloyd collected insurance money. Earlier he married Burnham's daughter under an assumed name of George Joseph Smith. Mrs Smith was found dead in the bathtub, and a verdict of accidental death was recorded. Smith collected insurance money. Burnham complained to the police. It was further revealed that Smith has married Munday a year earlier who also died under similar circumstances, the insurance money having been collected by Smith. All were drowned in boarding houses with the women lying supine with their heads under the water at the sloping end of the bath tub, with their legs sticking out of the other end. The bodies did not show any signs of violence. No shouting was heard in any case.

Inspector Neil experimented with a bathing suit-clad police woman who got into a bathtub identical to those used by Smith. He tried to force her under water. Water was splashed everywhere. Neil could not hold the girl under the water for more than a few seconds at a time, though he was strong. Then he picked up her legs and pulled, when the body was supine. As her head slid under water, she became unconscious immediately. She recovered after 30 minutes resuscitation. Smith confessed his guilt and was hanged in 1915.

DEATH OF NEWBORN INFANTS: In precipitate labour, the baby may fall into lavatory pan or bucket and die. Microscopy of the lungs and examination of the fluid in air-passages may be helpful. Foreign material inhaled into the lung parenchyma or passages may be seen and compared with a sample of fluid from bucket or lavatory pan. Chemical analysis of fluid in the air-passages, e.g., for soap or disinfectant agents present in the fluid in the lavatory or bucket is helpful.

Accidental drowning is very common.

HYPERVENTILATION DEATHS: For swimming for a longer time than normal under the water, the swimmer may hyperventilate before jumping into the water, due to which CO_2 tension is very much lowered. While swimming under the water, oxygen is utilised and CO_2 is produced, but the CO_2 tension does not rise sufficiently to irritate the respiratory centre and cause air-hunger, due to its abnormally low starting point. He may suddenly lose consciousness and drown.

DROWNING IN SKIN AND SCUBA DIVING: In skin diving simple mask and fins are used. The hazards are similar to those of swimming. SCUBA (self-contained underwater breathing apparatus) diving enables prolonged independent stay under the water. Serious accidents are caused by equipment failure, environmental factors, or human factors, e.g., exhaustion, panic, pre-existing disease, improper use of equipment. Hazards of scuba diving are drowning, barotrauma (pressure changes associated with descent or ascent), bends (Caisson's disease), acute pulmonary oedema, emphysema, pneumothorax, air embolism, etc. In scuba diving, frequently there is entrapment of air within the lungs on rising from the depths, producing fatal or non-fatal extra-alveolar air syndrome. Air escapes from the alveoli and may result in interstitial emphysema, pneumothorax or air embolism. This is caused by disproportionate expansion of air-containing alveoli, as compared to the adjacent fluid-filled vascular changes during too rapid an ascent.

SUICIDAL DROWNING: In India, drowning is a common method of committing suicide, especially amongst women, and more particularly in localities nearby the sea or river or canal. In case of a woman, the body is usually fully dressed. Suicides usually remove some of their outer clothing or shoes before leaping into the water. In a non-swimmer, a naked body suggests suicide. Suicides may drown themselves in very shallow water, or even by putting the head in a pail or cistern. If a body is found with heavy weights attached to it, it must be either homicide or suicide, and with children homicide alone. The nature of the weights, whether they are tied by ligature or fixed in clothing or found in the pockets are important. Sometimes, suicides tie their hands or legs together, and in such cases the manner of tying, and the knot of the rope or ligature should be examined to determine whether they could have been made by the suicide himself. Suicidal drowning may be preceded by the swallowing of the poison, cutting the throat or other suicidal attempts. Injuries may be caused during fall, especially if the bodies are found in the wells.

HOMICIDAL DROWNING: Murder by drowning is very rare, except in the case of infants and children. A person may be pushed into a river or into the sea. Marks of strangulation or throttling or severe violence applied to the head are presumptive of homicide. Bruises are strongly suspicious. **Homicidal drowning in shallow water is possible, if the assailants hold the victim's head in such a position as to cover the nostrils and mouth.** Signs of struggle or marks of violence on the body are likely to be found in such cases. If a person is taken unawares or rendered senseless and defenseless by alcohol or hypnotic drugs, and head is submerged in water for 5 to 10 minutes, no marks of violence will be found on the body.

NATURAL DEATH: The victim may suffer from cardiovascular catastrophe (common cause) and involuntarily fall in water. A person may collapse from natural disease while on boat, or a river bank. A pre-existing condition may be exacerbated due to physical exertion of swimming or struggling or by the effects of cold.

INJURIES ON DROWNED PERSONS: Wounds may be produced before, at the time of, or after immersion. Before immersion, they may be of accidental, suicidal or homicidal origin. In marine, air or rarely road transport accidents, the victims may be injured or killed before entering the water. Persons falling from docks, bridges or ships may strike hard objects, such as rocks or stone or some solid obstruction. It is difficult or impossible to know whether these injuries are antemortem. After immersion, injuries may be produced from the striking of the body into rocks, coral or marine structures. As the body floats along the bottom, abrasions may occur on the head, face, backs of the hands, knees and the toes. The body may be hit by boats, ship's propeller, which may produce often parallel, long and deep cuts and amputation. Bodies that have been suspended in shallow water may show injuries from being dragged against the bottom. Aquatic life (fish, crabs, turtles, lobsters, eels, crustaceans, etc.) attack and destroy soft parts of the face, i.e., eyelids, lips, nose, ears, penis, scrotum, and also anus. **The lesions are circular or oval and punched-out. Immersion of body in water for several hours may cause leaching out of blood from antemortem wounds. There may be no bleeding around these injuries, and as such can be mistaken for postmortem injuries.**

Probable Duration of Submersion: The rate of decomposition in an immersed body is reduced to half and doubles when it is removed from water and exposed to air. The time of floatation of body varies greatly. In salt water, bodies float earlier than in fresh water. Very obese persons, women, children and infants float more readily than thin or heavily-framed persons. **The body floats in about 12 to 18 hours in summer, and 18 to 36 hours in winter in India.** In cold countries the body floats in about two days to one week or more, depending on temperature of the water. The epidermis and nails are loosened and the skin of the hands and feet may be peeled off like glove or stocking in two to four days. The body usually floats with the spine uppermost, though obese persons and some women may float face up due to fat and gas in the breast and abdomen. In advanced decomposition, the body usually floats belly up. A drowned body will not move more than a few hundred metres from the initial position, unless there are strong currents. After floating it may drift a considerable distance from the site of death.

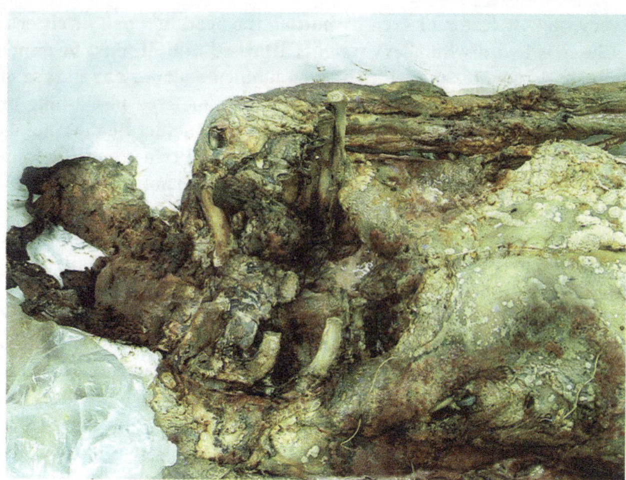

Fig. (13–48). Body recovered from river bed bank and kept in a cold storage for few days covered with fungus on whole body.

Long preservation of body and recovery from damp area show fungal growth **Fig. (13–48)**.

SEXUAL ASPHYXIAS

Sexual asphyxias (autoerotic asphyxia; asphyxiophilia) are very rare. **Partial asphyxia caused by pressure on carotid vessels, or partial obstruction of air-passages causes cerebral disturbances and may lead to hallucinations of an erotic nature in some men.** The degree of asphyxia produced by mechanical means is controlled, but in some cases death occurs accidentally. These cases are associated with some form of abnormal sexual behaviour, usually masochism and transvestism. The victims are almost always males, and usually young. The scene is usually the victim's own house; the bedroom, bathroom, basement or attic are usually selected, and the door is locked from the inside. Adult males with homosexual preferences tend to carry out the procedure in pairs as a means of protection from accidental death.

Methods: (1) Hanging is the most frequent form seen in sexual asphyxias. The neck is protected by a padding between the neck and the ligature. The ligature is passed around the neck in the form of a running noose, the free end of which is tied to a limb, or to a fixed object. The weight of the body is used to control the pressure. The free end of the ligature may be tied to the wrists or ankles, which are usually tied together. The noose can be tightened by extending the arms or legs, and when consciousness is lost, the relaxation of the limbs release the pressure on the neck. In some cases, a running noose may be passed upwards to some fixed point. There are indications that death is unintentional, for the individual is often found incompletely suspended with his feet on the ground or close to an object, such as a chair or stool, that would have allowed him to release the constriction. Evidence of previous episodes of similar activity may be found on the neck, such as old scars. Such persons are usually found naked, partly naked, or may be wearing women's dress. There may be padding of the brassieres to simulate breasts; female undergarments, and even sanitary pads, wigs and make-up may be worn. Frequently, they tie their arms, legs and sometimes waist and genitalia (bondage) with a rope, string, wire, padlocks, chain, etc. In addition to bonds and restraints, there is frequent evidence of self-mutilation, such as puncture wounds, cuts or burns, or one may find weights, clamps, or pincers attached to the genitalia or breasts. Erotic or pornographic literature or attractive female nude photographs are spread out within view, and there may be evidence of recent emission of semen. Sometimes, alcohol, cocaine or narcotics or some inhalant may be found at the scene. The person may blindfold himself or may arrange a mirror to watch the events or camera to make a photographic record. Many of these cases are misdiagnosed as suicidal hangings, and rarely as homicides. It is rarely seen in females, in whom foreign bodies may be found adjacent to or in the vagina or ropes tied around the genitalia and breasts. (2) Sexual gratification may be obtained by electrical stimulation. For this, electrodes are applied to the genitals or on abdominal wall, usually with a low voltage supply from a battery or transformer. (3) Other methods include, covering the head in a plastic or some impervious bag, which may be secured around the neck by an elastic band or a ligature to achieve partial anoxia. This ligature may form part of a system of bondage, which is also attached to the genitalia. In addition, lengths of chain with padlocks are often applied. It is sometimes combined with the inhalation of sniffing substances such as glue, ether, amyl nitrate, etc., and soaked pads with one of the sniffing substances are found with the bag. In these cases the head and face are pale, with few petechial haemorrhages in the eyelids. The interior of the bag contains abundant droplets of moisture. (4) Carbon tetrachloride, trichloroethylene, aerosal sprays, paint thinners, petrol, ethylene chloride, amyl acetate, etc. are inhaled either directly from the container or by re-breathing after placing in a plastic bag, which may cause death by hypoxia. (5) Less commonly death may occur from haemorrhage due to rectal trauma associated with foreign body insertion, or from peritonitis following perforation of the bladder after insertion of foreign bodies into the penis.

SCENE: The scene should be examined for: (1) Evidence of abnormal sexual behaviour, e.g., masochism, transvestism. (2) Evidence that the act had been practiced previously, such as grooves in the rafter or door from ropes, or verbal communications with others regarding the nature of activities, diaries, etc. (3) Evidence of attempts to conceal the act by some method to prevent a ligature from leaving marks around the neck. (4) No evidence to suggest a suicidal act.

CHAPTER

14 ANAESTHETIC AND OPERATIVE DEATHS

FM 2.19: Investigation of anaesthetic, operative deaths: Describe and discuss special protocols for conduction of autopsy and for collection, preservation and dispatch of related material evidences.

Anaesthetic deaths are very rare. Only one in ten thousand persons die totally as a result of anaesthetic. Anaesthetic deaths may be divided into two groups.

(A) DEATHS WHICH OCCUR DURING THE ADMINISTRATION OF AN ANAESTHETIC BUT WHICH ARE NOT DUE TO ANAESTHETIC: (1) The injury or disease which necessitate the operation is sufficiently serious to cause death, though the anaesthetic may have precipitated the death. (2) A patient suffering from a serious disorder, e.g., valvular disease of the heart, may have to undergo an operation for another disease or injury, in which the operation or anaesthetic may have only precipitated death. (3) The patient may be suffering from undiagnosed serious lesion, e.g., coronary artery arteriosclerosis which could have been an important contributory factor in causing death. (4) Surgical shock and exhaustion may be the major factors in causing the death of patient under anaesthesia. This can occur when the pre-operative condition of the patient was poor, or operation has been unduly prolonged. (5) A surgical accident during the administration of anaesthesia, e.g., damage to a large blood vessel or aneurysm may cause death.

(B) DEATHS WHICH ARE THE DIRECT RESULTS OF THE ADMINISTRATION OF AN ANAESTHETIC: (1) INEXPERIENCE: Most deaths occur due to inexperience and failure to adopt precautions when clearly indicated, e.g., mishaps due to intubation (e.g., aspiration of vomit, kinked tubes, etc.), and bronchoscopy. Each may cause vagal inhibition if there is inadequate depth of anaesthesia. Breathing circuit disconnections cause death. **(2) TECHNICAL MISHAPS:** Equipment failure or mislabelling of oxygen and anaesthetic gases may go undetected and may not be identified as a cause of resulting deaths. Explosions and fires may occur in the operating theatre through the ignition by an electric spark of the inflammable vapour caused by a mixture of air or oxygen with anaesthetic gas. The most dangerous mixtures are cyclopropane-oxygen and ether-oxygen. The ignition may come from the spark of a surgical diathermy electrode, from a faulty electrical appliance, from X-ray apparatus, from static electricity, etc. (3) Death may result from **respiratory failure** due to an inadequate supply of oxygen: (a) from a depression of the respiratory centre, which may be caused by an overdose of an anaesthetic agent, over-premedication, administration of relaxant drugs, such as curare, which causes paralysis of the respiratory and throat muscles, (b) from obstruction of the respiratory tract from laryngeal spasm (due to pre-existing asthma, hypersensitivity to drugs, aspiration of gastric contents and fluid overload), with progressive hypoxia, bronchiolar spasm, impaction of loose bodies, e.g., swabs or dentures in the larynx, trachea and bronchi, or by reactionary haemorrhages from an operative site in the nasopharynx. The tongue may fall back and obstruct the opening of the larynx. Deaths due to regurgitation of vomited matter are probably caused by hypoxia. Rupture of the lungs may occur from excessive pressure to the airway. Positive pressure ventilation will rapidly convert a simple pneumothorax into a tension pneumothorax. The use of nitrous oxide will cause a pneumothorax to expand rapidly, leading to death. (4) The most common cause of sudden death under general anaesthesia is **acute neurogenic cardiovascular failure,** which may occur in all types of operation. It usually occurs under light anaesthesia, e.g., when an operation is started before the patient is properly anaesthetised or when traction is exerted on the viscera or peritoneum, or when an instrument is passed into the larynx or trachea of a lightly anaesthetised patient. Severe shortage of oxygen during deep anaesthesia may be due to inadequate ventilation and can result in sudden death due to heart failure.

Deaths due to hypovolaemia may occur due to: (a) failure to recognise or to make adequate provisions for preoperative hypovolaemia, (b) vasodilation converts a compensated hypovolaemia into an uncompensated fatal form, (c) inadequate volume replacement for intraoperative losses may contribute to death from surgically induced haemorrhage, (d) replacement of large quantities of blood lost, leads to deficiencies in clotting factors of blood and shock with liberation of fibrinolysins which may cause death from uncotrollable haemorrhage.

Cardiac arrest during the induction of anaesthesia or while the surgical procedure is in progress may be due to inadequate preanaesthetic medication, obstruction of the airway from aspiration of food, vomitus or instruments, insufficient oxygenation, excessive CO_2 in the inspired air, too rapid induction of the anaesthesia, an overdose of the anaesthetic agent, or hypersensitivity of the individual to the anaesthetic agent employed.

Cardiac arrhythmias during anaesthesia may result from pre-existing disease, abnormal reactions to drugs, unskilful anaesthesia, surgical stimulation, or a combination of these. Increased catecholamine level (from endogenous or exogenous sources) may precipitate arrhythmias especially in combination with hypoxia, hypercarbia and halothane and from injection of adrenaline. Electrolyte disturbances, especially of extracellular potassium and magnesium predispose to dysrhythmias. Myocardial contractility may diminish due to metabolic disorders, electrolyte imbalances, hypoxia, hypothermia, anaesthetic drugs and acute myocardial ischaemia.

COMPLICATIONS OF ANAESTHESIA: Common complications are: hypoxaemia, aspiration of foreign material, atelectasis, pneumonia, pulmonary oedema, pneumothorax, bronchospasm, air embolism, oxygen intoxication and neurological sequelae. A variety of unexplained and untoward anaesthetic events may lead to minor complications to a fatal outcome, or a living death with termination of all conscious, volitional activity, or a paraplegia, or blindness, etc. All complications are not related to errors. They may result from the patient's disease or the patient's response to the anaesthetic drug or technique or may be unrelated to anaesthesia.

CAUSATIVE FACTORS: (1) **"Physiologic"**, e.g., insufficient oxygen or inadequate blood supply. (2) **"Pharmacologic"**: toxic or untoward effects of anaesthetic drugs and techniques. Some effects are of the minor histaminoid type and others are life-threatening bronchospasm and acute hypotension. Their incidence is about 0.2% of all anaesthetics. (3) **"Physical"**: trauma from electricity, heat, explosion, direct pressure or tension. (4) **"Malfunction"** or misuse of apparatus, instrument and anaesthetic agents.

MALIGNANT HYPERTHERMIA is a very rare inherited condition seen during general anaesthesia using halothane and succinylcholine, in which the body temperature increases suddenly to 40° to 45°C. with muscle rigidity, followed by severe metabolic disturbance and death. It occurs in approximately 1: 14,000 general anaesthetics, with mortality of 60 to 80%. The basic condition is an autosomal dominantly inherited trait associated with sudden uncoupling of oxidative phosphorylation, accompanied by massive energy production from the muscles. In 70% of carriers, creatine phosphokinase and aldolase activities are elevated, though the basic abnormality appears to be a defect in calcium transfer and phosphorylation within the muscle fibres.

AUTOPSY: Brain should be fixed and sections examined microscopically. Distal parts of cerebellar folia and Sommer's area of hippocampal gyrus show pallor, and rapid loss of Purkinje cells can be seen within a few hours. Hepatitis may follow the use of halothane. Nephrotoxicity and even death may occur from methoxyflurane.

DAMAGES: The assessment of responsibility for damage or injury is difficult. Often it is impossible to judge fairly because: (1) All facts are rarely ascertained. Usually no one is fully aware of everything that occurred at the moment of disaster. (2) The time interval between the anaesthesia and the clinical evidence of damage may be long. (3) With some complications, the association with anaesthesia is not clear. (4) With many complications, the nature takes place over an extended time period and the information is disseminated slowly, e.g., malignant hyperthermia.

METHODS OF INVESTIGATIONS, EXAMINATION AND STUDY: The following aspects should be taken into consideration by the pathologist when investigating an operative or anaesthetic death.

(1) History (A) The patient's condition of health at the time of admission to the hospital and at the time of administration of anaesthesia, state of health prior to the present illness/condition, the report of preanaesthetic medication, time of induction, total time of anaesthesia, unusual or untoward events during anaesthesia, the details of corrective measures adopted, the sequence of terminal events. (B) The details of surgical procedure, the usual risk involved in the procedure, whether informed consent taken, the details of surgical procedure actually done, the findings of the surgeon, implants used if any. (C) Any known allergies and diseases like ischaemic heart disease, diabetes, thyrotoxicosis, muscular dystrophies, Addison's disease, Cushing syndrome; details of all medications like dose, mode of administration, details of infusions/transfusions used, untoward reactions, corrective measures. A list of the relevant and potentially toxic chemicals associated with each of these periods should be obtained. A thorough review of the hospital chart and discussions with the surgical and anaesthetic team should be made.

(2) Conditions requiring surgery: Some surgical conditions are on high risk, e.g., resection of the aortic aneurysm and repair in which the surgeon may not be able to control the bleeding. Rarely, surgical errors cause death, e.g., ligation of the coronary artery while implanting a heart valve prosthesis.

(3) Other pre-existing conditions: Some contraindications to operative procedures are not easy to identify, and even if they are identified, their seriousness may not be appreciated, such as symptomless coronary artery disease may prove fatal due to increased anoxia by the anaesthetic agents. Other conditions, e.g., brown atrophy of the heart, anaemia, bronchitis, emphysema, interstitial pulmonary fibrosis, myxoedema, thyrotoxicosis, hypertension, etc., may contribute to death.

(4) Pre-anaesthetic medications: Errors in relation to pre-operative medication are: giving wrong medication, over-medication, or no medication, which may precipitate death.

(5) Anaesthetic agents: Inadvertent mixing of the anaesthetic gases may cause death. It is important to get information about the anaesthetic agent used, its quantity and the method of administration. The duration of time the patient remains under anaesthesia and the management of the anaesthetic should be noted.

(6) Burn or explosion: Deaths from anaesthetic explosions occur rarely.

(7) Shock and haemorrhage: Haemorrhage and shock should be evaluated with other findings of the case.

(8) Blood transfusion: Blood transfusion reactions and incompatibilities should be investigated.

(9) Resuscitative measures: The measures adopted should be noted.

(10) Equipment: With appropriate qualified individuals, all the equipment including the valves and containers should be checked to ensure the correct mixing of components in right proportion. Devices attached to and inserted into the body should be examined. Anaesthetic machines, gas supply, compatibility of connections and all sophisticated hardware of operating theater must be subjected to most rigorous inspection. Airway obstruction from faults in the connection tubing, leaks, disconnection, misconnection and abnormal posture of the neck is another danger. Flowmeter errors occur. Inadvertent use of wrong substance or the connection with an empty cylinder may occur.

Chloroform and halothane are hepatotoxic and chloroform may rarely produce ventricular fibrillation. Barbiturates, such as thiopentone may give rise to cardiorespiratory failure if quantity used has been excessive. Trichloroethylene and atropine have been involved in fatalities, the usual mode being sudden circulatory failure. Nephrotoxicity and even death may occur from methoxyflurone. Halogenated hydrocarbons like cyclopropane, trichloroethylene and halothane cause cardiac irritability. They sensitize myocardium to the action of adrenaline.

AUTOPSY: Attendance of clinician at autopsy is important. Full clinical information is essential. Surgical and anaesthetic devices introduced into the patient should not be removed before autopsy. In deaths from inhalation anaesthesia, the odour of the anaesthetic agent may be detected at autopsy. Examine *in situ* all the cavities. Measure the contents or fluids and preserve for analysis. Examine sites at surgical intervention *in situ* and describe in detail. Dissect all the organs and inspect every surgical suture. Engorgement of the dependent parts of the viscera is usually seen in cases of prolonged anaesthesia.

Introduction of some surgical and anaesthetic devices like laryngoscope for airways, indwelling catheters/needles, intravenous cannulae, wound drains, chest tubes, etc., during and subsequent to surgery are likely to interfere with the findings. Their proper placement and patency should be assessed. Exclude any cardiovascular disorder including occult conditions like myocarditis. Collect specimens for assessing the severity of disease for which the operation was done.

Brain: Hippocampal gyrus and the cerebellum show changes of hypoxia. Findings include: diffuse, severe leucoencephalopathy of cerebral hemispheres with sparing of the immediate subcortical connecting fibres. Demyelination and obliteration of axon and sometimes infarction of the basal ganglia is seen. Damage is limited to white matter.

CAUSE OF DEATH: An unsuspected cause of death may be detected, e.g., pulmonary fat or air embolism or evidence of asphyxia from aspiration of regurgitated material. Venous air embolism can occur during intravenous infusions, and through cerebral venous sinuses when they are opened in sitting posture during neurosurgery. The finding of internal haemorrhage, peritonitis and retained swabs and instruments, or evidence of hypersensitivity reactions are obvious.

Some conditions are not detected at autopsy, e.g., vagal inhibition, fall in blood pressure, arrhythmias of the heart, spasm of the coronary arteries, spasm of the larynx, etc. Blood should be collected for grouping, cross-matching and culture, and exudate for bacteriology. Take samples of all organs for microscopic examinations.

HISTOPATHOLOGY: A full range of specimens for histological examination should be taken to exclude occult condition, such as a lymphoma or myocarditis and to investigate the severity of the disease for which the surgical procedure was being performed.

TOXICOLOGICAL EXAMINATION: Collect: (1) One lung. A lung is mobilised and the main bronchus tied off with a ligature. The hilum is then divided and immediately the lung is placed in a nylon bag which is sealed. Plastic bags are not suitable. (2) 2 gm. of fat from the mesentery. (3) 10 gm. of skeletal muscle. (4) 100 gm. of brain from the cerebral hemispheres. (5) 100 gm. of liver. (6) 100 gm. of kidney. (7) Urine. (8) Blood should be collected under liquid paraffin. Specimens collected in case of inhaled anaesthetic should be kept in containers with as little head space as possible. They should be sealed and immediately refrigerated or frozen. Alveolar air should be collected with a needle and syringe under water by puncturing the lung before the chest is opened. Gaseous or volatile anaesthetics are easily lost if specimens or tissues are collected in routine fashion. To avoid losses due to exposure of tissues to the air, it may be necessary to obtain samples by biopsy techniques prior to autopsy. This may have to include *in situ* encapsulation or freezing, or direct transfer of specimens from the body into hermetically sealed containers, analysing solutions or even directly into the gas liberating module of an analysing instrument. Gases from cavities, heart, and blood vessels should be obtained by filling the body cavity with water and using a rubber dam to trap the gases before cutting the organs.

Extraneous specimens like residual solutions, medication containers, samples of gases used in anaesthesia, samples of the operating room air may have to be collected in some cases.

The analysis helps in: (1) detecting and estimating the quantity of the drug given, (2) estimating overdose of premedications of anaesthetic agents.

The fatal concentration of some of the anaesthetic agents in blood are:

Chloroform: 40 to 60 mg%
Ethyl chloride: 40 mg%
Diethyl ether: 180 mg%
Trichloroethylene: 50 mg%
Divinyl ether: 50mg%
Halothane: 20 mg%

A number of absorbed toxicologically pertinent agents are not actually demonstrated in postmortem tissues. Failure to find them does not exclude the possibility that they had a bearing on the cause of death. Toxicological investigations are generally unrewarding except where overdose with specific drugs, such as 'barbiturates or adrenaline, is involved. **Usually, the function of autopsy is to discover or exclude natural disease and mechanical blockage.** Discussion between pathologist, surgeon and anaesthetist may arrive at an amicable conclusion.

Finally, the pathologist should carry out retrospective evaluation of the case with appropriate disciplines.

LOCAL ANAESTHETICS: Deaths usually occur from overdosages or allergic reactions, hypersensitivity and idiosyncrasy. The important factors influencing the toxicity are: (1) The susceptibility of the patient. (2) The patient's general condition. (3) The rate of administration of anaesthetic agent. (4) The vascularity of the area injected. (5) Total dose. (6) Accidental intravascular injection. (7) Adrenaline used along with local anaesthetic agent can cause tachycardia, palpitation, sweating, high blood pressure and ventricular fibrillation.

The incidence of severe reactions to local anaesthesia is about 0.05% of which very few are fatal. The hazards of local anaesthesia are: (1) Overdosage of either the anaesthetic or vasoconstrictive agent. (2) Rapid absorption from highly absorptive areas or due to local vasodilatation. (3) Accidental injection into a vessel. (4) Hypersensitivity reactions.

There may be general effect on the CNS, which is either (1) excitory causing convulsions, or (2) depressive causing respiratory paralysis. Very rarely the heart may be directly affected, or when abnormally high concentration is injected directly into a nerve, permanent loss of function may occur.

Blood, brain, liver and tissue from the site of injection should be preserved for chemical analysis. In some cases hypersensitivity reactions may be obvious.

SPINAL ANAESTHESIA: Hypotension due to paralysis of sympathetic outflow is a common complication. The effects may be very severe in old persons, in those with pre-existing heart disease or in association with haemorrhage. Coronary insufficiency may be precipitated and there may be either cardiac or respiratory arrest. Death may occur suddenly due to cardiac inhibition following an unnatural stimulation of the vagus nerve. There may be diffusion upwards of the agent beyond the lower cord affecting vital centres. Lumbar puncture headache occurs in about a quarter of persons recovering from spinal anaesthesia. Rarely, there may be permanent paralysis of the muscles of one eye. Chronic adhesive arachnoiditis is a common complication and if it involves the cauda equina, dysfunction of the bladder and rectum may appear. Contamination of syringes and ampoules by sterilising and cleaning agents, such as phenols and detergents cause paraplegia. Sepsis may be introduced into the spinal canal.

In the case of local, spinal, caudal or intravenous anaesthetic agents, the concentration of the anaesthetic should be determined and also whether the agents were mixed in the correct proportions.

COMPLICATIONS OF SURGICAL PROCEDURES: All surgical operations, with or without anaesthesia, have some morbidity and mortality. Wound infections, fluid and electrolyte variations, pulmonary and renal problems, and cardiac arrest occur in any and all types of surgery. Severe burns from electrosurgery and explosions from electrocautery of the poorly prepared bowel may occur. Post-operative events, such as delayed haemorrhage, pulmonary emboli, and nosocomial infections are related to surgical care. Surgical complications may be delayed for weeks or months. Artificial plastic or metallic devices implanted in the body may fail to function properly after many years of good service, e.g., artificial heart valve.

Most deaths during or shortly after a surgical operation and general anaesthetic are not due to defects in the surgical technique or the anaesthetic procedure, but are due to other factors as described earlier. To evaluate a fatality occurring in these circumstances, the answers have to be found out for the following questions. (1) Was the death due to the natural disease for which the operation was being carried out, or was it due to the effects of the surgical procedure or anaesthetic? (2) Would the patient have died, without operation or anaesthetic? (3) Was the operation and anaesthetic essential to save the life of the patient? (4) Was there any defect in the surgical or anaesthetic technique? (5) Did the patient have any predisposing conditions, which made him susceptible to death from the operation or anaesthetic? (6) Was the death due to some natural condition entirely unrelated to the disease for which the operation was being performed and which was unsuspected at the time of operation? (7) Was the patient such a 'poor risk' that only the urgency of the clinical condition made the operation and anaesthetic necessary?

The examination of the operation site may be difficult due to the presence of haemorrhage, adhesions, oedema, sepsis and by surgical sutures and alteration of the anatomy by the surgical procedure. Sometimes, it becomes difficult to distinguish defects due to postmortem changes from abnormalities present during life, e.g., a sutured stomach or intestine may appear to have broken down, but the defect may be due to post mortem autolysis.

AUTOPSY: (1) Photograph the complete body. (2) Remove dressings and note the amount of blood, pus or other body fluid soaking the dressing. (3) Describe surgical wounds. (4) Perform tests for air embolism and pneumothorax before opening the body. Collect samples of air from air embolism for analysis. (5) Open the body. Remove the drainage tube after tracing and locating its internal end. (6) Examine in situ all the cavities. Note the amount of blood or fluid and preserve for analysis. (7) Examine sites of surgical intervention in situ and describe in detail. (8) Take a photograph of the operated site. (10) Inspect every

surgical suture for leakage, oozing, etc. (9) Describe and photograph any abnormal findings, e.g., ligation of big vessels or ducts, slipped ligature, sponges, packs, instrument left in the body, trauma to adjacent organs, removal of parathyroids during thyroidectomy, fat embolism, etc. (10) Examine all organs for disease, injury, malformations, etc. (11) Examine the air-passages for the presence of regurgitated gastric contents, foreign bodies like broken teeth, cotton plug, etc. Note injury to the larynx due to intubation or oedema of glottis. (12) Examine lungs for oedema, emphysema, collapse, chronic obstructive lung disease, embolism, etc. (13) Examine endocrine organs, especially thyroid and suprarenals. (14) Look for ligation of arteries, veins, ureters, bile ducts, perforation of large blood vessels and removal of vital organs or parts of organs. (15) Engorgement of dependent parts of the viscera is usually seen in cases of prolonged anaesthesia.

In most cases, there is no technical defect, and cause of death remains obscure after autopsy. A complete clinical history and consultation with the surgeon and anaesthetist is necessary. Most of the operation and anaesthetic deaths are of physiological nature. The opinion must be based on exclusion and reasoning, for functional lapses like fall in blood pressure, cardiac arrhythmia, spasm of the glottis, vagal inhibition, etc., cannot be demonstrated. Pre-existing natural disease, especially heart disease and respiratory insufficiency due to lung disease may be the factors in causing death. In persons already shocked from trauma, haemorrhage, etc., the contribution of this condition must be evaluated.

CHAPTER

15

IMPOTENCE AND STERILITY

FM 3.22: Define and discuss impotence, sterility, frigidity, sexual dysfunction, premature ejaculation. Discuss the causes of impotence and sterility in male and female.
FM 3.23: Discuss sterilization of male and female, artificial insemination, test tube baby, surrogate mother, hormonal replacement therapy with respect to appropriate national and state laws.
FM 3.24: Discuss the relative importance of surgical methods of contraception (vasectomy and tubectomy) as methods of contraception in the National Family Planning Programme.
FM 3.26: Discuss the national guidelines for accreditation, supervision and regulation of ART clinics in India.
FM 4.12: Discuss legal and ethical issues in relation to stem cell research.

Impotence is the inability of a person to perform sexual intercourse. Sterility (infertility) is the inability of the male to beget children, and in the female the inability to conceive children. About 10 to 15% of all married couples are involuntarily sterile. A person can be sterile without being impotent, or he can be impotent without being sterile, or both may co-exist. **Frigidity is the inability to initiate or maintain the sexual arousal pattern in the female. Ejaculation which occurs immediately before or immediately after penetration is termed premature ejaculation. Sexual dysfunction is an impairment either in the desire for sexual gratification or in the ability to achieve it.**

Legal issues: The question of impotence and sterility may arise in: (A) **Civil:** (1) Voidable marriage, (2) adultery, (3) disputed paternity, and legitimacy, and (4) claim for damages where loss of the sexual function is claimed as the result of an assault or accident. (B) **Criminal:** (1) Rape, (2) unnatural offences, where impotency is pleaded as a defence.

Examination: The examination should be undertaken only when asked by the Court or the police officer, not below the rank of subinspector. Before examining a male alleged to be impotent, a **complete history of the previous illness, especially with reference to nervous and mental condition, and his sexual history should be obtained.**

History: (A) Habits: (1) (a) Smoking, (b) alcohol, (c) drugs (hallucinogenic drugs like cannabis can cause impotence). (2) Diabetes (when complicated by peripheral neuropathy). (3) Trauma; head injury and spinal injury. (4) Venereal disease (syphilis in its tertiary stage can affect the posterior column of spinal cord which can cause impotence). (5) Hypertension (ganglion blocking drugs can cause impotence). (6) Occupation (painters, compositors and workers handling lead are likely to develop lead neuropathy). (B) Sexual history: (1) Sexual development. (2) Marital state (number of children). (3) Sexual deviation.

Medical examination: A complete medical examination, including central nervous system should be carried out. Pulsation in the peripheral arteries should be tested. Blood pressure and pulse rate should be measured. **The condition of the testes, epididymis, cord and penis should be noted and the private parts tested for sensation.** The penis is supplied by nerves from the second, third and fourth sacral segments through the pudendal nerve and pelvic plexus. Glans penis is supplied by dorsal nerves (sensory) which are branches of pudendal nerve. Erectile function is governed by parasympathetic input (excitatory) through erigentes nerve, the branches of which supply corpora cavernosa. Sympathetic input (inhibitory) is through nerve supplied by thoracolumbar plexus. Deep pudendal arteries supply glans and shaft of penis. Venous drainage is by penile veins. The length of the penis is measured from mons to the tip of glans, and circumference about middle of the shaft. Sexual organs are well developed by 16 years in females and by 17 to 18 years in males. The size of penis (flaccid) is about 2.5-4 cm during infancy, 5 cm children by pubertal age, 6 to 7 cm at puberty and slightly more by 15 to 16 years; fully developed to adult size by 17 years. The length of flaccid penis in adults is about 8.5 to 10.5 cm and the diameter 3 to 5 cm. When erect, the length is 13 to 15 cm. The penis varies greatly in size. The size of the penis has less constant relation to general physical development than that of any other organ of the body. The axis of the erect penis averages 26° to the horizontal ranging from 16° to 36°. **The prostate and seminal vesicles are palpated per rectum. In cases of sterility in the male, examination of the seminal fluid is essential.** Pressure should be made on the vesicles, and matter expressed is brought to the meatus by pressing the finger along the urethra and examined for spermatozoa.

Bulbocavernosus reflex test: Squeezing of the glans, immediately causes the anus to contract, if there is adequate nerve sensation in the penis.

Opinion: An opinion regarding potency must depend upon a man being like, or unlike other men. An opinion of diminished potency or impotency cannot be given, unless there is marked deviation from normal. **If the male external genitals are normal, it cannot be said that the person is impotent. In such cases, the opinion should be given in the negative form, stating that from the examination of the male, he finds nothing to suggest that the person is incapable of sexual intercourse.** Proof of potency or impotency is largely inferential. In the case of the female, the defect usually of the vagina is likely to be clearly seen.

THE CAUSES OF IMPOTENCE AND STERILITY IN THE MALE

(1) Age: The power of erection and therefore of coitus, may be present at a much earlier age than puberty. **Poor physical development of the penis is a common cause of impotence, and therefore the medical examiner should depend more on the development of the private parts of the person than on his age.** In cases of precocious development, as in gonadal or adrenal tumours, Mc Cune Albright syndrome, the sexual organs may show advance development as compared to the body as a whole. In advanced age, the power of erection and the ability to perform the coitus may diminish or disappear, but there is no specific age at which such loss of power occurs. **Spermatozoa are not usually found before the age of puberty, but may be found in the semen of very old men.** As long as live spermatozoa are present in the seminal fluid, the individual must be presumed to be fertile. Boys of 9 years, and old people of 94 having children have been recorded.

(2) Developmental Defects and Acquired Abnormalities: Absence of penis excludes coitus and **non-development of penis** may prevent the sexual act. In case of partial amputation, sexual act may not be possible. Certain malformations of external genitals, e.g., intersexuality, hypospadiasis and epispadiasis may prevent intercourse, and even when intercourse is possible, the seminal fluid may not reach the vagina, because of the abnormal position of the urethral orifice, but such individuals are not necessarily sterile. Double penis **Fig. (15–1)** and the penis adherent to the scrotum may cause difficulty in sexual intercourse. Loss of both testicles cause complete sterility after a certain time, but may not produce impotence. **If the testes are removed before puberty impotence is the rule, but if the testes are removed after puberty, potency is retained.** The removal of one testis does not affect either potency or fertility. Cryptorchids are not necessarily either sterile or impotent, but sterility is common. With both testes present a man may be sterile due to azoospermia.

(3) Local Diseases: Large hernias, elephantiasis or large hydroceles, phimosis, paraphimosis and adherent prepuce may cause temporary impotence by mechanical obstruction to sexual intercourse. Temporary impotency may be caused by acute disease of the penis, such as gonorrhoea, sores on the glans, etc. Diseases of the testicles, epididymis or penis, such as cancer, sarcoma, tuberculosis, syphilis, trauma, etc., may cause sterility, impotence or both. **Fracture pelvis with injury to parasympathetics, fracture spine at L-4 and 5 level with injury to sacral segments of spinal cord (erigentes nerve, genital branch of genito-urinary nerve) and brain damage can result in impotence. Bilateral lumbar sympathectomy causes impotence.** Tumours or injury of cauda equina, and spina bifida produce impotence. Lithotomy operation may damage ejaculatory ducts and produce sterility. **Exposure to X-rays causes temporary azoospermia.** When spermatic cords are blocked due to operation or disease, ligated or cut, sterility results.

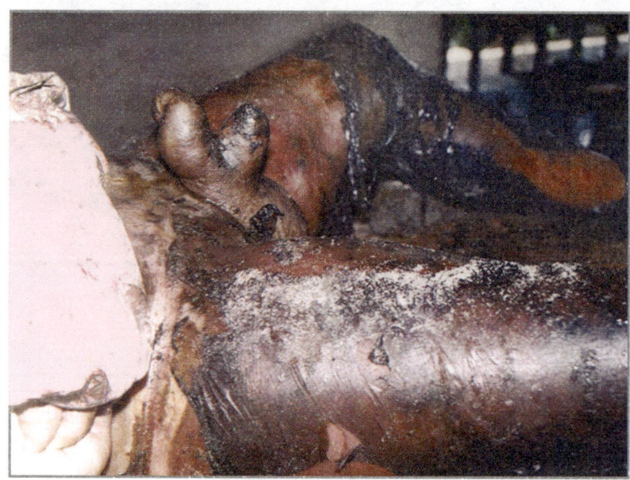

Fig. (15–1). Double penis.

(4) General Diseases: Temporary impotence is common during the course of any acute illness; in convalescence, normal function is rapidly regained. General diseases causing anaemia and debility, e.g., diabetes, pulmonary tuberculosis, chronic nephritis, etc., may cause temporary impotence. General ill-health may be associated with diminished fertility. **Endocrine disease may produce sexual infantilism and impotence.** Certain conditions of the central nervous system, such as hemiplegia, paraplegia, syringomyelia, locomotor ataxia, disseminated sclerosis, may cause impotence, but this is not always so. Lack of sexual power is common in those suffering from paranoia, tabes dorsalis and general paralysis of the insane. Occasionally, the reverse effect, i.e., **satyriasis or excessive sexual desire is seen.** Impotence may also be produced by excessive masturbation. Temporary impotence is found in neurasthenia. **Alcoholism, anabolic steroids, heroin and cannabis can cause erectile dysfunction. Heavy smoking causes impotence due to thrombosis in the penile arteries.** Antihypertensives, opiates, psychotropics and tranquilisers, etc., affect the neurotransmitters at the nerve endings resulting in impotence. Occupational exposure to lead may lead to sterility. Orchitis following mumps especially in adolescence may cause atrophy of the testes and may occasionally lead to sterility rather than impotence.

(5) Psychic Causes: Emotional disturbances are a common cause of temporary impotence. Fear of impotence or fear or inability to complete the act (first night impotence or honeymoon impotence in the bridegroom) are common causes of temporary impotence but usually they are soon overcome. Disgust of the sexual act or dislike of the partner may cause temporary or permanent impotence. Anxiety, guilt sense, timidity, depression, excessive passion and sexual overindulgence produce temporary impotence. **Quoad hoc** (as far as this) **is an individual who may be impotent with one particular woman but not with others. Aversion to females in general (sexual avulsion disorder) is defined as a persistent, recurrent aversion to and avoidance of all genital sexual contact with a sexual partner.**

Causes of erectile failure: Andrological research over the past years has proved that in 75 to 85% cases, there will be some organic causes. Nocturnal penile tumescence have revealed that a **majority of cases of impotence have organic causes** (Shabsigh, R. et. al, Mueller, S.C., et. al and Chiu, R.C, et. al.). **Vasculogenic impotence is one of the most frequent causes of erectile failure (about 40%).** Vasculogenic impotence may be due to poor arterial inflow into the penis due to arteriosclerotic narrowing of the arteries supplying penis. Diabetes, hypertension, pelvic and genital injuries can cause reduction in blood flow (arteriogenic impotence), or excessive venous leakage of blood from the penis which can occur in adult life after years of normal sexual life or due to congenital anomalies (venogenic impotence) or both. Other causes are diabetes mellitus (15 to 20%), psychogenic (12%), neurogenic (7%) and due to injuries to the spine, pelvic or perirenal injuries and pelvic surgeries causing injury to the nerves of the penis, endocrinologic, such as testosterone deficiency, luteinising hormone and prolactin, hypothyroidism, Cushing's syndrome, trauma, etc.

DIAGNOSTIC PROCEDURES: For the functional testing of erectile capability papaverine is injected i.v. which induces vascular changes similar to those which occur after stimulation of cavernous nerves, i.e., increased arterial flow, decreased venous flow, and sinusoidal relaxation. The techniques to assess the arterial and venous systems before and after injection of pharmacologic agents include, evaluation of the penile arteries with duplex ultrasonography during papaverine-induced erection, pudendal arteriography, pharmacocavernosometry, and cavernosonography.

Parmacological testing method in sexual dysfunction: Papaverine 15 mg and phentolamine 0.5 mg injections at the lateral sides of penis into cavernosum differentiates psychogenic and organic dysfunction. Person is asked to stand up after 2 minutes of injection and observed for 30 minutes for degree of erection. Early response is seen in psychogenic case. Arterio/cavernogenic requires 0.5 mg papaverine and 3 ml phentolamine. Organic causes require very high doses. Nowadays, sildenafil 50 mg is commonly used to test potency and Doppler ultrasonography is performed to find organic vasculopathies.

Treatment: Ultrasonogram and penis angiogram can make accurate study of penile blood supply. Microvascular surgery, epigastric dorsal artery bypass grafting can cure vascular problems. Leakage of blood from penile veins can occur in adult life after years of normal sexual life, which can be corrected by tying and removing deep dorsal vein of penis.

CAUSES OF IMPOTENCE AND STERILITY IN THE FEMALE

(1) **Age**: As the woman is the passive agent in the sexual act, the **age has no effect on potency**. Sexual desire is not completely lost in old age. A woman is usually fertile from puberty to the menopause.

CASE: A girl of 6 years and 6 months delivering full term baby has been reported. Kennedy records a case in which a woman gave birth to her twenty-second child when she was 63 years old after which she still continued to menstruate.

(2) **Developmental Defects and Acquired Abnormalities**: The vagina is sometimes absent in malformed females and Turner type intersexuals which makes a female completely and permanently impotent and sterile. Impotence may result from **some organic defects of the genitals,** e.g., total occlusion of the vagina, adhesion of the labia, and the tough imperforate hymen, which can be cured by surgery. Vaginal injury or severe infection may lead to stricture, and kraurosis vulva in old women may cause narrowing of the vagina. The conical cervix and absence of uterus, ovaries or Fallopian tubes produce sterility but not impotence. Occlusion of the vagina does not indicate sterility as long as the internal organs are healthy.

(3) **Local Diseases: Diseases of the genital organs do not cause impotence but may produce sterility,** e.g., gonorrhoea involving the cervix, uterus, ovaries and Fallopian tubes. Hyperaesthesia of vagina, prolapse of the uterus or bladder, and vulval or vaginal tumours, elephantaisis produce temporary impotence. Sterility may result from disease of the ovaries, obstruction of the Fallopian tubes or neck of the uterus, rectovaginal fistula, rupture perineum, disorder of menstruation, leucorrhoea, acid discharges from the vagina, etc.

(4) **General Diseases: As the woman is the passive agent in sexual act, general diseases do not cause impotence.** Occupational exposure to lead or exposure to X-rays lead to sterility. Drug dependence may also lead to sterility.

(5) **Psychic Causes**: Psychic factors may lead to impotence as in males. **In males, the impotence is passive leading to non-erection, but in females it is of an active nature, leading to vaginismus. Vaginismus is a spasmodic contraction of the vagina due to hyperaesthesia. It is a classical example of a psychosomatic illness.** Anatomically, it may affect the perineal muscles exclusively, or may be felt as a varying constriction of the levator ani, right up to the vaginal fornices. There is usually a definite cramps-like spasm of the adductor muscles. **Physiologically, these muscle groups contract spastically instead of their rhythmic contractual response to orgasmic experience. Hysterical hyperaesthesia co-exists with this condition, which in some cases may be more prominent than the spasm itself.** The hyperaesthesia starts at the vaginal introitus, but in extreme cases it may be present all over the vulva and even over adjacent part of the abdomen and thighs. **Any attempt at intercourse will cause painful reflex spasm of the levator ani, perineal muscles, adductor muscles of thighs and erector spinal muscles.** The spastic contraction of the vaginal outlet is completely involuntary reflex, stimulated by imagined, anticipated, or real attempts at vaginal penetration. **In a fully developed state, constriction of the vaginal outlet is so severe that penetration by the penis is impossible.** If an attempt is made to examine the hymen by passing a glass rod through hymenal orifice, sphincter muscles of the vagina contract due to which the rod is tightly grasped, and such severe pain is caused that she may scream. In a severe case, the legs cannot be separated sufficiently for the examination of the vulva and occasionally she may rise in a bow-shape, so that she rests only on her head and heels. It can occur with equal severity in the woman who has borne children as in the virgin. Normal female anatomy of female genitalia is shown in **Fig. (15–2)**.

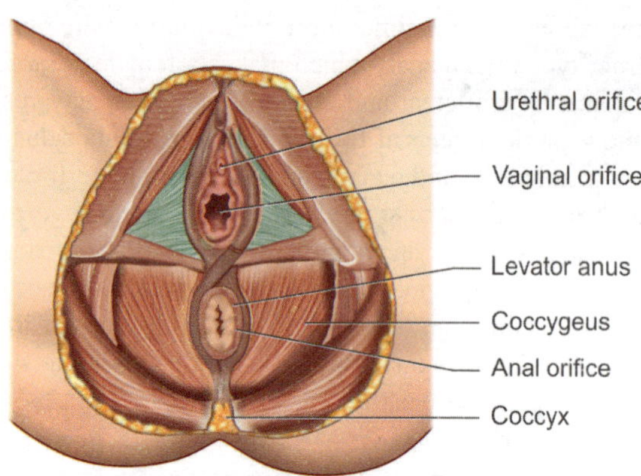

Fig. (15–2). The muscles of the pelvic floor.

Aetiology: (1) Male sexual dysfunction (wife's high levels of sexual frustration developing secondary to husband's impotence). (2) Psychosexually inhibiting influence of excessively severe control of social conduct due to religious orthodoxy. (3) Specific incidents of prior sexual trauma. (4) Stimulus derived from attempted heterosexual function by a woman with prior homosexual practice. (5) Secondary to dyspareunia. Severe laceration of the broad ligament, pelvic endometriosis, ulceration or fissures in the vagina, if untreated may lead to increasingly painful coitus and vaginismus. (6) Rarely, personal dislike or a general feeling of disgust at the idea of coitus. Anxiety, stress, fear of pain, guilt complex, etc. can cause strong contractions of paravaginal muscles at the time of intercourse.

Psychotherapy is beneficial. **Psychological causes affect fertility adversely. A woman may be sterile or impotent with a particular man but not with another.** Both environment and nutrition have some influence upon conception.

Conception is possible without penetration of the vagina by the penis due to **deposition of semen on the vulva which leads to "*fecundation ab extra*"**, the insemination occurring due to passage of spermatozoa from the external genitalia to the uterus. Rhythmic contraction of genital passage and pelvic floor muscles help in it.

Frigidity is usually psychological. It can develop in a female who does not experience orgasm in sexual intercourse. Dislike of the partner, neurological disorders, hypothyroidism, use of sedatives or depressants, menopause, etc., can cause frigidity.

STERILISATION

STERILISATION is a procedure to make a male or female person sterile, without any interference with potency. It is direct when it is intended to make the person operated upon sterile. It is indirect when it is the unintended result of an operation for some other purpose such as for preserving the life or health.

TYPES: (1) COMPULSORY: It is performed on a person compulsorily, by an order of the State. It may be carried out on mental defectives and others from a strictly eugenic point of view or as a punishment for sexual criminals. It is not done in India.

(2) VOLUNTARY: It is performed on married persons with the consent of both the husband and wife. It is performed for.

(A) THERAPEUTIC: This is performed to prevent danger to the health or life of the woman due to a future pregnancy. (B) EUGENIC: Sterilisation performed to prevent the conception of children who are likely to be physically or mentally defective. The object is to improve the race by preventing the transmission of disease and hereditable defects. (C) CONTRACEPTIVE: It is performed to limit the size of the family, i.e., for family planning.

METHODS: Sterilisation may be: (1) surgical. (2) radiological. (3) chemical, and (4) mechanical.

The methods of permanent sterilisation are: (1) vasectomy in male, (2) tubectomy in female, and (3) exposure to deep X-rays in both sexes. The methods of temporary sterilisation are: (1) coitus interruptus, (2) loop, (3) oral hormonal pills, (4) foam tablets, (5) diaphragm, spermicidal jellies, and condom.

Guiding Principles: To avoid legal complications, the following precautions should be taken. (1) The written consent of both wife and husband should be obtained for contraceptive sterilisation. (2) It is not unlawful if performed on therapeutic or eugenic grounds after obtaining true and valid consent. (3) It is preferable to have a check up after vasectomy. The person should be advised to abstain from sexual intercourse for about three months or until the seminal examination shows absence of spermatozoa on two successive occasions. (4) The pills containing hormonal substances may be harmful rarely, and so necessary precautions have to be taken to avoid any complications.

ARTIFICIAL INSEMINATION

The artificial introduction of semen into the vagina, cervix or uterus to produce pregnancy is called artificial insemination.

Types: (1) If the semen of the woman's husband is used, it is known as 'artificial insemination homologous' or "artificial insemination husband" (A.I.H). (2) If the semen of some person other than the husband is used, it is known as "artificial insemination donor" (A.I.D). (3) 'Pooled' donor semen is composed of donor semen to which semen from the husband has been added (A.I.H.D.).

Biological Aspects: Semen is obtained by masturbation and one ml. is deposited by means of a syringe in or near the cervix. The timing of insemination is important as the life span of the spermatozoa in the female reproductive tract is short. The time of maximum fertility coincides with ovulation. The ovum can survive in a fertilised form for 12 to 24 hours after it leaves ovary. The usual time taken by sperms to travel from vagina to tubes is 6 to 24 hours. The power of sperms to fertilise is usually retained for about 48 hours. Because of the problem of timing, insemination on several successive days in the month increases the chances of pregnancy. The success rate is 30 to 40% pregnancies within three to four months of the start of treatment. The use of frozen semen for AI.D. is becoming increasingly common. This is done by addition of glycerol, slow cooling, rapid freezing and storage at minus 196°C.

Indications: (1) When the husband is impotent. (2) When the husband is unable to deposit the semen in vagina due to hypospadiasis, epispadiasis, etc. (3) When the husband is sterile. (4) When there is Rh incompatibility between the husband and wife. (5) When the husband is suffering from hereditary disease.

Precautions: Certain recommendations have been made when a donor is used. They are: (1) Consent of the donor and his wife is essential. (2) The identity of the donor must remain secret. (3) The donor should not know to whom the semen is donated and the result of insemination. (4) The donor must be mentally and physically healthy and should not be suffering from any hereditary or familial disease. He should be screened with all available tests including chromosomal studies for possible genetic defects. (5) The donor must not be a relative of either spouse; he should have had children of his own. (6) The race and characteristics of the donor should resemble those of the husband of the woman as closely as possible. (7) The donor should be of the same blood group as that of the husband. (8) There should not be any Rh incompatibility between the donor and recipient. (9) The physician should have permission to use his own best judgement in selecting the donor. (10) The couple should be psychologically fit and emotionally stable. (11) The woman to be inseminated and her husband must give consent in writing that an unknown donor should be used. (12) A witness must be present, when insemination is done. (13) It is usually wise to use "pooled" semen. When husband's semen is mixed with that of a donor, there is the technical possibility that the husband may, in fact be the father of the child. (14) The physician who administers the artificial insemination should avoid delivering the child. This will avoid the necessity of either falsifying the birth records or disclosing the true paternity in those records. (15) Usually, a single donor's semen is not used to produce more than ten children.

Legal Problems: There is no statutory law in India for artificial insemination. Artificial insemination with the semen of the husband is justifiable and unobjectionable, since the child is actually the biologic product of both husband and wife, but it does not constitute evidence of proper consummation of marriage. The following are the legal aspects of A.I.D. as applicable to India.

(1) Adultery: The donor and recipient cannot be held guilty of adultery in India, as S. 497, I.P.C. requires sexual intercourse as necessary part of adultery. It has been decriminalized. It can be a ground for divorce.

(2) Legitimacy: The husband is not the actual father of the child, and as such, the child is illegitimate and cannot inherit property.

(3) Nullity of Marriage and Divorce: Mere A.I. is not a ground for nullity of marriage or divorce, because sterility is not a ground for it. However, if A.I. is due to impotence, it is a ground. Consent of husband has no bearing on this. When A.I. was done due to the impotence of the husband, the wife may ask for nullity or divorce, even if a child was born out of A.I. If A.I. is done without the consent of the husband, he can sue his wife for divorce and the doctor for damages.

(4) Natural Birth: If a child is born naturally sometime after the birth of a child by A.I., the status of the child born after A.I. remains illegitimate unless it is adopted, and the status of the natural born child remains legitimate. But, if the parents do not declare A.I., the child remains to be a natural child for practical purposes.

(5) Unmarried Woman or Widow: An unmarried woman or widow may have a child from A.I. but that child would be illegitimate.

(6) Incest: There is risk of incest between the children born by A.I and children of the donor, but this is not an offence in India.

COMPLICATIONS: The husband may feel humiliation of his deficiency from the presence of the child of someone else and may develop psychiatric symptoms. If the child is mentally retarded or physically deformed, the father may develop bitter feelings, for he may be held responsible for this deformity by other persons. A neurosis may develop in the mother, based on the fact that the child belongs to her alone. She may also develop an obsession to know the donor, and to have a second child from the same donor. The child may suffer mental trauma if he learns his past history.

THE DELHI ARTIFICIAL INSEMINATION (HUMAN) ACT, 1995: The main purposes of this legislation are: (1) to allow the issueless couples to have a child through A.I. and give it a legal status, (2) to control spread of HIV through A.I., (3) to regulate the donation, storage, sale or supply of human semen/ovum for A.I., (4) to make obligatory on the part of the medical practitioners: (a) not to indulge in segregating the XX or XY chromosomes, (b) not to disclose the identity of the donor/ recipient, (c) to prohibit to carry on semen bank without registration.

ASSISTED REPRODUCTIVE TECHNIQUE (ART): In India, there is no law on issues relating to ART. The following is the code of conduct for ART as formulated by Indian Council of Medical Research (ICMR). (1) ART clinic has to get approval from the appropriate accreditation authority. (2) The ART clinic is not commercial party in donor programme or surrogacy. (3) No ART procedure can be done without the spouses informed consent. (4) The sperm donor and surrogate should not be a relative or a friend of the couple. (5) Sex selection is not permitted. There should be pre-implantation diagnostic testing of parents for genetic abnormalities. (6) The consent of the couples for the use of embryos is a must. (7) Biological parents must adopt a child born through surrogacy. (8) The sale or transfer of human embryos outside the country is prohibited. (9) Donors should be screened for HIV and hepatitis B and C infections. (10) The records have to be maintained and regularly chequed to guard against tampering.

TEST TUBE BABIES (in vitro fertilisation; I.V.F): The techniques available are: (1) The ovum is removed from the ovary through the abdominal wall and is fertilised by the sperm of her own husband in a small laboratory dish in an artificial medium. At the stage of blastocyst, the embryo is returned to the uterus through the uterine cervix, which gets implanted in the endometrium. (2) Similar re-implantation of one of her own ova fertilised externally by donor sperm. (3) Implantation in an infertile woman of another woman's ovum fertilised by the sperm of the first woman's husband. (4) Implantation in an infertile woman's uterus, of a donor ovum fertilised by donor sperm.

SURROGATE MOTHERHOOD: A surrogate mother is a woman who by contract agrees to bear a child for someone else. It is intended to help a couple, of whom the woman is infertile, but the male has no reproductive deficiency. Artificial insemination with the semen of the barren woman's husband is carried out in a hired woman (womb leasing). Surrogate pregnancy can also be done with donated sperm or donated egg or donated embryo. After surrogate birth, the baby is returned to its biological father and his wife. The baby should be legally adopted by the couple. Another method is to remove a mature healthy ovum from the wife and fertilise it in 'vitro' with the husband's semen, and implant the embryo in the womb of a hired woman. Surrogate pregnancy can also be done with donated sperm or donated egg or donated embryo. According to the guidelines of Indian Council of Medical Research (ICMR), the genetic or biological parents names should only be mentioned in the birth certificate. In the birth registration, the hospital concerned should clearly indicate that the child was conceived through surrogate motherhood or by IVF procedure and pass on the information to the registrar concerned. The legal problems of surrogate motherhood are those of artificial insemination donor.

CLONING: It is the technique of producing a genetically identical duplicate of an organism artificially. Clone is an organism that has same genetic information as another organism. A clone is said to be all descendents derived asexually from a single individual.

The procedure is known as Somatic Cell Nuclear Transplant (SCNT). Nucleus is removed from an egg cell and nucleus from a somatic cell is introduced into it. The resultant structure is triggered chemically or electrically to develop into an embryo. This is implanted in a surrogate mother. In India, human cloning is officially banned.

Therapeutic cloning aims to develop medical therapies for which the cloned embryos grown only up to 14 days can harvest the stem cells that will be useful in treating certain diseases.

EMBRYONIC STEM CELL RESEARCH: Stem cells are unspecialized and undifferentiated cells capable of self-proliferation, migration and differentiation. Human embryonic stem cells (HESCs) are derived from inner cell mass of human blastocysts and its major source is use of spare or supernumerary embryos either fresh or frozen created during in-vitro fertilization to extract HESCs. India has allowed establishment of new HESC lines with spare, supernumerary embryo. Ethical issue plaguing the embryonic stem cell research is value of human life and dignity since embryos are considered potential person. Indian legal system provides for protection of rights of foetus from potential harm through Section 312 to 326 IPC and 416 CrPC. But Indian Legal and either issues are: (1) Duty of care. (2) Non-abandonment. (3) Protection of people. (4) Confidentiality except legally justified breach. (5) Informed consent.

CHAPTER 16

VIRGINITY, PREGNANCY AND DELIVERY

FM 3.18: Describe anatomy of male and female genitalia, hymen and its types. Discuss the medicolegal importance of hymen. Define virginity, defloration, legitimacy and its medicolegal importance.
FM 3.19: Discuss the medicolegal aspects of pregnancy and delivery, signs of pregnancy, precipitate labour superfoetation, superfecundation and signs of recent and remote delivery in living and dead.

VIRGINITY

A virgin *(virgo intacta)* is a female who has not experienced sexual intercourse. Defloration means loss of virginity.

Legal issues: The question of virginity arises in case of (1) defamation, (2) rape.

Legally, **marriage** is a contract between man and woman, which implies physical union by coitus. **Divorce** (S.13, Hindu Marriage Act), means, dissolution of previously valid marriage. **It can be obtained on the ground of adultery, bigamy, unnatural sex practices, desertion, cruelty and in cases of incurable insanity, leprosy or venereal diseases.**

Genitals: The **labia majora** are the two elongated folds of skin projecting downwards and backwards from the mons veneris. They meet in front in the anterior commissure and in back in the posterior commissure in front of the anus. In a virgin they are thick, firm, elastic and rounded, and lie in apposition so as to completely close the vaginal orifice. The **labia minora** (4 cm. long) are two thin folds of skin just within the labia majora. The labia minora are soft, small, pink, and sensitive. The lower portions of labia minora fuse in midline and form a fold called **fourchette**. Anteriorly they divide to enclose clitoris and unite with each other in front and behind the clitoris to form prepuce and frenulum respectively. The depression between fourchette and the vaginal orifice is called **fossa navicularis**. The **clitoris** is small and the vestibule is narrow. The vestibule is the triangular surface which extends from the clitoris above to the anterior margin of the hymen below, and laterally to the labia minora. It is usually concealed by the labia. Urethral opening is 2.5 cm. behind the clitoris, and immediately in front of vaginal opening. **Vulva** includes the mons veneris (pad of fat lying in front of the pubis), clitoris, labia majora and minora, vestibule, hymen and urethral opening. The **perineum** is the wedgeshaped area between the lower end of posterior wall of vagina and the anterior anal wall.

The **vaginal passage** is a pocket irregular in shape, rather than cylindrical tube. It is about 7.5 cm. long, shorter on its anterior wall (6 cm.), and longer on the posterior wall (9 cm.). It is collapsed to form a slit crosswise of the body. Distended it forms a gourd-shaped balloon, wider at the top and possibly lopsided because of the greater size of one lateral pocket or fornix. The width at the upper end is 3 to 4 cm. in nullipara, and 6 to 7 cm. in the parous woman. Bladder lies anteriorly, levator ani muscles laterally, perineal body and rectum lie posteriorly, and pouch of Douglas superiorly to the vagina. The vagina is narrow and tight, the mucosa is rugose, reddish in colour, sensitive to touch, and its walls are approximated. After frequent sexual intercourse (about fifteen to twenty sexual acts) the vaginal rugae become less marked, and the vagina lengthens into the posterior fornix, and the full length of the examining finger can be passed into the posterior fornix. The rugosity is removed only by first birth, but rarely it is absent even in a virgin. The cervical canal is nearly at right angle to the vagina when bladder and rectum are empty. In a virgin the posterior commissure and fourchette are intact. With repeated injury fourchette may become an irregular thickened scar. Fourchette is usually lacerated during child birth. A single intercourse does not alter the parts much, except rupture of the hymen.

When a virgin is placed in lithotomy position with legs wide apart, the vagina remains closed and only the edges of labia minora are seen slightly protruding from between the closed labia majora. In women who have borne children labia are open and the vaginal canal is exposed.

Hymen: The hymen is a fold of mucous membrane about one mm. thick, situated at the vaginal outlet. The average adult hymen consists of folds of membrane having annular or crescentic shape, the broadest part lying posteriorly. The diameter of hymenal orifice in children is roughly 1 mm. per year till it reaches about 10 mm. in a prepubertal girl and at puberty 1.2 cm. Wooden conical measures can be used for measuring circumference of hymen. **At ten years of age, the tip of the small finger and at puberty one finger can usually be passed into the vagina. More than one cm. diameter in a prepubertal child is seen commonly in abused girls. With repeated injury, the fourchette may develop an irregular thickened scar**. Up to the age of 3 to 4 years the hymen is often annular, fleshy and fimbriated. From then until the onset of puberty, it is usually a thin delicate almost translucent membrane with a width of tissue of about 4 mm at 6'O clock position. **The normal preadolescent hymen is essentially a two-dimensional structure located two to three cm. inside the vaginal introitus.** In children, hymen appears as a tense membrane when the thighs are separated. **At about puberty, hymen enlarges and gradually appears as a series of folds. The structure of hymen varies considerably. It may be thick, tough and fleshy or rigid, fibrous, unyielding structure, or it may be thin consisting of elastic tissue and be easily distensible. The normal hymen may lie between these two extremes.** Recognisable, though not severe haemorrhage occurs, when hymen is ruptured. In infants, a small swab can be passed through the hymenal orifice into the vagina without causing rupture.

Types Fig. (16–1): (1) **Semilunar** or crescentic (commonest type)**:** the opening is placed anteriorly. Notches or clefts are seen at 10 and 11° clock position, which may be equal in size or more prominent on one side. (2) **Annular:** opening is oval and situated near the centre of the membrane. (3) **Infantile:** a small linear opening in the middle. (4) **Cribriform:** several openings. (5) **Vertical:** the opening is vertical. (6) **Septate:** two lateral openings occur side by side, separated partially or completely by thin strip of tissue. (7) **Microperforate:** tiny opening with large posterior component. (8) **Fimbriated.** (9) **Imperforate Fig. (16–2):** no opening, (10) **Denticular:** look like a set of teeth surrounding vaginal opening.

Fimbriated hymen: The margin of the hymen is sometimes fimbriated (wavy or undulating or markedly irregular) and **shows multiple notches which may be mistaken for artificial tears.** Natural notches are usually symmetrical, occur anteriorly, do not extend to the vaginal wall and are covered with mucous membrane. Tears caused by sexual intercourse or by foreign body are usually situated posteriorly at one or both sides, or in the midline, and usually extend to the vaginal wall and are not covered with mucous membrane.

Causes of Rupture of Hymen: (1) **An accident,** e.g., a fall on a projecting substance or by slipping on the furniture or fence or while playing at seesaw. In these cases tearing takes place through the lateral margins of the labia into the vaginal wall, perineum, perineal body and hymen, and usually injuries on other parts of the body will be seen. Such hymenal tears are never associated

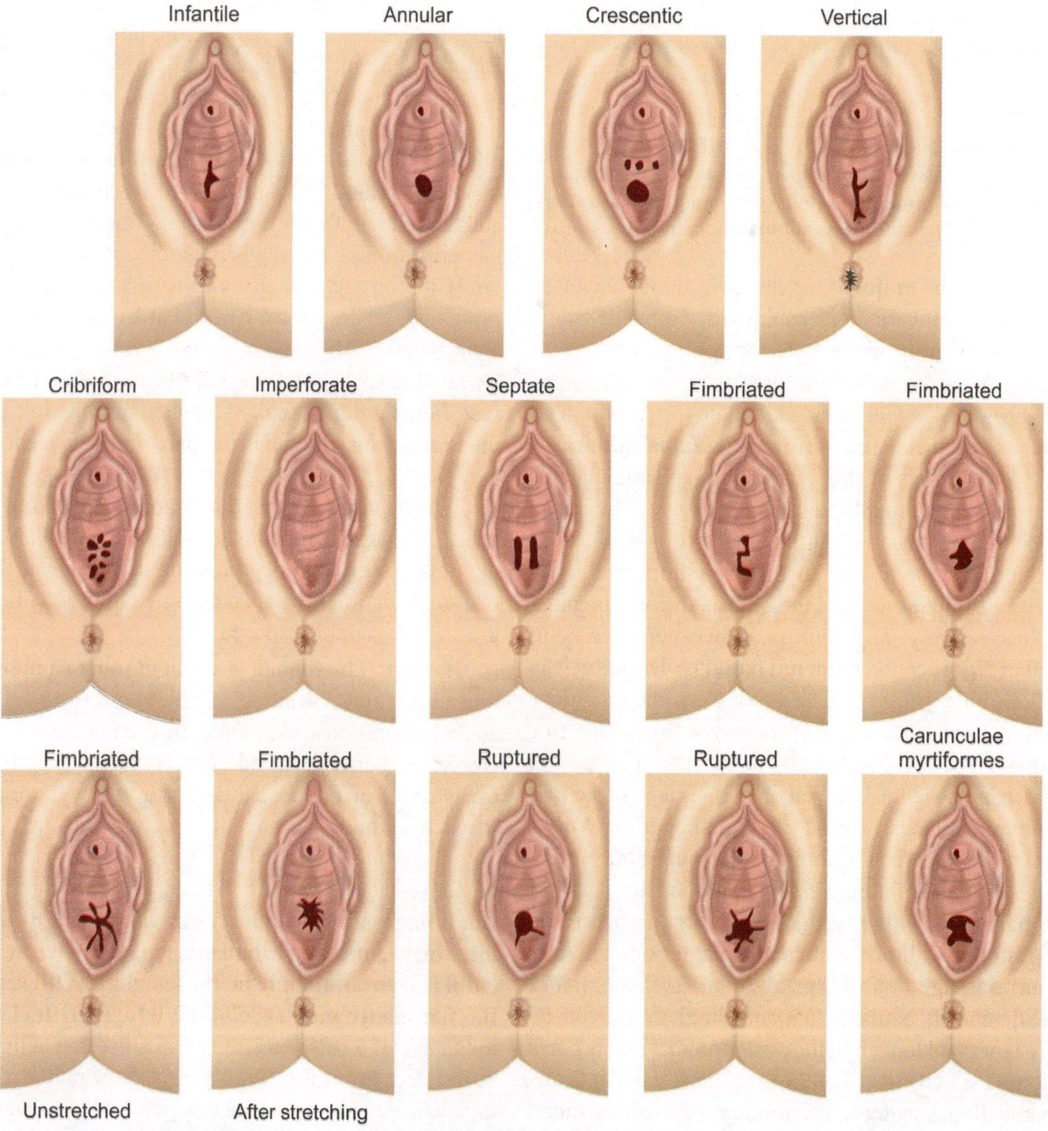

Fig. (16–1). Types of hymen.

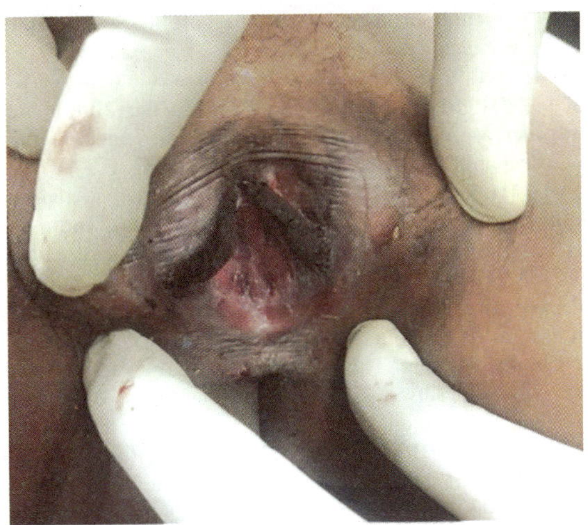

Fig. (16–2). **Imperforated hymen in a 18-year-old girl in Mayer-Rokitansky-Küster-Hauser syndrome.**

Courtesy: **Dr Radhey Khetre, Associate Professor, GMC, Aurangabad MS.**

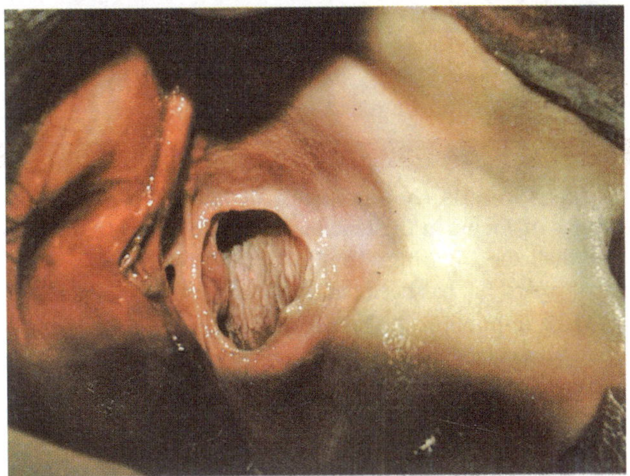

Fig. (16–3). **Thick muscular hymen in a 48-year-old female who had two children by caesarean section.**

with abrasion and bruising of the margins. Accidental straddle injuries usually involve periurethral tissues, labia, hymen and mons. Separation of thighs forcibly in children will not rupture the hymen, unless perineum is ruptured. Hymen does not rupture by riding, jumping, dancing, etc. (2) **Masturbation,** especially with some large foreign body. Hymen is not injured in most cases because manipulation is usually limited to the parts anterior to the hymen. Labia minora and clitoris are enlarged in such cases. The vaginal orifice may be dilated and edges of the hymen may show scratches. (3) **Surgical operation** and gynaecological examination. (4) **Foreign body,** e.g., sola pith introduced into vagina for rendering very young girls fit for sexual intercourse (*aptae viris*). Vaginal stretching, through the insertion of increasingly larger objects (sex toys, vegetables or household objects) may be performed. (5) **Ulceration** from diphtheria, fungus or other diseases. (6) **Scratching** due to irritation of the parts from lack of cleanliness. (7) Sanitary **tampon** may sometimes rupture the hymen.

Breasts: In a virgin the breasts are firm, elastic and hemispherical with a small undeveloped nipple surrounded by an areola which is pink in fair complexioned women and dark-brown in dark women. The breasts become large and flabby by frequent handling, but are not affected by single act of coitus. Occasionally, milk may be found in the breasts of virgins.

Medicolegal Aspects: The presence of unruptured hymen is a presumption, but is not an absolute proof of virginity. The diagnosis of virginity is difficult and in many cases a physical examination of the genital organs may not be helpful. With an intact hymen, there are true virgins and false virgins. The hymen is present always in a virgin in some form or other, but very rarely may be absent congenitally.

The hymen is usually ruptured at the time of the first coitus, and at first only presents a torn appearance. **Hymen may not be ruptured even after repeated acts of coitus, if it is loose, lax, folded and elastic, or thick Fig. (16–3), tough and fleshy, which permit displacement, distortion and stretching without rupture.** Cases have been recorded of women having sexual relations, of pregnant women and even prostitutes in whom the hymen was intact.

The principal signs of virginity: (1) An intact hymen. (2) A normal condition of the fourchette and posterior commissure. (3) A narrow vagina with rugose walls. These signs taken together, may be regarded as evidence of virginity, but taken singly they cannot be so regarded Table (16–1).

Table (16–1). **Difference between virginity and defloration**

	Trait	Virginity	Defloration
(1)	Hymen:	It is intact, rigid and inelastic; the edges are distinct, smooth and regular with a narrow opening hardly allowing a small finger to pass.	It may be torn or intact; in the latter case it is loose, elastic, with a wide opening allowing passage of two or more fingers.
(2)	Labia majora:	They are apposed to each other, fully developed and completely close the vaginal orifice.	They are not apposed to each other, not prominent and at the lower end vaginal orifice may be seen.
(3)	Labia minora:	They are in contact and are covered by labia majora.	They are not in contact and are exposed and separated from labia majora.
(4)	Fourchette:	Intact.	Torn or intact.
(5)	Fossa navicularis:	Intact.	Disappears.
(6)	Vestibule:	Narrow.	Wide.
(7)	Vagina:	It is narrow, the rugae more folded, and the vault more conical.	After repeated intercourse it usually grows in length, and the rugae are less obvious.

In women who are used to coitus, and in those who have borne children, the hymen is destroyed and small, round, fleshy projections or tags, known as carunculae hymenales or myrtiformes are formed round the hymenal ring.

PREGNANCY

Pregnancy is the condition of having a developing embryo or foetus in the female, when an ovum is fertilized by a spermatozoon. It is most likely to occur between the ages of 14 and 45 years, but has been reported much earlier and later.

M.L. importance: The question of pregnancy has to be determined in the following conditions. (1) When a woman pleads pregnancy to avoid attendance in Court as a witness. Pregnancy itself is not an excuse, unless it is so far advanced that delivery is likely to occur soon, or when she or the child is likely to suffer risk by such attendance. (2) If a woman sentenced to death is found to be pregnant, the High Court shall commute the sentence to imprisonment for life (S.416, Cr.P.C.). (3) When a woman feigns pregnancy soon after death of her husband to claim succession to property. (4) When a woman alleges that she is pregnant in order to get greater compensation when her husband dies through the negligence of some person. (5) In cases of divorce, the woman may claim to be pregnant to receive more alimony. (6) To assess damages in a seduction or breach of promise of marriage case. (7) When a woman blackmails a man and accuses that she is pregnant by him, to compel marriage. (8) In allegations that an unmarried woman, widow or a wife living apart from her husband is pregnant. (9) When pregnancy is alleged to be motive for suicide or murder of unmarried woman or widow. (10) In cases of alleged concealment of birth or pregnancy and infanticide.

Consent: The written consent of the woman should be taken after explaining the reason for the examination and its possible consequences.

DIAGNOSIS OF PREGNANCY: The signs and symptoms are usually classified into three groups: (1) The presumptive signs. (2) The probable signs. (3) The positive signs.

(I) PRESUMPTIVE SIGNS: (1) AMENORRHOEA: This is the earliest and one of the most important symptom of pregnancy. The periods may be missed for some time in unmarried woman after illicit intercourse simply from fear and nervousness. In married woman the periods may stop for some time, when there is an intense desire for pregnancy. Women who have never menstruated may become pregnant, and pregnancy may also occur in a woman during the amenorrhoea of lactation. Menstruation may occur for first 2 to 3 months after conception, until decidua vera and decidua reflexa are fused.

(2) CHANGES IN BREASTS: Breast changes are quite characteristic in primigravidas but are of less value in multiparas. A sense of tenseness and tingling in the breasts is frequent in early weeks. After the second month, breasts begin to increase in size and become nodular due to hypertrophy of the mammary alveoli. As they become still larger, the superficial veins are seen more distinct and enlarged, the nipples more deeply pigmented and more erectile and the areola which is pink in the virgin, gradually becomes dark-brown. Around the nipple, the sebaceous glands become enlarged by the end of second month to form small rounded dark coloured tubercles (MONTGOMERY'S TUBERCLES). COLOSTRUM is secreted usually in the third month, which can be expressed from the breasts by gentle massage. Colostrum is thin, yellowish fluid consisting of fat globules and large phagocytic cells filled with droplets of fat. After six months, striae are seen especially in primiparae due to the stretching of the skin.

(3) MORNING SICKNESS: It usually appears about the end of the first month and disappears 6 to 8 weeks later. Nausea and vomiting are usually present in the morning, and pass off in a few hours. It varies greatly in severity and is not reliable.

(4) QUICKENING: From about the 16th to 20th week, the pregnant woman feels slight fluttering movements in her abdomen, which gradually increase in intensity. These are due to movements of the foetus, and their first appearance is known as "quickening".

(5) PIGMENTATION OF THE SKIN: The vulva, abdomen and axillae become darker due to the deposit of pigment, and a dark line extends from the pubis to beyond the umbilicus, the so-called linea nigra.

(6) CHANGES IN THE VAGINA: The mucous membrane of the vagina changes from pink to violet, deepening to blue as a result of venous obstruction, after the fourth week. This is known as Jackquemier's sign or Chadwick's sign. The anterior wall of the vagina is flattened. The tissues become softer, the secretion of the mucus is increased, and pulsation can be felt at an early period.

(7) URINARY DISTURBANCES: During the early weeks of pregnancy, the enlarging uterus exerts pressure on the bladder and produces frequent micturition. This gradually disappears after few months, as the uterus rises up into abdomen, and reappears a few weeks before term when the head descends into the pelvis.

(8) FATIGUE: Easy fatigue is very frequent.

(9) SYMPATHETIC DISTURBANCES: Salivation, perverted appetite and irritable temper are common.

(II) PROBABLE SIGNS OF PREGNANCY:

(1) ENLARGEMENT OF THE ABDOMEN: During pregnancy, abdomen gradually enlarges in size after the twelfth week. By the end of third month, the uterus fills the pelvis, and between third and fourth months appears over the brim. At the fifth month, it is midway between the symphysis and umbilicus. At the end of sixth month, it is at the level of the umbilicus, and at the seventh month it is midway between the umbilicus and the xiphisternum, and at the end of the eighth month and early ninth month it reaches the xiphoid cartilage. Subsequently, the uterus sinks into pelvis and tends to fall forward to about 32 weeks height due to its weight Fig. (16–4). The umbilicus becomes level with the skin by about the seventh month. Striae gravidarum are pinkish or slightly bluish, curved, irregular, depressed lines arranged more or less concentrically, sometimes radially around umbilicus, gradually becoming broader and deeper near inguinal ligament. They also appear on the buttocks and front of thighs. They are seen in late pregnancy (6th to 7th month) and around the time of delivery, become paler with time, and after a year or so appear as white scars (linea albicantes). They are caused by rupture of subcuticular elastic fibres, due to gradual distension of abdomen.

(2) UTERUS: Hegar's sign is positive at about the sixth week. If one hand is placed on the abdomen and two fingers of other hand in the vagina, the firm hard cervix is felt and above it the elastic body of the uterus, while between the two the isthmus is felt as a soft compressible area. This is the most valuable physical sign of early pregnancy.

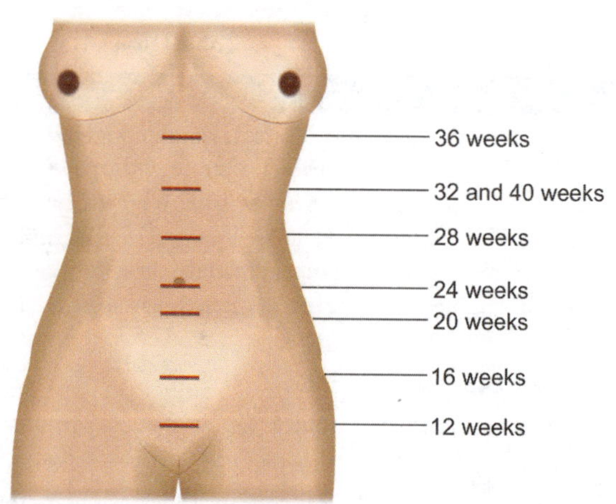

Fig. (16–4). Fundal heights during pregnancy.

(3) CERVIX: From the second month, the cervix progressively softens from below upward, which is well marked by fourth month. This is known as **Goodell's sign.** There is shortening of the cervix towards the last months of pregnancy. The orifice becomes circular instead of being transverse, and admits the point of finger to greater depth.

(4) INTERMITTENT UTERINE CONTRACTIONS (Braxton-Hick's sign): Intermittent, painless uterine contractions are difficult to be observed before the third month, but are easily felt after the fourth month. Each contraction lasts about a minute and relaxation for about two to three minutes. They are present even when the foetus is dead.

(5) BALLOTTEMENT: It means to toss up like a ball. This is positive during the fourth and fifth months of pregnancy as the foetus is small in relation to the amount of amniotic fluid present. To obtain vaginal ballottement, two fingers are inserted into the anterior fornix and a sudden upward motion given. This causes the foetus to move up in the liquor amnii and after a moment, the foetus drops down on the fingers like a ball bouncing back. External ballottement can be obtained by imparting a sudden motion to the abdominal wall covering the uterus; in a few seconds the rebound of the foetus can be felt. This can be negative if the amniotic fluid is scanty.

(6) UTERINE SOUFFLE: This is a soft blowing murmur, which is synchronous with the mother's pulse. It is heard by auscultation on either side of the uterus just above inguinal ligament, towards the end of fourth month. It is due to increase of blood flow through the uterine vessels.

(7) BIOLOGICAL TESTS: They are based on the reaction of test animals to chorionic gonadotropins contained in the pregnant woman's blood or urine. They are: (1) The rapid rat test. (2) The Aschheim–Zondek test. (3) Freidman test. (4) Hogben or female toad test. (5) Male frog test. (6) Galli-Mainini test. They are also positive in hydatidiform mole, chorionic epithelioma and ectopic pregnancy.

(8) IMMUNOLOGICAL TESTS: The hormone chorionic gonadotropin (HCG) and human chorionic somatomamnotropin (HCS) are secreted by the syncytial trophoblastic cells into the fluids of the mother. It can be detected in maternal blood on about the eighth day after impregnation. The rate of secretion rises rapidly to reach a maximum about seven weeks after conception, and decreases to a relatively low volume by 16 weeks after conception. HCG is a glycoprotein and acts on same receptors as LH. These tests utilise antibodies to react with another substance for the detection of HCG. Because they are convenient and very reliable (accuracy 98%), they have replaced bioassays for routine screening. An early morning urine specimen will contain the highest level of HCG and is preferable for testing. **Tests are positive 12 to 15 days after implantation.**

(1) INHIBITION (INDIRECT) LATEX SLIDE TEST: A simple rapid test employs polystyrene latex particles coated with a purified preparation of human chorionic gonadotropin as the antigen and antiserum to HCG. A drop of antiserum is mixed with a drop of urine on a glass slide for 30 seconds. Then, 2 drops of the sensitised latex particles are added and mixed with the combination of antiserum and urine. The slide is gently agitated for two minutes. If HCG is present in the urine it will combine with the anti-HCG antibody. This will leave no antibody free to combine with the latex HCG and there will be no agglutination of the latex particles (positive test). If there is no HCG in the urine, the antibody will be free to combine with the latex HCG and cause agglutination of the latex particles (negative test).

(2) DIRECT LATEX SLIDE TEST: In this the latex reagent consists of particles coated with anti-HCG antibodies. This reagent is mixed directly with the urine. If HCG is present in the urine it will combine with the antibodies and cause agglutination of the latex particles (positive test). If no HCG is present in the urine, there will be no agglutination of the latex particles (negative test).

(3) Haemagglutination inhibition tube test.

Radio immunoassay and ELISA test can detect pregnancy with high degree of accuracy.

(III) Positive Signs of Pregnancy:

(1) Foetal Parts and Movements: Active foetal movements are felt by placing the hands on the uterus from 16 to 18 weeks and may be seen by fifth month. Foetal parts such as head and limbs can be distinctly felt after 24 weeks of gestation.

(2) Foetal Heart Sounds: They are important and definite sign of pregnancy. They are heard between 18 to 20 weeks for the first time. The sounds are like the ticking of a watch placed under a pillow. They can be monitored and recorded accurately by an electronic foetal monitor. Their rate is usually about 160 at fifth and 120 at the ninth month. They are not synchronous with the mother's pulse.

Foetal heart sounds are not heard: (1) when the foetus is dead, (2) when there is excessive quantity of liquor amnii, (3) when abdominal wall is very fat, (4) when examination is made before 18 weeks of pregnancy.

(3) Placental Souffle: This is a soft murmur heard over the placental site, the rate of which corresponds to that of foetal heart sounds.

(4) Funic or Umbilical Souffle: This is a blowing murmur synchronous with foetal heart sounds and supposed to be produced in the umbilical cord.

(5) Radiological examination: At about fifteen to sixteen weeks, foetal parts can be detected with certainty, but occasionally parts are detected as early as ten weeks. **The shadows to be searched in the pelvis of the mother are:** (1) Crescentic or annular shadows of the skull. (2) A series of small dots in a linear arrangement of the vertebral column. (3) A series of fine curved parallel lines of the ribs, and (4) Linear shadows of the limbs. Usually the skull and spine are seen at fifteen to sixteen weeks.

At a later stage X-ray examination may be of value in the diagnosis of a twin pregnancy, **Fig. (16–5)** foetal death or abnormality, hydatidiform mole, etc.

Radiological signs of foetal death are: (1) Spalding's sign **Figs. (16–6 and 16–7)**. (2) Collapse of the spinal column due to absence of muscle tone. (3) Presence of gas in the heart and great vessels.

(6) Ultrasonography: This is done by employing three dimensional scanning with ultrasound. **Gestational sac is seen as white ring by sixth week,** and distinct echoes from the embryo within the gestational ring by seven weeks. **Foetal**

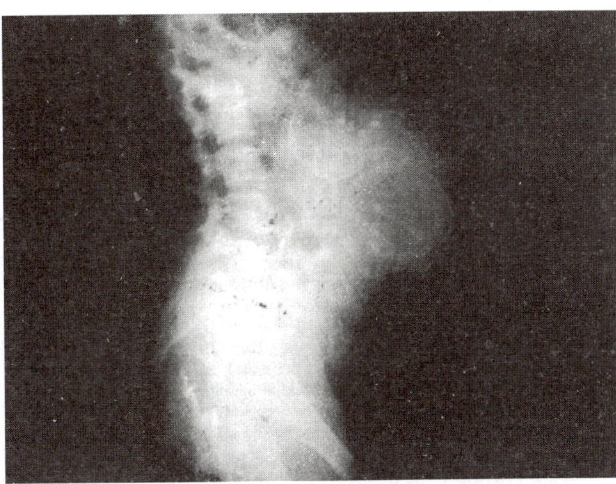

Fig. (16–5). Twin pregnancy.

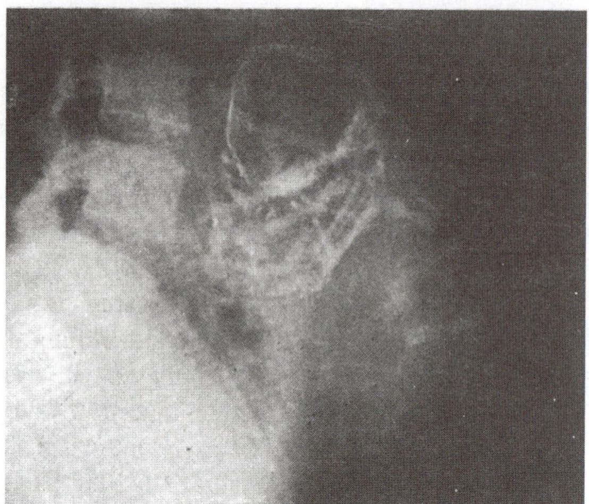

Fig. (16–6). X-ray photograph of the abdomen showing twin pregnancy. One foetus is dead and crumpled and shows Spalding's sign.

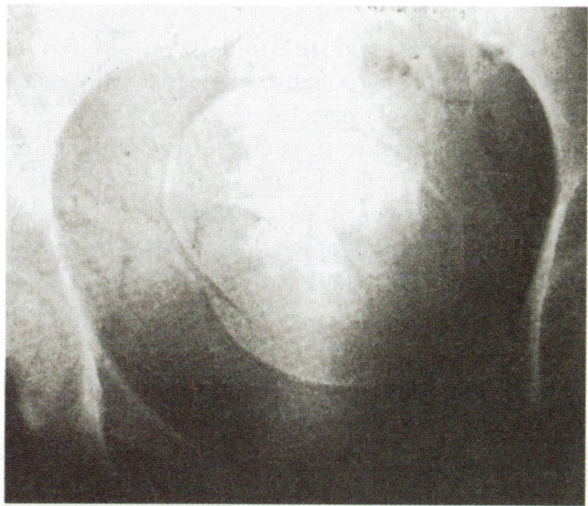

Fig. (16–7). X-ray photograph of the pelvis showing a dead foetus. The bones of the cranial vault show loss of alignment and overlapping (Spalding's sign).

heart beat can be made out by tenth week, sex of baby by thirteenth week, and foetal head and thorax by fourteenth week. In 8 to 14 weeks, crown-rump length of the embryo allows accurate estimation of gestational age. Early identification of dead embryo, multiple pregnancy, vesicular mole, placental site, foetal anomalies, hydramnios and foetal growth is possible. Scanning of abdomen and infant brain will reveal (1) intracranial haemorrhage and damage to brain, (2) bony injuries, periostitis and osteomyelitis, (3) cerebral oedema. The sex of the unborn should not be disclosed.

Signs of Pregnancy in the Dead: The presence of an embryo, foetus, placental tissue, membranes or any other product of conception is a positive proof. The uterus is thickened and increased in size. A well-formed corpus luteum is found in one of the ovaries. Even in an exhumed body which has been reduced to a skeleton, foetal bones will be found in the remains.

The Period of Gestation:

(1) The Average Period: The usually accepted average is 280 days from the first day of the last menstrual period, so that the actual period of gestation is about 266 days. **In most women, the period of gestation is forty weeks or ten times the normal intermenstrual period, which is usually 28 days.**

(2) The Maximum Period: The law does not lay down any fixed limit of gestation. Each case is decided on its own merits. Mc Keown and Gibson have well documented cases up to 328 days, and from an extensive study have concluded that for medicolegal purpose, a period of 354 days from the coitus to livebirth is not impossible. The maximum period according to some authors ranges from 315 to 322 days. As a rule, the longer the gestation, the larger the infant.

(3) The Minimum Period and Viability: Children born at or after 28 weeks of uterine life are viable, i.e. are born alive and able to survive. Children born after 180 days of uterine life may be viable and capable of continuing an independent life apart from their mothers. Infants born at still shorter periods have sometimes survived and grown-up.

Posthumous Child: It is a child born after the death of its father, the mother being conceived by the said father. Legal issues involved are: legitimacy, inheritance of property, compensation case for slander against the mother.

SUPERFECUNDATION: It means the fertilisation of two ova which have been discharged from the ovary at the same period by two separate acts of coitus committed at short intervals. The incidence of twin pregnancies is about one-and-half percent, and of these about 70% are binovular twins resulting from separate fertilisation of two ova formed in the same menstrual cycle. **Development of twins in utero is parallel but not equal, depending on the relative blood supplies from the separately formed placentae.** Both ova do not always develop to maturity. One foetus may be aborted early or die and retained until the labour that expels the other. **The dead foetus may be flattened by pressure and may not be recognisable, and is referred to as foetus compressus or foetus papyraceus.** The spermatozoa causing fertilisation may be from different men. The rare cases wherein two ova are fertilised by a white and black person or persons with entirely different blood groups are the only certain examples of this condition.

SUPERFOETATION: This means the **fertilisation of a second ovum in a woman who is already pregnant.** Ovulation may occur during first trimester of pregnancy until decidua vera comes into apposition with decidua reflexa and decidual cavity gets obliterated. Fertilisation of newly released ovum may occur following coitus. Later, **two foetuses are born either at the same time showing different stages of development, or two fully developed foetuses are born at different periods varying from one to three months.** Cases where a second fully developed child was born a considerable time after the first have been explained on the assumption of twin pregnancy, in which the second child did not develop either due to diminished blood supply or some other cause. On the birth of the normally developed child, the second foetus received proper nourishment and is born later as mature child. **Evidence is accumulating which indicates that superfoetation is not only a possibility but a reality.** Its occurrence in a bipartite or double uterus is certainly possible.

PSEUDOCYESIS (spurious or phantom pregnancy): It is usually observed in patients nearing the menopause or in younger women who intensely desire children. Most of the women suffer from some form of psychic or hormonal disorder.

Such patients may present all the subjective symptoms of pregnancy (amenorrhoea, morning sickness) associated with a considerable increase in the size of the abdomen which may be due to abnormal deposition of fat or to tympanites or contraction of diaphragm pushing forward the entire abdominal wall or occasionally due to ascites. **Changes in breast are sometimes present and in many cases, the woman may imagine foetal movements.** In some cases, pregnancy had gone to "full term" and frank labour pains occurred which ceased abruptly when the patients were told that they were not pregnant. **Clinical examination (if necessary under anaesthesia) and X-ray examination will solve the problem. It is possible for a woman to be pregnant and not to know it. In rare cases pregnancy may progress to full term without the woman being aware of the fact.**

Ectopic pregnancy: Bleeding occurs in fallopian tube due to trophoblastic invasion into the wall. Haemorrhage may occur into the layers of broad ligament. Rupture usually occurs after 6 weeks of pregnancy. Death occurs due to haemorrhagic shock or air embolism.

MATERNAL DEATHS

When a women dies during pregnancy of delivery look for:

(1) Air embolism within large veins and heart.

(2) For amniotic embolism, remove heart and lungs en bloc, incise the main pulmonary trunk, right and left pulmonary arteries and their branches and look for thrombotic and amniotic emboli (meconium, vernix, and lanugo hair). Lethal amniotic fluid embolism is most commonly associated with relatively small tears in the uterus, cervix or vagina where there may not be complete disruption of the well. Search carefully for tears and placental remains.

(3) Abnormal placentation is an important factor associated with haemorrhage. Open the uterus from funds to display the placenta. If the placenta is less than 350 g. it has adverse effect on pregnancy.

(4) In pre-eclamptic toxaemia, a major abnormality is seen in uterine vasculature. Fibrinoid necrosis associated with a large number of lipophages in the vessel wall are seen, the latter being cuffed by mononuclear cells.

(5) Take swabs from cervix and placenta, and blood for culture.

AMNIOTIC FLUID EMBOLISM: Most cases of amniotic fluid emboli occur during active labour due to tear in amnion, and shortly after delivery. Mortality rate is about 80%. Pelvic trauma of parturition, including rupture of uterus, instrumental interference in late pregnancy may allow opening of the sinuses in the placental bed with consequent escape of amniotic fluid. It can also occur in first and second trimester abortions, and following abdominal trauma and amniocentesis. The amniotic fluid enters into the maternal venous circulation with resultant pulmonary microvascular obstruction. The solid elements are rarely found in the liver, kidney and brain. On reaching the lung, this material is presumed to produce severe transient vasospasm of the pulmonary vasculature, pulmonary hypertension, right heart failure, bronchoconstriction and hypoxia. The exact mechanism of death is not known. In 50% of cases death occurs in the first hour. If death does not occur immediately, it causes disseminated intravascular coagulopathy, and fibrin deposition in many organs. In addition to the solids, the actual fluid itself may cause the allergic response that may cause severe collapse and death. The diagnosis is histological and depends upon the demonstration of mucin, foetal squamous cells, meconium, lanugo hair, vernix, fat globules, cells from chorion and amnion in the pulmonary vasculature in sections of the lung stained with H & E. Laboratory studies show decreased fibrinogen, elevated levels of fibrin split products, prolonged partial thromboplastin and prothrombin times, and thrombocytopaenia. Immunohistochemical techniques have also been used in the lung sections to demonstrate human keratin, amniotic fluid derived mucin and isolated trophoblastic cells.

Death may be caused due to: (1) Haemorrhage (antepartum or post-partum). (2) Embolisation (amniotic, fluid, air). (3) Infections. (4) Eclampsia. (5) Aggravation of natural diseases.

LEGITIMACY AND PATERNITY

Legitimacy: Legitimacy is the legal state of a person born in lawful marriage. If a person is born during the continuance of a legal marriage, or within 280 days after the dissolution of the marriage by divorce or death of the husband, his birth is presumed to be legitimate (S.112, I.E.A).

Illegitimacy: The child becomes illegitimate or **bastard,** if it can be proved that the husband could not possibly be the father of child by producing evidence that the alleged father is: (1) under the age of puberty, (2) physically incapable to beget children, because of illness or congenital or acquired deformities, (3) did not have access to his wife during the time that the child was begotten, (4) the blood groups of the child and the alleged father are not compatible.

The question of legitimacy arises in:

(1) Inheritance: A legitimate child only can inherit the property of his father.

(2) Affiliation Cases: A woman may allege a particular man to be the father of her illegitimate child and file a case in the Court for fixing the paternity (Affiliation cases). If the paternity is fixed on a certain person, he becomes responsible to support the child. A First Class Magistrate can sanction a **monthly allowance of any sum depending upon the circumstances of the case** for the maintenance of such child (S. 125, Cr.P.C.) Luxury is not taken into consideration, but only the necessities of life like food, clothing and lodging, etc., are considered. DNA fingerprinting will positively fix or exclude paternity.

(3) Supposititious Children: It means fictitious children. A woman may pretend pregnancy and delivery and later produce a living child as her own, or she may substitute a male child for female child born of her, or for an abortion. This is done for obtaining money or for the purpose of claiming property. Other legal issues involved are blackmailing a man or bringing a charge of breech of promise of marriage against a man. In such cases, the woman should be examined for signs of pregnancy and delivery. The medical evidence is useful only when the age of the supposititious child does not correspond to the date of the pretended delivery. DNA fingerprinting will be conclusive.

(4) Paternity: The question of paternity arises in contests over legitimacy, posthumous births, or supposititious children. It may be determined from:

(a) Parental likeness: The child may resemble the father in feature and figure and also in gesture and other personal peculiarities. Such evidence even when it is positive is regarded only as corroborative.

ATAVISM (Atavis = grandfather): The child does not resemble its parents, but resembles its grandparents. This is due to inheritance of characteristics from remote instead of from immediate ancestors, due to a chance recombination

of genes. Any mental or physical characteristic or tendency or disease peculiar to a remote ancestor may be inherited.

(b) Developmental Defects: Disease or deformities may sometimes be transmitted from parents to children.

(c) Blood Group Tests or Paternity Tests: Blood groups are transmitted from the parents to the children.

(d) DNA fingerprinting.

DELIVERY

Delivery means the expulsion or extraction of the child at birth. The question of delivery arises in (1) abortion, (2) infanticide, (3) concealment of birth, (4) feigned delivery, (5) legitimacy, (6) nullity of marriage, (7) divorce, (8) chastity, and (9) blackmail.

Signs of Recent Delivery in the Living:

(1) General Indisposition: For the first two or three days the woman is pale, exhausted and ill-looking with increase in pulse and slight fever.

(2) Breast Changes: These are full, enlarged and tender with a knotty feeling, and colostrum or milk may be expressed. The areolae are dark, nipples enlarged, and superficial veins prominent, striae gravidarum and Montgomery's tubercles are present. The presence of colostrum corpuscles in milk strongly indicates that delivery has taken place within a few days.

(3) The Abdomen: The abdominal walls are pendulous, wrinkled and show linea albicantes, especially in flanks. They are irregular, white or silvery subcutaneous scars. They are simply evidence of previous prolonged distension of the abdomen. They are not formed always and if formed they may disappear.

(4) The Perineum: It is sometimes lacerated and the age of tear may be of value in fixing the date of the delivery.

(5) The Labia: They are tender, swollen and bruised or lacerated.

(6) The Vagina: It is smooth-walled, relaxed, capacious and may show recent tears which usually heal by the seventh day. The rugae begin to reappear about the third week.

(7) The Uterus: Immediately after delivery, the contracted and retracted body of uterus feels like hard muscular tumour, the upper border of which lies about three cm. below the umbilicus. It then diminishes in size by about one-and-half cm. a day. On the sixth day, it is midway between the umbilicus and pubis, by 12th day 5 cm. above the pelvic brim, by 14th day at the level of the pubic symphysis and returns to normal condition in nine weeks. Uterus becomes normal in weight in 6 to 8 weeks.

(8) The Cervix: It is soft and dilated and its edges torn and lacerated transversely. The internal os begins to close in the first 24 hours. The external os is soft and patent and admits two fingers. At the end of a week one finger is admitted with difficulty and is closed in two weeks.

(9)The Lochia: It is a discharge from the uterus which lasts for two or three weeks. It has a peculiar sour, disagreeable odour. During the first 4 to 5 days, the discharge is bright-red and contains large clots (lochia rubra). During the next four days, it becomes serous and paler in colour (lochia serosa). After the ninth day colour becomes yellowish-grey or turbid (lochia alba) until its final disappearance.

(10) Intermittent Uterine Contractions: They are usually present for the first 4 to 5 days.

(11) If blood or urine gives a **positive pregnancy test,** it is strong corroborative evidence that pregnancy has recently terminated. They are likely to be negative in a week or ten days.

The above signs are more characteristic of a full term delivery than of a premature one.

In self-delivery scratches may be found on the neck of a newborn infant due to fingernails of the mother trying to assist birth by pulling on the neck.

SIGNS OF RECENT DELIVERY IN THE DEAD: All the local signs mentioned above may be present. The findings in the internal genitalia will vary with the period of gestation and the time after delivery at which death occurred. It is flabby for a day or two, and then gradually shrinks and resumes its firmness. Immediately after delivery the uterine wall is 4 to 5 cm. thick. The uterine cavity is almost obliterated by apposition of the anterior and posterior walls; its total length is 20 cm. and the length of its cavity 15 cm. In the first 2 or 3 days after delivery, the length is 17.5 cm. and breadth 10 cm. At the end of a week 13 to 14 cm. long and 5 cm. in thickness, and at the end of a fortnight it is less than 12 cm., and returns to normal size, i.e., 7 to 8 cm. length, 5 cm. in breadth, and 2 cm. in thickness in about 6 weeks. After delivery at term, the uterus weighs about 1000 g.; at the end of first week 500 g.; at the end of second week about 350 g.; at the end of 6 weeks 100 to 120 g. Shortly after delivery, the placental site appears as an irregular, nodular elevated area 15 cm. in diameter and is covered with clotted blood, lymph and portions of decidua. The placental site measures 3 to 4 cm. in diameter at the end of the second week, and only one to two cm. at the end of six weeks. The ovaries and Fallopian tubes are usually congested, but may become normal within a few days. A large corpus luteum is usually found in one of the ovaries. For the first few days after delivery, the peritoneum covering the lower part of the uterus is arranged in folds which soon disappears. Soon after delivery, the bladder shows oedema and hyperaemia and frequently submucous extravasation of blood.

Table (16–2). Difference in the uterus of parous and nulliparous women

	Trait	Parous uterus	Nulliparous uterus
(1)	Size:	9 cm. long; 6.5 cm. wide. Larger and thicker.	7 cm. long; 4.5 cm. wide. Smaller and thinner.
(2)	Weight:	80 to 120 g.	40 to 60 g.
(3)	Length:	The body is twice the length of cervix.	The body and the cervix have the same length.
(4)	Fundus:	The top of the fundus is convex and on a higher level than the line of broad ligament.	Upper surface of fundus less convex and on same level as broad ligament.
(5)	Cavity:	The walls are concave from inside forming a wider and rounded cavity.	The walls are convex from inside forming smaller and triangular cavity.
(6)	Cervix:	Irregular, and edges show scars. External os is transverse, irregular, and fissured. It may admit tip of the finger; the internal os is not well-defined.	Regular, no scars. External os is rounded and appears as a small hollow in the centre of cervix. The mucous membrane is smooth and intact and orifice closed. Internal os circular, well-defined.

SIGNS OF REMOTE DELIVERY IN THE LIVING: A previous pregnancy usually leaves permanent marks on a woman, especially when it has gone to full term. If however, there has been one pregnancy only and if this has not been of full duration, little or no indication of the previous pregnancy state may be left.

(1) ABDOMEN: The abdominal walls tend to be lax and show multiple white scars on the lateral aspects. Linea nigra is commonly present.

(2) BREASTS: The breasts are lax, soft and pendulous, frequently wrinkled if the woman has nursed her baby, and occasionally show linea albicantes. The nipples are enlarged, the areolae dark, and Montgomery's tubercles are usually present.

(3) VULVA: The vagina is partially open as the labia do not completely close the orifice. The perineum may show the scar of an old tear. The vaginal rugae are absent and walls are relaxed.

(4) UTERUS: As in Table 16–2.

SIGNS OF REMOTE DELIVERY IN THE DEAD: The uterus is larger, thicker and heavier. The walls are concave from inside forming a wider and rounded cavity. The body of the uterus is twice the length of the cervix.

CHAPTER

17

ABORTION

FM 3.27: Define, classify and discuss abortion, methods of procuring MTP and criminal abortion and complication of abortion. MTP Act 1971.
FM 3.28: Describe evidences of abortion—living and dead, duties of doctor in cases of abortion, investigations of death due to criminal abortion.

Legally, abortion (miscarriage) means the premature expulsion of the foetus from the mother's womb at any time of pregnancy, before full term of pregnancy is completed.

Classification: (1) Natural: (a) Spontaneous. (b) Accidental. **(2) Artificial:** (a) Therapeutic. (b) Criminal.

Natural Abortion: Abortion may occur at any time due to natural causes. **Abortion occurs in 10 to 15% of all pregnancies and is most common about the second or third month. Within the first week, ovum may be passed off without being recognised.** In abortions during the first two months of pregnancy, the embryo is expelled intact, covered by the decidua vera. In later months, the foetus is born first, followed by the amniotic sac and placenta, and later on the decidual tissues. **The products are expelled days or weeks after the death of the embryo.**

CAUSES: (1) Defect in the ova, including chromosomal defect is the most common cause of abortion in the first trimester. (2) Developmental defect of the foetus (common cause). (3) Low implantation of zygote. (4) Disease of decidua or placenta. (5) Rh incompatibility. (6) Retroverted uterus. (7) Submucous uterine fibroid. (8) Malformed uterus. (9) Uterine hypoplasia. (10) Hypertension. (11) Diabetes mellitus. (12) Hormonal deficiency. (13) Sudden shock, emotional disturbances. (14) Syphilis. (15) Nephritis. (16) Arsenic or lead toxicity. (17) Drug toxicity.

Accidental: A general shakeup in advanced pregnancy can produce abortion, but if the ovum is healthy, abortion will not occur.

Artificial Abortion: (1) Legal or Therapeutic Abortion (MTP Act): Abortion is justifiable only when it is done in good faith to save the life of the woman, if it is materially endangered by the continuance of pregnancy. The World Medical Association, adopted a resolution on therapeutic abortion, known as **Declaration of Oslo (1970).**

(2) Criminal Abortion: A criminal abortion is the induced destruction and expulsion of the foetus from womb of the mother unlawfully, i.e., when there is no therapeutic indication for the operation. It is resorted to mostly by widows and unmarried women. **It is usually carried out before the third month.** A case of criminal abortion is investigated only when the woman dies, and rarely when someone gives the information to the police.

Unsafe abortion means, abortion not provided through approved facilities, and/or persons.

ABORTIONISTS: They can be divided into three main groups: (1) The expert or medically qualified abortionist. (2) The semi-skilled abortionist, such as midwives, nurses, chemists, etc., who have a fair knowledge of anatomy and pregnancy but who have not the facilities available to the qualified person. (3) The unskilled abortionist.

LEGAL ASPECTS: Under Sec. 312, I.P.C. whoever voluntarily causes criminal abortion is liable for imprisonment up to three years, or fine or both and if the woman is quick with child the imprisonment may extend up to seven years. It is necessary that the woman should be pregnant and that abortion should be carried with her consent. Both the person causing the abortion and the woman are liable for punishment. If the means used do not succeed, it is punishable under Sec.511, I.P.C. with imprisonment up to half of the punishment under Sec. 312. Under Sec. 313, if the miscarriage is caused without the consent of the woman, the imprisonment may be up to ten years or life. Under Sec. 314, if a pregnant woman dies from an act intended to cause miscarriage, the offender is liable to be punished with rigorous imprisonment up to ten years and also fine up to two lakh rupees. Under Sec. 315, a person doing an act intended to prevent the child from being born alive or to cause to die after its birth, is liable to be punished with imprisonment up to ten years or fine or both. Under Sec. 316, causing death of quick unborn child by any act amounts to culpable homicide, and the punishment may extend up to ten years imprisonment.

THE MEDICAL TERMINATION OF PREGNANCY ACT, 1971

Indications: Under this Act, pregnancy can be terminated under the following conditions. **(1) Therapeutic:** When the continuation of pregnancy endangers the life of woman or may cause serious injury to her physical or mental health. **(2) Eugenic:** When there is risk of the child being born with serious physical or mental abnormalities. This may occur. (A) If the pregnant woman in the first three months suffers from: (1) German measles, (incidence of congenital defects 10 to 12%). (2) Smallpox or chicken pox. (3) Toxoplasmosis. (4) Viral hepatitis. (5) Any severe viral infection. (B) If the pregnant woman is treated with drugs like thalidomide, cortisone, aminopterin, antimitotic drugs, or if she consumes hallucinogens or antidepressants. (C) Pregnant woman is treated by X-rays or radio-isotopes. (D) Insanity of the parents. **(3) Humanitarian:** When pregnancy has been caused by rape. **(4) Social:** When pregnancy has resulted from the failure of contraceptive methods in case of a married woman, which is likely to cause serious injury to her mental health. **(5) Environmental:** When social or economic environment, actual or reasonably expected can injure the pregnant woman's health.

Rules: (1) Only a qualified registered medical practitioner possessing PG degree or diploma in Ob & G, or who has assisted in performing 25 cases of MTP, or has 6 months of experience as a house surgeon in Ob & G department in a recognised hospital will be eligible to perform MTP. MTP (amendment) Bill, 2014 allows homoeopathy and ayurvedic practitioners to conduct medical termination of pregnancy. Chief Medical Officer of the district is empowered to certify that a doctor has the necessary training to do abortions. (2) The pregnancy should be terminated in Government hospitals, or in the hospitals recognised by the Government for this purpose. (3) Non-governmental institutions may take up abortion if they obtain a licence from the Government or district level committee constituted by government with chief medical officer or district health officer as chairperson of the committee. (4) The consent of the woman is required before conducting abortion; written consent of the guardian is required if the woman is a minor or a mentally ill person. Consent of husband is not necessary. (5) Abortion cannot be performed on the request of the husband, if the woman herself is not willing. (6) The woman need not produce proof of her age. The statement of the woman that she is over eighteen years of age is accepted. (7) It is enough for the woman to state that she was raped, and it is not necessary that a complaint was lodged with the police. (8) Professional secrecy has to be maintained. The Admission Register for the termination of pregnancies is secret document, and the information contained therein should not be disclosed to any person. (9) If the period of pregnancy is below 12 weeks, it can be terminated on the opinion of a single doctor. (10) If the period of pregnancy is between 12 and 20 weeks, two doctors must agree that there is an indication. Once the opinion is formed, the termination can be done by any one doctor. (11) In an emergency, pregnancy can be terminated by a single doctor, even without required training (even after twenty weeks), without consulting a second doctor, in a private hospital which is not recognised. (12) The termination of pregnancy by a person who is not registered medical practitioner (person concerned), or in an unrecognised hospital (the administrative head) shall be punished with rigorous imprisonment for a term which shall not be less than two years, but which may extend to seven years. Where a doctor acts under the provisions of the act, various sections of the I.P.C. referring to abortion will not apply to him. The doctor is protected from any legal action for any damage caused or likely to be caused in terminating the pregnancy, provided he has acted in good faith and exercised proper care and skill. Though the Act does not state that it is "abortion on demand", the provisions are extremely liberal for any woman to obtain termination of pregnancy.

Confidentiality: The owner/head of the hospital should maintain an admission register for recording details of MTP. A number should be assigned to each patient. The name of the patient should not be entered in any case sheet, operation theater register or any other record. The entries in the registers shall be made serially for every year. The register is a secret document, which should be kept under safe custody for five years. In all other documents, the number assigned to each patient in the M.T.P. register should be used as a reference number. A certificate can be issued to an employed woman.

The form of consent, certified opinion of the doctors and the intimation of MTP should be placed in an envelope and sealed and serial number of the pregnant woman written and marked secret. The name of the doctor and date of termination should be written. These envelopes should be under the safe custody of head of hospital/owner. A monthly statement should be sent to the Director of Health Services.

THE METHODS OF PROCURING CRIMINAL ABORTION

Methods: The methods commonly used for terminating an unwanted pregnancy, can be roughly divided into three periods: (1) Up to the end of the first month, the woman may take violent exercises, hot baths and purgatives. Extreme violence may lead to internal injury. (2) Up to the end of the second month, when suspicion becomes certainty, abortifacient drugs are used. (3) About the third or fourth month, after failing to procure abortion by the above methods, mechanical interference is done either by the woman herself or by some other person.

(I) Abortifacient Drugs: Every common drug has been used at some time in an attempt to produce criminal abortion. They either produce congestion of the uterine mucosa and then uterine bleeding, followed by contractions of the uterine muscle and expulsion of the foetus, or they cause the uterine contractions by stimulating the myometrium directly. **There is no drug which when taken by the mouth causes abortion without endangering the life of the woman.**

(1) Drugs Acting Directly on the Uterus: (A) Ecbolics: They increase uterine contraction but do not relax or dilate the cervical canal and external os, which is necessary to expel the foetus. **Ergot** is most commonly used and has a uterine action which increases as pregnancy advances, but its toxic circulatory side-effects result in arterial spasm and gangrene of the extremities. It frequently fails during the earlier months of pregnancy. **Hydrastis canadensis** has an action similar to but less intense than ergot. **Quinine** has a direct action upon the uterus or uterine nerves, but its action is not certain. **Lead** in the form of pills made from diachylon (lead oleate), or lead plaster is commonly used. It causes tonic contractions of the uterus and also has a direct toxic effect on the cells of the developing ovum. **Death of the foetus may occur in doses which do not seriously affect the mother.** Symptoms of lead poisoning may occur before abortion takes place. **Pituitary extract** has a specific oxytocic effect on uterine muscle. Its effect is significant only near the term. Synthetic oestrogens do not have any abortifacient effect except perhaps in very large doses. Decoctions of cotton root bark, nitrobenzol, picrotoxin and strychnine are also used.

(B) Emmenagogues: They produce or increase the menstrual flow. **They act as abortifacient when given in large and repeated doses.** The chief of these are savin, borax, apiol, rue, laburnum, oestrogens, sanguinarin, senecio, caulophyllin, hellebore, etc.

(2) Irritants of the Genitourinary Tract: They produce reflex uterine contractions, e.g., oil of pennyroyal, oil of tansy, oil of turpentine, cantharides, etc. They may produce severe inflammation of the kidney in large doses. **Potassium permanganate** is applied to the vaginal vault in 120 to 300 mg. tablets, crystals or solution. It produces acute localised punchedout ulceration with raised edges and a granular black base and causes severe haemorrhage due to erosion of small arterial vessels.

(3) Irritants of the Gastrointestinal Tract: Any substance which causes irritation of the colon may produce hyperaemia and contractions of uterus. Saline cathartics, such as magnesium sulphate or drastic purgatives, such as aloes, calomel, castor oil, croton oil, jalap, colocynth, phenolphthalein, rhubarb, senna, scammony, podophyllum, elaterium or gamboge are commonly used. The commonly used emetic is tartar emetic.

(4) Drugs having Poisonous Effects on the Body: (A) Inorganic irritants, e.g., lead, copper, iron, mercury and antimony. (B) Organic irritants, e.g. cantharides, unripe fruit of *papaya*, unripe fruit of pineapple, seeds of carrot, *moringa*, etc., juice of calotropis, bark of plumbago rosea, caryophyllus, *methi,* saffron, etc.

(II) General Violence: It acts directly on the uterus, or indirectly by producing congestion of pelvic organs, or haemorrhages between uterus and membranes. **It may be successful in those in whom there is some natural irritability of the uterus,** but in others who are not naturally predisposed to abort, even violence of a severe degree fails to produce abortion.

Methods: (1) **Severe pressure on the abdomen** by kneading, blows, kicks, jumping, tight lacing, etc. and massage of the uterus through the abdominal wall.

(2) Violent exercise, e.g., horse riding, cycling, jumping from a height, severe jolting as driving over a rough road, running upstairs and downstairs and carrying or lifting heavy weights. Death may occur from rupture of liver, spleen or intestines.

(3) Cupping: A mug is turned mouth downwards over a lighted wick and placed on the hypogastrium and the mug is pulled, which results in partial separation of the placenta. This is usually practised in advanced pregnancy.

(4) Very hot and cold hip baths alternately.

(III) Local Violence: The choice of the method and its results will depend upon the skill of the operator Fig. (17–1).

(1) Syringing: The ordinary enema syringe with a hand-bulb is commonly used to inject fluid into the uterus, the hard nozzle being inserted into the cervix. Sometimes, **Higginson's syringe is used. The suction valve is placed in a bowl of fluid and pressure applied on the bulb. Due to imperfect filling of the bulb, a mixture of air and fluid is forced into the uterine cavity at a pressure higher than that present in uterine veins. The fluid detaches part of the amniotic sac and placenta from the uterine walls, followed by haemorrhage, uterine contraction and abortion.** Soap water is often used as an injection material. **Irritating substances may be added to the water,** such as lysol, cresol, corrosive sublimate, alum, inorganic acids, potassium permanganate, formalin, turpentine, arsenic compounds, lead compounds, etc. A necrotic pseudo-membrane may form in the vagina and cause severe damage to cervix. These substances may be absorbed through the vaginal and uterine mucosa and cause toxaemia, shock and death. **Extensive tissue destruction may lead to infection and fatal haemorrhage. Death may result from air embolism.** The risk of air embolism increases as pregnancy advances and emboli may enter the brain through the placental venous plexus or the abdominal or thoracic veins which anastomose with the vertebral venous plexus. In early pregnancy, antiseptic fluid may enter the peritoneal cavity via fallopian tubes causing shock and chemical peritonitis and may also cause widespread venous thrombosis and uterine infarction. Rough insertion of the syringe into the cervix, or rapid injection of cold or unduly hot fluid, may **cause sudden death from vagal inhibition. Fear, apprehension and nervous tension act as more potent mechanism for cervical shock.** Douches of hot or cold water may be applied to the vagina or water may be projected with considerable force towards the uterine os. The injection of fluid can be self-administered or carried out by an abortionist.

(2) Rupturing of the Membranes: The membranes are ruptured by introduction of an instrument, e.g., a uterine sound, catheter, probe, stick, pencil, penholder, umbrella rib, knitting needle, crochet needle, curtain rod, nail, hairpin, piece of

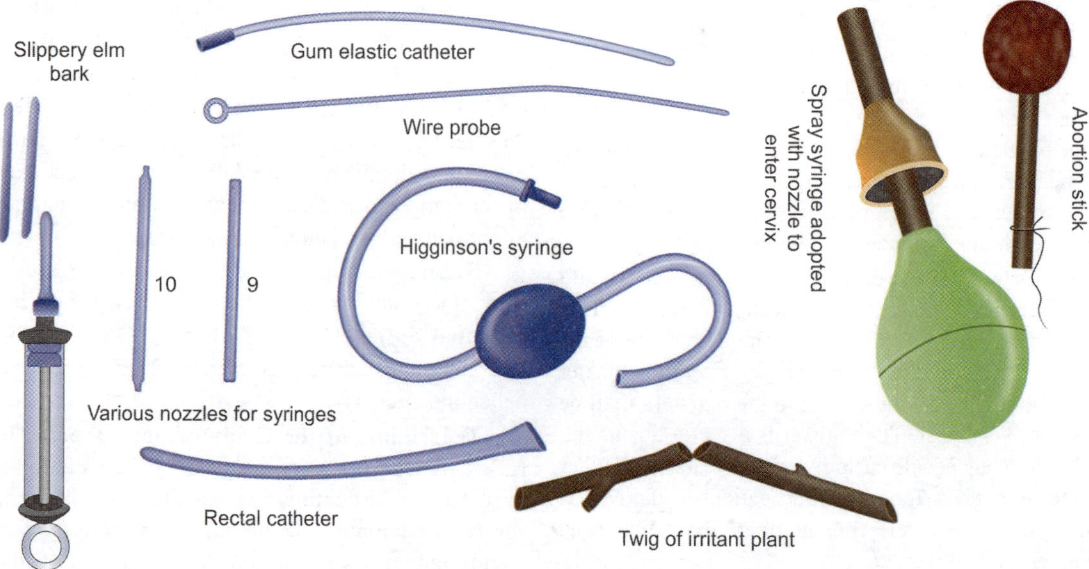

Fig. (17–1). Common instruments used to procure criminal abortion.

wire, glass rod, screwdriver, douche cannula, etc., into the cavity of the uterus. **Abortion usually occurs from few hours to two to three days, due to escape of liquor amnii but occasionally may not occur for days or weeks.** Instruments or parts of the instruments can break after introduction into the uterine cavity or perforation of vaginal or uterine wall. This can be done by the woman herself or by an abortionist.

(3) Syringe Aspiration: A large syringe attached to a catheter or length of a plastic tubing **can produce suction within the uterus sufficient to rupture the chorionic sac and precipitate abortion.**

(4) Dilation of the Cervix: Foreign bodies left in the cervical canal, such as pessaries, laminaria tent (a dried stalk of a seaweed) or seatangle tent (cylinder 8 cm. long and a diameter of 3,4 or 8 mm) or obturator, **dilate the cervix, irritate the uterine mucosa and produce marked congestion and uterine contractions, with expulsion of the foetus.** A white thread is attached to one end for easy removal. They are used after 8 weeks of pregnancy in nulliparous women and in cases with rigid cervix. **The cervical canal may be dilated by introducing a compressed sponge into the cervix and leaving it there.** The sponge swells from moisture in the uterine segment with expulsion of the foetus. **Slippery elm bark** is obtained from a tree grown in Central and North America. It occurs in soft flat pieces of varying length and width and about three mm. in thickness. **The pieces are cut to the desired length and breadth and inserted into the cervical canal.** They absorb moisture and within a few minutes, a jelly-like layer is produced on each side of the bark, which is as thick as the bark itself, due to which cervical canal is dilated.

(5) Abortion Stick: **This is a thin wood or bamboo stick, from 12 to 18 cm.** long. This stick is wrapped round at one end or for the greater portion of its length with cotton-wool or a piece of cloth, and soaked with juice of marking nut, calotropis, jequirity, asafoetida or paste made of arsenious oxide, arsenic sulphate, mercuric chloride and red lead, etc. **It is introduced into the vagina or os of uterus by professional abortionists *(dhais)* and retained there till uterine contractions begin. Instead of this stick, a twig of some irritant plant, e.g., calotropis, nerium odorum, cerbera thevetia, plumbago rosea or zeylanica, etc. is used. In some cases irritating juice is directly applied to the os, or a piece of cloth saturated with irritating juice, or paste is introduced into the vagina.**

(6) Air Insufflation: Air is introduced into vagina and uterus by various means, e.g., pumps, syringes, douche tips, and oral-genital contact.

(7) Electricity: The negative pole is placed over the cervix in the posterior vaginal vault, and positive over the sacrum or lumbar vertebrae. When current is passed (110 volts), uterus contracts and may expel its contents.

(8) Curettage: Some criminal abortions are produced by dilation and curettage under general anaesthesia.

(9) Pastes: Pastes containing soap, myrrh resinoid, thymol, potassium iodide, or mercury (Utus, Foetex, Indulabo, Interruptin pastes) are injected from a collapsible tube with a uterine applicator. Ten to thirty ml. is injected into the uterus through the external os. **The principle is to detach parts of placenta from the uterine wall, similar to the syringing method.** They produce necrosis and infection of the uterine wall similar to that produced when soap water is injected into the uterus in a large quantity. Failure rate is high and infection can occur.

METHODS OF THERAPEUTIC ABORTION: (1) Mifipristone (RU 486) inhibits the action of progesterone. This causes breakdown of endometrium and detachment of embryo from the uterine wall. After 36 to 48 hours misoprostol (prostaglandin) is given which produces uterine contractions and the products are expelled within four hours. The procedure resembles a normal abortion. It is not very effective after seven weeks.

(2) ELECTRICAL VACUUM ASPIRATION: This is done during the first three months of pregnancy. The cervix is dilated and the cannula is introduced into the uterine cavity. Between 8 to 12 weeks of pregnancy, a nine mm. cannula is sufficient. A negative pressure of 0.4 to 0.6 kg/sq.cm. is produced in the uterine cavity by means of a vacuum pump for evacuation of the contents. The cannula is moved gently up and down over all sides of the uterine cavity. The contents are broken up by aspiration, and are collected in a bottle connected to the cannula. Aspiration usually takes 3 to 5 minutes. Ease of performance, less haemorrhage and diminished danger of perforation of uterus are the advantages of this method.

(3) Dilatation of the cervix and oxytocic infusion, or a direct injection of ten units of oxytocin into the uterus.

(4) Dilation of the cervix and evacuation of the uterus by curettage, during the first three months.

(5) Low rupture of the membranes.

(6) Utus paste is injected through a cannula into the cervical canal.

(7) PROSTAGLANDINS: Prostin E_2 (PGE_2), and prostin F_2 (PGF_2) induce labour and abortion. They can be given intravenously or orally. Intra-amniotic injection of 25 mg. prostaglandin F2 is used for second trimester abortions.

(8) AMNIOTIC FLUID REPLACEMENT THERAPY: This method is useful after twelfth week of pregnancy, or in cases of intrauterine death. With long needle, amniotic fluid is removed and replaced with equal volume of 20% saline or 50% glucose. Abortion usually occurs in 24 to 48 hours after injection.

(9) MANUAL VACUUM ASPIRATION: A hand-held vacuum syringe and flexible plastic cannula are used. The products are aspirated by suction into the syringe. Sedation or anaesthesia are not required.

(10) ABDOMINAL HYSTEROTOMY: This method is preferred after 14 weeks of pregnancy.

ABORTION AND THE MEDICAL PRACTITIONER: Sometimes, an abortionist produces an incomplete abortion and sends the woman to the doctor as a case of genuine abortion. A woman may insert a tablet of potassium permanganate into the vagina which causes acute localised ulceration with profuse bleeding due to erosion of small arterial vessels. The patient then visits a doctor who may be led to believe that she is threatened with abortion and may evacuate the uterus. Sometimes, a woman may go to a doctor with the complaint of displacement of the uterus, and the unsuspecting doctor may pass a sound, which may result in abortion.

SUSPICION OF CRIMINAL ABORTION: It should be suspected when: (1) the deceased is pregnant and deeply cyanosed, (2) instruments to procure an abortion or abortifacient drugs are found at the scene of death, (3) the underclothing appears to be disturbed after death, (4) fluid, soapy or blood-stained is coming out of the vagina.

EVIDENCE: The evidence of criminal abortion is obtained from: (1) The victim's or deceased's medical history and her whereabouts prior to death. (2) The clinical or autopsy examination. (3) The examination of aborted material if available.

PROOF: The following points should be proved to convict the abortionist: (1) that the dead woman was pregnant, (2) that the accused was responsible for the act which resulted in the interruption of the pregnancy, (3) that the accused acted for the purpose of producing an illegal abortion, and (4) that death occurred as the result of the attempt to

interrupt the pregnancy. The findings depend upon the mode of abortion practised and the time which has passed between its performance and death.

EVIDENCE OF ABORTION

IN THE LIVING: In the living, abortion cases come to the doctor: (1) when a woman alleges abortion after a blow or quarrel in order to inflict severe penalty on the accused, (2) when a woman is charged with abortion but wishes to conceal it.

Signs of injury to the abdomen or body and any diseases predisposing to natural abortion should be noted. **The signs of recent abortion are essentially those of recent delivery, but they depend on the length of pregnancy.** The signs are modified depending on the time that has passed between abortion and examination.

In abortion during the first two to three months of pregnancy, the signs are ill-defined and consist of haemorrhage, slight softening of external os and vaginal walls, and slight enlargement of the uterus, which disappear in few days. The breast changes of pregnancy in the case of primipara are useful. During the fourth and fifth months of pregnancy, the haemorrhage is more marked, and the internal os may admit a finger. The os is not injured in abortions of less than six months of pregnancy. The genital organs are much softened and tags of membrane may be found in the uterus. The general condition of the genital tract and the injuries can be made out by visual examination with a speculum. The vaginal canal may show erosions or lacerations. Cervix may show marks of valsellum forceps, fissures or lacerations, indicating use of an instrument.

The organisms causing uterine sepsis following evacuation are: Cl. welchii, E. coli, Streptococcus pyogenes, Staphylococcus aureus and anaerobic Streptococci. Strong antiseptics produce surface tissue necrosis which encourages bacterial growth. In fatal cases, the sepsis usually involves the endometrium, especially the placental site and pieces of retained products. The myometrium, tubes and adjacent pelvic organs and peritoneum are also infected. Material and liquid from the vagina, uterine cavity and blood should be collected for chemical and bacteriological examination. Urine and vomit should be preserved for chemical analysis.

Expelled material: The material alleged to have been expelled from the uterus should be examined for products of conception. If recognition is not possible, the material should be placed in water to dissolve the blood. A portion should be examined microscopically to know whether it is a blood clot, foetus, polyp or fibroid. In the case of blood clot, grouping and precipitin test should be done to know whether it is compatible with the woman's blood groups. In the case of a foetus, the age should be determined. Vaginal contents are removed by pipette and examined for chemicals. Expelled material (placental and foetal) is very useful in fixing absolute identification of accused person by DNA profiling.

Evidence at the Scene: The doctor should make a note of: (1) Condition of the bed-linen (blood-stained, soiled, etc.). The arrangement of clothing should be noted, especially the underclothing. The soaked clothes may smell of carbolic soap or dettol. (2) Any signs of recent interference of pregnancy. (3) Any evidence of discarded linen, dressings, cotton-wool, swabs, bowls, etc. (4) Presence of any known abortifacient drug. The presence of a second person is indicated by the absence of instruments at the scene, if subsequent autopsy reveals that death was due to an instrumental abortion.

(1) Abortion by the Drugs: The gastrointestinal tract must be examined for evidence of irritant poisoning. If such evidence is found, the whole tract and its contents together with other organs of the body should be preserved for analysis. The urinary tract should be examined for signs of inflammation, such as might be produced by cantharides or turpentine. The vagina and cervix should be examined for erosions and inflammation due to local application of irritant and caustic substances, such as phenol, lysol, mercuric chloride, potassium permanganate, arsenic, formaldehyde and oxalic acid. A necrotic pseudomembrane may form in the vagina and severe damage to cervix may occur. They should be preserved for analysis.

(2) Instrumental Abortion: Signs of injury to the abdomen or body may or may not be present. **The abdomen is opened, and before removing any parts from the cavity, the peritoneum, pelvic organs and floor are examined for punctures, ruptures, haemorrhage or inflammation. If embolism is suspected, the presence of air in the large veins and in the heart should be looked for, before the organs are removed.** The great veins of the abdomen should be inspected for air bubbles and then pelvic veins. Appreciable delay allows absorption of air. Air bubbles in cerebral veins are artefacts caused by removing calvarium. The uterus may be crepitant and bubbles may be seen under the serosal surface or even under the parietal peritoneum of the pelvis. On opening uterus, gas bubbles may be seen in the wall of the placental bed.

Pelvic dissection: To obtain bloodless field, all internal organs except pelvic organs are removed and pelvis elevated by placing a block under the sacrum. Make an incision just outside the labia majora and extend it backwards to include the anus, and forwards up to the symphysis pubis Fig. (17–2). Pubic rami on both sides are cut with a saw, and the central wedge is removed. The peritoneum is cut along the brim of the pelvis and all pelvic viscera, including uterus, vagina, anus, rectum and bladder are removed. The organs are examined externally and then opened, adopting the incisions so as to avoid an injured part. The uterus and pelvic organs are pale, if death occurs due to hemorrhage, but may be congested if death occurs during menstruation. The uterus is opened first by a classical caesarean incision. This will facilitate the collection of any fluid retained in the lower uterine segment. Then the uterus is opened in its long axis and the colour, size and texture noted. If the chorionic sac is still present, its integrity and the attachment to deciduae are noted. Products of conception are sought and the state of the placental bed noted. **If evacuation was done by curetting, endometrium may show evidence of scooping.** The presence of chorionic villi will indicate abortion. Next, the cervical canal is opened and examined for injuries. The vaginal canal, and especially the posterior fornix should be examined for signs of lacerations, bruising, perforations and inflammation and foreign material. Note state of dilatation of cervical canal. **Wounds of the cervix occur in about 50% of the cases,** which may be groove-like, parallel notches of the cervical canal, tenaculum marks on the external orifices, cavitation of the wall, fissures, lacerations and perforations. **The perforations of the vagina and uterus are of different sizes and**

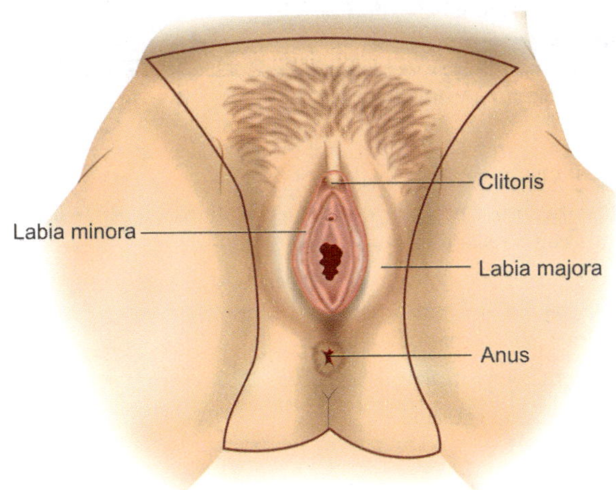

Fig. (17–2). Incision for removal of the female external genitalia.

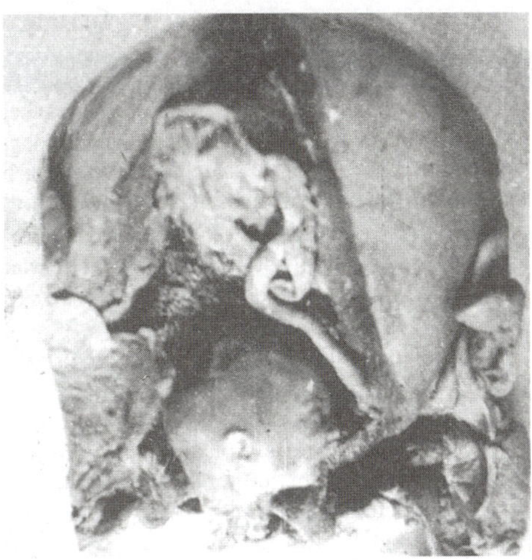

Fig. (17–3). Criminal abortion (five months pregnancy). The severed foetal head is retained in the uterus.

forms varying from a small ragged, stellate opening about one cm. in diameter to much larger tears of stellate, oval or irregular shape. Sometimes, one or more perforations may be present in the fundus. Open the urethra into the bladder, and then open the anus and rectum. **Ragged, stellate or irregular tears of small or large intestine, mesentery, omentum and bladder may occur. Caecum, sigmoid and rectum are usually involved.** Segments of the intestine, omentum or mesentery may enter the uterine cavity. The nature of injury may indicate whether the instrument is penetrating and sharp-pointed or blunt-poined, but the exact nature cannot be made out. Sometimes, foreign bodies may be found in the genital tract which should be preserved. If abortion stick has been used excoriation, bruising or perforation of upper part of vagina or uterus can occur. Gross injury when present indicates lack of skill or knowledge of the parts Fig. (17–3).

Infection: In skilled hand, instrumentation may leave little or no evidence of any kind, but **infection if present is suspicious of interference, unless the foetus is macerated or products are retained. Septic endometritis, infection of uterine walls, broad ligments, pelvic connective tissues may be seen, even without apparent damage. In uterine infection, uterus becomes swollen, spongy and discoloured.** The serosal surface may be brownish and endometrium may be ragged, foul-smelling and even purulent. Signs of septicaemia may develop with an enlarged, soft spleen, prominent lymph nodes and hepato-renal failure. In extreme cases, the kidneys may show bilateral cortical necrosis. Cl. welchii may cause fulminating septicemia within 18 to 24 hours. In clostridial septicaemia skin may be bronze coloured, having a mottled or raindrop appearance. **In natural abortion, infection is rare.** In self-practised interference the damage is great, but when done by another person the damage is slight. Rarely, self-instrumentation may not cause any damage. Material and fluid from the vagina, uterine cavity, and blood from both ventricles should be collected for chemical and bacteriological examination. Tissue from the uterus, ovaries and other organs must be taken for histological examination. This is especially important in cases where there is no evidence of foetal parts or placental remains. Bacteriological examination should also be done on possible instruments of abortion. Fluid from the cut surface of the lung and pulmonary blood should be collected for fatty acid estimation and for phenolic derivatives depending on the agent used. A full photographic record should be maintained Table (17–1).

(3) Abortion by Syringing: There may be fluid in the vagina and soiling of clothes. **The mucous plug in the cervix is usually displaced or disintegrated.** Corrosion or tissue damage may be seen due to the use of antiseptics. The cervical canal may be dilated and injured. **Foamy-red or dark-red fluid may be seen between the uterine wall and foetal membranes with partial detachment of the placenta.** The injected fluid enters the uterine sinusoids under pressure and the fluid and bubbles of gas can be detected in the venous system extending from the sides of the uterus up to right heart. **The right side of the heart, the superior and inferior vena cavae, and pulmonary conus contain foamy blood and are "ballooned out" and have a characteristic elastic feel. When fatal venous air embolism has occurred, the inferior vena cava, uterine, ovarian and pelvic veins present a beaded appearance due to the air within their lumens.** The large abdominal veins should be examined for the presence of air by gently moving aside the bowel before the thoracic cavity is opened and the internal mammary vessels are incised. Segmentation of the coronary vessels is seen due to gas bubbles. **In air embolism, collapse occurs in about two minutes and death in ten minutes.** Delayed death may occur when the victim is at rest and the air is temporarily locked in the uterus. When the woman moves about, utero-placental detachment increases and air enters uterine sinusoids. Perforation may occasionally result. In self-induced cases, the woman may be found dead in a posture consistent with recent use of a syringe. Usually the apparatus is by her side, but she may have had time to dispose it off.

FABRICATED ABORTION: Rarely, when a woman is assaulted, she may try to exaggerate the offence by alleging that it caused her to abort. She may acquire a human foetus, or an animal foetus to support the charge.

CASE: A woman claimed that she had been assaulted while pregnant, and as the result of violence had aborted. The products of the alleged abortion were sent, which on examination was found to be 'foetus' of a dog. The forelegs and tail had been clipped off and the remains bottled.

Table (17–1). Difference between natural and criminal abortion

Trait	Natural abortion	Criminal abortion
(1) Cause:	Predisposing diseases	Pregnancy in unmarried woman or widow.
(2) Infection:	Rare.	Frequent.
(3) Marks of violence:	Not present on the abdomen.	May be present on abdomen.
(4) Genital organs:	Injuries are not present	Injuries, such as contusions, lacerations, perforations, etc., may be seen in uterus or its contents and vagina.
(5) Toxic effect of drugs:	Absent.	Erosions and inflammation of vagina and cervix due to local application of irritant and caustic substances may be present. The GI or urinary tract may show signs of irritation.
(6) Foreign bodies:	Not present in genital tract.	May be present in genital tract.
(7) Foetus:	Wounds absent.	Rarely wounds may be present.

Doctor's Duties in a Case of Criminal Abortion: (1) The doctor should keep all the information obtained by him as a professional secret. (2) He must ask the patient to make a statement about the induction of criminal abortion. If she refuses to make a statement, he should not pursue the matter. (3) He must consult a professional colleague. (4) He must treat her to the best of his ability. (5) If the woman's condition is serious, he must arrange to record the dying declaration. (6) If the woman dies, he should not issue a death certificate, but he should inform the police.

MEDICOLEGAL IMPORTANCE OF PLA-CENTA: (1) It gives an idea of the length of gestation. (2) In criminal abortion, often pieces are retained in the uterus. (3) The transfer of poisons, bacteria, antibodies, etc. across the placenta may result in death, disease or abnormalities of the foetus.

TRAUMA AND ABORTION: Trauma may rarely cause an abortion in the absence of serious or life-threatening injury to the mother. Often it is difficult to establish a causal relationship between trauma and abortion. An abortion occurring within a few days of the trauma may be in progress at the time of injury. Trauma producing embryonic injury may not cause abortion for several weeks or even months. Most of such complications occur without any trauma. Travel in the absence of trauma does not increase the incidence of abortion. Because of the above inconsistencies, it is often difficult to answer whether trauma, such as traffic accident, a fall, an assault, etc. can cause abortion. Without any known cause abortion may occur, the foetus may die, or the placenta separate. Rupture of membranes or premature separation of placenta may occur in some cases, directly due to trauma.

The following criteria suggest a causal relationship between trauma and abortion. (1) The traumatic event was followed within twenty-four hours by a process that ultimately led to abortion. (2) The foetus and placenta should be normal. (3) The appearance of the foetus and placenta should be compatible with the period of pregnancy at which the traumatic event occurred. (4) Factors known to cause abortion should be absent, such as: (a) abnormalities of the uterus including congenital defect of uterine development, leiomyomas, endometrial polyps and incompetent cervical os; (b) a history of repeated abortion without any cause; (c) chronic infections in the mother, e.g., syphilis, or toxoplasmosis involving the uterus; (d) history of exposure to abortifacients, e.g., X-ray, lead, folic acid antagonists; (e) a physical attempt to induce abortion. (5) Adherent clot or a depression of the placental surface.

FOETAL INJURIES: Trauma may cause foetal injury or death. The age of the injury should correspond with the time passed after trauma. Soft tissue injuries heal in the uterus. In the case of fractures, the process can be dated by X-ray. A relationship may be established, if the age of fracture coincides with the traumatic event. Fractures of the skull and long bones can occur during delivery. To differentiate birth trauma from accidental trauma, X-rays are very helpful.

MEDICOLEGAL QUESTIONS: The doctor should be able to answer the following questions after autopsy. (1) Was the deceased pregnant recently? (2) Was there any evidence of abortion? (3) Was there any evidence of criminal interference by instruments or the use of drugs? (4) Was the cause of death related to abortion?

INSTRUMENTAL ABORTION: The following questions arise in the case of instrumental abortion.

(1) HAS ANY INSTRUMENT BEEN USED, AND IF SO, WHEN? The presence of any injuries in the vagina, cervix, uterus or its contents and dilation of the cervix or injection of fluid will indicate the use of an instrument. If the abortionist is skilled, the injuries are likely to be minimal. The age of the injuries should be determined by microscopic examination. Gross injuries indicate lack of skill or knowledge of the parts. Recent dilation of the cervix may be difficult to differentiate from cervical relaxation during passage of the foetus. The injected fluid may be washed out by the floodings of an abortion. In such case, the contents of the fluid, e.g., soap, phenol, potassium permanganate, etc., can be detected in the blood obtained from the inferior vena cava and the pulmonary arteries. In the absence of injuries, the development of infection should arouse suspicion of interference, unless the foetus is macerated or products are retained.

EVIDENCE ON THE TIME OF INTERFERENCE: The timing of the passing of an instrument can be better judged from the course of complications rather than of abortion itself. Vagal inhibition will produce instantaneous death. Death from air embolism occurs within seconds or a minute but delayed collapse and death may occur, probably due to delay in separation of the placenta. In such cases, an abortion may have been carried out in the house of the abortionist, but the patient may reach her own home before she collapses and dies. In haemorrhage, death occurs after some hours, depending on the amount of bleeding. Clostridial infection may develop within 24 hours and due to other bacteria in a day or two. Mixed infections associated with phlebitis or pyaemia may last for weeks. If placental remains are responsible, death may occur after several days, and if due to sepsis after weeks or months. When abortifacient drugs have been used, the timing of administration can be estimated from the development of toxic signs or symptoms. Due to the unreliability of the witnesses, in most cases it is not possible to estimate the interval between instrumentation and death.

(2) WHAT KIND OF INSTRUMENT WAS USED? The nature of the injuries may indicate whether the instrument is penetrating or non-penetrating and sharp-pointed, blunt-pointed, hard-nosed, or soft-nosed, but the exact nature cannot be made out. Injecting instruments usually do not produce injuries. Marks produced by surgical forceps, tenaculum, etc., during treatment may cause confusion. The doctor who attended on the patient should be shown the specimen to exclude any marks made by him.

(3) HOW MAY ANY INJURIES PRESENT BE INTERPRETED? The doctor should determine the type of instrumental interference, i.e., dilating, perforating, injecting, etc., from the available facts. Necrosis and infection may supervene in areas of bruising and internal laceration of the cervix or uterus, which may cause difficulty in interpretation.

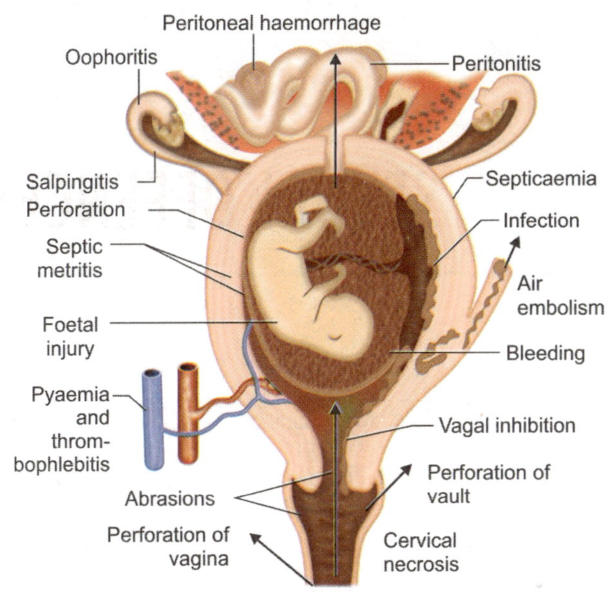

Fig. (17–4). Complications of criminal abortion.

(4) WAS INSTRUMENTATION SELF-INDUCED OR ASSISTED?

Gross damage indicates self-instrumentation and minor injuries or absence of injuries indicate skilled assistance.

(5) HOW DID DEATH OCCUR?

The causes of death could be Fig. (17–4):

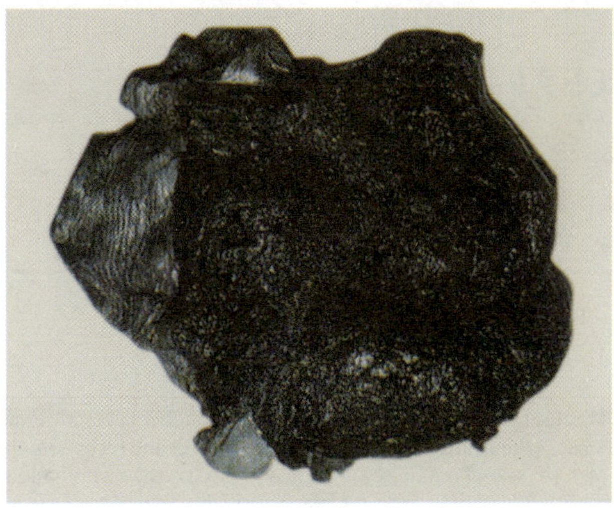

Fig. (17–5). Gas gangrene in uterus following criminal abortion.

(A) **Immediate Deaths**:(1) Vagal inhibition. (2) Air embolism. (3) Haemorrhage. (4) Fat embolism. (5) Amniotic fluid embolism. (6) Rarely poisoning.

(B) **Delayed Deaths** (onset within 48 to 72 hours): (1) Septicaemia. (2) Pyaemia. (3) Confined local infection and toxaemia. (4) General peritonitis. (5) Tetanus. (6) Gas gangrene **Fig. (17–5).**

(C) **Remote Deaths:** (1) Jaundice and renal failure. (2) Bacterial endocarditis. (3) Pulmonary embolism.

CHAPTER

18 SEXUAL OFFENCES

FM 3.13: Describe different types of sexual offences. Describe various sections of IPC regarding rape including definition of rape (Section 375 IPC), Punishment for Rape (Section 376 IPC) and recent amendments notified till date.
FM 3.14: Sexual offences: Describe and discuss the examination of the victim of an alleged case of rape, and the preparation of report, framing the opinion and preservation and dispatch of trace evidences in such cases.
FM 3.15: Sexual offences: Describe and discuss examination of accused and victim of sodomy, preparation of report, framing of opinion, preservation and dispatch of trace evidences in such cases.
FM 3.16: Sexual offences: Describe and discuss adultery and unnatural sexual offences—sodomy, incest, lesbianism, buccal coitus, bestiality, indecent assault and preparation of report, framing the opinion and preservation and dispatch of trace evidences in such cases.
FM 3.17: Describe and discuss the sexual perversions fetishism, transvestism, voyeurism, sadism, necrophagia, masochism, exhibitionism, frotteurism, necrophilia.

Classification: (I) Natural offences: (1) Rape. (2) Incest. (3) Adultery. **(II) Unnatural offences:** (1) Sodomy. (2) Tribadism. (3) Bestiality. (4) Buccal coitus. **(III) Sexual paraphilias:** (1) Sadism. (2) Masochism. (3) Necrophilia.(4) Fetichism. (5) Transvestism. (6) Exhibitionism. (7) Masturbation. (8) Frotteurism. (9) Undinism, etc. **(IV) Sex-linked offences:** (1) Stalking. (2) Voyeurism. (3) Sexual harassment. (4) Trafficking. (5) Indecent assault.

RAPE

S. 375, I.P.C.: A man is said to commit "rape" if he—(a) **penetrates his penis, to any extent, into the vagina, mouth, urethra or anus of a woman or makes her to do so with him or any other person**; or (b) **inserts, to any extent, any object or a part of the body, not being the penis, into the vagina, the urethra or anus of a woman** or makes her to do so with him or any other person; or (c) **manipulates any part of the body of a woman so as to cause penetration into the vagina, urethra, anus or any part of body** of such woman or makes her to do so with him or any other person; or (d) **applies his mouth to the vagina, anus, urethra of a woman or makes her to do so** with him or any other person, under the circumstances falling under any of the following seven descriptions: (1) Against her will. (2) Without her consent. (3) With her consent, when her consent has been obtained by putting her or any person in whom she is interested, in fear of death or of hurt. (4) With her consent, when the man knows that he is not her husband and that her consent is given because she believes that he is another man to whom she is or believes herself to be lawfully married. (5) With her consent when, at the time of giving such consent, by reason of unsoundness of mind or intoxication or the administration by him personally or through another of any stupefying or unwholesome substance, she is unable to understand the nature and consequences of that to which she gives consent.(6) With or without her consent, when she is under eighteen years of age. (7) When she is unable to communicate consent.

Explanation: (1) For the purposes of this section, **"vagina" shall also include labia majora**. (2) Consent means an unequivocal voluntary agreement when the woman by words, gestures or any form of verbal or non-verbal communication, communicates willingness to participate in the specific sexual act: Provided that a woman who does not physically resist to the act of penetration shall not by the reason only of that fact, be regarded as consenting to the sexual activity.

Exception: (1) **A medical procedure or intervention shall not constitute rape**. (2) Sexual intercourse or sexual acts by a man with his own wife, the wife not being under fifteen years of age, is not rape.

S. 376 I.P.C: (1) Whoever, except in the cases provided for in sub-section (2), commits rape, shall be punished with **rigorous imprisonment of either description for a term, which shall not be less than ten years, but which may extend to imprisonment for life,** and shall also be liable to fine.

(2) Whoever (a) being a police officer, commits rape (i) within the limits of the police station to which such police officer is appointed; or (ii) in the premises of any station house; or (iii) on a woman in such police officer's custody or in the custody of a police officer subordinate to such police officer; or (b) being a public servant, commits rape on a woman in such public servant's custody or in the custody of a public servant subordinate to such public servant; or (c) being a member of the armed forces deployed in an area by the Central or a State Government commits rape in such area; or (d) being on the management or on the staff of a jail, remand home or other place of custody or of a women's or children's institution, commits rape on any inmate of such jail, remand home, place or institution; or (e) being on the management or on the staff of a hospital, commits rape on a woman in that hospital; or (f) being a relative, guardian or teacher of , or a person in a position of trust or authority towards the woman, commits rape on such woman; or (g) commits rape during communal or sectarian violence; or (h) commits

rape on a woman knowing her to be pregnant; or (i) commits rape, on a woman incapable of giving consent; or (j) being in a position of control or dominance over a woman, commits rape on such woman; or (k) commits rape on a woman suffering from mental or physical disability; or (l) while committing rape causes grievous bodily harm or maims or disfigures or endangers the life of a woman; or (m) commits rape repeatedly on the same woman, shall be punished with rigorous imprisonment for a term which shall not be less than ten years, but which may extend to imprisonment for life, which shall mean imprisonment for the remainder of that person's natural life, and shall also be liable to fine.

Whoever commits rape on a woman under 16 years, shall be punished with rigorous imprisonment for not less than 20 years, which may extend for life, meaning for that person's for that person's remainder of natural life and also fine.

S 376A, I.P.C: Whoever, commits an offence punishable under sub-section (1) or sub-section (2) of section 376 and in the course of such commission inflicts an injury which causes the death of the woman or causes the woman to be in a persistent vegetative state, shall be punished with rigorous imprisonment for a term which shall not be less than twenty years, but which may extend to imprisonment for life, which shall mean imprisonment for the remainder of that person's natural life, or with death.

S 376AB, I.P.C: Whoever commits rape on a woman under 12 years, shall be punished with rigorous imprisonment of not less than 20 years, but may extend for life, meaning for that person's remainder of natural life and with fine or with death.

S 376B, I.P.C: Whoever has sexual intercourse with his own wife, who is living separately, whether under a decree of separation or otherwise, without her consent, shall be punished with imprisonment of either description for a term which shall not be less than two years but which may extend to seven years, and shall also be liable to fine.

S 376C, I.P.C: Whoever, being: (a) in a position of authority or in a fiduciary relationship; or (b) a public servant: or (c) superintendent or manager of a jail, remand home or other place of custody or a women's or children's institution; or (d) on the management of a hospital or being on the staff of a hospital, abuses such position or fiduciary relationship to induce or seduce any woman either in his custody or under his charge or present in the premises to have sexual intercourse with him, such sexual intercourse not amounting to the offence of rape, shall be punished with rigorous imprisonment of either description for a term which shell not be less than five years, but which may extend to ten years, and shall also be liable to fine.

S 376D, I.P.C: Where a woman is raped by one or more persons constituting a group or acting in furtherance of a common intention, each of those persons shall be deemed to have committed the offence of rape and shall be punished with rigorous imprisonment which may extend to life which shall mean imprisonment for the remainder of that person's natural life, and with fine.

S. 376DA: Where a woman under 16 years is raped by one or more people constituting a group, each of those people shall be deemed to have committed offence of rape (imprisonment for life, which shall mean for the remainder of that person's natural life and fine).

S. 376DB: Where a woman under 12 years is raped by one or more people constituting a group, each of those people shall be deemed to have committed offence of rape (imprisonment for life, which shall mean for the remainder of that person's natural life and fine or with death).

S 376E, I.P.C: Whoever has been previously convicted of an offence punishable under section 376 or section 376A or section 376D, 376DA and 376DB and is subsequently convicted of an offence punishable under any of the said sections shall be punished with imprisonment for life which shall mean imprisonment for the remainder of that person's natural life, or with death.

COMMENT: "Will" and "consent" are different. Will is a psychological desire, consent is a legal concept. Every act done against the will of a person is done without her consent, but an act done without the consent of a person is not necessarily against her will. Sexual intercourse with an unconscious woman is both against her will and without her consent. A girl under 12 years is incapable of giving consent to sexual act under Sec 90, I.P.C, and as such, even if the sexual intercourse cannot be said to be "against the will" of the girl, the accused will be guilty of rape. The woman must have voluntarily participated in the sexual act, after the exercise of intelligence and also her choice between resistance and assent, for the consent to be valid. Submission is not necessarily consent, though a consent necessarily involves submission. Whether the alleged consent by the victim was mere passive submission or willing consent depends on the circumstances of each case. The material facts to be considered are the conduct and behaviour of the victim. It is not rape where a woman initially objects, but subsequently gives her consent to sexual act. A woman may be willing for sexual intercourse, but may not give consent for fear of detection or social stigma.

S. 100, I.P.C: " *Seventhly*–An act of throwing or administering acid or an attempt to throw or adminster acid which may reasonably cause the apprehension that grievous hurt will otherwise be the consequence of such act". In this the right of private defence of the body extend to causing death.

S. 166B, I.P.C: Punishment for a doctor for refusal to provide medicolegal examination and treatment of sexual assault victim (imprisonment up to 1 year or fine or both).

S. 176(1A), Cr.P.C: If any person dies, or disappears, or rape is alleged to have been committed on any woman during the custody of the police, or any other custody authorized by the court, in addition to police inquest, an inquest shall be held by Judicial magistrate and body is sent for autopsy.

S.228–A, I.P.C.: Whoever prints or publishes the name or any matter which may make known the identity of victim of rape (offences under S. 376 and 376A to E) shall be punished with imprisonment extending to two years.

S. 294, I.P.C.: Whoever to the annoyance of others (a) does any obscene act in any public place or (b) sings, recites or utters any obscene song, ballard or words, in or near any public place shall be punished with imprisonment up to 3 months, or with fine or with both.

S.326–A, I.P.C.: Voluntarily causing grievous hurt by use of acid, etc. Imprisonment of not less than 10 years may extend to life and fine of 10 lakh rupees.

S.326–B, I.P.C.: Voluntarily throwing or attempting throw acid (imprisonment of not less than 5 years, may extend to 7 years and fine).

S.354, I.P.C.: Assault or use of criminal force to woman with intent to outrage her modesty (imprisonment not less than one year may extend to 5 years and fine).

S. 354–A, I.P.C: SEXUAL HARASSMENT: (1) Physical contact and advances involving sexual overtures, (2) a demand or request for sexual flavours, (3) making sexually colored remarks, (4) showing pornography and (5) imprisonment of 1 to 3 years or with fine or both.

S. 354–B, I.P.C: Assault or use of criminal force to woman or compelling her to be naked with intent to disrobe (imprisonment of not less than 3 years, may extend to 7 years and fine).

S. 354–C, I.P.C: VOYEURISM: Imprisonment of not less than 1 year; may extend to 3 years and fine; for second and subsequent offences imprisonment of 3 to 7 years.

S. 354D, I.P.C: STALKING: Whoever follows a woman and contacts or attempts to contact such woman to foster personal interaction repeatedly, despite a clear indication of disinterest by such woman, or monitors the use by a woman of the internet, e-mail or any other form of electronic communication, (imprisonment up to 3 to 5 years and fine).

S.370, I.P.C.: TRAFFICKING OF PERSON: Whoever for the purpose of exploitation (a) recruits, (b) transports, (c) harbours, (d) transfers, (e) receives a person, by (1) using threats, (2) using force or coercion, (3) by abduction, (4) by fraud or deception, (5) by abuse of power, (6) by inducement, including giving payments or benefits commits the offence of trafficking (imprisonment for 7 to remainder of that Person's natural life).

Explanation: Exploitation includes prostitution or other forms of sexual exploitation, slavery or forced removal of organs. (consent of the victim is immaterial).

S. 370A, I.P.C: Whoever knowingly that a minor has been trafficked, engages such minor for sexual exploitation will be punished with imprisonment for not less than five years, but may extend to 7 years and fine.

S.493, I.P.C.: Cohabitation caused by a man deceitfully inducing a belief of lawful marriage is punishable with imprisonment up to 10 years.

S. 498, I.P.C.: Enticing or taking away or detaining with criminal intention a married woman is punishable with imprisonment up to 2 years or fine or both.

S. 509, I.P.C.: Whoever intending to insult the modesty of any woman, utters any word, makes any sound or gesture, or exhibits any object, intending that such word or sound shall be heard, or that such gesture or object shall be seen by such woman, or intrudes upon the privacy of such woman, shall be punished with simple imprisonment up to 3 years and also fine.

S. 53-A, Cr.P.C: (1) When a person is arrested on a charge of committing an offence of rape or an attempt to commit rape, and there are reasonable grounds to believe that an examination will afford evidence as to the commission of the offence, it shall be lawful for a registered medical practitioner employed in a hospital run by the government or by a local authority and in the absence of such a practitioner within the radius of 16 km from the place where the offence has been committed, by any other R.M.P. acting at the request of a police officer not below the rank of a sub-inspector to examine the arrested person with use of reasonable force as required. (2) The doctor has to examine the person without any delay and prepare a report giving following particulars, namely the name, age and address of the accused, brought by whom, injury over the body if any with complete description of all the materials taken from the body of accused for further investigations. (3) The report should precisely state all the reasons for each conclusion arrived at. (4) The exact time of commencement and completion of the examination. (5) The report should be forwarded without delay to the investigating officer who shall forward it to the magistrate.

S. 164, A, Cr.P.C: (1) When during investigation, medical examination of victim of rape/attempted rape is to be done, such examination shall be conducted by a RMP employed in a government hospital or a local authority and in the absence of such a practitioner, by any other RMP, with the consent of such woman or of a person competent to give such consent on her behalf and such woman should be sent to a RMP within 24 hours from the time of receiving the information relating to the commission of such offence. (2) The RMP should examine her, without any delay and prepare a report giving the following particulars, namely the name, age and address of the woman, brought by whom, injuries over the body, general mental condition and detailed description of all materials taken for investigation. (3) The report should precisely state all the reasons for each conclusion arrived at. (4) The report shall specifically record that the consent of the woman or of competent person on her behalf to such examination had been obtained. (5) The exact time of commencement and completion of the examination shall be noted. (6) The report should be forwarded, without delay to the investigating officer, who shall forward it to the magistrate. (7) Nothing in this section shall be lawful if examination is done without consent of the woman.

157, Cr.P.C: The statement of victim of rape and indecent assault should be recorded by a woman police officer at the victim's residence or at the place of her choice in the presence of her parents or guardians.

S. 161, Cr.P.C: The statement of a woman against whom an offence under S. 376A to E and S. 509 I.P.C is alleged to have been committed shall be recorded by a woman police officer or any woman officer.

164(5A), Cr.P.C: Statement of victim should be taken by judicial magistrate and recorded by audio-video electronic means in presence of advocate of accused.

S-176, 1 (A), Cr.P.C: (a) Any person dies or disappears, or (b) rape is alleged to have been committed on any woman, while such person or woman is in the custody of the police or in any other custody authorised by the magistrate or the court, under this code in addition to the inquiry or investigation held by the police, an inquiry shall be held by the judicial magistrate or the metropolitan magistrate.

273, Cr.P.C: Victim of rape or other sexual offences if below 18 years should not be confronted with the accused.

The judicial magistrate or metropolitan magistrate or executive magistrate or police officer holding an inquiry or investigation under subsection 1-A, shall within 24 hours of the death of a person, forward the body to the nearest civil surgeon or other qualified medical person appointed by the government for examination, unless it is not possible to do so for reasons to be recorded in writing.

S. 327(2), Cr.P.C: **The inquiry into and trial of sexual assault or an offence under S. 376 and 376 A to E of I.P.C., shall be conducted *in camera* (in secret) and forbids the disclosure of the identity of the victim. It means the judge and staff along with both parties and their lawyers will be inside the court room.** However, if the judge thinks fit on an application made by either of the parties, may allow a particular person to have access to, or remain in the room used by the court.

S. 327(3), Cr.P.C: The trail of rape case should be conducted in camera by a woman judge. Produce to trail or rape should not be published without previous permission by court.

357C, Cr.P.C: All hospitals, public or private, whether run by the Central Government, the State Government, local bodies or any other person, shall immediately, provide the first-aid or medical treatment, free of cost, to the victims of any offence covered under (voluntarily causing grievous hurt by use of acid, etc.) section 326A, 376, 376A, 376B, 376C, 376D or section 376E (Rape) of the Indian Penal Code, and shall immediately inform the police of such incident.

S. 375B, Cr.P.C: Additional compensation to be given by state over and above fine paid by convicted persons in cases of gang rape and vitriolage.

53–A, I.E.A.: In a prosecution for an offence under S.354 & S.354, A to C, subsection 1 or 2 of S.367 and 367 A to E of I.P.C. or for attempt to commit any such offence, where the question of consent is in issue, evidence of the character of the victim or of such person's previous sexual experience with any person shall not be relevant on the issue of such consent or the quality of consent.

S.54, I.E.A.: In criminal proceedings, the fact that the accused person has a bad character is irrelevant, unless evidence has been given that he has a good character, in which case it becomes relevant. **Exception:** This section does not apply to cases in which the bad character of any person is itself a fact in issue.

S. 114A, I.E.A: In a prosecution for rape under clause 'a' to 'm' or clause 'n' of subsection (2) of S. 376 I.P.C, where sexual intercourse by the accused is proved and the question is whether it was without the consent of the woman alleged to have been raped and such woman states in her evidence before the court that she did not consent, the court shall presume that person did not consent.

Explanation: In this section sexual intercourse shall mean any of the acts mentioned in clauses a to c of section 375, I.P.C.

S.26, 154, 157, 164, 176, 198, 273, 309, 327, 357, Cr.P.C and S. 54, 114, 146, 155 I.E.A deal with the trial of rape cases.

Statutory Rape: It is sexual intercourse with a girl below 18 years of age even with her consent. It is neither violent nor physically coerced.

Gang rape or group rape occurs, when a group of people participate in the rape of a single victim. Each of the persons shall be deemed to have committed gang rape.

Date Rape: It is sexual intercourse with a woman, who is given a drink containing a sedative **drug like GHB (gamma hydroxybutyrate), rohypnol (flunitrazepam), ketamine, etc.** in a party without her knowledge. These drugs are called rape/club drugs.

Marital Rape: It is forceful sexual intercourse with wife who is living separately from him under a decree of separation, or any custom or usage without her consent.

Consent: A woman of eighteen years and above can give valid consent for sexual intercourse. The consent must be free and voluntary, and given while she is of sound mind and not intoxicated. The consent should be obtained prior to the act. Even a prostitute cannot be forced to have intercourse against her will.

Consent is not valid: (1) When it is obtained by fraud, as by impersonation of the husband or by misrepresentation of facts. (2) When it is obtained by putting her or any person in whom she is interested, in fear of death or hurt. (3) When obtained from a woman who is of unsound mind, or is in a state of drunkenness. (4) When the woman is below 18 years of age.

Presumption and Proof of Consent: Consent or its absence can be presumed from the accompanying circumstances of each case. **The chief evidence of lack of consent is sign of resistance, which is naturally expected from a woman unwilling to a sexual intercourse forced upon her. Such a resistance may cause the tearing of clothes, and injuries on the body, and even on her private parts.** It is necessary to prove that maximum resistance was offered by the woman, and that all means had been tried to prevent sexual intercourse, e.g., shouting, crying, beating, biting, etc. **The woman may surrender from fear or exhaustion, which case it is regarded as rape.** Women who faint due to fear, or are made helpless due to their clothes being thrown on their face, or who have been drugged or unconscious from any cause, and children may not be able to resist. **The resistance offered depends upon the type of woman, her age, development and on the social status.** In most cases of rape physical injury involves hitting or slapping the victim, pressing the neck, knocking her to the ground, and/or forcibly tearing her clothes. Even though the rapist may not employ physical methods or a visible weapon in his track, the victim is convinced she is in mortal danger and reacts by doing whatever appears most likely to preserve her life. Often this involves non-violent submission to her assailant.

What Constitutes Rape? The slightest penetration of the penis within the vulva, such as the minimal passage of glans (tip) between the labia with or without emission of semen or rupture of hymen constitutes rape. Completed act of intercourse is not necessary. It is an essential part of proof in a rape, that there should have been not only an assault but actual penetration. **Rape can be committed even when there is inability to produce a penile erection.** Rape can occur without causing any injury, and as such **negative evidence does not exclude rape. The doctor should mention only the negative facts, but should not give his opinion that rape has not been committed.** Corroboration by eye witnesses or circumstantial evidence is necessary in such cases.

Exception: A husband cannot be guilty of rape on his wife, if she is above fifteen years, because in marriage the wife consents to the husband's exercising the marital right of intercourse during the continuation of legal marriage.

Burden of Proof: The prosecution has to prove all elements of the offence. In many cases of rape, there are no signs of injury or intoxication by stupefying drugs, and the entire allegation of lack of consent is based on fear and on fraud. According to S. 114-A I.E.A., if the victim states in her evidence before the Court that she did not consent, the Court shall presume that she did not consent in a custodial situation or when she is a victim of gang rape. **The burden of proof of the consent rests on the accused.** Under the law, **rape can only be committed by a man, and a woman cannot rape a man, although she may be guilty of an indecent assault upon him.**

Age of the Accused: The Court decides the question of his potency from the evidence in the case. Even old men commit rape on young girls.

TYPES OF SEXUAL OFFENCES: (1) Normal well adjusted men who behave abnormally when under the influence of alcohol. This is probably the commonest type of rapist. (2) Sexually deviated but psychologically non-deviated offenders. (3) Sexually and psychologically deviated offenders. Compulsive and emotionally disturbed. (4) Sexually non-deviated but psychotic, defective, or suffering from brain damage, etc.

Age of the Victim: No age is safe from rape, as children of one year or less, and old women of 85 years have been raped. **Children are more frequently raped than adults** as they cannot offer much resistance, and also due to false belief that venereal diseases are cured by sexual intercourse with a virgin.

EXAMINATION OF THE VICTIM

Objects: The objects of medical examination are: (1) To search for physical signs (injuries) that will corroborate the history given by the victim. (2) To search for, collect and preserve all physical (trace) evidence for laboratory examination. (3) To treat the victim for any injuries and against venereal disease or pregnancy, and prevention or lessening of permanent psychological damage.

The scene of alleged offence may be examined if it appears desirable. The police should advise the victim not to change clothes, bathe, or douche prior to the medical examination.

The victim of rape may go directly to the doctor, who should examine her after obtaining her consent, and after examination he should inform the concerned police station, so that the due legal process can be set in motion.

To bring a charge or rape against a boy, his age should be more than seven years.

The union health ministry has asked all hospitals to **set up a designated room for forensic and medical examination of victims of rape.**

General Procedure: The following is an outline of a planned procedure. (1) **The victim should be examined when there is requisition from investigating police officer or the Magistrate. The Court or the police has no power of forcing a woman for medical examination against her will.** (2) The written, witnessed consent of the woman for examination, collection of specimens, taking of photographs, treatment, and for the release of information to the police, and if she is under twelve years, or of unsound mind, the consent of her parents must be taken in writing.

(3) The victim should be identified by the escorting police constable, whose name and number should be recorded. Identification marks should also be noted. (4) The name of the victim and her parent, marital status, residence, occupation, time, date, year, place of examination and by whom requisition is given should be noted. Date and time is important because the interval between the alleged incident and the examination

is material. (5) The victim is examined in the presence of a third person, preferably a female nurse or a female relative of the woman, whose name should be recorded. This is necessary to avoid himself being accused. (6) The examination should be carried out without delay. Minor degrees of injury may fade rapidly, and swelling and tenderness of vulva may disappear in few hours. Detection of spermatozoa from the genital tract also diminishes with time delay. (7) Statements of the victim and of others with her are recorded separately of: (a) preliminary affairs; whether she knows the accused? whether she was given food or drink prior to the act which affected her consciousness? Whether she was put under any threat? (b) date, time and place of alleged offence, (c) location: inside or outside, wet or dry weather, (d) number of alleged assailants, (e) alcohol or drugs involved with details, (f) restraints, or weapons and their use, (g) details or struggle or resistance: injuries sustained by victim (when, how and where on the body), (h) injuries sustained by the assailant, due to scratching, bites, etc., (i) exact relative positions of the parties, (j) type and number of sexual acts, (k) use of condoms or lubricants, (l) use and disposal of sanitary pads or tampons, (m) was any pain experienced either at the time of the incident or subsequently, (n) did ejaculation take place during the act, either within the vagina or outside, (o) the appearance of any discharge, (p) was there bleeding from the vagina, (q) calls for help, and (r) recent consenting intercourse if the alleged victim is a married woman, (s) whether consciousness was lost at any time during the incidence, (t) details of events after the alleged assault: changed or washed clothing; bathed, douched, defecated or urinated prior to the examination; washed, brushed or combed hair; alcohol or drugs taken, treatment taken, (u) the time of the first complaint, and if there was any undue delay, the reason for such a delay. The victim may complain of severe abdominal pain after a gang rape due to unaccustomed weight of many men atop her in a short time, or forceful sexual intercourse. This must be taken down verbatim. The degree of agreement of various statements will be strong proof of their truth or the contrary. It also indicates the position of any injury or bruising, which although present, may not be obvious externally on examination. (8) Previous history with regard to sexual experience, menses, vaginal discharge, venereal disease, pregnancies, pelvic operations, etc. should be recorded. (9) The age should be determined and the height and weight recorded. (10) The physical development should be noted in order to determine her capacity for struggle and resistance. In the case of children, bodily development, especially of the breasts and genitalia should be noted. (11) An attempt at undressing the woman should not be made, but she should be asked to undress herself. (12) If the victim is in menstrual period, a second examination should be done after stoppage of menstruation. (13) Her general demeanour (distressed or calm, dishevelled, dazed or shocked, intoxicated, excited, agitated, withdrawn, tearful, cooperative or aggressive, hysterical, stoic, etc.); emotional and mental state should be observed while she tells her story. Elevated pulse may reflect emotional stress or major trauma. (14) If it appears that she is under the influence of alcohol or drugs, it must be noted and sample of blood, and urine should be collected. (15) The gait should be observed; whether she complains of pain on walking, on micturition or defecation. The pain leads to guarded gait, the victim walking with legs apart and slow paces.

The answers to the following questions have to be found from the examination of the victim. (1) Whether there is evidence of recent sexual intercourse? (2) Whether there is evidence of previous sexual intercourse? (3) Whether the physical signs present confirm the use of force or of stupefying drugs? (4) Whether the physical findings are consistent with the history? (5) Whether the medical evidence confirms the allegation? (6) Whether all the relevant specimens have been collected to confirm the allegations and to assist in identifying the parties involved?

Examination Proper: (1) Clothes: Find out whether the clothes are those worn at the time of assault, or changed. Ideally, each item of clothing should be removed by the patient in the presence of the doctor. The patient should be standing on a clean sheet of paper and anything that falls, e.g., earth, buttons, hair, fibres, gravel, leaves, etc. should be preserved. **Each item of clothing should be examined for various stains (blood, seminal, mud, earth, grease, grass, etc.), soiling, tears and loss of buttons,** and the site and type of damage. Semen is often found on clothing, bedding, carpets, car seats, etc. It can also be found on almost any other article, depending on the movements of the victim and the suspect. Seminal stains will be found on underclothing due to drainage from the vagina, especially if an upright position is adopted soon after ejaculation has occurred. **If the offence has been committed in an open place, corroboration can sometimes be obtained by finding grass, leaves, mud, etc., on the buttocks or on the back.** The clothes should be dried, stored in a clean paper bag and sent to the laboratory. In certain cases, stains may be present on pieces of material or handkerchief used by the victim after assault for cleaning purposes. **Suspicious stains should be preserved for chemical analysis. Vulval pads and vaginal tampons should be preserved,** whether worn at or after the time of the incident. **Clothes are very important in corroborating or contradicting her story.** Foreign hair, fibres, etc., found on clothes or on the skin surface must be preserved and compared with those found on the accused.

(2) General Examination: The victim should be completely undressed and examined using ultraviolet light to detect seminal stains. All areas of soiling must be noted and swabbed with plain cotton swabs. Any loose hair or other foreign substances found on skin surface should be collected. Large and closeup photographs of the injuries, especially of the sexual area should be taken. The whole body must be examined for marks of violence, especially scratches or bruises, lacerations and areas of tenderness resulting from struggle as regards their appearance, extent, situation and probable age. **Petechiae on the face or conjunctivae indicate partial asphyxia** caused during forcible restraint or with intent to make the victim unconscious or silence her. Marks of violence, especially bruises and scratches may be found: (1) about the mouth and throat, produced while preventing her from calling for help. Bruising of the lips and even tearing of the inner aspect may be found, due to blows or rough handling, (2) about wrists and arms where the man seized her, (3) on the back, especially shoulders and buttocks from pressure on gravel or hard ground, (4) on the thighs and buttocks from struggle to achieve intercourse. Both inner and outer side of thighs may be bruised and scratched, esp. inner aspect of upper thigh, (5) on breasts by rough handling, (6) true bite marks and love-bites may be usually found on the breasts, which are often manually squeezed and manipulated, causing discoid bruises of one to two cm. on any part, especially around the nipples, neck, face, shoulders, chest wall, and also on the lower abdomen and upper parts of thighs. The nipples may be bitten off. Suction lesions may appear as circular or oval areas of bruising, in which there are many intradermal petechial haemorrhages produced by sucking the skin into the mouth due to rupture of small vessels from reduced air pressure. The lips may produce semilunar marks at the periphery, and teeth may produce indentations or abrasions. **Marks of general violence are likely to be found in one-third cases.** Absence of general injuries may be due to: (1) Submission of the victim due to fear of injury or death, etc. (2) The force used or the resistance offered is insufficient to produce an injury. (3) Bruises may not be noticed for 48 hours following the assault. (4) A delay in reporting the incident during which minor injuries will fade or heal. The age of injuries should be noted.

The extent and nature of the general injuries should correspond to the victim's description of the assault. If the throat has been gripped, or if a severe blow is struck on the head, the victim's capacity for resistance becomes greatly reduced. Fingernail clippings, or scrapings from beneath the fingernails should be placed in envelopes marked right and left, labelled and sent to the laboratory.

(3) HAIR: The pubic hair should be combed out, as non-matching male pubic hair and foreign material may be present. In the case of the deceased victim, fifteen to twenty pubic hairs are pulled with forceps and placed in a separate envelope, so that root characteristics are available for comparison. In the living victim, fifteen to twenty hairs are cut, not pulled. Hair samples from the head should be taken from the front, top, back, left side and right side. In the pubic region, the hairs on the pubic bone area can differ from hairs in the area of the vagina or scrotum. Therefore, both these areas are sampled as comparative standards. All samples should be carefully retained, packed, sealed and labelled and then sent to the laboratory. Foreign hair or other foreign substance if found should be placed in clean envelopes, sealed and labelled. If the hair is intact, tandem repeat analysis on the root can be performed. If no root is present, mitochondrial DNA typing can be done on the shaft.

(4) SEMINAL STAINS: If the pubic hair is matted, the entire matted hair should be cut away as close to the skin as possible. The pooling of seminal fluid in the vagina is a sign of recent sexual intercourse but this pooling rapidly disappears, if an upright posture is adopted soon after ejaculation has taken place as semen will drain out of vagina. Swabs must be taken from the area of the introitus and perineum (as seminal fluid may leak out of the vagina) before hymen is examined. After examining the hymen, a low vaginal swab should be taken by gently separating the labia minora, without touching the labia or the perineum. Accesible tampons should be removed. Then, a small vaginal speculum should be introduced into the vagina and a high vaginal swab should be taken under direct vision through the speculum. These swabs should be taken before any digital examination of the vagina is attempted. When there is gross external injury and in very young children anaesthesia may be needed before speculum is introduced. A swab of the cervical mucus can be taken if the offence was committed more than 48 hours back. Some mucus should be taken as far up the vagina as possible by means of glass rod, cotton swab or spatula, or the contents are aspirated from the posterior fornix (10 ml. of normal saline can be instilled in the posterior fornix) by means of blunt-end pipette and examined immediately for living sperms. Smears should be prepared immediately, and allowed to dry on the slides, otherwise the sperms will disintegrate. It is then fixed by heat. The slides can also be fixed in a fixative containing equal quantities of absolute alcohol and ether. Clearly label slides by etching the patient's name on them, using a diamond pencil. The material may be taken from anywhere in the vagina, but the cervical canal gives the best results. A second swab is inserted in a small amount of normal saline, which is examined for the presence and motility of spermatozoa. A third swab is air-dried and placed in clean dry test tube and is used for acid phosphatase determination. Areas of seminal soiling will show fluorescence by the use of ultraviolet lamp. Any soiled area, especially on external genitals, tops of thighs, buttocks, abdomen and hands should be swabbed with a cotton swab moistened with saline, air-dried and placed in a sterile container. Dried seminal stains found on external genitals and thighs should be scraped with a blunt knife, sealed in a packet and sent to the chemical examiner. The presence of spermatozoa in the vaginal secretion of children and grownup virgins is a positive sign of sexual intercourse.

(5) BLOOD STAINS: The presence or absence of blood stains about the vagina and legs should be noted. Determine whether such stains could be due to menstruation. Profuse bleeding from the vagina will wash out all the seminal contents and spermatozoa are not found.

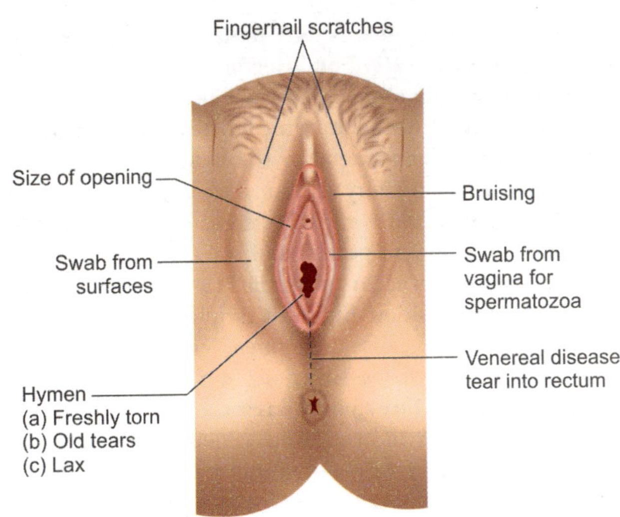

Fig. (18–1). Examination for evidence of rape.

(6) VENEREAL DISEASE: The presence of any discharge due to gonorrhoea, or inflammation of the parts, or signs of syphilis, should be noted. The degree of normal cleanliness of woman should be noted. In unclean woman, there may be superficial areas of erythema, irritation and sometimes abrasions. Redness from chronic inflammation or due to irritation by a chronic discharge must be differentiated from the effect of recent injury. Other sexually transmitted diseases are: Chlamydia, trichomoniasis, herpes simplex, HIV and human papilloma virus.

(7) Local Examination: The Genitals: The woman is placed on a table in good light, with her legs drawn up and widely open (lithotomy position). If the separation of thighs is painful, and in cases of gross external injury and in very young children cocaine solution should be applied to the parts. The examination of genitalia should be thorough, for much depends upon it **Fig. (18–1)**.

Genital injuries are present in about one-fifth cases because: (1) The alleged sexual act may consist of only rubbing or touching the genitalia. (2) The victim is sexually experienced. (3) The elasticity of genitalia and hymen in a post-pubertal female. (4) The use of lubricants.

Rape on Virgin: Firstly, pubic area should be examined and entire matted area should be cut as close to the skin surface as possible. Next, the entire area should be combed and any loose hair removed should be retained for laboratory examination. Next, the tops of thighs, labia and perineum should be inspected and injuries noted. At this stage, swabs must taken from the area of introitus and perineum.

Hymen: Both labia majora and minora should be inspected before labial retraction. The labia are separated by gentle traction to examine the hymen. At this stage, a low vaginal swab should be taken by gently separating labia minora and passing the swab into vaginal canal. **Rupture of hymen occurs with the first intercourse which is the main evidence of rape in the virgin.** As the penis enters the genitals, it tends to compress the labia both anteriorly and laterally, producing bruising of both the labia minora and the labia majora. The amount of bruising will depend upon the force used. Further penetration forces the penis backwards, because the symphysis pubis prevents anterior movement, and **the hymen is torn posteriorly. Usually tears due to digital penetration or insertion of tampons do not extend to the margin of the hymen, while tears due to penile penetration extend to the margin, but tears caused by full finger penetration can extend to the hymenal margin.** The character and extent of injury varies in different cases depending upon (1) the nature of the hymen, (2) disproportion between penis and vagina, (3) extent of penetration, and (4) amount of force used. **Tearing usually occurs posteriorly at the sides, between 5 and 7 'O clock position, but most frequently in the middle line of the hymen, because the hymen lies suspended across a potential space,** whereas anteriorly the periurethral tissues buttress the hymen. **More than two tears are unusual. Several hymenal lacerations indicate first sexual intercourse.** Any object passing through the hymenal orifice which is larger than its original opening will cause a "V" shaped cleft or clefts. One deep tear may be seen at 6 O' clock position or few tears usually in the posterior half of the membrane. **In prepubertal children, the posterior tear of the hymen may involve fourchette, producing a deep "U" shaped defect.**

Soon after the act, the margins of the torn hymen are sharp and red which bleed on touch, the tissues round about them are tender. **In 8–24 hours, margins are oedematous swollen with sero-sanguineous oozing;** for 2 to 3 days, there may be pain, congestion with oozing of blood stained fluid. On third day slight oedema and swelling is seen without oozing. After three to four days, the edges of tear are congested and swollen, which completely heal in a week, but they do not unite. **With healing, over a period of months V shaped tears become rounded and appear as U shaped defect.** Rupture of the hymen due to sudden stretching can be caused by agents other than the penis, such as fingers, and therefore evidence of local injury is not proof of penetration. **Frequently, in the absence of frank hymenal tearing, there is abrasion and bruising of the hymen and the vaginal orifice.**

In **fimbriated hymen**, a moistened swab can be used to visualise the edges of the hymen. If the hymenal opening is not seen, application of a few drops of warm sterile water or saline on to the hymen will reveal hymenal edges. Anterior concavities in the hymen are congenital and do not change with age, but posterior and lateral concavities and attenuation (reduction in the width of hymenal tissue) increases in frequency with age.

Examination of hymen: The hymen can be closely examined by: (1) Glaister-Keene rods or globes Fig. (18–2) which are glass or plastic rods with a diameter of 6 mm., having a globe at one end and varying in size from one to two-and-half cm. A rod is warmed to body temperature and passed through the hymenal orifice, spherical head first. Then it is passed round the posterior surface of hymen, which is slightly stretched by separation of labia minora. In this way, the edges of the hymen become slightly everted. By slowly rotating the sphere around the edges, natural notches are easily differentiated from tears, recent or old. This method does not cause either pain or injury. (2) Foley's catheter or an inflatable balloon which contains a small electric light is introduced into the vagina in order to transilluminate the hymen. (3) Pass a finger into the rectum above the perineal body, and push the posterior vaginal wall forwards and downwards. This pushes the hymen forwards which is clearly seen entirely, lying against

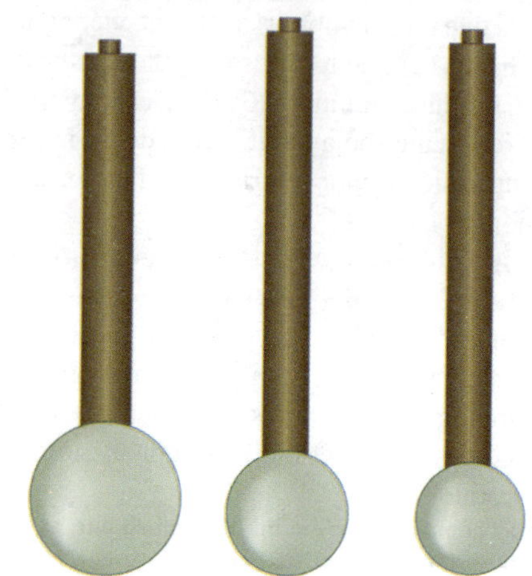

Fig. (18-2). Solid glass spheres for examination of hymenal edges.

the posterior vaginal wall. (4) Hymenoscope gives excellent trans-illumination of hymen to detect tears. After examination of hymen, a low vaginal swab should be taken, gently separating the labia minora.

Toluidine blue dye test: It is used in the identification of genital and perianal injuries, which are not revealed even by colonoscopy. After examination of posterior fourchette apply 10% aqueous solution of toluidine blue dye to posterior fourchette and fossa navicular is with a swab. After about 15 seconds, remove excess dye with lubricant, such as K-Y jelly or 10% acetic acid and gauze. Dye uptake is considered positive and affirms injury when there is residual blue colouring of the lacerations or its borders. The patient may experience stinging at the site of application.

Labia: The labia may be red and inflamed with slight oedema of the vaginal introitus, if it is the first sexual act, or if there is disproportion between the male and female genitalia. If the labia majora are drawn apart, thin tears in the folds of skin between the labia majora and labia minora may be seen sometimes, due to the labia minora being inverted towards the vaginal orifice, causing contraction on their junction with the labia majora. Injury to labia is not common, but **fingernail scratches may be present on the labia, particularly the labia minora and upper parts of thighs.** Swelling and tenderness of the labia minora may indicate sexual activity. Redness of the labia minora may be due to uncleanliness. **Swelling and congestion of the mucosa at the introitus, the clitoris and the labia minora are caused by genital stimulation, but they may also be caused by digital stimulation or masturbation.** These signs usually fade in one to two hours. **Small tears (few mm in length) may be seen in the regions of fourchette and fossa navicularis produced by excessive stretching of the skin. The fourchette is fragile and may tear during first intercourse. Fossa navicularis disappears. The posterior commissure often ruptures at first intercourse,** especially if there is much disproportion in the size of the penis and vagina. **Bruising and lacerations of external genitals may be present with redness, swelling and inflammation. Clitoris is red swollen and oedematous.**

Vagina: A small vaginal speculum should be gently introduced into vagina and a high vaginal swab should be taken under direct vision. With the speculum in site, the interior of vagina should be inspected for signs of abrasions, bruising and laceration of vaginal walls or vault, and a high vaginal swab and a swab of cervical mucus taken. Abrasion and bruising of the hymen and vaginal orifice may be seen in the absence of hymenal tear, due to digital or penile penetration. **Bruising of the vagina is seen as dark-red area against overall redness of the vaginal mucosa, and within twenty-four hours the colour becomes deep-red or purple. It is more frequently seen on the anterior vaginal wall in the lower third, and on the posterior wall in the upper third.** Bruising of this nature is more consistent with penetration of the penis, than with digital penetration. **Abrasion of the vaginal mucosa is more frequent in digital penetration.** These types of injuries can occur during consenting sexual intercourse. In rape or digital penetration without consent, where preliminary stimulation has not taken place, initial lubrication will be lacking due to which more severe local bruising or abrasion can result. **Frank laceration of the vaginal wall or vault is rare following sexual intercourse in women of child-bearing age, but it can occur in very young children and in the atrophic post-menopausal vagina.** In an adult, digital or penile penetration does not produce tears of the vaginal wall or perineal body, but may be produced in old women, or if there is gross disproportion between the penis and the vagina, or in cases where large foreign bodies have been inserted into the vagina, such as sticks, large vibrators, dildos, etc. **In young children and in adults when intercourse takes place in 'standing erect' position, tears of the vaginal wall or perineal body may occur.** Vault injuries vary from minimal mucosal trauma to extensive lacerations. They are not seen in anterior fornix. Posterior laceration of vaginal wall may result from consenting intercourse where there has been (a) marked disproportion between penis and vagina, (b) in very active and enthusiastic copulation, (c) in cases where there has been complete abstinence from intercourse for a considerable length of time.

Cervix: **Abrasion of the cervix and vagina occur almost invariably due to vaginal penetration, and usually due to digital rather than penile penetration.** It can be caused by the insertion of a tampon. **Erosions are seen as bright-red areas on the overall redness of the cervix and are usually situated around the external os with well-defined margins which may bleed on contact.** Colposcope (binocular microscope) which gives 5 to 30 times magnification can be used to directly visualise cervix.

The majority of adult rapes are associated with a sudden forcible dilation of vagina resulting in some degree of local injury. **Bruising, abrasion or laceration of genitalia are at all times consistent with forcible intercourse with a consenting woman, and do not necessarily indicate rape.** A second examination of the victim should be made, for bruising may take a little time to come to the surface, especially in the lower vagina.

Injuries caused by instruments: All the injuries of the labia and vagina found in cases of sex assaults are not due to rough manual and penile connection. **Tears in the deeper parts of vagina, and gross lacerating wounds of the vault are not likely to occur during sexual intercourse, but are often caused by sexual perverts using instruments. Lacerations may be seen in the posterior fornix of the right side of the vault, and less frequently in the left side. The acts may be separate incidents, or they may follow coitus.** In making the examination, it is better to note down the condition found diagrammatically.

Vaginal examination: **In all cases where there are no fresh injuries, vaginal examination should be carried out to assess** (1) the laxity of the vaginal orifice, (indicating previous penetration), (2) the length of the vagina into the posterior fornix, (elongation indicates previous sexual intercourse on a number of occasions), (3) the number of fingers that can be introduced through the hymenal orifice, (4) elasticity of the hymen and to determine the degree of penetration which would be possible without its rupture, (5) the areas and the degree of the tenderness complained of by the patient, if the state of hymen permits. **In most young women, a finger may be passed into vagina with intact hymen,** which is felt as a constricting ring round the tip of the finger. **If the vaginal opening is enough to admit two fingers easily, sexual intercourse is possible without rupture of hymen.** Two finger test was banned by Supreme Court of India in 2013, holding that it violated the right of rape survivors to privacy. The circumference of the hymen can be measured by a measuring cone. **A circumference of 9 to 10 cm. is considered the least necessary for sexual intercourse.**

Rape on Deflorate Women: In deflorate women even without childbirth, the hymen is completely destroyed, the vaginal orifice dilated and the mucous membrane wrinkled and thickened. **Complete penetration can occur in such women without any evidence except semen. The only proof in fact, that the penetration has occurred is presence of spermatozoa in the vagina.** Therefore, absence of injuries under certain circumstances, does not exclude even complete penetration. **In a married woman, marks of violence to the genitalia are less likely to be found but they must be looked for, because usually rape is associated with greater violence than sexual intercourse with consent.**

If the woman offers resistance, local injury will be present. The vagina may show some deep injury, laceration or bruising with effusion of blood and swelling and inflammation of the vulva, even when no marks of violence indicating a struggle may be found externally. When older women are raped, senile atrophy and friability of their genitalia results in bruising and extensive vaginal lacerations and perineal trauma. Spontaneous rupture of the vagina can also occur. In women who have been used to sexual intercourse, injuries from rape usually disappear or become obscure in 3 to 4 days. When there has been much violence, the signs may persist longer. **The presence of violence in other parts of the body is the chief evidence of the crime.**

Rape on Children: **In young children there are few or no signs of general violence,** for the child usually has no idea of what is happening, and also incapable of resisting. In an older child, typical grasping injuries and bruises from blows may be found. **The hymen is deeply situated, and as the vagina is very small, it is impossible for the penetration of the adult organ to take place. Usually, the penis is placed either within the vulva or between the thighs. As such, the hymen is usually intact** and there may be little redness and tenderness of the vulva.

It tends to compress the labia both anteriorly and laterally producing bruising of labia minora and majora. Further attempt at penetration, penis. As the penis enters the genitals, is forced backwards, because the symphysis pubis prevents anterior movement and the **hymen is torn posteriorly. As the penis advances into the vagina, additional pressure is put on the anterior and lateral structures and the hymenal tear extends into or through the perineal body and often involves the anterior wall of the anorectal canal.** As a general rule, the younger the child, the more prominent the tissues of labia majora, and more likely that they can be contused, abraded and lacerated, particularly in the anterior half. **Circumferential tears of the mucosa of the vestibule are common.** As the age and size of the child increases, the pattern of injury will become less marked but the circumferential tears of the vestibular mucosa are found up to the age of six years or more. **Full penile penetration produces extensive haematoma affecting particularly the anterior half and frequently tears of the anterior and posterior vaginal walls. Anterior tears can involve the bladder and the posterior tears the anorectal canal. Vaginal vault may rupture, and there may be vaginal herniation of abdominal viscera.** The hymen may be entirely destroyed or may show lacerations. Bleeding will be brisk from the skin and mucosa but may be slight from the perineal body.It normally stops within 5 to 10 minutes, but may restart if the child moves or if the wound margins are wiped. **Blood may be oozing from the injured parts, or clots of blood may be found in the vagina.** There may be mucopurulent discharge from the vagina. Any attempt to separate the thighs for examination causes great pain, because of the local inflammation. The child walks with difficulty due to pain. **The absence of marks of violence on the genitals of the child, when an early examination is made is strong evidence that rape has not been committed.**

In digital penetration of the infant vagina, there is frequently some scratching, laceration or bruising of the labia, hymen and fourchette and injury to the cervix, but the circumferential tears are absent. The hymen shows a linear tear in the posterior or posterolateral quadrant, which may extend into the posterior vaginal wall and on to the skin of the perineum, and may involve the perineal body. Ano-rectal canal is rarely involved. Bruising in the margins of tear and of anterior vaginal wall are common, but vaginal vault injury is rare. Speculum examination should not be performed on the prepubertal child.

AUTOPSY: Before transporting the body from the scene, paper bags should be placed on the hands to preserve any trace evidence and the body wrapped in a clean white sheet. Clothing should be examined while it is still on the body. Any material removed from clothing should be preserved. Examine the hands for foreign material and nail clippings preserved. After undressing, collect trace evidence and examine for injuries. Obtain samples of head hair. 15–20 pubic hair are pulled with forceps and preserved. Take photographs of bite marks with a scale present in picture. The autopsy incision should be similar to that described for abortion, and the uterus, cervix and vaginal canal should be examined for injuries as in the case of criminal abortion. Dissect this block of tissue separately. The vagina is opened with large scissors avoiding injuries to the posterior fornix, and all injuries should be noted and photographed. The cervix, uterus and anus are examined in the same way. Injuries may be of all types, from reddening or swelling to complete disruption of the vaginal canal. Vaginal injuries, especially by instruments, may continue into the abdominal cavity, either through the posterior fornix or lateral vaginal walls. Candles, bottles, bananas, broken glass, etc. may be found in the vagina.

CORROBORATIVE SIGNS OF RAPE

(1) SEMINAL FLUID: The thighs, pubic hair and vagina of the victim should be examined. The presence of spermatozoa in the vagina is proof of sexual connection, but not of rape. Sometimes ejaculation may occur while the man is in the mounting position and seminal fluid may enter vagina; their absence is no proof that sexual connection has not taken place, for they may have been removed by washing or by discharges, or there may not have been an emission, or it may have been aspermic due to vasectomy or naturally or condom was used, or ejaculation occurred outside. The woman may rapidly wash the vagina with strong antiseptic solutions due to fear of impregnation. This may completely remove all seminal material or introduce factors that interfere with the detection of the constituents of seminal material. Emission may take place without penetration. The presence of fresh seminal stains on the person or clothes of a woman provides strong evidence of intercourse, attempted or committed. Semen is lost from the vagina of the living victim due to drainage, dilution with vaginal fluid and phagocytosis of sperms by neutrophils and mononuclear cells. Rarely, a used condom containing semen may be found in the vagina. The end should be tied to retain the contained fluid and placed in a paper bag. Any external sanitary napkin or internal tampon is collected for analysis. The number of semen donors can be determined with the use of Y-chromosome STR (DNA fingerprinting) markers.

(2) VAGINAL DISCHARGES: If any fluid is coming out from the vulva, it should be picked up with clean pipette and preserved. Vaginal discharges may arise from local infection, from worms or unclean habits. If the assailant is suffering from venereal disease, he may transmit it to his victim, which is strong corroborative evidence of intercourse. In gonorrhoea an inflammation with an abundant mucopurulent discharge will be seen in two to four days (occasionally a week), while in syphilis an indurated ulcer on the external genitals may appear in about three weeks. In the case of adults, smears should be taken from the cervix and urethra for gonococci which are kidney-shaped, intracellular, Gram-negative diplococci. In the case of children, smears should be taken from the vagina. An initial negative smear may be of value, if a positive smear is obtained within a few days of the assault. A blood sample should be taken for serological examination for syphilis. An initial negative reaction may be of value, if a positive reaction is obtained after six weeks. Sometimes, the sores on the genitals may be due to chancroid. Smears from sores or bubo fluid, when stained show the Ducrey's bacillus which is Gram-negative streptobacillus with rounded ends.

(3) STRUGGLE: Signs of active resistance may be present. The fingernails may be broken or bent due to scratching the accused. A broken fingernail can be matched to its source by direct physical match or by stria on undersurface of nail which are as individual as fingerprints. Under the nails, debris may be present, e.g., blood, fibres, hair and skin fragment from the accused. Other signs of struggle may also be present.

FINDINGS RELATED TO TIME OF ASSAULT

(1) SEMINAL FLUID: The spermatozoa deposited in the vagina lose motility within one to six hours, and at the end of six hours usually no motile sperms are found. Sperms may be recovered up to 24 hours from the vagina.

(2) VENEREAL DISEASE: The presence of V.D. is useful in determining the time of sexual assault.

(3) WOUNDS: If the age of any wound present is consistent with the alleged time of rape, it will be of value.

The evidence collected by medical examination of the victim and accused, may either confirm or contradict the allegations made by her.

SPECIMENS TO BE COLLECTED FROM VICTIM: The objects of collecting specimens are: (1) To obtain confirmation of the allegations. (2) To attempt to establish a link between the victim and the scene. (3) To attempt to establish a link between the victim and the assailant.

SAFE (sexual assault forensic evidence) kit or PERK (physical evidence recovery kit) is designed for collection and preservation of trace evidence in case of sexual assault.

(1) Hair: (a) Ten hairs cut close to roots from different locations on the head. (b) Pubic hair combings. (c) Avulsed pubic hair. (d) Loose hairs found anywhere on the body (to compare and identify foreign hairs). (e) Matted pubic hair (for spermatozoa, lubricants, etc.) (2) Finger scrapings (for blood or tissue from the accused). (3) Any foreign matter. (All of them to be packed in separate polythene bags). (4) Blood 5 ml. (plain) for grouping and 5ml (EDTA) for DNA profile. (5) Blood 5 ml. (sodium fluoride and potassium oxalate) for alcohol and drugs and venereal disease. **Blood samples should be refrigerated, but must not be frozen, which causes the cells to lyse.** (6) Urine (sodium fluoride) for alcohol and drug screening. (7) Saliva for secretor grouping. (8) Swabs from any body surface which has been kissed, licked, sucked or bitten for saliva. All the swabs should be packed without any transport medium and refrigerated. (9) Genital swabs from introitus, vagina and cervical os. Vaginal speculum should be used to obtain a swab from cervical os. (10) Swabs from any soiled areas of skin. (11) Condoms, if used during intercourse. (12) Sanitary towels, tampons worn after intercourse. (13) Swabs can be used to collect vaginal epithelial cells for DNA study. All bottles, tubes and packages should be sealed and labelled. The date and time of examination, time of collection, identification of victim/accused, case number and place of examination recorded.

IDENTITY OF THE ACCUSED: Blood, semen, urine, saliva, hair, and general debris present on the clothing or person of the victim may help the identity of the accused by comparing with the known materials from the accused. The presence of V.D. is also helpful.

To **summarise,** evidence of rape is obtained from: (1) marks of violence on the person of the victim and the accused, (2) marks of violence about the genitals, (3) the presence of stains of semen, or of blood on the clothes and the body of the victim or accused, (4) the presence of seminal matter in the vagina, and (5) the existence of gonorrhoea or syphilis in both the parties. The evidence will vary, according to circumstances.

Bays and Chadwick (1993) reviewing literature, proposed that a markedly enlarged hymenal opening for age with associated findings of hymen disruption including absent hymen, hymenal remnants, healed transection or scars in the absence of an adequate accidental or surgical explanation, would be diagnostic of sexual abuse.

Opinion: **Rape is not a medical diagnosis, it is only a legal definition. Medical proof of intercourse is not legal proof of rape.** The report should contain negative as well as positive findings. **The doctor should never make a diagnosis of rape. He may give opinion that there are signs of recent vaginal penetration, recent sexual intercourse, general physical injuries, and/or intoxication, and that the signs are consistent with the history given. Rape is an accusation easily to be made, and hard to be proved, and harder to be defended by the party accused.** Independent corroboration of the victim's story may be obtained by an eyewitness, evidence acquired at the crime scene, and from the body of the victim or accused. **Since many rapes are not witnessed, circumstantial evidence is offered in most cases.**

False Charges: Sometimes, false charges are made by a consenting woman, when the act is discovered by the parents or someone else, when she becomes pregnant, or for purposes of revenge or blackmail.

NATURE OF FALSE ALLEGATIONS: False allegations often contain less common elements, such as: (1) She cannot describe the assailant because she kept her eyes closed. (2) Assailant was a total stranger or a person whom she can describe in vague and nonspecific terms. (3) She offered resistance but was forcibly overcome as the assailant was large or powerful. (4) She was assaulted by more than one person, but cannot offer descriptions. (5) She cannot describe details and sequence of the sexual activities to which she was subjected.

EVIDENCE: False allegations (simulated rape) are suggested by: (1) She cannot recall where the crime took place. (2) Crime scene does not support her story, i.e. no footprints or disturbance of the ground. (3) Damage to her clothing is inconsistent with any injuries she reports. (4) Confirming laboratory findings are absent. (5) Undue delay in reporting. (6) Uncertainty about consent.

Pattern and Nature of Injuries: In false allegations: (1) Injuries are not serious and are made either by fingernails or by sharp instrument. The parents may injure the genital organs of the child by introducing a blunt instrument or thumb into vagina or place irritants, such as chillies within the vagina to simulate rape. Adult women may stain their garments with a solution of starch or white of egg to simulate seminal stains, and with the blood of an animal. (2) Injuries do not involve sensitive tissues, such as genitals, nipples, lips. (3) Location and angles of injuries are inconsistent with defence wounds. (4) Hesitation marks may be present. (5) Fingernail scrapings of victim reveal her own skin tissue.

COMPLICATIONS OF RAPE: (1) Death may occur from (a) shock due to fright and emotion or by blunt force injuries, (b) haemorrhage from injuries to genitals and perineum, (c) suffocation if mouth and nostrils are closed by the hand or cloth or by strangulation. (2) Mental derangements, convulsions and epileptic fits. Psychological trauma is much more when the victim knows the rapist. (3) It may disrupt the victim's physical, social and sexual life.

RAPE TRAUMA SYNDROME: It consists of those behavioural, somatic and psychological reactions that occur as a result of forcible rape or attempted forcible rape. It is generally regarded as a post-traumatic stress disorder. Burgess, et al., define a rape trauma syndrome in two stages: (1) Immediate or acute (disorganisation) phase, characterised by emotional reactions of several kinds, e.g., tension symptoms together with feelings of guilt and humiliation. (2) A long-term (reorganisation) phase, during which the victim readjusts her life as far as possible. During this phase, she may suffer from nightmares and various phobias.

RAPE CRISIS CENTRES (established in the West) provide: (1) Counselling to the victim and her relatives, (2) educate public on rape related issues and to reform the law, (3) reform the institution which deal with the victims. These centres are largely staffed by volunteers, non-professional women, or who have been close to someone who was raped.

MEDICOLEGAL QUESTIONS

(1) RAPE AND RESISTANCE: In ordinary conditions, it is not possible for a man to have sexual intercourse with a healthy adult female in full possession of her senses against her will. The woman may not be able to offer marked resistance from terror or from an overpowering feeling of helplessness, or when her movements may have been obstructed by her clothing. The social status, physical development, and type of woman should also be considered, for a woman used to look after herself is less likely to be terrified than a woman who has led a sheltered life. When a woman is overpowered by two or more men she cannot resist much, and marks of violence may not be marked.

(2) RAPE UNDER NARCOTICS OR DURING SLEEP: Rape may be committed without the knowledge of the woman while she is under the influence of narcotics, such as opium, cocaine, hyoscine, alcohol, etc., while under the influence of an anaesthetic, while in a state of coma, and possibly while in a hypnotic trance. When a woman takes an aphrodisiac or alcohol voluntarily in order to increase sexual feeling or encourage petting and becomes a victim of sexual intercourse, the question of consent depends on the extent to which she had become affected. If she is conscious, she can refuse consent. In such cases, complete history should be taken and blood, and urine should be preserved for chemical examination. On emerging from light anaesthesia, patients (especially neurotic) may have hallucinations or dreams of an erotic or fearful nature and genuinely believe that the doctor or dentist had sexual intercourse

with them while they were unconscious. It is as difficult to put a woman under the influence of chloroform by force as to rape her. There is no drug which can produce immediate unconsciousness when placed in front of the face of person. It is impossible to have complete sexual intercourse with a woman during her natural sleep without her knowledge.

DATE RAPE DRUGS (DRUG-RELATED SEXUAL ASSAULT WITH DATE RAPE DRUGS): Sexual assault with pre-meditated planning after mixing of sedative drugs in spiked soft or hard drinks to facilitate resistance free solo or group sexual activities is usually known as 'date rape'. In majority of the cases alcohol is usual base for these drinks or sometimes soft drinks.

The drugs with sexual assault are alcohol, flunitrazepam, with other benzodiazipines and gamma-hydroxybutyrate (GHB), ketamine and scopolamine. In a typical case, a sexual offender stealthily mixes the drink of unsuspecting person with a sedative drug for the purpose of drugging. The victim after consuming 2–3 standard drinks of alcohol (one drink is roughly 15 g. of alcohol) starts enjoying the atmosphere of social gathering. At this stage, the drug mixed drink is given to the **unsuspecting person. The victim may not remember events experienced while under its effect.** The sedative effects appear in 15 to 20 minutes and last for 4 to 6 hours. Victims are disinhibited showing least resistance. Victims report loss of memory during and after these incidents. They wake up in unfamiliar places, inappropriately dressed and often with the sense but not the actual recollection of having had sex.

Rave party: High energy all night dance parties and clubs known as "raves" have fast music, beem lights and get together of teenagers and young adults. The use of alcohol, MDMA, Ketamine, GHB, rohypnol and LSD are part of party. Death may be caused due to overdose, pontine haemorrhage, cardiac toxicity and arrhythmias. Blood and urine are samples for screening.

(3) RAPE BY PERSONATION OF THE HUSBAND: This is possible when the woman is sleeping. Rarely the victim may be awake, but lying in the dark.

(4) RAPE BY FRAUD OR MISREPRESENTATION: Fraudulent sexual connections occur from time to time (S. 493, I.P.C.).

CASE: (1) A music master had sexual intercourse with a girl under the pretence that her breathing was not quite right and that he had to perform an operation to produce her voice properly.

(2) The parents of a girl of 16 engaged a choirmaster of a church to give her lessons in singing and voice production. On the second singing lesson the master told her that she was not singing well and not getting her notes properly and asked her to lie down on a settee. He then removed a portion of her clothing and placed an instrument which was not working on the lower part of her abdomen and asked her to take deep breath three times. He looked at the instrument and pretended to write something in a book. He then dropped on to her and proceeded to have sexual intercourse. She said "what are you going to do"? He told her not to worry as he is going to make an air-passage and that her parents have arranged it. The girl did not resist. A few days later again he had sexual intercourse with her. She told the parents about the incident. He was prosecuted and sentenced to seven years imprisonment.

EXAMINATION OF THE ACCUSED

General Procedure: The procedure of examination of the accused is similar to the victim. It is better to examine the accused after the victim, and to look specifically for any injuries, which she says she has inflicted. If possible the accused should be examined by the same doctor who has examined the victim, for better correlation between the injuries found on the female, such as bite marks, fingertip bruises, comparison of size and build and the physical features of the accused.

Procedure: (1) **The consent of the accused should be taken, and it should be explained to him that the report will be furnished to the police and courts, which may go against him, and that he has right to refuse consent.** Accused can be examined without the consent **(S. 53(A) Cr.P.C.)** on the request of police officer. (2) He should be identified by the escorting police constable, and identification marks should be recorded. (3) The examination must be begun without delay as the signs of the act disappear rapidly. (4) A general medical history should include details of all past illnesses, surgical operations, serious accidents, medication, and consumption of alcoholic drinks. **No attempt should be made to obtain any history of the specific incident.** It should be found out whether the accused had consenting intercourse with any person within the previous 24 hours; when did he had the last bath; when was the last change of clothing and his explanations for the injuries found on his body. (5) The exact time, date, month and place of examination should be noted.

GENERAL EXAMINATION: (1) The age, development of genital organs and physical power of the accused should be noted and compared with that of female to determine the possibility of his overpowering her. (2) His mental state and general behaviour (dazed or shocked, distressed or calm, co-operative or aggressive) should be observed. (3) If he appears to be under the influence of alcohol or drugs, it must be recorded. (4) The clothes should be examined for: (a) tears and loss of buttons, (b) hair, fibres and foreign matter, (c) cosmetic contact traces, e.g., facepowder or lipstick stains, (d) blood stains, (e) mud and other stains, grass, etc., and (f) seminal stains. Particles of earth or fibres trapped between the uppers and soles at the welt of shoes will identify the suspect with the scene. Trousers will often show soiling at the knees from grass and earth. Loose hair from the victim may be caught in the zip fly. Blood and seminal stains may be present on the inside of the trouser fly and the inside of the underwear. The clothing may have physiological fluids or hairs from the woman on its surface. (5) Nail scrapings should be examined for blood, epithelial cells, fibres, etc. (6) Marks of struggle, such as bruises, scratches and teeth-bite marks on the face, neck, hands, chest, trunk, buttocks, upper limbs, thighs and genitals should be noted, caused during struggle from the resistance offered by the victim. The age of the injuries should be determined. (7) Note the matting of pubic hair due to emission of semen. (8) Female hair on the face, body or clothes of accused or of feminine pubic hair in his prepucial fold indicates commission of the offence. The hair should be preserved. (9) Existence of venereal disease must be looked for.

Examination of the genitals: (1) Note the development of genital organs with special reference to the potency. (2) **Note any scratches or abrasions and bruising on genitals caused by the victim during struggle for prevention of intercourse.** Forceful penetration against the resistance into a virgin hymen, may produce **tears or bruising of the fraenulum of the prepuce in the uncircumcised, and abrasion of the glans penis in both the uncircumcised and the circumcised.** Such injuries are more common in sexual assault involving very young children, because of the disparity in the size between the penis and the vagina. **Reddening of the glans especially the rim, often patchy is more common.** Dried blood stains may be found on the shaft of the penis, the scrotum and the adjoining skin. (3) Suspect's penis is washed with saline, and the material is stained with Papanicolaou's stain. **Vaginal and cervical cells and Barr body identification suggest recent intercourse.** (4) **Examine**

the glans for vaginal cells. This is done by cleaning the organ with a filter-paper and exposing the paper to vapours of Lugol's iodine. The paper becomes brown if vaginal epithelial cells are present, because of the glycogen. The test is positive up to fourth day. (5) **Smegma:** If accused is not circumcised, foreskin may be retracted and the presence or absence of smegma (cheesy secretion of sebaceous glands, consisting mainly of desquamated epithelial cells) on corona glandis should be noted. **The absence of smegma may indicate that intercourse might have been performed but presence of smegma rules out possibility of complete penetration** because smegma gets rubbed off during intercourse. Smegma will also be removed by bathing or washing. Smegma usually requires about 24 hours to collect.

DNA from the victim can be recovered from the swabs of the penis using STR up to 24 hours after intercourse if the individual did not bathe. Analysis identifies X chromosome and 8 STR loci.

Specimens to be Collected from Accused: (1) Swab from coronal sulcus (after retracting the prepuce), prepuce, penile shaft and urethral orifice, for they may reveal infecting organisms or blood that may also be present on the victim's swabs. (2) Blood for grouping. (3) Pubic hair combings and avulsed pubic hair. (4) Matted pubic hair. (5) Head hair. (6) Loose hair found anywhere on the body. (7) Nail scrapings.

Priapism is persistent abnormal erection of the penis, usually without sexual desire, and accompanied by pain and tenderness. It is seen in diseases and injuries of the spinal cord and certain injuries to the penis.

Formication is voluntary sexual intercourse of the unmarried.

INDECENT ASSAULT: Indecent assault is any offence committed on a female with the intention or knowledge to outrage her modesty. Outrage means gross violation of decency, morality or feelings. **Usually the act involves the sexual parts of either, or is sexually flavoured.** In such assaults, a man may try to kiss a woman, press or fondle her breasts, touch or expose the genitalia or thighs, try to put a finger in her vagina, play with vulva, etc. This is usually committed against children, or adolescent girls and rarely on adult or old women. Men may encourage children to handle or masturbate their sexual organs. **Indecent offences between two or more male persons include** such offences as friction of penis on the gluteal folds, handling of the male genitalia, mutual masturbation, etc. or intercrural connection (penile friction between the inner thighs and external genitalia). **Stripping naked a female patient for medical examination is regarded as an assault. Such assaults are punishable under** S. 354, I.P.C., **up to one to 5 years imprisonment and fine.** In such cases, medical examination is of little value. Abrasions or bruises may sometimes be present due to struggle.

Modesty is an attribute associated with female human beings as a class. It is a virtue which attaches (to) a female owing to her sex. knowledge that modesty is likely to be outraged is sufficient to constitute the offence without any deliberate intention of having such outrage alone for its object. The culpable intention of the accused is the crux of the matter. The reaction of the woman is very relevant, but its absence is not always decisive.

SEXUAL HARASSMENT: It is an unwelcome sexual gesture or behaviour whether directly or indirectly as: (a) sexually coloured remarks, (b) physical contact and advances, (c) showing pornography, (d) a demand or request for sexual favours, (e) any other unwelcome physical, verbal, non-verbal conducts being sexual in nature. S. 354A, (imprisonment up to 3 years).

WIFE BATTERING: A battered wife is a woman who has received a deliberate, severe and repeated demonstrable physical injuries from her husband. The involved men below the age of forty suffer from personality or neurotic disorders, while those over forty suffer from psychiatric disorder. Domestic discord, often in families with numerous children, drunkenness and demands for dowry are usually responsible. Faulk has categorised these men into five groups: (1) Dependent passive. (2) Dependent suspicious. (3) Violent and bullying. (4) Dominating. (5) Normal, stable and affectionate (498 A, I.P.C).

CHILD SEXUAL ABUSE: Paedophilia is a psychological disorder in which an adult experiences a sexual preference for prepubescent children. Paedophilia crimes may be committed within a family or among acquaintance group, or by strangers. It includes: (1) sexual assault, (2) sexual molestation (non-penetrative activity with a minor, such as exposing to pornography or to sexual acts of others), (3) sexual grooming, such as making a minor accepting of their advances. The effects of child sexual abuse include depression, post-traumatic stress syndrome, anxiety, physical injury, transmission of venereal disease.

PROTECTION OF CHILDREN FROM SEXUAL OFFENCES ACT, 2012 (POCSO): It is an Act to protect children from offences of sexual assault, sexual harassment and pornography and provides for establishment of special courts for trial of such offences. It recognizes forms of penetration other than peno-vaginal penetration, criminalizes act of immodesty, watching or collecting of pornographic content involving children and makes abetment of sexual abuse an offence. It is mandatory for everyone whoever comes to know about crimes under this Act to inform the police.

INCEST

Incest means sexual intercourse by a man with a woman who is closely related to him by blood (prohibited degrees of relationship), e.g., a daughter, granddaughter, sister, stepsister, aunt or mother. Incest between father and daughter and brothers and sisters are common. **These cases usually have psychological features. In India, incest as such, is not an offence.**

Incest occurs (1) between mental defectives who are unable to understand the prohibitions against it, or whose feelings are too strong to inhibit them behaving in this way; (2) where alcohol removes the natural inhibitions; (3) in case of cerebral disease, such as general paralysis, senile cerebral degeneration, etc. (4) where a brother and sister have been separated since childhood or for a long period and meet later as strangers; (5) where close relations have to live in intimacy.

Adultery: Sexual intercourse with the wife of another man, without the consent or connivance of that man constitutes adultery. In such case, the wife shall not be punishable as an abettor. It has decriminalized. It can be a ground for divorce. (S. 497, I.P.C).

UNNATURAL OFFENCES

Voluntary sexual intercourse against the order of nature with any man, or woman, or animal is an unnatural sex offence (S. 377, I.P.C.). Explanation: Penetration is sufficient to constitute the offence. These offences are punishable with imprisonment for life or up to ten years and also with fine. **Homosexuality means persistent emotional and physical attraction to members of the same sex.**

SODOMY

Sodomy is the anal intercourse between two males, or between a male and female. This used to be practiced in a town called Sodom. It is also called **buggery.** It is called **gerontophilia** when the passive agent is an adult, and **paederasty,** when the passive agent is a child, who is known as **catamite.** **A paedophile is an adult who repeatedly engages in sexual activities with children.** Aggression and sadism are inherent components of paedophilia. The Greeks of the "Golden Age" also practised it, and it is sometimes referred to as **Greek love.** It can be heterosexual or homosexual. When practised between two men, they may alternately act as active and passive agents. **Any degree of penetration or any attempt at penetration just into the anal margin, are punishable. Proof of emission is not necessary.** Sodomy between two adult males or a male and female in private with consent is not an offence, if the consent is free, voluntary in nature and devoid of any duress or coercion. Anal sex has been recognized as a sexual choice of the individual rather than any mental abnormality. Only the active agent is punished when the offence is committed without consent. It is difficult to be performed against the will of the person, unless the person is drugged or very drunk, for **slightest resistance is sufficient to prevent the offence**. The crime is frequent among sailors, prisoners, in hostels, military barracks, etc. for they are thrown together for long periods. False charges may be made for blackmail, and men may be tricked into homosexual relationship by men disguising as women. This type of homosexuality is seen among all levels of the society.

Eunuchs: In India, a class of male prostitutes called **"Eunuchs", act as passive agents in sodomy.** Among them there are two groups. (1) **Hijrahs,** and (2) **Zenana,** who live separately. **In hijrahs before puberty penis and scrotum are removed by making a clean sweep with a knife at a secret ceremony. The resulting scar becomes contracted and invaginated and is mistaken for female genitalia.** They possess a typical feminine appearance, high pitched voice, abundance of fat round the hips, tendency to genu valgum, broad hips, absence of hair on body and face, and absence of genital organs. Their speech and gait is feminine, they adopt feminine names, and their instincts, passions and expressions correspond to those of female, due to the resulting hormonal imbalance. **The genitalia of the zenana are intact.**

Examination of Passive Agent: General Procedure: The routine medical examination of the passive agent of sodomy should follow similar pattern as in the case of alleged victim of rape. Consent must be obtained and general history taken. Enquire about the victim's bowel habits, including previous constipation, use of laxatives, enemata or suppositories, and any surgical operation or instrumentation of the bowel, previous acts of anal intercourse, their frequency and the last act of anal intercourse.

History: The specific history should include: (1) the date, time and place of alleged act, (2) the position in which sodomy was performed, (3) details of struggle or resistance, (4) the use of any lubricant, (5) the degree of penetration, (6) ejaculation during the act, (7) pain experienced either at the time of the incident or subsequently, (8) any bleeding, (9) defecation after the alleged act, (10) whether changed the clothes, (11) whether bathed or washed the anal area after the act.

The clothing should be examined as in the case of the victim of rape. The crutch area of the underwear and trousers should be examined for the presence of blood, seminal or faecal stains. General injuries together with scratches, especially on the back and buttocks should be looked for. **The examination must be carried out in the presence of a third person either in the lateral position or better in prone or in the knee-elbow position.** Swabs must be taken from the anal verge and the skin of the perineum. A small, unlubricated proctoscope should be passed, and swabs should be taken from the lower rectum and anal canal, through the lumen of the instrument. Lower rectum and anal canal must be inspected for injuries or for mucosal abnormality.

Anal examination: Salient features: (1) Up to 24 hours anal muscle is oedematous, abraded and bruised with oozing of blood. Oozing, congestion and oedema are present for 2 to 3 days. Anal muscle is found dilated, irritable and tender to touch. (2) Digital examination may show loss of elasticity and tone. **If only one finger is admitted with discomfort and there are no scars, it indicates that full act has not taken place. If two fingers are admitted with slight discomfort and there are no scars, then it is possible that the act could have taken place.** (3) **Haematoma is frequently seen,** either as a diffuse swelling of the anal margin, with obliteration of the normal anal skin folds, or as localised swelling. (4) **Linear abrasions,** varying in number and extending from the anal margin into the anus itself, either anteriorly, posteriorly or laterally with adherent specks of blood suggest recent act **Fig. (18–3).** (5) If sudden violence is used, there may be **triangular bruised-tear** at the posterior part of the anus with its base externally at anus. This can be seen by pulling outwards the skin of the buttocks. (6) Tearing of the sphincter ani is rare in adults and older children, but can occur in young children. (7) There may be anal prolapse. (8) Lesions are marked in children because of great disproportion in size between anal orifice of victim and the penis of the accused. If a moderate-sized penis is introduced without violence and with care, the anus may dilate sufficiently, and the act may be completed without leaving any trace. Signs of injury similar to those of penile penetration are produced if two or more fingers or large objects are introduced into the anus. (9) Normally, the anal orifice is slit-like, running anteroposteriorly and surrounding skin shows marked natural folds due to the act of corrugator cutis ani muscle. Anal fissures (longitudinal) may involve the external skin only, or may extend within the anal canal to the mucocutaneous junction, which is situated in adults from 2 to 2.5 cm within anal canal. Fissures are produced due to the overstretching of the skin. It is usually

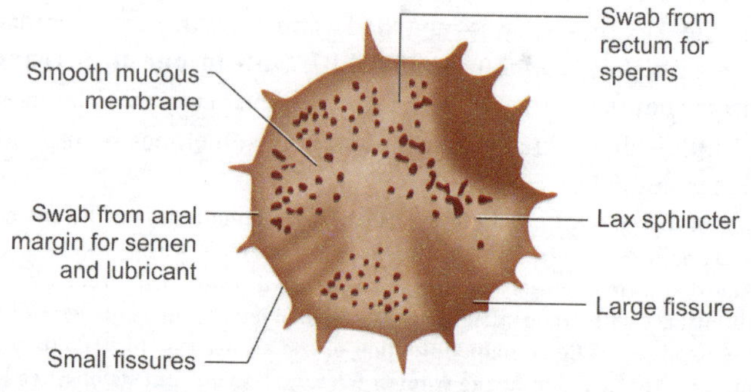

Fig. (18–3). **Examination for evidence of sodomy.**

single and frequently seen at the posterior quadrant. It is usually wedge-shaped, with the wider portion being situated laterally and the point being directed radially towards the anal canal Fig. (18–3). (10) Blood stains around the anus, on perineum and on clothes. (11) Faecal matter around the anus. (12) There is pain during walking, defecation and anal examination. (13) Signs of struggle, e.g., bruises and abrasions, if he is not a consenting party. (14) For 2 to 3 days, there may be pain, congestion with oozing of bloodstained fluid.

The smoothness of the anal margin skin, spasm of the anal sphincter, and the fresh appearance of abrasions may disappear in one to two days. Proctoscope may be used if necessary. **A fissure remains visible for many days and a perianal haematoma takes seven to ten days for absorption. Signs of first act of sodomy disappear in about ten days. If the act has been performed carefully, or if the passive agent is habituated, there may be no signs,** as the anus can undergo considerable distension without injury if it is dilated slowly. In the living, a lax anus, prolapsed mucosal rim and thickened anal margin may be genuine signs. Digital penetration of the anus by one finger may not result in injury, even in infants of less than one year. **Anal penetration by two or more fingers produce signs of injury that are similar to those of penile penetration.**

Diagnosis: The only proof of sodomy is the presence of semen in the anus. Opinion as to the cause of the dilation should be guarded and **it should only be stated that it is consistent with entry of a penis.**

Lubricant matter, seminal fluid or venereal infections found at the anus or recovered by swabs from the rectum is a strong evidence of the crime.

Habitual Passive Agent: The following signs may be present. (1) The shaving of the anal hair. (2) The skin about anus becomes smooth and thickened extending up into the anal canal to the mucocutaneous junction and sometimes into the upper anal canal. (3) **The muscle of the anus loses its tone and does not contract so readily when the skin around it is pinched.** (4) Slight depression of buttocks towards the anus due to absorption of fat. Funnel-shaped anus is very rare, and is usually an anatomical variant. (5) **Dilatation and laxity of the anus,** and an epithelisation of the wrinkled mucosa of this part. Lax (overstretched) anus is significant, but elastic (capable of dilation) has no value. (6) There may be anal fissures, scars, etc. (7) Absence of fine wrinkles in the anal mucosa. (8) Piles and fissures are very common in old sodomists. (9) Presence of venereal disease.

Lateral buttock traction test: A thumb is placed on each side of the anus and lateral traction is applied. In persons who are not accustomed to sodomy, there will be reflex constriction of the anal sphincter. In a habitual sodomite a complete relaxation of the sphincter occurs with dilation of the opening which may be four to five cm. in diameter through which rectum can be seen.

Specimens to be Collected: (1) Blood. (2) Urine. (3) Head hair. (4) Pubic hair. (5) Loose hair and fibres found anywhere on the body. (6) Swabs from any soiled areas of skin. (7) Swabs from the anal, perianal and lower rectum, if necessary with the aid of a proctoscope. (8) Rectal washing with sterile saline. (9) Nail scrapings.

Active Agent: The routine medical examination of the accused of sodomy should follow similar pattern as in the case of alleged accused in rape. (1) **The only evidence commonly found is the peculiar smell of anal glands transferred to the penis, and traces of faecal matter and lubricant on the organ.** (2) **Abrasions on the prepuce, glans penis, tearing of fraenum or swelling or redness of penis.** (3) Faecal soiling, blood and foreign hairs are likely to be found in the area of coronal sulcus. (4) The urethral swab may show faecal material and organisms similar to those found on the anal verge swabs from the passive agent, which corroborate penetration. (5) Blood and seminal stains. (6) Presence of venereal disease. Smears should be taken from the external meatus after applying pressure on the undersurface of the penis along the urethra for gonococci. (7) Marks of violence on the body. (8) The clothes may show seminal stains or a mixture of semen and faeces. (9) In habitual sodomites, penis may be elongated and constricted at some distance from the glans with twisted urethra.

Swabs should be taken from shaft of penis, coronal sulcus and glans. Transmission of AIDS may occur after only a few sexual acts in homosexuals, eunuchs and prostitutes.

Gay clubs, i.e. association of homosexuals are present in some countries like U.K., U.S.A., etc.

BUCCAL COITUS: (Coitus per os or sin of Gomorrah). According to the Bible, this sin was common in a town called Gomorrah. In this type of sexual offence, the **male organ is introduced into mouth of another male or female, but usually of a young child.** Rarely, erythema, petechiae and faint teeth marks and abrasions may be seen on the penis. Death may result from aspiration of semen or impaction of the penis in the hypopharynx. The diagnosis is made by finding semen in the respiratory tract or stomach of the victim. **Spermatozoa can be found in the mouth up to nine hours** provided: (1) the victim has not cleaned the teeth nor taken a hot drink after the incident, and (2) careful swabbing has been done by rubbing around inside mouth, under tongue gum margins and between teeth. The victim's mouth is rinsed with distilled water, which can be expectorated into a sterile container, centrifuged and examined. **It is punishable under S. 377, I.P.C.** if absence of consent.

The **male prostitutes** will submit to homosexual acts either as oral or anal inserters or receivers and even perform intercourse in the armpits (playing the bagpipes). The submammary fissures and intercrural folds are sometimes used.

TRIBADISM: Female homosexuality is known as tribadism, lesbianism or sapphism. According to Greek mythology, women of Isle of Lesbos practised this perversion.

Sexual gratification of a woman is obtained by another woman by simple lip kissing, generalised body contact, deep kissing, manual manipulation of breasts and genitalia, genital apposition, friction of external genital organs, sucking of breasts or external genitalia, etc. In some cases enlarged clitoris is used as organ of passion or some artificial penis or phallus may be used. The external genitals may show scratch marks, abrasions or teeth marks. **Many lesbians are masculine in type, possibly because of endocrine disturbances and are indifferent towards individuals of the opposite sex. The practice is usually indulged in by women who are mental degenerates or those who suffer from nymphomania (excessive sexual desire).** It is the result of interactions of biological, psychological, developmental and sociologic factors. It may lead to interference with young girls. Lesbians who are morbidly jealous of one another, when rejected may commit homicide, suicide or both. **Tribadism is not an offence in India.**

BESTIALITY: Bestiality is the sexual intercourse by a human being with a lower animal. The animals involved include those that are kept on the farm or as pets in households. **Because of their convenient size, animals like calves and sheep are more often involved. A few of larger birds like chicken, ducks and geese are also involved.** Other animals used are cows, mares, she-asses and bitches. **Vaginal intercourse is the most common,** but intercourse may take place through the anus or any other orifice, e.g., nose. This is seen in persons suffering from mental abnormality. Persons who go out to graze cattle in the fields may be excited when alone with the animals. Sometimes, the act is committed due to the false belief that gonorrhoea is cured by intercourse with a she-ass. Dogs and cats are the common animals for females. Usually the animal manipulates the genitalia with its mouth, and actual coitus is very rare. Both the accused and the alleged animal are to be examined.

Signs in the Accused: (1) Animal faeces, vaginal secretion or hair may be present on the penis. There may be tearing of the fraenum. (2) Marks of injuries on the body due to kicks, teeth or claws of the animal. (3) Presence of animal hairs especially of its external genitals on the person or the clothes. (4) Stains of dung or animal blood on the person or clothes.

Signs in the Animal: (1) Presence of human spermatozoa in the vagina or anal canal of the animal is a positive sign. (2) Abrasions and lacerations with effusion of blood on the external genitals. (3) Presence of gonorrhoeal discharges in the animal. It is better that the animal is examined by a veterinary surgeon.

Female Genital Mutilation (circumcision): Female sexual mutilation is done by: (1) Excision of prepuce with or without part of clitoris. (2) Excision of clitoris with partial or total amputation of labia minora. (3) **Excision of any part of external genitalia with narrowing of vulval introitus,** often through stitching. Typically, it occurs below ten years, but is done in all age groups in sub-saharan Africa and areas of Arabian peninsula. It is performed in Christians, Muslims, Jews and Atheists.

The procedure is a part of a religious practice of Dawood Bohra community. It is done most secretively when the girls are 5 to 6 years old called khatna. The community believes the clitoral head to be unwanted skin and a source of sin that will make women stray out of their marriage. The tradition aims to curb sexual drive in women and exert control.

Male Sexual Assault: Males are raped by other men by forcing to submit to anal intercourse, oral sex, masturbation of the offender and other sexual acts.

SEXUAL PARAPHILIAS

Paraphilias (Sexual perversions; Sexual deviations) are persistently indulged abnormal and unorthodox sexplay by using objects or parts of body, or fantasies in which complete satisfaction is sought and obtained without sexual intercourse. Perversions are acts which are socially prohibited or unacceptable, or biologically undesirable. The person must have experience in the perversion for a period of six months or more, and the behaviour must cause significant distress or impairment in social, occupational or other significant areas of the individual's functioning. The perverted behaviour is really a repulsively abnormal and frequently cruel form of tension release that by its nature tends to operate under compulsion. Most cases of sexual perversion involve early conditioning influences beyond the range of immediate knowledge. Sexual paraphilics are usually psychopaths suffering from mental aberrations and conflicts, sociosexual maladjustments, psychosexual imbalances and abnormalities. **The mental state of the accused should be determined in all such cases by a psychiatrist.**

URANISM: It is a general term for sexual perversions which includes sexual gratification by fingering, fondling, licking and sucking of the genitalia of opposite sex.

SADISM: (active algolagnia): (algos = pain; lognia = lust or craving). The term is derived from the name of a French nobleman, the Marquis de Sade, infamous for his crimes and writings. Many of his stories were about sexuality, cruelty, and torture. In sadism, **sexual gratification is obtained or increased from acts of physical cruelty or infliction of pain upon one's partner.** It is seen more commonly in men. To obtain sexual gratification the sadist may bite, beat, whip, produce cuts, cigarette burns, etc., or ill-treat or torture his sexual partner in many other cruel ways. Extremely sadistic attacks may be made in which the victim's nipples may be bitten off, articles such as a bottle, candle or sticks are inserted into the vagina, cigarettes or lighters may be used to burn the skin, or blows which may rupture internal organs or cause fractures. **It develops due to early experiences of brutality in relation to sex.** Many are sociopathic, some schizoid and others inadequate personalities.

LUST MURDER: In extreme cases of sadism, murder serves as a stimulus for the sexual act and becomes the equivalent of coitus, the act being accompanied by erection, ejaculation and orgasm. The typical lust murder is characterised by: (1) Periodic outbreaks, due to the patient's recurring compulsion or sudden outbursts of sexual desire. (2) Cutting or stabbing of the breasts, genitalia or the lower abdomen, usually with sucking, licking or mouthing of the wounds and biting of the skin. In some cases, there is desire to drink the blood and eat the flesh. (3) Erection and ejaculation may sometimes be followed by sexual intercourse with the dying or injured victim. (4) His behaviour is usually normal until the next outbreak. Many rape murders result from an aggressive sexual reaction to inner fear. **In true lust murders, mental disease is quite frequent.** Every murder committed during a sexual act is not a lust murder. The murder may be the result of anger, jealousy, revenge, etc.

NECROPHILIA: (philia = to defile or foul). In this condition, there is a **desire for sexual intercourse with dead bodies.** It is said to have sadomasochistic foundation and that decomposition, foul smell, and coldness act as stimulants. There is also no danger of rejection or resistance. **The offence is usually committed on a newly buried corpse or a body awaiting burial.** The corpse may be mutilated following intercourse. Murder for the purpose of necrophilia is very rare. **Necrophilia and necrophagia are punishable under S. 297, I.P.C. with imprisonment up to one year and/or fine.**

NECROPHAGIA: (necros = corpse; phagia = to eat): This is extreme degree of sadism in which the **person after mutilating the body, sucks or licks the wounds, bites the skin, drinks the blood and eats the flesh of his victim to derive sexual pleasure.**

MASOCHISM (Passive algolagnia): This term is derived from the name of Leopold von Sacher-masoch, an Austrian novelist. Being whipped by his wife used to be a stimulant for his literary work. **This condition is the opposite of sadism.** In masochism, **sexual gratification is obtained or increased by the suffering of pain**. Masochists get pleasure from being beaten, abused, tortured, humiliated, enslaved, degraded or dominated by their sexual partner, and they tend to place themselves repeatedly in self-defeating situations. Such painful stimuli may entirely replace the ordinary sex stimuli. It is usually found in males but it may be found in females, who may willingly expose themselves to the risks of severe bodily injury or murder at the hands of brutal husbands or lovers.

Sadism and masochism are rarely found in a pure state. They are usually found as a combination with one type dominant over the other. The combining of these practices is called **bondage.** They are found in all age groups and in all socioeconomic levels. The acts of cruelty or pain associated with sadomasochism may serve as a stimulant for, or as a complete substitute for sexual intercourse.

Algolagnia includes both sadism and masochism.

FETICHISM: A fetish is an abnormal stimulus or object of sexual desire. Fetichism means the use of such objects for sexual gratification. In this, recurrent, intense sexual fantasies, sexual urges or behaviour involving the use of living or non-living objects occur. In this, **the person experiences sexual excitement leading to orgasm from part of the body of a woman or some article belonging to her that normally has no sexual influence on the mind, e.g., underclothing, brassiere, petticoat, stocking, shoes, etc. which act as substitute for the female love object.** The fetish may be only incidentally associated with human body, e.g., a flower. In some cases, a picture of the fetish object provides sufficient stimulus. Sometimes, the act of stealing the articles provides adequate sexual satisfaction, though often the fetish article is stored to the satisfaction of the fetish, or touching it gives him sex pleasure, or he may masturbate into the object. **It is almost exclusively seen in males.** It is harmless, but rarely it may drive the person to obtain his fetish object through violence, or other criminal act, e.g., objects may be stolen, or women may be attacked either as part of robbery with violence, or because the fetish provides the trigger for rape or indecent assault.

TRANSVESTISM OR EONISM: The term is derived from the name of Chevelier d' Eon Beamont, a Frenchman, who preached this. A transvestite (trans = opposite; vesta = clothing) is a person whose **whole personality is dominated by the desire to be identified and thought of as a member of the opposite sex. His dress, manner, occupational interests and associations are all designed to increase his feeling of being a woman.** Sexuality with him is relatively unimportant, except as it promotes his feelings of feminity. There are varying degrees of transvestism. **It is usually found in the males who obtain sexual pleasure by wearing female dress.** Psychologically, it may depend upon an individual's erotic attraction for opposite sex. Only small percentage are homosexuals. Rarely, it develops out of a fetishistic interest in clothing or some part of opposite sex. **Many cases are associated with sadomasochism. There is no hormonal disturbance or genital abnormality.**

Transsexualists are persons who have an obsessional desire to become members of the opposite sex and seck surgery for anatomical alteration.

SEXUAL ORALISM: It is the obtaining of sexual pleasure from the **application of the mouth to the sexual organs.** It is seen both in heterosexuals and homosexuals. **Anilingus (rimming) is the kissing, licking and sucking of the anus by a sexual partner. Cunnilingus (mouth job) is the kissing, licking and sucking of a female's genitals by her partner.** During these procedures there may be repeated thrusting of the tongue over the mandibular incisors which may cause injury to the tongue or ulceration of the lingual frenulum. **Fellatio** (irrumination; blow job) is the **stimulation of the penis by the partner's mouth.** Non-consensual fellatio may result in bruising (petechial and confluent) on the soft palate and the junction between the soft and hard palates, laceration of the frenula and bruising and abrasion of the lips.

MASTURBATION: Masturbation (onanism: ipsation; autoeroticism) **is the deliberate self-stimulation which effects sexual arousal.** Mild masturbatory exercises are common both to men and women and are of little importance. **Techniques are largely manual, by moving the penis against a bed or other object.** Urethral insertions and anal stimulation and anal insertions are rare. Hollow articles like bottles, test tubes, etc., are sometimes used, or articles made of rubber and plastic which simulate the female genitalia are used.

In females, a finger is gently and rhythmically moved over clitoris or labia minora or steady pressure is applied over these parts with several fingers or whole hand. The genitalia may be rubbed against a pillow, a bed or some other object. Sometimes, women may insert fingers, wooden rods, glass tubes, metallic bars, bananas, etc., or dildo (object serving as an erect penis substitute) made of rubber or plastic into the vagina. Masturbation is an offence only when practised openly, e.g., in telephone booths, lavatories, etc.

EXHIBITIONISM: An exhibitionist is one who, over a period of six months or more, **experiences recurrent, intense, sexually arousing fantasies, sexual urges or behaviour, including the exposure of one's genitals to an unsuspecting stranger.** It usually occurs before adulthood. It is done mostly by males, often to children or the persons of the opposite sex. The pervert adopts a childish method of attracting attention to himself, to experience sexual gratification at the time of the exhibition, without physical contact. In some cases, the act is premeditated. Occasionally, women may expose themselves in public. Majority of them are psychopathic or suffer from compulsion neurosis and suffer from alcoholism, epilepsy, senile dementia, GPI, etc. **It is an obscene act punishable under** S. 294, I.P.C. with **imprisonment up to three months or fine.**

Flashing is the display of bare breasts by a woman with an up-and-down lifting of the shirt, blouse or bra, or a man exposing his genitals. **Mooning** is the display of bare buttocks by pulling down trousers and underwear. In either case, these may not be any sexual desire, but may be done for getting attention. Streaking is the act of taking off one's clothes and running naked through a public place. It is purely an attention getting act.

VOYEURISM OR SCOPTOPHILIA: It is the **counterpart of exhibitionism.** Voyeur (the socalled **Peeping Tom) is defined as one who, experiences recurrent, intense, sexually arousing fantasies, sexual urges or behaviours involving the act of observing an unsuspecting person who is naked, in the process of disrobing, or engaged in sexual activity.** Most often, the victim is a stranger. Masturbation at the scene or later to the memories of watching the unsuspecting stranger is normally the source of sexual pleasure. The onset is usually before the age of fifteen and may be chronic in nature. **This perversion occurs in case of severe sociopathic personality disorder.** To many males, observation of a female who is undressing may be erotically more stimulating than observing her when she is fully nude. Usually such persons do not commit a major sex crime, but sometimes they may assault the victim, or commit a murder. It is rare in females (S. 354, C.I.P.C.).

TROILISM: It is sexual practice involving 3 persons, 2 of one sex and one of the opposite sex. It is an extreme degree of voyeurism. **A perverted husband gets sexual satisfaction inducing his wife to sexual intercourse with another man and by watching the same.**

MIXOSCOPIA: It is a form of voyeurism in which **sexual gratification is obtained by the sight of others engaged in sexual intercourse.**

OEDIPUS COMPLEX: It is sexual desire of son towards his mother. **Electra complex** is sexual desire of daughter towards her father. **Pharoan complex** is sexual desire of brother towards his sister. Such persons are psychopaths with history of some mental trauma in the early life.

FROTTEURISM: Frotteurism (frottage; toucherism) is **contact with another person in order to obtain sexual satisfaction. Sexual satisfaction is obtained by rubbing his private parts against a female's buttocks, thighs, breasts or genital area in crowds.** Fantasy is an extensive component, i.e. they think that touching behaviour will not offend victims and also victims will find it pleasurable. If they attempt intercourse they have a premature ejaculation or they are impotent. It is an uncommon perversion often seen with other paraphilias. **It is punishable under** S. 290, I.P.C **with fine up to 200 rupees.**

PLAY PIERCING: Fig. (18–4) It is a form of sex play, often performed alone as a means of stimulating genitals. Disposable hypodermic needles are used, though pins, sewing needles or even nails may be used. The application of removable clips (often metal) may cause localised swelling or minor trauma. Hypodermic needles are frequently inserted into labia majora and minora, usually in large numbers bilaterally. Clitoris and prepuce are also involved (sado-masochistic experience).

BOBBIT SYNDROME: This is a type of perversion in which the female partner amputates the penis of her male partner with a sharp-cutting weapon.

Zoophilia: Sexual satisfaction is obtained from fondling of animals.

Undinism: In this the sexual pleasure is often obtained by witnessing the act of urination by some one of the same or opposite sex. In some cases pleasure is obtained by being urinated upon by the loved one or in urinating on him or her, but this is rare.

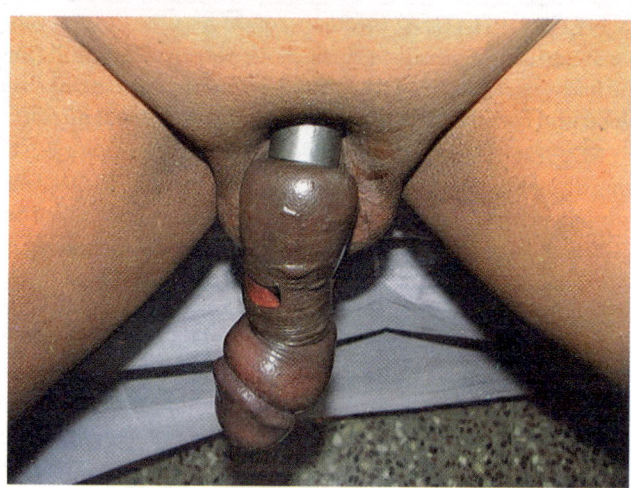

Fig. (18–4). Penile strangulation. Metallic ring seen at the base of penis in a case of sexual perversion.

Courtesy: **Dr K. Tamil Mani, Chennai**

Pyromania: In most cases of pyromania, there is an underlying psychosexual disorder. Some have a latent form of sadism, and others obtain sexual stimulation or satisfaction while seeing the flames and destruction of a building.

Caprolalia: Sexual excitement is obtained by using obscene language.

Caprolagnia: Sexual excitement is associated with sight or smell of faeces or defecation.

Urolagnia: Sexual excitement is associated with the sight or thought of urine or urination.

Narcism (Narcissism): Self-love, which may or may not include genital excitation.

Pygmalionism: It is falling in love with an object made by him.

Sexting: Transmitting sexually explicit messages or materials including nude photos and videos of themselves or others. It is punishable with imprisonment and fine.

Telephone Scatologia: Obscene telephone calls are made usually by heterosexual males, who call known or unknown females to carry out sexually provocative conversations.

SEMINAL FLUID

LEGAL ISSUES: Seminal stains have to be detected in cases of rape or attempted rape, sexual murder of the female, sodomy and bestiality. Fertility of the semen has to be proved in civil cases, e.g., disputed paternity.

CHARACTERISTICS: Semen is greyish-yellow, thick, jelly-like and sticky when fresh, and has a characteristic odour. The quantity of seminal fluid in a single emission is two to five ml. and contains about 60 to 150 million sperms per ml., of which 90% are motile at the time of ejaculation. Spermatozoa constitute about 10 to 20% of the volume of the semen. Semen contain lipids, fructose, proteins and a number of enzymes. Prostate secretes mainly acid phosphatase, spermin and zinc, while seminal vesicles secrete choline which help in identification of seminal fluid. The fluid is alkaline with a pH of 7.4.

The stains are usually found on the clothing, but may be found on the person of either the victim or the accused. They may also be found on bed clothes, on floor or on the grass where the offence was committed. Seminal stains have to be differentiated from those due to starch, pus, leucorrhoeal discharge and egg albumen.

COLLECTION OF MATERIAL: (1) Fluid from the vagina is collected with a pipette or throat swab inserted with or without the aid of a speculum, or vaginal washing is done, which is concentrated by centrifugation. (2) Dried stains could be removed by scraping with a clean scalpel blade. (3) Thin dried stain is collected with a wet throat swab. (4) A portion of cloth containing the stain is cut out, dried and preserved. (5) The pubic hair should be plucked and placed in a small

container. (6) Stains on smooth, impervious surface should be gently scraped off with the point of a knife into a glass container.

(I) PHYSICAL EXAMINATION: Seminal stains when dry have a greyish-white or yellow-grey colour and show an irregular, map-like outline. The cloth is stiffened as if starched. A fresh stain on a non-absorbent material appears translucent. After a month it becomes yellow to brown. When examined under filtered ultraviolet light, they show a fluorescence of a bluish-white colour (due to choline), which is not specific as other albuminous materials such as nasal, leucorrhoeal discharges and detergents also fluoresce. Fluorescence depends on choline of semen. It is masked by blood and disappears if the stain is soaked in water. Fresh stains have a characteristic odour.

(II) CHEMICAL EXAMINATION

(1) Florence Test: The stain is extracted by 10% hydrochloric acid, and a drop is placed on a glass slide and allowed to dry. A coverslip is placed over this, and a drop of Florence solution (potassium iodide, iodine, and water) is allowed to run under the coverslip. If semen is present, **dark-brown crystals of choline iodide appear immediately. They are rhombic or needle-shaped crystals resembling haemin but are larger, arranged in clusters, rosettes, crosses, etc.** Choline originates from the seminal vesicles. The test is not proof of seminal fluid, but only of presence of some vegetable or animal substance. A negative reaction is proof that the stain is not seminal.

(2) Barberio's Test: A saturated aqueous or alcoholic solution of picric acid when added to spermatic fluid produces **yellow needle-shaped rhombic crystals of spermine picrate.** The reaction probably depends on the presence of prostatic secretion.

(3) The Acid Phosphatase Test: The prostatic secretion element of seminal fluid contains 500 to 1000 times greater acid phosphatase than any other body fluid. Human red cells, semen of higher apes, and juice of cauliflower have acid phosphatase level similar to that of human semen. **Undiluted semen has an acid phosphatase activity of 340 to 360 Bodansky units or 2500 to 3500 Angstrom units per ml.** The concentration of acid phosphatase gradually falls with time in vaginal secretions, and positive reactions are found for periods of thirty six hours, with gradual disappearance in 72 hours, but is little changed if the body is refrigerated. 5 to 10 ml. of normal saline solution is placed in the vagina with a syringe. The fluid is then removed and placed in a sealed tube and refrigerated for enzyme examination. **Concentration in excess of hundred Bodansky units with or without motile sperms indicate that ejaculation occurred within twelve hours of examination. Dried seminal stains which have not undergone putrefaction retain acid phosphatase activity for weeks or months,** although enzymatic activity decreases slowly with time. The concentration is slowly reduced when the stain is left at room temperature and exposed to light. Heating of the specimen to 60°C. or over destroys it within five minutes. Low levels of acid phosphatase are present in vaginal secretions. In humans, acid phosphatase content is greater than in animals. **This test is conclusive in the absence of demonstrable sperms or in aspermia.**

(4) Creatine Phosphokinase: Spermatozoa contain a high concentration of creatine phosphokinase, which is more than double, than found in any other body fluid. Normal seminal fluid contains 385 to 1400 units of CPK/ml. **Levels over 400 are almost diagnostic of seminal stains.** The enzyme is stable and can be demonstrated even in old stains of six months.

(5) IMMUNOLOGICAL METHOD: MHS-5 produced from seminal vesicles and Mab 4 E6 can be detected on the sperm cells and in the ejaculated fluid. Prostate specific antigen (PSA, P30) is a glycoprotein produced by prostate and is found in seminal plasma (normal and aspermic semen), male urine and blood, but not in any tissues or fluid of the female. Undiluted semen contains 300 to 4200 μg per ml, with a mean of 1200 μg per ml. of PSA. It is found in vaginal fluid up to twenty seven hours after sexual intercourse, but sometimes may be detected up to forty seven hours. Tests for P_{30} have replaced the quantitative analysis for acid phosphatase. A positive PSA finding is a reliable indicator of semen, regardless of the presence of spermatozoa or elevated acid phosphatase level.

Fluorescent in situ hybridisation (FISH) has been suggested as a sensitive and specific test for detection of male epithelial cells in the post-coital vagina up to one week. Y-chromosome positive epithelial cells have been identified in vaginal swabs even in cases with no ejaculation.

(6) CHOLINE AND SPERMINE TEST: Liquid semen and dried seminal stains can be identified by a thin layer chromatographic technique. The test is based on the unique combination of choline and spermine which is present only in semen. Spermine is found in testes, pancreas, liver, spleen, brain, blood, bone marrow and body fluids, but its concentration is lower than in semen. One microlitre of semen present can be detected by this method.

Zinc (from prostate) is present in a concentration of 140 mg/ml in contrast to 1.2 mg/ml.

The sensitivity of detection and identification has been enormously enhanced by amplification techniques, such as PCR (polymerase chain reaction). Y chromosome short tandem repeat (STR) markers have been successfully used to analyse mixed stains with a male component.

After vasectomy, chemical and enzymatic tests for semen remain positive, though no sperms will be present.

(III) MICROSCOPIC EXAMINATION: A small piece of the stained fabric is moistened with a few drops of 1% hydrochloric acid or 3% acetic acid in a watch glass for half to one hour when the stains are fresh, or two to four hours when old. Dilute acids, bases and detergents can be used to free spermatozoa from dried seminal stains. **The central portion of the stain usually contains the largest number of sperms.** Slides are prepared by rubbing the piece of fabric on them. Films are dried in the air without heat or fixed for one minute in methyl or ethyl alcohol and then stained. The slide is stained with methylene blue for 15 to 30 minutes and counterstained with eosin for two minutes. **The posterior half to one-third of head is stained deep-red or pink, while the anterior half or two-third appears unstained or is faintly stained with basic dye. The tail is stained pink** Fig. (18–5). Alternatively, staining with haemalum two to five minutes, and eosin two to five minutes is satisfactory. **Old stains (even several years) may give positive results, but the older they are, the less is the chance of finding intact sperms. Complete sperms have been found on clean cotton material after five years.** In the vagina, sperms are continually removed by phagocytosis, lysis, agglutination or degeneration as a result of local physico-chemical reactions. The slide should be etched with a glass marking pencil. Human spermatozoa vary from **50 to 55 microns in length and consist of head, neck and tail. The head is oval and flattened when seen in front and pear-shaped in profile. It is five microns in length and three-and-half microns in its greater diameter. The neck is very short. The tail is long and tapered to a fine point. Sperms of**

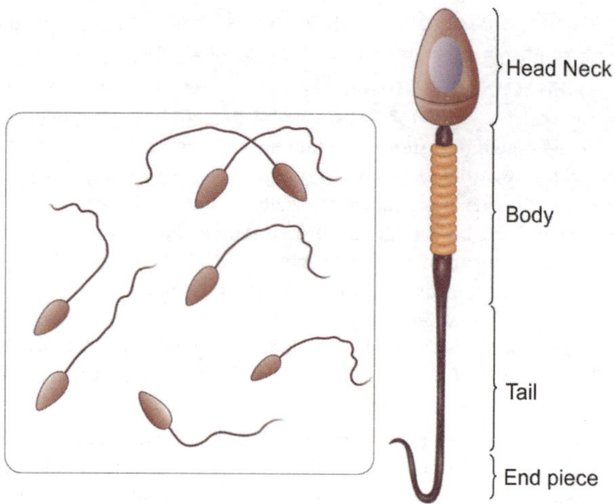

Fig. (18–5). **Human spermatozoa.**

various animal species differ in their morphology, even among closely related species.

Spermatozoa are easily found in stains that dry rapidly. The head resists decomposition for some time, and as such, few heads of spermatozoa may be found in decomposed stain. They undergo disintegration within a few months, but may be found up to five years. With an ultrasonic apparatus, maximum recovery of complete spermatozoa is readily obtained.

Motility of Sperms: A drop of mucus removed from vagina is placed on a glass slide, and diluted with a drop of normal saline and examined for motile spermatozoa. When semen is kept at room temperature, full motility persists for about three hours; 50% are motile by eight hours, and 10% for 24 hours. If the specimen is kept at body temperature, motility persists for several hours. **In living persons, motile sperms are usually seen up to six hours and rarely 12 hours after ejaculation into the vagina. Mobility of sperm in female genitalia is one to 4 mm per minute. Complete sperms are seen up to twenty six hours, and occasionally up to two to three days.** Then they separate into heads and tails. Broken sperms are found up to one week in vagina and cervix and up to one to two weeks in uterus. In the dead, sperms are destroyed by decomposition, but not by drainage or the action of the vaginal secretion. Willmott (1975) reviewed the literature and reported that sperm head had been found in the vagina up to nine days and in the cervix up to twelve days. In the anus, they have been found up to two days, and in the mouth up to nine hours after intercourse. After death intact sperms may be found up to two days in vagina, and one week in cervix and uterus.

Precipitin Test: Species identification can be done by precipitin test and personal identification can be done by DNA analysis.

Group of Seminal Fluid: The semen of the secretors contain ABO groups, PGM, AK, HLA, LDH, Gm, Km and GLO.

Enzyme typing: PGM and peep A found in semen and vaginal secretions are two enzyme markers commonly used in the genetic profiling of semen. PGM can be detected till 6 hours and peep A till 3 hours.

PROOF OF SEMEN: The only absolute proof of semen is the finding of at least one unbroken spermatozoon, or electrophoretic LDH isoenzyme detection of sperms. Positive identification of a sperm should not be made only on the basis of recognising "sperm head". In the absence of spermatozoa, a stain which gives characteristic fluorescence in ultraviolet light, positive precipitin test, high level of acid phosphatase and a high creatine phosphokinase and p30 can be considered to be due to semen.

In vaginal smear, bacteria, fungi, trichomonas, yeast, monilia, naked nuclei from vaginal epithelial cells and foreign substances are usually present, which may obscure or simulate sperm head or even entire spermatozoa. If there is any doubt whether some object in the smear is a sperm, the probability is that it is not.

Single photon fluorimetry has been used to differentiate between different semens. DNA amplification techniques, such as PCR and Y-chromosome short tandem repeat (STR) markers can separate and identify different semens.

CHAPTER

19

INFANT DEATHS

FM 2.27: Define and discuss infanticide, foeticide and stillbirth.
FM 2.28: Describe and discuss signs of intrauterine death, signs of livebirth, viability of foetus, age determination of foetus, DOAP session of ossification centres, hydrostatic test, sudden infants death syndrome and Munchausen's syndrome by proxy.
FM 3.29: Describe and discuss child abuse and battered baby syndrome.

Infanticide Act of England: According to the Infanticide Act of England (1938), **infanticide means the unlawful destruction of a child under the age of one year. Only the mother can be charged with the offence when the circumstances justify** it, such as when the infant is killed by its mother while suffering from disease of the mind (psychotic disturbance or depression) due to the effect of stress, associated with her pregnancy, delivery, puerperium or lactation. In such cases, the mother may not be held wholly responsible for killing the infant.

Law in India: **In India,** there is no such special Act, and as such **there is no distinction between the murder of newborn infant and that of any other individual.** **Foeticide** is the killing of the foetus at any time prior to birth. **Filicide** is the killing of a child by its parents. **Neonaticide** is the deliberate killing of a child within 24 hours of its birth. **Infanticide does not include the death of foetus during labour, when it is destroyed by craniotomy or decapitation.**

Motive: Infanticide is rare and usually committed by a young unmarried woman or widow. **Infanticide is usually committed at the time of, or within a few minutes or hours after the birth.** The alleged mother should be examined for signs of recent delivery and her mental condition should be noted.

Child: In case of the child, the points to be decided are: (1) Whether the child was stillborn or deadborn? (2) Whether the infant has attained viability or not? (3) Whether the child was born alive? (4) If born alive, how long did the child live? (5) What was the cause of death?

STILLBIRTH: **A stillborn child is one, which is born after twenty-eighth week of pregnancy, and which did not breathe or show any other signs of life, at any time after being completely born. The child was alive in utero, but dies during the process of birth.** Stillbirths occur more frequently among illegitimate and immature male children in primiparae. The incidence is about five percent. **It is common in obstructed labour due to contracted pelvis. Signs of prolonged labour,** i.e., oedema and bleeding into the scalp, a caput succedaneum, and severe moulding of the head indicate stillbirth, or death from natural causes shortly after birth. Squames and/or meconium within the alveoli does not indicate stillbirth. Meconium staining of the body merely indicates that foetal distress has occurred before or during delivery. Lungs are dark-red. **It is born in sterile condition, and as such, putrefaction occurs from without inwards,** whereas in case of newborn child which lived for some time, the bacteria inside the body may cause putrefaction to start in the abdomen.

Common causes of stillbirth are: prematurity, anoxia of various types, birth trauma especially intracranial haemorrhage due to excessive moulding, placental abnormalities, toxaemias of pregnancy, erythroblastosis foetalis, and many types of congenital defects.

DEADBIRTH: **A deadborn child is one which has died in utero**, and shows one of the following signs after it is completely born.

(1) Rigor mortis at delivery.

(2) Maceration Fig. (19–1): Maceration is a process of aseptic autolysis, and is the usual change. This occurs when the dead child remains in the uterus for about three or four days surrounded with liquor amnii but the exclusion of air. If air enters the liquor amnii after death of the foetus, putrefaction occurs instead of maceration.

Features: **The earliest sign of maceration is reddening or brownish-pink colour of skin with peeling and slippage, which can be seen in 12 hours after the death of the child in utero. Gas in great vessels (aorta in 12 hours) of foetus indicates foetal death (Robert's sign).** The surface is slimy,

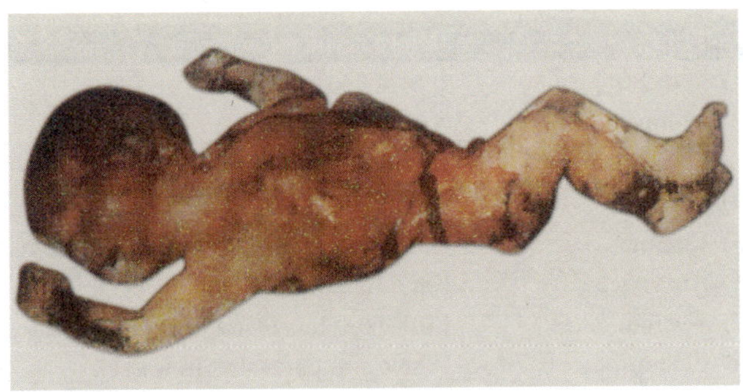

Fig. (19–1). Severely macerated foetus.

blistered, desquamated and rarely jelly-like. The body of a macerated foetus is soft, flaccid and flattens out when placed on a level surface. It has a sweetish, disagreeable odour. **Large blebs appear at 24 hours,** which contain a red serous or serosanguineous fluid. **The epidermis detaches easily** and leaves moist and greasy areas. The tissues are reddish due to haemolysis and oedematous. The abdomen is distended. The serous cavities may contain a turbid reddish fluid after 48 hours. **The bones are flexible and readily detached** from the soft parts. The joints become abnormally mobile. **All the viscera become soft and oedematous and lose their morphology, but lungs and uterus remain unchanged for a long time.** The umbilical cord is red, smooth, thickened and soft. The skull bones are separated and the brain has a greyish-red pulpy appearance. After several weeks, dehydration results in the formation of foetus papyraceus. Collapse of the vertebral column occurs. The placenta must be examined for infarcts as possible reason for foetal death.

Spalding's Sign: Loss of alignment and overriding of the bones of the cranial vault occur due to shrinkage of the cerebrum after death of the foetus. In the early stage, there is only loss of alignment without overriding. The sign will develop earlier with a vertex presentation than with a breech. **It may be detected within a few days (about 7 days) of death of the foetus, but often takes much longer time, sometimes even two to three weeks.**

(3) Mummification: Mummification occurs when the foetus dies from deficient supply of blood, when liquor amnii is scanty, and when no air enters uterus.

Viability of the Infant: Viability means the physical ability of a foetus to lead a separate existence after birth apart from its mother, by virtue of a certain degree of development. **A child is viable after 28 weeks of intrauterine life. In India, age of viability is not defined in law.**

The world's smallest baby boy was born on October 1, 2018 in Japan. As the mother was having hypertension, caesarean section was done after 24 weeks and five days of pregnancy. The baby weighed 258 grams with a length of 22 cm. Nearly seven months later he weighed over 2 kg. The smallest surviving girl was born in Germany in 2015, weighing 253 grams.

Livebirth: It means that **the child showed signs of life when only part of the child was out of mother,** though the child may not have breathed or completely born. The causing of death of such a child is regarded as homicide.

SIGNS OF LIVEBIRTH

Legal aspects: In civil cases, **any sign of life after complete birth of the child is accepted as proof of livebirth,** e.g., hearing a cry, seeing movement of the body or limbs, muscle contractions, etc. The muscles may twitch for some time after death, and therefore it is not safe to assume that twitching of muscles indicate life. A child may cry either in the uterus or in the vagina, which may be heard by bystanders or even outside the room of delivery. This occurs only when the membranes have ruptured and air has entered the uterus. The law presumes that every newborn child found dead was born dead until the contrary is proved. In criminal cases, **signs of livebirth have to be demonstrated by postmortem examination of the child.** Internal examination may provide strong, but not definite evidence of a livebirth.

Autopsy: External: Examine clothes and wrappings. Foot prints may be recorded. Determine the age. Examine for marks of violence. Foreign bodies may be found in mouth and upper respiratory tract. Eyes should be examined for icterus. Note the site, extent and character of caput succedaneum. Note evidence of malformation if any. Examine for evidence of birth injuries. Note the length of umbilical cord and whether it has been cut, torn or attached to placenta. Examine the cord for abnormal twists and knots. The region of umbilicus should be examined for signs of sepsis. If placenta is still attached record its measurements, weight and general appearance. If it is much smaller, it may be contributing factor in death. Disease of decidual vessels and extensive infarction may cause foetal death in utero.

Internal: (I) Shape of the Chest: Before respiration, the chest is flat and its circumference is one to two cm. less than the abdomen at the level of the umbilicus. **After respiration, the chest expands and becomes arched or drum-shaped.**

(II) The Position of the Diaphragm: The abdomen should be opened before the thorax, and the highest point of the diaphragm is noted, which is found about the level of fourth or fifth rib if respiration has not taken place, and at the **level of the sixth or seventh rib after breathing.** The position is affected by gases of decomposition.

(III) Lungs: Breathing causes important and permanent changes in the lungs, the extent of which depends on the physical strength and period of respiration Table (19–1).

(1) Volume: Unrespired lungs appear smaller, being collapsed on to the hilum when the thorax is opened. **Fully respired lungs fill the pleural cavities,** and the medial edges overlap the mediastinum and part of the pericardium.

Table (19–1). Difference in lungs before and after respiration

Trait	Before respiration	After respiration
(1) Weight:	1/70 of body weight.	1/35 of body weight.
(2) Volume:	Normal or small.	Larger, and cover the heart.
(3) Consistency:	Dense, firm, non-crepitant.	Soft, spongy, elastic, crepitant.
(4) Margins:	Sharp.	Rounded.
(5) Colour:	Uniformly reddish-brown or bluish-red.	Mottled or marbled appearance.
(6) Air vesicles:	Not inflated.	Inflated.
(7) Section:	Little frothless blood exudes on pressure.	Abundant frothy blood exudes on section.
(8) Floatation:	Whole and parts sink in water.	Expanded areas or whole float in water.

(2) Margins: Before respiration the margins are sharp, which become rounded even when the breathing is feeble. Feeble or brief respiration will affect only the margins. The edges of lungs including interlobar fissures are more rounded. In minimally respired lung, the anterior margin shows partial expansion; lingula, anterior or diaphragmatic margin and medial edge of lower lobe are sometimes pinker and more expanded than the posterior parts. Glistening bullae appear along the margins when there has been a struggle to breathe due to some mechanical obstruction.

(3) Consistency: Before respiration, the lungs are dense, firm, and non-crepitant like liver. After respiration they are soft, spongy, doughy, elastic and crepitant. The lungs are also crepitant in putrefaction and after artificial inflation.

(4) Colour and Expansion of the Air Vesicles: Before respiration, lungs are uniformly reddish-brown, bluish or deep-violet, according to the degree of anoxia. The surface of the lobules is marked with shallow furrows. On section, interior of the lung is uniform in colour and texture, and little frothless blood exudes on pressure. After respiration, the air cells become distended with air, usually about the anterior surfaces and margins, and then on the remaining portions of the lungs. As the air vesicles expand, they become raised slightly above the surface, and may be seen as polygonal or angular areas on the surface of the lung, giving it a fine mosaic appearance. As **the blood becomes aerated in the expanded area, the colour becomes a light-red, or pink, and the whole lung has a mottled or marbled appearance, with rose-coloured patches of expansion and aeration alternating with the collapsed dark bluish-red areas.** Even a single good breath can expand some of the foetal pulmonary tissues. Robust or prolonged breathing may lead to total expansion. If there is complete expansion of the lungs, they usually float and support the heart on the surface of the water. On section, frothy blood exudes from the cut surfaces on slight pressure. **Bloodstained froth in bronchi and bronchioles indicates that respiration has taken place.** Exposure to air will brighten the colour of the foetal lungs, but the air cells are not distended. Mottling is absent in artificially inflated lungs, and on section the exposed surface will exude little blood but no froth.

(5) Gas: If the air present is due to respiration, part of air will be expelled and will rise to the surface as a stream of minute dots. In putrefaction, bubbles of gas are seen under the pleura which can be moved from place to place by stroking with the finger. Interstitial blebbing indicates decomposition.

(6) Blood in the Lung Beds: The amount of blood in the lungs **after respiration is about twice that in circulation in the stillborn.**

(7) Weight: (a) Static Test or Fodere's Test: The lungs are ligated across their hila and separated. **The average weight of both lungs before respiration varies from 30 to 40 g., and after respiration from 60 to 66 g.** The increase in weight is due to the increased flow of blood.

(b) Ploucquet's Test: The blood flow in the lung beds is so increased after breathing that their **weight is almost doubled from 1/70 of the body weight before respiration to 1/35 after respiration.** The increase in weight is not constant and is not a reliable indication of breathing.

(8) The Hydrostatic Test (Raygat's test): It is based on the fact that on breathing, the volume of the lungs is increased, which more than compensates the weight of the additional blood, due to which their specific gravity is diminished. **The specific gravity of the lungs before respiration varies from 1040 to 1050, and after respiration about 940.** A ligature is tied on the bronchi, and lungs separated. Each lung individually is placed in water. If they float, each lung is cut into twelve to twenty pieces and placed in water. A small piece of liver may serve as control. If the liver floats, the test is of no value. **If these pieces float, they are each squeezed in between thumb and index finger under the surface of water, to see if any bubbles of air escape, and if they still persist to float,** or they are taken out of water, wrapped in a piece of cloth and squeezed by putting a weight to remove the tidal air. **The pieces are again placed in water, and if they continue to float, due to the presence of residual air, it indicates that respiration has taken place.** If the pieces sink after pressure, respiration has not taken place. If some pieces float while others sink, it shows feeble respiration. A small piece of liver may serve as control. **A piece of lung is rolled gently between the finger and thumb very near to the ear. A crackling crepitant noise indicates a significant degree of respiratory activity.** If the liver floats, test is useless. **The hydrostatic test is not of much value,** because the lungs of the liveborn who have lived for few days may sink, and the lungs of the stillborn may float. It can simulate a false sense of scientific validity.

Fallacies of hydrostatic test: The expanded lungs may sink from: (1) **Disease,** e.g. acute oedema, pneumonia, congenital syphilis, etc. (2) **Atelectasis** (non-expansion) of the lungs due to: (1) Air not entering the lungs due to feeble respiration, but aeration of lungs may occur through the mucosa of trachea and bronchi. (2) Complete absorption of air from the lungs by the blood, if circulation continued after stoppage of respiration. (3) More air being expelled from the lungs during expiration than what is inhaled during inspiration, if the respiratory movements are very feeble. (4) Obstruction by an alveolar duct membrane.

The unexpanded lungs may float from: (1) Putrefactive gases: The putrefied lungs are soft and greenish. Bubbles of gas may be seen on surface of the lung, which are large and not uniform, project considerably from the surface, and the gas in them can be pushed readily from place to place, and bubbles collapse on pricking. Signs of decomposition of the body will be seen. **(2) Artificial inflation:** The foetal lungs may be artificially inflated by blowing air through a tube, catheter or cannula passed into the trachea or by the mouth-to-mouth method. In such cases, the lungs can be inflated only partially and the stomach contains air but not intestines. They do not show marbled or mottled appearance. On section little blood and no froth exudes. External cardiac massage and administration of oxygen, completely negate its value.

Hydrostatic test is not necessary when: (1) The foetus is a monster. (2) The foetus is macerated or mummified. (3) The foetus is born before 180 days of gestation.(4) The stomach contains milk. (5) The umbilical cord has separated and a scar has formed.

Signs of the struggle to breathe: The victims of the "struggle to breathe" may be stillborn or they die shortly after delivery.

The gross changes in both the groups are similar. The sequence of changes, as the struggle to breathe develops is as follows: (1) Dark fluid blood (due to raised CO_2), haemoconcentration, "pseudo-clots". (2) Cyanosed, expanded lungs. Expansion due to (a) inhaled liquor amnii or vernix, (b) obstructive emphysema, (c) oedema with or without air or liquor amnii. (3) Tardieu's spots on pericardium, pleura and thymus. (4) Liver swelling due to congestion of whole lobule. (5) Distension of large bowel with meconium. (6) Ascites. (7) Retroperitoneal oedema.

Respiration Before and During Birth: A child may breathe: (1) while it is in the womb, after the rupture of the membranes **(vagitus uterinus)**, (2) while its head is in the vagina **(vagitus vaginalis)**, (3) while its head is protruding from the outlet. A child which has breathed in the uterus or vagina may die from natural causes, before it is completely born. Therefore, **proof of breathing is not proof of livebirth**. In the newborn child, the respirations may not be strong or deep enough to expand the air cells, and the child may live for some time on oxygen absorbed from the respiratory cells of the alveolar ducts. Some air may pass into the cells, but may not be sufficient to distend the fibrous tissue. This air may be subsequently absorbed by the blood, or may be lost. The child may live for many hours or even one or two days with only small portion of its lung tissue expanded. When the air cells have been distended once, they never return to the foetal condition. For the above reasons, the hydrostatic test fails in a small percentage of cases.

Microscopic Examination of the Lungs: Microscopic examination is of value in determining the extent of respiration, and the presence of pulmonary disease or abnormality, which may have caused or contributed to the death. The thoracic contents are removed intact by cuts with a scalpel by "no touch" technique of Osborn (1953), to eliminate artifacts. They are fixed for 48 hours and sections are taken of the whole lung in cross-sections. At four months pregnancy, the parenchyma of the lung has gland-like structure with a cuboidal or columnar cell lining. After fifth month, the air sacs contain amniotic fluid. The thin-walled adult type of alveolus is formed before full term. At full term, the normal foetal lung is almost completely atelectatic but many of its terminal bronchioles and vesicles are partly expanded by amniotic fluid. **The foetus towards term normally makes respiratory movements which fill the alveoli with amniotic fluid. This material is not stained with haemotoxylin and eosin, giving the impression that alveoli have been well expanded by air.** With respiration, the alveoli further expand and the fluid is partly expelled through the bronchi and partly absorbed back into the pulmonary circulation. It was thought that if respiration has not taken place, the alveoli appear as hollow gland-like structures lined by cuboidal or columnar epithelium. This is not correct, for the changes in the type of cell which lines the air sacs does not occur with the onset of respiration. **If the child has lived only for a few minutes, microscopy cannot always provide clear evidence of extrauterine respiration. Obstruction of the lower bronchial tree by hyaline duct membrane causes respiratory failure.** Its development and clinical features are obscure, but its presence is evidence that death is due to natural cause. The struggle to breathe may result in: (1) incomplete lung expansion, (2) suboxia and cyanosis, (3) petechial haemorrhages mainly subpleural, (4) oedema of the mediastinum and often of the lung.

Fallacies: Microscopic examination of the lungs is not helpful because in a child who has breathed, diffuse atelectasis may be seen, and in a stillborn child open apparently aerated alveoli. A gland-like appearance of the alveoli does not exclude livebirth but only indicates prematurity. Tardieu's spots may be present both in stillbirth and livebirth and also in bronchopneumonia.

Tests for foetal lung maturity are: lecithin, creatine and fat cells.

(IV) Changes in the Stomach and Intestines: Air is swallowed into the stomach during respiration. **The stomach and intestines are removed after tying double ligatures at each end. They float in water if respiration has taken place, otherwise they sink.** This is known as **Breslau's second life test, or stomach-bowel test.** This test is not of much value because air may be swallowed by the child in attempting to free the air-passages of fluid obstructions in cases of stillbirth. It is useless when there is decomposition.

In a stillborn child or one dying shortly after birth, the stomach will contain grey-white gastric mucin mixed with swallowed amniotic fluid. Sometimes, the infant may swallow maternal blood during delivery. **When dissected under water, the stomach shows mucus, saliva and air bubbles if respiration has taken place, and only mucus if breathing has not occurred. Blood, meconium or liquor amnii in the stomach indicate that the child was alive at or shortly before birth.** If milk is present in the stomach, it is a positive evidence that the child has lived for some time after birth.

(V) CHANGES IN THE MIDDLE EAR (Wreden's Test): Before birth, the middle ear contains gelatinous embryonic connective tissue but no air. With respiration, the sphincter at the pharyngeal end of eustachian tube relaxes and air replaces the gelatinous substances in few hours to five weeks. Middle ear must be opened under water by removing tegmen tympani. A bubble of air comes out if test is positive. This is not at all reliable.

Livebirth is probable when: (1) All the lobes of the lungs are fully expanded with or without obstructive emphysema. (2) There is oedema of the lungs, especially gross. (3) An alveolar duct membrane is present and has widespread distribution in the lungs. (4) Pulmonary atelectasis due to obstruction by an alveolar duct membrane is present. (5) Contusions of the lungs are present.

Stillbirth is probable in the presence of: (1) Maceration of the infant. (2) Flooding of the lungs with liquor amnii, and especially evidence of phagocytosis of meconium by the cells lining the air sacs. (3) Desquamation of bronchial epithelium. (4) Distention of large bowel with meconium indicating a struggle to breathe.

(VI) Changes in child after birth: Several changes occur in the child after birth, which are helpful in estimating the length of time the child lived after birth.

(1) Blood: Nucleated red cells usually disappear from the blood within 24 hours. Foetal haemoglobin (synthesised mainly in liver) which is about 80% to 90% before birth rapidly decreases to 7 to 8 percent at third month.

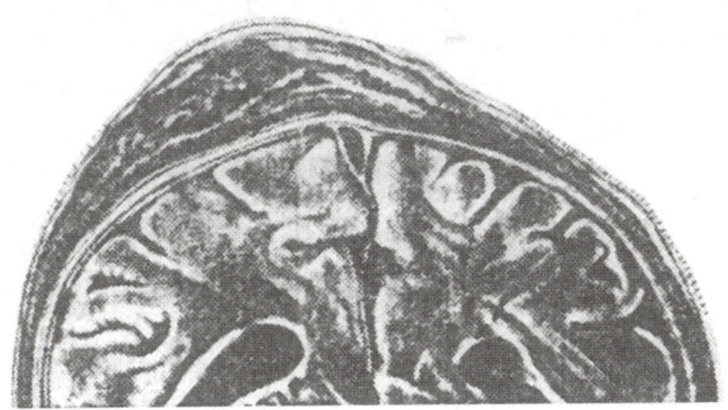

Fig. (19–2). Caput succedaneum.

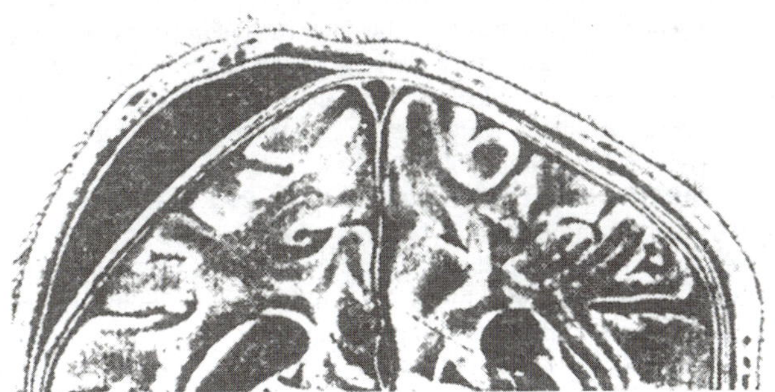

Fig. (19–3). Cephalhaematoma over the right parietal bone.

(2) Meconium: **It is the green viscid substance consisting of thickened bile and mucus. The meconium is completely excreted from the large intestine in the first 24 to 48 hours after birth, but in a breech presentation and also in severe anoxia, the meconium may be excreted completely before birth.** Meconium stains are brownish-green and stiffen the cloth. The reaction is acid.

(3) Caput Succedaneum Fig. (19–2): **This is an area of soft swelling that forms in the scalp over the presenting part of the head in vertex presentations. It is associated with head moulding.** The elevated rounded area of the caput succedaneum corresponds to the portion of the scalp surface that is exposed within the opening of the dilated cervix during labour. The scalp in the area of the caput is swollen to three to four times its normal thickness. **The localised area of oedema and congestion is due to local interference with venous return produced by the pressure of the rigid cervical ring.** Most commonly, the caput occurs asymmetrically over the crown of the head, in the parietal region. **With breech presentations, similar swellings occur over the buttocks and scrotum or labia.** The caput succedaneum gradually diminishes often disappearing within 2 to 4 days after birth.

Cephalhaematoma: **This is a localised accumulation of blood deep to the scalp, between the periosteum and bone surface.** It is caused by tearing of diploic veins due to mechanical trauma. It has been associated with higher birth weight and instrumental delivery**. The haematoma is limited to the periosteal sheath of single bone, commonly the right parietal bone, and never crosses a suture line.** Cephalhaematoma is rare, occurring in less than one percent of newborns, and **varies in size from one to 5 cm.** The haematoma swelling often tends to increase during the first day or two after birth, as more and more blood accumulates, It shows the usual colour changes common with the bruises and disappears in about 15 days. Neonatal jaundice may be increased because of the extra load of blood pigment Fig. (19–3).

(4) Skin: At first skin is bright-red, which becomes darker on second or third day, then brick-red, yellow and normal in about a week. **Physiological jaundice is seen by third day** due to relative insufficiency of enzymes required for conjugation and excretion of bilirubin. Vernix caseosa covers the skin, mostly in the axilla, inguinal region and folds of the neck, buttocks and persists for one or two days. Sometimes it may be absent at birth and it is removed by washing. **Vernix caseosa is a white cheesy substance consisting of sebaceous secretion and epithelial cells. It protects foetal skin against maceration while in liquor amnii.** The skin of the abdomen exfoliates during the first three days after birth.

(5) Air in G.I. Tract: Air moves along the gastrointestinal tract at the same speed in full term infants as in premature ones. **The air reaches stomach after fifteen minutes; small intestine after one or 2 hours;** colon after 5 to 6 hours; and rectum after 12 hours. Bacterial gas formation and resuscitation attempts may be a source of error.

(6) Umbilical Cord: The blood clots in the cut end 2 hours after birth, and the vessels begin to be closed in about 24 hours. **The cord attached to the child shrinks and dries in 12 to 24 hours,** but this appearance is also seen in the body of a stillborn infant, and an **inflammatory ring forms at its base in 36 to 48 hours. It mummifies on second or third day.** Mummification of the cord also occurs after death if exposed to air but does not occur if the child is submerged in water immediately after birth. **The cord falls off on the fifth or sixth day and leaves an ulcer, which heals and forms a scar in 10 to 12 days.**

Placenta: If a placenta is found with the body, it should be examined. If placenta is absent, the length of the remaining umbilical cord should be measured. Examine the cord to see whether a ligature has been applied and to know whether it has been cut or torn. **A torn cord is usually ragged.**

(7) Circulation: Contraction of the umbilical arteries starts in about ten hours and are completely closed by third day. The umbilical vein and ductus venous are closed on the fourth day. The ductus arteriosus closes by tenth day, and foramen ovale by second or third month.

CAUSES OF DEATH: (I) NATURAL CAUSES: (1) Immaturity. (2) Debility due to lack of general development. (3) Congenital diseases, e.g. syphilis and specific fevers, such as smallpox, plague, etc. affecting the mother, or disease of the child's internal organs, such as lungs, heart, brain, etc. (4) Malformations. (5) Haemorrhage from the umbilical cord, genital organs, stomach, rectum, etc. (6) Post-maturity. (7) Pre-eclamptic toxaemia. (8) Disease of the placenta or its accidental separation from the uterine wall. (9) Placenta praevia or abnormal pregnancy. (10) Neonatal infection. (11) Intrapartum or antepartum anoxia. (12) Cerebral birth trauma. (13) Erythroblastosis.

(II) UNNATURAL CAUSES: These may be: (1) Accidental, and (2) Criminal.

(I) ACCIDENTAL CAUSES: (A) DURING BIRTH: (1) PROLONGED LABOUR: Severe compression of the head against contracted or deformed pelvis may cause intracranial haemorrhage and death with or without fissured fracture of the parietal bones of the skull. Extradural haemorrhage is rare. Subdural haemorrhages are common and usually bilateral. They are usually caused by rupture of the bridging veins, but may also occur less commonly from tears of the falx cerebri.

Rarely, haemorrhages occur from ruptures of the internal or great cerebral veins. Tentorial tears may be bilateral and haemorrhage occurs into the subdural space either above or below the tentorium. In such cases, the head of the child shows evidence of well-developed moulding and caput succedaneum. Fractures and dislocations of the limb bones and clavicles may be found.

(2) PROLAPSE OF THE CORD OR PRESSURE ON THE CORD: They produce death by asphyxia. The cord is liable to be compressed by the foetal head, especially in breech presentations. On postmortem examination, blood, meconium, liquor amnii or vernix caseosa may be found in the bronchial tubes.

(3) TWISTING OF THE CORD ROUND THE NECK OR KNOTS OF THE CORD: It causes compression but no abrasions or ecchymoses and cause death by strangulation.

(4) INJURIES TO THE MOTHER: Heavy blows or kicks on the mother's abdomen or falls from a height may cause concussion of the brain of the child with or without fracture of skull or rupture of blood vessels or organs. Rarely, powerful uterine contractions may fracture the cranial bones of the foetus.

(5) DEATH OF THE MOTHER: The child can be saved if it can be delivered within five to ten minutes of the mother's death.

(B) AFTER BIRTH: Suffocation: It may result when the membranes cover the head during birth, or if the face is pressed accidentally in the cloth or submerged in the discharges, such as blood, liquor amnii or meconium. A child can survive in the membranes for 20 to 30 minutes.

PRECIPITATE LABOUR: Labour terminating in a very short time than that taken on the average, either in a primipara or multipara is called precipitate labour. **In this delivery occurs suddenly and rapidly without the knowledge of the mother. All the three stages of labour are merged into one. The foetus is normal or premature. It is possible in multiparae with large roomy pelvis, but is extremely rare in primiparae.** A woman may be delivered unconsciously during fits or periods of coma, hysteria, hypnosis, under the influence of narcotic drugs, anaesthetics, and even deep drunkenness. It is highly improbable that any primiparous woman would be delivered during ordinary sleep without being aroused. **Sometimes, a woman may not be able to distinguish the sense of fullness produced by the descent of a child from the feeling of bulky evacuation. The child may die from (1) suffocation** by falling into a lavatory pan, **(2) head injury** and fracture of the skull with subdural haemorrhage often bilateral, by a fall on a hard floor, if the woman was standing, and **(3) haemorrhage from the torn end of the cord.**

If the birth occurs in the toilet bowl or into a bucket containing liquid, the infant will inhale the liquid and blood, and meconium and vaginal mucus are found in the air-passages. Microscopic examination of the lungs will show the foreign particles contained in the drowning fluid. In accidental falls, the haemorrhages are usually subdural and often bilateral. The average length of the cord is 50 cm. which is not sufficient to allow the child to fall to the ground, and is sufficiently strong to withstand the weight of the foetus without breaking. **The cord is torn most commonly at the foetal end than the placental end, but is not torn in its middle or the placenta is expelled with the child. Caput succedaneum and moulding of the head are absent.** Foreign materials, such as mud, sand, gravel may be found in the hair or injured scalp of child. The fractures of the skull are usually fissured and limited to parietal bones, but may extend to frontal and squamous part of temporal bones Table (19–2). Fractures due to forceps lie at points normally gripped by the instrument and are usually "gutter" or "pond" type.

Medicolegal Importance: (1) The mother or her relatives may be accused of killing the infant, while the death may be due to injury, haemorrhage or asphyxia from precipitate labour. (2) In a case of murder, death of the child may be attributed to precipitate labour.

(II) CRIMINAL CAUSES: These may be (1) acts of commission, and (2) acts of omission.

(A) ACTS OF COMMISSION: They are acts done positively to cause the death of the infant. Numerous injuries may be found on the body, especially around the face, head and neck, due to attempts at self-delivery. There may be multiple circumferential abrasions around the whole surface on the neck caused due to fingernails. They should not be mistaken for homicide.

(1) Suffocation: The child's nose is closed with two fingers and the lower jaw is pushed up with the palm to occlude the airway. Other methods are placing a pillow or towel over the child's face and pressing down, or pushing the face down into bedclothing. The amount of force to produce smothering is so minor that there is no evidence of trauma. Overlaying, or forcing mud, rag or cotton-wool into the mouth are other methods.

(2) Strangulation: Throttling or strangulation by ligature is also common, and in the latter case the ligature is frequently left *in situ*. Sometimes, umbilical cord is used as a ligature to simulate accident. Abrasions on the neck may be caused by the frantic efforts of the mother to deliver herself.

(3) Drowning: It is rare, but the body of a dead foetus may be thrown into a well, tank, etc.

(4) Burning: Infanticide by burning is rare, but it may be used as a mode of disposal.

(5) Blunt head injury: Dashing the head against a wall or the floor by holding the feet is rare. In such cases, there may be bruising of the ankles and feet, where they were firmly gripped. Blows on head may be produced with a blunt weapon. Subdural and subarachnoid haemorrhages are common and are usually accompanied by fractures (depressed or comminuted) of the skull and contusions and lacerations of the brain and scalp. In infants, extradural haemorrhages are limited to single bones because of the adherence of the dura to the skull along the suture lines.

(6) Fractures and dislocation of cervical vertebrae: These may be caused by twisting the neck.

(7) Wounds: The child may be killed by stabs, incised wounds, cut-throat, etc.

(8) Poison: Rare

(B) ACTS OF OMISSION OR NEGLECT: A woman is guilty of criminal negligence, if she does not take ordinary

Table (19–2). Difference between head injury due to labour and blunt force

Trait	Head injury due to labour	Head injury due to blunt force
(1) Bruises:	May be present on the presenting parts of the scalp.	Found anywhere on the scalp.
(2) Lacerations:	Not present on the scalp.	Present on the scalp.
(3) Fractures:	Fractures are fissured; usually of parietal bones and run downwards at right angles to the sagittal suture.	Extensive comminuted and depressed fractures of the skull bones affecting vault or base.
(4) Brain:	Usually not injured.	Contusions, lacerations and haemorrhage.

precautions to save her child after birth. The following acts of omission amount to crime. (1) Failure to provide proper assistance during labour may cause death by suffocation or head injury. (2) Failure to clear the air-passages which may be obstructed by amniotic fluid or mucus. (3) Failure to protect the child from exposure to heat or cold. (4) Failure to supply the child with proper food. (5) Failure to tie the cord after it is cut usually does not cause death by haemorrhage. Tearing of the cord within the uterus during delivery may cause massive haemorrhage and foetal death.

THE ABANDONING OF INFANTS: (1) If the father or mother of a child under the age of twelve years, or anyone having the care of such child, leaves such a child in any place with the intention of abandoning the child, shall be punished with imprisonment up to seven years. (2) If the child so exposed or abandoned is a girl child, the person doing so, shall be punished with rigorous imprisonment for a term which may extend to ten years and shall also be liable to fine which may extend to one lakh rupees (Sec. 317, I.P.C.).

CONCEALMENT OF BIRTH: (1) Whoever, secretly buries or otherwise disposes off the dead body of child, whether such child dies before or after or during its birth, intentionally conceals the birth of such child, shall be punished with imprisonment up to two years. (2) If the child whose dead body is so disposed off is of a girl child, the person committing such offence shall be punished with rigorous imprisonment for a term which may extend to 2 years or fine or both (Sec. 318, I.P.C).

CHILD ABUSE: Child abuse is the physical, sexual or emotional mistreatment or neglect of a child. It can occur in child's home, or in the organisations, schools or communities the child interacts with.

Types: (1) Child neglect, (2) emotional and psychological abuse, (3) sexual abuse, (4) physical abuse, (5) chemical abuse (intentional poisoning).

BATTERED BABY SYNDROME OR NON-ACCIDENTAL INJURY OF CHILDHOOD: It is also known as child abuse syndrome, Caffey's syndrome, and maltreatment syndrome in children. The typical form of this condition is very rare in India. **A battered child is one who has received repetitive physical injuries as a result of non-accidental violence, produced by a parent** or guardian. In addition to physical injury, **there may be non-accidental deprivation of nutrition, care and affection.**

Classical features: The classical features of syndrome are **obvious discrepancy between the nature of the injuries and explanation offered by the parents, and delay between the injury, and medical attention which cannot be explained. The constant feature is repetition of injuries at different dates, often progressing from minor to more severe.**

Features: (1) **Age**: Usually less than three years old, though it may occur at any age. (2) **Sex**: Slightly more in males (55 to 63%). (3) **Position in family**: One child of a family, commonly the eldest or the youngest and often unwanted, such as the result of pregnancy before marriage, failure of contraception or an illegitimate child. (4) **Socio-economic factors**: Parents tend to be young between 20 to 30 years, and belong to lower social class and lower education. The family is usually isolated. There is often a history of family disharmony, long-standing emotional problems or financial problems. Many of the fathers have criminal records, or unemployed or socially unstable. Many mothers have multiple social and psychiatric problems with a chaotic and violent home background. The mother is of lower I.Q., often pregnant or in the premenstrual period at the time of battering. Unhappy childhood experiences are common in both parents and many battering parents were "battered children" themselves. Most of the parents suffer guilt-amnesia. (5) **History**: There is obvious difference between the nature of the injuries and the explanation given by the parents, which may change on several times of repetition, each time the child is taken to a different doctor. (6) **Treatment:** There is always delay between the injury and medical attention. (7) **Precipitating factors**: Violence is precipitated by actions of the child itself, e.g., crying, refusal to be quiet, persistent soiling of napkins, etc.

INJURIES: Direct manual violence is the commonest method of injury. SURFACE INJURIES: Soft tissue injuries are very common and may be seen almost anywhere on the child's body. The head, face and neck show bruises, abrasions and lacerations of different ages. Multiple bruises are seen on brows, cheeks, mouth and neck. Laceration of the mucosa inside the upper lip, often tear of the fraenulum is the most characteristic lesion. This may extend laterally and separate the inner surface of the lip from the base of the gums. This injury results from a blow on the mouth or due to other efforts to silence a screaming or crying child. Multiple bruises of various ages all over the body from rough handling, beating, kicking or throwing the infant are common. Bruises may be seen on either side of the chest, behind the axillae and down the anterior chest wall, where the child has been gripped roughly, between two adult hands and shaken. Caffey (1974) described the effects of shaking a child as a major cause of subdural haematoma and intraocular bleeding in battered babies, the so-called "infantile whiplash syndrome". Recent research has thrown doubt on the common acceptance of this mechanism. Some pathologists believe that impact to the head is necessary. In such cases, bruises are produced in areas where the child is held by the hands, but there are no external injuries to the head or fractures of the skull, but there may be traction lesions of the periosteum of the long bones without fracture. Permanent brain damage may be caused due to habitual, prolonged shaking. BITE MARKS may be found on the cheeks, shoulders, chest, abdomen, arms, legs and buttocks. Bruises are usually present around the elbows and knees due to gripping of the child, so as to shake or pull him, or hurl him into cot or against furniture, etc. Slap marks may show clear lines of petechial haemorrhages. Knuckle punches show as rows of three or four roughly round bruises. Bruising caused by belts, straps, canes, pieces of wood, hair brushes may be seen frequently on the buttocks and thighs. Pinch marks may appear as butterfly-shaped bruises with one wing caused by thumb larger than the other. Subgaleal haematoma resulting from vigorous pulling on the scalp is characteristic. Bald patches on the scalp due to pulling out the hair (traumatic alopecia) is very characteristic. EYES: Retinal separation, lens displacement, retinal haemorrhages, vitreous haemorrhages, subconjunctival haemorrhages, and subhyaloid haemorrhages and black eye have been found. VISCERAL INJURIES: Subdural haemorrhage is found in about 40% of fatal cases. Crushing or compressing force applied to the abdomen produce either "bursting" injuries of the liver or spleen, or perforations of distended hollow viscera including the stomach, intestine or urinary bladder. The second part of the duodenum and jejunum may be completely transected. Deceleration or whipping forces produced by punches or blows, tear the mesentery and can lead to disruption of the small intestine. Extensive internal injuries may be present with minimal external signs of injury. BURNS: Stubbing of cigarette ends upon the skin produce small circular, pitted burns which are pink or red when fresh. When healing, they tend to be silvery in the centre with a narrow red rim. The child may be made to sit upon a hot stove or electric radiator or he may be dipped in very hot fluids. SKELETAL INJURIES: Skull fractures are common. in occipito-parietal area. The fractures are multiple, depressed and wide. Large periosteal haematomas are common because periosteum is readily stripped in infants. Bleeding under the periosteum causes calcification, which is seen on X-ray as an extra line of opacity running alongside the affected length of bone. The violent forces applied to the limbs involve pulling and twisting, both capable of producing epiphyseal

separation and periosteal shearing. Transverse and spiral fractures of long bones result from compression, bending and direct forcible blows. Anteroposterior compression of the chest causes fractures of ribs in midaxillary line. Violent squeezing of the chest from side to side causes fractures at the costochondral junctions. Multiple rib fractures also occur along the posterior angles of the ribs. After one to two weeks, callus is formed, and on X-ray" a string of beads " appearance is seen in the paravertebral gutter (NOBBING FRACTURES). Avulsion of the metaphyses or chipping of the edges of the metaphyses or epiphyses may occur, with small fragments seen isolated on X-ray. Before autopsy, a whole body X-ray should be taken to detect old fractures and especially metaphyseal and epiphyseal injuries in various stages of healing. Head injury is the most common cause of death followed by rupture of an abdominal organ.

DIAGNOSIS: **The diagnosis depends upon (1) nature of injuries, (2) time taken to seek medical advice, and (3) recurrent injuries. Differential diagnosis has to be made from scurvy, congenital syphilis, osteomyelitis, leukaemia, rickets, juvenile osteoporosis with stress fractures, paralytic disease with fractures, infantile cortical hyperostoses and osteogenesis imperfecta. Radiological manifestations of trauma and especially the metaphyseal lesions are specific to the battered baby syndrome (Hospital addiction syndrome).**

MUNCHAUSEN'S SYNDROME (Hospital addiction syndrome): Munchausen syndrome is feigning illness or injury by adults and going from hospital to hospital for unnecessary investigations and treatment. These patients appear to be compulsively driven to make their complaints. The person is aware that he is acting an illness, but he cannot stop the act. There is continuity, ranging from exaggerated claims of infirmity to actual self-induced illness. It is a psychiatric factitious disorder, wherein those affected feign disease, illness or psychological trauma to draw attention, sympathy or reassurance to themselves.

MUNCHAUSEN'S SYNDROME BY PROXY (MSbP): This term is used to describe the **actions of one person (usually mother) who inflicts harm against another person (usually an infant or small child) in an attempt to gain sympathy and attention for both her own and child's suffering.** It is a variation which is a peculiar and dangerous type of child abuse usually involving the mother, in more than 90% cases, in which children are brought to doctors for induced or fabricated signs and symptoms of illnesses with a fictitious history. The sex ratio is almost equal. It has been described in children of few weeks of age to 16 years, but is most common in the first two years of life. More than 50% mothers have personal abnormal illness behaviour in the form of factitious or somatoform disorder. **Often the parental illness alternates with that of the child; the self-injurious behaviour of the parent may wax and wane as the factitious illness of the child waxes and wanes. The child is admitted frequently in the hospital for medical evaluation for the non-existent conditions.** At the extreme end, life-threatening injuries are masqueraded as being legitimately contracted. Rosenberg (1989) gave four diagnostic criteria: (1) Illness produced or alleged, or both by a parent. (2) Repeated requests for medical care of a child, leading to multiple medical procedures. (3) Parental denial of knowledge of the cause of symptoms. (4) Regression of symptoms when the child is separated from the parents.

Method of simulation or production of illnesses: (1) The mother pricks her finger and adds blood to the urine of the child and takes the sample to the doctor. (2) The child's nose is closed with two fingers and the lower jaw pushed up with the palm to block the airway. (3) A pillow or towel is put over the face of the child and the face is pushed down into bed clothing.(4)The mother gives insulin to the child and takes to hospital with hypoglycaemia. (5) Vomiting: allegation or by ipecacuanha. (6) Diarrhoea: laxatives, salt poisoning. (7) Convulsions: allegation or by theophylline, insulin, psychotropic drugs. (8) Bleeding: anticoagulants, phenolphthalein poisoning, exogenous blood. (9) CNS depression: barbiturates, benzodiazipines. (10) Fever: alleged. (11) Rash: scratching or intoxication.

Fabrication may impact child's physical and emotional development.

SUDDEN INFANT DEATH SYNDROME

Sudden infant death syndrome (SIDS), or **cot death or crib death** is defined as the **sudden and unexpected death of seemingly healthy infant, whose death remains unexplained even after thorough case investigation,** death scene examination, review of clinical history and complete autopsy.

Features: (1) **Incidence:** 0.6 per thousand livebirths. (2) **Age:** 2 weeks to 2 years, but most deaths take place between one and 7 months, with a peak at 2 to 4 months. (3) **Sex:** There is slight increase in males. (4) **Twins:** There is increased risk (threefold) amongst members of a twin pair. Most twins are premature and of low birth weight. (5) **Geographical distribution:** The occurrence is worldwide. (6) **Time of death:** Death always occurs during sleep at all times of night with a moderate increase in the early morning hours. (7) **Prematurity** has a higher risk. (8) **Socio-economic** standard of the family is usually low. (9) **Cigarette smoking and drug abuse** by pregnant women increase the risk.

The child is either quite well when put to the bed, or may have only a minor upper respiratory tract infection (cold or snuffles), or minor gastrointestinal disturbance. **Cot deaths are major cause of death in infants in the first six months of life.**

AUTOPSY: **In about 15% of cases, some pathological condition may be found, such as frank pneumonia, congenital heart disease, Down's syndrome or a tracheobronchitis. The only constant findings are multiple petechial haemorrhages on the visceral surfaces of the heart, lungs and thymus (70 to 75%), which are agonal in nature, perhaps from terminal respiratory efforts against a closed glottis. Bloodstained fluid at the mouth and nose is present in about 50% cases. A small amount of milky vomit in the trachea and main bronchi, and shedding of individual tracheobronchial epithelial cells are commonly found. Many infants show froth in the air-passages and facial pallor. Petechial haemorrhages in the face or eyes may be seen. The hands are often clenched around fibres from the bed clothes. The lungs show patchy or uniform purplish discolouration of the surface and are firm in consistency with congestion, oedema, patchy alveolar collapse and increase in weight. The alveolar walls are thickened and are infiltrated with lymphocytes and occasional neutrophils and monocytes. Peribronchiolar cell infiltration is the main finding. Laryngitis, tracheitis, bronchitis, bronchiolitis, pneumonitis and pleuritis either individually or in various combinations may be found. In the majority of cases, the extent of the pathology present is rarely sufficient to cause death. It is a diagnosis of exclusion. Chemical examination of viscera and laboratory examination should be carried out.**

Theories: Various theories have been advanced, but **there is no single cause of cot death, and death may result from a number of causes which combine and act via a common pathway of cardiorespiratory failure, while a child is passing through a vulnerable period of development.** Probable mechanism of deaths may be due to electrolyte imbalance, conductive disorders, respiratory distress laryngospasm metabolic disorders, overlaying, viral infection, prominent tracheobronchial secretions.

CHAPTER

20

BLOOD STAINS

FM 3.20: Discuss disputed paternity and maternity.

Collection of Blood Stains: (1) A clean piece of white filter paper or a piece of clean white cloth or gauge or cotton swab may be used, allowing blood to soak into it, then drying it at room temperature. A control filter paper, etc. should also be sent for examination. (2) If the object is porous, a portion of unstained area should also be taken. (3) If the object is non-porous and particularly if it is metallic, stains can be removed by scraping and placed in small glass containers. They should not be placed in envelopes where they will be reduced to powder. (4) Stains on clothing may be scraped off or a fragment of the material cut. (5) If blood is liquid, a sample can be pipetted and placed in a bottle and refrigerated.

Solvents: The solvents for blood stains are: (1) 10% solution of potassium cyanide. (2) 10% solution of glycerine in distilled water. (3) A weak solution of ammonia. A coloured solution is obtained immediately with any of the above solvents. Otherwise, the material must be covered and left for from 12 to 24 hours at room temperature.

Preservation of Blood Stains: The stained article is allowed to dry at room temperature. No extra heat should be used as this will cause deterioration of the stain. **If the stained clothes are not dried, putrefaction sets in, and it becomes difficult or impossible to know whether the blood is of human or animal origin.** The stained object should be identified by initializing the object and dating it. If this is not possible, a tag or other device will have to be identified and attached. **For packing bloodstained articles, polythene bags or air-tight containers must be avoided,** because the residual moisture may get trapped and give rise to bacterial growth leading to destruction of the stains. **Each garment should be wrapped separately and should not come in contact with other clothing. While folding the garment, care should be taken to avoid two stains touching each other, as they could belong to two different sources. A clean paper should be kept between each stain.**

All kinds of stains should be sent to the State Forensic Science Laboratory for examination.

SUBSTANCES RESEMBLING BLOOD STAINS

(1) RUST STAINS: On knives and steel weapons they resemble dried blood stain, but they do not have a dark and glazed appearance and do not fall off in scales, when the opposite side of the blade is heated. They do not stiffen the cloth, and are soluble in dilute hydrochloric acid. Tests for iron are positive.

(2) SYNTHETIC DYE STAINS: They are changed to yellow by nitric acid, and the original colour is restored by a strong solution of alkali.

(3) MINERAL STAINS: They generally contain oxides of iron, red lead or red sulphide of mercury.

(4) VEGETABLE STAINS: Certain fruits, e.g., mulberry, gooseberry, currants, jambans, etc., produce stains which resemble blood stains. On microscopic examination, vegetable cells and detritus are seen. Henna, catechu, *pan juice,* tobacco, and the barks, leaves and fruits of some trees produce red stains resembling blood stains. Most of them contain tannin, which becomes black if a drop of ferric chloride is added.

(5) OTHER STAINS: Spots of grease, resin, tar and pitch especially on dark fabrics may resemble old blood stains. The tests for blood are negative.

STAINS ON CLOTHING: In the case of clothing, type of garment, its colour and consistence should be noted and if the garment is torn, the position of the tears should be noted. Whether the clothes were dry, damp or wet when received should be noted. Both the outer and inner surfaces of the garments should be examined. The position of all stains should be given correctly by a description of the stain in its relation to the manner in which a garment is usually worn, e.g., a stain on the trousers should be described as being above, behind, or to the outer side of the knee. Stains may also be described in relation to the pockets, the buttons, or the seams of a garment. The size and the shape of the stain should be noted. If the stain is in the form of a smear, its general direction should be noted. Blood stains are extremely resistant to washing by water. The dried blood on a dead body or article will remain intact for quite a long time, even though the body has been totally submerged. Invisible blood stains can be detected by spraying luminal on the cloth or stained material with an atomiser inside a dark room. The stained area will luminesce if blood is present in those areas.

EXAMINATION OF BLOOD STAINS

(I) GENERAL: (1) STAINS FOUND AT THE SCENE OF THE CRIME: One of the important aspects of the visit to the scene of crime is searching for and interpretation of bloodstains. Relatively minor blood smearing may also provide significant evidence, such as a smear on the door handle. Heel prints or shoe prints on bloodstained area of the body, help in the identification of the assailant.

The distribution and amount of blood at the scene of the crime may give valuable information about the manner of death, whether it was suicidal or homicidal, and whether the victim struggled or moved about after his injuries. **The vessels usually go into spasm for a second or two after the injury and therefore the site of blood staining may not be site of infliction of injury.** When much blood is present, it suggests serious injury during life, but if a large vessel is cut, bleeding can occur after death. The collection of a pool of blood near the body during life indicates that the deceased fell unconscious and remained immobile after the injury. **A blood clot of the size of a clenched fist is roughly 500 ml.**

The spread of blood on clotting, on floor in an area of one square foot indicates loss of 100 ml of blood. Usually the amount of blood present at the scene cannot be measured, and the amount present is likely to be overestimated because of the highly coloured nature of blood. A trail of blood stains will indicate that the victim was wounded at some distance from the place at which the body is found. The victim's person and clothing show dried blood streaks running from the wounds towards his feet. It can happen when the victim is attacked while running or in case of suicide. If a victim is injured while he was on the floor, the dried blood streaks usually run down his sides. Blood coming from the arteries of a living person will be scattered in a fine spray over surfaces upon which it has fallen. A major vessel, such as the common carotid when cut can spray blood up to a distance of half a metre. Blood spray at the scene of violence is usually due to waving of the weapon, rather than direct spray from blood vessels. Venous bleeding is a slow steady flow, causing a pool if the victim is at rest, and separate widely spaced drops, if the victim walks about. The shapes adopted by blood spots may be drops, smears, splashes, spurts, trails, and pools.

THE DIRECTION OF THE FALL OF BLOOD ON TO A SURFACE: If it drops vertically on to flat surface, the stains are circular and the pattern is distinct according to the distance travelled. If the height does not exceed a few centimetres, the drop appears as a round spot. If it has travelled thirty cm. or more, it shows prickly edges, the projections growing finer and larger in number with the increase in length. When the height is still greater, ray-like splashes break out from the drop, and may be seen up to a distance of 15 to 20 cm. Splashes of blood striking a surface obliquely may appear like spears or exclamation marks, depending on the velocity and angle of the fall; the pointed end indicates the direction of the motion. If projected on to a wall by an upward sweep of an injured hand, the dots point upwards; or if by a downward sweep, downwards. If the long axis of the stains lie horizontally, it is possible to tell whether the drops fell in a forward or backward direction Fig. (20–1). Discontinuous spots of blood on the walls of the room indicate splashing of blood from the victim, the assailant, or the weapon, or spurting of blood from a cut artery. Blood which has run down a surface before clotting, shows thickening of clot at its lower margin. When blood falls upon porous articles or clothing, such as linen or cotton, it is absorbed, and spreads. It may be possible to see clear drag marks. Smears caused by fingers or palms are helpful in identification. A photograph of blood stains at the scene of a crime is useful.

(2) PART OF THE BODY FROM WHICH STAIN IS DERIVED? MENSTRUAL BLOOD is usually found on female garments, diapers or pieces of cloth. It is dark and fluid, has a disagreeable smell and the reaction is acid. On microscopic examination, it shows endometrial and vaginal epithelial cells, and number of microorganisms consisting of groups of bacilli and cocci. Trichomonas vaginalis or monilia may be present. It contains fibrinolysins and elevated levels of LDH4 and LDH5. If the blood is from the **NOSE,** mucus and hair from the nose may be found. **VOMITED BLOOD** is of chocolate colour and acid in reaction due to the action of gastric juice. Blood due to **HAEMOPTYSIS** is bright red and frothy, with alkaline reaction. In blood due to **RAPE,** semen and pubic hair may be found. Blood stains due to **BOILS AND SORES** show a smeared appearance without definite drops of blood, and may contain pus cells and bacteria.

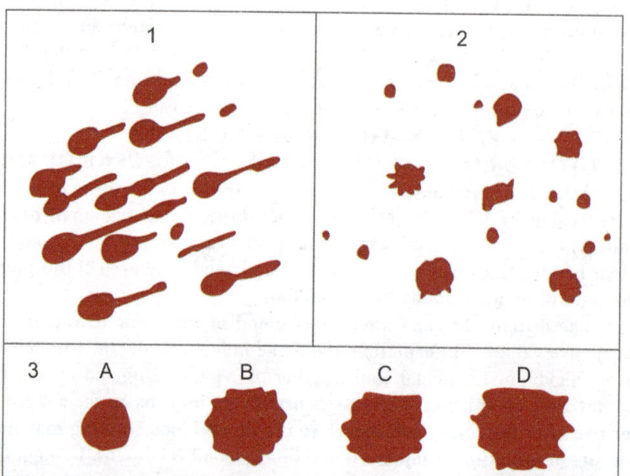

Fig. (20–1). (1) Spurting (indicating direction). (2) Blood falling vertically. (3) Drops of blood from various heights: (A) Up to 1.5 metres. (B) 1.5 to 3 metres. (C) 3 to 5 metres. (D) 5 to 7 metres.

(3) AGE OF BLOOD STAINS: Fresh stains on light coloured clothes are of bright-red colour, which gradually changes to reddish-brown in 24 hours, and brown within a few days, which may become black after a long time. Fresh stains are moist and sticky, and on drying, they stiffen the cloth because of the proteins. On many metallic articles, blood stains appear as dark shining spots or smears, and when dry, show fissures and cracks. In ordinary conditions, a drop of blood dries in an hour or two. If blood is collected in pools, it may take 12 to 36 hours to dry, depending upon the size and depth of the pool formed. The recently shed arterial blood is bright-red and venous blood dark-red. The solubility of blood stains in water and other liquids depends mainly on the age of the stains and the type of material on which it is found. The fresher the blood, the more easily it is dissolved. The solubility gradually diminishes with age. The age can also be determined by the spread of the soluble ingredients like chlorides into surrounding material. Fluorescence decreases as the stain becomes older due to the increasing amount of haematin. It can only be stated that the stain is very fresh, recent, some weeks, months, or very old.

(4) SEX AND AGE OF PERSON: Sex can be determined from the presence of sex chromatin in the leucocytes, if the cells can be identified. At birth, the blood forms a thinner and softer coagulum. The presence of foetal haemoglobin indicates that the blood is derived from a child.

(5) LIVING OR DEAD BODY: Blood which has effused during life can be removed in scales on drying, due to the presence of fibrin. Blood which has flowed after death tends to break up into a powder on drying.

(6) SOURCE OF BLOOD: If the victim and assailant are of different blood groups, it is helpful in establishing the identity. If the stains are on the inner side of the garment, they usually belong to the victim, but if found outside they may belong to the victim or accused.

(II) CHEMICAL EXAMINATION: The chemical tests depend on the presence in the blood stains of an enzyme peroxidase, which in the presence of hydrogen peroxide, oxidises the active ingredient of the reagent and produces the characteristic coloured compound.

(1) BENZIDINE TEST: Cut out a small piece of stained material or tease out fibres from the stained fabric and place it on porcelain tile. Add a drop of saturated solution of benzidine in glacial acetic acid, and then a drop of 10 volumes hydrogen peroxide. If blood is present, dark blue colour is produced immediately.

A positive reaction is given by blood of almost any age, blood that has been exposed to heat or cold, and blood stains treated with cleaning agents. This is the best preliminary test for blood and it detects blood when present in a dilution of one part of blood in three lakhs. A positive reaction is not proof of the presence of blood, but a negative reaction rules out of the presence of blood. A weaker reaction is obtained from certain other substances, e.g. pus, saliva, milk, rust, formalin, certain vegetable and animal juices, oxidising agents, bacteria, etc.

(2) PHENOLPHTHALEIN TEST (KASTLE-MEYER TEST): To a solution extracted from the stain with distilled water, add ten to twenty drops of phenolphthalein reagent (phenolphthalein 2g. + sodium hydroxide 20g. + zinc+ distilled water 100 ml), and then a drop or two of 10 volumes hydrogen peroxide. If blood is present, a pink or purple colour develops immediately. The test is more specific for blood than benzidine test, but comparatively less sensitive. Traces of copper give positive reaction.

The tests employing guaiacum (deep blue) and leucomalachite green are rarely used in medicolegal work.

(III) MICROSCOPIC EXAMINATION

Red Corpuscles Fig. (20–2): Intact red cells are seen only when the stains are fresh or when a blood clot is available. The

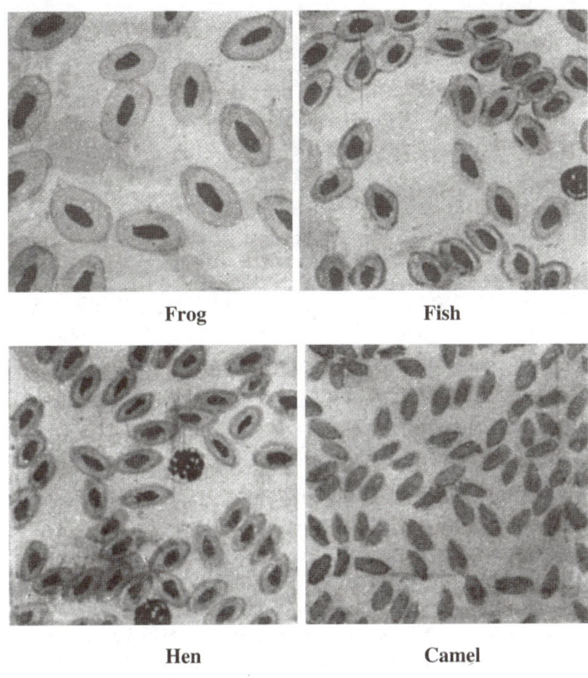

Fig. (20–2). Red blood corpuscles.

red cells become unrecognisable when dried. A small piece of stain is cut out and soaked in a watch glass with two or three drops of Vibert's fluid (sodium chloride 2 g., mercuric chloride half g., distilled water 100 ml.), or normal saline for 30 minutes. It is then teased with needles and examined under high power. If the stain is not dissolved, dilute solution of ammonia or 2% hydrochloric acid can be used. **Red blood cells are circular, biconcave, non-nucleated discs in all mammals except camels. In camels, they are oval and biconvex but non-nucleated. In birds, fishes, amphibia, and reptiles, they are oval, biconvex and nucleated.** Pus cells, epithelial cells, bacteria, faecal matter, etc., are sometimes found mixed with blood.

(IV) MICROCHEMICAL TESTS: Microchemical tests are based on the property of heme (iron) part of haemoglobin to form characteristic coloured crystals with certain reagents.

(1) HAEMIN CRYSTAL TEST (TEICHMANN'S TEST): A small crystal of sodium chloride and two to three drops of glacial acetic acid are placed on a small piece of the suspected stain on a glass slide. A coverslip is applied and the acid is evaporated by heating over a small flame. It is examined under the microscope after cooling. **Faint yellowish-red to brownish-black rhombic crystals of heamin or haematin chloride arranged single or in clusters are seen if blood is present Figs. (20–3 and 20–4).** Bubbles of gas are given by haematin crystals, on addition of a drop of hydrogen peroxide. The reaction is negative if the stain is old, is washed or treated by chemicals, presence of too much salt, moisture in acid and over-heating.

(2) HAEMOCHROMOGEN CRYSTAL TEST (TAKAYAMA TEST): Place a small piece of suspected material on a glass slide and add 2 to 3 drops of Takayama reagent (sodium hydroxide, pyridine, glucose), and cover with a coverslip. **Pink, feathery crystals of haemochromogen or reduced alkaline haematin arranged in clusters, sheaves, etc., appear in one to six minutes.** Slight warming of the slide hastens the reaction.

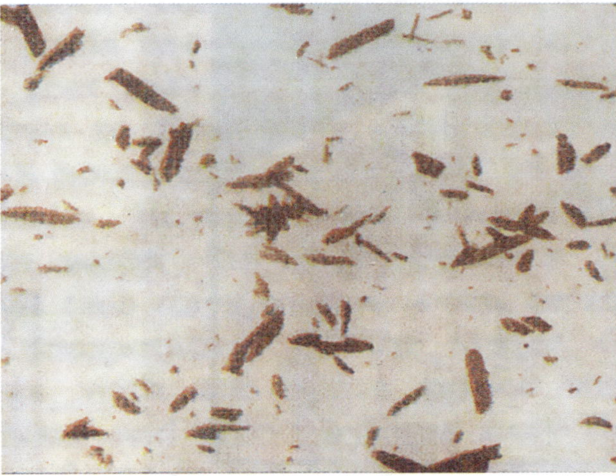
Fig. (20–3). Haemin crystals.

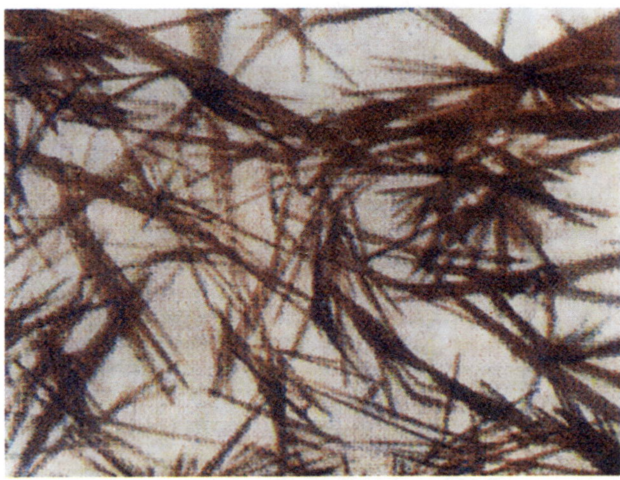
Fig. (20–4). Haemochromogen crystals.

The result is negative if crystals are not formed in 30 minutes. The test gives good result even with old stains. It is delicate and more reliable.

(V) SPECTROSCOPIC EXAMINATION: It is the most delicate and reliable test for detecting the presence of blood in both recent and old stains. Less than 0.1 mg. of blood is sufficient. The blood stain is dissolved in water, normal saline or dilute ammonia, and is placed in a small glass test tube which is then kept between the spectroscope and the source of the light. The extract of the blood must be dilute and if turbid it should be filtered. **The solution of the blood has the property of absorbing some of the rays from the spectrum, producing characteristic dark absorption bands, which vary with the type of the blood pigment present Fig. (20–5).**

SPECTRA OF HAEMOGLOBIN AND ITS DERIVATIVES: (1) OXYHAEMOGLOBIN is marked by two distinct bands in the yellow between the Fraunhofer lines D and E, the one nearer D being about half the breadth of the other and more defined.

(2) REDUCED HAEMOGLOBIN shows a broad band which lies between D and E.

(3) CARBOXYHAEMOGLOBIN has a spectrum similar to oxyhaemoglobin which remains unchanged after addition of ammonium sulphide, which reduces oxyhaemoglobin.

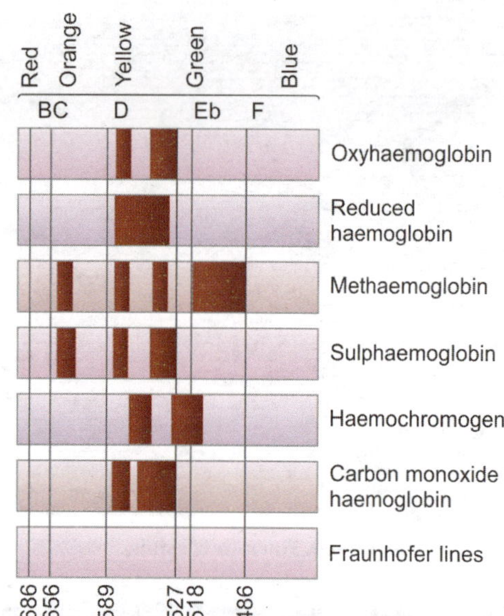

Fig. (20–5). Absorption spectrum of haemoglobin and its derivatives.

(4) METHAEMOGLOBIN spectrum is similar to oxyhaemoglobin with third dark band in the red between C and D, and the fourth between E and F, which is more indistinct.

(5) ACID HAEMATIN has a sharp band between C and D and a broad band between D and F which is not well-defined.

(6) ALKALINE HAEMATIN has a band between C and D.

(7) HAEMOCHROMOGEN or reduced alkaline haematin has a dense narrow band midway between D and E and a pale, broad band over E.

(8) CYANHAEMOCHROMOGEN has absorption bands, similar to those of haemochromogen, but slightly wider.

(9) ACID HAEMOTOPORPHYRIN gives a dark sharp and broad band between D and E.

(10) ALKALINE HAEMATOPORPHYRIN consists of four bands. One between E and F is darkest and broadest, two are between D and E, and the fourth between C and D.

Forensic Serology: It involves examination and analysis of a variety of blood and fluids which include blood, saliva, semen and urine.

(VI) SEROLOGICAL EXAMINATION: This determines whether the blood is derived from human being or from a lower animal.

(A) IMMUNOLOGICAL METHODS:

(1) PRECIPITIN TEST: PRINCIPLE: Blood serum contains proteins in colloidal suspension, and when human serum is injected into an animal, the animal becomes immunised against these proteins and antibodies develop in its blood. **If human serum is then brought into contact with this animal serum, the antibodies in the animal serum react with the proteins in the human serum and a visible precipitate forms.** The antibodies causing this reaction are known as precipitins and the animal serum is known as antihuman precipitin serum. A rabbit or a fowl is injected with human blood every third day for 3 to 5 injections. After this the animal is killed and the antiserum is collected. A suitable antiserum should react immediately or within a minute on the 1:1,000 dilution.

Technique: The presence of blood is determined first. An extract of stained material is prepared by soaking it in normal saline. No chemical should be added to extract the stain. The extract should be clear and may be filtered or centrifuged if necessary. The extract is diluted to 1: 100 with normal saline. **Two drops of undiluted antiserum are gently added to 0.75 ml. of diluted stain extract in a small tapering test tube held in a slanting position. The antiserum slowly settles down to the bottom, and at the junction of two fluids, a white ring with well-defined borders appears in the case of a positive reaction.** The ring is situated mostly in the antiserum. In the case of negative reaction no ring appears. A positive reaction should begin in ten minutes and should be read in half hour. **The results are qualitative and expressed as positive or negative.** For medicolegal purposes all doubtful reactions are read as negative.

Application of the Test: It is a specific protein test, and the reaction demonstrates the presence of albuminous substances obtained from any part of human body. **The origin of skin, flesh, bone or even secretions, such as saliva, milk and semen is determined by this test.**

(2) ANTIGLOBULIN CONSUMPTION TEST: (Haemagglutination inhibition test): When human globulin is mixed with antihuman globulin serum, the latter is absorbed and is no longer capable of agglutinating Rh positive red cells sensitised with incomplete anti-D. This detects globulins in dilutions of 1: 50,000

(3) GEL DIFFUSION: Wells are punched in an agar plate and antiserum and antigen are placed in adjacent wells. Diffusion will occur and precipitin bands will develop between wells containing corresponding antigen and antiserum. The advantage of this method is that there is no necessity to obtain clear antisera and stain extracts.

(4) DOUBLE DIFFUSION IN AGAR GEL: A piece of stained material or extract is placed in a central well cut in agar gel, while each of six wells surrounding this contains a drop of antiserum specific for the globulin of a particular species of animal. The advantage of this method is that the extract can be tested against different antisera simultaneously.

(5) PRECIPITATION-ELECTROPHORESIS: The gel is poured on microscopic slides in a layer one to two mm. thick, and wells punched after it has solidified. The extract of the stain is placed in the cathodic well and the antiserum in the anodic well. After 15 to 20 minutes of electrophoresis precipitin band will be visible between the wells where positive reactions have occurred.

(6) LATEX TEST: A saline extract of blood stain is mixed with dilute suspension of latex particles sensitised with antiserum. A positive reaction is shown by agglutination of the particles into clumps.

(B) ISOENZYME METHODS: These are based on the electrophoretic demonstration of the existence of enzymes in blood of the same species in multiple molecular forms known as isoenzymes. These methods are relatively less sensitive than immunological methods.

Blood groups ABO, MNS and Rh are determined in a blood stain by (1) Latte's crust method. (2) Absorption-elution technique. (3) Absorption-inhibition. (4) Latex method. (5) Enzymological methods.

AGGLUTINOGENS: The red cell antigens, representing over 400 serologically determined specificities, belong to a large number of blood group genetic systems with individual chromosomal loci. They are situated in the outer envelope of the red blood cells. They appear in the cells early in foetal life. They are also called isoagglutinogens or antigens.

AGGLUTININS: Isoagglutinins appear in the latter half of antenatal life. Agglutinins at birth may be derived from the mother by filtration through the placenta. They diminish or disappear during the first ten days of life, after which the infant produces its own agglutinins.

BLOOD GROUPS: Blood group antigen is attached to cell membrane of red cells, which appear early in foetal life. Agglutinins appear in the latter half of antenatal life. Landsteiner (1930) discovered ABO blood groups. The presence of blood group substances is shown by a clumping (agglutination) of the red cells when they are mixed with appropriate antisera. The antisera are prepared from human blood

which contain agglutinating bodies called antibodies which will detect the antigens on the red cells.

The genes which are present in the nuclei of all cells of the body control the formation of the antigens. On Mendelian principle, a person inherits one gene for each blood group from each parent, who themselves may be homozygous or heterozygous for the particular group. If the genes contributed by each parent are the same, the individual is called homozygous for the particular gene and if different, he is heterozygous.

The blood group systems currently in use are: (1) Red cell antigens. (2) White cell antigens. (3) Serum protein polymorphisms. (4) Red cell enzyme polymorphisms.

(I) RED CELL ANTIGENS:

(1) THE ABO SYSTEM: Human blood may be divided into four distinct blood groups, A, B, AB and O, depending upon the presence in the red cells of two agglutinogens which are designated by the letter A and B. The A, B and O characters are inherited by means of three allelomorphic genes, every individual having two chromosomes each carrying A, B or O, one from each parent. Thus the possible genotypes are AA, AO, BB, BO, AB, and OO. Group A type may thus be AA or AO. Since there is no true O antigen, group O individuals would be more precisely identified as group H individuals. H–h is inherited independently of the ABO system. The rare hh individuals (Bombay phenotype) lack A, B, or H antigens on their erythrocytes and in ABH substances in most secretions. Antigens of the ABO system can be detected even before birth. Their strength goes on increasing after birth, till about three years of age Table (20–2).

A and B are both "dominant" to O, and O is "recessive" to A and B, whereas A and B are equally dominant. AA the homozygote, cannot be serologically differentiated from AO, the heterozygote, and the same occurs with the genotypes, BB and BO, the serologically demonstrable blood groups (phenotype) in each case being A and B. The other phenotypes are AB and O. A has two subgroups A_1 and A_2. These are also found in group AB giving rise to subgroups, A_1B and A_2B. Subgroups A_3, A_4 and A_5 are weak and very rare. Anti-A or a and anti-B or b agglutinins are normally developed in the serum against whichever agglutinogens are absent from the red blood cells. There is no positive method of identifying the 'silent' gene O. **ABO group is not found in CSF. Group O is universal donor, and AB universal recipients.**

Gram-negative bacteria like E. Coli, Proteus, etc. may contain substances similar in property to A, B and O blood group substances and are likely to vitiate the tests.

TESTS FOR DETERMINING ABO GROUPING IN BLOOD STAINS: (1) Tube method: A drop of washed suspension of red cells is added to equal volumes of each of the antisera of A, B and O in separate tubes. The blood group can be identified when agglutination is seen by naked eye or microscope in the tubes. **(2) Tile Method:** A porcelian tile is used instead of tubes Tables (20–1 and 20–2).

(3) Absorption-inhibition method: The sample and antisera are allowed to react with each other for a longer period.

(4) Mixed agglutination test: The sample piece of stained cloth is cut into pieces of 2 to 3 mm and the fibres are separated. and added to tubes along with antisera of A, B, O types. The group can be known by the antisera which clumped to the cloth fibres.

(5) Absorption-elution technique: Test is similar to mixed agglutination, but the clumps are seen on the walls of the test tube and not on fibres. This test can be used for body tissues also.

Blood stains can be typed for the presence of ABO agglutinogens by absorption-elution, absorption-inhibition, mixed agglutination or ELISA method, or for agglutinins by the Lattes crust method.

(2) THE MNSs SYSTEM: Two further agglutinogens M and N, which are quite distinct and independent of the agglutinogens A and B, occur in human blood. The M and N factors are inherited as Mendelian dominants. They are present at birth. They form three groups, M, N and MN. Anti-M and Anti-N agglutinins are not normally developed in human sera but they may be present rarely. The agglutinogens, M and N are feebly antigenic. The subgroup S is closely allied to the MN system. The phenotypes are: MS, NS, MNS, MNs, MSs, NSs, NNSs.

Table (20–1). Determination of ABO groups

Known test sera		Unknown			
Groups	Agglutinins	O	A	B	AB
A	b	–	–	+	+
B	a	–	+	–	+
O	a & b	–	+	+	+

+ = Agglutination.
– = Absence of agglutination.

Table (20–2). ABO blood groups

Blood group	Agglutinogens	Agglutinins
A	A	Anti-B
B	B	Anti-A
AB	A and B	None
O	None	Anti-A and Anti-B

(3) THE P SYSTEM: P factor is present in about 75 percent of persons, but satisfactory anti-P serum is rare. The main possible genotypes are P_1P_1, P_1 P_2 and P_2 P_2. P seems to be transmitted as Mendelian dominant. It is weak and medicolegally unimportant.

(4) THE Rh SYSTEM: The Rhesus factor was detected originally by the use of serum from a rabbit which has been immunised against the red blood cells of the Rhesus monkey, and hence the term Rh factor. This factor is present in the red cells of 90 percent of Indians, who are known as Rh-positive, the remainder Rh-negative. Amniotic fluid contains Rh.

A complex of antigens is involved, six in number, named Cc, Dd, and Ee, each of which is capable of producing antibodies, although they are all not equally powerful in this respect. As the gene 'd' is amorphic, 'd' antigen is not produced and the symbol 'd' stands for the absence of D rather than the presence of d. The Rh antigens can be detected in a foetus after six weeks of pregnancy.

A member of each pair occupies one of three closely related genes in the relevant chromosome. Eight combinations are therefore possible, and 36 genotypes could result from them. The antibodies do not occur naturally in human serum. They are produced by the entry of a Rhesus antigen into blood, which is foreign to the individual, either due to blood transfusion or from a foetus in pregnancy.

About 150 mg. of blood-stained material or about 75 mg. of dried blood and the control free from stain should be available for grouping test. The agglutinogenic specificity of blood stains is retained, even though the red cells are not intact, **if the stains are properly preserved. ABO retain their agglutinogenic specificity indefinitely. MNS and Rh factors lose their specificity within 3 to 5 weeks.** The agglutinins present in the serum lose their specificity in the stains in a short duration. **Most of the enzymes in the stains lose their specificities within 3 to 5 weeks.**

SERUM LIPOPROTEINS: The Lp system has at present three phenotyes Lp (a+x–), Lp (a+x+) and Lp (a–x+). The Xm antigens are also serum lipoproteins.

The agglutinogens in the stain are retained for a longer time, even though the red cells are destroyed. The absorption-inhibition technique and absorption-elution method are employed for the grouping of such stains. By using mixed agglutination technique, stains on clothes or fibres can be grouped in about three year old stains.

Electrophoresis and immunoelectrophoresis can positively identify blood stains. Separation and migration of haemoglobin and its derivatives can be done by chromatography.

Group Specific Substances: The agglutinogens of the ABO system are also present in body tissues. In the tissues they appear in a lipoidal form. In about 80 percent of the people they appear in a water-soluble form, and can be demonstrated in all the body fluids except the cerebrospinal fluid. They are not found in nerve tissue, epithelium, skin appendages, bone and cartilage. **Persons who possess only the lipoidal form are known as 'non-secretors', while those who possess a water-soluble form are known as 'secretors'.** The capacity of secreting these antigens in body fluids is controlled by a pair of allelic genes Se and se, the former being dominant over the latter. **The individuals with genotype Se Se, and Se, se are color, and those with the genotype se se are non-secretors.** Secretors possess H antigen on their red cells irrespective of their blood group of the ABO system. However, the amount of H antigen is the highest on the red cells of O group persons. The ability to secrete agglutinogens into the body fluids remains constant throughout and is transmitted as a simple Mendelian dominant. The agglutinins, a and b are also present in the body fluids. M and N agglutinogens are widely distributed in the body tissues in a relatively water-soluble form. The group specific substances in dried stains can be identified by absorption technique. The Rh agglutinogens are widely distributed in the body tissues but are not found in the body fluids, except the amniotic fluid.

Medicolegal Aspects of Blood Groups: The application of blood groupings to medicolegal problems is based on the following principles: (1) A blood group antigen cannot appear in a child, unless present in one or other parent. (2) If an individual is homozygous for a blood group factor, it must appear in the blood of all his children. (3) If a child is homozygous for a blood group factor, the gene for the same must have been inherited by it from each of its parents. (4) The blood group characters are peculiar to the individual and are unchanged throughout life.

EXCLUSION OF PATERNITY: (1) First-order exclusion: Where the child has a blood group gene that is absent in both the mother and the putative father. (2) Second-order exclusion. Where the putative father is homozygous for a blood group gene, but the gene is not present in the child in question.

PHENOTYPE is the entire physical, biochemical and physiological makeup of an individual as determined both genetically and environmentally.

Blood Groups and Heredity: Brenstein postulated the mode of inheritance of ABO system. The ABO, MN and Rh factors are inherited according to Mendelian principles. **The rules of inheritance of ABO system are:** (1) Agglutinogen A or B cannot appear in the child unless it is present in one or both parents. (2) Agglutinogen A_1 or A_2 cannot appear in the blood of the child unless it is present in one or both parents. (3) The combination of A_1 B parent with A_2 child, and vice versa cannot occur. Conversely, the combination of A_2B parent with A_1 child and vice versa cannot occur. (4) An O parent cannot have an AB child and an AB parent cannot have O child. (5) Parents of AO and AO genotype may have a OO child. (6) Parents of AA or AO genotype may have a A child.

The rules of inheritance for MN system are: (1) Agglutinogens M and N, cannot appear in the blood of a child unless present in one or both parents. (2) A type M parent cannot produce a type N child and conversely an N parent cannot produce M child. (3) In matings where both parents are homozygous type M or N, the children are always of the same type as the parents. (4) In matings where one parent is type M and other type N, all children are type MN. (5) In matings where one parent is homozygous (M or N), and the other heterozygous (MN), the children are of parental types in 50 to 50 ratio. (6) In matings where the parents are both MN, children of all three types are possible.

Rules of inheritance of Rh groups are: (1) Rh negative parents cannot produce an Rh positive child. (2) Rh positive and mixed parents can have Rh positive and Rh negative children.

BLOOD GROUPS IN TISSUES

(1) BONE: The determination of blood groups from bone tissue is more difficult than from other body tissues. Bones not having extractable plasma proteins, such as burnt bones and bones after 5 to 10 years following death give negative serological results. Carbohydrates, glycolipids and glycoproteins can be extracted as blood group substances from the bone marrow. With fresh bone marrow and spongy bone, blood groups can be determined with a relatively high accuracy. Bone samples should be collected from the regions rich in red bone marrow, i.e., the proximal epiphysis of humerus and femur. In compact bone, blood group substances are thought to originate not only from bone cells but also from red cells in vascular systems. Mainly ABH blood groups are detected in the bone, but with compact bone, groups A or B are frequently misjudged as AB. MN, Gm, PGM, 6-PGD and esterase D (EsD) have also been detected.

(2) DENTAL TISSUE: Absorption-elution technique is preferred for blood grouping of dental tissues including dentine, cementum and dental pulp. Enamel contains only traces of blood group substances and grouping is very difficult. Blood grouping of a denture and dental calculus is possible if the denture has been used for a long period of time due to the accumulation of saliva. Cementum gives a weak reaction. Results are most accurate with dental pulp. Blood grouping of old teeth is possible if they are dry and not infected with bacteria. Heating at 200°C and over, destroys groups. Apart from ABO, PGM, AK, ADA, and 6–PGD can be identified from the dental pulp.

(3) HAIR: With absorption-elution technique, blood groups can be determined by a single hair shaft about six cm. in length. Blood grouping is practicable with scalp hair from foetuses and newborn infants and also with grey scalp hair. If hair is heated at 250°, it is impossible to detect blood groups. Hair left in water or soil for up to six months give good results. PGM, esterase D, 6 phosphoglucomate dehydrogenase, glyoxalase and a-L fucosidase (FUC) types have been detected from hair roots with sheath cells.

(4) NAILS: Three to six mg. is adequate to detect ABO groups. The human nails contain mainly ABH blood group antigens. MN blood groups have been detected in some cases. Marshall (1980) reported that proteins of human nail show a genetic variation with regard to both low-sulphur and high-sulphur protein fractions, which could serve as biochemical markers of individuality.

(5) SOFT TISSUES: The mixed agglutination technique (the mixed agglutination reaction, MCAR) is useful for detecting ABH antigens on tissue cell surfaces in all kinds of soft tissues. This technique is suitable for the direct determination of blood groups on cell fragments adhering to weapons, bullets and clothing. Decomposed muscle acquires blood group antigens different from native one, and also many bacteria have blood group antigens similar to human ABH antigens.

(II) WHITE CELL ANTIGENS: The Human Leucocyte Antigen (HLA) System consists of protein substances on the surface of a wide variety of tissues and organs, on tumours, white cells and platelets.

They are reported to be present on spermatozoa, but not on ovum, nor on the trophoblast. They are present on the placenta at term and in foetal tissue at six weeks. They are found both on lymphocytes and granulocytes. HLA-Dr antigen is present on B lymphoblastoid cell lines, monocytes and macrophages. The major human leucocyte antigens HLA–A, B, C, D, and DR are determined by a single chromosomal segment, the 'major histocompatibility complex' (MHC), which is situated on the short arm of human chromosome 6. In white cells 68 antigenic factors are present. Each parent contributes to a child one of the two chromosomes containing the HLA region. The presently known seven multiple loci with about 125 multiple allelism, and with a very high degree of polymorphism, provide a very good discriminating capacity. Only fresh blood samples are examined in solving the problems relating to parentage. In tissue grafts, the better HLA match between subjects, the better the chances of graft's survival. The presence of these antigens may be detected by using the white cells of the blood and a suitable antiserum that either agglutinates the white cells or damages them so that they are stainable with suitable dyes that do not affect the damaged cells. Other components of this system may be detected by observing the characteristic swelling reaction of lymphocytes that do not contain the antigen, when they are placed in contact with lymphocytes that do contain it.

(III) SERUM PROTEIN POLYMORPHISM: The serum protein groups which are subject to genetic variation include the Gm and Inv types of gamma globulin, the group specific components (Gc types), the haptoglobin (Hp) types, the transferrin types (Tfc), cerulospasmins and third complement component (C_3) and several lipoprotein systems. They are usually demonstrated by electrophoresis.

(1) SERUM HAPTOGLOBINS: Haptoglobins are haemoglobin-binding proteins found in human serum. Three genotypes are present Hp_{1-1}, Hp_{2-2} and Hp_{2-1}. The pattern of inheritance is identical to that of the MN groups.

(2) GC GROUPS: Inheritance is controlled by two alleles Gc 1 and Gc 2 giving the three phenotypes Gc 1–1, Gc 2–2 and Gc 2–1.

(3) AG GROUPS: This system of serum antigens is complex but two genes, Ag(x) and Ag(y) appear to be allelic. The possible phenotypes are Ag(x–y–), Ag (x–y+), Ag(x+y+). These factors are present at birth and not transmitted across the placenta.

(4) GM BLOOD SERUM POLYMORPHISM: In the newborn, the gamma globulin present is not its own, but has been transmitted from the mother across the placenta. As such, Gm and Inv. studies are useful in cases of mix up or exchange of babies in hospitals. The child's own gamma globulin begins to form from third month with disappearance of the Gm transferred from the mother. There are five types of immunoglobulins, IgG, IgM, IgA, IgD, and IgE which form a group of serum proteins to which all antibodies belong. Normal serum contains eight types of IgG molecules. Various Gm antigens designated Gm 1 to Gm 25 are so far determined by various allelic genes. IgG crosses placenta.

(5) ABNORMAL HAEMOGLOBINS: More than hundred variants of heamoglobin have been described. The abnormal haemoglobins are under direct genetic control. The specific mutation is known for more than 30 Hb variants. The abnormal haemoglobins C, D, E, G,H, I, J, K, M, S are designated in the order of their discovery. **Haemoglobin C and E are associated with thalassaemia.**

(IV) RED CELL ENZYME POLYMORPHISMS: More than 160 antigens, 150 serum proteins and 250 cellular enzymes have been found in human blood. A large number of enzymes, which catalyse the various vital biochemical reactions are also present in the blood, mainly in the plasma. Phosphoglucomutase (PGM) and adenylatekinase (AK) are of established value in paternity testing. Adenosine deaminase (ADA), red cell acid phosphatase (EAP), serum cholinesterase (SCE), 6–phosphogluconate dehydrogenase (6-PGD), glutamate pyruvate transaminase (GPT), esterase D (Es D), and glyoxalase I (GLO), may also be used. They are usually demonstrated by starch gel electrophoresis technique. These enzymes do not persist for more than one month in stained material.

Paternity can be excluded by ABO grouping alone in about 18%, and if MNSs system is added in about 60%. Red cell antigens and serum proteins exclude 82%. If red cell enzymes are included, exclusion will be 94%. By testing a number of HLA systems, the exclusion is 98.5%. DNA fingerprinting will positively fix or exclude paternity.

Medicolegal Application of Blood Groups: (1) Disputed Paternity: The question of disputed paternity arises in the Court in the following conditions. (1) When a child is born in lawful marriage, but the husband denies that he is the father of the child. (2) When a child is born out of lawful marriage, and the mother accuses a certain man of being the father of the child, while the man denies the accusation. (3) When a woman pretends pregnancy and delivery and obtains a child claiming it as her own, in order to obtain a share in her husband's property. (4) In suits for nullity of marriage.

Many cases can be solved by means of the blood groups of the parent and the child. In the case of the adults, 5 ml. of venous blood is taken and placed in plain tube. Neither party should have had a blood transfusion within three months, before taking the sample. The infants should preferably be at least six months of age, but not less than two months before testing is performed. One ml. of blood should be obtained by a heel or earprick, or venepuncture into a plain tube. The testing of the mother, child and putative father, i.e., the man whose potential paternity is under investigation, should be done in the same laboratory, by the same person, on the same day, and using the same batch of reagents and antisera.

However, tests have their limitations. They may exclude a certain person as the possible father of the child, but they cannot definitely establish paternity. They can only indicate its possibilities. The exclusion of putative father is based upon the principle that a specific agglutinogen cannot appear in a child unless it was present in one of its parents, e.g. if the agglutinogen A is present in a child but not in its mother. If two men are alleged to be the fathers of the child, and if one of them shows the agglutinogen A in his blood and the other does not, the person possessing agglutinogen A, must be the father. If both men have agglutinogen A, no positive opinion regarding the paternity can be given. The blood groups in current use in the investigation of cases of doubtful paternity are: ABO, MNS, Rh, Kell, Lutheran, Duffy and Kidd. The P system and the Lewis system have been well studied but are not used because of their complexity or instability.

(2) Disputed Maternity: When the same child is claimed by two women, or when two children are interchanged either by accident or by design in maternity home or hospital, or supposititious child, and when a woman kidnapping a child and claiming to be the mother of that child, blood grouping tests are helpful.

(3) Crimes: Blood stains may be found on clothing and person of suspect. If the accused alleges that the stain is of his own blood, it will have similar blood group systems and haptoglobins. If the victim has similar characters, the test is not conclusive. If there is difference in blood group of the stain and the accused's blood, then the stain is of some other person's blood. If the characteristics of the victim's blood coincide with those of the stain, an association is established between the suspect and the victim. Blood stains may be present at the scene of house-breaking, e.g. on a broken window, if the culprit has cut himself. If the character of these stains are similar to that of blood of the suspect, it establishes association. Blood stains may be present under the fingernails of assailant in a case of throttling. If there has been a struggle, blood stains derived from the accused may be found under the fingernails of the victim due to scratching. Vehicles which have caused injury can be identified when they show blood resembling that of the victim.

Blood does not adhere readily to swiftly moving metallic objects, e.g. it is difficult or impossible to detect blood on a bullet which has passed through a body; sharp knives which have made a deep gash in a body may show little or no evidence of blood. In every case of murder a sample of blood (preferably from the heart) for identification should be placed in a container and labelled.

Stains on clothes due to crushing of bugs, fleas, louse, mosquitoes, etc., are common. These stains are small in size and sharply angular in outline and are usually found on the inside of the garment. If the insects are crushed, fragments of the hair or scales of the insect and eggs may be found on microscopic examination.

(4) Stains due to Body Fluids: The blood group agglutinogens can be demonstrated in stains on clothes due to semen, sweat, saliva, nasal secretion, urine or faeces in persons who are "secretors". This may be a corroborative evidence of the accused.

(5) Identity: The specificity of various blood group combinations is like that of the fingerprints. When an individual has some rare blood group, he can be identified with certainty. But when they are of common type, they are not of use.

(6) Cause of Death: In certain cases, cause of death can be established, e.g., incompatible blood transfusion. Various P (I.C) poisons can be detected in the blood.

HAZARDS OF BLOOD TRANSFUSION: Some type of reaction will occur in about one to 2% of patients who receive blood transfusion. The antigens of the ABO and Rh systems commonly produce transfusion reactions. In the case of other antigens a number of incompatible transfusions may be required to stimulate sufficient antibodies and cause a reaction. (A) **IMMUNOLOGICAL REACTIONS:** (1) Intravascular haemolysis. (2) Extravascular haemolysis. (3) Sensitivity to white blood cells, platelets and plasma components. **(B) NON-IMMUNOLOGICAL REACTIONS:** (1) Circulatory overload. (2) Coagulation defects. (3) Hyperkalaemia. (4) Citrate toxicity. (5) Infections and transmission of syphilis, hepatitis, toxoplasmosis, AIDS, etc. (6) Air embolism. (7) Hypothermia. (8) Rigors.

The commonest mistakes in blood transfusions are: (1) clerical error, (2) confusing terms, such as "group A serum" instead of "anti-B serum", (3) failure of the staff to check the reference on the bottle against the actual laboratory report on compatibility, (4) the presence of similarly named patients in the ward.

Samples to be preserved are: (1) Sample of blood transfused. (2) Sample of blood of the recipient before and after transfusion. At autopsy, (1) kidneys (2) Blood (3) Urine.

Death occurs due to anaphylaxis, renal failure, electrolytes imbalance or circulatory overload.

INVESTIGATIONS: (1) HAEMATOLOGICAL EXAMINATION: In case of intravascular haemolysis, the serum of a post-transfusion sample of blood will show the presence of haemoglobin and methaemalbumin. Haptoglobins will be reduced. In extravascular haemolysis, there is an increase in the quantity of unconjugated bilirubin.

(2) URINE: In intravascular haemolysis, haemoglobin will be found in urine. Urobilin, urobilinogen, and red cell casts may be found.

(3) SEROLOGICAL EXAMINATION: A two percent red cell suspension in saline of the patient's blood may show agglutinates. Coomb's test is positive. Ig A specific antibodies will be found in the patient's blood in sensitivity reaction to donor leucocytes, platelets and plasma factors. There may be eosinophilia.

(4) BACTERIOLOGICAL EXAMINATION: Residual donor blood may show microorganisms, which can be confirmed by culture.

(5) AUTOPSY: In acute intravascular haemolytic reactions, haemoglobinuric nephrosis is seen. The tubules will show acute necrosis and casts of haemoglobin. Lungs will be oedematous in cases of circulatory overload. Air in the right ventricle indicates death due to air embolism.

VARIOUS STAINS: SALIVA: It contains enzymes like ptyalin, glucose 6-phosphate dehydrogenase, various proteins, lipids, chlorides, thiocyanate ions, etc. The stains are identified from the presence of amylase and buccal epithelial cells. Amylase activity can be measured by the starch-iodine test or Phadebas test. ABO grouping and species origin can be carried out.

VOMITUS: It will contain food material and reaction is acid.

FAECES: The stains can be identified from odour, presence of undigested muscle and vegetable fibres and cells, E. coli, urobilinogen and stercobilin.

URINE: The stains can be identified from the presence of urea, uric acid and creatinine. Blood group antigens can be detected in secretors.

VAGINAL SECRETION: It consists of white coagulated material consisting of shed vaginal epithelium and Doderlein's bacilli. **Leucorrhoeal** stains contain epithelial cells.

VOMITUS: It has low pH and contains food stuff.

DNA FINGERPRINTING

DNA fingerprinting (DNA typing, DNA identification, or genetic typing) is a technique involving chemically dividing the DNA into fragments which form a unique pattern and then matching that "identity profile" with the pattern obtained from similarly testing a suspect's blood specimen. The chances of two people having the same sequence is about one A million billion. Even in siblings, the chances are only one in ten thousand million. With recent advances, even twins can be differentiated. This method is as unique as fingerprints to an individual. Dr. Alec Jeffreys in 1985, developed DNA fingerprinting. It was first used to help solve two murder cases.

Human body consists of about six thousand billion cells which constitute tissue and organ systems. Every living cell has genetic material contained in units called chromosomes, which are located in nucleus. DNA is present only in nucleated cells. Each human somatic cell has 23 pairs of chromosomes of which 23 are derived from biological father, and 23 from the mother, due to fertilisation of ovum with sperm. Genes are arranged along the length of each chromosome, which are responsible for various functions of the body. Each gene carries instructions for the production of a particular protein which performs a particular function. Genes are also responsible for transmission of heredity. The genes are made up of chemical molecules called deoxyribonucleic acid (DNA). The human genome contains about 6 x 10^9 DNA molecules per diploid genome.

The core of the chromosome is a very long and extremely thin thread of DNA. A single human chromosome is about 1/12,500 cm. long. The DNA molecule in this chromosome is about 2.5 cm. in length, compacted into the chromosome by successive coiling.

The total DNA in a cell is about 108 cm. in length. Each chromosome consists of two long linear DNA molecules, the polymers being hydrogen bonded via specific nucleotide pairing and coiled as a double helix which is spiral in nature, and looks like a spiral staircase. The helix is structurally stabilised by nuclear proteins called histones, the complex of DNA and histones being referred to as chromatin. Chromatin may be condensed to varying degree of compactness and in its most compact form is seen microscopically as chromosomes at the metaphase stage of each cell cycle. The chromosomes are continuous strands of DNA ranging from 50 to 500 million molecules per chromosome, encoded in this. DNA is also found in mitochondria which have originated from mother.

Each nucleotide is composed of phosphate, deoxyribose sugar, and organic nitrogenous base. The bases are adenine (A), guanine (G), cystosine (C), and thymine (T). The bases of one strand are connected to the bases of the other strand by hydrogen bonds, while adjacent nucleotides are linked with each other by covalent bonds. Adenine combines only with thymine and guanine combines only with cytosine. The DNA molecule resembles a twisted rope ladder with four kinds of stair-steps, e.g., A-T, T-A, C-G, or G-C. There are three hydrogen bonds between G and C, and 2 bonds between A and T.

A single DNA molecule consists of 50 to 500 million base pairs. The two strands of DNA helix run in opposite direction. The base sequence of one strand is always complementary to the sequence on the other. Each segment of DNA in a chromosome which codes for a particular protein is called a gene. In the human genome there are about 10,000 genes, accounting for about 5% of the entire cellular DNA. In between the active base pairs which code for a particular protein, there are large number of redundant/inactive base pairs forming 95% of DNA, which is considered as "junk DNA'. In junk DNA short sequences of base, repeat themselves over again like a stutter (repetitive DNA), e.g. GCTA, GCTA, GATA, GATA, etc. The regions containing repetitive DNA demonstrating hypervariability from person to person are called "satellite DNA", which shows an extremely high degree of variability, and these variants are called "variable number tandem repeats" (VNTR) or "minisatellites". There are more than 1500 VNTR's in the human genome. Selected regions of VNTR are broken into fragments using special enzymes (restriction endonucleases), which are individualistic in nature and establish 100% identity.

DNA is much more resistant to environmental degradation than most other biological molecules, such as proteins, blood groups, serum enzymes, etc. DNA is a robust molecule which can tolerate remarkable range of temperature, pH and other factors. DNA mixed with detergents, oil, gasoline and other adulterants does not alter its typing characteristics. Improper preservation and storage of samples can result in the fragmentation of DNA molecule and can lead to problems in the analysis. When the sample is contaminated with bacteria, DNA will be degraded.

The various techniques in use at present are: **(1) RFLP METHOD:** DNA can be extracted from any body fluid or tissue in which nucleated cells are present. All the samples should be frozen at minus 20°C before use. The samples (blood, bone marrow, semen, hair roots, tooth pulp, tissue from any organ, or skin) are usually examined. The separation of DNA involves (1) disruption of cells and fractionation of cellular organelles, (2) dissociation of DNA from proteins by the use of salt solution or detergent, (3) addition of an extractant to phase-separate the bulk of the protein from the DNA, (4) use of enzymes or differential precipitation to remove the RNA and polysaccharides. The isolated DNA is quantitated by ultraviolet spectrophotometry. DNA is completely digested with restriction enzymes called restriction endonucleases. (that have evolved to prevent bacteria from infection by certain bacteriophages). These enzymes recognise the specific sequence in the double strand DNA and cut the DNA at this site into various fragments, called as restriction fragment length polymorphism (RFLP). RFLP's are produced due to variations in human DNA. These variations in restriction fragment lengths is due to presence of variable number of tandem repeats (VNTR). Most of repeated DNA are arranged as short sequences repeatedly contiguously in tandem, hence called VNTR. When the process is repeated with several enzymes, each of which cuts at different sites, enough information is gathered to construct a detailed genetic fingerprint of a person. Several restriction endonucleases are in use, e.g., Eco-R-1, PsT-1, Hin F-I (obtained from E. coli), Sau 3A-1 (obtained from Staphylococcus aureus), Hae-III (obtained from Haemophilus influenzae). PsT-1 (a six-base cutter) is commonly used, which recognises the sequence CTG, CAG.

Digested DNA is run on agarose gel electrophoresis. The different restriction fragments are separated varying in length between 0.5 to 25 kb, which varies from one individual to another. The smaller fragments move much faster through the gel than the larger one. The gel is later stained with ethedium bromide for 40 minutes which tightly binds to DNA and fluoresces under UV light.

From the agarose gel, DNA is transferred to nylon membrane using capillary transfer technique of Southern. The result is a mirror-image replica of fragment distribution. Vacuum blotting of transfer is used more commonly as it is less time consuming. DNA is then fixed by heat at 80°C or cross-linked by the cation of UV irradiation.

Next hybridisation is done which is the pairing of two complementary single strands of DNA to form double stranded DNA. It involves the addition of a probe to the nylon membrane. A probe is a single-stranded recombinant DNA segment, or synthetic DNA, which is designed to go to a particular predetermined locus on a particular chromosome. It is usually tagged with a radioactive marker, such as P_{32}. The probe scans all the DNA fragments and wherever it encounters its complementary sequence, it will hybridise with it, thereby making the fragment radioactive. Usually four probes are used one at a time, due to which four different regions of the DNA would be analysed Fig. (20–6).

In the Centre for DNA Fingerprinting and Diagnostics (CDFD), Nacharam, Hyderabad-76, A.P. India, BKm probe is used, which is a multilocus probe isolated from the female banded krait, as a minor satellite DNA. More than 36 hypervariable VNTR are detected by BKm.

The label incorporated into the probe permits to localise these sites. After hybridisation, the membranes are washed with 0.05% SDS which removes loosely bound probe. The membrane is then wrapped in the saran wrap and placed in the X-ray cassette holder along with X-ray film, and kept at 80°C. Exposure time depends upon the specific activity of the probe ranging from few hours to days (up to 10 days). X-ray films are then developed and fixed in the respective reagents and finally wahsed in water and dried. This autoradiograph is a permanent record, in which grey to black bands are seen where the radioactive probes had hybridised to fragmets bearing complementary sequences. The series of bands seen on the film is called an "autorod", which represents the DNA fingerprint of that individual from whom the DNA had been obtained. The pattern of bands is unique to each individual.

(2) POLYMERASE CHAIN REACTION (PCR): This technique is used when a very small amount of DNA or a partially degraded biological material is available. A small amount of DNA is amplified more than a million-fold using thermal TAQ polymerase. It is particularly useful for diagnostic purposes. DNA is isolated and split apart, by heating the sample to more than 94°C. Later, the temperature is lowered, during which small segments of DNA (primers) bind specifically to the DNA which has the polymorphic regions of interest. The primers act as the starting point for the DNA duplication process. The temperature is again raised to 72°C which causes DNA polymerase (TAQ polymerase) to extend the primers and copy the two separated strands of DNA. The TAQ polymerase utilises nucleotides by inserting them opposite the appropriate base, thereby ensuring the integrity of DNA's base pair complementarity. The cycle is repeated for 30 times or more which synthesises more than a million copies of DNA. Detection of amplification products for VNTR polymorphism is done by electrophoresis, followed by visualisation by fluorescent detection or silver staining. PCR technique can analyse 36 samples at a time. It is sensitive and quicker method but less specific than RFLP.

PCR is now widely being used by all laboratories, as it is very sensitive, reaction is highly specific, easily automated and capable of amplifying minute amounts of samples even if the biological material is degraded.

In case of MLPs the probe used detects variations at several genetic regions simultaneously. The band pattern produced on X-ray plate produces a strip of 30 to 40 dark bands.

SLPs analyse only single hypervariable location in human DNA. These play a very major role in forensic practice as **they have far greater detection sensitivity than the MLPs.** Each SLP detects just two bands (one maternal and one paternal). **The sensitivity is such that a single hair root can be identified.** Results can also be obtained from degraded DNA (often found in forensic samples) as SLP detects the remaining, non-degraded alleles among the DNA fragments. As they detect only two bands/SLP, using single SLP reduces the probability to 1/10000 population as compared to 1 in 10^{12} MLP. Using multiple SLPs is therefore the practice now a days. SLPs are human specific, MLPs detect DNA fingerprint in all vertebrates. **80% of forensic work depends on SLPs.**

Multilocus or single locus probes are either cloned probes or synthetic oligonucleotides.

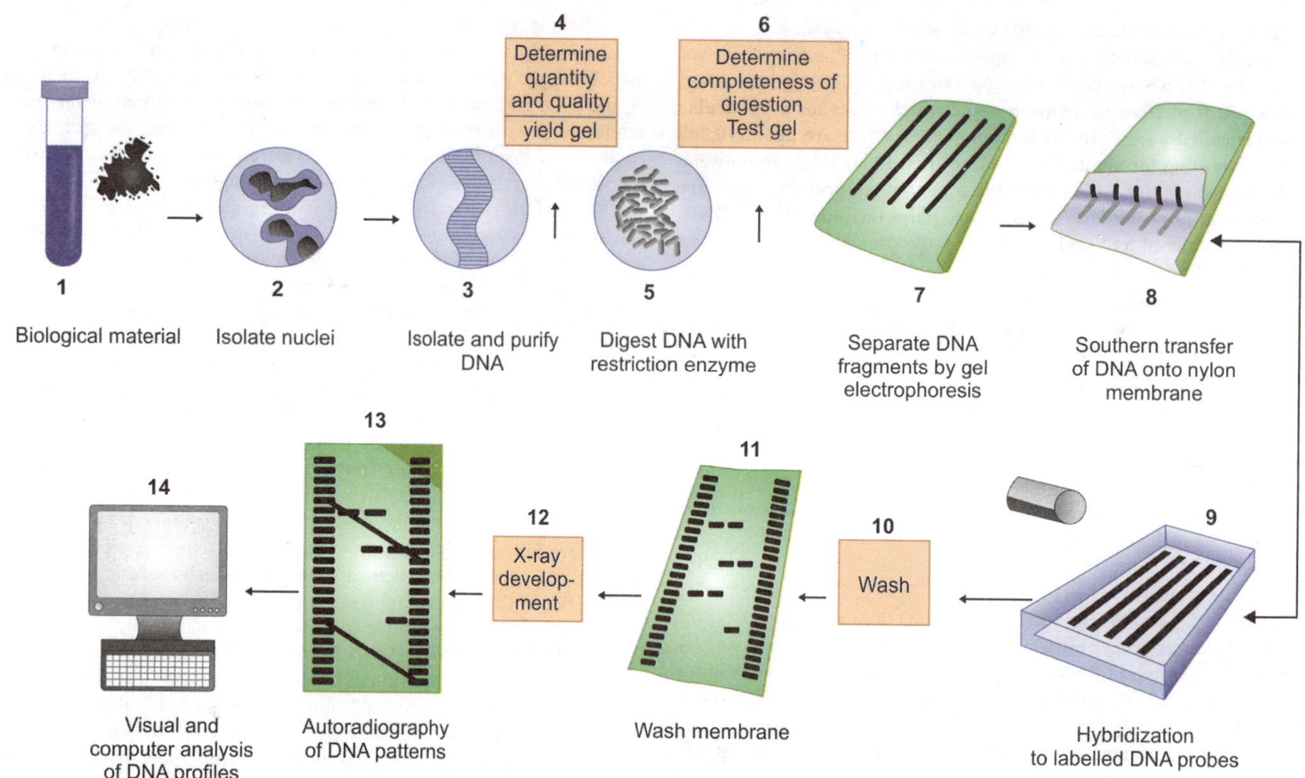

Fig. (20–6). Restriction fragment length polymorphism (RFLP) analysis used for DNA profiling testing.

The main disadvantages of RFLP method are: (1) The samples have to be in good condition to be analysed. (2) Fragments isolated/identified by this method are in the ranges of 2 to 20 Kbps.

The advantages of PCR over the RFLP are: (1) It is relatively simple and easily carried out in the laboratory. (2) The results are obtained within few days. (3) It permits analysis of extremely tiny amounts of DNA. The disadvantages are: (1) It is susceptible to contamination. (2) Most PCR loci have fewer alleles than the VNTR areas utilised in RFLP. (3) Some of the PCR loci are functional genes.

Most of the forensic work using SLPs, MLPs are the method of choice if the sample being tested is in a good amount and condition. A single MLP, by detecting numerous hypervariable loci simultaneously, yields a large amount of information in less time. Band pattern of SLP is simple (only two bands per SLP), hence easy to analyse; amount of sample needed is very small as detection is highly sensitive. But to increase specificity a large number of SLPs are to be used. Therefore time taken is very much.

VNTR: This method uses another set of probes which detect specific variable number tandem repeats of a sequence. These also remember the minisatellite in that they consist of a repeated sequence with the number of copies of the sequence varying from one person to the other. However, where there are usually many minisatellites of a given type in a genome, there is only one VNTR of each type. These probes therefore produce simpler banding patterns. Several VNTR probes are used, each of which recognises one VNTR site, to characterise a DNA sample. After the frequencies of the various bands produced by each VNTR probe have been established for each ethnic group, these can be used to calculate the probability of any particular combination of patterns occurring in each individual. The basic method is similar to the RFLP method.

(3) SHORT TANDEM REPEATS (STR) ANALYSIS: STR technology is used to evaluate specific regions (loci) within nuclear DNA. STR is a term that describes any short, repeating DNA sequence. This technique is the most prevalent. It uses highly polymorphic regions that have short repeated sequences of DNA (the most common is 4 bases repeated, but there are 3 and 5 bases repeats in use). Because different people have different numbers of repeat units, these regions of DNA can be used to discriminate between individuals. These STR loci are targeted with sequence-specific primers and are amplified using PCR. The DNA fragments that result are then separated and detected using electrophoresis. The polymorphisms displayed at each STR region are by themselves very common. Typically each polymorphism will be shared by about 5 to 20% of individuals. When looking at multiple loci, it is the unique combination of these polymorphisms to an individual that makes this method discriminating as an identification tool. The more STR regions that are tested in an individual, the more discriminating the test becomes. Different STR based DNA profiling systems are in use in different countries. The odds that two individuals will have the same 13-loci DNA profile is about one in one billion. Whichever system is used, many of the STR regions under the test are the same. These DNA profiling systems are based around multiplex regions, whereby many STR regions will be under test at the same time. Compared to PCR based systems, multiplex STRs are more simple and direct at the allele detection stage and are slightly more vulnerable to missing alleles, Fig. (20–7).

For forensic purposes STR typing is the recommended method, which must involve the study of at least 13 core loci.

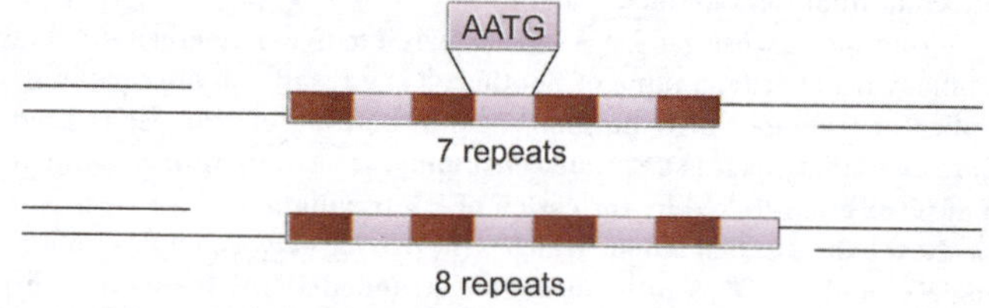

Fig. (20–7). Short Tandem Repeats (STRs).

(4) AMPLIFIED FRAGMENT LENGTH POLYMORPHISM (AmpFLP): This technique relied on variable number tandem repeats (VNTR) polymorphism to distinguish various alleles, which were separated on a polyacrylamide gel using an allelic ladder. Bands could be visualised by silver staining gel. As the analysis is done on a gel. very high number repeats may bunch together at the top of the gel, making it difficult to resolve. Due to its low cost and ease of setup and operation, AmpFLP is popular in low income countries.

(5) MITOCHONDRIAL DNA ANALYSIS (mt DNA): For highly degraded samples, it is sometimes impossible to get a complete profile of the 13 CODIS STRs. In these situations, mitochondrial DNA (mtDNA) is sometimes typed as there are many copies of mt DNA in the cell, while there are only 1 to 2 copies of the nuclear DNA. Mitochondrial DNA analysis can be used to examine the DNA from samples that cannot be analysed by RFLP or STR. While older biological samples that lack nucleated cellular material, such as hair, bones, and teeth cannot be analysed with STR and RFLP, it can be analysed with mt DNA. In the investigation of cases that have gone unsolved for many years, mt DNA is extremely valuable. All mothers have the same mitochondrial DNA as their daughters. This is because the mitochondrion of each new embryo comes from the mother's egg cell. The father's sperm contributes only nuclear DNA. Comparing the mtDNA profile of unidentified remains with the profile of a potential maternal relative can be important technique in missing person investigations.

(6) Y-CHROMOSOME ANALYSIS: The Y-chromosome is passed directly from father to son, so the analysis of genetic markers on the Y chromosome is especially useful for tracing relationships among males or for analysing biological evidence involving multiple contributors, such as gang rape.

This technique is more rapid and can be done in 2 to 3 days. It can be performed on small quantities of DNA. It is possible to run the products from several STR loci simultaneously on one gel as long as the fragment sizes do not overlap.

Rapid DNA: ID microchip-based genetic detectors are used at crime scene. These can display profile and can be uploaded in centeral data base.

SAMPLES (BIOLOGICAL) ENCOUNTERED IN FORENSIC PRACTICE

Sterile uncontaminated gloves should be used while collecting samples for DNA analysis. (1) BLOOD: Stains on cloth/wood/metal/plastic/floor titles/wall paper/newspaper/food. (2) SEMEN: Stains on cloth/paper/furniture/floor tiles, anal/vaginal/buccal/penile swabs, vaginal aspirates, fur/matted hair (pubic/axillary/scalp, etc.) (3) HAIR: Head/body/pubic/scalp. (4) TISSUE: Bonemarrow/muscle/spleen/fingernail scrapings. (5) MOUTH: Swabs. (6) FOETUS: Muscle biopsy/chorionic villous samples. (7) SALIVA STAINS: Cigarette butts/envelopes/also nasal mucus stains.

COLLECTION AND FORWARDING OF FORENSIC SAMPLES FOR DNA FINGER-PRINTING: The samples collected at the scene of crime along with the control samples should be sent to the DNA typing laboratory within the minimum period of time.

(1) LIQUID BLOOD: In cases of paternity, maternity disputes, biological relationships, etc., or as control samples in criminal cases, 2 to 5 ml. of i.v. drawn blood should be collected in sterile leakproof preferably screw-capped tubes containing heparin or EDTA as anticoagulant. EDTA extracts metallic ions, prevents clotting, inhibits enzymes in blood or microorganisms which may breakdown DNA during storage. The sample should be mixed thoroughly but slowly, and placed in a container containing ice, or a thermos flask. The sample tube should be sealed and labelled containing the names of the source of the blood sample, the name of the doctor collecting the blood sample, time and date of collection, name of forwarding authority, etc. The samples should reach the laboratory within 24 to 48 hours. If the person is suffering from visible genetic disorder, it should be mentioned in the forwarding letter of advice.

A blood-soaked dried gauze can be used for many years, if required. It is sealed in polythene bag or paper bag and sent at room temperature. In cases of crimes, a blood clot can be transferred by using a clean cotton cloth. Dried blood stains on weapons, garments, etc. can be left intact and entire object submitted. Dried blood stains on large immovable articles can be scraped into a clean piece of paper, or the stain can be lifted from the surface using adhesive tape, or sample can be eluted by rubbing the stained area with cotton swab moistened with distilled water. The swab is air-dried without heat.

(2) SEMEN, VAGINAL SWABS: Sterile cotton ear buds can be used as swabs. After collection, these swabs should be completely air-dried, and placed in a dry sterile tube, sealed and labelled with necessary information. Other relevant information about the sample should be sent separately along with the sample. In gang rape cases, 3 to 4 vaginal swabs should be collected from different areas of vagina and sent in separate tubes. The surrounding areas of the private parts of victim should be swabbed with wet cotton swabs moistened with sterile water. These swabs should be packed in separate vials. The clothes worn by the victim at the time of the offence, should be air-dried and packed in papers. The sample should not be dried under direct sunlight or by any artificial method. If there is delay in dispatching the samples to the lab, the vaginal swabs should be stored at 4°C in a refrigerator. The cloth material should be stored at room temperature. The vaginal smeared slides should be packed individually and sent at room temperature to the lab. Dried stains on immovable articles can be collected as in the case of blood stains. The blood samples of the accused should be collected in a glass bottle as described earlier.

(3) SALIVA: Saliva in liquid state or stained area, as much as possible should be sent in dried condition.

(4) STAINS FROM SCENE OF CRIME: Stains from body fluids at the scene of crime or large objects should be swabbed with sterile cotton buds moistened with sterile water, air-dried and placed in a clean bottle and sent to lab at room temperature.

(5) BLOOD/SEMEN stains from individuals or in field conditions: Blood/semen from the individuals could be collected in sterile conditions and spread on sterile bandage cloth folded several times so as to make it absorb all the body fluid. This should be air-dried in shade and placed in a clean envelope, sealed, labelled and sent to lab at room temperature. Liquid semen found in the vagina or elsewhere should be recovered with a fine pipette, placed in a small plain tube and frozen.

(6) URINE: Urine about 10 ml should be freezed, or stain as available should be sent in dried condition.

(7) HAIR: Hair(10 to 20) can be picked up by using a forceps without damaging the root.

(8) VISCERAL SAMPLES: In mutilated bodies, samples of 100 g. of muscle should be dissected using sterile instruments and placed in a sterile glass or polypropylene tube containing normal saline, as a preservative. If available, a 20% solution of dimethyl sulphoxide (DMSO) saturated with sodium chloride can be used as preservative. In cases of mass disasters, air crashes, bomb blasts, etc., where several pieces of body are found, sufficient amount of muscle may be collected individually and sent as separate exhibits. In exhumations when dry tissues are present, they should be placed in a sterile tube without preservative and sent at room temperature to the lab.

In case of foetus, the placenta should be removed and only foetus sent in normal saline or DMSO. The jar containing foetus should be placed in a thermocole box containing ice and sent to the lab.

(9) BONES AND TEETH: Femur and humerus yield more bone marrow and are preferred. If skull containing teeth are found, molar teeth from upper and lower jaws should be detached and sent. If molar teeth are not available, other teeth may be sent. Bones should be packed in clean paper or cloth. No preservative is necessary. Teeth should be placed in a clean polythene cover. Skull containing teeth, which has been used for superimposition test is not useful for DNA analysis. As such few teeth should be extracted from upper and lower jaws before cleaning for superimposition.

(10) FINGERNAIL SCRAPINGS: The palm of the victim should be placed on a clean polythene sheet, and the inner portion of the fingernails scraped with a toothpick, etc. and placed in a polythene sheet.

SAMPLE PRESERVATION: Freezing is simplest procedure. For long storage –70°C up to 5 weeks; up to 5 days storage in ice. The tissue samples should be wrapped in aluminium foil, placed in plastic bags

and frozen. Fixation by formaldehyde is not recommended. Dried stains should be collected in clean envelops and maintained dry or frozen.

AUTHENTICATION AND FORWARDING: Blood samples in cases of paternity disputes and in cases where they are used as control samples for identification purposes should be collected in the presence of judicial officer. The samples should be sealed, and a specimen of the seal on paper, should be sent along with the samples for verification. The identification card and the forwarding note should be filled, certified and sent to the lab along with the samples. In persons who had blood transfusion within three months preceding the date of collection, the samples are not useful.

The material can be forwarded to the lab by Executive or Judicial Magistrates, S.I. of Police or above ranks, Asst. Civil Surgeons and above rank.

Forensic Applications: (1) Murder: The blood on a weapon can be matched against the blood of the victim. Blood stains on the clothing or the person of the accused in a case of murder can be matched with the blood of the victim. Hair roots found on a weapon can be matched against the blood of the victim and accused.

(2) Sexual crimes: In sexual crimes, the seminal DNA obtained from the vaginal aspirates or swabs, or from the skin or clothing of the victim is printed and compared with the DNA prints obtained from blood samples of the suspects. **There is no need to match semen against semen. A salivary stain or a hair transferred from the accused to the victim can be used for comparison.** If they match, the suspect is criminal, otherwise not. If a condom is recovered it should be frozen intact. Seminal stains and vaginal epithelial cells will identify the victim and assailant. This technique has particular use in cases of serial rapists in matching evidence obtained from different cases.

(3) Paternity disputes: In paternity dispute cases, the blood of the child, mother and alleged father are printed for DNA. A child will have 50% DNA from mother and 50% from father. **The bars in the child's code are matched first with the patterns of the mother. The remaining bars are then matched with the patterns of the father.** If they correspond, he is the father. The parents should not have had a blood transfusion within three months, before taking the sample. Mutation of the genes (non-inherited germline) in a child can give rise to wrong results in paternity testing.

(4) Disputed maternity.

(5) Exchange of newborn in hospitals.

(6) Identification of **mutilated remains** as in cases of accidents, mass disasters, bomb blasts, burnt bodies, putrefied bodies, etc. The DNA fingerprint obtained from such remains can be compared with previous prints if available or with that of the close blood-relatives of the deceased, which can establish links between family members.

(7) Extortion cases: Saliva samples from envelopes, face masks, nasal secretions, saliva from cigarette butts, etc.

(8) Identification of bodies in exhumation cases.

(9) For tracing pedigrees and for establishing family relationship.

(10) For species identification and sexing.

(11) It is useful to know if male or female components are present in the sample. The amelogenin locus will show one band in female and two bands in male.

(12) All cases of biological identification.

(13) To exonerate a falsely implicated person of any crime.

(14) In hit-and-run traffic accidents matching DNA from blood of victim from bloodstains on a vehicle.

(15) Diagnosis of inherited disorders in prenatal and newborn babies.

(16) To determine how the races migrated from one region to another.

The test can be done even on very old stains or specimens.

PROBLEMS: Problems associated with profiling are: (1) The technique is essentially an autoradiographing technique in the sense that the radioactive probes activate X-ray film. If the hybridization is improper/if activation is less, the band pattern might change. (2) Improper preservation and storage of sample can result in fragmentation of DNA molecule, and can lead to problems in analysis. (3) When sample is contaminated with bacteria, DNA will be degraded. (4) Mutation of genes in a child can give rise to wrong results in paternity testing. (5) Recent DNA typing methods do not discriminate monozygotic (uniovular) twins. In such cases, DNA sequence of bone marrow derived B lymphocytes have to be studied. (6) The scientists interpretation of the band pattern might be inaccurate due to inability to visualise the patterns properly. (7) Unlike the fingerprints, which can be enlarged and shown in the Court, allowing the judges to make up their minds about points of resemblance, DNA profile are very minute. Resolution may be very faint, hence the expert's evidence is taken on trust and faith.

There are yet no proper International guidelines. Each lab has its own control/standardization methods. As the test is a fairly complicated procedure requiring stringent control measures, labs may make mistakes. Court is unlikely to understand in any detail the principles of the process. In DNA profiles/fingerprints everything is taken on trust. Expert witnesses put an interpretation upon an autoradiograph, assert odds of random matches, explain apparent non-matches.

CASES: (1) A Ghanian boy living in U.K. emigrated to Ghana to join his father. When he decided to return to U.K. the immigration authorities, suspecting a replacement/substitution refused entry. Conventional blood and genetic marker tests showed that the mother and the boy were related, but the possibility that the woman was the boy's aunt could not be ruled out. DNA test carried out by Jeffrey proved that the boy and the woman were in fact mother and son.

(2) Loraine Benson was murdered near Raynes Park station in London just before Christmas'88. Several items were submitted to FSL including a man's hanky, stained with blood. The blood stain proved to be Loraine's. A nasal mucosal stain was also found on hanky which was profiled. This was not Loraine's. No semen/alien blood stains was detected. Early in February '89, a rape attempt occurred close to the murder scene. A suspect, Dumme, was arrested after a chance fingerprint was found and tallied. Police thought him to be a likely suspect. His blood sample was profiled. This matched with the profile obtained from the mucosal stain on the hanky. Dumme pleaded guilty.

(3) A rape victim thought that she had recognized the assailant from her school days. After positive identification at an identification parade, a blood sample was sent for DNA analysis and compared with DNA profile obtained from rapist's semen. The suspect was eliminated. However the DNA banding proved similar, thereby suggesting that a close relative of the suspect could be the assailant. A sample from the brother of the suspect proved positive and he pleaded guilty.

This case is particularly interesting as it proved highly protective for an innocent man. Traditional blood grouping test might well have produced results quite similar to his brother. That and a positive identification based on past acquaintance could have put him in real danger of miscarriage of justice.

Several convictions have occurred in India, in which DNA fingerprinting has been accepted as evidence under S.45, of Indian Evidence Act.

CHAPTER

21

ARTEFACTS

FM2.14: Describe and discuss examination of clothing, preservation of viscera on postmortem examination for chemical analysis and other medicolegal purposes, postmortem artefacts.

Artefact is any change caused or feature introduced in a body after death (accidental or physiologically unrelated finding to the natural state of the body), **that is likely to lead to misinterpretation of medicolegally significant antemortem findings. Artefact is a structure or substance not normally present but produced by some external agency or action. Misinterpretation may lead to wrong cause and manner of death and miscarriage of justice.** The responsibility of autopsy pathologist is very great. Often the doctor is the chief source of evidence upon which legal decisions are made, and the freedom or imprisonment, or the life or death of an accused person depends on his evidence. Therefore, **the doctor should learn to draw conclusions logically and correctly,** instead of forming hasty judgement. The autopsy pathologist should be able to distinguish them from the significant antemortem changes. Further, if the doctor misinterprets the artefacts, he will have a tough time in the Court during cross-examination, for a lawyer aware of these pitfalls, may attempt to discredit his evidence.

(A) ARTEFACTS INTRODUCED BETWEEN DEATH AND AUTOPSY

(I) Agonal Artefacts: (1) Regurgitation and aspiration of gastric contents is a common agonal artefact. It may be seen in natural deaths, as a terminal event, or due to handling of the body, or due to resuscitation. (2) One of the effects of asphyxia is to cause vomiting due to medullary suboxia. As a result, the air-passages may be filled at the end of asphyxial event by inhaled vomit. The findings, especially in infants should not be assumed to be the cause of asphyxia ; it is more likely to be the result. In case of choking, particles may be drawn into the bronchioles, which distinguish the condition from those cases in which food is forced up the oesophagus and falls in the larynx after death. (3) **Oesophagogastromalacia** is rarely seen in persons who die within hours or days after receiving severe head injury with cerebral damage. This occurs due to autodigestion; stomach contents are spilled into left chest cavity or left subphrenic area. The tissue affected is grayish-white to black and very friable. It may occur immediately before or shortly after death. It is an agonal or postmortem artefact.

(II) Resuscitation Artefacts: (1) The injection marks of resuscitation are usually found in the cardiac region or on the extremities. In intracardiac injection, heart may show contusion and blood may collect in the pericardium. Some of the injection marks may be associated with postmortem bruises. (2) A defibrillator applied to the chest may produce a ring-like contusion. Superficial skin burns resembling the shape of conductive material and skeletal muscle necrosis can be caused by trans- thoracic defibrillator. (3) External massage may cause bruising of the anterior chest wall, haemorrhage into subcutaneous tissues and pectoral muscles, symmetrical, parasternal fractures of several ribs and sometimes of sternum. The sternum fractures through the middle of the body and manubrium. There may be associated tears of the lungs with release of free air into the tissues. Haemorrhages in the lungs are usually associated with remote parenchymal and subpleural hexagonal foci of aspirated blood. There may be rupture of atria and ventricles. Anterior pericardial or mediastinal contusion, sometimes haemopericardium, and rarely epicardial haematoma or myocardial contusion may be seen. Lacerations of the liver occur due to direct manipulation of the liver area and also by a push and pull effect on the liver ligaments and the diaphragm. Less commonly, the spleen is lacerated due to the same mechanism. In most of these cases, fracture sites do not show haemorrhage and intercostal muscles do not show contusions. In such cases, the lungs show bone marrow or fat emboli in about 20% of cases. (4) Vigorous resuscitation with a thoracotomy and internal cardiac massage, produces air embolism. (5) When positive pressure breathing apparatus (respirator) is used for resuscitation, it produces acute emphysema, sometimes with subpleural blebs, air in the mediastinum or tension pneumothorax. The administration of oxygen by mask or tube may cause rupture of oesophagus and lung. (6) Contusions of soft tissues of the neck may be mistaken for homicidal strangulation. The introduction of i.v. cannulae into veins in the neck may cause large haematomata and more diffuse bleeding into the tissues alongside the larynx. These resuscitation injuries may be mistaken for those due to assault or from steering-wheel impact injuries. In such cases, history is very important. (7) Damage to the mouth, palate, pharynx and larynx can occur from attempts to introduce a laryngoscope. The oesophagus can be perforated by incorrectly inserted airway. (8) Oesophageal intubation can produce gastric dilatation. (9)

Endotracheal intubation can cause contusions, lacerations, abrasions and petechiae in laryngeal and tracheal mucosa and in some cases in mouth, epiglottis and pharynx. Contusions and lacerations of the pharynx or oesophagus with perforation can occur. (10) Pneumothorax may develop from placing a subclavian or internal jugular central venous catheter (11) Pulmonary artery wedge catheter can cause haemothorax, pneumothorax and pulmonary artery tear. (12) A cervical neck collar used to stabilise the head and neck may produce linear impressions in the skin of the neck which may resemble a ligature furrow. (13) A chest tube may be placed through a pre-existing stab wound or gunshot wound. (14) Sometimes, more than one incision may be made to insert chest tubes. These should not be confused with inflicted stab or incised wounds from an assault. (15) After death, extremities may be bound by string to facilitate transport, producing marks resembling abrasions. (16) Medical tape after removal, can abrade the skin in a linear fashion, and resembles a ligature abrasion. Mouth-to-mouth breathing may cause contusions of the face, neck, and damage to the lips and inner gums, when the face and neck have been gripped by a hand.

(III) Artefacts due to the Handling of the Body: (1) Occasionally, fractures of the ribs or the bones of extremities, or of cervical spine may occur by rough handling of bodies, especially if there is severe osteoporosis. They are commonly produced during attempts to straighten the limbs contracted due to rigor mortis. Bleeding is usually absent in such postmortem fractures. (2) Contusion of the occipital region may be caused, if the head of corpse is allowed to fall on a hard surface during handling. (3) Fresh abrasions may be produced due to dragging of the body which were originally free from them, during the transfer of the body from the scene of crime. (4) **Undertaker's fracture is a subluxation of the lower cervical spine due to tearing of the intervertebral disc at about C6–C7.**

(IV) Artefacts Related to Rigor Mortis: (1) The handling of the body may cause breaking of the rigor at least partially, which may mislead the doctor in the estimation of the time of death. (2) The onset and duration of the rigor may be altered by atmospheric conditions like extreme heat or cold, or antemortem conditions like muscular state, exhaustion, wasting diseases, and hyperthermia due to infections. (3) Rigor affecting the heart may simulate concentric hypertrophy of the heart. (4) Rigor in stomach may accentuate the rugae or fix a point of contraction so as to give a pseudo-hourglass, which is readily removed by traction. (5) Rigor in pylorus causes it to be unduly firm and contracted.

(V) Artefacts Related to Postmortem Lividity: (1) The colour of the postmortem stains is usually bluish-purple. Certain poisons may change the colour of the hypostatic area, e.g., cherry-red colour in CO poisoning, bright-red colour in HCN poisoning, brown or chocolate colour in poisoning by nitrites, potassium chlorate and aniline, dark-brown colour in phosphorus poisoning. The postmortem stains are of pink colour in bodies exposed to cold and in refrigerated bodies. (2) Patches of haemorrhage, sometimes quite large and confluent, can occur in the tissues behind the oesophagus at the level of the larynx. These lie on the anterior surface of the cervical vertebrae and are caused by distension and leakage from the venous plexuses that lie in this area, and can be mistaken due to strangulation. (3) 'Banding' of the oesophagus may be seen, especially when the tissues are congested. These bands are pale areas in the mucosa caused by postmortem hypostasis being prevented from settling by the external pressure of adjacent anatomical structures, including parts of the larynx, trachea, and aortic arch. It is commonly seen in routine non-traumatic autopsies. (4) Large petechiae or ecchymoses, sometimes with raised blood blisters may be seen in the dependent skin of persons who have died a congestive death, or when upper part of the body hangs down after death. They are commonly seen over the upper part of front of chest and on the back of the shoulders. The face may show haemorrhages when the head is dependent.

(VI) Artefacts due to Burns: (1) Heat ruptures may resemble lacerated or incised wounds. (2) Heat haematoma may simulate extradural haemorrhage. (3) An unburnt groove around the neck due to tightness of the clothes, e.g. collar, may resemble a strangulation mark. In severely burnt bodies, fat droplets may be found in the pulmonary vessels, which should not be mistaken for antemortem pulmonary fat embolism. (4) Radiant heat reaching the body after death may cause loosening or drying and tanning of the skin.

(VII) Artefacts in Firearm Wounds: (1) Drainage wounds may be mistaken for firearm wounds. (2) In decomposition, there may be peeling of skin and loss of hair and gunpowder from the skin around an entrance wound. The margins of an entry wound may become ragged due to disintegration of the tissue at the margins, and it becomes difficult to distinguish entrance wound from exit. (3) Cleaning, excision, suturing or surgical extension of entry wound will remove gunpowder and alter size, shape, etc. causing difficulty in differentiating entry and exit wound. (4) Use of trocar for embalming through gunshot wound may alter the track making interpretation difficult. (5) Sometimes, unexpectedly a bullet may be found in the body, which may be densely encapsulated due to old injury, whereas the actual cause of death may be something else.

(VIII) Artefacts due to Animal and Insect Bites (Anthropophagy): (1) Rodents gnaw away tissue over localised areas, which are usually circular or wedge-shaped, with finely serrated margins, showing irregular edges by nibbling and leave long grooves. (2) The bites by dogs are clear-cut, with deep impressions of teeth in small area. Individual punctures may resemble stab wounds. (3) Cat bites are usually very small and round. Face and neck are usually involved in the recumbent body. They may sometimes resemble knife wounds, especially in bones. (4) Marks produced by insects (ants or roaches) are dry, brown with irregular margins, and are usually seen in moist parts of the body, e.g., ears, armpits, groin, scrotum, anus, etc. They resemble antemortem abrasions. As they become dry, they resemble brush burns. They do not show vital reaction. Extensive linear ant lesions around the neck resemble ligature abrasion. (5) Rarely, injuries, caused by crabs, may simulate stab wounds. (6) Postmortem injuries produced from the bumping of the body into rocks, coral or marine structures should be distinguished from antemortem trauma. (7) Similarly, fractures caused by fall into the water from a height due to the body striking forcibly against some solid object, or mutilation from boat propellers, or loss of fingers, toes, eyelids, lips, genitals or rarely whole portions of the body occurring from the attacks of marine animals should also be distinguished. (8) Leeches, which become attached to

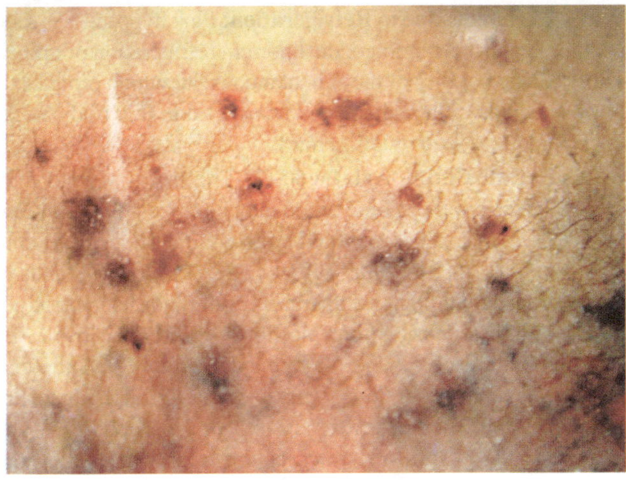

Fig. (21-1). **Ant bites.**

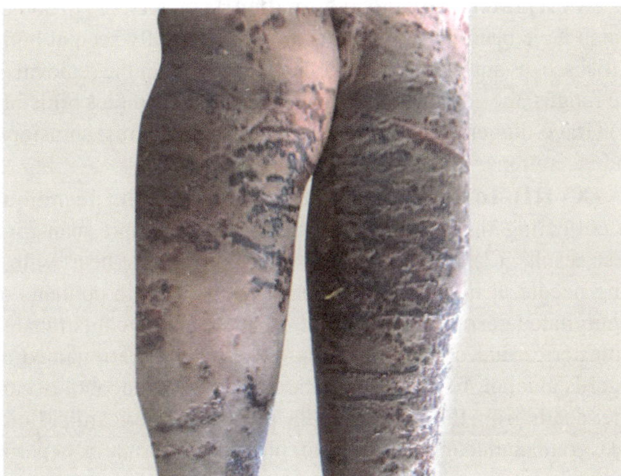

Fig. (21–2). **Ant bites on legs.**

Courtesy: **Dr K Tamil Mani, Chennai**

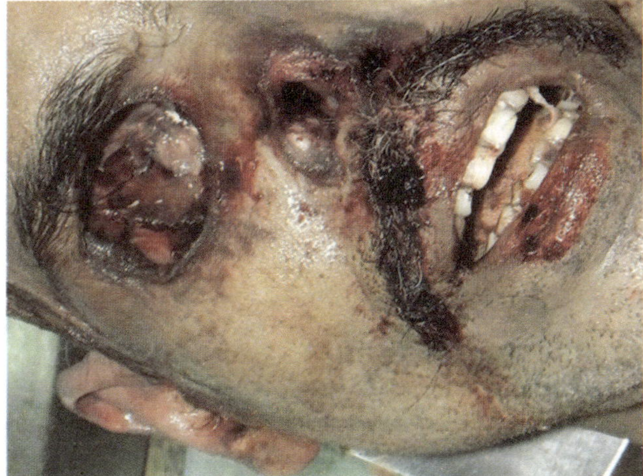

Fig. (21–3). **Rodent bites.**

the skin around the eyes, and detach when the body is removed from the water may produce haemorrhagic lesion simulating a black eye. (9) Crabs and other crustaceans, turtles and fish tend to gnaw the soft tissues around the eyes, ears, mouth, genitals,

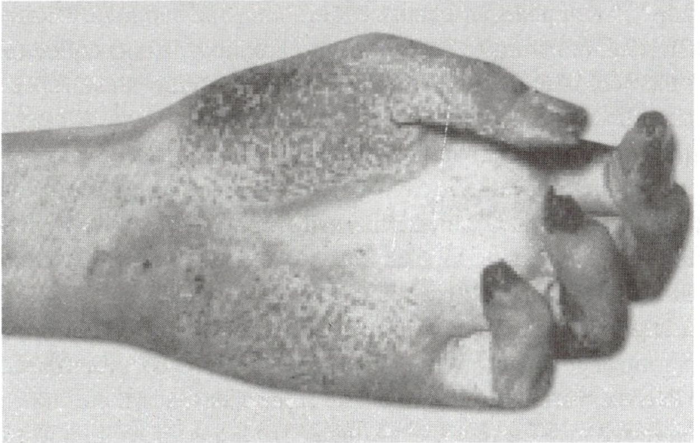

Fig. (21–4). **Erosion of the skin by rodents.**

anus and edges of the surface wounds of the body. Any animal attacking the dead body usually selects those areas where the skin is broken. Antemortem wounds are thus greatly enlarged.

(IX) Artefacts in Brain: (1) Flattening of the convolutions of brain is seen in cases of oedema of the brain, which is generalised. Regional flattening of the cerebral convolutions is a postmortem artefact, which is seen in those parts of the brain which are in contact with the cranium, especially the occipital lobes. (2) Grooving of the unci is seen in cases of raised intracranial pressure. Uncal grooving is also found in normal brains as an artefact. (3) Rough removal of the brain may cause artificial damage to the ponto-medullary region or to the midbrain-pons junction.

(X) Artefacts in Liver: (1) The undersurface of the liver in contact with transverse colon shows greenish colouration due to putrefaction. (2) The liver surface is also stained due to bile.

(XI) Postmortem Haemorrhage: (1) Before the blood clots, a postmortem injury may damage a blood vessel and produce haemorrhage. (2) After death, blood may collect in the pleural cavities due to wounds produced on the chest wall and the lung tissue. **Intercostal veins bleed much more than arteries.** (3) After death, blunt impact may lacerate blood vessels and displace red cells into the tissue spaces. Patches of haemorrhage, sometimes large and confluent can occur in the tissues behind the oesophagus on the anterior surface of the cervical vertebrae, due to distension and leakage from the venous plexuses that lie in these areas.

(XII) Artefacts Related to Hair: The beard may appear to grow after death in some cases, whereas the growth of hair stops immediately after death. The cause of this postmortem apparent growth of beard is the shrinkage of the skin, due to which greater part of the hair shaft is exposed above the epidermis.

(XIII) Artefacts due to Decomposition: (1) Intense localised lividity of skin due to hypostasis, or displacement of internal pools of blood by pressure of gases of decomposition produces pseudo-bruising which may simulate antemortem bruises. (2) Internal hypostasis with haemolysis of red cells may resemble haemorrhage, especially in the meninges, kidneys and retroperitoneal tissues. (3) In a dead body lying on its back, blood accumulates in the posterior part of the scalp due to gravity. In advanced decomposition, due to lysis of red cells and breakdown of the vessels, blood seeps into the soft tissues of the scalp. This appears as a confluent bruising and cannot always be differentiated from true antemortem bruising. Blood collecting in the occipital areas of brain due to gravity may cause rupture of small venules in decomposing bodies with very thin localised film of blood in subarachnoid or subdural areas of occipital lobes. (4) Bloody fluid may be found in the mouth and nose in decomposed bodies, which is marked in conditions which produce pulmonary oedema. In such cases, the cause of death should not be mistaken for haemorrhage. (5) Accumulation of blood in the tissues of the neck in drowning may simulate antemortem haemorrhage due to strangulation. (6) The blood becomes darker in decomposition, due to which the brain, lungs, heart, etc. appear congested, which may be mistaken for signs of asphyxia. (7) Due to decomposition, gases collect in the tissues, cavities, and hollow viscera under considerable pressure, and subcutaneous tissues become emphysematous. These changes may cause a false impression of antemortem obesity. (8) A deep groove simulating ligature mark of strangulation may be seen around the neck in decomposed bodies and also in mummification, if the deceased has been wearing buttoned shirt at the time of death. (9) Air in the right side of the heart due to decomposition may be mistaken for air embolism. Oxygen in right heart will indicate air embolism, because it is not present in appreciable quantity, if the gases were those of decomposition. In cases of air embolism, the volume of air is much larger than that due to decomposition. (10) Blebs formed due to putrefaction may be mistaken for blebs from burns. (11) Regurgitated gastric juices may cause tanning of the skin of the face and neck, which may simulate antemortem burning. (12) Separation of sutures of the skull in a child due to gases of decomposition within the brain, and bursting of the abdomen with protrusion of the abdominal viscera due to advanced decomposition should not be mistaken for trauma. (13) In advanced decomposition, small miliary granules or plaques one to 3 mm. in diameter may be seen on serous or endothelial surfaces of the body, such as pleura, peritoneum, pericardium and endocardium. They resemble grayish-white colonies of bacteria growing on surface of an agar. They consist of calcium, fat, endothelial cells and bacteria, and should not be mistaken for inflammatory lesions or the effect of a poison. (14) Lungs may show postmortem bacterial colonies. (15) The pancreas is one of the most vulnerable organs to postmortem autolysis, because of the action of its own enzymes. At first it is softened and haemorrhagic. Later, it may resemble haemorrhagic pancreatitis. Histological changes of necrosis are usually seen within a few hours after death. Inflammatory reaction and fat necrosis are absent in such cases. (16) Fissures or splits in the skin formed due to putrefaction may simulate antemortem lacerations or incised wounds. (17) Small round holes produced by maggots may simulate bullet holes. (18) Excessive flaccidity of vaginal orifice with effusion of bloody fluid and spontaneous detachment of portions of mucous membrane of vagina may simulate antemortem sexual assault.

(XIV) Artefacts due to Chemicals: In automobile accidents or airplane crashes, exposure to gasoline causes postmortem detachment of epidermis. On exposure to air, the underlying dermis has a yellow to brown colour as drying occurs. They resemble thermal burns or abrasions. They occur particularly when the fire is put out with water.

(XV) Artefacts due to Refrigeration: Pink hypostasis is seen in bodies kept in cold storage. Postmortem refrigeration of infants usually causes solidity of the subcutaneous fat, which produces a prominent crease where there was a normal skin fold of the neck, which resembles strangulation mark.

(XVI) Embalming Artefacts: (1) The trocar wound may simulate a stab wound. Some blood may be forced out of injured blood vessels due to pressure and collect in the tissues and may be mistaken for antemortem haemorrhage. (2) The skin tends to become transparent due to embalming and minor haemorrhages become visible, which may sometimes create problems. (3) A homicidal stab wound may be enlarged by the embalmer to approach an artery or he may pass a trocar through a gunshot wound. This will modify the dimensions of the wounds. (4) The trocar may also disturb the track of the weapon or bullet and produce false tracks. (5) The blood will clot and produce multiple clots within the pulmonary vasculature.

(XVII) Interment and exhumation Artefacts: (1) In bodies which have been buried, fungus growth is usually seen at body orifices, eyes and at the sites of open injuries. After the removal of the fungus, the colour of the underlying skin resembles bruising. (2) Grave-diggers can produce postmortem fractures, abrasions, and lacerations.

(XVIII) Toxicological Artefacts: (1) Faulty technique in collecting the sample, especially blood sample, can give false results. (2) When blood is collected from the heart with a long needle, it may be contaminated with stomach contents or regurgitated oesophageal contents. (3) If blood is contaminated with pericardial or pleural fluids, false results are obtained as regards alcohol, because significant diffusion of alcohol occurs after death, from the stomach to the pleural and pericardial fluid. (4) Certain anticoagulants used for blood, e.g., formalin, heparin, methenamine, and EDTA give a positive test for methanol. (5) Decomposition of the tissues after death produces ethyl alcohol and other higher alcohols. Many of the bacteria can produce alcohol, the values of which are less than 200 mg%. (6) Decomposition also causes an increase of concentration of CO in the blood up to 19%. (7) Significant amounts of cyanide are also produced due to decomposition. (8) In cases of death due to burns, significant amounts of cyanide may be found in the blood, possibly due to inhalation of hydrogen cyanide. (9) Many substituted phenols are found in decomposing tissues, especially P-hydroxyphenyl derivatives. (10) In buried bodies, arsenic may be imbibed from the surrounding earth. Keratin tissues absorb arsenic by external contamination due to which, the concentration in hair and nail may be much greater than the concentration of arsenic in the contaminating fluid.

(B) ARTEFACTS INTRODUCED DURING AUTOPSY:

(I) Air in Blood Vessels: Pulling of the dura in the sagittal line will cause the air to enter the blood vessels at the top of the brain. Similarly air may enter the veins of the neck during the reflection of the skin. This may lead to erroneous diagnosis of air embolism.

(II) Skull Fractures: Fractures of skull usually in the middle fossae may be produced due to partial sawing and forceful pull of the skull cap or due to partial sawing and then using chisel and hammer to loosen the skull cap. This may produce additional fractures or may cause extension of already present antemortem fractures. In such cases, differentiation between antemortem and postmortem fractures may become very difficult.

(III) Visceral Damage: (1) Rough handling of the brain during removal may produce tears of the midbrain. (2) Rough handling of the liver during removal may produce tears of the diaphragmatic surface, which simulate antemortem lacerations. (3) If the neck structures are pulled too hard during autopsy to drag out the thoracic viscera, they may be torn, and also transverse intimal tears may be produced in the descending aorta.

(IV) Extravasation of Blood: (1) In case of suspected cranial injury, the body should be opened, and the cardiovascular system decompressed by opening the heart before the head is opened. If blood has not been drained from vessels of the head, damage to the dura and the dural venous sinuses on removal of skull cap, may lead to an escape of blood into the subdural space, simulating an antemortem subdural haemorrhage. (2) Large blood vessels may be cut, while opening the thoracic and abdominal cavities, and considerable amount of blood escape into the pleural and peritoneal cavities. (3) Air may be drawn back into the circulation and enter coronary vessels and give false impression of air embolism. (4) During autopsy, the handling of organs and the incision of the vessels may result in extravasation of blood into the tissues. (5) The removal of the neck structures *en block* as in routine autopsies, may produce artefacts in the neck tissues which resemble bruises seen in the case of throttling. Therefore, the neck structures should be dissected *in situ* and in a bloodless field.

(V) Fracture of Hyoid Bone: (1) When the tongue and neck structures are firmly grasped and pulled upon while removing the neck organs, the hyoid bone and thyroid cartilage may be fractured, especially in old persons. Surrounding the fracture regions, haemorrhages are not seen. (2) Osseous union between the segments of hyoid may be unilateral. Such unilateral mobility or artefact by dissection may lead to the erroneous impression of antemortem fracture.

(VI) Injury to Blood Vessels: While dissecting the neck structures, if toothed dissecting forceps is used, it may damage the intima of the carotid artery which resembles a tear, as is seen in case of strangulation.

(VII) Toxicological Artefacts: They may be introduced due to: (1) Contamination of viscera with stomach contents during autopsy, or by putting all the organs in one container, or by using contaminated instruments or containers. (2) Faulty technique in collecting the sample. (3) Faulty storage or use of preservatives.

CHAPTER

22

FORENSIC SCIENCE LABORATORY

FM 6.1: Describe different types of specimen and tissues to be collected both in the living and dead: Body fluids (blood, urine, semen, faeces saliva), skin, nails, tooth pulp, vaginal smear, viscera, skull, specimen for histopathological examination, blood grouping, HLA typing and DNA fingerprinting. Describe Locard's exchange principle.
FM 6.2: Describe the methods of sample collection, preservation, labelling, dispatch, and interpretation of reports.
FM 7.1: Enumerate the indications and describe the principles and appropriate use for:

- DNA profiling
- Facial reconstruction
- Polygraph (Lie detector)
- Narcoanalysis
- Brain mapping
- Digital autopsy
- Virtual autopsy
- Imaging technologies

Forensic science is **the study and application of scientific examination and evaluation of evidence, for legal purposes.** Forensic sciences include: (1) Forensic medicine. (a) Forensic pathology. (b) Forensic psychiatry. (2) Forensic toxicology. (3) Forensic immunology. (4) Forensic odontology. (5) Forensic anthropology. (6) Forensic police sciences. (a) Criminalistics, wherein evidence, such as blood stains, glass, soil, clothing and firearms is compared, identified, individualised and interpreted. (b) Questioned documents examination involves the scientific examination of handwriting, typewriting, printing ink, paper, or other aspects of a document for the purpose of determining various legal questions asked about the document. (c) Trace evidence. (d) Ballistics. (7) Other forensic science specialities, which include voice print examination, polygraph technology, fingerprinting, etc.

ORGANISATION: Such institutes should provide three major categories of service: clinical, pathological and laboratory. In addition, it should have stores, exhibit room, workshop and library. Usually only laboratory services are provided by the forensic science laboratory.

CLINICAL SERVICES: They include examination of victims of assault, sexual crime, drunkenness, etc.

PATHOLOGY SERVICES: They include chemical analysis, toxicology, serology, biology, photography, fingerprints, ballistics, etc.

MUSEUM: Every laboratory should establish a museum containing fingerprints, bullets and cartridge cases, tyre tread patterns, animal hair, soils, typewritten specimens, inks, rope and cordage, cloth, photographs of various crystal poisons, etc.

STAFFING: (1) Director, medical or scientific. (2) Clinical services. Physician and obstetrician. (3) Pathology services: Pathologist. (4) Laboratory services: Biologist, physicist, serologist, microanalyst, photographer, fingerprint expert, ballistic expert, etc. (5) Others: Librarian, liasion officer.

Functions: (1) To examine, compare and evaluate physical evidence, so as to link a suspect to the victim, or to the scene of a crime. In most cases, the laboratory supplements the work of police investigator in order to convert suspicion into a reasonable certainty of either guilt or innocence. (2) Protection of the innocent, e.g., a person arrested for selling narcotics, is set free if the chemical analysis of the material shows it to be harmless. **It determines facts, which are not subject to the bias and prejudice and other human failings of the eyewitness.** (3) Training of the police investigators as to what constitutes physical evidence, how it is to be found, collected, preserved and delivered to the laboratory.

It is not a solution for all the difficulties that confront the police in searching out crime; **it is merely an aid in crime detection. Its results are more often rather negative than positive.**

Material: The items which are most commonly handled by the laboratory and which frequently serve as evidence are knives, blunt instruments, blood and seminal stains, chemical substances, poisons, fingerprints and footprints, hair, fibres, firearms, bullets, cartridge cases and wad, tools and tool marks, broken glass, paint chips, oil, grease, petroleum products, soils, clothing, pieces of papers, cigars, cigarette stumps, matches, documents and fragments of various materials. Sometimes, laboratory technicians are called to the scene of a crime to collect specimens with which investigating officers are not qualified to deal.

Criminal Investigation: All criminal investigation is concerned either with people or with material objects. **Only people commit crimes but they invariably do so through the medium of objects. It is these objects that together constitute**

physical evidence. The main objective of crime investigation is to recognise, collect, preserve, analyse, interpret and reconstruct all the physical evidence collected (by hands or cellotapes) from the scene of crime. **The term physical evidence (trace evidence) includes any and all objects, living or non-living, solid, liquid or gas, and the relationship between all objects as they relate to the problem in question, e.g., a crime.** A knife, burglar tool, wood splinters, tool marks, firearms, bullets, blood and seminal stains, saliva, pus, milk, poisons, sputum, vomit, fingerprints, hair, fibres, glass, paint, oil, grease, chemicals, signature, teeth marks, handkerchief, footwear, dust, debris, soil, vegetable matter, like grass, seeds, pollen, microscopic fragments of all types, bacteria and even an odour are all physical evidence. The microscopic evidence persists at the scene of a crime long after all the visible and obvious evidence has been removed, and may solve the problem. **When there is even a reasonable chance of finding significant evidence, it should never be neglected, even when the crime was committed long back. Physical evidence can be obtained from the scene of crime, the victim and the suspect and his environment. Physical evidence is useful in two ways:** (1) **It is often the decisive factor in determining guilt or innocence.** It can do this by supplying the demonstrable facts, thus resolving discrepancies in ordinary testimony. (2) **It can be a material aid to link a suspect, a weapon or a scene to a crime.** Evidence should be marked or labelled so that it can be positively identified. Date, time, place, from whom and by whom it was taken or found, should be recorded. The chain of evidence must be intact and complete. Evidence should be preserved in the same condition in which it was found. The forensic scientist must routinely work with forensic scientists of various other disciplines in the investigation of a criminal matter or civil dispute.

Locard's Exchange Principle: When any two objects come into contact, there is always a transfer of material from each object on the other. Traces from the scene may be carried away on the person or tools of the criminal, and at the same time, traces from all or any of these may be left at the scene. Wherever a criminal goes, whatever he touches, and whatever he leaves will serve as silent evidence against him, e.g., fingerprints, footprints, hair, fibres from clothes, broken glass, tool marks, paints, scratches, blood or seminal stains, etc. **It is actual evidence, and its presence is absolute proof of the crime. The evidence of eyewitnesses may be wrong as a result of their partisanship, faulty memory, or defective observation. Physical evidence cannot be wrong and completely absent. Only its interpretation can be wrong. Only human failure to find it, study and understand it, can diminish its value.** The laboratory must be devoted to this study and understanding. Large numbers of criminals escape because the physical evidence is not fully understood and utilised. More laboratory failures are due to inadequate collection of existing evidence, than are caused by the failure of the laboratory to examine it properly. **All laboratory findings are related to a probability, and a single piece of evidence is rarely sufficient in itself to establish proof of guilt or innocence.**

Control Sample: It means specimens of material, e.g. vegetation or soil from the scene, sample of blood, hair, fingerprint, etc. from the victim for comparison with any questioned material from the crime scene. Blood stains found on garment, soil, etc. will require unstained samples to rule out the false positive test due to substrate interference.

ILLUSTRATIONS: The following are some of the illustrations of the usefulness of forensic science laboratory in criminal investigations. The following paragraphs should be correlated with the appropriate chapters.

(1) PERSONAL IDENTITY: The main problem of the criminal investigator is the establishment of personal identity of the criminal. Fingerprints, foot prints, hair, blood, semen, etc., are unique to the individual.

The criminal may be identified indirectly through the tool he used, the gun he fired, the clothes he wore, writing he made, the soil, glass, paint, etc., he removed from the scene of crime. No two objects are ever completely identical. In physical evidence, the term identity must be understood to signify practical and determinable identity only.

(2) BLOOD: In murder, assault, rape, etc., blood from the victim may be present at the scene of the crime, and on the person and clothing of accused and weapons. The distribution and appearance of bloodstained areas on the victim and his clothing may be used to interpret and reconstruct details of the crime. The criminal may be injured in the course of struggle or accidentally either by fall while moving in the dark, or by protruding nail, or broken window glass, in the act of breaking into a house. Blood groups are very useful in cases of disputed paternity.

(3) SEMEN: Stains may be found on the clothes of the accused and victim, pubic hair and person, on the bedding, mattress, floor or ground on which the offence was committed or on the piece of cloth used by the culprit or the victim for wiping after the offence. Ultraviolet light is useful in fluorescence tests, such as examining stains on garments.

(4) FIREARMS: A bullet recovered from a dead body can be examined to determine the type of gun which fired it , and the type of ammunition fired. By careful study of the markings on the bullet, the gun which fired it can be determined.

(5) FINGERPRINTS: A criminal can be identified especially by means of latent prints left at the scene of a crime, on a weapon, or in another incriminating location. Fingerprints are also useful in identification of dead bodies, persons suspected of operating under aliases, amnesia victims, etc.

(6) HAIR: Traces of certain elements are deposited in our hair because of diet, drug intake and atmospheric conditions. The proportions of these differ considerably in different persons and these can be measured through neutron activation analysis. Hair from a criminal may be pulled out by objects at the scene. Similarly, hair from the victim may adhere to the criminal's person, clothing or weapon. In a sexual offence, hair from the victim may be found on the genitals of the accused and vice versa. Hair found sticking to a motor vehicle involved in an accident are useful in the identity of vehicle. Animal hair are very important in case of bestiality, and cattle thefts.

(7) FIBRES: The fibres may be of animal, vegetable, mineral, and synthetic origin. A crime against person often involves contact between the criminal's clothes or weapon on one side and the victim's clothes on the other. Even in burglary, or theft, the criminal often handles or touches several objects in the premises, due to which clothing fibres are transferred from the criminal to the scene of crime and vice versa, because the clothes constantly carry loose fibres. If it is found that a fibre from one source exactly matches one from another source, there is definite probability that the two sources have come into contact with each other.

(8) POISONS: In a suspected case of poisoning, the identification of the poison is necessary. It must be remembered that the presence of injuries or a disease sufficient to account for death does not rule out the possibility of poisoning.

(9) WEAPONS AND TOOLS: A wide variety of tools are used in the commission of crimes, e.g., knives, screwdrivers, bars, saws, pliers, cutters, hammers, drill, etc. Some of these leave marks which are very characteristic, and by which the tool may be quite accurately identified.

The tool may also carry traces from the scene in the form of paint, oil, particles of wood or scratches from nails or other hard objects, and these may lead to the detection of crime. The examination of the wound will indicate the type of the weapon used, and the microscopic evidence can connect the weapon with the perpetrator or perhaps even with wound.

(10) CLOTHES: Fibres, paint, grease or dust may be found on the suspect's clothes in a burglary, and stains of semen or blood on the clothes of both the victim and the assailant in sexual offences.

(11) GLASS: In hit-and-run traffic accident, cyclist's rear lamp may be broken, the glass fragments of which may be found on bumper or other parts of the vehicle. Also, traces of glass from the headlamp of the vehicle may be found at the scene. The burglar in trying to enter the house may break window glass, the fragments of which may be carried in his clothes, etc. The refractive index, specific gravity and exposure to ultraviolet light of the glass fragment help to identify their probable source. The composition of glass can be checked chemically or by spectroscopic examination.

(12) WOOD: If a piece of wood from the handle of the tool used by the criminal is found at a scene, it can be identified by matching it with the handle of the tool seized from the suspect. Particles or splinters of the wood found on the suspect's clothes or tool should be compared with the wood of the door or window broken for the forced entry. Faults, marks, bruises and other individual pointers assist in matching a piece of wood with another piece from which it has been separated. Paint and external factors also indicate a relation between broken pieces. Microscopical examination of the cell structures is useful in identification of sawdust.

(13) METALS: Most evidence which is metallic in nature is in the form of tools and weapons. Like wood, metal pieces from the tool used by the criminal may be found at the scene of the crime, and metal fragments from the door and window fittings, and from the boxes and safes, may be recovered from the criminal's clothing or tool. Metallic fragments can be examined chemically or with the spectroscope and can be identified with a specimen sample of the metal.

(14) TOOL MARKS: The two main types of tool marks are compression and scrap marks with a combination of both and also cutting marks. Every tool has its own peculiarities and the wear causes an individuality which are transmitted to the object on which the tool has been used. The density, pigment distribution, spectrographic analysis to determine the chemical composition of the mineral constituents of paint samples, and microscopic examination give positive proof.

(15) PAINT: In a road accident, flakes of paint from the vehicle may be found on the ground or on the person, animal or object hit by it, and traces of paint from the object may be seen on the vehicle. A burglar may carry on his body, tool or clothing, paint from the wall or doors of the house which he has burgled or from the safe which he has broke open.

(16) DUST AND DIRT: A criminal invariably carries soil in varying quantities on his feet or footwear, from the earth on which he has walked, and on his body or clothing, from the ground on which he has lied down during the commission of the crime, or fallen in the course of a struggle. Soil usually consists of mineral constituents, decomposed organic matter, broken leaves, pollen, grains, etc., capable of direct identification.

(17) VEGETABLE MATERIAL: Anyone committing a crime out of doors is likely to get plant material on his clothing, the identification of which will connect him with the scene. Algae and fungi are usually found on damp walls, in buildings, the soils, on vegetation and on domestic articles. The burglar climbing the damp wall or fallpipe may get smears of green algae. Seeds, portions of leaf, bark and other vegetable fragments are useful and can be identified to belong to particular areas of country. Grass fragments, particularly uncommon types, pollen, weeds and seeds are identifiable with their particular source of origin.

(18) STRINGS AND ROPES: The criminal may have brought his tools to the scene tied up in a bundle with string or cord, and may have left it behind. If it is identical in structure, size, shape, and appearance with another found in the suspect's possession, it is of great value.

(19) TYRE MARKS: It may be possible to trace a car by means of its tyre marks. A tyre mark should be compared with a test mark and not directly with the tyre.

(20) DOCUMENTS: Questioned documents may necessitate: (1) Physical and chemical examination including a study and identification of: (a) writing materials, e.g., paper, pen, ink, pencil, typewriter, (b) erasures, obliterations, and alterations, (c) order and age of writing, typing or other markings, (2) identification of the authorship of the writing. The individual should be asked to write something for the purposes of comparison with a questioned document. Infrared light will assist in the examination of closed letters, questioned documents, etc.

(21) SPEECH: Computer Speech Lab (CSL) facilitates comparison of two voices, one that of the suspect and the other known by means of a combination of words and sentences selected from speech. It uses computers to compare pitch, frequency, intensity and micro-tremors in the voice of a person. It can help in cases like kidnap for ransom, threats, obscene calls, terrorist threats, extortion, etc. Voice mails and gunshots also can be analysed.

(22) PHOTOGRAPHY: Photography provides life-like reproductions which serve to refresh memory, and are a useful evidence. In the forensic sciences photographs are used (1) as a means to record a phenomenon observed, and (2) to reveal that cannot normally be seen. The first category includes the recording of simple matching techniques, photomicrography, and photomacrography. The second category includes the effect of infrared and ultraviolet radiations which helps in seeing things which are not seen in ordinary light, such as faint letter marks, and the production of radiographs using X-rays.

(23) LIE DETECTION: (A) Polygraph: It is an instrument used to detect lies. Keeler polygraph, and Stoelling deceptograph are in common use. **Polygraph makes a continuous record of blood pressure, pulse, respiration, muscular movements and electrodermal reaction changes in response to stimuli in the form of questions. It is based on the theory, that when the person tells a lie in answer to a question, and there is fear that lie will be detected, the emotion of fear results in stimulation of sympathetic nervous system which results in certain physiological changes (psychosomatic reactions), some of which may be easily recorded.** There is relative rise in blood pressure and recovery, pulse rate increases, slowing down of the breathing, erratic breathing, and many times suppression of involuntary muscular movements, and lowering of the galvanic skin resistance of the individual due to increased activity of sweat glands.

In pre-test interview, the test questions are framed with the mutual consent of the subjects and to the satisfaction of examiner, that they are adequate to serve the purpose of the particular examination. **A basic explanation of the attachments in the polygraph is given to the subject.** An attempt is made to answer the subject's questions regarding the procedure. **The questions are framed in such a way that they are clearly understood by the subject and they call for only 'Yes' or 'No' as answer. The questions usually number ten. Relevant and irrelevant questions are mixed up.** The control questions are put to reduce the natural nervousness, the natural stigma of the issue at stake, and the natural slight resentment of the accusatory nature of the matter involved in the investigation. A question is asked every 20 to 25 seconds, and polygraph chart recorded in 3 to 4 minutes. Usually, the same test is repeated twice or thrice as a check on any possible error. **An experienced and competent polygraph examiner can correctly detect truth or lie in about 80 to 90% cases.** The few errors that do occur favour the innocent, since the known mistakes in diagnosis almost always involve a failure to detect lies of deceptive subjects. Offenders, suspects, complainants, witnesses and informants are examined by this method to test truth of their statements. It is also useful in civil cases, e.g., paternity cases, insurance claims, pre-employment screening by banks and other institutions.

(B) Narcoanalysis: ("truth serum" drugs): This is based on the principle, that at a point very close to unconsciousness, the subject will be mentally incapable of resistance to questioning, and incapable of inventing the falsehoods that he has used to conceal his guilt. The methods used are: (1) Half mg. of scopolamine hydrobromide, s.c., followed by one-fourth mg. every twenty minutes, for an average of 3 to 6 injections, until the subject reaches the proper stage for questioning. (2) Sodium amytal or sodium pentothal (truth serum) 2.5 to 5% solution i.v. at a rate not to exceed one ml., until the proper stage is induced. (3) 0.1g. sodium seconal, one and half hours before induction; 45 minutes later 15 mg. morphine sulphate and half mg. scopolamine hydrobromide are given s.c To save time all three drugs may be given intravenously. It depresses CNS, lowers B.P. and slows heart rate. **In a state of relaxation, the suspect is susceptible to suggestion and reveals repressed feelings or memories. The drugs will remove inhibitions, but not self-control. As such, the subject may be able to tell lies, fabricate or confabulate due to the hallucinatory effect of the drug. This method is risky to the subject. Large number of false negatives are common.**

(C) Hypnosis: Many people cannot be hypnotised and many cannot be hypnotised to a deep level. It does not often enhance memory. Hypnotised witnesses (1) produce more fabricated recollections, (2) are more influenced by interviewer's misleading comments and questions, and (3) more confident in the accuracy of their recollections, than are non-hypnotised witnesses, even when their recollections are false.

(D) Word Association: Changes in reaction time of the subject's reply to word stimuli, either visual or auditory, or by stereotype of answers, or by exhibition of uncoordinated physical movements, have been employed in attempts to detect deception.

(E) Brain Mapping (Brain fingerprinting): It is a technique that measures recognition of familiar stimuli by measuring electrical brain wave responses (P_{300}) to words, phrases, or pictures that are presented on a computer screen. **It is based on the theory that the suspect's reaction to the details of an event or activity will reflect if the suspect had prior knowledge of the event or activity. It detects evidence stored in the brain.**

Technique: Modern brain scanning technique consists of electroencephalography (EEG), magneto encephalography (MEG), positron emission tomography (PET), magnetic resonance imaging (MRI and functional MRI) and computed tomography (CT). The equipment called **"electro-cap"** with 19 electronic sensors is fixed on the suspect's shaven scalp for recording EEG. The suspected person is questioned about the crime and also shown the visuals of the crime scene (victim, weapon, time, place and how he committed the crime, etc. along with irrelevant words, photographs, etc.) on a video monitor under computer control to stimulate his brain and encourage a reaction on a computer monitor. Apart from his verbal replies another computer keeps track of the neuro-impulses (brain waves, chemical responses) emitted whenever the visual is seen. Electrical brain responses of the suspect are measured non-invasively through electrocap equipped with sensors. A specific wave response called MERMER (memory encoding related multifaceted electroencephalographic response) is elicited when the brain processes the relevant information it recognises. This pattern occurs within about a second after the stimulus presentation and can be detected using EEG amplifiers and a programmed computer. Probes contain information that is known only to the perpetrate and investigators and none else. **Probe stimuli** are relevant to investigated situation, but the subject denies knowing. Target stimuli are relevant to the investigation situation and are known to the subject. **When the details of the crime the perpetrator would know are presented, a MERMER is emitted by the brain of a perpetrator, but not by the brain of an innocent suspect. It depends on eognitive brain responses.** A computer analyses the brain responses to detect the MERMER. Each stimulus appears for a fraction of a second. Three types of stimuli are presented, targets, irrelevants and probes. The targets elicit a MERMER. Most of the non-target stimuli are irrelevant and do not elicit a MERMER. Some of the non-target stimuli are relevant to the situation and are called probes. and does not depend on the emotions and is not affected by emotional responses. Similarly, when the information tested is information known only to members of a particular organisation group, e.g. terrorist group, the information present indicates affiliation with the group in question. **It is used in crime detection, screening employees, especially in military and foreign intelligence and counter-terrorism, insurance fraud, etc. It is said to be 99% accurate.**

Constitution of India: According to Article 20 (3) of constitution of India no person accused of any offence shall be compelled to be a witness against himself. The Supreme Court (2010) held that no individual should be forcibly subjected to narco-analysis, polygraph and brain mapping tests on accused, suspects and witnesses without their consent as they violate the right against self-incrimination. **Even when the subject had given consent to undergo any of these tests, the test results by themselves could not be admitted as evidence because "the subject does not exercise conscious control over the responses during the administration of the test.** However, any information or material that is subsequently discovered with the help of voluntary administered test results can be admitted, in accordance with Section 27 of the Evidence Act."

CHAPTER

23

FORENSIC PSYCHIATRY

FM 5.1: Classify common mental illnesses including post-traumatic stress disorder (PTSD).
FM 5.2: Define, classify and describe delusions, hallucinations, illusion, lucid interval and obsessions with exemplification.
FM 5.3: Describe civil and criminal responsibilities of a mentally ill person.
FM 5.4: Differentiate between true insanity from feigned insanity.
FM 5.6: Describe the Indian Mental Health Act, 1987 with special reference to admission, care and discharge of a mentally ill person.

Psychiatry deals with the study, diagnosis and treatment of mental illness. Forensic psychiatry deals with application of psychiatry in the administration of justice. Mental illness or unsoundness of mind can be defined as a disease of the mind or the personality, in which there is derangement of the mental or emotional processes and impairment of behaviour control. The intelligence is weakened or perverted, but the insane person may not show physical weakness. The law has not defined insanity. **The term is used for those persons who are unable to adopt themselves to the ordinary social requirements, due to mental disease. The law is most frequently concerned with "mental impairment" and not "mental illness."** Different kinds and degrees of mental impairment are required for different legal issues.

A psychologist is a person without medical qualifications who has a degree in psychology which concerns the study of normal and abnormal mental functioning usually by means of tests of intelligence, personality, etc. A psychiatrist is a person with a medical degree.

Application: Forensic psychiatry is involved to determine responsibility for crimes, sexual psychopathy (rape) and other sexual problems, such as homosexuality, transvestism, pedophilia, fetishism, competence in contract actions, competence to testify, ability to give informed consent to treatment, competency to stand trial, testamentary capacity, malingering, etc.

Legal and Ethical Issues: (1) During admission, treatment and discharge. (2) To evaluate his ability to consent when he commits a crime. (3) To differentiate between psychosis and neurosis. (4) To differentiate between true and feigned mental illness. (5) To nominate his representatives. (6) Validity of marriage.

ABNORMAL MENTAL STATES: An abnormal mental state may be due to a functional psychosis, to substance misuse, to an abnormal metabolic state, such as hypoglycaemia, or due to less common problems, such as learning disability, organic brain disease or head injury. In abnormal mental state, the effects of stress anxiety, fear or anger may coexist with intoxication (hallucinogenics and stimulants) of some kind and the behaviour, demeanour and appearance should be observed.

Common terms used in psychiatry:

ABRECATION: Reviving and bringing into consciousness, forgotten and other traumatic experiences or repressed emotions from unconscious level by catharsis.

AFFECT: Emotion, feeling or mood, e.g., lability of mood, cyclothymia, flattening, incongruity and inappropriateness of affect.

AFFECTIVE DISORDER: Psychiatric disorder in which the chief feature is a relatively prolonged affective change of an abnormal degree, i.e., depression and mania.

APHASIA: The loss of ability to express meaning by the use of speech or writing (motor aphasia), or to understand spoken or written language (sensory or auditory aphasia).

COGNITION: It refers to **higher mental faculties, such as memory, intelligence, concentration, orientation, etc.**

CONFABULATION: A false memory that the patient believes to be true.

DELIRIUM: It is a disturbance of consciousness in which orientation is impaired, the critical faculty is blunted or lost and thought content is irrelevant or inconsistent. In the early stage the patient is restless, uneasy and sleepless. He then completely loses self-control, becomes excited and talks furiously. Delusions and sometimes hallucinations are present. It usually occurs in physical diseases, in which there is continuous high temperature, and sometimes due to overwork, mental stress or drug intoxication. A person may become impulsive and violent and may commit suicide. **Such person is not responsible for his criminal acts.**

DELUSION: Delusion is a false and firm belief in something which is not a fact, and which persists even after its falsity has been clearly demonstrated. A normal person can have a delusion, but is capable of correcting it by his reasoning power, by his past experience and by being convinced by others. A secondary delusion arises from some morbid experience. Delusion in insane person is a symptom of brain disease. **It is under the control of emotional but not rational forces.** They are found in epileptic, affective and schizophrenic psychoses. Delusions are not seen in anxiety neurosis and other neurotic illnesses.

Types: (1) Grandeur or exaltation: A man imagines himself to be very rich while in reality he is a pauper. They are seen in delirium tremens. **(2) Persecution (paranoid):** The person imagines that attempts are being made to poison him by his nearest relatives like wife, sons or parents. They are seen in paranoid schizophrenia, dementia and depression. Delusions of grandeur and persecution are often present together in the same person. **(3) Reference:** The person believes that people, things, events, etc., refer to him in a special way. He believes that even strangers in the street are looking at him and are talking about him, or items in the radio or newspapers are referring to him. **(4) Influence:** They occur in schizophrenia. The person complains that his thoughts, feelings and actions are being influenced and controlled by some outside agency, like radio, hypnotism, telepathy, etc. **(5) Infidelity:** A man imagines his wife to be unfaithful while in fact she is chaste. **Athello syndrome:** The person has **delusions of infidelity** about his wife or mistress and assaults her. If she confesses due to severe pressure he explodes into violent acts and he may attempt or commit murder. **(6) Self-reproach (self accusation):** The person blames himself for the past failures and misdeeds which are often of no importance. **(7) Nihilistic:** The person declares that he does not exist or that there is no world, etc. **(8) Hypochondriacal:** The person believes that there is something wrong with his body, though he is healthy. **(9) Other types** are of jealousy, of religion, etc.

M.L.Importance: Delusion is never an isolated disorder, but is merely an indication of deep-seated, widespread disorder. For this reason, **such person cannot be regarded as fully responsible for his antisocial acts.** Suicide is a major risk. There may be a combination of murder and suicide.

EROTOMANIA: Erotomania is a delusion in which the person believes that someone is deeply in love with him/her. The erotomanic develops an obsession for a particular person and starts believing that the other person is reciprocating. The person is usually of a higher status, famous or superior at work, but can also be a complete stranger. The erotomanic tries to get close with the person through telephone calls, letters, gifts, visits, etc. The person is otherwise normal.

EMPATHY: The degree to which the observer is able to enter into the thoughts and feelings of the patient and establish good contact.

FUGUE: A state of altered awareness during which an individual forgets part or whole of his life, leaves home and wanders. It may occur in hysteria, depressive illness, schizophrenia and epilepsy.

HALLUCINATION: Hallucination is a false sense perception without any external object or stimulus to produce it. They are purely imaginary, and may affect any or all the special senses.

Types: (1) Visual: A person imagines of being attacked by a lion when no lion exists. **(2) Auditory:** A person hears voices and imagines that a person is speaking to him when no one is present. **(3) Olfactory:** A person smells pleasant or unpleasant odour when none is present. **(4) Gustatory:** A person feels sweet, sour, bitter, good or bad taste in the mouth, though no food is actually present. **(5) Tactile (haptic):** A man imagines rats and mice crawling into his bed, when there are none. They are common in alcohol withdrawal syndrome and in chronic cocaine poisoning. **(6) Psychomotor:** A man will have feeling of movement of some part of the body in the absence of such movement. **(7) Command:** The patient is ordered by hallucinatory voices to do things/acts, which may be frightening or dangerous. They may be pleasant, but more often they are unpleasant. A person suffering from unpleasant hallucinations may be incited to commit suicide or homicide. **(8) Microptic or macrotopic:** Any object appears usually smaller or bigger. **(9) Sexual:** A person feels sexually satisfied from unfounded self-imaginative objects.

Visual hallucinations are the commonest in organic mental disorders, while the auditory hallucinations are the commonest in functional disorders. Visual hallucinations are present in delirium tremens, focal CNS lesions, toxic disturbances, schizophrenia and drug withdrawal syndromes; auditory in schizophrenia, delirium, psychotic mood disorders, and toxic and metabolic encephalopathies; gustatory in organic brain diseases and temporal lobe epilepsy; olfactory in organic brain disease and major depressions and tactile in cocainism. Hallucinations occur in fevers, intoxications, and insanity.

ILLUSION: Illusion is a false interpretation by the senses of an external object or stimulus which has a real existence, e.g., when a person sees a dog and mistakes it for lion, or hears the notes of birds and imagines them to be human voices, or imagines a string hanging in his room to be snake, or may mistake the stem of a tree for a ghost in the dark. A sane person may experience illusion, but is capable of correcting the false impressions. An insane person continues to believe in the illusions, even though the real facts are clearly pointed out. Illusions are a feature of psychoses, particularly of the organic type.

IMPULSE: This is a sudden and irresistible force compelling a person to the conscious performance of some action without motive or forethought. A sane person is capable of controlling an impulse. An insane person having no judgement and no reasoning power, and no capacity to understand the facts, may do things on impulse. These are usually seen in imbecility, dementia, acute mania, and epilepsy.

Types: (1) Kleptomania: An irresistible desire to steal articles of little value. **(2) Pyromania:** An irresistible desire to set fire to things. **(3) Mutilomania:** An irresistible desire to mutilate animals. **(4) Dipsomania:** An irresistible desire for alcoholic drinks at periodic intervals. **(5) Sexual impulses:** Compulsive urge to perform sexual intercourse which may often be in a perverted way. **(6) Suicidal and homicidal impulses.**

OBSESSION: In this, a single idea, thought, or emotion is constantly entertained by a person which he recognises as irrational, but persists in spite of all efforts to drive it from his mind. It is a disorder of content of thought. Any attempt to resist makes them appear more insistent, and yielding is the almost inevitable outcome. It is a borderline between sanity and insanity. They usually occur in neurotic people, well able to discharge the ordinary responsibilities of life. These ideas are usually associated with some sort of dread or fear. **The person experiences anxiety and to control anxiety, he indulges in repetitive acts, i.e., compulsive acts.** A wife may continuously believe her husband to be unfaithful in spite of proof to the contrary. A person may go to bed at night after securely bolting the door of his room, but he soon gets up to see he has done so. A sane person may repeat it once or twice, but an insane person does not sleep, and spends the whole night in frequently seeing whether the door is bolted.

Obsessional acts are usually carried out on the basis of obsessional impulses or fears, e.g., obsessional cleaning and washing because of morbid fear of dirt.

PHOBIA: It is an **excessive or irrational fear of a particular object or situation.** Phobias may develop to almost any object or situation. Acrophobia is morbid fear of high places. Agarophobia is fear of being in a large open space. Nyctophobia is morbid fear of darkness. Claustrophobia is fear of staying in a closed or confined space. Mysophobia is morbid fear of filth or contamination. Xenophobia is fear of strangers.

LUCID INTERVAL: This is a period occurring in insanity, during which all the symptoms of insanity disappear completely. The individual is able to judge his acts soundly, and **he becomes legally liable for his acts.** The period of lucid interval varies from person to person and from time to time in the same person, and as such one cannot be certain about the time when a person passes again in the state of insanity. Therefore **if he commits an offence, he cannot be completely held responsible, because it is very difficult to know, whether he was suffering from some mental abnormality at the time of committing the offence (Table 23–1).** In mania and melancholia lucid intervals are common.

Insight: Awareness of one's own mental condition.

Mood: Pervasive emotion or feeling which is sustained.

Oneiroid States (oneirophrenia): It is a dream-like state, which may last for days or weeks. The patient suffers from mental confusion, amnesia, illusions, hallucinations, disorientation, agitation and anxiety. It occurs in delirium and early schizophrenia.

Twilight State (psychomotor automatism): It is **a state of diminished awareness of acts of relatively short duration, of which he has no recollection.** The patient may do some unaccustomed automatic acts sometimes in an aggressive way, and may suffer from visual hallucinations. It is usually seen in epilepsy.

Personality: Personality is considered as an **integrated organisation of attitudes, perceptions, emotions, behaviours and habits that characterise a person's distinctive way of relating to others and to himself.**

Hysteria: It is characterised by **self-dramatisation, excessive emotionality and attention seeking behaviour.** Egocentric and demanding interpersonal relationships are typical of this condition.

PSYCHOPATH: Psychopath or sociopath is a person who is neither insane nor mentally defective, but fails to conform to normal standards of behaviour. Psychopaths have abnormal personality, persistently behave in an antisocial or disruptive manner, and are unable to appreciate the moral implications of their actions. **It is not a ground for an insanity defence, but may provide a plea of diminished responsibility.**

Antisocial acts include shop-lifting, theft, house breaking, arson, sexual offenses and murder. It is also recognised as Antisocial Personality Disorder [DSM-5301.7 (F60.2)].

Symptoms and Criteria for Antisocial Personality Disorder: According to the DSM-5, there are four diagnostic criterion, of which criterion A has seven sub-features.

(A) Disregard for and violation of other rights since age 15, as indicated by one of the seven sub-features:
- (1) Failure to obey laws and norms by engaging in behaviour which results in criminal arrest, or would warrant criminal arrest
- (2) Lying, deception, and manipulation, for profit or self-amusement
- (3) Impulsive behaviour
- (4) Irritability and aggression, manifested as frequently assaults others, or engages in fighting
- (5) Blatantly disregards safety of self and others
- (6) A pattern of irresponsibility and
- (7) Lack of remorse for actions (American Psychiatric Association, 2013)

The other diagnostic criterion are:

(B) The person is at least age 18

(C) Conduct disorder was presented by history before age 15

(D) The antisocial behaviour does not occur in the context of schizophrenia or bipolar disorder (American Psychiatric Association, 2013)

The consensus is there is very little in the way of effective treatment for Antisocial Personality Disorder (APD). Individuals with APD may have to be contained by the criminal justice system, through some combination of incapacitation (incarceration), supervision and monitoring (parole, probation, or house arrest), or informal monitoring by local law enforcement to contain their harmful behaviours to others to the greatest extent possible.

In this there is a failure of maturation of the personality, the individual retaining a child-like selfishness. They have no abnormality of thought, mood or intelligence, but their behaviour is unacceptable. Lack of emotional response, an unswerving desire for the gratification of their desires and complete lack of conscience are characteristic of psychopathic personality. Frustration of any whim is not tolerated and is met with aggression, completely devoid of any regret or remorse. Immediate violence including murder can arise from any challenge to their egotism. They can plan and implement their antisocial acts in an efficient way. **The basic defect appears to be moral, rather than psychological or neurological.**

Types: (1) Predominantly aggressive. (2) Predominantly inadequate (in education, training, behaviour, etc.) (3) Predominantly moral and mental deficiency.

PSYCHOSES: They are characterised by a withdrawal from reality; a living in a world of fantasy. These mental illnesses supervene upon a normally developed mental faculty. There is deterioration in the personality and progressive loss

Table (23–1). Difference between lucid interval in insanity and head injury

Trait	Insanity	Head Injury
(1) History:	Of insanity present.	Of injury to the head.
(2) Preceding symptoms:	Of insanity.	Of concussion.
(3) Following symptoms:	Of insanity.	Of cerebral irritation and compression of the brain.
(4) Occurrence:	Frequent.	Only once.

Table (23–2). Difference between psychosis and neurosis

Trait		Psychosis	Neurosis
(1)	Nature:	A disease entity with a physical basis which is determined genetically.	A reaction to stressful circumstances due to adverse childhood experiences.
(2)	Severity:	Major.	Minor.
(3)	Empathy:	Absent.	Present.
(4)	Contact with reality:	Absent.	Present.
(5)	Insight:	Absent.	Present.

of contact with reality. Such persons incorrectly evaluate the accuracy of their perceptions and thoughts and make incorrect inferences about external reality, even in the face of contrary evidence. Delusions and hallucinations are common. Certain drugs, such as alcohol, heroin, morphine, cannabis, cocaine and LSD used habitually may produce psychoses. Psychosis may occur in epilepsy, cerebral tumours, cerebral trauma, pregnancy/childbirth Table (23–2).

(1) THE PSYCHOTIC KILLER: Such person is either: (a) incapable of knowing the nature of the act (as in cases of organic disorder), or (b) his judgement is faulty (due to delusions and hallucinations). Murders are common in depression. Schizophrenics commit murders due to delusions of persecution. Morbid jealousy associated with alcoholism may lead to murder of the spouse due to delusions of infidelity. Rarely maniacs and hypomaniacs commit murders due to delusions.

(2) THE PSYCHOPATHIC KILLER: The killing may be unintentional due to loss of control. Over- controlled murderer is one who has a high level of control over his aggression, but commits a murder due to an explosive response. After the aggressive act, he returns to his rigidly controlled behaviour. In some, normal emotional responses may be almost absent.

NEUROSES: The patient suffers from emotional or intellectual disorders, but he does not lose touch with reality. They occur mostly in the form of anxiety, depression or hysteria. The effects may be mild or may cause considerable distress to the patient, but they are not associated with severe affective change, nor with disturbances of thought Table (23–2).

NEURASTHENIA: It is a condition of nervous exhaustion due to physical or mental conditions. There is an abnormal fatigue and irritability of the nervous system.

MUTISM: There is complete loss of speech. It is seen is hysteria, catatonic schizophrenia, depression, organic brain lesion and malingering.

CAUSES OF INSANITY: (1) Hereditary, e.g., Huntington's chorea and amaurotic family idiocy. (2) Environmental factors, e.g., faulty parental attitude and lack of mental hygiene. (3) Psychogenic, e.g., unsuccessfully repressed mental conflicts. (4) Precipitating, e.g., financial and business worries, frustrations and disappointments in sexual affairs, death of close relative, etc. (5) Organic, e.g., head injury, atherosclerosis, senile degeneration, myxoedema, pernicious anaemia, etc.

CLASSIFICATION

The World Health Organisation has recommended in the International Classification of Diseases (1992) the following.

(A) Organic mental disorders include dementia in Alzheimer's disease, vascular dementia and dementia in other diseases, organic amnesic syndrome, delirium not induced by alcohol and other mental, personality and behavioural disorders due to brain disease, damage or dysfunction.

(B) Mental and behavioural disorders due to psychoactive substance use.

(C) Schizophrenia.

(D) Mood disorders.

(E) Neurotic stress-related and somatoform disorders.

(1) Anxiety disorders.
(2) Obsessive-compulsive disorder.
(3) Reaction to stress and adjustment disorders.
(4) Dissociative (conversion) disorder.
(5) Somatoform disorders.

(F) Behavioural syndromes associated with physiological disturbances and physical factors.

(1) Eating disorders.
(2) Non-organic sleep disorders.
(3) Sexual dysfunction not caused by organic disorder or disease.
(4) Mental and behavioural disorders associated with puerperium.
(5) Abuse of non-dependence producing substances.

(G) Personality disorders.

(1) Specific personality disorders.
(2) Habit and impulse disorders.
(3) Gender identity disorders.
(4) Disorders of sexual perversion.

(H) Mental retardation.

(I) Disorders of psychological development.

Intelligence Quotient (I.Q): (Binet-Simon test). It is the intellectual capacity of a person in relation to his chronological age, which is expressed as a percentage. Normal adult I.Q. is 90 to 110%.

Mental retardation: Earlier, under the term **amentia, three groups, idiocy, imbecility and feeble- mindedness (morons) were recognised, which is now replaced by the term 'mental retardation' and includes mental subnormality and mental handicap.** It refers to below average general intellectual functioning with typical onset in infancy or birth that must occur before 18 years of age. It signifies a condition of retarded, incomplete or abnormal mental development. It is characterised by incomplete maturation of attention, perception, cognition and social adaptability. It results from environmental, genetic, endocranial, metabolic, infective, toxic causes and birth trauma. **Oligophrenia** refers to feeble mindedness, mental subnormality or mental retardation.

It is graded according to IQ levels as: (1) **mild:** IQ 50 to 70. (2) **moderate** IQ 35-55. (3) **severe:** IQ 20 to 40, (4) **profound**: IQ below 25.

PSYCHOSIS ASSOCIATED WITH ORGANIC DISEASES

Mental illnesses which arise from some structural brain damage are called organic psychoses. The organic psychoses are characterised by lability of mood, failure of memory, deterioration of intellect, irritability, irrational anger, confusion, loss of social inhibitions, etc., which may lead such persons into unacceptable behaviour and even sudden violence.

DEMENTIA is a condition in which there is degeneration of mental faculties after they have been fully developed. Memory, intellect and judgement are impaired. (1) PRESENILE DEMENTIA: It may be seen before 65 years. Pseudodementia is associated with schizophrenia. (a) Alzheimer's disease. (b) Pick's disease. (c) Creutzfeldt-Jacob disease. (d) Huntington's chorea.

(2) SENILE DEMENTIA: It is caused due to arteriosclerosis and old age. It usually starts after 65 years. A feeling of loneliness, of being unwanted, loss of prestige and death of a close relative cause the onset of

the disease. The patient is confused, judgement and memory is impaired. Delusions, hallucinations and emotional outbursts are common.

(3) CEREBRAL TUMOURS: Mental symptoms may occur at any stage of growth of cerebral tumours involving prefrontal, frontal, temporal and parietal lobes.

(4) CEREBRAL TRAUMA: It can precipitate any type of mental illness.

(5) DRUG-INDUCED PSYCHOSIS: Dependence on barbiturates, amphetamines, cannabis, heroin, cocaine, etc., leads to psychosis. Cocaine, LSD, amphetamines and mescaline can produce clinical symptoms similar to schizophrenia.

(6) TOXIC PSYCHOSIS: Heavy metals, such as arsenic and mercury may produce mental degeneration.

(7) DEFICIENCY STATES: Deficiency of cyanocobalamin (pernicious anaemia), nicotinic acid (pellagra), 5-hydroxytryptamine (phenylketonuria), and hypoglycaemia produce mental degeneration.

(8) GENERAL PARALYSIS OF THE INSANE: This is a chronic progressive condition leading to paralysis and dementia. It is usually associated with menigovascular syphilis and tabes dorsalis. There is a chronic psycho-organic syndrome characterised by temperamental and personality changes. The memory is impaired and thought retarded.

(9) EPILEPTIC PSYCHOSIS: Short transitory fits of uncontrollable mania occur. There is general impairment of the mental faculties with loss of memory and self-control. Auditory and visual hallucinations are followed by delusions of persecution. Moral sensibility is lost and sometimes they are dangerous to themselves and to others. There may be progressive dementia.

(A) PRE-EPILEPTIC INSANITY: Instead of epileptic aura, the patient may occasionally develop violent fits of mania or extreme depression of mind. Hallucinations and delusions are common during this stage, and such persons may commit assault or other criminal acts.

(B) POST-EPILEPTIC INSANITY: The stupor following epileptic fit is replaced by automatic acts, of which the patient has no recollection. The patient is confused and terrified by visual and auditory hallucinations and delusions of persecution, and may commit crimes like thefts, incendiarism, sexual assaults and murders. These crimes are involuntary, automatic and unpremeditated. The patient never attempts to conceal them at the time of committing, but may try to conceal them on regaining consciousness. Automatic action tends to be of the same type in each attack. The action is usually habitual, e.g., a man walks into a shop, picks up something and walks out again, afterwards being arrested for theft, or one who exposes himself in a public place and is arrested for indecent conduct; or a person cutting something may inflict incised wounds or kill a child; or a person accustomed to firearms may shoot somebody.

TWILIGHT STATE: In this condition the field of consciousness is narrowed for a short time, followed by amnesia. The patient may do some automatic act and is aggressive and suffers from visual hallucinations. It is seen usually in epilepsy and rarely in hysteria, punchdrunkenness and head injury.

(C) PSYCHOMOTOR EPILEPSY (temporal lobe, masked or psychic epilepsy): In this, instead of epileptic fit, the patient suffers from temporary and transient seizure of maniacal excitement with loss of consciousness. It is likely to cause disturbed sensations and sounds, and to give rise to automatic behaviour. The patient may commit crimes without any motive.

(10) ALCOHOLISM: (A) Alcoholic blackouts. (B) Delirium tremens. (C) Alcoholic hallucinosis. (D) Korsakov's psychosis. (E) Delusions of jealousy.

FUNCTIONAL PSYCHOSES: Mental illnesses which have no neurological basis are called functional psychoses. The functional psychoses are characterised by disorders of thought which have no physical basis. (a) In schizophrenic psychoses, disorders of the thought process are dominant. (b) In affective psychoses, mood abnormality is dominant. This is a disease of hereditary origin affecting young adults and forms a major group of all psychiatric illnesses.

SCHIZOPHRENIA: It is a condition of split personality, in which the patient loses his contact with his environment. It is primarily a disorder of thinking (cognition). This disorder can be in form, stream, possession or content of thought. It is characterised by splitting of different psychic functions. (1) Disorders of behaviour: withdrawal from reality, preoccupation with the self (narcissism), attribution of feeling of strangeness to outside influence (depersonalisation), and feelings that his mind and body are under control (passivity of feeling). (2) Disorders of thought: confused thoughts leading to thought block, devious thinking leading to incoherence of speech often with newly formed words (neologism). (3) Disorders of affect: depression, elation, inappropriate moods, lability of mood, anxiety and blunting of emotions. (4) Delusions: of grandeur, paranoid, hypochondriac and influence. (5) Hallucinations: commonly auditory, sometimes visual and tactile. (6) Personality deterioration: affecting his work, family and social relationships. It is the commonest type of insanity in homicidal crimes, especially where the victim is a stranger. The impulses are not sudden and the crime is usually preceded by much complaining and planning.

(1) SIMPLE SCHIZOPHRENIA: It begins in early adolescence. There is a gradual loss of interest in the outside world from which he withdraws. There is an all-round impairment of mental faculties. He becomes emotionally flat and apathetic and has difficulty in forming social relationships. Complete disintegration of the personality occurs later.

(2) HEBEPHRENIA: It begins in adolescents or young adults. Thinking process is disturbed. Wild excitement, illusions, hallucinations and bizarre delusions are present. Often conduct is impulsive and senseless. Ultimately the whole personality may disintegrate completely.

(3) CATATONIA: This is characterised by alternating stages of depression, excitement and stupor; impulsive suicidal or homicidal attacks and auditory hallucinations are common. This phase lasts for few hours to few days followed by a stage of stupor which begins with lack of interest, concentration and general indifference.

(4) PARANOID SCHIZOPHRENIA (paranoia, paraphrenia): Paranoid is the term used to describe all delusions of being affected in some harmful or persecutory way. Paranoia is the mild form, and is common in males. Paranoid schizophrenia develops insidiously in the fourth decade. It is characterised by suspiciousness, delusions of persecution and auditory hallucinations. At first delusions are indefinite, but later they become fixed on some person. The patient usually retains his memory and orientation. When delusions affect his behaviour, he is often a source of danger to himself and others. In paraphrenia, delusions and hallucinations are present, but the personality is relatively intact.

(5) SCHIZO-AFFECTIVE PSYCHOSIS: This is an atypical type of schizophrenia in which there are mood disturbances. Attacks of elation or depression, unmotivated rage, anxiety, panic, etc., occur.

(6) PSEUDO-NEUROTIC SCHIZOPHRENIA: It may start with overwhelmingly permanent neurotic symptoms.

Psychosis due to pregnancy and child birth: During pregnancy, delusions and dislike or hatred towards husband may occur, and tendency to suicide may develop. Postpartum psychosis may result in mania with a tendency to homicide, due to which she may kill her infant. Late in puerperium depression with a tendency to suicide may develop. Lactational psychosis is characterised by mental confusion, hallucinations, delusions and depression, which may lead to suicide or infanticide.

POST-TRAUMATIC PSYCHOSIS: Brain damage at birth or during early childhood may cause mental subnormality or epilepsy. Organic headache may persist for a long time. Confusional and delirious states may occur.

PSYCHOSIS DUE TO GENERAL DISEASES: Acute infectious diseases may cause confusional state and sometimes depression with suicidal tendency after recovery. Thyroid deficiency, pellagra and beriberi may produce psychosis.

AFFECTIVE TYPES: These diseases are of hereditary origin affecting young adults, and form a major group of all psychiatric illnesses.

MANIC-DEPRESSIVE PSYCHOSIS shows wide swings of mood from euphoric elation to deepest depression, quite out of proportion or often totally unrelated to external circumstances. The two extremes of these moods are hyperactive, excitant at one and depressive stupor at the other. The primary disturbance is of affect. It occurs periodically. Isolated attacks of mania and depression may occur in the same patient and some show attacks of one type only.

(1) MANIC PHASE: This is a condition of exaltation of the emotions and the intellect. (A) Acute mania: It is characterised by euphoria or irritable mood, excitement, loss of self-control, flight of ideas and great muscular activity. Mood is elated, attention is fleeting and there is high degree of distraction. (B) Hypomania: It is the mildest form in which there is an exaggerated sense of self-importance. Offences, such as petty theft, deception, indecent assault, and fraud may be committed.

(2) DEPRESSIVE PHASE (MELANCHOLIA): It is an intense feeling of depression and misery without any cause. The sadness of mood is reflected in posture, movements and facial expression. He retires from his usual social activities, avoids friends. Suicide is well planned and is of great danger to the patient. He may kill relatives, especially dependent young children. Homicidal and suicidal tendencies co-exist. They have feelings of self-reproach and guilt, and marked psychomotor disturbances.

TYPES: (1) Endogenous. (2) Reactive and neurotic. (3) Involutional. (4) Puerperal.

NEUROSES: This forms a group of personality disturbances resulting from reactions to life situations. They may occur singly or in combination.

(1) ANXIETY NEUROSIS: It results from autonomic stimuli. The patient has spells of dyspnoea, choking, palpitation, insomnia, faintness, trembling, headache, chest pain, etc. The person is apprehensive and depressed and worries about his health. Intolerance of noise, children and spouse may be seen.

(2) HYSTERICAL NEUROSIS: It is common in young females, but may occur in old ladies whose nervous system starts degenerating. The symptoms commence when faced with unpleasant life situations. The patient shows deafness, blindness, loss of smell, anaesthesia, paraesthesia, paralysis, aphonia, etc. Convulsions may occur. In the dissociative type, change in the patient's level of consciousness and identity are observed.

(3) PHOBIC NEUROSIS: Phobias are specific fear which the patient recognises as irrational. They often act as defence mechanisms that protect the patient from unpleasant life situations. The different types are: acrophobia (high places), agoraphobia (open spaces), claustrophobia (closed spaces), necrophobia (dead bodies), nyctophobia (darkness), phonophobia (sound), pathophobia (disease), thanatophobia (death), toxiphobia (being poisoned), etc. It interferes with daily life.

(4) OBSESSIVE-COMPULSIVE NEUROSIS: Anxiety, depression and fear are present in varying degrees. Obsessional thought may be associated with a whole range of objects. Doubt may exist whether doors are locked or lights switched off.

(5) DEPRESSIVE NEUROSIS: It resembles manic-depressive psychosis but the degree of depression is less, and mental retardation, delusions and hallucinations are absent. There is risk of suicide.

PERSONALITY DISORDERS: Personality is the characteristic pattern of an individual's attitudes, behaviours, beliefs, feelings, thoughts and values, i.e., the sum of a person's emotional, cognitive, and intellectual attributes. The person is said to suffer from a personality disorder, when the behaviour is inappropriate to the situation. Psychopathic personality refers to a special derangement of the mind. The important features are: (1) Lack of normal conscience. (2) Absence of normal feelings for other people, such as love, affection, sympathy, etc. (3) A tendency to antisocial impulsive acts. (4) Failure to learn from experience and to be prevented from crime by punishment. (5) Freedom from any other form of mental disorder. The symptoms usually appear in early childhood, but become pronounced in adulthood, and gradually diminish in later life. Sexual perversions and crimes are common.

SEXUAL DEVIATION: It may be a symptom of an underlying psychiatric disorder, such as schizophrenia, senile dementia, personality disorder. The person indulges in sexual perversions and unnatural sex practices.

DRUG DEPENDENCE: Drug addicts have a wide range of personalities. Most of them are emotionally unstable, immature, impulsive, angry with society, and unable to achieve their goals or face difficult situations in life. About 10% suffer from psychopathic personality disorders. Alcohol, cannabis, cocaine, morphine and heroin may produce a variety of mental conditions.

CONFUSIONAL STATES: They occur sometimes from excess of physical or mental fatigue, acute infectious diseases, childbirth and other stresses of life. Visual and auditory hallucinations are common. Recovery is the rule.

DIAGNOSIS OF INSANITY

In typical case of insanity the diagnosis is easy, but in early stages, especially when he has no permanent delusions, and in borderline cases, the correct diagnosis becomes difficult. The object of the clinical examination is to form an opinion about the patient's mind and the degree of responsibility.

(1) Preliminaries: Note the name, age, sex, and address of person. Time of beginning and end of each examination should be noted.

(2) Family History: Enquire into the mental condition of the patient's parents and siblings and whether any of them suffered from chorea, epilepsy, or frank mental illness, etc.

(3) Personal History: (1) History of previous mental disease in the parents. (2) Factors connected with environment, such as parents and homes, over-protection as a child, rejection, strictness, inferiority complex, discrimination by parents, emotional maladjustments during childhood, emotional fixation during adolescence to parents. (3) Psychogenic factors, such as repression, emotional conflict and anxiety states. (4) Organic diseases, like cerebral vascular accidents, head injury, acute fevers, advanced renal and cardiac disease, senile degenerative condition, toxaemias, etc. (5) Drug dependence to opium, pethidine, barbiturates, alcohol, cannabis, etc. (6) Domestic difficulties. (7) Emotional shock. (8) Frustration in life, love, sex, etc.

(4) Physical Examination: (1) Observe the patient's manner of dressing and walking, bearing and gestures. (2) Examine for the presence of deformities and malformations in the head or body. (3) Note the pulse rate and body temperature, both of which may be increased. (4) The tongue may be furred. (5) The skin is dry and wrinkled and the hands and feet moist. A complete and detailed physical examination should be carried out to exclude any disease.

(5) Mental Condition: The following observations should be recorded. (1) General appearance: Naked, dressed properly, improperly, dirty or clean habits, and facial expression, whether vacant, grimacing, mask-like or makes faces. (2) Talk: Mutism, aphonia, distraction, irrelevant, neologism (coining his own vocabulary), echolalia (repeating identical words uttered by another person), perseveration (repetition of an act monotonously), wandering speech and talkative. (3) Speech: Coherent, incoherent, aphasia, lalling, lisping, drawling, slurring, stammering. (4) Writing: Agraphia, flight of ideas, obscene or insulting language, unintelligible. (5) Behaviour: Stereotypy, perseveration, mannerism, impulsive, lazy, stupor, automatic obedience, negativism, seclusive, echopraxia (copying all actions of another), etc. (6) Mood: Emotion, euphoria, joy, anger, elation, exaltation, apathy, irritable, touchy, etc. (7) Memory: Good, bad, concentration, appreciation, grasp, etc. (8) Sleep: Insomnia, hyposomnia, somnambulism, somnolentia. (9) Walking and gait: Stealthy, hurried, etc. (10) Attitude and posture: Proud, peculiar, over-erect, aggressive, worried, etc. (11) Sex behaviour: Towards same sex and opposite sex. (12) Attention: Attentive, inattentive, fluctuating, etc. (13) Thought process: Retardation, preoccupied, ambivalence, double orientation, power of orientation, etc. (14) Thought content: Delusions, hallucinations, illusions, obsession, self-consciousness, etc.

(6) Other Investigations: Additional evidence can be collected from pathological examinations of the blood, urine and CSF, and X-ray and electroencephalographic recordings.

Observation: The person should be kept under observation in a general hospital or general nursing home, or psychiatric hospital or nursing home, or in any other suitable place, which **should not exceed ten days, but with the permission of the Magistrate, he may be detained for further periods of ten days, up to a maximum of 30 days.**

Table (23–3). Difference between real mental illness and feigned mental illness

	Trait	Real mental illness	Feigned mental illness
(1)	Onset:	Gradual.	Sudden.
(2)	Motive:	Absent, e.g., no history of commission of crime.	Present, e.g., commission of crime.
(3)	Predisposing factors:	Usually present, e.g., history of insanity in parents, or of sudden monetary loss, grief, etc.	Absent.
(4)	Signs and symptoms:	Uniform and present whether the patient is being observed or not.	Present only when conscious of being observed; variable and always exaggerated, and do not resemble any particular mental disease.
(5)	Mood:	Excited, depressed or fluctuating.	May overact to show abnormality in mood
(6)	Facial expression:	Peculiar, e.g., vacant look or fixed look of excitement.	No peculiarity; frequently changing, exaggerated and voluntary.
(7)	Insomnia:	Present.	Cannot persist; patient sleeps soundly after a day or two.
(8)	Exertion:	Can stand exertion of fatigue, hunger and sleep for several days without breaking down.	Cannot stand exertion for more than a few days and breaks down.
(9)	Habits:	Dirty and filthy.	Not dirty and filthy.
(10)	Skin and lips:	Dry, harsh.	Normal.
(11)	Frequent examination:	Does not mind.	Resents for fear of detection.

Violent and criminal persons should be kept in a prison. The person should be watched during different times of the day, when he is alone, in company and while he is working, eating, reading or writing, and when he is unaware of the fact of being observed.

Certification: A certificate should not be issued after single examination. **Three examinations on different days and different hours are usually recommended,** with the possibility of more, because a person may behave peculiarly at a single examination, either due to the effect of drugs, or due to delirium caused by fever. The certificate should contain a clinical description of the patient, and indicate the reasons for the diagnosis of the specified disorder.

Feigned Mental Illness: Mental illness may be feigned by criminals to evade sentence of death or long terms of imprisonment, by soldiers and policemen to leave the service, and by businessmen to avoid contracts **Table (23–3).**

THE MENTAL HEALTH CARE ACT, 2017

An Act to provide for mental health care and services for people with mental illness and to protect, promote and fulfill rights of such people during delivery of mental health care and services. The Mental Health Care Act, 1987 is repealed.

Independent patient or an independent admission refers to admission of person with mental illness, to a mental health establishment (MHE), who have the capacity to make mental health care and treatment decisions or requires mental support in making decisions. Every major person shall have a right to make **an advance directive in writing,** the way he wishes to be cared for and treated for a mental illness and the person he wants to appoint as his **nominated representative** for his care and treatment. In case of a minor, the legal guardian has the right to make an advance directive in writing. All admissions in MHE, shall, as far as possible, be independent admissions except when such conditions exist as to make supported admission unavoidable. MHE should be registered with central or state mental health authority.

Admission, treatment and discharge:

(1) Independent admission and treatment: Any major person who considers himself to be a mentally ill person and desires to be admitted to any MHE for treatment, may request the medical officer in-charge of MHE to be admitted as independent patient. The Medical Officer (M.O.) of MHE should admit the person, if he is satisfied that the person requires admission and will benefit from treatment, and the request for admission is his own free will without any undue influence. The consent of a relative or care-giver is not necessary. An independent may get himself discharged without consent of medical officer.

(2) Admission of minor: In case of minors, the nominated representative should apply to M.O. in-charge of MHE. Such minor may be admitted if two psychiatrists or one psychiatrist and one mental health professional have independently examined the minor and both independently conclude that the minor has a mental illness and requires admission with regards to his health, well-being or safety. Such minor should be accommodated separately from adults. The nominated representative or an attendant appointed by him should stay with the minor for the entire duration of the admission. If the nominated representative requests discharge of minor, he should be discharged.

(3) Admission and treatment of a person with mental illness with high support needs up to 30 days: The in-charge of MHE should admit every such person upon application by nominated representative of the person, if the person has been independently examined on the day of admission or on the preceding 7 days by one psychiatrist and one mental health professional or medical practitioner and both independently conclude based on examination and information provided by others that the person has a mental illness of such severity that admission is necessary. Admission will be limited for 30 days after which the person may continue to remain admitted in MHE, as an independent patient and has a right to leave MHE.

(4) Admission and treatment of a person with mental illness, with high support need be beyond 30 days (supported admission

beyond 30 days): If a person with mental illness requires continuous admission and treatment beyond 30 days or has been discharged, he will be admitted if the nominated representative applies and if two psychiatrists have independently examined the mentally ill person in the preceding 7 days and both independently conclude that the person has a mental illness of a severity that he requires admission and treatment. Such admission should be reported to the concerned Board and will be limited to 90 days in the first instance, which may extend to 120 days and thereafter 180 days each time by the Board.

(5) Duties of police officer in respect of people with mental illness: Every officer in-charge police station should take under protection any person found wandering at large, whom the officer has reason to believe has mental illness and is incapable of taking care of himself or to be a risk to him or self or others due to mental illness. Such person should be taken to the nearest MHE for assessment of the person's health care needs. The in-charge of MHE should arrange assessment of the person and the needs of the person with mental illness and act as per provisions of admissions.

(6) Report to magistrate of person with mental illness in private residence who is ill treated or neglected: The officer in charge of a police station who has reason to believe that any person has mental illness and is being ill treated or neglected, or if any person reports to the police officer of such case, should report to the Magistrate. The Magistrate may order to produce the mentally ill person before him and may order in writing that the person is sent to a public MHE for assessment and treatment if necessary or to admit for not more than 10 days to carry out an assessment. The in-charge of MHE should submit a report to the Magistrate and the person should be dealt with in accordance with the provisions of admissions.

(7) Prisoners with mental illness: A mentally ill prisoner can be admitted into any psychiatric hospital, by an order passed by an appropriate authority under Prisoners Act (1900), Air Force Act (1950), Army Act (1950), Navy Act (1957), or under Section 330 or 335 of Cr.P.C (1973).

(8) People in custodial institutions: If it appears to the person in-charge of custodial institution (beggar homes, orphanages, women's protection homes, children's homes) that any resident of institution has a mental illness, he should take such resident to nearest MHE. The in-charge of MHE should assess the person with mental illness and treatment required according to the provisions of admission and treatment.

(9) Admission of an escaped mentally ill person: He can be taken into protection by any police officer at the request of in-charge of MHE and shall be sent to the MHE immediately.

Mental illness and judicial process: If during any judicial procedure before any court, proof of mental illness is produced and challenged by other party, the court should refer the same to further scrutiny to the concerned Board, which should submit the opinion to the court.

Leave of absence: The in-charge of MHE may grant leave to any person admitted for mental illness for such duration that he may consider necessary.

Restraint and seclusion: Mentally ill person should not be subjected to seclusion or solitary confinement. Physical restraint may only be used when it is the only means available top prevent imminent and immediate harm to person concerned or to others for a period necessary to prevent risk of significant harm. It should be authorized by psychiatrist in-charge of treatment. He should be kept in a place where he can cause no harm to himself or others under supervision of medical personnel at the MHE.

MENTAL DISORDER AND RESPONSIBILITY

Responsibility, in the legal sense means the liability of a person for his acts or omissions, and if these are against the law, the liability to be punished for them. The law presumes that every person is mentally sound until the opposite is proved. The type and degree of mental disorder which shall free a person from civil or criminal responsibilities is greatly controversial. Section 328 to 339 of Cr.P.C. 1973, relate to provisions as to accused persons of unsound mind, including fitness to stand trial and the subsequent procedures.

CIVIL RESPONSIBILITY

The question of civil responsibility arises in the following conditions.

(1) Management of Property and Affairs of Mentally ill Person: If any relative or friend of an alleged mentally ill person possessing property gives an application, the Court may direct inquiry whether the person is of unsound mind and incapable of managing his property and affairs. The medical evidence is given in the form of a certificate, which should state, "that unsoundness of mind is of such a degree as to make him incapable of managing his property and affairs". In case of doubt, it is safer to give an opinion in favour of sanity. **If on inquiry, a person is found incapable of managing his property and affairs, but is not dangerous to himself or to others, the Court appoints a manager to look after his property, granting him necessary power.** The Court may order the sale or disposal of the property of the mentally ill person for the payment of his debts and expenses. The Court may order a second inquiry, if it is reported that unsoundness of mind had ceased and will order all proceedings in the unsoundness of mind to cease.

(2) Mental illness and Contracts: **A contract is invalid if one of the parties at the time of making it was incapable of understanding what he was doing due to mental illness.** Contract entered into with a mentally ill person may be valid, if the other party can show that he did not know that the other party was mentally ill, and that the contract is a fair contract. Mental illness which develops subsequent to the contract does not make it invalid, unless performance of services becomes impossible. A mentally ill person is responsible for the payment of the simple necessities of life, such as food, shelter, clothing, medical care, etc., but he is not responsible if the order is grossly excessive or unreasonable, or if the seller has taken undue advantage of his mental illness. The mental disorder of partner does not itself dissolve the partnership, unless steps be taken for dissolution. A person who is usually of unsound mind, but occasionally of sound mind, may make a contract when he is of sound mind. A person who is usually of sound mind, but occasionally of unsound mind, may not make a contract when he is of unsound mind.

(3) Mental illness and Marriage Contract: A marriage is considered invalid, if at the time of marriage, either party (1) is incapable of giving valid consent due to mental illness, or (2) though capable of giving valid consent, has been suffering from such a kind or degree of mental disorder as to be unfit for marriage and procreation, or (3) has been suffering from recurrent attacks of unsoundness of mind or epilepsy.

(4) The Competence of Mentally ill Person to be a Witness: **A mentally ill person is not incompetent to testify, unless he is prevented by his lunacy from understanding the question put to him and giving rational answers to them** (S.118, I.E.A.). A person of unsound mind who suffers from delusions, but is able to tell what he has seen, and who understands the obligation of an oath, is competent to give evidence. A mentally ill person is competent to give evidence during the period of lucid interval.

(5) Consent and Mental Illness: **Consent to certain acts like sexual intercourse or hurt is not valid,** if such consent is given by a person who from unsoundness of mind, is unable to understand the nature and consequences of that act.

(6) Mental Illness and Testamentary Capacity: Testamentary capacity (testament = will) is **the mental ability of a person to make a valid will.** "Will" denotes any testamentary document (S.31, I.P.C.).

Requirements: The requirements for a valid will are as follows. A written and properly signed and witnessed document must exist. **The testator must be major, and of sound disposing mind, at the time of making the will.** Force, undue influence, or dishonest representation of facts, should not have been applied by others. A sound disposing mind is a mind which has capacity of recollecting, judging and feeling the relations, connections and obligations of his family and blood relations. **Holograph will is one which is written by a testator in his own handwriting.**

Medical Examination: Doctors are sometimes called upon to witness the execution of the will of a sick person. The doctor should proceed in the usual way: physical examination, mental state including intelligence testing, and laboratory investigations. **The testator is said to be of sound mind if he is capable of disposing of his property with understanding and reason.** The following tests are recommended to find out whether the testator is of sound and disposing mind. (1) Ask the testator preliminary questions, e.g., about his relatives, their number and the degree of social contact with them; his opinions on family, friends and business partners; his age, politics and hobbies. (2) Ask general questions for testing awareness as regards time, place, etc. (3) Ask him about the nature, extent and value of his properties, and the manner of distribution desired by him. If any unusual or unjust distribution is to be made, find out whether it is intentional, and if so the reasons for it, and whether he is able to repeat the main provisions of will. (4) Test the patient's powers of concentration by simple sums of arithmetic, etc. (5) Ask all other persons to leave the room, and then ask the patient whether there was any pressure or influence on him by any one. The doctor should exclude any disease, infirmity, pain, strain, influence of drug or drink or any insane delusion, which are bound to affect a normally sound and disposing state of mind. Drugs or their withdrawal, may cause changes in consciousness, reasoning ability, perception of reality and memory, affecting an individuals testamentary capacity. **The most common symptom of absence of legal capacity is impairment of memory.** Prejudices, dislikes and hatred, however ill-found, or however strongly entertained cannot be classed as due to mental illness delusions. Dislike of ones relatives without reason is not necessarily proof of want of capacity. **The most important thing to determine is, whether at the time of making the will, the testator understood the business in which he was engaged, and knew how he wanted to dispose of his property.**

Valid will: (1) A person affected by delusions due to unsoundness of mind, can make a valid will, if the delusion is not related in any way to disposal of the property, or the persons affected by the will. (2) Persons can make valid wills during lucid interval. (3) A will is considered valid even though the testator committed suicide shortly after making a will, if there is no other evidence of mental disorder. (4) Persons of extreme age and feeble health with defective memory can make a valid will, unless their mind has become so impaired, that they are unable to understand its nature and consequences. (5) A person suffering from motor or sensory aphasia, agraphia (failure to communicate by writing), and alexia (failure to understand by reading), or who is deaf, dumb or blind, can make a valid will, if he knows what he does by it, if he can make clear by gestures that he wishes to make a will, and is able to understand the meaning of questions put to him in this connection. (6) An eccentric person can make a valid will, if there is no other mental derangement or a delusion.

Invalid wills: (1) Wills made by persons in extremis (at the point of death) may be regarded with suspicion, because at that time a clear mind is unusual. (2) A will executed by a dying person during delirium would be invalid. (3) Partial drunkenness does not invalidate a contract or will, but when drunkenness has caused a temporary loss of reasoning powers, the person cannot make a valid will.

An executor is appointed under the will by the testater to carry out terms after his death.

CRIMINAL RESPONSIBILITY

The law: **The law presumes that every person is sane and responsible for his actions. The defence has to prove that the accused is mentally ill. The law also presumes that for every criminal act, there must be criminal intent or mind, mens rea** (guilty state of mind; mens = mind; rea = criminal) motivating it. **Actus reus** means the actual forbidden physical act causing death. **If unsoundness of mind is proved, the accused person is found "not guilty", and is ordered to be kept in a psychiatric hospital or other suitable place of custody.**

Tests for determining criminal responsibility.

(1) MC NAUGHTEN RULE (THE RIGHT OR WRONG TEST; THE LEGAL TEST): English Courts, in dealing with the responsibility of the mentally ill person in criminal cases, are guided by the rules laid down after the Mc Naughten trial in 1843. Daniel Mc Naughten a 29 year old Scotsman, was probably suffering from paranoid schizophrenia. For many years he had a delusion that spies sent by Catholic priests, with the help of Tories (the party then in power in England), were constantly following him, harassing him and hatching a conspiracy against him. He also, probably, had auditory hallucinations with Tories accusing him of crimes of which he said he was not guilty. Therefore, he decided to kill the Tories Prime Minister, Sir Robert Peel, making elaborate plans for the criminal act. On 20th January 1843, he shot Sir Peel's Private Secretary, Edward Drummond, in the back, mistaking him for the Prime Minister. During the trial, he admitted that he 'was driven to desperation by persecution'. Ten physicians (nine for defence and one for prosecution) found him of unsoundness of mind. He was found 'not guilty on grounds of mental illness', and was sent to Bethlem Mental Hospital for life. The verdict lead to unprecedented public outcry. Queen

Victoria, summoned the House of Lords to a special session. The Lord Chancellor, Lord Lyndhurst put to a panel of 14 judges, 5 hypothetical questions designed to clarify the legal position. The answers, given on 19th June, 1843, came to be known as the 'Mc Naughten Rules'.

The most important of these rules is as follows. **"An accused person is not legally responsible, if it is clearly proved, that at the time of committing the crime, he was suffering from such a defect of reason from abnormality of mind, that he did not know the nature and quality of the act he was doing, or that what he was doing was wrong".**

This legal test has also been accepted in India as the law of criminal responsibility and is included in **Sec. 84, I.P.C.** which is as follows: **"Nothing is an offence which is done by a person, who at the time of doing it, by reason of unsoundness of mind, is incapable of knowing the nature of the act, or that he is doing what is either wrong or contrary to law".**

COMMENT: CLEARLY PROVED: The unsoundness of mind must be directly related to the offence in such a way as to satisfy the Court that the mental abnormality had a direct causative relationship to the offence, and that the offence would not have occurred if there was no mental abnormality.

DEFECT OF REASON: It is necessary to show that the intellectual or cognitive faculties of the accused were so disordered, that his reasoning powers as to facts and actions were not functioning normally.

ABNORMALITY OF THE MIND: When an unsoundness of mind defence is used, it must be clearly established that a defect of reason resulted from the 'abnormality of the mind'. The 'abnormality of the mind' is a legal, and not a psychiatric concept. The English Law recognizes as abnormality of the mind, any disease which is capable of producing mental dysfunction. The law is not concerned with the brain but with the mind, as the term is used in lay terminology meaning reason, memory and understanding. However, when mental dysfunction is attributable to external factors (e.g., alcohol and drugs consumed voluntarily), this is not called as the abnormality of the mind. It is usually assumed to mean one of the major functional or organic psychoses.

NATURE AND QUALITY: It refers to the physical nature of the act.

WRONG: A crime is an act declared by the law of the land to be an offence at a particular time. It is a behaviour which is in violation of the law and is punishable. A crime consists of two main elements. (1) The actus reus (i.e., the guilty act which is against the criminal law). (2) The mens rea (i.e., the intent). Both these elements must be present before the accused can be said to have committed certain crimes.

The rule concerns itself with the ability of the accused to distinguish between 'right' and 'wrong' with reference to the particular crime. If at the time of the commission of the crime, the accused had the capacity to know that his act was wrong, he will be fully responsible, even if he was mentally ill, and unable to refrain from doing the act at that time. If a person commits a crime under the influence of a delusion due to unsoundness of mind, he is judged as though the delusionary facts were real.

Examples: (1) If due to a delusion due to unsoundness of mind, a person thinks that another man is attempting to kill, and he kills that man in self-defence, he has no criminal responsibility. (2) If under the influence of a delusion due to unsoundness of mind, a person thinks another to be a wild animal and kills him, he has no criminal responsibility, because he does not know the physical nature of the act. (3) If under the influence of a delusion due to unsoundness of mind, a person thinks that he is the State Executioner, and that he has to execute the victim as a part of his job, he is exempt from punishment. (4) If under a delusion due to unsoundness of mind, a person thinks that another person has caused a serious injury to his character and fortune and kills him, he becomes responsible, because under the law no one can kill a person in revenge.

The defect of Mc Naughten rule is that, for deciding that a person is of unsoundness mind, **only intellectual factors (reason) are taken into consideration, but not the emotional and volitional factors, delusional beliefs, hallucinations and the ability of the individual to control the impulses.**

(2) DURHAM RULE (1954): "An accused person is not criminally responsible, if his unlawful act is the product of mental disease or mental defect". The term mental disease referred to mental disorder while the term mental defect referred to mental retardation. In this the causal connection between the mental abnormality and the alleged crime should be established.

(3) CURREN'S RULE (1961): "An accused person is not criminally responsible, if at the time of committing the act, he did not have the capacity to regulate his conduct to the requirements of the law, as a result of mental disease or defect".

(4) THE IRRESISTIBLE IMPULSE TEST (NEW HAMPSHIRE DOCTRINE): "An accused person is not criminally responsible, even if he knows the nature and quality of his act and knows that it is wrong, if he is incapable of restraining himself from committing the act, because the free agency of his will has been destroyed by mental disease".

(5) THE AMERICAN LAW INSTITUTE (ALI) TEST (1972): "A person is not responsible for criminal conduct, if at the time of such conduct, as a result of mental disease or defect, he lacks adequate capacity either to appreciate the criminality of his conduct, or to adjust his conduct to the requirements of the law".

(6) THE FEDERAL RULE (U.S.A.): An accused person is not criminally responsible if at the time of commission of the acts constituting the offence, the defendant, as a result of severe mental disease or defect was unable to appreciate the nature and quality or the wrongfulness of his acts.

MENTAL ILLNESS AND MURDER: Medical examination: In criminal cases where mental illness is pleaded as a defence, the defence has to prove it **S.105, I.E.A**. The opinion of the medical witness must be based on his own personal observations. The doctor should obtain detailed history from the accused person and from other sources, and then carry out physical examination and investigations. The following factors which are helpful, should be taken note of: **(1) History:** History of the accused and his family with regard to mental disease. **(2) Motive:** There is no motive. **(3) Preparation:** Prearrangement or preplanning are absent. **(4) Accomplices:** Not present. **(5) Nature of crime:** A mentally ill person may kill several persons including his friends and relatives. **(6) Conduct of the criminal at the time of the crime:** A mentally ill person does not try to destroy evidence. **(7) Conduct of the criminal after the crime:** A mentally ill person may even notify police about the crime.

Sections 328 to 339 of Cr.P.C. deal with provisions as to accused persons of unsound mind including fitness to stand trial and the subsequent procedures. **The law considers the state of mind only at the time of the alleged offence and not generally.** The mental status of responsibility at the time of the alleged offence has to be determined.

Competency to stand trial: A plea of unsoundness of mind is advanced (1) in bar of conviction if the accused was of unsound mind when the alleged crime was committed, (2) in bar of the trial when the accused is of unsound mind and cannot plead, (3) in bar of infliction of capital punishment when a condemned prisoner is of unsound mind. An individual who is unable to understand the nature and the object of the proceedings against him, to consult with his lawyer with a reasonable degree of rational as well as factual understanding of the proceedings against him or follow the proceedings of a trial with a reasonable degree of rational understanding and to assist in the preparation of his own defence may not be subjected to a criminal trial. The capacity to stand trial is determined at the time of the actual trial. The interval between the alleged offence and the time of trial may be days, months or years.

Psychiatrist's opinion: The psychiatrist conducts the examination of the alleged mentally ill person at some time after the alleged crime, and before the trial. The psychiatrist's task becomes difficult with the increase in the interval between the alleged crime and his examination. Psychiatric prediction has limited reliability. **An opinion of the present mental state of an individual usually carries the lowest risk of error; an opinion about a recent past mental state has greater risk of error, and an opinion about the future carries the greatest error and least reliability. The greater the interval between commission of crime and psychiatric examination, the lower will be the reliability of the opinion for legal purposes.** The opinion of the psychiatrist about the mental state of an accused at a previous period of time depends on his knowledge about the accused's present clinical condition, past history obtained from relatives and medical sources, his behaviour before, during and after the act in question, and his knowledge of, course and natural history of the disorder of mind of the accused. Therefore, at the very best the psychiatrist's views concerning the accused's degree of responsibility and self-control at the time of alleged offence will be matters of inference. **If he finds evidence of frank psychosis, epilepsy or other illness accepted as disease or disorder of mind, he can justifiably infer that such illness played a part in the offence with which the accused is charged.** There is probably greater difficulty in giving a defensible opinion with respect to a causal relationship between a retrospectively established mental illness and a particular criminal act. He will also be required to show that the accused either fulfils the requirements of the Mc Naughten rules, or that his illness has caused a substantial impairment of his responsibility.

Legal consideration: All the mental disorders do not free a person from criminal responsibility for his acts. If the disorders impair the cognitive faculties of the accused, i.e., the faculty of understanding the nature of his act and its consequences, he is not held responsible. Cognition includes all aspects of perceiving, thinking and remembering. If mental illness affects only the emotions and the will, but not the cognitive faculties, the person is held responsible for his acts. **The law recognises a guilty intent, the mens rea, as an essential part of the crime. Only those persons who are completely incompetent, demented or wild are considered to lack the ability to have a guilty intention.** The most serious problem for Courtroom presentation of psychiatric and psychological evidence is the inherent uncertainty of the field itself. There is often a confusion between findings and opinions in the individual patient. Genuine disagreement between experts is common, even in areas of diagnosis and prognosis. When a medical witness deposes regarding the existence, characters, and extent of the mental disease, the Judge has to decide whether the disease justifies an acquittal on the ground of unsoundness of mind. The question whether in given circumstances, a man was sane or mentally unsound is for the Court to decide.

Doctrine of Diminished Responsibility: Diminished responsibility is a term used for border-line mental state. It recognises that there are different degrees of mental disorder, and **in general a defence of diminished responsibility requires evidence of a state of mind bordering upon but not amounting to unsoundness of mind.** This includes certain organic states, depressions, obsessional states and some paranoid and psychopathic states.

The defence of diminished responsibility is usually applied for people with a lesser degree of mental abnormality (whether arising from a condition of arrested development or any inherent causes or induced by disease or injury) that could be brought within the Mc Naughten rules. On the other end, this defence is also not used for simulated mental illness, mild character defects, bad temper, jealousy, hatred, drug use, racial characteristics, low intelligence, poor judgement, political fanatism and similar unfavourable personal feelings. Such person may be punished for culpable homicide not amounting to murder.

AUTOMATISM: Automatism is conduct that is performed by a person whose consciousness is impaired to such an extent, that he is not fully aware of his actions. There may be no consciousness at all of the actions in question, or there may be awareness that falls below the level of normal consciousness. **It is an apparently purposeful, and complex behaviour which occurs without conscious control, and for which there is amnesia later.** This alteration of consciousness may be produced by organic factors or by non-organic factors, such as stress or shock. **The main factors producing automatism recognised by the criminal Courts are: (1) Epilepsy (mentally ill automatism). (2) Concussion or cerebral disease. (3) Hypoglycaemia, and (4) Somnambulism (non-mentally ill automatism).** However, the concept of automatism is very vague and unsatisfactory. The Indian law has no special provision for automatism.

SOMNAMBULISM: It means, **walking during sleep. It is characterised by aimless wandering with incomplete arousal from sleep, attended with acute anxiety. A person leaves his bed and walks in the house or out of the house without any awareness of his actions, but rarely injures himself. He is not asleep but in a state of dissociated consciousness, in a hallucinatory state, unrelated to his immediate environment.** It is similar to an automatism. Such persons are usually well-adjusted in life, socially well-behaved, and not aggressive. A large percentage of adults have psychiatric problems attended with acute anxiety. There may have been immediate stress or concealed mental conflict preceding the walk. The crime is not wilful or premeditated. The mental faculties are partially active and are so concentrated on one particular idea, that he may solve a difficult problem or commit a crime, e.g., theft or murder. He may commit suicide, fall in a well or meet with an accident. There is no recollection of the event, but in some cases, the events of one fit are remembered in a subsequent fit and carried out similarly. **Such person is not criminally responsible for his acts.**

SOMNOLENTIA (semisomnolence): It is often **called sleep-drunkenness and is midway between sleep and waking.** It is a condition of prolonged transition from sleep to waking, with partial alertness, disorientation drowsiness, poor coordination and sometimes excited or violent behaviour. If such a person is suddenly aroused from a deep sleep, he may commit some crime due to confusion of the mind, especially when he is having a dream at that time. Such person is not **criminally responsible for his acts.**

Impulse: Some crimes are committed due to an impulse, in which the person loses self-control, such as sudden violent anger. Such persons are **criminally responsible**, unless unsoundness of mind is present.

Hypnotism or Mesmerism: This is a **sleep-like condition produced by artificial means or by suggestions.** During a hypnotic trance, a person may perform acts suggested by the hypnotist, but does not remember them afterwards. **A hypnotised person usually cannot be tricked into doing some immoral or dishonest act.** Medical hypnosis is safe and is used in the treatment of many conditions of ill-health including states of depression and other mental disorders.

Delirium: A delirious person may commit criminal acts due to delusions and hallucinations. **He is not legally responsible for the acts committed during delirium**.

DRUNKENNESS: An act done by a person, who is incapable of knowing the nature of the act due to intoxication is **not an offence, if the thing which intoxicated him was administered to him without his knowledge or against his will** (Sec. 85. I.P.C.). An intoxicated person (voluntary drunkenness) is **criminally responsible, if he had the intention or knowledge of committing a crime** (S.86, I.P.C.). Thus, if a person commits criminal abortion due to which the woman dies, the abortionist may be guilty of murder, for he intended to commit an unlawful act. **Mental disorder brought about by drugs or delirium tremens due to drink, frees one of criminal responsibility.**

A person is not responsible for his criminal acts done during post-traumatic automatism, twilight states and oneroid states.

CHAPTER 24 GENERAL CONSIDERATIONS

FM 8.1: Describe the history of toxicology.
FM 8.2: Define the terms toxicology, forensic toxicology, clinical toxicology and poison.
FM 8.3: Describe the various types of poisons, toxicokinetics, and Toxicodynamics and diagnosis of poisoning in living and dead.
FM 8.4: Describe the Laws in relations to poisons including NDPS Act, medicolegal aspects of poisons.
FM 8.8: Describe basic methodologies in treatment of poisoning: decontamination, supportive therapy, antidote therapy, procedures of enhanced elimination.
FM 8.9: Describe the procedure of intimation of suspicious cases or actual cases of foul play to the police, maintenance of records, preservation and dispatch of relevant samples for laboratory analysis.

Toxicology is the science dealing with properties, actions, toxicity, fatal dose, detection and estimation of, interpretation of the results of toxicological analysis and treatment of poisons. **Forensic toxicology deals with the medical and legal aspects of the harmful effects of chemicals on human beings. Poison is a substance (solid, liquid or gaseous), which if introduced in the living body, or brought into contact with any part thereof, will produce ill-health or death,** by its constitutional or local effects or both. The definition of poison is vague and unsatisfactory for (1) a substance which is harmless in small quantities may act as poison, and cause death when taken in large amount, and (2) bacterial toxins are not regarded as poisons in ordinary sense of the term. **Clinical toxicology deals with human diseases caused by, or associated with abnormal exposure to chemical substances. Toxinology refers to toxins produced by living organisms which are dangerous to man,** e.g., poisonous plants, the venom of snakes, spiders, bees, etc., and bacterial and fungal toxins.

HISTORY: The early history of poisons is described in the ancient Indian Shastras, Egyptian Papyri, Sumerian, Babylonian, Hebrew and Greek records. Menes Pharohs I (3000 B.C.) is said to have studied many poisons. The Ebers Papyrus (1500 B.C.) contains information extending back many centuries. Of the more than eight hundred recipes given, many contain recognised poisons, such as hemlock, aconite, opium, lead, copper and antimony. Atharva Veda (1500 B.C.) describes poisons. A detailed description of various poisons and their treatment was given in Agnivesa Charaka Samhita (Seventh Century, B.C.) In Kalpasthana, Chikitsasthana and Uttarasthana of the Shastras, symptoms and antidotes of poisons are given in detail. Susruta (350 B.C.) described how the poisons were mixed with food and drink, unointment oils, perfumes, medicines, bathing water, snuff, or sprinkled over clothes, shoes, beds, jewellery or put in the ears, eyes, etc. Kautilya in his Arthashastra (about second century B.C.) states that the art and science of poisoning was extensively studied as a separate branch, and used both as an offensive and defensive measure against the enemy. Gradually, there arose a class of 'professional poisoners', who could ingeniously mask the bitter taste or strange odours of the poisons with sweet-tasting and pleasant substances. In 82 B.C. Sulla issued the Lex Cornelia in Rome, which appears to be the first law against poisoning, and it later became a regulatory statute directed at careless dispensers of drugs. Hippocrates added a number of poisons in fourth century B.C. in Greek medicine. In the mythology and literature of Greek history many references to poisons and their use are found. Theophrastus (fourth century B.C.) included numerous references to poisonous plants in De Historia plantarum. Dioscorides, a Greek physician, in the Court of Emperor Nero, attempted at a classification of poisons which remained a standard for sixteen centuries. The Greeks and later the Romans made considerable use of poisons, often political. In the seventh, eighth and ninth centuries Avicenna, Rhazes and Jaber, the Arab pharmacologist-physicians developed the art and science of pharmacology and therapeutics. With the spread of Muslim rule over Europe and Asia, the use of this science also spread. Bhoja-prabhanda (980 A.D.), has a reference to the inhalation of medicaments before surgical operations, and an anaesthetic called "sammohini" is said to have been used in the time of Buddha.

The Italians brought the art of poisoning to its zenith prior to the Renaissance period and extended into that period. Paracelsus created the basic scientific discipline of toxicology in the late Middle Ages. Orfila (Spanish chemist, 1787 to 1853), was the first to attempt a systematic correlation between the chemical and biologic information of the poisons known then. He improved on the work of others and carried on his own experimentation on animals. He pointed to the necessity of chemical analysis for legal proof of lethal intoxication and he devised methods for detecting poisons. He published several books on poisoning. At about the same time Marsh, Magendie, Tardieu, Ambrose Pare, Stas, Scheelle and Reinsch made valuable contributions. Robert Christison (1779 to 1882) was markedly influenced by Orfila and produced à major work on poisons (1845). Rudolf Kobert, also wrote a textbook on toxicology in the style of Orfila (1893).

THE LAW ON POISONS

(1) THE POISONS ACT, 1919: It regulates the import, possession and sale of poisons.

(2) THE DRUGS AND COSMETICS ACT, 1940: It regulates the import, manufacture, distribution and sale of all kinds of drugs. One of its main features is the control of the quality, purity and strength of drugs. Any patent or proprietary medicine should display on the label or container, either the true formula or a list of ingredients contained in it. This Act empowered the Central Government to form a Drugs Technical

Advisory Board, and to establish a Central Drugs Laboratory, to help and advice both the Central and State Governments.

(3) THE DRUGS AND COSMETIC RULES 1945: They were framed under the Drugs Act, 1940, to regulate the importation of drugs, the functions and procedures of the Central Drugs Laboratory, the appointment of licensing authorities, and the manufacture, distribution and sale of drugs. These rules have classified drugs into Schedules as follows. (i) Schedule C: Biological and special products. (ii) Schedule E1: List of poisonous substances under Ayurvedic, Siddha and Unani system of medicine. (iii) Schedule F, part 1: Vaccines: Part II: Antisera: Part III: Diagnostic antigens. Schedule G contains about 65 drugs e.g., aminopterine, antihistamines, bleomycin, insulin, etc., which must be labelled with the word "caution". Schedule H contains several prescription drugs to be sold by retail on the prescription of registered medical practitioner only. Schedule I: contains a list of 51 diseases for the cure of which no drug can be advertised.

The supply of any drug on a prescription must be recorded at the time of supply in a prescription register specially maintained for the purpose. The following particulars must be entered. (1) Serial number of the entry, (2) the date of supply, (3) the name and address of the prescriber, (4) the name and address of the patient, (5) the name of the drug or preparation and the quantity, (6) the name of the manufacturer, the batch number and the date of expiry of potency in the case of Schedule C and L drugs, and (7) the signature of the qualified person supplying the medicine. Both Schedule H and L drugs must not be sold by retail, except on a prescription by a registered medical practitioner.

(4) THE PHARMACY ACT, 1948: It was passed in order to make better provision for the regulation of the profession of pharmacy and to constitute Central Council of Pharmacy and State Councils of Pharmacy. The object of this Act is to allow only the registered pharmacists to compound, prepare, mix or dispense any medicine on the prescription of a medical practitioner. This does not apply to the dispensing by a doctor for his own patients.

(5) THE DRUGS CONTROL ACT, 1950: It provides for the control of sale, supply and distribution of drugs, the issue of cash memo for sale, marking of prices, and exhibiting list of prices and stocks. It gives power to fix the maximum price of any drug, which may be charged by a dealer or producer.

(6) THE DRUGS AND MAGIC REMEDIES (Objectionable Advertisement) Act, 1954: The object of the Act is to ban advertisements which offend decency or morality, and to prevent self-medication and treatment which cause harmful effects. Advertisements of magic remedies for procuring abortion or prevention of conception, increase of sexual potency, correction of menstrual disorders, and treatment of venereal diseases is completely prohibited.

(7) THE MEDICINAL AND TOILET PREPARATIONS (EXCISE DUTIES) ACT, 1956: It provides for the levy of and collection of duties of excise on medicinal and toilet preparations containing alcohol and narcotic drugs.

(8) NARCOTIC DRUGS AND PSYCHOTROPIC SUBSTANCES (NDPS) ACT, 1985: It repeals three acts: (1) The Opium Act, 1857. (2) The Opium Act, 1878. (3) The Dangerous Drugs Act, 1930. The Act consolidates and amends the existing laws relating to narcotic drugs, strengthens the existing laws relating to narcotic drugs, strengthens the existing controls over drugs of abuse, enhances the penalties particularly for illegal trading offences, makes provision for exercising effective control over psychotropic substances, and makes provision for the implementation of international conventions relating to narcotic drugs and psychotropic substances. A psychotropic drug is one that alters mental function by its action. A narcotic drug means Cocoa leaf, Cannabis, Opium, Poppy straw and includes all manufactured drugs. "Psychotropic substance", means any substance, natural or synthetic, or any natural material or any salt or preparation of such substance or material, included in the list of psychotropic substances specified in a Schedule to the Act. This schedule lists 77 psychotropic substances, e.g., LSD, amphetamine, tranquilisers, barbiturates, benzodiazepines, methaqualone, ketamine, psilocybine, phencyclidine, mescaline, etc.

Cultivation of poppy, cannabis and coca plants require licence.

(9) PREVENTION OF ILLICIT TRAFFIC IN NARCOTIC DRUGS AND PSYCHOTROPIC SUBSTANCES ACT, 1988. If a person produces, possesses, transports, imports, exports, sells, purchases, or uses any narcotic drug or psychotropic substance except ganja, he shall be punishable with imprisonment.

Drug	Small		Commercial
Cocaine	2 gm		100 gm
Heroin	5 gm		250 gm
Opium	25 gm		2.5 kg
Charas/Hashish	100 gm		1 kg
Ganja	1 kg		20 kg
Punishment	6 m and 10K	10 years and 1 lakh	10–20 years and 1–2 lakh

Death sentence for repeat offenders

Medicolegal Aspects of Poisons: Sections, 85, 86, 176, 177, 193, 201, 202, 284, 299, 300, 304A, 306, 309, 320, 324, 326 and 328 I.P.C. and S.39, 40 and 175, Cr.P.C. deal with offences relating to administration of poisonous substances. Sections 270 to 278, I.P.C. deal with adulterated foods and drugs.

The intention with which any act is committed is an important element in law. Accurate definition of poison is not absolutely necessary in law, for **administration of any substance with the intention of causing injury or death, and which causes injury or death as a result, is legally sufficient for awarding punishment,** whether the substance is one which can be called poison or not. The law does not make any difference between murder by means of poisons and murder by other means. **Deliberate administration of poison proves the intention of the accused to cause death, or other such bodily injury which is sufficient to cause death, and will bring culpable homicide within the scope of murder.** Sec. 284, I.P.C. deals with negligent conduct with respect to poisonous substances. "Whoever does, with any poisonous substance, any act in a manner so rash or negligent as to endanger human life, or to be likely to cause hurt or injury to any person, or knowingly or negligently omits to take sufficient care to guard against probable danger to human life, shall be punished with imprisonment up to six months, or with fine or both". Whoever administers to or cause to be taken by any person, any poison or any stupefying, intoxicating or unwholesome drug, or other thing with intent to cause hurt to such person, or with intent to commit or to facilitate the commission of an offence, shall be punished with imprisonment up to ten years and also fine (Sec.328, I.P.C.). Adulteration of drugs is punishable with imprisonment up to 6 months or fine or both (S. 274, I.P.C.). Administering poison to a person with criminal intent is by itself a criminal offence, whether actual hurt is caused or not.

EPIDEMIOLOGY: Poisoning both accidental and intentional are a significant contributor to mortality and morbidity throughout the world. According to WHO, three million acute poisoning cases with 2,20,000 deaths occur annually. Of these 90% of fatal poisoning occur in developing countries particularly among agricultural workers. Acute poisoning forms one of the commonest causes of emergency hospital admissions. Pattern of poisoning in a region depends on variety of factors, such as availability of the poisons, socioeconomic status of the population, religious and cultural influences and availability of drugs.

The exact incidence of poisoning in India is uncertain due to lack of data at central level as most cases are not reported, and as mortality data are a poor indicator of incidence of poisoning. It has been estimated that about 5 to 6 persons per lakh of population die due to poisoning every year. There are more than four thousand species of medicinal plants growing as herbs, shrubs and trees in India, many of which are poisonous when administered in large doses. The toxic principles belong to alkaloids, glycosides, toxalbumins, resins, cannabinoides and polypeptides. Suicidal and homicidal cases of poisoning are common in India, as poisons can be easily obtained and many poisonous plants grow wild, e.g., datura, oleanders, aconite, nux vomica, etc. Many Indians consider the taking of life by bloodshed a greater crime than poisoning, strangling, etc. Accidental poisoning occurs from the use of philters or love potions, and quack remedies containing poisonous drugs, and snake bites. A love philter is a drug which is supposed to increase the love between the giver and taker. All aphrodisiacs such as cantharides, arsenic, alcohol, opium, cocaine and cannabis, are supposed to act as love philters. In India, the common poisons are insecticides and pesticides, such as organophosphates, chlorinated hydrocarbons, aluminium phosphide, carbamates and pyrethroids. Other poisons are corrosives, sedatives, alcohol, datura, oleanders, calotropis, croton and cleaning agents. In children kerosene, pesticides, drugs and household chemicals are commonly involved.

The commonest cause of poisoning in India and other developing countries is pesticides, the reasons being agriculture based economics, poverty and easy availability of highly toxic pesticides. Occupational poisoning due to pesticides are also common in developing countries, due to unsafe practices, illiteracy, ignorance and lack of protective clothing. In India, organophosphates form the largest bulk of pesticide poisoning. Since 1985, aluminium phosphide poisoning has been reported as the commonest cause of intentional poisoning in northern parts of India, viz., Haryana, Punjab and Rajasthan.

Among the adults, females predominate in all age groups, with an evident preponderance in the second and third decades of life. Acute poisoning in children is almost entirely accidental, while in adults it is mainly suicidal.

Mortality varies from country to country depending on the nature of the poison and availability of facilities and treatment by qualified persons.

OCCUPATIONAL AND ENVIRONMENTAL TOXICOLOGY: Occupational toxicology deals with the chemicals found in the place of work. Persons working in various industries may be exposed to various agents during the synthesis, manufacture or packaging of these substances or through their use during the occupation. Under the Workmen's Compensation Act, 1923, if workman contracts any disease specified therein as an occupational disease peculiar to that employment, such as anthrax, primary cancer of the skin, pathological manifestations due to X-rays, radium, etc., poisoning by lead, arsenic, mercury, phosphorus, etc., it is deemed to be an injury by accident for purpose of compensation.

HAZARDOUS MATERIALS are substances that can potentially cause adverse health effects in individuals through contact with skin or mucous membrane or absorption through skin, respiratory or gastrointestinal absorption. They include chemicals, biological agents and radioactive substances, which may be in the solid, liquid or gaseous state.

Potential toxic exposures on the farm include a wide assortment of pesticides, noxious fumes, solvents, corrosive agents, fertilisers, envenomations (bites by snakes, scorpions, bees and wasps, centipedes, spiders, ticks, marine animals, caterpillars, etc.), and natural toxic aerosols.

Anthracosis, asbestosis (and its complications, such as pulmonary adenocarcinoma and mesothelioma), silicosis, brucellosis occur due to occupational exposure. Gas and wood stoves, chemically treated furniture and fabrics and domestic pest control are some of the examples of non-occupational exposures.

ENVIRONMENTAL TOXICOLOGY: It deals with potentially harmful impact of chemicals present as pollutants of the environment, to living organisms. Environment includes all the surroundings of living organisms, especially the air, soil and water. A pollutant is a substance present in the environment due to human activity, and which has harmful effect on living organisms. More than 60,000 chemicals are said to be in common use. With advances in technology, pollution is increasing. The main causes of pollution are the production and use of industrial chemicals, increased use of insecticides, etc., in agriculture and production and use of energy. Threshold limit values (TLV) for about 600 chemicals commonly used have been prepared in USA.

All substances causing methaemoglobinaemia, and smoke inhalation can cause upper airway obstruction, lower airway obstruction, bronchospasm, pulmonary oedema and tissue hypoxia. Smoke may contain acrolein (aldehyde), ammonia, CO, cyanide, oxides of nitrogen, hydrogen sulphide, sulphur dioxide, hydrogen chloride, chlorine, phosgene, isocyanates, etc., depending on the material burnt. Acute respiratory failure may occur due to atelectasis, airway obstruction, or pulmonary oedema. Toxin-induced effects may contribute to adult respiratory distress syndrome (ARDS), sepsis, pneumonia, leading to prolonged illness or delayed death. Toxic combustion products depress CNS by acting as anaesthetic agents.

ECOTOXICOLOGY: It is concerned with the toxic effects of chemical and physical agents on living organisms, especially in populations and communities within defined ecosystems. It includes the transfer pathways of those agents and their interactions with the environment.

Poison Information Centres: **National Poisons Information Centre has been established in AIIMS, New Delhi.** It uses a computer software on poisons (INTOX) compiled by WHO. National Institute of Occupational Health at Ahmedabad has also a centre. Regional centres are located in Chennai and Cochin (POISINDEX). These centres provide toxicity assessment and treatment recommendations over the telephone throughout the day for all kinds of poisons.

Prevention: (1) Education is a major component of any poison prevention programme. (2) All drugs and toxic substances should be kept in locked cabinets. (3) All household poisons must be kept separate from food. (4) All products, pesticides and medicines should be kept in their original containers. (5) Keep caps and tops on bottles properly closed. (6) Do not keep household cleaners on the floor, under the kitchen sink, or in low cupboards that a child can easily open. (7) The label should be read before using the drug. (8) No drug should be given or taken in the dark. (9) All drugs whether expired or otherwise, should be disposed in a safe manner. (10) Drugs in child-proof packages only should be purchased. (11) Children should be taught not to eat plants or berries. (12) Wherever cooking gas is used, adequate ventilation should be provided. (13) In persons showing suicidal tendencies, special care should be taken. (14) In chemical factories air-pollution should be prevented. (15) The workers in all factories should be properly educated, and safety equipment provided.

NATURE OF POISONING: **(1) Ideal Homicidal Poison:** The characters of an ideal homicidal poison should be: (i) cheap, (ii) easily available, (iii) colourless, odourless and tasteless, (iv) capable of being administered, either in food, drink or medicine, without producing any obvious change to prevent suspicion, (v) highly toxic, (vi) signs and symptoms should resemble a natural disease, or the serious ill-effects should be delayed sufficiently long for the accused to escape suspicion, (vii) there should not be any antidote, (viii) there should be no postmortem changes, (ix) should not be detected by chemical tests, or other methods, and (x) must be rapidly destroyed or made undetectable in the body.

Organic compounds of fluorine (used as rodenticides), and thallium satisfy several of the above criteria. Arsenic and aconite are commonly used.

(2) Ideal Suicidal Poison: The characters of an ideal suicidal poison should be: (i) cheap, (ii) easily available, (iii) highly toxic, (iv) tasteless or of pleasant taste, (v) capable of being easily taken in food or drink, and (vi) capable of producing painless death. **Opium and barbiturates satisfy several of the above criteria. Organophosphorus compounds, aluminium phosphide and endrin are commonly used as suicidal poisons.**

(3) Stupefying: Datura, cannabis indica, chloral hydrate.

(4) Abortion: Calotropis, oleanders, aconite, croton, semecarpus, cantharides, ergot, lead, arsenic, mercury, potassium permanganate, etc.

(5) Accidental: Household poisons **Table (24–1).** Non-accidental poisoning may occur as an extension of the syndrome of child abuse, usually in children below 30 months.

(6) Rare: Bacteria, insulin.

(7) Cattle Poisoning: The usual motive is destruction of cattle of an enemy, or to obtain the hides. The usual poisons are abrus precatorius, oleanders, calotropis, organophosphorus, arsenic, aconite, strychnine, zinc phosphide, nitrate, etc.

(8) Arrow Poisons: Abrus precatorius, croton oil, calotropis, aconite, strychnine, curare and snake venom.

(9) Aphrodisiacs: Cantharides, cocaine, cannabis, opium, strychnine, arsenic.

CLASSIFICATION: Poisons may be classified according to the chief symptoms which they produce. **(I) Corrosives:** (1) **Strong acids:** (a) **Mineral or inorganic acids:** Sulphuric, nitric, hydrochloric. (b) **Organic acids:** Carbolic, oxalic, acetic, salicylic. (2) **Strong alkalis:** Hydrates and carbonates of sodium, potassium and ammonia. (3) **Metallic salts:** Zinc chloride, ferric chloride, copper sulphate, silver nitrate, potassium cyanide, chromates and bichromates.

(II) Irritants: (1) **Agricultural.** (2) **Inorganic:** (a) **Non-metallic:** Phosphorus, iodine, chlorine, bromine, carbontetrachloride. (b) **Metallic:** Arsenic, antimony, copper, lead, mercury, silver, zinc. (c) **Mechanical:** Powdered glass, diamond dust, hair, etc. (3) **Organic:** (a) **Vegetable:** Abrus precatorius, castor, croton, calotropis, aloes. (b) **Animal:** Snake and insect venom, cantharides, ptomaine.

(III) Systemic: (1) Cerebral: (a) **CNS depressants:** Alcohols, general anaesthetics, opioid analgesics, hypnotics, sedatives. (b) **CNS stimulants:** Cyclic antidepressants, amphetamine, caffeine, methylphenidate. (c) **Deliriant:** Datura, belladonna, hyoscyamus, cannabis, cocaine, etc. **(d) Psychotropic** (1) antidepressants (amphetamines, tricyclics, MAOI, etc.), **(e) Neuroleptics (antipsychotics):** Phenothiazines, thioxanthines, butyrophenones, etc. **(f) Hallucinogens (psychedelics):** LSD, phencyclidine, etc. **(2) Spinal: (a)Stimulant:** strychnine. (b) **Depressant;** Gelsemium. **(3) Peripheral:** Conium, curare. **(4) Cardiovascular:** Aconite, quinine, oleander, tobacco, cyanide. **(5) Asphyxiants:** CO, CO_2, hydrogen sulphide.

(IV) Miscellaneous: Food poisoning, botulism.

Poisons may also be classified according to their morbid anatomic manifestations. (1) No morphologic changes are present which can be attributed to direct chemical action by the toxic agent, e.g., acute CNS depressants (alcohols, sedatives, hypnotics, tranquilisers, salicylates); chemical asphyxiants (carbon monoxide, hydrogen cyanide); organophosphates and most alkaloids. The abnormalities seen at autopsy result from shock and terminal anoxia. (2) Systemic lesions are produced without injury at the portal of entry, e.g., acute haemolytic poisons (arsine, nitrobenzene). (3) Injury is present at portal of entry without systemic injuries, e.g., corrosives, chlorine, sulphur dioxide. Death may be caused by local tissue changes (pulmonary oedema) or acute vasomotor collapse. (4) Local and systemic injuries are present, e.g., heavy metals.

Criminal Offences: The administration of a poison is a criminal offence whenever: (1) it is with intent to kill, (2) with intent to cause serious injury, (3) used recklessly even though there is no intent to kill, (4) for stupefying to facilitate a crime, e.g., robbery or rape, (5) to procure an abortion, (6) to annoy the victim, (7) to throw poison on another person with intention to injure him.

Poisoning may result from: (1) The administration of a poison for criminal purposes. (2) The swallowing of poison in mistake for harmless substance. (3) The inhalation through ignorance or accident, of the vapours of a poison. (4) The incorrect preparation of medicines containing a poison. (5) The accidental taking of a large dose of medicine containing a poison. (6) Excessive self-medication. (7) Addiction to drugs. (8) Bite by a poisonous animal. (9) Food infected with bacteria or their toxins.

Routes of Administration: In order of rapidity of action: (1) Inhaled in gaseous or vapourous form. It usually involves a volatile substance, gas, dust, smoke or aerosol. Volatile solvents, such as benzene, toluene, xylene, acetone, methylene chloride, methyl chloroform, and carbon tetrachloride poisoning in industrial exposures; solvent sniffing among adolescents, or accidents in the home; gases such as CO, hydrogen sulphide and methane in industries; smokes and dusts of industrial origin may involve lead, mercury, silicon, asbestos and beryllium. (2) Injection into blood vessels. (3) Intramuscular, subcutaneous and intradermal injection. (4) Application to a wound. (5) Application to a serous surface. (6) Application to a bronchotracheal mucous membrane. (7) Introduction into stomach. (8) Introduction into the natural orifices, e.g., rectum, vagina, urethra, etc. Some drugs can be given by rectal route to produce a systemic effect, e.g., aspirin, barbiturates, chloral hydrate, chlorpromazine, etc. (9) Application to unbroken skin. Organic phosphates, nicotine, some organic solvents and lewisite gas can penetrate the skin and produce intoxication and death. Other substances which are absorbed through the skin are: phenol and its derivatives, endrin, methyl salicylate, mercury, tetraethyl lead and alkylated compounds, cantharidin, hydrocyanic acid, hormones, such as oestrogen, progesterone, testosterone and desoxycorticosterone, vitamin D and K.

FATE OF POISONS IN THE BODY: The greater part of a poison is thrown out of the body as a result of vomiting and purging. The portion absorbed is mainly deposited in a less soluble form in the liver, which either partially metabolises or completely destroys it. The unaltered portion enters into the general circulation and acts on the body as a whole, or on the particular organs with which it has special affinity, provided the poison is not destroyed or made harmless by the kidneys and muscles. Some inorganic poisons like arsenic and antimony are retained in certain tissues, such as nails, hair, bones, etc., for a considerable time. Certain

Table (24–1). Common household poisons

Preparation	Toxic substance
(A) Domestic Poisons:	
(I) Cosmetics:	
(1) Cuticle remover:	Potassium hydroxide; trisodium phosphate.
(2) Depilatories:	Barium sulphide; thallium.
(3) Hair wave lotions:	Thioglycollate salts; perborates; bromates.
(4) Nail polish removers:	Acetone.
(5) Suntan lotions:	Denatured alcohol; methyl salicylate.
(6) Baby powder:	Boric acid.
(II) Kitchen:	
(1) Baking powder:	Tartaric acid 50%.
(2) Baking soda:	Sodium bicarbonate.
(3) Dish washing compounds:	Sodium polyphosphates; sodium carbonate; sodium silicates.
(4) Fire extinguishing fluids:	Carbon tetrachloride; sodium carbonate; methyl bromide.
(5) Matches:	Antimony; phosphorus; sesqui-sulphide, potassium chlorate.
(III) Rat Poisons:	
(1) Rat paste:	Aluminium phosphide; zinc sulphide; zinc phosphide; arsenious oxide; red squill; thallium sulphate, phosphorus, barium carbonate, strychnine, norbromide, warfarin, sodium fluoroacetate.
(2) Rodine:	Yellow phosphorus.
(IV) Roach powder:	Sodium fluoride.
(V) Sanitary:	
(1) Deodorant tablets:	Formaldehyde; naphthalene.
(2) Drain cleaners:	Sodium hydroxide.
(3) Disinfectants:	Phenol; bleaching powder (calcium hydrochlorite).
(VI) Miscellaneous:	
(1) Insecticide spray:	D.D.T., Gammexane, etc.
(2) Moth balls:	Naphthalene.
(3) Marking ink:	Aniline.
(4) Ink remover:	Sodium hypochlorite 5%
(5) Anti-rust products:	Ammonium sulphide; hydrofluoric acid; naphtha; oxalic acid.
(6) Cleaning solvents:	Petroleum hydrocarbons; carbon tetrachloride; trichloroethylene.
(7) Flourescent lamps:	Beryllium
(8) Furniture polish:	Turpentine; petroleum hydrocarbons.
(9) Paint remover:	Sodium hydroxide; lead acetate.
(10) Shoe polish:	Aniline; nitrobenzene.
(11) Hair bleach:	Potassium permanganate; hydrogen peroxide.
(12) Toys (paints):	Lead.
(13) Fireworks:	Arsenic; mercury; antimony; lead; phosphorus; thiocyanate.
(14) Crayons (chalk):	Salts of arsenic, copper, lead.
(15) Crayons (wax):	Paranitroaniline.
(B) Garden poisons:	
(1) Insecticides:	Organophosphorus compounds; chlorinated hydrocarbons; nicotine; tar oils.
(2) Fungicides:	Lead arsenate; copper compounds; organic mercurials, lime, sulphur.
(3) Weed-killers:	Sodium chlorate; arsenious oxide, and arsenites; dinitrocresol; paraquat.
(C) Therapeutic poisons:	
(1) Antiseptics:	Iodine, benzoin.
(2) Tonic tablets:	Iron.
(3) Tonic syrup:	Strychnine.
(4) Sleeping tablets:	Barbiturates.
(5) Headache tablets:	Aspirin.
(6) Cough remedies:	Codeine.
(7) Throat tablets:	Potassium chlorate.
(8) Pep tablets:	Benzedrine.
(9) Others:	Antidepressants; tranquilisers.

poisons like chloroform, phosphorus, nitrates and acetic acid disappear by evaporation or oxidised or destroyed in the body and no trace of them can be detected in the viscera or tissues if postmortem is delayed.

Poisons which delay putrefaction are heavy metals, carbolic acid, zinc chloride.

Poisons which hasten putrefaction are chronic alcoholism, hydrogen sulphide.

Poisons which are destroyed by putrefaction are aconitine, morphine.

Poisons which resist putrefaction are corrosives, barbiturates, organophosphates, cyanide, datura, heavy metals.

Drugs Secreted into the Stomach: (1) Acids: Salicylic acid, barbital, probenecid, p-Hydroxypropiophenone, phenylbutazone, thiopental. **(2) Bases:** Theophylline, antipyrine, aminopyrine, quinine, levorphanol, acetanilid, aniline, phencyclidine, dextromorphan, tolazoline. Narcotics, cocaine and amphetamines can be found in high concentrations in stomach even when given parenterally.

Routes of Elimination: The absorbed portion of poison is mainly excreted by the kidneys and to some extent by the skin. Other routes are bile, milk, saliva, mucous and serous secretions. The unabsorbed portion is excreted in the vomit and faeces.

Levels of consciousness:

Grade 0 : Fully conscious.
Grade 1 : Drowsy but responding to verbal command.
Grade 2 : Maximum response to minimal painful stimuli.
Grade 3 : Minimal response to maximum painful stimuli.
Grade 4 : No response to painful stimuli, loss of all reflexes including the pharyngeal, laryngeal and corneal.

The most painful stimulus is probably rubbing one's knuckles over the patient's sternum. This hurts more than pressing the eyeball and is potentially less dangerous.

Pharmacokinetics is the study of action of a drug in the body over a period of time including processes of absorption, distribution, localisation in tissues, biotransformation and excretion. Pharmacodynamics **is the action of drugs on living organisms.**

ACTION OF POISONS: (1) LOCAL: The local action by coming in direct contact with the part. (1) Chemical destruction by corrosives. (2) Congestion and inflammation by irritants. (3) Effects on motor and sensory nerves, e.g., tingling of skin and tongue by aconite, dilation of pupils by belladonna or datura.

(2) REMOTE: Remote action produced either by shock acting reflexly through severe pain caused by corrosives, or by poison being first absorbed into the system through the blood, and then exerting a specific action on certain organs and tissues, e.g., cantharides acting on kidneys produces nephritis, nux vomica acting on the spinal cord causes tetanic convulsions.

(3) COMBINED: Drugs like carbolic acid, oxalic acid, phosphorus, etc., have local and remote actions.

CAUSES MODIFYING ACTION OF POISONS

(1) QUANTITY: More the quantity, more severe are the toxic effects. A large quantity of poison taken orally may cause excessive vomiting, causing its rapid elimination and decreased toxicity, e.g., alcohol, copper sulphate, etc. The action of a poison varies with the dose, e.g., a very large dose of arsenic may produce death by shock without causing irritant symptoms, while moderate doses produce irritant symptoms and small doses produce therapeutic action.

(2) FORM: (a) PHYSICAL STATE: Poisons act most rapidly when gaseous and less when liquid. In case of solids, the action depends on their solubility.

(B) CHEMICAL COMBINATION: The action of a poison depends upon the solubility or insolubility resulting from a chemical combination, e.g., silver nitrate and hydrochloric acid are both strong poisons, but when combined, form an insoluble salt of silver chloride which is harmless. A substance may be harmless in metallic state but its salt may be toxic, e.g., arsenic is not poisonous but its salts are poisonous. Certain poisons which are not soluble in water may become dissolved in the acid secretion of the stomach and absorbed into the blood, e.g., lead carbonate and copper arsenite.

(C) MECHANICAL COMBINATION: The action of a poison may be altered if combined mechanically with inert substances, e.g., small dose of concentrated mineral acid produces corrosive action, but the same dose largely diluted with water is harmless.

(3) MODE OF ADMINISTRATION: The rapidity of the action is in the order described under routes of administration. As a rough guide if the active dose by the mouth is considered as unit, the rectal dose is about one-and-half to two, and the hypodermic dose about one-fourth. A lethal dose is usually ten or more times the maximum medicinal dose.

The rate of absorption from the alimentary canal is variable. Absorption by the stomach occurs more rapidly when the stomach is empty than when it is full. Absorption may be hastened if nature of stomach contents is such as will dissolve the poison, e.g., action of phosphorus will be hastened if oil is taken immediately after it is swallowed. Gastroenterostomy hastens the entry of poisons into the small bowel. Sleep, narcosis and trauma causing gastrointestinal stasis will retard it. Retardation during gastrointestinal absorption, dilution and alteration during digestion, or metabolism by the action of the liver render some poisons almost inactive and greatly reduce the potency of others. The skin is on the whole a bad absorptive organ.

(4) CONDITION OF THE BODY: (a) AGE: Age has a considerable effect upon the dosage of drugs. Poisons have greater effect at the two extremes of age. A child under two years of age has not yet fully developed the drug-metabolising enzymes of the liver, and does not have an effective blood-brain barrier, and as such is much more susceptible to the effect of most drugs. There are some drugs of which children can take more than their proportionate dose, e.g., mercury and belladonna. There are some of which they cannot take even a proportionate dose e.g., morphine.

(B) IDIOSYNCRACY: It may be defined as the inherent personal hypersensitivity to the agent in question. Certain people are sensitive for certain drugs and even articles of diet, e.g., shellfish, eggs and fruit. The symptoms usually occur in the skin as an urticaria, but may be of a more general nature with dyspnoea, rigors, fever, diarrhoea, haemorrhage from the bowel and albuminuria. Fatal cases are comparatively rare, but symptoms may be alarming or dangerous. Iodine, bromine, opium, belladonna, cocaine, aspirin, penicillin, and mercury are common examples of drugs to which many people are allergic.

(C) HABIT: The effect of certain poisons decrease with habituation. Tolerance is the ability of an organism to show less response to a specific dose of a chemical than it showed on a previous occasion from the same dose. It results from a decreased reaction between the chemical and the biologic effector substance. Opium preparations frequently taken, lose much of their effect after a time, and require to be administered in increased doses. Addicts can tolerate quantities of the drug which would endanger life if they had been initial doses. Tolerance is seldom a natural phenomenon. The same effect of habit occurs from the use of tobacco, alcohol, cocaine, morphine and other alkaloids. It is more usually a feature of natural substances, less of synthetic drugs, such as sulphonal, barbiturates, chloral, etc. Tolerance for mineral substances is limited, but it occurs in connection with arsenic to a certain extent.

(D) STATE OF HEALTH: A healthy person tolerates better than a diseased. General debility, senility, chronic or disabling disease may cause death of a person to a dose that is ordinarily safe, e. g., CO may kill at a blood saturation of only 25 to 30%. In some diseases, larger doses of certain drugs may be given without harmful effects, e.g., opium in tetanus, delirium tremens and mania, and strychnine in paralysis, while in other diseases certain drugs cannot be given even in small doses, e.g., opium in granular kidney and bronchial asthma and mercury in chronic nephritis.

(E) SLEEP AND INTOXICATION: The action of a poison is delayed if a person goes to sleep soon after taking it. The action is also delayed if one takes a poison in an intoxicated condition.

(F) CUMULATIVE ACTION: Poisons which are eliminated slowly may accumulate in the body when given in repeated doses for a long time and may ultimately produce symptoms of poisoning.

TYPES OF POISONING: (1) Acute poisoning is caused by an excessive single dose, or several smaller doses of a poison taken over a short interval of time. **(2) Chronic poisoning** is caused by smaller doses over a period of time, resulting in gradual worsening. The poisons which are commonly used for the purpose of chronic poisoning are arsenic, antimony, phosphorus and opium. **(3) Subacute poisoning** shows features of both acute and chronic poisoning. **(4) Fulminant poisoning** is produced by a massive dose. In this death occurs rapidly, sometimes without preceding symptoms.

Parasuicide (attempted suicide, or pseudocide) is a conscious, often impulsive, manipulative act, undertaken to get rid of an intolerable situation. Drug ingestion is the

Table (24–2). Toxidromes

Toxidrome	Poisons (Drugs)	Clinical findings
Anticholinergic	Antihistamines, antiparkinsonian drugs, atropine, scopolamine, amantadine, antipsychotic drugs, antidepressants, antispasmodics, skeletal muscle relaxants, many plants (especially Datura), and fungi (e.g., Amanita muscaria).	Hyperthermia, dry skin, dilated pupils (mydriasis), vasodilation causing flushed skin, hypervigilant, hallucinating, delirium with mumbling speech, tachycardia, myoclonus, urinary retention, decreased bowel sounds.
Cholinergic/ Anticholinesterase	Organophosphates, carbamates, parasympathomimetic drugs, and some mushrooms.	Confusion, CNS depression, salivation, lacrimation, urinary and faecal incontinence, vomiting, sweating, fasciculations, seizures, miosis, pulmonary oedema, tachy/bradycardia.
Sympathomimetic/ Withdrawal	Cocaine, ecstacy, amphetamines, caffeine, theophylline.	Paranoia, delusions, tachycardia, hypertension, hyperpyrexia, hyperreflexia, sweating, mydriasis, seizures, arrhythmias.
Opioid	Morphine, pethidine, fentanyl, codeine, methadone.	Miosis (pin point pupil), hypotension, bradycardia, hypothermia, CNS depression, pulmonary edema, respiratory depression, hyporeflexia, coma, rarely convulsions.
Sedative/Hypnotics	Barbiturates, benzodiazepines, ethanol.	Miosis, hypotension, bradycardia, hypothermia, confusion, CNS depression, hyporeflexia, coma.

commonest form. Most persons are psychologically disturbed. There is no actual intention to die.

DIAGNOSIS OF POISONING: (1) IN THE LIVING: There is no single symptom, and no definite group of symptoms, which are absolutely characteristic of poisoning. The closest resemblance to disease, may be produced by thallium poisoning. The symptoms of a disease may simulate acute poisoning, e.g., the sudden onset of intestinal obstruction may be mistaken for irritant metal poisoning. A detailed clinical history is of great importance.

Suspicion of Poisoning: The following conditions should arouse suspicion of poisoning. (1) The symptoms appear suddenly in a healthy person. (2) The symptoms appear immediately or within a short period after food or drink. (3) The symptoms are uniform in character, and rapidly increase in severity. (4) When several persons eat or drink from the same source of poison in the food or drink at the same time, all suffer from similar symptoms at or about the same time. (5) The discovery of poison in food taken, in the vomit or in the excreta is strong proof of poisoning.

Symptoms: The following groups of symptoms are suggestive of poisoning. (1) The sudden onset of abdominal pain, nausea, vomiting, diarrhoea and collapse. (2) The sudden onset of coma with constriction of pupils. (3) The sudden onset of convulsions. (4) Delirium with dilated pupils. (5) Paralysis, especially of lower motor neurone type. (6) Jaundice and hepatocellular failure. (7) Oliguria with proteinuria and haematuria. (8) Persistent cyanosis. (9) Rapid onset of the neurological or gastrointestinal illness in persons known to be occupationally exposed to chemicals.

Collect: (1) Stomach wash (entire quantity). (2) 10 ml. blood. (3) Urine, as much as possible. 100 mg. of sodium fluoride for 10 ml. blood acts both as a preservative and as an anticoagulant.

Symptoms of Chronic Poisoning: (1) The symptoms are exaggerated after the administration of suspected food, fluid or medicine. (2) Malaise, cachexia, depression and gradual deterioration of general condition of the patient is seen. (3) Repeated attacks of diarrhoea, vomiting, etc., are seen. (4)When the patient is removed from his usual surroundings, the symptoms disappear. (5) Traces of poison may be found in the urine, stool or vomit.

A detailed history of the quality and quantity of the poison administered, the character of the symptoms with reference to their onset, and the time that passed between the taking of the poison and the development of symptoms, the duration of illness, the treatment given, and the time of death, should be obtained from the relatives of the deceased. **A toxidrome is a constellation of findings, resulting from any given poison. It serves to clue the clinician into the correct diagnosis** Table (24–2).

DIAGNOSIS OF POISONING IN THE DEAD: Collect all information from the inquest report, medical records if available, and from the relatives of the deceased.

(I) Postmortem Appearances: External: (1) The surface of the body and the clothes may show stains or marks of vomit, faeces or the poison itself. **The colour changes in the corroded skin and mucous membrane are:** (a) sulphuric and hydrochloric acid: grey, becoming black from blood; (b) nitric acid: brown; (c) hydrofluoric acid: reddish-brown; (d) carbolic acid: greyish-white; (e) oxalic acid: grey, blackened by blood; (f) cresols: brown, leathery; (g) caustic alkalis: greyish-white; (h) mercuric chloride: bluish-white; (i) zinc chloride: whitish; (j) chromic acid and **potassium chromate:** orange, leathery. **(2) Colour of postmortem staining:** The skin may be dark-brown or yellow in phosphorus and acute copper poisoning; cherry-red in poisoning by carbon monoxide; chacolate-coloured in cases of death from poisoning by nitrites, aniline, nitrobenzene, acetanilide, bromates, chlorates, etc. due to the formation of methaemoglobin. **(3) Smell about the mouth and nose:** Substances which may be recognised by their odour are: (a) Garlicky: Organophosphates, arsine gas, arsenic, phosphorous. (b) Fishy or musty: Aluminium phosphide, zinc phosphide. (c) Sweet or fruity: Ethanol, chloroform, nitrites. (d) Kerosene-like: Organophosphates, Carbamates. (e) Bitter almond: Cyanides. (f) Rotten egg: Sewer gas, hydrogen sulphide. (g) Burnt rope: Cannabis products. (h) Burnt coal: CO. (i) Moth balls: Camphor, naphthalene. (j) Phenolic substances. (k) Putrid: Anaerobic infections. (4) **The natural orifices,** e.g., mouth, nostrils, rectum and vagina may show the presence of poisonous material or the signs of its having been used. (5) **Injection marks** should be looked for with care. (6) **Skin** should be examined for lesions, e.g., hyperkeratosis and pigmentation may be found in chronic arsenical poisoning. Jaundice may occur in poisoning from phosphorus, senecio, and in susceptible persons by potassium chlorate. (7) Any evidence of **marks of violence,** such as bruises, or wounds of any nature, may suggest some form of death other than poison.

The bodies of persons poisoned are not more rapidly decomposed than those of others. Some poisons may delay the action of the putrefactive bacteria to some extent.

Internal: There is no special routine particular to poisoning cases. All organs must be examined and all contents preserved.

(1) Smell: On opening the body, note any peculiar smell. The skull should be opened first to detect unusual odours in the brain tissues, because such odours are masked by the opening of the body cavities. This is useful in cyanide, alcohol, phenol, cresol, ether, chloroform and camphor poisoning.

(2) Mouth and Throat: Examine the tongue, mouth and throat for any evidence of inflammation, erosion or staining. Areas of necrosis of the pharynx may be seen in death associated with agranulocytosis caused by amidopyrine, thiouracil, dinitrophenol, sulphonamides and barbiturates.

(3) Oesophagus: Corrosive alkalis produce marked softening and desquamation of the mucous membrane. In acute cantharidin poisoning, the mucous membrane is often swollen and engorged and may show patches of ulceration. Perforation of oesophagus may occur in poisoning from paraquat and fluorides.

(4) Upper Respiratory Tract: Examine the larynx, trachea and bronchi for evidence of volatile irritants or inhaled poisonous matter. Oedema of glottis, and congestion and desquamation of mucous membrane of the trachea and bronchi may be seen in corrosive acid or alkali poisoning when it enters the respiratory tract.

(5) Stomach: Toxic substances may be held in high concentrations in the rugae and crypts of the mucosa, or even in the blood in the actual stomach wall. The pathway of acids and alkalis in food-filled stomach starts along the lesser curvature of the stomach and leads to the pylorus, which explains the location of greatest damage in food-filled stomach **Figs. (24–1 to 24–3).** Stomachs without food tend to have significant injury in the lower half to two-thirds and may have sparing of the fundus. The colour and appearance may be normal, though poison is present.

(a) Hyperaemia: Hyperaemia of the mucous membrane caused by an irritant poison is usually patchy and of a deep crimson colour. The ridges are more involved in poisoning than in disease. The mucous membrane is often covered with a sticky secretion and shows small haemorrhagic foci. Redness of mucous membrane of the stomach is found after death, but is usually limited to the posterior wall. In this case, there is no thickening of mucous membrane, nor any thick mucus over its surface. Redness of the mucosa is also found during digestion, in asphyxial deaths due to general venous congestion, and when

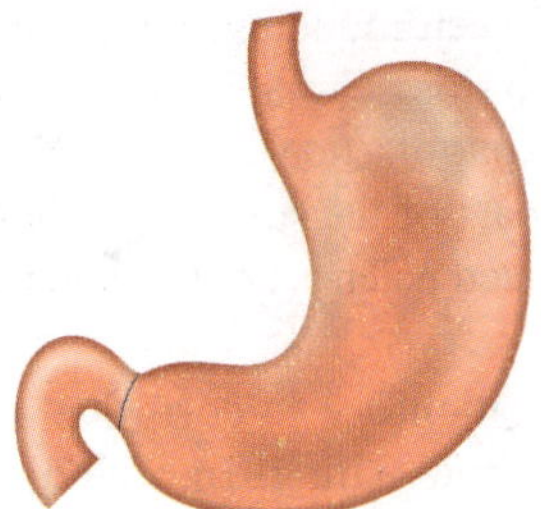

Fig. (24–1). Magenstrasse is the term applied to the pathway acidic agents follow.

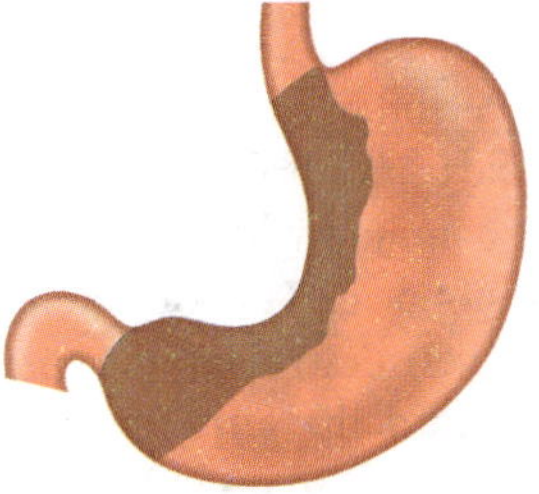

Fig. (24–2). Coloured region indicates the area of greatest injury caused by acid ingestion in a food-filled stomach.

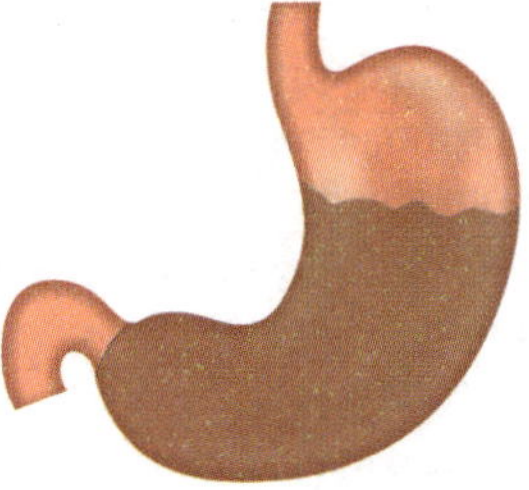

Fig. (24–3). Coloured region indicates the area of greatest injury caused by acid ingestion in an empty stomach.

it is exposed to atmosphere. Hyperaemia caused by disease is uniformly spread over the whole surface and not in patches. Putrefactive changes will alter the colour of a healthy stomach, but the destructive changes of poisoning are usually present. Histological examination helps in cases of doubt.

Colours other than red may be present due to various causes. Mercury usually causes a slate-coloured stain; arsenic may show white particles adherent; strong sulphuric, acetic or hydrochloric acids, and concentrated oxalic acid are likely to blacken or char the wall; nitric acid may cause yellow colour, carbolic acid may produce buff or white colour and shrivelling; cresols produce brown colour; copper produces a blue or green colour. The colour may also be due to bile when there will be no signs of inflammation, or to fruit juice or food, when it is uniform and without signs of inflammation.

(b) Softening: Corrosives and irritants produce immediate contraction of the muscularis, due to which the superficial epithelium is damaged, while the depths of the glands are protected by compression of their necks by the spasm. Excess of mucus is secreted by the glands due to the neighbouring irritation. If life is prolonged, the poison passes deeper and deeper. Spasm of the pylorus holds a poison at this point, which is the site most often involved. Softening of mucous membrane of stomach, is usually caused by corrosive poisons, chiefly alkaline corrosives. It is also seen in mouth, throat and oesophagus. In disease, it is limited to stomach and is usually found at its cardiac end. Softening due to putrefaction begins in most dependent parts and affects all the coats of the stomach without detachment of its mucosa, and softened patch is not surrounded by an inflamed area.

(c) Ulcers: Ulceration due to corrosive or irritant poisons **appears as an erosion with thin, friable margins. The surrounding mucosa is softened due to inflammation, and there is diffuse hyperaemia.** An ulcer from disease is usually seen on the lesser curvature and the margins are well-defined, thickened and indurated.

(d) Perforation: Perforation is occasionally observed, when the strong mineral acids have been taken, especially sulphuric acid; it is much less common with other acids. Ammonia can cause perforation of stomach. **The stomach, in such cases is blackened and extensively destroyed, the aperture is irregular, the edges sloughing, and the adjacent tissues easily torn. The acid escapes into the abdomen and causes peritonitis.** Perforation by irritant poisons is rare. In chronic gastric ulcer, it is oval or rounded and has a punched-out appearance and may show chronic adhesion to neighbouring organs.

In autolysis from postmortem digestion, the change is confined to the stomach alone, and it is commonly found only at the cardiac end. The opening is large and irregular, with rough and pulpy edges. The surrounding mucous membrane is softened and gelatinous. Peritonitis is not seen.

The Contents of the Stomach: The ligatured stomach should never be sent for analysis without being opened, as putrefaction may obscure changes in the mucous membrane, and the gases produced may result in the lid of the jar being forced off in transit. **The stomach is opened along its greater curvature in a clean porcelain dish.** The wall is examined for fragments of poison adhered to it, such as powdered poisons, fragments of capsules, starch from tablets, fragments of leaves or fruit, cantharides, etc. The contents must be carefully observed and written notes made, regarding the volume, colour and contents, including food. The presence of seeds, leaves, capsules and foreign bodies, such as nails, pins, glass, etc., must be noted.

The cells of plants in the alimentary canal, retain their characteristic shape, dimensions, surface ornamentation and other characters, which can be identified in vomit or material from gastrointestinal tract, by microscopic examination.

(6) The Duodenum and Intestines: A strongly acid reaction is of greater significance here than in the stomach contents. Sodium hydroxide can rarely cause perforation of duodenum. Ulceration beyond the pylorus is usually due to natural disease. The only characteristic change which occurs in the intestine is seen in **mercury poisoning. This change which usually involves the ascending and transverse colons, is a diphtheritic colitis, which may resemble the enteritis of acute bacillary dysentery.**

A normal gastrointestinal tract rules out poisoning by corrosive acids and alkalis, phenols, mercury and arsenic.

(7) Liver: Substances, such as arsphenamine, phosphorus, chloroform, trinitrotoluene, carbon tetrachloride and senecio, may produce liver necrosis. Arsenic, carbon tetrachloride, amanita phalloides, yellow phosphorus and rarely ferrous sulphate produce a fatty liver. Jaundice may be produced by phosphorus, senecio and potassium chlorate, due to acute haemolytic anaemia.

(8) Respiratory System: Oedema of the glottis and congestion and desquamation of the mucous membrane of the trachea and bronchi may be seen in corrosive poisoning when the acid or alkali has entered the respiratory tract. The lungs show non-specific signs of congestion and oedema.

(9) Kidneys: Parenchymatous degenerative changes are commonly found in irritant metal poisoning, and in cantharidin poisoning. Extensive necrosis of proximal convoluted tubules may be found in deaths from poisoning by mercuric chloride, phenol, lysol and carbon tetrachloride.

(10) Heart: Subendocardial haemorrhages in the left ventricle occur in most cases of acute arsenic poisoning.

(11) The **bladder,** and in females the **vagina and uterus** should be particularly examined, for poison is occasionally introduced into the body by these routes. In criminal abortion, it may be necessary to send the vagina and uterus for analysis.

Many poisons, such as alkaloids do not produce characteristic tissue changes. The presence of wounds or of a disease sufficient to cause death, does not rule out the use of poison. A poison can cause death without leaving any naked eye changes, and proof of poisoning must be obtained from other sources, or from chemical examination. **No poison kills without producing some symptoms of illness, if no signs after death.** Therefore, enquiry as to symptoms in life is very important. **The conclusion that death was caused by poison depends on evaluation of clinical, toxicologic and anatomic evidence.**

(II) Chemical Analysis: If a refrigerator is available, all organic substances should be kept in it as soon as possible after removal from the body. Chemical compounds should not be added, as they may confuse the issue. Decomposition may produce substances not in the original stomach, but allowances can almost always be made for these without confusion.

The specimens of blood, urine, bile and vitreous should be placed in glass containers, but not in plastic containers, as these fluids can leach out plastic polymers from the wall of a plastic container, which may mask some compounds and interfere with analysis.

Blood is the specimen of choice for detection of poisons, as it gives the best indication of the quantity of drug exerting an effect on the person at the time of death. The urine concentrates the drug or poison in many cases. It is suitable for single direct spot test, because there is no protein-binding to prevent extraction. The concentration of poisons found in urine is not important in evaluating the quantity ingested or the toxicity. In delayed deaths, the poison may be found in urine, when none is found in viscera.

The muscle, especially of thigh is well preserved in advanced decomposition. Levels of drugs in the muscle more accurately reflect blood levels than the liver or kidney.

Postmortem diffusion of the drugs occur from the stomach into the liver, mainly the left lobe. Diffusion also occurs in the base of left lung, spleen and pericardial fluid and to a lesser degree into heart, aorta and inferior vena cava.

In a living person, the concentration of a poison is lower in the venous blood as compared to arterial, because tissues may take up the compound from the arterial supply. Portal blood has higher

concentration of a poison that is being absorbed from the intestine. After death, variation in concentration is caused by uneven destruction by enzymatic and microbiological activity and from diffusion from sites of higher concentration. Postmortem levels of many poisons are unreliable because the barriers formed by living cell membranes breakdown after death, and molecules can easily move through the tissues into blood vessels.

THE ANALYTIC PROCEDURE

For toxicologic analysis, poisons can be divided into five groups.

ANALYSIS: Toxicological analysis of biological tissues involves: (1) Separation of the drug from the biological tissue. For this, the contents of stomach are diluted in water, and the solid viscera are cut into small pieces and macerated in water. Then a solvent is used to extract the poison. (2) Purification of the drug. This is done by additional extraction procedures using alkaline and acid solutions. (3) Analytical detection and quantitation. This is done by thin-layer chromatography (TLC), gas chromatography (GC), gas chromatography-mass spectrometry (GC-MS), and rarely UV spectrophotometry. Except for gas chromatography-mass spectrometry, none of the methods is totally specific. If a method of analysis other than GC-MS is used for initial identification, then often it is easier to make positive identification and even quantitation using the GC-MS.

GROUP I. GASES: Gases are separated from blood or lungs by simple aeration procedures and specific tests applied. Air samples collected at scene of exposure give better results.

GROUP II. STEAM VOLATILE POISONS: They include both organic and inorganic substances, which are separated from biological materials by steam distillation from an acidic or basic medium, e.g., ethyl and methyl alcohol, phenol, chlorinated hydrocarbons, benzene, amphetamines, nicotine, yellow phosphorus, etc.

Steam distillation of a sample of finely minced tissue containing tartaric acid separates volatile acidic and neutral substances. The residue is made alkaline and redistilled, which separates volatile basic substances. Individual qualitative tests are carried out on suitable portions of the distillate. If some volatile compound is identified in distillate, a fresh weighed sample of tissue is used for quantitative analysis.

GROUP III. METALLIC POISONS: (1) In Dry Ashing Procedure, the weighed and minced tissue is dried in an oven and then placed in muffled furnace at 450°C until all the organic matter is destroyed. The remaining ash is leached with mineral acids and resulting solutions subjected to qualitative and quantitative analysis for individual metals. Arsenic, antimony and mercury are volatile at 450°C and would be lost in such procedure.

(2) The Wet Ashing Procedure employs a mixture of nitric, sulphuric and perchloric acids to oxidise the organic matter. The remaining solution is the ash which is used for analysis of various metals.

GROUP IV. NONVOLATILE ORGANIC POISONS: This group includes all compounds that are alcohol and water soluble. (1) Compounds which may be extracted from an acidic aqueous medium by chloroform or ether include organic acids and organic neutral compounds, such as barbiturates, acetanilid, phenacetin, etc. (2) Compounds which may be extracted from a basic aqueous medium by chloroform or ether include organic bases, such as cocaine, quinine, strychnine, phenothiazines, imipramine, nicotine, demerol, etc. (3) Compounds which may be extracted from aqueous solution, which is faintly alkaline with ammonia or sodium bicarbonate, by chloroform with 10% ethanol include morphine, dionin, dilaudid, etc.

For the above substances 200 to 500 g. of tissue is finely ground, and treated with alcohol, filtered and alcohol evaporated, and process repeated and a final residue is obtained and tests, such as TLC, GC, GC-MS carried out to find out specific poison.

GROUP V. MISCELLANEOUS: This includes all substances which are not classified in any of the above four groups, such as non-metallic inorganic substances and water and alcohol insoluble organic compounds. For identification, special individual procedures for each substance must be employed.

Cause of Death: The blood level of the drug or chemical is useful to determine the cause of death, in correlation with clinical and anatomic findings. A lethal level does not by itself establish the cause of death. **The blood level of a drug need not always be in the lethal range for it to reflect the cause of death, especially in a treated case. When the presence of a highly toxic material is established even in trace amounts, the inference that the poisoning is cause of death is justified.**

Toxic and Lethal Drug Levels: **Fatal concentrations of poisons vary depending upon:** (1) analytical techniques which vary widely both in method and accuracy, (2) site of sampling, (3) fatal level being attributed to one substance without considering the levels of other toxic substances that the deceased may have taken, and of which the pathologist or analyst may not be aware. **Many victims who die due to poisoning, have lower blood concentrations of the responsible agent than those usually regarded as fatal. The causes for this may be:** (1) Unusual susceptibility to the drug; (2) combinations of drugs can interact in an additive fashion; (3) some pre-existing natural disease may have contributed to death; (4) rapid but not complete absorption of drug; (5) metabolic degradation of the drug during a prolonged survival in which respiratory complications and hypoxic encephalopathy maintain coma and act as the immediate causes of death.

If low levels are found in viscera, consider: (a) Poly-pharmacy. (b) Time lapse after ingestion with resulting metabolism of drug. (c) Positional asphyxia. (d) Intravascular sickling in certain haemoglobinopathies. (e) Postictal respiratory failure. Death may occur one to two weeks after ingestion of drugs from apparent unrelated causes, e.g., (a) Bronchopneumonia. (b) Therapeutic from tracheostomy. (c) Hepatitis. (d) Fungal or bacterial endocarditis. (e) Encephalomalacia. (f) Haematologic problems.

Toxicity: The **"therapeutic index",** or the ratio of the toxic to the effective dose of a drug, indicates the relative toxicity of drugs. Toxicity of the chemicals have been devised depending on the amounts which produce harm Table (24–3).

The **lethal dose is the dose that kills.** "Minimal lethal dose" is the smallest dose that has been recorded as fatal to a healthy person. **The usual lethal dose of a poison is ten times the therapeutic dose.**

YOUNG'S RULE: The dose of a drug for a child is obtained by multiplying the adult dose by the age in years and dividing the result by the sum of the child's age plus 12.

INTERPRETATION OF TOXICOLOGICAL RESULTS: The following factors should be considered in the interpretation of the result of toxicological analysis. (1) Age and weight of the deceased. (2) Presence of a natural disease condition. (3) Presence of traumatic lesions. (4) Degree of tolerance of the individual. (5) Hypersensitivity reaction.

PUTREFACTION AND TOXICOLOGIC ANALYSIS: In postmortem decomposition, many poisons present in the tissues undergo chemical changes, and cannot be detected such as chloral hydrate, sodium nitrite, cocaine and aconite. Putrefaction of normal tissue may produce substances which give chemical reaction similar to those obtained from toxic compounds. Most volatile compounds are lost due to putrefaction, but ethyl alcohol and cyanide may be produced from normal tissue. Neurin, muscarin, mydalein, etc., are produced due to putrefaction, the toxicity of which is equal to the well-known alkaloids. In an embalmed body, it is very difficult to detect and identify most volatile poisons.

Table (24–3). Toxicity rating (Gosselin, et. al)

< 5 mg/kg	6 (super toxic)
5 to 50 mg/kg	5 (extremely toxic)
50 to 500 mg/kg	4 (very toxic)
0.5 to 5 g/kg	3 (moderately toxic)
5 to 15 g/kg	2 (slightly toxic)
>15 g/kg	1 (non-toxic)

Organophosphorous compounds, endrin, barbiturates, cyanide, yellow oleander, strychnine, CO, datura, fluoride, nicotine endrine, and heavy metals can be identified in putrefied bodies.

Failure to Detect Poison: In some cases, no trace of poison is found on analysis, although from other circumstances, it is almost or quite certain that poison was the cause of illness or death. **The possible explanations of negative findings are:** (1) The poison may have been eliminated by vomiting and diarrhoea, e.g., in irritant poisons. (2) The whole of the poison has disappeared from the lungs by evaporation or oxidation. (3) The poison after absorption may be detoxified, conjugated and eliminated from the system. (4) Some vegetable alkaloidal poisons cannot be definitely detected by chemical methods. (5) Some drugs are rapidly metabolised, making extraction difficult. (6) Some organic poisons especially alkaloids and glucosides may by oxidation during life, or due to faulty preservation, or a long interval of time, or from decomposition of the body, may deteriorate and cannot be detected chemically. (7) Biological toxins and venoms which may be protein in nature cannot be separated from body tissues. Immunoassay procedures can detect these compounds. (8) If the poison acts slowly and death is delayed following production of irreversible organic changes (e.g., hydrogen sulphide or cyanide), the poison may be completely excreted. (9) Sometimes, decomposition products makes the detection difficult or impossible. (10) Treatment may alter the poisonous substance. (11) Many drugs may be present in very small amount and these may require considerable amount of viscera for their identification. (12) The wrong or insufficient material may have been sent for analysis.

False positive results: (1) Many poisons enter the body regularly in small amounts with food, water or air. (2) Due to decomposition: (a) Gases (methane, H_2S, CO_2, mercaptan). (b) Alcohol. (c) CO. (d) Cyanide. (3) Cyanide (burns). (4) Anticoagulants used for blood (methanol, formalin, EDTA, heparin). (5) Regular intake of arsenic, mercury and lead by food and water. (6) Therapeutic use of arsenic, strychnine, sedatives and tranquilisers. (7) Nicotine in the blood of smokers. (8) Chemical burns due to gasoline (in automobile and aircrash accidents). (9) Faulty technique of sample collection. (10) Contamination of blood with stomach contents, pleural or pericardial fluids.

(III) Experiments on Animals: This is not an ideal test, for signs and symptoms may be due to other causes. Absence of signs and symptoms may be due to insusceptibility of the animal to the particular poison, e.g., rabbits are insusceptible to belladonna, hyocyamus and stramonium; pigeons are not affected by opium. **Cat and dog are affected by poisons almost in the same way as human. For tissue and stent studies white pig were also considered as good.** They may be fed with the suspected food, or with the poison after it is separated from the viscera and the symptoms noted.

(IV) Moral and Circumstantial Evidence: Such evidence may consist of motive, the evidence of witness about the recent purchase of the poison, his behaviour before and after the commission of the offence, and the recovery of the poison from the possession of the accused.

TYPES OF DRUG FATALITIES: Drug-related deaths can be: (1) Primary drug fatalities are those in which death is due to the toxic or adverse effect of the chemical agent, with or without the contributory influence of pre-existing, unrelated natural disease. (2) Secondary drug fatalities are those arising from medical complications of drug abuse, such as viral hepatitis and bacterial endocarditis. (3) Drug associated fatalities are those caused by homicidal, accidental and suicidal violence arising directly or indirectly from activities related to the obtaining and use of illicit drugs.

Drug Automatism: According to this hypothesis, the patient develops a state of toxic delirium after ingesting one or several doses of a drug (usually depressant drugs, alcohol, or a combination of these), and in the delirious or automatism state, takes additional doses of the drug without realising it. It is difficult to prove or disprove this hypothesis.

DUTIES OF A MEDICAL PRACTITIONER IN A CASE OF SUSPECTED POISONING: The duties are: (I) **Medical:** Care and treatment of the patient. (II) **Legal: Assist the police to determine the manner of death.** (1) Note preliminary particulars of the patient, i.e., age, sex, address, date and time, identification marks, etc. (2) **In case of suspected homicidal poisoning, the doctor must confirm his suspicion before expressing an opinion. For this he must:** (a) Obtain history of route of exposure, quantity consumed, time elapsed since ingestion, etc. Collect vomit and urine, and submit for analysis. (b) Carefully observe and record the symptoms in relation to food; any change in the colour, taste or smell of the food or drink; other persons affected at the same time; the condition of the patient; explanation offered by the patient for the symptoms, and statements of other persons present which appear to be relevant. (c) Consult in strict confidence senior practitioner and keep him informed about the case. (d) Move the patient to hospital. If the patient refuses to be moved, the doctor should engage nurses of his confidence, who should administer themselves the medicine and food, and allow no one to be with the patient alone, and maintain detailed records of the condition of the patient and of the treatment. (e) If a particular person is suspected, attempts should be made to outwit him by changes of diet and the alteration of meal times. Such person should be allowed to visit the patient only in the presence of a nurse or doctor. (f) Suspicion may arise when a person insists on preparing all the food and serving the patient personally, and also if the person insists on throwing away all the food which the patient leaves. (g) The doctor should keep detailed records of the number of his visits, the symptoms and signs observed, and treatment given from time to time. (3) Once the suspicions are confirmed, he should request the removal of the patient to hospital. If the victim is an adult who retains his mental faculties, it might be desirable to speak to him about the steps to be taken. (4) **Any suspected articles of food, excreta, and stomach wash samples should be preserved.** Full or empty bottles, capsules, paper packets, or liquids lying about should be collected and preserved. Any recent stains on bedclothes, furniture, etc., should be preserved if possible. **Non-compliance is punishable under S. 201, I.P.C.** if it is proved that the doctor did it with the intention of protecting the accused. (5) **If a private practitioner is convinced that the patient** is suffering from homicidal poisoning, he is bound under S. 39, Cr. P.C. to inform the police officer or Magistrate. Non-compliance is punishable under S. 176, I.P.C. (6) If he is sure that patient is **suffering from suicidal poisoning, he is not bound to inform the police,** since S. 309 of the I.P.C. is not included in the section of the I.P.C for which information has to be given under S.39, Cr.P.C. (7) If the practitioner is summoned by the investigating police officer, he is bound to give all information regarding the case that has come to his notice under S. 175, Cr. P.C. If he conceals the information, he is liable to be prosecuted under S. 193 and 202, I.P.C. If he gives false information, he is liable to be charged under S. 177, I.P.C. (8) **A Government medical officer is required to report to police all cases of suspected poisoning, whether accidental, suicidal or homicidal attended in the** hospital. (9) If the condition of the patient is serious, he must **arrange to record the dying declaration.** (10) If the patient dies, he should not issue a death certificate, but he should inform the police. (11) **In case of food poisoning, public health authorities must be notified.**

TREATMENT OF POISONING

(I) Immediate resuscitative measures in comatose patients should be adopted to stabilise respiration, circulation and to correct CNS depression (ABCD of resuscitation). (A) **Airway:** Opening up and cleaning up the airway (oral cavity, nostrils) of secretions, vomit or any other foreign body might be life saving. Protecting and securing the airway by means of endotracheal intubation may be necessary. (B) **Breathing:** If the arterial blood gas cannot be maintained in spite of establishing an effective airway, then graduated supplemental oxygen therapy either by a ventimask or through endotracheal tube should be administered. (C) **Circulation:** I.V. fluid administration may be life sustaining line. (D) **Depression of CNS** should be corrected. An unconscious patient should be turned to lie on one side to stop the tongue blocking the throat and to allow fluid to come out of the mouth (recovery position). Most of the poisoning cases, whether they are conscious or unconscious recover with supportive care alone.

(II) Removal of Unabsorbed Poison from the Body. (1) Inhaled Poisons: If the poison is inhaled as a gas, the **patient must be removed into fresh air, artificial respiration and oxygen** (6 to 8 litres per minute) should be given. The air-passages should be kept free from mucus by postural drainage or by aspiration. Nikethamide 2 ml. i.v. should be given if necessary. Give aminophylline 250 to 500 mg. if there is severe bronchospasm and diuretics if there is pulmonary oedema.

(2) Injected Poisons: If the poison has been injected subcutaneously from a bite or an injection, **a tight ligature should be applied immediately above the wound, which must be loosened for one minute after every ten minutes, to prevent gangrene.** The wound should be excised, the poison sucked out, and the poison neutralised by suitable chemical substance. Local vasoconstriction can be produced by injection of adrenaline. Immersion of the extremity in water at 10°C. slows capillary blood flow and limits absorption.

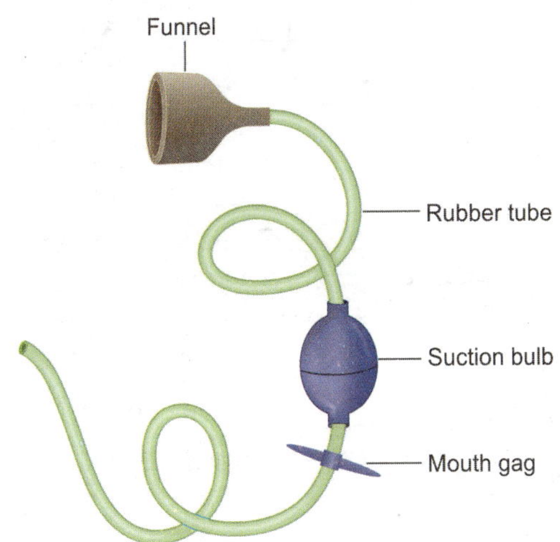

Fig. (24–4). Stomach pump.

(3) Contact Poisons: Patient's contaminated clothes, contact lenses and jewellery should be removed immediately. If poison is applied to the skin or wound, or is inserted into the vagina, rectum or urinary bladder, it should be **removed by washing with water for 30 minutes or should be neutralised by specific chemical.** Eyes should be irrigated with normal saline for at least 15 minutes.

(4) Ingested Poisons: GASTRIC LAVAGE: **It is useful any time within 2 hours after ingestion of a poison.** It is done using a stomach tube (Ewald's or Boa's, tube) or ordinary soft, non-collapsible rubber tube of one cm. diameter and one-and-half metre length, with a **funnel attached at one end, and a mark about 50 cm. from the other end, which should be rounded with lateral openings to avoid any injury when it is being passed** Fig. (24–4). At about the midpart of the tube there is a suction bulb, used to pump out the stomach contents. A wooden mouth gag has a hole at its mid-part to allow the passage of the tube through it. One end of the gag is pointed so that it can be forcefully inserted by the side of the mouth in non-cooperative patients. **Dentures must be removed and a mouth gag is placed** in right position in between the teeth of two jaws, so that the teeth do not bite the tube. Care should be taken in unconscious persons, who are likely to regurgitate and then aspirate stomach contents into respiratory tract and die from asphyxia. Patient should be lying on his left side or prone with head hanging over the edge of the bed, and face down supported by an assistant, so that the mouth is at a lower level than larynx, so that any fluid which may leak out through the sides of the tube will not trickle down inside the larynx and trachea Fig. (24–5). The end is lubricated with olive or sweet oil, liquid paraffin or glycerine, and is **passed into the stomach by depressing the tongue with two fingers or tongue depressor, and slowly passing it downwards through the pharynx and oesophagus into the stomach, till the 50 cm. mark is reached. If there are no marks on the tube, the tube should be passed for a distance equal to that measured between the bridge of the nose and the tip of the xiphoid process.** Force must not be used to insert the tube. Absence of coughing and of breath sounds in the funnel will confirm that the tube has not entered into the trachea. Whenever in doubt, test by keeping the free end of the tube just below a water surface. Air from the stomach is usually

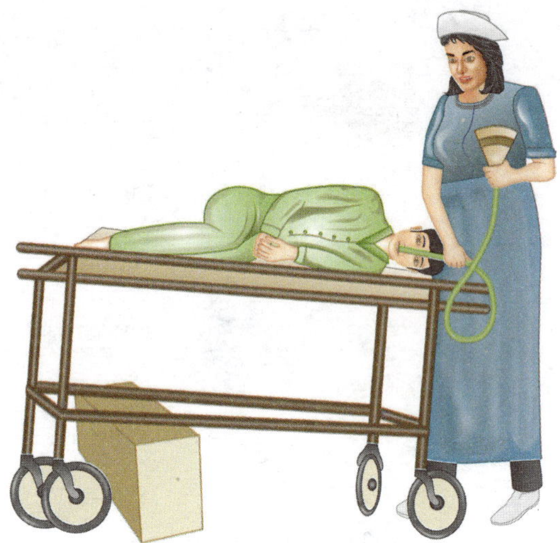

Fig. (24–5). Position of patient for gastric lavage.

expelled completely in 2 to 3 expirations, whereas air from the lungs causes bubbling at each expiration. **About one-fourth litre of warm water (35°C) should be passed through the funnel held high up above the patient's head.** When funnel is empty, compress the tube below it between the finger and thumb and lower it below the level of the stomach, and its contents will be emptied by syphon action on releasing the pressure on the rubber tubing. **If stomach pump is used, applying suction on the bulb will siphon the stomach contents. Stomach contents can be aspirated by a 20 ml. syringe. Preserve this for chemical analysis.** If there is any bleeding, abandon the procedure. Gastric lavage may be done with water ; 1:5000 potassium permanganate; five per cent sodium bicarbonate ; four percent tannic acid; one percent sodium or potassium iodide; one to three percent calcium lactate; saturated lime water or starch solution, or 0.9% saline. **Next, use about half litre of suitable solution and repeat till no further particulate matter is seen and clear and odourless fluid comes out.** This indicates that there is no further interaction between the antidote and poison. **At this stage, the stomach is not completely emptied but a small quantity of the fluid containing the antidote or activated charcoal suspension (one gm/kg body weight, or/and a cathartic) is left behind in the stomach, so that it may neutralise whatever small quantity of the poison is left behind.** Ryle's tube or a number 10 to 12 French catheter can be used for infants and children, and about 25 cm. is necessary to reach the stomach. **After a recent heavy meal, the bulky contents are first removed by emetics.** Stomach wash is better than emesis because of the discomfort caused to the patient in vomiting.

In poisoning with salicylates, phenothiazines, tricyclic antidepressants, antihistamines, lavage can be done up to 12 to 18 hours after ingestion of the poison.

Contraindications: The only absolute contraindication is corrosive poisoning (except carbolic acid), owing to the danger of perforation. In the following conditions stomach wash can be done by taking proper precautions. (1) **Convulsant poisons,** as it may lead to convulsions. Lavage should be done after controlling the convulsions. (2) **Comatose patients,** because of the risk of aspiration of fluid into the air-passages. The airway should be sealed by cuffed endotracheal tube (8 to 9 mm) and lavage done. (3) **Volatile poisons,** which may be inhaled. (4) Upper alimentary disease, e.g., oesophageal varices. (5) In patients with marked hypothermia, and haemorrhagic diathesis.

Complications: (1) Laryngeal spasm. (2) Aspiration pneumonitis. (3) Perforation of stomach. (4) Cardiac arrhythmias. (5) Vagal inhibition.

EMETICS: Emetics should be used only if there is difficulty in obtaining or using a stomach tube. Vomiting can be produced only if the medullary centres are still responsive. Due to the danger of inhaling gastric contents, vomiting should only be induced when a conscious patient is lying on his side with the head dependent. **Ipecacuanha powder one to 2 g. or 30 ml. of ipecac syrup for adults,** 15 ml (1 to 12 years), 10 ml (9 to 12 months), 5 ml (6 to 9 months) followed by several glasses of water **induces vomiting in 90 to 95% of patients within 20 to 30 minutes.** Syrup of ipecac contains cephaeline and emetine. It induces vomiting by local activation of peripheral sensory receptors in the GIT, and stimulation of vomiting centre. **The dose is repeated if vomiting does not occur in half an hour.** This is the only and best method of producing vomiting. Ingestion of excessive amount of salt water may cause fatal hypernatraemia. **Household emetics, i.e., mustard powder (one teaspoon) and common salt are not effective and can lead to complications.** Apomorphine, copper sulphate, tartar emetic and zinc sulphate are absolete. Some physicians consider ipecac to be obsolete.

Contraindications: Same as for stomach wash and (1) severe heart and lung diseases, (2) advanced pregnancy, and (3) after ingestion of a CNS stimulant, because further stimulation associated with vomiting may produce convulsions.

Tickling throat: Make patient lie face down or sit well forward with the head lower than the chest, and ask the patient to touch the back of the throat with his fingers or with your own finger or a blunt object, such as a spoon handle or a wooden tongue depressor. **This is usually ineffective.**

(III) ADMINISTRATION OF ANTIDOTES: Antidotes are substances which counteract or neutralise the effects of poisons. Common modes of action of antidotes are: (1) Inert complex formation, e.g., chelating agents for heavy metals, dicobalt edetate for cyanide. (2) Accelerated detoxification, e.g., thiosulphate for cyanide. (3) Reduced toxic conversion, e.g., ethanol for methanol. (4) Receptor site blockade, e.g., naloxone for opiates; atropine for organophosphates at muscarinic receptor sites. (5) Toxic effect bypass, e.g., 100% oxygen in cyanide poisoning.

(I) MECHANICAL OR PHYSICAL ANTIDOTES: They **neutralise poisons by mechanical action or prevent their absorption.** **(1) Activated charcoal** is a fine, black, odourless and tasteless powder. It is produced by the destructive distillation of various organic materials, usually from wood pulp, and then treating at high temperatures with a variety of activating agents, such as steam, CO_2, etc., to increase its adsorptive capacity. The particles are small, but the surface area is very large. Each gram of activated charcoal has a surface area of 1,000 square metres. **It can be used by mixing with water to form a soup-like slurry (8 ml. of water per gram of charcoal). Superactivated charcoal has double the adsorbing surface area. It acts mechanically by adsorbing and retaining within its pores organic, and also to a less degree mineral poisons, and thus**

delays the absorption from the stomach. Barbiturates, atropine, benzodiazepines, quinine, strychnine, phenothiazines, digitalis, amphetamines, antidepressants, antiepileptics, antihistamines, chloroquine, cimetidine, tetracycline, theophylline, pyrethrins, aluminium phosphide, ergot, beta blockers, meprobamate, phenyl butazone, quinidine, glutithimide are well adsorbed. **In multiple doses it significantly increases the total body clearance of opium, cyanide and phenobarbital.** Phenol, salicylates, kerosene, paracetamol are moderately adsorbed. It is not useful in poisoning with corrosives, heavy metals, cyanide, hydrocarbons and alcohol. **The initial dose is 60 to 100 g. in adults and 15 to 30 g. in children using 8 ml. of diluent per gram of charcoal.** Adsorption may lead to release of the offending chemical as the pH of the environment changes during the passage of the material through the gastrointestinal tract. Repeat doses of 50 g. every four hours can be given in poisoning by aspirin, phenobarbital, theophylline, phenothiazines, antihistamines, tricyclic antidepressants, and carbamazepine, up to 2 days. (2) **Demulcents are substances which form a protective coating on the gastric mucous membrane and thus do not permit the poisons to cause any damage,** e.g., milk, starch, egg-white, mineral oil, milk of magnesia, aluminium hydroxide gel, etc. Fats and oils should not be used for oil-soluble poisons, such as kerosene, phosphorus, organophosphorus compounds, DDT, phenol, turpentine, aniline, acetone, carbontetrachloride, etc. (3) **Bulky food** acts as a mechanical antidote to glass powder by imprisoning its particles within its meshes, and thus prevent damage being effected by the sharp glass particles.

MULTIDOSE ACTIVATED CHARCOAL: It facilitates the passage of substances from plasma into the intestinal lumen (by creating a concentration gradient between the blood and bowel fluid), **where the concentration of toxin has been significantly lowered by intraluminal charcoal adsorption, and significantly decreases the half-life of several drugs.** Initial loading dose is 1 to 2 g/kg. Repeat doses of 0.5 to 1 g/kg are given at 4 to 6 hours intervals. It can also be administered by continuous infusion of 0.25 to 0.5 g/kg/hour through a nasogastric tube.

CHARCOAL HAEMOPERFUSION: This is useful even with highly protein-bound substances that have a large volume of distribution and are lipid-soluble. They include barbiturates, salicylates, paraquat, phenytoin, theophylline, chloral hydrate, digitalis, glutethimide, methaqualone, methotrexate, pentobarbital, carbamazepine, theophylline and paracetamol. **Blood is circulated extracorporeally from an arterial source through a filter filled with adsorptive materials, i.e., charcoal coated with various polymers** (acrylic hydrogel is commonly used), **or resins and then back to the patient's venous side. The circuit is heparinised and primed with saline.**

(2) CHEMICAL ANTIDOTES: They counteract the action of poison by forming harmless or insoluble compounds or by oxidising poison when brought into contact with them. (1) **Common salt decomposes silver nitrate by direct chemical action, forming the insoluble silver chloride.** (2) **Albumen precipitates mercuric chloride.** (3) Dialysed iron is used to neutralise arsenic. (4) Copper sulphate is used to precipitate phosphorus. (5) **Potassium permanganate has oxidising properties.** 1:5000 solution is used in poisoning for opium and its derivatives, strychnine, phosphorus, hydrocyanic acid, cyanides, barbituric acid and its derivatives, atropine and other alkalis. **When it reacts with the poison in the stomach, it loses its pink colour. The wash must be continued till the solution coming out of the stomach is of the same pink colour as the solution put in.** (6) A solution of tincture iodine or Lugol's iodine 15 drops to half a glass of warm water precipitates most alkaloids, lead, mercury, silver, quinine and strychnine. (7) Tannic acid 4%, or tannin in the form of a strong tea or one teaspoonful of tannic acid in water tends to precipitate apomorphine, cinchona, strychnine, nicotine, cocaine, aconite, pilocarpine, lead, silver, aluminium, cobalt, copper, mercury, nickel and zinc. (8) Alkalis neutralise acids by direct chemical action. It is safer to give little weak solution of an alkaline hydroxide, magnesia or ammonia. Bicarbonates should not be given, because of the possible risk of rupturing the stomach due to liberated CO_2. (9) Acids neutralise alkalis by direct chemical action. Only those substances which are by themselves harmless should be given, e.g., vinegar, lemon juice, canned fruit juice. Neutralisation of acids with alkali and vice versa should be avoided because exothermic reaction of neutralisation can cause additional injury.

Universal antidote: So-called universal antidote consisting of activated charcoal, or burnt toast 2 parts, magnesium oxide one part and tannic acid or strong tea one part **is not recommended.**

(3) PHYSIOLOGICAL OR PHARMACO-LOGICAL ANTIDOTES: They act on the tissues of the body and produce symptoms exactly opposite to those caused by the poison. They are used after some of the poison is absorbed into the circulation. Their use is somewhat limited and not without danger. **These agents act on the principle of antagonism by interfering with another's action upon the enzymes, tissue cells or opposing nerve systems.** Most of the known antidotes are only partial in their action. **Atropine and physostigmine are two real physiological antidotes, as both of them affect nerve endings and produce opposite effects** on the heart rate, state of the pupils, and glandular secretory activity. Other examples are: cyanides and amyl nitrite; barbiturates and picrotoxin or amphetamine; strychnine and barbiturates.

Chelating Agents: Chelating agents (metal complexing agents) **are used in the treatment of poisoning by heavy metals.** They have a greater affinity for the metals as compared to the endogenous enzymes. **The complex of the agent and metal is more water-soluble than the metal itself, resulting in higher renal excretion of the complex.** They can form stable, soluble complexes with calcium and certain heavy metals.

(A) B.A.L. (British anti-lewisite; dimercaprol; dimercaptopropanol): It is primarily used in arsenic, mercury and lead poisoning. It is also used in antimony, bismuth, copper, gold and thallium poisoning. Many heavy metals have great affinity for sulphydryl (SH) radicles and combine with them in tissues and deprive the body of the use of respiratory enzymes of tissue cells. **Dimercaprol has two unsaturated sulphydryl groups which combine with the metal, and thus prevent union of arsenic with the SH group of the respiratory enzyme system. The compound formed by the heavy metal and dimercaprol is relatively stable, which is carried into the tissue fluids, particularly plasma, and is excreted in the urine. In severe poisoning a dose of 3 to 4 mg/kg. is given. Each ml. contains**

50 mg. 3 ml of 10% BAL and 20% benzyl benzoate in arachis oil is injected deep i.m. fourth hourly for the first two days, and then twice daily for ten days or till recovery. It should not be used when liver is damaged. BAL may induce haemolysis in the G6PD deficient individuals.

(B) E.D.T.A. (ethylenediaminetetraacetic acid; calcium disodium versenate; edathemil; edetic acid; versene): It is a chelating agent and is effective in lead, mercury, copper, cobalt, cadmium, iron and nickel poisoning. It is currently used almost exclusively for lead poisoning. Intramuscular administration causes pain. **The usual dose is 25 to 35 mg/kg. body weight in 250 to 500 ml. of 5% glucose or normal saline i.v. over a one to 2 hour period twice daily for five days, and may be repeated after two to three days.** It forms chelates with lead which are water-soluble, non-toxic, non-ionised, non-metabolised and excreted intact in the urine.

(C) PENICILLAMINE (cuprimine; dimethyl cystine): It is a hydrolysis product of penicillin. It has a stable SH group. **It is given in a dose of 30 mg/kg. body weight up to a total of 2 g. per day in 4 divided doses orally for about 7 days.** One to 3 g. can be given in slow normal saline drip daily for 2 to 4 days. **It is the chelating agent of maximum efficiency for copper, lead and mercury.**

(D) DMSA, succimer (Meso-2, 3-dimercapto-succinic acid): It is used in lead, mercury and arsenic poisoning. It is superior to EDTA in the treatment of lead poisoning, as it does not lead to redistribution of lead to the brain. It is less toxic to the kidneys. It can be given in patients with G6PD deficiency. **It is given in a dose of 10 mg/kg orally every 8 hours for 5 days, followed by the same dose every 12 hours for 14 days.** A combination of succimer and EDTA is said to be more effective.

DMSA and DMPS possess the same dithiol (sulphydryl) chelating grouping as dimercaprol and the molecules are more hydrophilic. They have a better therapeutic index.

(E) DMPS: (2,3-dimercaptopropane 1-sulfonate) is effective in the treatment of mercury, lead and arsenic poisoning. Dosing regimen is same as DMSA.

(F) DESFERRIOXAMINE: It contains trivalent iron as a chelate and is **very useful in acute iron poisoning. 8 to 12 g. is given orally daily to absorb iron in the stomach.** 2 g. in 5% of laevulose solution is given i.v. to bind absorbed iron, repeated twelve hourly if necessary. It is also used to promote removal of radioactive heavy metals.

(IV) Elimination of Poison by Excretion: Indications: (1) Severe poisoning. (2) Progressive deterioration in spite of full supportive care. (3) When there is high risk of serious morbidity or mortality. (4) When normal route of excretion of the toxic compound is impaired. (5) When the poison produces delayed but serious toxic effects. (6) When the patient is having cardiovascular, respiratory or other diseases that increase the hazards.

(1) RENAL EXCRETION: It may be improved by giving large amounts of fluid, tea or lemonade orally. Forced diuresis may cause pulmonary or cerebral oedema. Urinary acidification is not recommended.

(2) PURGING: Thirty g. sodium sulphate with large amounts of water, hastens the elimination of poison in the stool. Magnesium sulphate should be avoided, since sufficient may be absorbed to produce central nervous system depression in cases of renal failure. To remove unabsorbed material from the intestinal tract, poorly absorbable material, such as liquid petroleum which is a solvent for fat-soluble agents is effective. Sorbitol 50 ml of 70% solution is a better purgative, but in young children it may cause fluid and electrolyte imbalance.

(3) WHOLE-BOWEL IRRIGATION: Whole bowel irrigation involves the use of a polythylene glycol with electrolyte lavage solution which is a non-absorbable, osmotically active compound. This is administered usually by nasogastric tube (0.5 litres/ hour to children less than 5 years of age and 2 litres/ hour to adults) continuously until the rectal effluent is clear. It takes about 4 to 6 hours. It is useful in patients who have ingested large quantities of substances that are difficult to remove, e.g., iron and lithium overdose, sustained release preparations, cocaine, heroin, etc.

(4) DIAPHORETICS: In most cases, it is doubtful whether this speeds up the excretion of toxic agents. In most cases application of heat (blankets, hot water bottles), and administration of hot beverages (hot tea, hot milk, hot lemonade) will cause increased perspiration. Profuse perspiration will be produced by five mg. of pilocarpine nitrate, s.c. and a less marked effect may be produced by cutaneous irritation and cutaneous vasodilation produced by alcohol, salicylates and antipyretics.

(5) FORCED ALKALINE DIURESIS, achieving a urinary pH of 7.5 to 9 promotes, excretion of drugs that are weak acids, such as salicylates, phenobarbital, chlorpropamide, methotrexate, etc. A solution of sodium bicarbonate 50 to 100 mEq. added to one litre of 0.45% saline may be administered at the rate of 250 to 500 ml/hr for the first 1 to 2 hours. Alkaline solution and diuretics should be administered to maintain a urinary output of 2 to 3 ml/kg/hr.

(6) PERITONEAL DIALYSIS: Alcohols, long-acting barbiturates, chloral hydrate, lithium, salicylates, bromides, inorganic mercury, quinidine, theophylline, and sodium chlorate are effectively removed by peritoneal dialysis. For adults, the exchange is usually 2 litres; for children under 5 years, 200 ml. It is only 10 to 25% as effective as haemodialysis. Exchange transfusion especially in children is useful in barbiturate, CO and salicylate poisoning.

(7) HAEMODIALYSIS: It is very useful for removing ethanol, methanol, ethylene glycol, chloral hydrate, lithium, trivalent arsenic, acetaminophen, bromides, phenobarbital, salicylates, fluoride, sodium chlorate, digitalis, methaqualone, boric acid and thiocyanates.

(8) HAEMOPERFUSION: Large volumes of patient's blood are passed over an adsorbent substance to remove toxic substances. Activated charcoal and resins are commonly used as sorbents. It is useful in poisoning from barbiturates, paraquat, acetaminophen, digitalis, carbamazapine, meprobamate, methaqualone, theophyllin, etc. It removes many of the toxins that are not removed by haemodialysis.

(9) PSYCHIATRIC CARE: Any patient, who shows suicidal tendencies, should get psychological assessment and support as early as possible.

(V) SYMPTOMATIC TREATMENT: It refers to the adoption of general measures to support the life of the patient and to lessen suffering. The symptoms should be treated on general lines.

(VI) FOLLOW-UP: Adequate follow-up is necessary to treat the complications if any. In suicidal cases, psychiatric treatment is necessary.

CHAPTER

25

AGRICULTURAL POISONS

FM 9.5: Describe general principles and basic methodologies in treatment of poisoning: decontamination, supportive therapy, antidote therapy, procedures of enhanced elimination with regard to organophosphates, carbamates, organochlorines, pyrethroids, paraquat, aluminium and zinc phosphide.

More than thousand chemicals are currently used as insecticides and pesticides. They can be classified as follows depending on the toxicity.

(I) VIRTUALLY HARMLESS: (1) Phenoxyacetic acid plant hormones, e.g., M.C.P.A., D.C.P.A., T.C.P.A. They are used for dock and thistle control. (2) Copper oxides, oxychlorides, used as fungicides. (3) Lime-sulphur washes, used as orchard fungicides. (4) Petroleum washes, used as orchard insecticides. (5) Tar-oil emulsion, used as orchard ovicides.

(II) COMPARATIVELY HARMLESS: (1) Sulphuric acid (20%), used as weed-killer. (2) Sodium chlorate used as mass herbicide for roads and rail tracks.

(III) MILDLY TOXIC: (1) Chlorinated hydrocarbon insecticides: (a) DDT. (b) Gammexane. (c) Methoxachlor. (d) Chlordan, aldrin and dieldrin. They are used to control fly, louse, tick, as agricultural insecticides and cattle disinfestors.

(IV) HIGHLY TOXIC: (1) Arsenical compounds: (a) Sodium arsenite. (b) Lead and calcium arsenate. (c) Paris green. They are used as weed-killers and orchard insecticides. (2) Nicotine, sulphates, tannates. They are used as horticultural insecticides. (3) Hydrocyanic acid, KCN, NaCN. They are used as a disinfestor and raticide. (4) Dinitro compounds, e.g., D.N.P. (dinitrophenol), D.N.O.C. (dinitro-orthocresol). They are used as selective weed-killers, ovicides and insecticides. (5) Organic polyphosphates: (a) HETP (hexaethyltetraphosphate). (b) TEPP (tetraethyl-pyrophosphate). (c) OMPA (octamethylpyrophosphoramide). (d) Parathion (diethyl nitrophenyl thiophosphate). They are used as insecticides and acaricides.

CLASSIFICATION: (1) INSECTICIDES OF VEGETABLE ORIGIN: They are nicotine, pyrethrins and rotenone.

(2) CHEMICAL INSECTICIDES: (I) Inorganic: They are phosphorus and compounds of antimony, arsenic, barium, mercury, thallium, zinc and fluorides.

(3) SYNTHETIC ORGANIC CHEMICAL INSECTICIDES: They can be divided into: (1) Phosphate esters. (2) Carbamates. (3) Chlorinated hydrocarbons: (a) Indane derivatives (chlordane, heptachlor, aldrin, dieldrin, endrin, diendrin). (b) Chlorobenzene derivatives: (DDT, chlorophenothane). Fatal dose: 150 mg/kg. body weight. (c) Benzene hexachloride (lindane, gammexane). Fatal dose: 15 g. (d) Chlorinated camphenes. (toxaphene, strobane). Fatal dose: 2 g.

ORGANOPHOSPHORUS POISONS

They are esters of phosphoric acid and form two series of compounds.

(A) Alkyl phosphates: (1) HETP. (2) TEPP (Tetron). (3) OMPA. (4) Dimefox. (5) Isopestox. (6) Malathion (Kill bug; Bugsoline). (7) Sulfotepp. (8) Demeton. (9) Trichlorfon.

(B) Aryl phosphates: (1) Parathion (nitrostigmine) (Follidol; Kill phos; Ekato). (2) Paraoxon. (3) Methyl-parathion (Metacide). (4) Chlorthion. (5) Diazinon (Diazion; Tik 20). They are available as dusts, granules and liquids.

Absorption: They are absorbed **by inhalation, through the skin, mucous membranes and the gastrointestinal tract.** They are widely distributed in the body and readily cross placenta. Excretion is prolonged over a week. When sprayed in air, absorption in the plants occurs through leaves and stems.

Metabolism occurs in the liver. **Detoxification occurs via cytochrome P_{450} monooxygenase.** The aryl organophosphates require liver activation to become toxic. Excretion of metabolites occurs in the urine.

They are mixed with a solvent, usually aromax, which is responsible for kerosene-like smell in the body cavities, stomach contents, vomit, froth, etc. Some of the solvents used are odourless.

Action: Acetylcholine is produced at the myoneural junction, and acts as a chemical signal transmitter at synapses (neurotransmitter) which is hydrolysed to choline and acetic acid spontaneously. Hydrolysis is greatly increased by cholinesterases, which are present in plasma and on the membranes, or within the cytoplasm of many cells. **Organophosphorus compounds are powerful inhibitors of carboxylic esterase enzymes, including acetylcholinesterase (true cholinesterase found in red cells, nervous tissue and skeletal muscle) and pseudocholinesterase (found in plasma, liver, heart, pancreas and brain). Organophosphorus compounds bind firmly to the esterase enzyme, inactivating it by phosphorylation, at the myoneural junctions and synapses of the ganglions.** A proportion of the enzyme inhibited by a single dose is restored to activity within a few hours, but some remains permanently inactivated and can only be replaced by the synthesis of new proteins. Phosphorylated acetylcholinesterase loses an alkyl group, due to which the enzyme cannot spontaneously hydrolyse and becomes permanently inactivated. They are called **cholinesterase inhibitors. Organic phosphates inhibit AChE in all parts of the body, due to which acetylcholine accumulates at the parasympathetic, sympathetic and somatic sites. This produces a syndrome of overactivity due to unhydrolysed acetylcholine with continued stimulation of local receptors and eventual paralysis of nerve or muscle.** The inactivation of cholinesterase enzymes becomes irreversible after 24 to 36 hours. **Symptoms appear in both the sympathetic and parasympathetic nervous system. Mild poisoning usually occurs when cholinesterase activity is 20 to 50% of normal; moderate poisoning occurs when activity is 10 to 20% of normal, and severe poisoning when activity is less than 10% normal.** Small repeated exposures may gradually depress the cholinesterase activity to very low levels, often resulting in minimal symptoms.

Signs and Symptoms: They are similar to those resulting from overdosage of acetylcholine, pilocarpine, physostigmine or muscarine. They have three distinct toxic actions. (1) **A muscarine-like effect which potentiates postganglionic parasympathetic activity.** (2) **Nicotine-like stimulation followed by paralysis** of postganglionic and somatic motor nerves. (3) **Central nervous system stimulation followed by depression.** They depend on the balance between stimulation of muscarinic and nicotinic receptors in the autonomic nervous system and skeletal muscle neuroreceptors. The dose received, route and rate of absorption, and other individual factors influence this balance. Onset of systemic symptoms is most rapid following inhalation, and least rapid following absorption from the skin. **Involuntary muscles and secretory glands are affected first, then voluntary muscles and finally vital brain centres. Respiratory symptoms may resemble an attack of asthma.** With massive ingestion or inhalation, symptoms may begin within five minutes, or may be delayed for half to one hour and are at a maximum in two to eight hours. **Signs and symptoms appear when the cholinesterase level drops to 30% of its normal activity.** The respiratory or gastrointestinal symptoms are more marked depending on the route of entry. Ocular exposure causes persistent miosis.

(I) Muscarinic manifestations: These symptoms can be easily remembered by the acronym **SLUDGE: Salivation, lachrymation, urination, defecation, gastrointestinal distress, and emesis.** (1) **Bronchial tree:** Bronchoconstriction, increased bronchial secretions, dyspnoea, cyanosis, pulmonary oedema. (2) **G.I.T.:** Anorexia, salivation, nausea, vomiting, cramps, diarrhoea, faecal incontinence, tenesmus. Pancreatitis may develop. (3) **Sweat glands:** Increased sweating. (4) **Salivary glands:** Increased salivation. (5) **Lacrimal glands:** Increased lacrimation. (6) **C.V.S.:** Bradycardia or tachycardia, arrhythmias, conduction blocks, hypotension. (7) **Pupils:** Miosis, occasionally unequal or dilated. (8) **Ciliary body:** Blurred vision. (9) **Bladder:** Urinary incontinence.

(II) Nicotinic manifestations: (1) **Striated muscle:** Initial stimulus results in contraction. Later there is paralysis due to persistent depolarisation. Muscle weakness is due to accumulation of acetylcholine. Muscular fasciculations, cramps, weakness, areflexia. (2) **Sympathetic ganglia:** Hypertension, tachycardia, pallor, mydriasis.

(III) CNS manifestations: Restlessness, emotional lability, headache, tremors, anxiety, drowsiness, confusion, slurred speech, ataxia, generalised weakness, coma, convulsions, depression of respiratory and cardiovascular centres.

In some cases, only muscarinic or nicotinic or CNS effects are seen, but most cases show a combination of all three. **Nicotinic effects are seen in 10 to 20% cases only.**

Mild poisoning (Cholinesterase activity 20 to 50% of normal): Signs and symptoms are: nausea, malaise, fatigue, minimal muscle weakness, cramping without diarrhoea.

Moderate poisoning (Cholinesterase activity 10 to 20% of normal): SLUDGE and/or tremors, weakness, fasciculations, confusion, lethargy, anxiety.

Severe poisoning (Cholinesterase activity less than 10% of normal): SLUDGE, and respiratory insufficiency, weakness, fasciculations, coma, paralysis, seizures, autonomic dysfunction.

Porphyrinaemia, resulting in **chromodachryorrhoea (shedding of red tears)** due to accumulation of porphyrin in the lachrymal glands is seen very rarely.

Intermediate Syndrome: In some cases after one to four days muscle weakness and paralysis characterised by motor cranial nerve palsies, weakness of neck flexor and proximal limb muscles, and acute respiratory paresis are seen due to prolonged cholinesterase inhibition and muscle necrosis. It does not respond to oximes or atropine.

Delayed Sequelae: Delayed peripheral neuropathy can occur one to 5 weeks after exposure to certain compounds, such as parathion, malathion, trichlorfon, etc. It begins with paraesthesias and pain or cramps in the calves followed by ataxia, weakness, and toe drop. It rapidly progresses to a flaccid paresis which can ascend similar to Guillain-Barre syndrome. Reflexes are diminished. The disease may progress for 2 to 3 months, and muscle wasting occurs.

Fatal Dose:

TEPP 50 mg. i.m. or 100 mg. orally.

OMPA 80 mg. i.m. or 175 mg. orally.

Parathion 80 mg. i.m. or 175 mg. orally.

HETP 60 mg. i.m. or 350 mg. orally.

Malathion and diazinon one g. orally.

Fatal Period: Death usually occurs within 24 hours in untreated cases, and within ten days in those treated cases when treatment is not successful. In non-fatal cases, the acute effects last for six to thirty hours which disappear in 2 to 3 days, but may sometimes persist for two weeks. Complete recovery occurs in ten days in patients treated early, unless hypoxic encephalopathy intervenes.

Cause of Death: Death is caused by paralysis of respiratory muscles, respiratory arrest due to failure of respiratory centre, or intense bronchoconstriction. Late death, as long as 15 days after acute ingestion may be caused by ventricular arrhythmias.

Diagnosis: (1) Five ml of heparinised blood should be collected for **cholinesterase determination.** Serum is separated and both refrigerated. Alternatively, samples can be frozen for cholinesterase. **The average normal values of cholinesterase are 77 to 142 in the red cells and 41 to 140 in the plasma. RBC cholinesterase level of less than 50% of normal indicates**

poisoning. The plasma cholinesterase is more sensitive and will fall more rapidly and before that of red cells. Thus, if there is dissociation of the two, i.e., **if the plasma is down and red cells relatively little changed, the amount of exposure is less. The plasma value will approach normal in 7 to 10 days.** In untreated cases, plasma cholinesterase levels may require 4 weeks to normalise. The cholinesterase at the motor end-plate can be demonstrated histochemically in muscles kept at room temperature for one to two days, and up to several months in the tissues stored at 4 to 6°C. Fixation of tissue with phosphate buffered formalin and cold acetone for 24 hours or the embalming of the body does not affect the cholinesterase activity at the myoneural junctions.

(2) **Diagnosis may be confirmed** by giving 2 mg. of atropine. In a normal person this causes marked atropinisation, but in a case of poisoning by organophosphorus, symptoms are relieved without atropinizing. Estimations of cholinesterase are confirmatory.

Treatment: (1) The patient is removed from the source of exposure, the contaminated clothing removed and the exposed areas are washed with soap and water, followed by ethanol and water, or some alkaline solution. If eye is contaminated irrigate the conjunctival recesses, cornea, bulbar conjunctiva, internal and external palpebral surfaces. (2) The airway should be kept patent. Tracheostomy may be required. (3) When the poison is ingested, the **stomach should be washed with 1:5,000 potassium permanganate solution.** (4) **Activated charcoal** 1 g./kg. Ipecac should not be used. A cathartic, e.g., sorbitol or magnesium citrate can be given once, unless diarrhoea has occurred. (5) **Avoid physostigmine, endorphonium chloride and succinylcholine.** (6) **Atropine sulphate arrests the muscarinic effects of postganglionic parasympathetic (peripheral) activity (muscarinic receptor antagonist) and arrests CNS effects. It has no effect on nicotinic actions.** It is ineffective on respiratory centre in the presence of severe asphyxia and also if B.P. falls, Heart rate exceeding 140 beats/min should be avoided. **2 to 4 mg. is given i.v. (paediatric dose 0.05 mg/kg.) as a test dose. If there is no effect this dose may be doubled every 10 to 15 min. until muscarinic symptoms are relieved. Atropine should be continued until the tracheobronchial tree is cleared of the secretions and most secretions are dried, but not pupillary status. The average patient requires 40 mg per day, but as much as 1000 mg/day has been used.** It can be given in continuous infusion. Tachycardia is not a contraindication. **Once signs of adequate atropinisation occur, the dose should be adjusted to maintain this effect for at least 24 hours. When cyanosis is present, maximal oxygenation should be achieved before atropine is given** for avoiding increased risk of ventricular tachyarrhythmias associated with hypoxia. (6) **Specific cholinesterase reactivators like diacetyl monoxime (DAM), or 2-pyridine aldoxime methiodide (pralidoxime iodide, 2- PAM), or pralidoxime chloride (Protopan, 2-PAM chloride) or pyridine aldoxime methane sulphonate (P2S) act by competing for the phosphate moiety of the organophosphorus compound and release it from the cholinesterase enzyme. DAM crosses the blood-brain barrier and can regenerate some of the CNS cholinesterase.** Its action is marked at nicotinic sites, often improving muscle strength within 10 to 40 min. It also decreases muscarinic and CNS symptoms. **The adult dose is one to 2 g. i.v., either as a 5% solution given over 5 min., or in 150 ml. of saline and infused over half-an-hour. This can be repeated in one hour** if muscle weakness and fasciculations are not relieved. **This dose should be repeated at 6 to 12 hours intervals for 24 to 48 hours to** ensure distribution to all affected sites. **Maximum dose should not exceed 12 g. in a 24 hour period.** Alternatively, two-and-half percent solution can be given as continuous infusion of half g./hour. If signs and symptoms of cholinergic excess persist, continued dose may be necessary until symptoms subside. **Pralidoxime and atropine work synergistically, and should be used together. Oximes reactivate inhibited cholinesterase, remove the block at neuromuscular junction, prevent formation of phosphorylated enzyme, and directly detoxify organophosphates.** They do not cross blood-brain barrier. They should be started as early as possible, although they may be beneficial when given after 24 to 36 hours of exposure. They are given until the patient is clinically well and not requiring atropine. **Pralidoxime decreases the amount of atropine required and also potentiates the action of atropine.** Oximes are ineffective or minimally effective for: dimefox, dimethoate, ciodrin, methyl diazinon, methyl phenocapton, phorate, schradan and wepsyn. (7) **Obidoxime chloride is more potent, but its toxicity is slightly greater.** Dose: 250 mg. i.v. or i.m. It can be given if oximes are not available. (8) HI-6 and H10-7 appear to have activity against all known organophosphates. (9) Convulsions can be controlled with i.v. diazepam 10 to 20 mg. at a rate of 0.5 ml (5 mg. per minute), repeated if necessary after 30 to 60 minutes. This may be followed by i.v. infusion to a maximum of 3 mg/kg. of body weight over 24 hours. If convulsions persist, use i.v. phenobarbital 10 to 20 mg/kg body wt. or i.v. phenytoin 18 mg/kg. For status epilepticus, general anaesthesia may be used. **Diazepam decreases anxiety and counteracts some aspects of CNS toxicity which are not affected by atropine.** (10) Pulmonary oedema and bronchospasm should be treated with oxygen, intubation, atropine and positive pressure ventilation. (11) Antibiotics to prevent pulmonary infections.

Prophylaxis: The precautions to be taken are: (1) Protective clothing consisting of overall of white cotton, a white cloth hood to cover the head and neck, rubber apron, gloves and boots, eye-shields and respirator. (2) The face and the hands should be thoroughly washed after spraying with soap water or he should take a bath on the farm itself. (3) **Not more than 2 hours spraying a day should be done by a worker, and he should not work for more than 6 successive days on spraying.** A person suffering from cold, bronchitis, etc. should not be engaged in spraying operation. (4) The workers should be properly instructed and their work supervised. (5) The workers should not smoke, chew or drink in the spraying area. (6) Spraying machines, tanks, containers, hoses, etc. should be thoroughly washed at the end of the work and before repairs are carried out. (7) Stop spraying immediately if you get a rash or feel sick, if your eyesight troubles you or you begin to sweat more than usual or feel unusually thirsty or have a headache.

Postmortem Appearances: Signs of asphyxia are found. The face is congested and there is cyanosis of the lips, fingers and nose. Bloodstained froth is seen at the mouth and nose. The stomach contents may smell of kerosene. The mucosa of the stomach is congested with submucous petechial haemorrhages. Respiratory passages are congested and contain frothy haemorrhagic exudate. The lungs show gross congestion, excessive oedema and subpleural petechiae. Heart is sometimes soft and flabby. The internal organs are congested. The brain is congested and oedematous; meninges are congested. Petechial haemorrhages are present. The cholinesterase in erythrocytes and at myoneural junctions is below normal. **Organophosphorus can be detected in putrefied bodies.**

Chronic Poisoning: It is seen in persons engaged in pesticide spraying of crops, due to inhalation or skin contamination. Symptoms include weakness, anxiety, gait disorders, muscle cramps, paraesthesias, drowsiness, confusion, irritability and psychiatric manifestations.

Risk Groups: Certain groups of people are at risk. (1) Those who are engaged in the manufacture and packing of the compounds. (2) Those who use these compounds as sprays or dusts in the open as insecticides. (3) Children of users. (4) Research workers. (5) Suicide is very common. (6) Homicide is rare.

Hazards to consumers of sprayed crops appear to be very slight as they rapidly breakdown into non-toxic substances. Poisoning usually occurs from cutaneous absorption, ingestion or inhalation.

CASE: (1) In one case, one drop of parathion fell on the skin of forearm, which was not washed for two minutes, caused death.

(2) A child of nine weeks died after having been given deliberately two drops of parathion (Seifert, 1954).

CHEMICAL TEST: In parathion poisoning, P-nitrophenol is excreted in the urine. Sodium hydroxide added to steam distillate of urine gives a strong yellow colour.

CARBAMATES

They are derivatives of carbonic acid. They are marketed in the form of dusts or solutions, such as aldicarb (Temix), aminocarb (Matacil), aprocarb (Baygon), carbaryl (Sevin), carbofuran (Furaxdan). Absorption occurs through all routes. Carbaryl, carbofuran, methomyl (Lannate) and propoxur are highly toxic. Aldicarb, carbendezim and triallate are moderately toxic. **They are also anticholinergic and inhibit carboxylic esterase enzymes by carbamylation.**

Signs and Symptoms: Symptoms begin in 15 minutes to 2 hours. Carbamates differ toxicologically from organophosphates: (1) **They will spontaneously hydrolyse from the cholinesterase enzymatic site within 24 to 48 hours, whereas organophosphates will not.** (2) **They do not effectively penetrate into the CNS, and as such CNS toxicity is limited. All other clinical manifestations are similar to organophosphates.**

Fatal dose: 3 to 6 g.

Treatment: Atropine is the specific antidote. Pralidoxime may diminish the severity of symptoms and help prevent some morbidity. It improves respiratory functions and patient's well-being.

ORGANOCHLORINES

Classification: The organochlorine (chlorinated hydrocarbons) can be divided into four categories: (1) DDT and analogues: DDT, methoxychlor. (2) Benzene hexachloride: gamma hexachlorobenzene (Lindane). (3) Cyclodienes and related compounds: aldrin, chlordane, chlordecone, dieldrin, endosulfan, endrin, hepatachlor, isobenan, mirex. (4) Toxaphene and related compounds. **All of these pesticides are absorbed through skin, orally and via inhalation.** DDT is the least well absorbed. These agents are highly lipid soluble. They are partially metabolised in the liver and directly excreted in the urine, faeces and milk.

Action: They interfere with nerve impulse transmission. CNS is first stimulated and then depressed.

Fatal Dose: DDT; 30 g.; gammexane 15 g. Lindane 15 g; chlordane 30 g.

ENDRIN

Endrin is a polycyclic, polychlorinated hydrocarbon belongs to the group of cyclodiene insecticides. It is a stereoisomer of dieldrin. It is soluble in aromatic hydrocarbons and ketones, sparingly in alcohols, but is not soluble in water. Its taste is bitter. It melts at 245°C. It is also called **"plant penicillin"**, because of its broad spectrum of activity against various insect pests. It is sold in the market under the trade names of Endrin-We-16, Endox-DB 50, Endtox EC-20, Endrex, Tafdrin, etc. These products contain about 20 to 50% of endrin mixed with petroleum hydrocarbon, such as aromax, which smells like kerosene. It is commonly used as sprays or as dusts, diluted with inert clays. Endrin is rapidly metabolised and eliminated and does not persist in body tissues.

Symptoms: These begin within 1 to 6 hours. They are salivation, nausea, vomiting, abdominal pain, rarely diarrhoea, hoarseness of voice, coughing, froth at the mouth and nose, dyspnoea, headache, giddiness, restlessness, hyperirritability, dilated pupils, incoordination, ataxia, mental confusion, tremors, tonic and clonic convulsions, coma and death due to respiratory failure. In non-fatal cases, most of the persons feel well after twenty-four hours.

Chronic Poisoning: Long term exposure to some of these compounds results in cumulative toxicity characterised by loss of weight, weakness, ataxia, tremors, mental changes, oligospermia and increased tendency to leukaemias, purpura, aplastic anaemia and liver cancer.

Fatal Dose: 5 to 6 g. By ingestion it is 3 times as toxic as aldrin, dieldrin and 10 times as toxic as DDT.

Fatal Period: One to several hours.

Postmortem Appearances: The mouth and stomach contents smell of kerosene. Signs of asphyxia are present. Endrin resists putrefaction and can be detected in the viscera quite some time after death.

Treatment: (1) Clothing should be removed and skin washed with soap and water. (2) Gastric lavage, or the stomach evacuated by emetics and cathartics. (3) Give activated charcoal. (4) **Cholestyramine is a non-absorbable bile acid binding anion exchange resin, which increases the faecal excretion of organochlorines.** It is given 16 g. per day in divided doses for several days. (5) **There is no specific antidote.** (6) Maintain and assure adequate airway, breathing and circulation. (7) If the mental state is altered give dextrose, naloxone and thiamine. (8) Control convulsions with diazepam followed by phenobarbital. If necessary general anaesthesia is given. (9) Calcium gluconate is useful.

Circumstances of Poisoning: Human poisoning occurs from occupational or accidental exposure to endrin. Suicide is very common. Homicide is rare, but it is sometimes given mixed with food or sweets, or alcohol is used to conceal the smell. Accidental deaths are very rare.

CHLOROPHENOXYACETATES: They are plant harmone used as weed-killers. They include 2, 4, -D, MCPA, mecoprop, dichloroprop (DCPP), 2, 4, 5-T. They irritate skin, mouth, GIT and damage muscles, nerves and brain. They are absorbed through skin, lungs and GIT.

SYMPTOMS: Symptoms include: redness and irritation of skin and eyes, burning in mouth, coughing and choking, pain in abdomen, vomiting, diarrhoea, confusion, muscle weakness, twitchings, hypotension, fast breathing, convulsions, coma and death in few hours. If patient survives for more than a few hours, liver and kidney damage occurs.

TREATMENT: Symptomatic.

CHLORATE

It is used as a weedkiller, in match heads and in fireworks. Sodium salt (resembles table sugar) is more toxic than potassium salt. Fatal dose is about 20 to 30 g. It is a powerful oxidising agent, and it attacks all body cells. It reacts with thiol groups on red cells and may cause it to lyse. It oxidises haemoglobin to methaemoglobin. It is also a potent nephrotoxin. Haemolysis may liberate large quantities of potassium ion making the serum level sufficiently high to reach fatal levels.

SYMPTOMS: They develop 1 to 4 hours after ingestion. They include: nausea, vomiting, diarrhoea, abdominal pain, shallow breathing, blood, protein and haemoglobin in urine, oliguria or anuria and renal failure, haemolysis, jaundice and hepatic failure, methaemoglobinaemia which may reach 40% or more, agitation, generalised weakness, muscular twitchings or convulsions, and death due to renal failure. On skin and eyes, it causes irritation, redness, burns and ulcers.

TREATMENT: (1) Stomach wash. (2) Methylene blue 25 ml. 1% sol. i.v. (3) Sodium thiosulphate 2 to 5 g. in 200 ml. of 5% sodium bicarbonate as a drink. (4) Ascorbic acid 1 g. every 4 hours as a drink or by slow i.v. injection. (5) Peritoneal dialysis or haemodialysis. (6) Symptomatic.

PARAQUAT

It is a bipyridylium compound and used as herbicide and weed-killer. It is sprayed on weeds before planting crops. It is inactivated when in contact with soil. It is produced commercially as a brownish concentrated liquid of the dichloride salt in 10 to 30% strength, under the trade name, 'Gramoxone' and for horticultural use, as brown granules called "Weedol" at about 5% strength. Deaths occur due to ingestion. Deaths by inhalation while spraying are very rare.

ACTION: Paraquat undergoes a NADPH (nicotinamide adenine dinucleotide phosphate) dependent reduction to form the free radical, which reacts with molecular oxygen to reform the cation and produce a superoxide free radical and hydroxyl radical (OH), which disrupt cellular function, structure and cell death. Concentrated solutions corrode G.I. mucosa.

ABSORPTION AND EXCRETION: Absorption is mainly through GI tract and occurs through inhalation, skin or eye contact is minimal. 5 to 10% of the dose is absorbed, and the rest is excreted in the faeces. It is distributed to all the organs, but the highest concentrations are found in the kidneys and the lungs, followed by muscles from which paraquat can redistribute back into the circulation as plasma concentration decreases. More than 90% of the absorbed paraquat is excreted unchanged in the urine within the first 24 hours but can be detected in urine up to three weeks after ingestion.

FATAL DOSE: 10 to 5 g.

FATAL PERIOD: 2 to 5 days.

SIGNS AND SYMPTOMS: Doses of less than 1.5 g. produce transient vomiting and diarrhoea which resolve within days. Ingestion of more than 50 mg/kg kill within 72 hours. LOCAL: Irritation and inflammation of skin, nails, cornea, conjunctivae and nasal mucosa. G.I.T.: Oropharyngeal ulceration and corrosion, nausea, vomiting, haematemesis, diarrhoea; painful mucosal ulceration, dysphagia, aphonia, perforation of oesophagus, mediastinitis and pneumothorax. KIDNEYS: Oliguria or non-oliguric renal failure due to acute tubular necrosis; proximal tubular dysfunction. LUNGS: Cough, haemoptysis, dyspnoea due to pulmonary oedema, haemorrhage or fibrosis. PANCREAS: Pancreatitis. LIVER: Centrilobular hepatic necrosis and cholestasis. C.V.S.: Hypovolaemia, shock, arrhythmias. C.N.S.: Late coma, convulsions, cerebral oedema. ADRENAL: Insufficiency due to necrosis. BONE MARROW: early; Polymorphonuclear leucocytosis; late: anaemia.

CAUSE OF DEATH: Death occurs from multi-organ failure or corrosive effects in the G.I. tract. Death from oesophageal perforation and mediastinitis can occur within 2 to 3 days of ingestion. In ingestions of less than 3 g. death occurs from 5 days to several weeks.

TREATMENT: (1) Gastric lavage may be beneficial if done within one hour of exposure. Emetics are contraindicated. (2) One litre of a 15 to 30% aqueous suspension of Fuller's earth or 7% bentonite are given to adsorb paraquat, followed by 200 ml. of 20% mannitol. If the adsorbent has not appeared in the stool within 6 hours of its administration, the dose of the cathartic should be repeated. (3) If the above adsorbents are not available, activated charcoal (1 to 2 g. /kg) can be given. (4) **Haemodialysis and haemoperfusion** is useful if done within 12 hours of ingestion. (5) Avoid oxygen therapy. (6) Remove all clothing and wash the patient thoroughly with soap and water. (7) Analgesics should be given for pain.

POSTMORTEM APPEARANCES: There may be ulceration around the lips and mouth. The mucosa of mouth may be reddened. Oesophagus may contain casts of shed epithelium. The stomach may show erosions and patchy haemorrhages or may be normal. The kidneys may show cortical pallor and diffuse tubular damage. If rapid death from acute hepatorenal failure does not occur, then progressive lung damage may cause death within the next two weeks. A hyaline is often seen. Diffuse pulmonary oedema and haemorrhages occur. Within a few days repair begins. Within the first week, the air spaces become occluded by mononuclear cells forming rounded-up fibroblasts. If patient continues to survive, the alveoli begin to fibrose, with reticulin and collagen being laid down to form a rigid, stiff lung. The lungs may be mistaken for a diffuse pneumonia. There may be a fibrinous pleurisy and sometimes slight bloody pleural effusion. The liver may show pallor, mottled fatty change and centrilobular necrosis.

PYRETHRINS AND PYRETHROIDS

Pyrethrins are extracted from crysanthemum plant. Pyrethroids are synthetic analogues. Toxicity is very low due to their rapid metabolism. They are used as insect repellents, insecticides and pesticides. They are available as sprays, dusts, powders, mats and coils. Pyrethrum, allethrin, D-allethrin, permethrin, deltamethrin, decamethrin, cypermethrin, fenvalerate, flavalinate are some of the examples.

ACTION: They prolong the inactivation of the sodium channel by binding to it in the open state.

FATAL DOSE: 1 gm/kg. body weight.

SIGNS AND SYMPTOMS: Skin contact causes dermatitis and blistering. Paraesthesias, nausea, vomiting, vertigo, fasciculations, hyperthermia, altered mental state, convulsions, pulmonary oedema and coma. Inhalation causes rhinorrhoea, sore throat, wheezing, and dyspnoea.

TREATMENT: (1) Stomach wash with activated charcoal. (2) Oils and fats should be avoided. (3) Atropine and oximes are contraindicated. (4) Skin should be washed with soap and water. (5) Give adrenaline 0.5 to 1 ml. of 1:1000, i.m. for allergic reactions. Antihistamines such as chlorphenamine or pyromethazine by slow i.v. injection after adrenaline injection.

DINITRO COMPOUNDS

Dinitro-orthocresol and dinitrophenol are commonly used weed-killers. They are also used to kill insects and fungi and to preserve wood. They act by greatly increasing the cellular metabolism of any cell with which they come in contact. They are absorbed orally, through the skin, and respiratory tract. Inhalation and ingestion may occur during spraying of crops. Fatal dose one to 2 g. and fatal period 4 to 15 days.

SYMPTOMS: They appear rapidly and resemble a thyrotoxic crisis. CONTACT: Yellow colour of the skin and hair and rashes. Burns of lips and buccal mucosa. CNS: Anxiety, restlessness, tiredness, insomnia, convulsions, coma. C.V.S: Tachycardia and arrhythmias. R.S.: Tachypnoea and pulmonary congestion. METABOLIC: Hyperpyrexia and intense perspiration. RENAL: Acute renal failure. HEPATIC: Acute liver necrosis. EYES: Severe irritation, redness, watering.

TREATMENT: Symptomatic.

FLUORIDES

USES: Sodium fluoride is used in rat poison and cockroach powders. Sodium silicofluoride, fluoroacetamide and fluoroacetate are used as rodenticides.

ACTION: Fluoride compounds react with acid in the stomach and form hydrofluoric acid which is corrosive. After absorption, fluoride ions bind calcium ions and to some extent potassium and magnesium ions and cause hypocalcaemia, hypokalaemia and hypomagnesaemia. Fluoride ions also inactivate proteolytic and glycolytic enzymes and act as general protoplasmic poison.

FATAL DOSE: 5 mg/kg. body weight.

SIGNS AND SYMPTOMS: Ingestion causes burning pain in the mouth and epigastrium, thirst, salivation, vomiting, diarrhoea, haematemesis and haematuria, coma and convulsions. Death may occur within minutes from respiratory and cardiac failure.

TREATMENT: (1) Calcium orally and intravenously. (2) Stomach wash with lime water or milk.

ALUMINIUM PHOSPHIDE

Uses: Aluminium phosphide (ALP) is a solid fumigant pesticide, insecticide and rodenticide. It is widely used as grain preservative. Phosphite and hypophosphite of aluminium which are non-toxic residues are left in the grains. In India it is available as white tablets of Celphos, Alphos, Quickphos, Phostoxin, Phosphotex, etc., each weighing 3 g. and has the capacity to liberate one gram of phosphine (PH_3). ALP has garlicky odour.

Action: On coming in contact with moisture ALP liberates phosphine. **Phosphine inhibits respiratory chain enzymes and has cytotoxic action.** It acts by inhibiting the electron transport resulting from preferential inhibition of cytochrome oxidase. **Phosphine is a systemic poison and affects all organs of the body.** The chemical reaction is accelerated by the presence of HCL in the stomach.

Absorption and Excretion: Phosphine is rapidly absorbed from the GI tract by simple diffusion and causes damage to the internal organs. **It is also rapidly absorbed from the lungs after inhalation.** After ingestion, some ALP is also absorbed and is metabolised in the liver, where phosphine is slowly released accounting for the prolongation of symptoms. Phosphine is oxidised slowly to oxyacids and excreted in the urine as hypophosphite. It is also excreted in unchanged form through the lungs.

Fatal Dose: 1 to 3 g.; 1 to 3 tablets. 1 to 2 g. Inhalation of phosphine at a concentration of 400 to 600 ppm is fatal within one hour.

Fatal Period: 6–12 hours. Majority die within twenty-four hours.

Signs and Symptoms: They depend on the dose and severity of poisoning.

Inhalation: Mild inhalation exposure produces irritation of mucous membranes and acute respiratory distress. Other symptoms are: dizziness, fatigue, tightness in the chest, nausea, vomiting, diarrhoea and headache. Moderate toxicity produces ataxia, numbness, paraesthesia, tremors, diplopia, jaundice, muscular weakness, incoordination and paralysis. Concentration of PH_3 in air higher than 0.3 ppm causes severe illness. Severe toxicity produces adult respiratory distress syndrome, cardiac arrhythmias, congestive heart failure, pulmonary oedema, convulsions, and coma.

Ingestion: Mild intoxication produces nausea, vomiting, headache and abdominal pain, and the patients usually recover.

In moderate and severe poisoning, systemic manifestations are early and progressive and mostly fatal. **G.I.T.:** Nausea, vomiting, diarrhoea, retrosternal pain. **C.V.S.:** Hypotension, shock, arrhythmias, myocarditis, pericarditis, acute congestive heart failure. **R.S.:** Cough, dyspnoea, cyanosis, pulmonary oedema, respiratory failure. **Hepatic:** Jaundice, hepatitis, hepatomegaly, **Renal:** Renal failure. **C.N.S.:** Headache, dizziness, altered mental state, restlessness, convulsions, acute hypoxic encephalopathy, coma. **Rare**: Muscle wasting and tenderness and bleeding diathesis, due to widespread capillary damage. Cardiogenic shock is the most common cause of death. Complications include pericarditis, acute congestive cardiac failure, acute massive gastrointestinal bleeding and ARDS. Mortality is high, 35 to 100%.

Treatment: (1) Gastric lavage with potassium permanganate is done after endotracheal intubation as it oxidizes phosphene to non-toxic phosphate and repeated 2 or 3 times. (2) **Give activated charcoal 100 g. orally mixed with sorbitol (not water) using 240 ml for every 30 g. to adsorb phosphine.** (3) Antacids reduce symptoms pertaining to the stomach and reduce absorption of phosphine. (4) **Liquid paraffin** is given for excretion of ALP and phosphine from the gut. (5) **There is no specific antidote.** (6) **Magnesium sulphate reduces organ toxicity, corrects hypomagnesaemia and arrhythmias.** The usual dose is one g. repeated for the next two hours, and then 1 to 1.5 g. every 6 hours for 5 to 7 days in the form of continuous i.v. infusion. (7) To treat shock 4 to 6 litres of fluids are to be administered during the first 3 to 6 hours; of this 50% must be normal saline. (8) **Low dose dopamine infusion, 4 to 6 microgram/kg/min is useful.** (9) **I.V. hydrocortisone 400 mg**

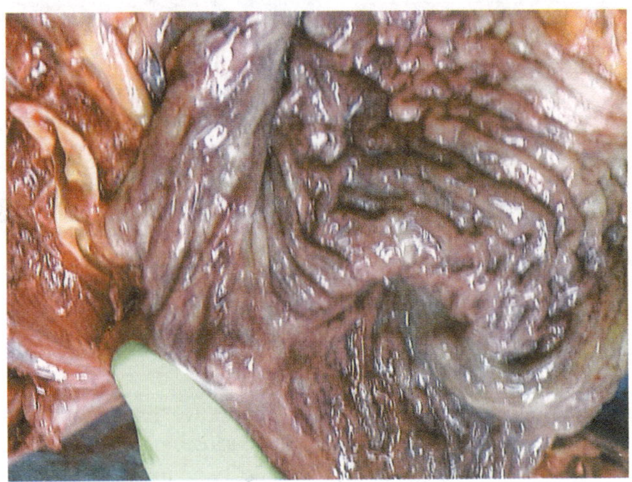

Fig. (25–1). Stomach in aluminium phosphide poisoning C.

Courtesy: Dr Manoj Kumar, Professor and Head, AIIMS, Patna, India.

every 4 to 6 hours is highly effective. It reduces the dose of dopamine. (10) Hypoxia is treated with oxygen. (11) Shock should be treated with fluids and hydrocortisone. (12) Metabolic acidosis should be corrected with i.v. sodium carbonate. Peritoneal or haemodialysis is useful.

Postmortem Appearances: Garlic-like odour is present at the mouth and nostrils and in the gastric contents. Blood-stained froth is found in the mouth and nostrils. Mucous membrane of the lower part of oesophagus, stomach and duodenum are congested. Decreasing congestion of the G.I. tract is seen in the small intestine Fig. (25–1). The lungs, liver, spleen, kidneys and brain are congested. Centrizonal haemorrhagic necrosis of the liver may be seen.

HISTOPATHOLOGY: (1) Stomach: Congestion, oedema, leucocytic infiltration, sloughing of gastric mucosa. (2) Lungs: Congestion, oedema, desquamation of respiratory epithelium, thickened alveoli, lymphocytic infiltration. Kidneys: Congestion, necrosis, tubular degeneration and regeneration. Adrenals: Congestion, haemorrhage, necrosis, area of lipid depletion in cortex. Heart: Congestion, oedema, fragmentation of fibres, focal necrosis, leucocytic infiltration. Brain: Congestion, oedema.

CHEMICAL TEST: (1) 5 ml. of gastric aspirate and 15 ml. of water are put in a flask and the mouth is covered with a filter paper impregnated with silver nitrate (0.1N). The flask is heated at 50°C for 15 to 20 minutes. If phosphine is present, the filter paper turns black. (2) A piece of filter paper impregnated with 0.1 N silver nitrate solution is used in the form of a mask through which the patient breathes for 5 to 10 minutes. The filter paper turns black, if phosphine is present. (3) The filter paper impregnated with $AgNO_3$ (0.1N) is used in the form of face mask and the patient is asked to breathe in and out of this filter paper for 15 to 20 minutes. Presence of PH_3 is indicated by the blackening of filter paper. In breath, the test is positive only in patients who have ingested more than 6 g. of ALP.

Poisoning is usually suicidal, occasionally accidental and rarely homicidal.

ZINC PHOSPHIDE

It is a steel-grey crystalline powder with a garlicky or fishy odour. Symptoms are similar to those of aluminium phosphide, but are usually slower to start because of the slow release of phosphine.

It is used to preserve grain and as rat poison. Some patients die due to pulmonary oedema within a few hours; most patients die within 30 hours of exposure, secondary to cardiovascular collapse due to a direct myocardial toxic effect.

FATAL DOSE: 2 to 5 g.

FATAL PERIOD: 24 hours.

TREATMENT: (1) Move patient to fresh air if there are poisonous gases or fumes. (2) Stomach wash followed by instillation of milk, starch or lavage with 3 to 5% of sodium bicarbonate to neutralise gastric acid. (3) Activated charcoal. (4) Purgatives.

POSTMORTEM APPEARANCES: Garlicky odour in stomach contents. Blood is cherry-red. Congestion and oedema of the lungs. Fatty degeneration and necrosis of the liver.

CHAPTER

26 CORROSIVE POISONS

FM 9.1: Describe general principles and basic methodologies in treatment of poisoning: decontamination, supportive therapy, antidote therapy, procedures of enhanced elimination with regard to: caustics inorganic—sulphuric, nitric, and hydrochloric acids; organic— carboloic acid (phenol), oxalic and acetylsalicylic acids.

Action: A corrosive poison **fixes, destroys and erodes the surface with which it comes in contact.** They act by extracting water from the tissues, and coagulate cellular proteins, and convert haemoglobin into haematin.

MINERAL ACIDS

ACTION: An exothermic reaction occurs when strong mineral acids, e.g. sulphuric acid comes into contact with moist skin. The heat together with corrosion causes coagulation necrosis. This crust may prevent further penetration of acid to deeper layers, but the acid can be absorbed resulting in systemic acidosis, haemolysis and decreased cardiac output. Damage is primarily superficial, which may result in sloughing of extensive areas of the lining of stomach and perforation, which may result in mediastinitis, sepsis, shock and death. Acids cause greatest damage to the stomach and pylorus. The oropharynx and oesophagus usually have minimal involvement. The hydrogen ions from the acid are neutralised fairly quickly and deep penetrating tissue destruction does not occur. Hydrofluoric acid causes liquefaction necrosis. They have no remote action. They act as irritants when slightly diluted, but as stimulants when well diluted. No trace of acid may be found if the victim survives for two days or more.

Corrosive mineral acids and alkalis are identified only in the gastrointestinal content.

SULPHURIC ACID

Characteristics: Pure sulphuric acid (oil of vitriol; H_2SO_4) is a heavy, odourless, colourless, non-fuming, hygroscopic, oily liquid, and has tendency to carbonise organic substances. Commercial sulphuric acid is usually brown or dark in colour. **It causes superficial burns after only one second of contact, and full thickness burns after 30 seconds.**

Signs and Symptoms: The lips are usually swollen and excoriated and brown or black streaks may be found extending from the angles of the mouth to the sides of the chin, and sometimes to the front of the neck due to flow of the acid. **There is corrosion of mucous membranes of mouth, throat and oesophagus,** immediate burning pain, stridor, drooling, odynophagia and dysphagia. Epigastric pain soon spreads all over the abdomen and thorax. **Pharyngeal pain is the most common presenting symptom.** Eructation, nausea and vomiting occur. The vomit is brown or black, mucoid, strongly acid, and may contain shreds of the charred wall of the stomach. Thirst is intense, but any attempt to drink causes vomiting. **Circulatory collapse may cause immediate death or may result from asphyxia due to oedema of the glottis. Teeth are chalky-white. Tongue becomes swollen, sodden and black.** The abdomen becomes distended and very tender. Constipation is severe, and there is tenesmus. The **voice becomes hoarse and husky.** The eyes are sunken and the pupils usually dilated. **The mind remains clear till death. If person recovers, late oesophageal, gastric and pyloric strictures and stenoses may develop.** Permanent scars may also appear in the skin and oropharynx.

Fatal Dose: 10 to 15 ml.

Fatal Period: 12 to 24 hours.

Cause of Death: (1) Circulatory collapse. (2) Spasm or oedema of glottis. (3) Collapse due to perforation of stomach. (4) Toxaemia. (5) Delayed death may occur due to hypostatic pneumonia, secondary infection, renal failure, or starvation due to stricture of oesophagus.

Complications: (A) Acute: (1) Upper airway obstruction and injury. (2) G.I. haemorrhage. (3) Oesophageal and gastric perforation. (4) Sepsis. (5) Tracheobronchial necrosis, atelectasis and obstructive lung injury. **(B) Chronic:** (1) Oesophageal obstruction. (2) Pyloric stenosis. (3) Vocal cord paralysis with airway obstruction.

Treatment: (1) Avoid gastric lavage or emetics. (2) **The acid should be immediately diluted and neutralised *in situ* by giving one-fourth litre of water or milk or milk of magnesia or lime water or soap suds or aluminium hydroxide gel, if the patient is seen within 30 minutes of ingestion. Alkaline carbonates and bicarbonates, which liberate carbon dioxide should not be used,** as they cause gastric distension and sometimes rupture. (3) Give a **demulcent:** olive oil, milk, egg-whites, starch water, mineral oil, melted butter. (4) Prednisolone 60 mg./day may be given in divided doses to prevent oesophageal stricture and for shock. It is generally not recommended due to increased risk of perforation. Later on 4 cm. diameter mercury-filled bougie should be passed daily if stricture develops. (5) In the first 24 to 48 hours of ingestion, the use of flexible fibre optic endoscopy is recommended to assess the extent of damage to oesophagus and stomach. If there are circumferential second or third degree burns, an exploratory laparotomy should be performed. If gastric necrosis is present, oesophagogastrectomy may have to be done.

(6) Tracheostomy, if there is oedema of glottis. (7) Give nothing by mouth. Nutrient substances are given by intravenous route for about a week. Then try liquids, soft food, and finally a regular diet. (8) Skin burns are washed with large amounts of water and a paste of magnesium oxide or sodium bicarbonate is applied. (9) Eye burns are irrigated with water or sodium bicarbonate solution for 10 to 15 minutes. A suspended i.v. bag that administers low pressure irrigation is ideal. (10) Symptomatic.

Postmortem Appearances: External: They depend on the quantity and strength of the acid used, and the time that the patient survives after taking the acid. Corrosion of mucous membranes of lips, mouth and throat, and of the skin over the chin, angles of the mouth, and hands is seen. **The necrotic areas are at first grayish-white, but soon become brown or black and leathery.** The clothing should be examined for burns and stains.

Internal: Internal changes are limited to the upper digestive tract, and the respiratory system. The upper digestive tract is inflamed and swollen by oedema and severe interstitial haemorrhage, even when corrosion is absent. When the acid is taken from a spoon, lips and mouth escape injury. **In acid burns, the squamous epithelium of the oesophagus is usually relatively resistant and superficial mucosal reaction is produced. Acids have their major effects on columnar epithelium of the stomach,** leading to superficial erosion and coagulation with eschar formation. Perforation of the oesophagus is rare. **The greater part of stomach may be converted into a soft, spongy, black mass which readily disintegrates when touched Fig. (26–1).** Sometimes, only the pyloric region is involved, because fluid pathway from oesophagus occurs usually along lesser curvature to the pylorus. Initial exposure of the pylorus to acid causes severe spasm, which promotes injury at this site. The mucosal ridges are more damaged than the intervening furrows. **In the damaged area, the mucosa or even the whole thickness of the stomach wall has a brown or black colour. The stomach contains altered blood from damaged mucosa and is dark brown or black from acid haematin and the wall is studded with acute erosions. Calcium oxalate crystals may be seen in the stomach contents or in scrapings from mucosa. Perforation may occur with the escape of gastric contents into the peritoneal cavity,** and if the patient lives for few hours, chemical peritonitis and corrosion of organs is seen. **Perforation of diaphragm may occur.** The duodenum may show similar but less intense changes, and the small intestine may show signs of irritation. **In many cases, little or no free acid can be found in the viscera, because the acid is converted to substances normally present in the body** especially if the victim has survived for 2 days or more. Corrosion or severe inflammation of the larynx and trachea may be present. Secondary toxic swelling of the liver and kidney is seen if person survives longer. Renal tubules show necrosis, primarily in proximal convoluted tubules.

Time course of injury: (1) Acute inflammatory stage occurs during first 4 to 7 days. Perforation and acidosis may occur at this early stage. (2) Granulation stage occurs between 4 to 7 days. (3) **Perforation most often occurs between 7 to 21 days,** because during this period the tissue is the weakest. (4) Cicatrisation stage starts at 3 weeks and may persist for years. Over-production of scar tissue results in stricture formation.

TESTS: For mineral acids or alkalis, the only material suitable for analysis is that found in the stomach. (1) Strong acid chars organic matter. (2) Barium nitrate or chloride solution produce a white precipitate of barium sulphate.

The Circumstances of Poisoning: Accidental poisoning results due to mistaking it for glycerine or castor oil or from inhalation of vapour in chemical factories. (1) Most cases are suicidal. (2) It is not used for homicide, because of its acid taste, almost immediate local action, and the physical changes which it produces in the food. (3) It is taken internally or injected into vagina as abortifacient.

VITRIOLAGE (vitriol throwing): **Throwing of sulphuric acid on another individual** is **known as vitriolage Fig. (26–2).** Jealous or disgruntled persons may throw a corrosive to disfigure and harm their enemies. **The burns are painless. They are penetrating burns** and the acid devitalises the tissues and predispose to infection. Repair is slow and the scar tissue causes contracture. Blindness may occur if the eyes are involved. **Death may result from shock or toxaemia, if extensive area is involved.** Sometimes, nitric acid, carbolic acid, corrosive alkali or juice of marking nut or calotropis is used to disfigure the face.

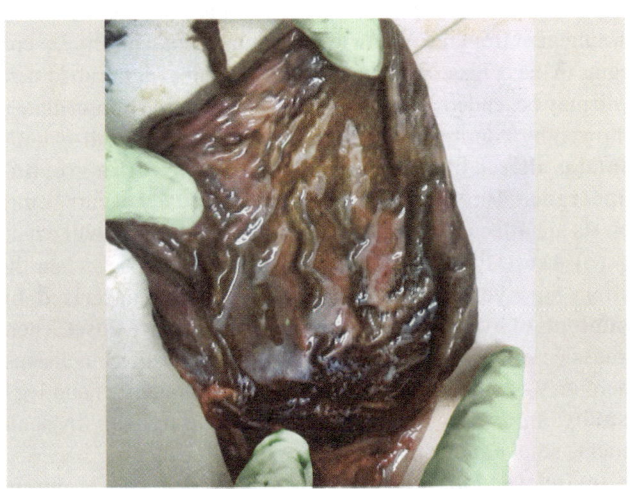

Fig. (26–1). Stomach in sulphuric acid poisoning.

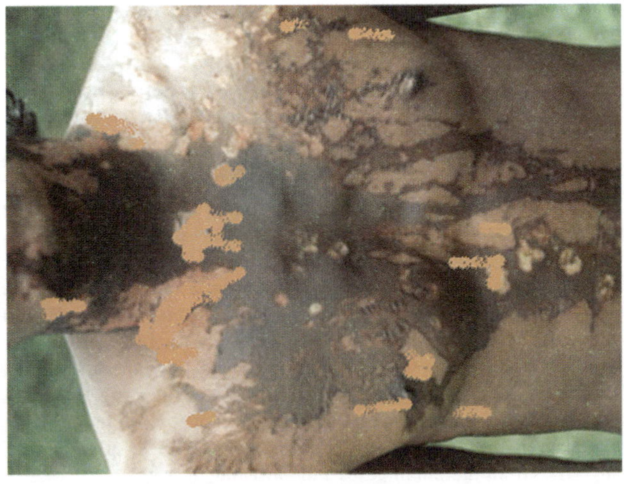

Fig. (26–2). Vitriolage.

Treatment: Wash the affected parts with plenty of water and soap or sodium or potassium carbonate. **Later, a thick paste of magnesium oxide or carbonate is applied.** The eyes are washed with water and irrigated with a dilute sodium bicarbonate solution. Later, a few drops of olive oil or castor oil are instilled into the eyes.

S.326, A.I.P.C: Causing permanent or partial damage by throwing or administering acid with intention and knowledge that it is likely to cause injury or hurt will be punished with imprisonment of not less than 10 years of life and fine. The fine should be given to person on whom the acid was thrown.

S.326, B.I.P.C: Person throwing acid or attempt to throw acid (any corrosive substance) which causes damage shall be punished with imprisonment for 5 to 7 years and also fine.

NITRIC ACID (HNO_3)

Nitric acid (aqua fortis; red spirit of nitre) is a clear, colourless, fuming, heavy liquid, and has a peculiar and choking odour. **In concentrated form it combines with organic matter and produces an yellow discolouration of tissue due to the production of picric acid (xanthoproteic reaction).**

Signs and Symptoms: They are those of poisoning by sulphuric acid. There is more eructation and greater abdominal distention owing to gas formation. **It causes yellow discolouration of the tissues,** including the crowns of the teeth and yellow stains on the clothing. Inhalation of fumes causes lachrymation, photophobia, irritation of air-passages and lungs producing sneezing, coughing, dyspnoea and asphyxia. **Colour of urine is brown.**

Fatal Dose: 10 to 15 ml.

Fatal Period: 12 to 24 hours.

TREATMENT: Same as for sulphuric acid.

Postmortem Appearances: They are those of sulphuric acid, but the tissues are stained yellow. In the oesophagus and stomach, corrosion of mucous membrane may not be accompanied by yellow discolouration, which may appear brown or brown-black due to acid haematin. **The stomach wall is soft, friable and ulcerated.** Perforation of the stomach is not common but extensive areas of the mucosa of the stomach or oesophagus are sometimes detached.

In death from inhalation of fumes, the larynx, trachea, and bronchial tubes are congested and lungs are oedematous.

TEST: The test is for the presence of nitrates. If strong ferrous sulphate solution and sulphuric acid are added to a solution containing nitric acid, a brown ring is formed at the junction of the two fluids.

THE CIRCUMSTANCES OF POISONING: Most cases of poisoning are the result of an accident or suicide. Homicide by this acid is rare.

HYDROCHLORIC ACID (HCL)

Hydrochloric acid (muriatic acid) is pungent, colourless, fuming liquid. It is a natural constituent of the fluid of the stomach and bowels.

Signs and Symptoms: It is less corrosive in its action than sulphuric acid. It does not usually corrode or seriously damage the skin, but it readily destroys mucous membrane. The mucous membrane is at first grey or grey-white, and later becomes brown or black, due to the production of acid haematin. Inhalation of fumes causes intense irritation of throat and lungs with symptoms of suffocation, coughing, dyspnoea and cyanosis. Constant exposure to fumes produces chronic poisoning characterised by coryza, conjunctivitis, corneal ulcer, pharyngitis, bronchitis, inflammation of gums and loosening of teeth.

Fatal Dose: 15 to 20 ml.

Fatal Period: 18 to 36 hours.

Treatment: Same as for sulphuric acid.

Postmortem Appearances: They are those produced by sulphuric acid, although corrosion is less severe. The stomach contains brownish fluid. The folds of the whole stomach mucosa are brownish. Perforation of the stomach is rare. Acute inflammation and oedema of respiratory passages and lung tissue are common.

TEST: A solution of silver nitrate produces a heavy, curdy, white precipitate of silver chloride.

The Circumstances of Poisoning: Most cases of poisoning are suicidal. A few are accidental or homicidal. Rarely it is injected into the vagina to produce abortion.

OXALIC ACID

Characteristics: Oxalic acid (acid of sugar, salt of sorrel, $C_2H_2O_4$) occurs in the form of colourless, transparent, prismatic crystals, and resembles in appearance the crystals of magnesium sulphate and zinc sulphate. In the form of oxalate, it exists as a natural constituent of many plants, e.g. spinach, rhubarb, cabbage, etc. **About 20 mg. is excreted in urine daily.**

Uses: It is used as a bleach to remove stains, or to clean brass or copper articles or leather, in calico-printing, and for removing writing and signature illegally.

Action: Local: Crystals of the acid and concentrated solution of more than 10% of oxalates are corrosive poisons. They rarely damage the skin, but readily corrode the mucous membrane of the digestive tract. They do not lose their poisonous properties when diluted. Less than 10% is a strong irritant, but cause serious systemic effects when absorbed. Urinary excretion persists up to 24 hours.

Systemic: (a) Shock: Large doses cause rapid death from shock. **(b) Hypocalcaemia:** Those who survive for a few hours develop hypocalcaemia, because it readily combines with the clacium ion in the body tissues and causes its withdrawal from them. **Death usually occurs within 12 hours. (c) Renal damage:** Oxalates produce **tubular nephrosis or necrosis and cause death from uraemia in 2 to 14 days.**

Fatal Dose: 15 to 30 g.

Fatal Period: 1 to 2 hours.

Signs and Symptoms: (a) Fulminating Poisoning: Large concentrated dose of 15 g. or more produce immediate symptoms and death within minutes. There is a burning, sour, bitter taste in the mouth with a sense of constriction around the throat and burning pain from the mouth to the stomach. Pain is very severe, begins in the epigastrium, but soon radiates all over the abdomen; there may be tenderness. Nausea and eructations are immediately followed by vomiting which may be persistent. **Vomit usually contains altered blood and mucus and has a "coffee-ground" appearance.** Thirst may be present. Death usually occurs before bowels are affected, but if life is prolonged diarrhoea will occur.

(b) Acute Poisoning: It occurs by a large dose, when the patient survives for a few hours, and is **characterised by symptoms of hypocalcaemia, and less by digestive upset.** There is muscle irritability and tenderness, tetany or usually convulsions. There may be numbness and tingling of the fingertips and legs. **Usually, signs of cardiovascular collapse appear.** In some patients stupor and coma occur.

(c) Delayed Poisoning: It is **characterised by the symptoms of uraemia.** The urine may be scanty or suppressed and may contain traces of blood, albumin and calcium oxalate crystals. There may be metabolic acidosis and ventricular fibrillation.

Treatment: (1) The stomach is washed out carefully using calcium lactate or gluconate, two teaspoonfuls in each lavage. (2) **The antidote for oxalate poisoning is any preparation of calcium, which converts the poison into insoluble calcium oxalate,** e.g., lime water, calcium lactate, calcium gluconate, calcium chloride, a suspension of chalk in water or milk. One-and-half g. of chalk will neutralise about one gram of oxalic acid. (3) **Calcium gluconate 10%, 10 ml. i.v. at frequent intervals.** (4) Dialysis or exchange transfusion for renal failure. (5) **Parathyroid extract 100 units i.m. in severe cases.** (6) Demulcent drinks. (7) The bowels may be evacuated by an enema or by castor oil. (8) Symptomatic.

Postmortem Appearances: Burns of the face and skin are rare. If the poison has been **used in strong solution, the mucous membrane of the tongue, mouth, pharynx and oesophagus will be whitened as if bleached and has a scalded appearance,** but is sometimes reddened by irritation. The inner surface of the oesophagus is corrugated and shows longitudinal erosions. The mucous membrane of the stomach is reddened or punctate from erosions or almost black. It may be softened in patches but perforation is very rare. **Numerous dark-brown or black streaks run along the length of the stomach over the mucous membrane, often with intercommunicating branches. The stomach contents are gelatinous and brownish** due to acid haematin formation. Sometimes, the whole stomach will become corroded. The intestines usually escape, but upper part of the duodenum may be affected. The kidneys are swollen by oedema, congested and the tubules are filled with oxalate crystals. The renal tubules are necrosed, primarily in the proximal convoluted tubules. If the effects are only narcotic, there will be congestion of the lungs, liver, kidneys and brain, without any local appearances.

TEST: A solution of barium nitrate gives a white precipitate of barium oxalate, which is soluble in hydrochloric acid or nitric acid.

The Circumstances of Poisoning: (1) Accidental poisoning is due to its being mistaken for magnesium sulphate, or sodium bicarbonate. (2) Suicidal poisoning is rare. (3) Homicidal poisoning is rare due to sour, acrid taste. (4) Rarely it is used to procure abortion by vaginal injection.

CARBOLIC ACID (phenol; C_6H_4OH)

Physical Characters: When pure, the acid consists of short, colourless, prismatic, needle-like crystals, which have a burning sweetish taste, which turn pink and liquefy when exposed to air. It has a characteristic 'carbolic' or phenolic smell. It is slightly soluble in water but is freely soluble in glycerine, ether, alcohol and benzene. **The commercial carbolic acid is a dark-brown liquid containing several impurities, chiefly cresol.** It is largely used as an antiseptic and as a disinfectant in various preparations.

Preparations: Lysol is a 50% solution of cresol in saponified vegetable oil. Phenol is about eight times more toxic than lysol. Dettol is a chlorinated phenol with turpineol. Important derivatives of phenol include cresol, creosote (coal tar), thymol, menthol and tannic acid.

Absorption: It is readily absorbed from the alimentary tract, respiratory tract, rectum, vagina, serous cavities, wounds and through the skin.

Excretion: Phenol is converted into hydroquinone and pyrocatechol in the body before being excreted in the urine. A trace is excreted by the lungs, salivary glands, skin and stomach. About 36 hours are required for complete excretion. It is partly detoxicated by liver.

Fatal Dose: 10 to 15 g.; 25 to 50 ml. of household phenol.

Fatal Period: 3 to 4 hours.

Signs and Symptoms: Poisoning by carbolic acid is known as **carbolism.**

Local: (1) Skin: It causes burning and numbness due to damage to nerve endings. **It precipitates protein and coagulates the cell contents and tends to stiffen the tissues and bleach them, so that hard, cracked, whitish surfaces are seen on the face and skin. Deep burns are black. It produces a white opaque eschar which is painless and falls off in a few days and leaves a brown stain.** There may be necrosis and gangrene of the tissue which becomes green-white or brown-white; the dead tissue sloughs readily. Lysol discolours the tissues a brownish-purple.

(2) Digestive Tract: Hot burning pain extends from the mouth to the stomach, which is followed by tingling and later anaesthesia. Deglutition and speech become painful and difficult. The lips, mouth and tongue are corroded, which soon become white and hardened Fig. (26–3). Nausea and vomiting are present in about 20% of cases.

(3) Respiratory Tract: Pulmonary and laryngeal oedema develop due to irritation. Breathing is slow and laboured, progressing to respiratory failure. When vomiting occurs, the poison may be aspirated into the lungs, causing bronchitis and bronchopneumonia.

Systemic Effects: Phenol is a depressant of the nervous system, especially the respiratory centre. Headache, giddiness, unconsciousness and coma occur. The temperature is subnormal, the pupils are contracted, breathing is stertorous, pulse is rapid, feeble and irregular, face covered with cold sweat, and there is **dusky cyanosis, respiratory alkalosis and metabolic acidosis.** Liver may be damaged. In severe cases haemolysis and methaemoglobinaemia is a characteristic feature. There is a strong odour of phenol in breath. Convulsions and lock-jaw sometimes occur.

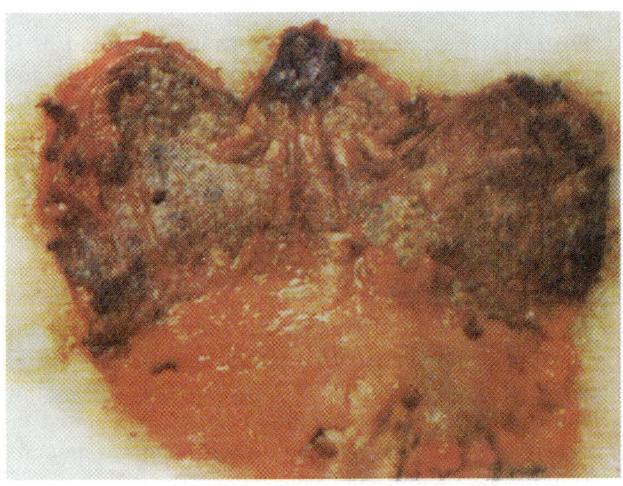

Fig. (26–3). Stomach in lysol poisoning.

Urine: It is scanty and contains albumin and free haemoglobin; suppression may follow. **It may be colourless or slightly green at first, but turns green or even black on exposure to air. In the body, phenol is partly oxidised to hydroquinone and pyrocatechol, which with unchanged phenol are excreted in the urine, partly free, and partly in unstable combination with sulphuric and glucoronic acids. The further oxidation of hydroquinone and pyrocatechol in the urine is the cause of green colouration. This is known as carboluria.**

Chronic Poisoning (Phenol Marasmus): It is characterised by anorexia, weight loss, headache, vertigo, dark urine and pigmentation of skin and sclera. **The hydroquinone and pyrocatechol may cause pigmentation in the cornea and various cartilages, a condition called oochronosis. Ochronosis is commonly associated with alkaptonuria** (an inborn error of metabolism), in which homeogentisic acid gets deposited in cartilages, ligaments and fibrous tissues.

Cause of Death: (1) Syncope. (2) Asphyxia due to (a) failure of respiration, (b) oedema of glottis, (c) complications, e.g., bronchopneumonia.

Treatment: (1) **An emetic often fails** due to the anaesthetic effect. (2) **The stomach should be washed repeatedly, carefully with plenty of lukewarm water containing activated charcoal, olive oil, castor oil, magnesium or sodium sulphate, or saccharated lime with which phenol combines and forms harmless products.** Soap solution or 10% glycerine may be used and the washing continued until the washings are clear and odourless. This is followed by administration of olive oil or vegetable oil to remove surface phenol and prevent deep penetration. (3) **When lavage is completed, 30 g. of magnesium sulphate or a quantity of medicinal liquid paraffin should be left in the stomach.** (4) **Demulcents.** (5) Saline containing seven g. of sodium bicarbonate per litre is given i.v. to combat circulatory depression, to dilute carbolic acid content of blood and to encourage excretion by producing diuresis. (6) **Haemodialysis, if there is renal failure.** (7) **Methylene blue i.v., if there is severe methaemoglobinaemia.** (8) If phenol falls on the body, contaminated clothing should be removed at once, skin washed with undiluted polyethylene glycol. If this is not available the area is washed with soap and water for at least 15 minutes. Olive oil, or methylated spirit or ten percent solution of ethyl alcohol act as solvents.

Postmortem Appearances: External: Corrosion of the skin, especially in tracks from the angles of the mouth on to chin, has a greyish or brown colour. The tongue is usually white and swollen, and there is smell of phenol about the mouth. **The mucous membrane of the lips, mouth and throat is corrugated, sodden, whitened or ash-grey and partially detached with numerous small submucous haemorrhages.**

Internal: The mucosa of the oesophagus is tough, white or grey, corrugated and arranged in longitudinal folds. The stomach mucosal folds are swollen and covered by opaque, coagulated, grey or brown mucous membrane. The intervening furrows are usually less damaged, dark-red and are not opaque. **The mucous membrane is thickened and looks leathery Fig. (26–3).** Often there is partial separation of necrotic mucosa, with severe congestion of underlying tissue. The stomach may contain a reddish fluid mixed with mucus and shreds of epithelium and smells of phenol. The duodenum and upper part of the small intestine may show similar but milder changes. **The liver and spleen usually show a whitish, hardened patch where the stomach has been in contact with them due to the transudation of phenol.** The kidneys show haemorrhagic nephritis in cases of delayed death. The brain is congested, may be oedematous. The blood is dark and semifluid or only partially coagulated. If vomit or poison has been inhaled, coagulation necrosis of the mucosa and severe congestion of the submucosa of the air-passages may be seen. Laryngeal and pulmonary oedema also occur.

TEST: Add a few drops of 10% ferric chloride solution to one ml. of urine. A bluish colour will develop. Salicylates also give positive results.

The Circumstances of Poisoning: (1) It is used for suicidal purposes. (2) Accidental poisoning. (3) It is rarely used for homicide because of its odour and taste. (4) It is sometimes injected into the vagina and uterus to produe abortion. (5) Its indiscriminate medical use sometimes causes poisoning.

FORMIC ACID

It is a colourless liquid with a pungent, penetrating odour. It is used in electroplating, tanning, rubber, textile and paper industry, airplane glue, stain remover, etc.

ACTION: It has a corrosive action (coagulation necrosis) on G.I. mucosa. It causes haemolysis leading to acute renal failure. ATP synthesis is diminished.

FATAL DOSE: 50 to 200 ml.

SIGNS AND SYMPTOMS: G.I.T.: Burning pain, salivation, vomiting, mucosal ulceration and corrosion, haematemesis. R.S: Acute respiratory distress. C.V.S: Tachycardia or bradycardia, hypertension or hypotension. BLOOD: Haemolysis. C.N.S: Drowsiness, coma, dilated pupils. SKIN: Blisters. Metabolic acidosis, shock and death.

TREATMENT: (1) Milk is given for dilution of acid. (2) Gastric lavage and emetics are contraindicated. (3) Folinic acid 1mg/kg i.v. at 4 hourly intervals for 6 doses. (4) Dialysis or exchange transfusion.

POSTMORTEM APPEARANCES: Corrosion and blackening of gastric mucosa and pulmonary oedema.

Poisoning is suicidal or accidental.

BORIC ACID

It is used as antiseptic and insecticide. 15 to 20 g. is fatal.

Symptoms: Generalised erythema resembling 'boiled lobster' appearance with massive areas of desquamation indistinguishable from toxic epidermal necrolysis or staphylococcal scaled syndrome is seen.

Detergent or chemical suicide: In Japan, it is a new method of committing suicide. Common household chemicals (bath sulphur with toilet bowl cleaner) are mixed to produce hydrogen sulphide gas in cars, closets or other enclosed spaces.

CAUSTIC ALKALIS

The chief poisons are ammonia, potassium hydroxide, sodium hydroxide, calcium hydroxide, ammonium carbonate, potassium carbonate and sodium carbonate.

Physical characters: They are extensively used in commerce. Most of these occur as white powders. Ammonia is a colourless gas with a very pungent, choking odour. Ammonium hydroxide is a liquid containing about 30% ammonia.

Action: They are the commonest cause of chemical burns. The hydroxyl ion produces a saponification of fat, soluble alkaline proteinases, cellular dehydration and an exothermic reaction.

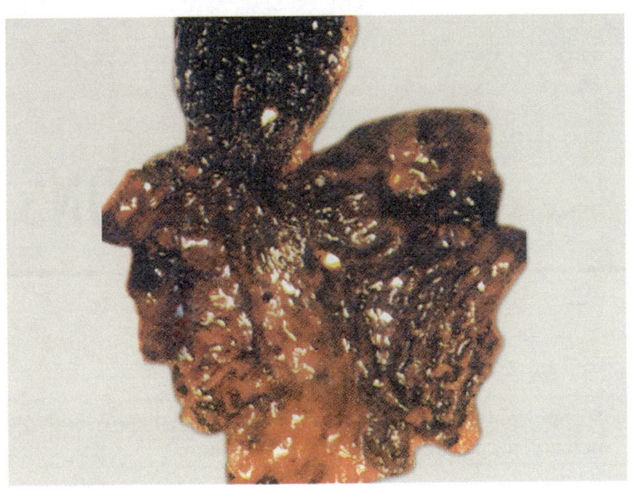

Fig. (26–4). Stomach in caustic soda poisoning.

The ion passes from molecule to molecule, denaturing each in turn, and burrows deeply, producing soft gelatinous, friable eschars (liquefaction necrosis). Ingestion of an alkali produces severe effects mainly on lining of oesophagus, while gastric involvement is less common. Therefore, **stricture formation is much more common with alkalis than with acids. Liquid alkali preparations tend to cause less damage to the oropharynx and oesophagus and more damage to the stomach.**

Signs and Symptoms: In general, the lesions caused by caustic alkalis have about the same extent and distribution as those due to acid corrosives. There is an acid caustic taste and a sensation of burning heat extending from the throat to the stomach. **Vomited matters are alkaline and do not effervesce on contact with the ground.** It is at first thick and slimy, but later contains dark altered blood and shreds of mucosa. **Purging is a frequent symptom,** accompanied by severe pain and straining. The motions consist of mucus and blood.

Contact with skin causes greyish, soapy, necrotic area. When strong alkali is ingested, abrasions, blisters and brownish discolouration are seen on the lips and the skin about the mouth. **The mucosa of the digestive tract is swollen, soft and a grey slough readily detached, lies over the inflamed tissues.** Haemorrhage into the tissue is also seen Fig. (26–4). Oesophageal stricture formation is a major long-term complication.

LYE (NaOH): It can produce transmural necrosis of the oesophagus after only one second of contact. Oesophageal stricture is common with occasional perforation.

PROPERTIES OF AGENTS: (1) Household bleaches (sodium hypochlorite) cause (1) oesophageal irritation but rarely cause strictures or serious injury. (2) Detergents (sodium tripolyphosphate) may produce serious tissue injury. Usually mild ulceration without stricture occurs. (3) Drain cleaners (sodium hydroxide) cause extensive damage to oesophagus and stomach. (4) Ammonium hydroxide 3% usually causes minor irritation, but higher concentrations can cause severe injury to the oesophagus and stomach.

MINIATURE (BUTTON) BATTERIES: They contain potassium hydroxide, which when swallowed can cause liquefaction necrosis following leakage from battery. Symptoms are mostly limited to GI tract.

Ammoniacal vapour when inhaled causes congestion and watering of the eyes, violent sneezing, coughing and choking. Sudden collapse and death may occur from suffocation due to inflammation and much swelling of the glottis or later from pneumonia.

Fatal Dose:

Potassium or sodium hydroxide 5 g.
Potassium carbonate 18 g.
Sodium carbonate 30 g.
Ammonia 15 to 20 ml.

Fatal Period: Usually 24 hours.

Treatment: (1) **Demulcents,** e.g. white of egg, or milk, or water 1 to 2 glasses may be given if the patient is seen within 5 to 10 minutes of ingestion. (2) **In mild cases the stomach can be washed carefully.** (3) **In poisoning by ammonia vapour, oxygen inhalation** should be given or the patient should be kept in an atmosphere made moist with steam. (4) Keep the airway patent. Tracheostomy may be necessary. (5) Give adequate parenteral analgesics. (6) Antibiotics to prevent infection.

POSTMORTEM APPEARANCES: The marks about the mouth become dark in colour and parchment-like after death. When a strong alkali is ingested, lips, mouth and throat show corrosion. Inflammatory oedema with corrosion and sliminess of the tissues of the oesophagus and stomach are prominent features. Alkalis most severely affect the squamous epithelium of the oesophagus, although stomach is involved in 20% cases. Mucosa may be brownish due to formation of alkali haematin. The duodenum and jejunum may show similar changes but of lesser intensity. In some cases, the alkali may be regurgitated and inhaled causing oedema of the glottis, pseudomembranous inflammation of the air-passages and a peribronchial pneumonia. Perforation of the oesophagus or stomach is rare but may occur in ammonia poisoning. Oesophageal stricture formation is common with alkalis than acids.

TEST: The caustic alkalis produce a brown precipitate with silver nitrate. The caustic carbonates produce a whitish-yellow precipitate and effervesce if an acid is added.

CIRCUMSTANCES OF POISONING: Poisoning by alkalis is rare. Accidental cases occur due to its being mistaken for medicine. Homicidal poisoning is rare, but few suicidal cases are seen. Sometimes, a solution of caustic soda is thrown with evil intention on the face and body of an enemy. Poisoning by ammonia is more common than other alkalis.

CHEMICAL BURNS: In chemical burns, the amount of tissue damaged depends upon the agent, its strength and concentration, the quantity of the chemical, the duration of contact, and the extent of penetration of the body by the chemical. Chemicals continue to act on tissue until they are either neutralised by another agent or inactivated by the tissue reaction.

Strong acids have a pH of less than 2. Alkalis injure the tissue if the pH is 11.5 or more. Alkalis produce more severe injury than acids, because they dissolve protein and saponify fat. They produce a liquefaction necrosis permitting deeper invasion of tissue with deep burns and marked oedema. Alkalis produce a soft, oedematous, translucent, soap-like, swollen eschar, red-brown from the absorption of altered blood pigment. The sloughs are mucilaginous. Charring is not seen.

Acids precipitate proteins, producing a coagulation necrosis with a hard eschar. Acids cause more damage to the stomach than the oesophagus. The burns are clearly demarcated, dry and hard. Oedema is mild. The burns are usually of second degree, but if contact is prolonged, third degree burns are caused, especially from concentrated sulphuric or nitric acid, and the scab is dark, leathery and dry. Hydrofluoric acid causes much deeper burns.

Prolonged contact with cement (pH 12.5 to 14) can produce chemical burns. Prolonged contact with hydrocarbons, such as gasoline, can cause chemical burns due to their irritant effect and their high lipid solubility. Chemical burns are also produced by phosphorus and phenol.

CHAPTER

27 METALLIC POISONS

FM 9.3: Describe general principles and basic methodologies in treatment of poisoning: decontamination, supportive therapy, antidote therapy, procedures of enhanced elimination with regard to arsenic, lead, mercury, copper, iron, cadmium and thallium.

ARSENIC

Metallic arsenic (black coloured) is not poisonous, as it is not absorbed from the alimentary canal. When volatilised by heat, arsenic unites with oxygen and forms poisonous vapour of arsenic trioxide.

POISONOUS COMPOUNDS: (1) Arsenious oxide or arsenic trioxide *(sankhya or somalkhar)*. This is the most common form of arsenic used, and is known as white arsenic or arsenic. It occurs in two forms: (a) white, smooth, heavy, crystalline powder, (b) white and opaque solid mass similar to porcelain. It has no taste or smell and is sparingly soluble in water. When the powder is added to water it floats on the surface, though it is three-and-half times heavier than water. It sublimes on heating. Arsenic is used in fruit sprays, sheep-dips, weed-killers, insecticides, rat poisons, fly papers, calico-printing, taxidermy, wall papers and artificial flowers, as mordant in dyeing and for preserving timber and skin against white ants. (2) Copper arsenite (Scheele's green) and copper acetoarsenite (Paris green or emerald green). (3)Arsenic acid. (4) Sodium and potassium arsenate. (5) Arsenic sulphide, orpiment and realgar. (6) Arsenic trichloride (butter of arsenic). (7) Arseniuretted hydrogen or arsine is a colourless gas with garlic-like, non-irritating odour. (8) Organic compounds, e.g., cacodylates, atoxyl, acetarson, tryparsamide, salvarsan, mepharsen, etc.

Action: Arsenic interferes with cellular respiration by combining with the sulphydryl groups of mitochondrial enzymes, especially pyruvate oxidase, and certain phosphatases. Its particular target is vascular endothelium, leading to increased permeability, tissue oedema and haemorrhage, especially in the intestinal canal. Locally it causes irritation of the mucous membranes and remotely depression of the nervous system. Arsenate causes its toxicity by uncoupling mitochondrial oxidative phosphorylation. It interferes with glycolysis.

Signs and Symptoms: (1) The Fulminant Type: Massive doses (3 to 5 g.) of arsenic when rapidly absorbed cause **death in one to three hours from shock and peripheral vascular failure** or may be delayed for many days when hepatorenal failure is the mode of death. All the capillaries are markedly dilated, especially in the splanchnic area with a marked fall of blood pressure. Arsenic also has a direct action on heart muscle. In this type gastrointestinal symptoms are absent.

(2) The Gastroenteric Type: This is the common form of acute poisoning, and resembles bacterial food poisoning. Symptoms usually appear half to one hour after ingestion, but may be delayed many hours especially when arsenic is taken with food. There is sweetish metallic taste. **G.I.T.:** Constriction in the throat and difficulty in swallowing; burning and colicky pain in oesophagus, stomach and bowel occur. **Intense thirst and severe vomiting which may be projectile are the constant symptoms. Purging (within 1 to 3 hours) is usually accompanied by tenesmus, pain, and irritation about the anus. The stools are expelled frequently and involuntarily, and are dark-coloured, stinking and bloody, but later become colourless, odourless and watery resembling rice-water stools of cholera** Table (27–1). **A garlicky odour of breath and faeces may be noted. Hepatic:** Fatty infiltration. **Renal:** Oliguria, uraemia; urine contains albumen, red cells and casts, pain during micturition. **C.V.S.**: Acute circulatory collapse with vasodilation, increased vascular permeability, ventricular tachycardia, ventricular fibrillation. **CNS:** Headache, vertigo, hyperthermia, tremors, convulsions, coma, general paralysis. A peripheral neuropathy that is more sensory than motor can occur in asymmetric, distal stocking-glove distribution after one to two weeks of acute or chronic exposures. **Skin:** Delayed loss of hair, skin eruptions. Death is usually due to circulatory failure.

(3) Narcotic Form: In this form, the **gastrointestinal symptoms are very slight.** There is giddiness, formication and tenderness of the muscles, delirium, coma and death. Rarely there is complete paralysis of the extremities.

Late sequelae of acute exposure include haematuria, and acute tubular necrosis. Anaemia, leucopaenia and thrombocytopaenia can occur.

Normal blood levels of arsenic <4 mg/l and urine <0.03 mg/l. Blood concentration level >1.5 mg/100 ml. indicates serious poisoning.

Arseniuretted hydrogen, when inhaled acts as a direct poison to the haemoglobin, producing haemolysis, haemoglobinuria and renal failure. Death is almost instantaneous.

Fatal Dose: 200 to 300 mg. arsenic trioxide.

Fatal Period: 1 to 2 days.

Treatment: (1) Emetics. (2) The stomach should be emptied and then thoroughly and repeatedly washed by the stomach tube with large amount of warm water and milk.

Table (27–1). Difference between arsenic poisoning and cholera

Trait		Arsenic poisoning	Cholera
(1)	Pain in throat:	Before vomiting.	After vomiting.
(2)	Purging:	After vomiting.	Before vomiting.
(3)	Stools:	Dark-coloured and bloody, later rice-watery.	Rice-watery, not bloody and passed in continuous involuntary jet.
(4)	Tenesmus and anal irritation:	Present.	Absent.
(5)	Vomited matter:	Contains mucus, bile and blood.	Watery without mucus, bile and blood.
(6)	Voice:	Not affected.	Rough and whistling.
(7)	Conjunctivae:	Inflamed.	Not inflamed.
(8)	Analysis of excreta:	Arsenic present.	Cholera vibrio present.
(9)	Circumstantial evidence:	Of arsenic poisoning may be present.	Other cases of cholera in locality.

The stomach should be washed out at intervals to remove iron compounds, and adherent arsenic. (3) **Butter and greasy substances prevent absorption.** (4) Alkalis should not be given as they increase the solubility of arsenic. (5) **Freshly precipitated hydrated ferric oxide and dialyzed iron are not recommended.** (6) Whole bowel irrigation. (7) Nasogastric suction to be done as arsenic is resecreted in gastrointestinal tract. (8) **B.A.L.** 400 to 800 mg. on first day, 200 to 400 mg. on second and third days, in divided doses every four hours and 100 to 200 mg. in two divided doses for 7 to 10 days or until urine level falls below 50 mg in a 24 hour specimen. (9) **Penicillamine may be used with BAL.** 100 mg/kg daily up to 1 to 2 g. in four divided doses for five days. (10) **DMSA (succimer) or DMPS can be used instead of BAL if available. They are superior to BAL.** (11) Demulcents lessen irritation. (12) Castor oil or magnesium sulphate to prevent intestinal absorption of arsenic. (13) Glucose-saline with sodium bicarbonate is helpful to combat shock and improve alkali reserve. (14) Haemodialysis or exchange transfusion may be given in cases of renal failure. (15) Chelation therapy is ineffective in arsine poisoning.

Postmortem Appearances: External: The eyeballs are sunken and the skin is cyanosed. The body may be shrunken due to dehydration.

Internal: The mouth, pharynx and oesophagus is usually not affected, but in some cases is inflamed or ulcerated. **The lesions are mainly found in the stomach. The mucosa is swollen, oedematous and red either generally or in patches,** especially **in the pyloric region. There may be lines of redness running along the walls or curved lines of submucous haemorrhages.** Usually groups of petechiae are seen scattered over the mucosa and sometimes large submucosal and subperitoneal haemorrhages. **The stomach mucosa resembles red velvet. Small acute ulcerations or large erosions may be found, especially at the pyloric end.** A mass of sticky mucus covers the mucosa in which particles of arsenic may be seen. Congestion is most marked along the crest of the rugae. The small intestine appears flaccid and contains large flakes of mucus with very little faecal matter. The mucosa is pale-violet and shows signs of inflammation with submucous haemorrhages along its whole length Fig. (27–1). The caecum and rectum show slight inflammation. **Sometimes, arsenic penetrates through the walls of the stomach and appears in liver, omentum and endocardium. If putrefaction has taken place, yellow streaks will be found in the subperitoneal layer of the stomach and to less extent of the intestines, due to absorbed arsenic which has been converted into sulphide.** In fulminating type, the stomach and intestines may not show any signs of inflammation. The liver, spleen and kidneys are congested, enlarged and show cloudy swelling and occasionally fatty change. The lungs are congested with subpleural ecchymoses. Nephritis, particularly of golmerular type is frequent. Haemorrhages may be found in the abdominal organs, mesenteries and occasionally in larynx, trachea and lungs. There may be oedema of brain with patchy necrosis or haemorrhagic encephalitis. The meninges are congested. **Subendocardial petechial haemorrhages of the ventricle are common in arsenic poisoning and may be found even when the stomach shows little sign of irritation. It is typical of arsenic poisoning,** although they are sometimes found in poisoning by phosphorus, barium and mercury, and in cases of heat stroke and in acute infectious disease, e.g., influenza or in traumatic asphyxia. In a few days fatty deposits occur in the heart, liver and kidneys, and kidneys show acute tubular necrosis.

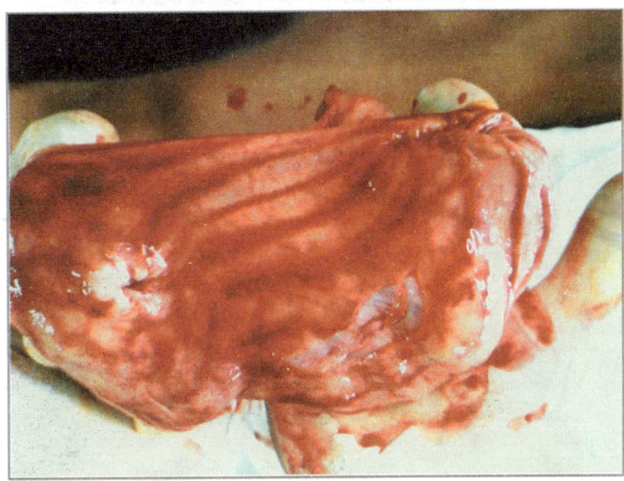

Fig. (27–1). The stomach mucus showing red velvet appearance with lines of redness running along the walls in arsenic poisoning.

In death due to acute arsenic poisoning, arsenic values in the liver and blood in excess of 1 mg. % are usually present. X-ray may show presence of arsenic in G.I. tract.

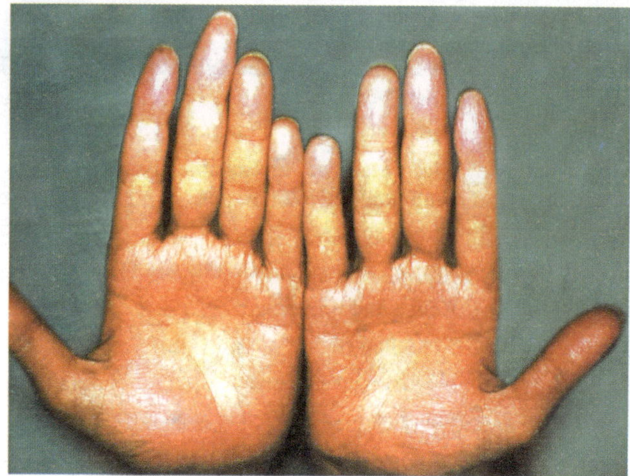

Fig. (27–2). Raindrop pigmentation of palms of hand in chronic arsenic poisoning.
Courtesy: **Dr. Ashok Rastogi, AIIMS, Patna.**

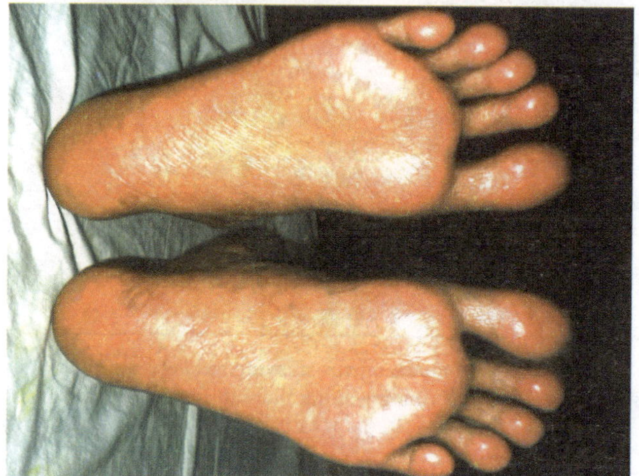

Fig. (27–3). Raindrop pigmentation on soles of feet in chronic arsenic poisoning.
Courtesy: **Dr. Ashok Rastogi, AIIMS, Patna.**

Chronic Poisoning: It may be due to accidental ingestion of repeated small doses by those working with the metal, or by taking food or drink in which there are traces of drug. It may be of homicidal nature due to repeated small doses, or may occur after recovery from one large dose.

C.N.S.: Polyneuritis, anaesthesias, paraesthesia, encephalopathy. **Skin:** Pigmentation consists of a finely mottled brown change mostly on the skin flexures, temples, eyelids and neck **(raindrop type of pigmentation),** which persists for many months **Figs. (27–2 and 27–3)**. There may be a rash resembling fading measles rash. In prolonged contact, hyperkeratosis of the palms and soles with irregular thickening of the nails and development of transverse white lines in the fingernails called **Aldrich-Mees lines** is seen. **Eyes:** Congestion, watering of the eyes, photophobia. **G.I.T.:** Nausea, vomiting, abdominal cramps, diarrhoea, salivation. **C.V.S. and kidneys:** Chronic nephritis, cardiac failure, dependent oedema. **Hepatic:** Hepatomegaly, jaundice, cirrhosis of the liver. **Haematologic:** Bone marrow suppression, hypoplasia, anaemia, thrombocytopaenia, leukaemia. **General:** Anaemia and weight loss, loss of hair, brittle nails. **R.S.:** Cough, haemoptysis, dyspnoea.

Arsenic is **teratogenic** and can result in lung and skin cancer, leukaemia, etc.

POSTMORTEM APPEARANCES: The stomach may be normal or may show a chronic gastritis. Some rugae may show patchy inflammatory redness. In some cases, patchy haemorrhagic gastritis with acute and chronic erosions are seen. The small intestine is dilated, reddened , with thickened mucosa. The liver may be fatty or there may be severe necrosis. There may be jaundice. The kidneys show tubular necrosis.

Treatment consists in removing the patient from the source of exposure and administration of B.A.L.

ORGANIC ARSENICAL COMPOUNDS: They contain arsenic either in trivalent or pentavalent combination. They are less toxic than inorganic compounds. Their chief toxic manifestations are immediate anaphylactic symptoms and later on skin reactions, agranulocytosis, hepatitis, jaundice and encephalitis.

Absorption: The average daily human intake of arsenic is half to one mg. contained in food and water. **It is absorbed orally (pentavalent arsenic), dermally (arsenite), by inhalation (arsine), or parenterally.** On absorption, it is bound to the protein portion of haemoglobin. Permissible limits of arsenic in ground water is 0.05 mg/litre.

DISTRIBUTION: Arsenic is normally present in almost all tissues. In the early stage, arsenic is found in greatest quantity in the liver, followed by kidneys and spleen. Arsenic does not cross blood-brain barrier well (brain has lowest level), but inorganic arsenic can cross the placenta. In cases in which life is prolonged, it is found in the muscles for days, in the bones and in the keratin tissues, hair, nails and skin for years. It replaces phosphorus in the bone where it may remain for years. Normally hair contains less than two parts per million arsenic. It can appear in hair and nails within hours of ingestion. Estimates of time of exposure can be made by measuring the distance of Mee's lines from the base of the nails or the length of hair from its growth site. In fatal cases, the concentration of arsenic in the liver is usually 1 mg % or more. Neutron activation analysis and atomic absorption spectroscopy helps in estimating concentration of arsenic in hair, nails, bone, etc.

ELIMINATION: It is eliminated mainly by the kidneys, in the form of methylated arsenic, but also in the faeces, bile, sweat, milk and other secretions. Breast milk does not contain significant amounts of arsenic. It may be found in the urine within half-an-hour of ingestion and excretion by urine is fairly continuous for about 10 to 12 days. Normal level in urine < 0.03 µg/l. In acute poisoning 24 hour excretion in urine is more than 100 µg. The arsenic is excreted into the epidermal tissues, such as hair and nails within hours of ingestion, and in cases of intermittent chronic poisoning, there will be successive deposits of arsenic in the hair and nails. The excretion of arsenic in a healthy person taking food rich in fish, especially shellfish, can be more than that seen in chronic poisoning. Arsenic is excreted into the stomach and intestines after absorption, even when given by routes other than mouth. It becomes fixed in cancellous tissues or bones, chiefly long bones.

Tolerance: Some people take arsenic daily as a tonic or as an aphrodisiac, and they acquire tolerance up to 0.3 g. or more in one dose. Such people are known as **arsenophagists.**

TESTS: Detection is done by atomic absorption spectroscopy. Marsh's test and Reinsch's tests are absolete.

The Circumstances of Poisoning:

(1) Homicide: **Arsenic is popular homicidal poison because:** (1) it is cheap, (2) easily obtained, (3) colourless, (4) no smell, (5) no taste, (6) small quantity is required to cause death, (7) can be easily administered with food or drink, (8) onset of symptoms is gradual, (9) symptoms simulate those of cholera. **The disadvantages** are: (1) it delays putrefaction, (2) can be detected in completely decomposed bodies, (3) can be found in bones, hair and nails for several years, (4) can be detected in charred bones or ashes.

(1) For homicide, it is given orally mixed with some articles of food like sweets, bread, milk, tea, cold drinks, etc. (2) Mass homicidal poisoning occurs when it is mixed with food or in a well. (3) Sometimes, it is given mixed with tobacco or cigars for homicide or to rob. (4) Suicide is rare because it causes much pain. (5) Accidental death may be due to admixture with articles of food, or from its improper medicinal use. Chronic poisoning results from drinking well water containing arsenic. (6) It is sometimes ingested or applied locally in the form of a paste or ointment to abortion sticks to produce abortion. (7) It is fed to the animal mixed with cattle fodder.

Postmortem Imbibition of Arsenic: In exhumations, the possibility of imbibition of arsenic from the stomach into neighbouring viscera and also contamination from the surrounding earth should be remembered. Arsenic found in the soil is usually an insoluble salt. **Keratin tissues absorb arsenic by contamination from outside.** The concentration in hair and nails thus contaminated is likely to be much greater than the concentration of arsenic in the contaminating fluid. **If arsenic is introduced into the stomach after death, the transudation occurs into the organs of the left side before those of the right** and the signs of inflammation and ulceration are absent.

MERCURY (QUICK SILVER)

It is liquid metal, bright silvery appearance and is volatile at room temperature. It forms two series of compounds: (1) mercuric, which are soluble and intensely poisonous; and (2) mercurous, which are much less soluble and therefore less active. Metallic mercury is not poisonous if swallowed, for it is not absorbed. If the mercury is breathed or swallowed as vapour, or if applied to the skin or mucous membrane in finely divided state it is absorbed.

POISONOUS COMPOUNDS: (1) Mercuric chloride ($HgCl_2$; corrosive sublimate), occurs as colourless masses of prismatic crystals, or as a white crystalline powder. It has no smell, but a styptic, nauseous, metallic taste. (2) Mercuric oxide (brick-red crystalline powder). (3) Mercuric iodide (scarlet-red powder). (4) Mercuric cyanide (white prismatic crystals). (5) Mercuric sulphide (cinnabar, sindoor). Artificial preparation occurs as red crystalline powder and is known as vermilion. (6) Mercurous chloride (calomel). (7) Mercuric nitrite. (8) Mercuric sulphate (white crystalline powder). (9) Sulphate of mercury (lemon-yellow powder). (10) Ammoniomercuric chloride. (11) Organic compounds of mercury. (12) Mercury thiocyanate (used in Diwali to produces a large winding snake–Pharaoh snake/serpent).

ACTION: The mercuric ion binds with sulphydryl groups of enzymes and cellular proteins, nucleic acids and mitotic apparatus interfering with enzyme and cellular transport functions. It is rapidly converted to mercuric ions in the blood which can lead to renal tubular damage. In the CNS, mercury acts mainly upon cerebellum, temporal lobe, basal ganglia and corpus callosum.

Acute exposure to elemental mercury vapour may produce corrosive bronchitis with fever, chills and dyspnoea. It may progress to pulmonary oedema and fibrosis. Sometimes, manifestations similar to Kawasaki disease (mucocutaneous lymph node syndrome) are seen especially in children.

SYMPTOMS: FIRST PHASE: Acrid metallic taste and feeling of constriction in the throat, hoarse voice, difficulty in breathing. The mouth, tongue and fauces become corroded, swollen and show a greyish-white coating. Hot burning pain in the mouth, extending down to the stomach and abdomen, followed by nausea, retching and vomiting. The vomit contains greyish slimy mucoid material with blood and shreds of mucous membrane. This is followed by diarrhoea with bloodstained stools and tenesmus. Circulatory collapse occurs soon. Inhalation of fumes produce nervous symptoms, e.g., ataxia, restriction of visual field, paresis and delirium.

SECOND PHASE: If the person survives, second phase begins in one to 3 days. Glossitis and ulcerative gingivitis appear within 24 to 36 hours. Severe infection, loosening of teeth and necrosis of the jaw may occur. In 2 to 3 days, renal tubules show necrosis and produce transient polyuria, albuminuria, cylindruria, uraemia and acidosis. Recovery may occur within 10 to 14 days. After many days membranous colitis develops and produces dysentery, ulceration of colonic mucosa and haemorrhage.

Intramuscular injection produces abscess with ulceration. i.v. injection may cause mercurialism in which thrombophlebitis, granuloma formation, pulmonary embolism and repeated haemoptysis is seen.

Normal levels of mercury: (1) Blood <10 µg/l. (2) Urine <20 µg/l. (3) Normal urinary excretion in 24 hours <50 µg/l.

Chronic exposure: (1) Blood >35 µg/l. (2) Urine >150 µg/l.

Organic mercurials, such as phenyl and methoxymethyl mercury, ethyl and methyl mercury are more toxic. Symptoms are mainly CNS and include ataxia, dysarthria, paraesthesias, neuropathies, mental deterioration and chorea.

Fatal Dose: 1 to 2 g. of mercuric chloride.

Fatal Period: 3 to 5 days.

Treatment: (1) Milk, egg-white, 5% salt-poor albumin **or 2 to 5% sodium bicarbonate may be used for gastric lavage to bind the mercury.** Sodium formaldehyde sulphoxylate is not recommended. Activated charcoal is of uncertain benefit. (2) Cathartics should not be given but **whole bowel irrigation** may be beneficial. (3) **Penicillamine** is used for less severe mercury vapour and inorganic mercury poisoning. It is given orally in a dose of 100 mg/kg every 6 hours (maximum one g/day) for 5 days in acute poisoning in children and 250 mg. four times a day for five days in adults. For chronic poisoning in children 25 to 40 mg (maximum one g/day) divided into two doses and for adults 250 mg twice a day is given until urine mercury levels are less than 50 µg/l. (4) **BAL is the chelating agent of choice.** Dosage regimen is same as for arsenic. (5) **BAL and penicillamine in combination should not be used as they may cause formation of a toxic compound.** (6) **Ca-EDTA should not be used, as it is nephrotoxic with mercury.** (7) Urine must be kept alkaline. (8) High colonic lavage with 1: 1000 solution of sulphoxylate twice daily. (9) Haemodialysis is indicated if there is significant kidney damage.

Postmortem Appearances: The mucosa of the gastrointestinal tract shows inflammation, congestion, coagulation and corrosion. If the person survives for few days, the large intestine shows necrosis due to the re-excretion of mercury into the large bowel. Acute tubular and glomerular degeneration or haemorrhagic glomerular nephritis is seen. The liver is congested and shows cloudy swelling or fatty change.

CHRONIC POISONING (Hydrargyrism): This may result from (1) continuous accidental absorption by the workers, (2) excessive therapeutic use, (3) from recovery from a large dose, and (4) if ointment is used as external application for a long time.

Chronic exposure to elemental mercury yields a classic triad of gingivitis, stomatitis, and salivation, tremors and neuropsychiatric changes. The symptoms are salivation, inflammation of gums and occasionally a blue line at their junction with teeth, sore mouth and throat, loosening of teeth, gastrointestinal disturbances, anaemia, anorexia, loss of weight and chronic inflammation of kidneys with progressive uraemia. Tremors (sometimes called **Danbury tremors) occur first in the hands, then progress to lips and tongue and finally involve arms and legs. The tremor is moderately coarse and is interspersed by jerky movements. The advanced condition** is called **hatter's shakes or glass-blower's shakes,** because they are common in persons working in glass-blowing and hat industries. The patient then becomes unable to dress himself. write legibly or walk properly. The most severe form is known as **concussio mercurialis,** in which no activity is possible. **Mercurial erethism** is seen in persons working with mercury in mirror manufacturing firms. **This term is used to refer to the psychological effects of mercury toxicity. These include anxiety, depression, shyness, timidity, irritability, loss of confidence, mental depression, delusions and hallucinations, or suicidal melancholia, or manic depressive psychosis (mad hatter), emotional instability, loss of memory and insomnia. Mercurialentis is a peculiar eye change due to exposure to the vapour of mercury.** It is due to brownish deposit of mercury through the cornea on the anterior lens capsule. Slit-lamp examination demonstrates a malt-brown reflex from the anterior lens capsule. It is bilateral and has no effect on visual acuity. Renal damage results in membranous glomerulonephritis with hyaline casts and fatty casts in the urine. Kidney is the primary target.

Acrodynia or pink disease (because it is characterised by a generalised body rash) is thought to be an idiosyncratic hypersensitivity reaction particularly seen in children. This can be caused by chronic mercury exposure in any form. The onset is insidious with anorexia, insomnia, sweating, skin rash and photophobia. Hands and feet become puffy, pinkish, painful, paraesthetic with peeling of skin. Teeth may be shed.

Treatment: (1) Removal of patient from further exposure. (2) Demulcents. (3) Saline purgatives. (4) Oral hygiene. (5) Chelation therapy: D-penicillamine 25 to 40 mg/kg/day (maximum 1g) for children in two divided doses and 250 mg 4 times a day for adults is given until urine mercury levels are less than 50 µg/L or BAL 100 mg i.m. 4th hourly for 2 days, followed by 100 mg every 8 hours for 8 to 10 days, or DMPS 5 mg/kg i.v. or 6 infusions of 250 mg/day, followed by 100 mg orally twice a day for 24 days or DMSA 30 mg/kg/day orally for 5 days, followed by 20 mg/day for 14 days. (6) For organic mercurials chelation is not very effective.

MINIMATA DISEASE is a type of organic mercurial poisoning due to eating of fish poisoned by mercury. This disease occurred as a disaster in Japan in 1956 by eating contaminated fish from Minimata Bay.

FATE AND EXCRETION: After absorption, the mercuric ion is distributed between blood cells and plasma. It then diffuses into the tissues where it rapidly binds to most protein sulphydryl groups. Mercury is impounded in all tissues, particularly in liver, kidneys, spleen and bones. Excretion is by kidneys, liver and colonic mucous membrane. It is also excreted in the saliva, milk, sweat and faeces, if the quantity is larger. It passes rapidly to the foetus in utero through the placental circulation. It is not a constituent of the human body. Normal blood mercury level is less than 4 µg/100ml.

TEST: If a piece of copper wire is introduced in the solution and a few drops of hydrochloric acid are added, a silver coating of mercury will be formed on the wire.

THE CIRCUMSTANCES OF POISONING: (1) Accidental poisoning by mercuric chloride may be due to the use of strong solution in washing abscess cavities or irrigating the vagina, uterus or rectum. (2) Sometimes, it is introduced into the vagina as a contraceptive or for producing abortion. (3) Homicidal and suicidal poisoning is rare.

LEAD

POISONOUS COMPOUNDS: It is a heavy steel-grey metal. Metallic lead and all its salts are poisonous. The principal salts which produce toxic effects are: (1) Lead acetate (sugar of lead); white crystals. (2) Lead carbonate (*safeda*): a white crystalline powder. (3) Lead chromate: a bright yellow powder. (4) Lead monoxide (litharge); pale brick-red or pale orange masses. (5) Lead tetroxide (red lead, vermilion, *sindur*); scarlet crystalline powder. (6) Lead sulphide is least toxic. Lead is used in storage batteries, solders, paints, hair dyes, electric cable insulations, pottery and ceramics and petrols.

ACTION: At the cellular level, lead interacts with sulphydryl groups and interferes with the action of enzymes necessary for haem synthesis, and for haemoglobin and cytochrome production. It interferes with mitochondrial oxidative phosphorylation, ATPases, calcium dependent messengers and enhances oxidation and cell apoptosis. It causes haemolysis.

FATAL DOSE: About 20 g. lead acetate; 40 g. lead carbonate.

FATAL PERIOD: 1 to 2 days.

ACUTE POISONING: The symptoms are: an astringent and metallic taste, dry throat, thirst, burning abdominal pain, nausea, vomiting, sometimes diarrhoea, peripheral circulatory collapse, headache, insomnia, paraesthesias, depression, coma and death.

Cerebellar ataxia is common in children in acute lead poisoning.

TREATMENT: (1) Gastric lavage with one percent solution of sodium or magnesium sulphate. (2) Demulcents. (3) The combination of B.A.L. and calcium disodium versenate or DMSA is effective. (4) Penicillamine. (5) Calcium chloride 5 mg. of a 10 percent solution i.v. causes deposition of lead in the skeleton from the blood. (6) Peritoneal or haemodialysis. (7) Symptomatic treatment.

POSTMORTEM APPEARANCES: Signs of acute gastroenteritis are seen. The mucosa of the stomach may by thickened and softened with eroded patches and may be covered with a greyish-white deposit.

CHRONIC POISONING (plumbism; saturnism): Causes: (1) Inhalation of lead dust and fumes by makers of white lead and makers and users of lead paints (most common source of exposure for children), smelters, plumbers, glass-polishers, printers, enamel workers, glass blowers, etc. (2) Continuous absorption of minute amounts from drinking water stored in lead cisterns, from tinned food contaminated with lead from the solder, and from constant use of hair dyes and cosmetics containing lead. (3) Absorption through raw or intact skin. (4) Use of *ghee* stored in brass or copper vessels lined inside with tin in which oleate of lead is formed and also by taking food cooked in tinned vessel. (5) Absorption of vermilion applied to the scalp. (6) Children can be chronically poisoned through chewing or licking toys, walls, furniture, etc. painted with lead-based compounds. Chronic poisoning results from a daily intake of one to two mg. of lead. **Lead vapour is more dangerous than dust. Lead is a typical cumulative poison.**

Signs and Symptoms: (1) Facial Pallor: The facial pallor particularly about the mouth is one of the earliest and most consistent sign. It seems to be due to vasospasm.

(2) Anaemia: There may be polycythaemia with polychromatophilia in early stages, but later there is anaemia which is associated with polychromasia, punctate basophilia, reticulocytosis, poikilocytosis, anisocytosis, nucleated red cells **(sideroblasts)** and an increase in mononuclear cells, whereas polymorphonuclear cells and platelets are decreased. The anaemia is probably due to decreased survival time of red blood cells and inhibition of haeme synthesis by interference with the incorporation of iron into protoporphyrin. **Punctate basophilia** or **basophilic stippling** means the presence of many dark **blue-coloured pinhead-sized spots in the cytoplasm of red blood cells, due to toxic action of lead on porphyrin metabolism. Reticulocytes and basophilic stippled cells result from the inhibition of 5 pyrimidine nucleotidase, an impaired ability to rid the cell of RNA degradation products and the aggregation of ribosome. Stippled red cells may also be seen in arsenic and zinc poisoning. Eosinophilia is more common than basophilic stippling.** Porphyrins excreted in urine may be 500 micrograms per day.

(3) Lead Line: **A stippled blue line, called Burtonian line, is seen on the gums in 50 to 70% of cases.** It appears due to subepithelial deposit of granules at the junction with teeth, only near dirty or carious teeth, within a week of exposure, especially on upper jaw. It is due to formation of lead sulphide by the action of hydrogen sulphide formed by decomposed food in the mouth. **A similar blue line may be seen in cases of poisoning by mercury, copper, bismuth, iron and silver.**

(4) Colic and Constipation: It is usually later symptom. Colic of intestines, ureters, uterus and blood vessels occur in 85% of cases. The colic occurs at night and the pain may be very severe. Individual attacks last only a few minutes, but may recur for several days or weeks. Constipation is usual but diarrhoea or vomiting may occur.

(5) Lead Palsy: It usually occurs late, and is seen in less than 10% of cases. There may be tremors, numbness, hyperaesthesia, and cramps before the actual muscle weakness. It is commoner in adults than in children, and men are particularly affected. The muscle groups affected are those most prone to fatigue. **Usually the extensor muscles of the wrist (wrist drop; radial nerve is affected) are affected, but the deltoid, biceps, anterior tibial (foot drop), and rarely muscles of eye or intrinsic muscles of hand or foot are affected.** The paralysis is associated with degeneration of the nerve and atrophy of the muscles. Recovery may be complete but is usually slow.

(6) Encephalopathy: Lead encephalopathy, in some form is said to be **present in almost every case of plumbism. It is common in children often associated with tetraethyl lead.** The symptoms are vomiting, headache, insomnia, visual disturbances, irritability, restlessness, delirium, hallucinations, convulsions, coma and death. Lead encephalopathy is usually irreversible and about 85% have permanent brain damage. Death occurs in about 25% cases.

(7) Cardiovascular System and Kidneys: Lead causes vascular constriction, leading to hypertension and permanent arteriolar degeneration. Chronic arteriosclerotic nephritis and interstitial nephritis occur.

(8) Reproductive System: Menstrual derangements, such as amenorrhoea, dysmenorrhoea, menorrhagia, sterility of both sexes, and abortion are frequent. Abortion occurs in pregnant women between 3 to 6 months.

(9) Other Systems: They are dyspepsia, anorexia, emaciation, general weakness, exhaustion, irritability, foul breath, headache, vertigo, loss of hair and drowsiness. Peripheral neuritis is rare.

Retinal stippling is noticed by ophthalmoscopic examination showing presence of greyish glistening lead particles in the early phase of poisoning.

Diagnosis: (1) History. (2) Clinical features. (3) X-ray evidence of increased radio-opaque bonds or lines at the metaphyses of long bones and along margins of iliac crest is seen in children. (4) Erythrocyte protoporphyrin (EP) commonly assayed as zinc protoporphyrin (ZPP) is usually below 35 μg/L, is not sufficiently sensitive at lower blood lead levels. (5) Basophilic stippling. (6) X-ray may show radio-opaque material in the G.I. tract, if lead is ingested during preceding 36 to 48 hours. (7) Porphyrinuria, mainly due to coproporphyrin III, is a valuable screening test. In the blood, levels above 20 μg%, and in the urine 150 μg. per litre is diagnostic.

Prophylaxis: To prevent chronic lead poisoning in factory workers, the following measures should be taken. (1) Maintenance of proper ventilation in factories. (2) Maintenance of personal hygiene of the workers and periodical medical examination. (3) A diet rich in calcium. (4) Small amount of sulphuric acid in water. (5) Weekly saline purgative.

Treatment: (A) Severe acute poisoning with encephalopathy: (1) BAL 4 mg/kg immediately (in childen). Repeat the same dose at 4 hourly intervals until blood lead levels fall below 40 μg/100 ml. Then reduce BAL to 12 mg/kg/day in 3 divided doses. (2) CaNa2 EDTA 75 mg/kg/day i.v. infusion. Reduce EDTA to 50 mg/kg/day as condition improves. (3) The above regimen is continued until patient is asymptomatic and can tolerate oral chelation with D-penicillamine 10 mg/kg/day or DMSA, 10 mg/kg/ dose t.i.d. for 20 days.

(B) Severe poisoning without encephalopathy: (BL more than 70 μg/ 100 ml): (1) BAL 12 mg/kg/day. (2) EDTA 50 mg/kg/day. (3) Discontinue BAL when blood level falls below 40 μg/100 ml. but continue EDTA for 5 more days. (4) Continue oral chelation until the BL falls below 15 μg/100 ml. or for 3 months.

(C) Moderate poisoning (BL between 45 to 75 μg/100 ml): (1) EDTA 50 mg/kg/day. (2) When BL falls below 40 μg/100 ml begin oral chelation.

(D) Mild poisoning (BL 20 to 35 μg/100 ml): D-penicillamine 30 mg/kg/day in 3 divided doses. Start with one-fourth of the calculated dose. Double this after one week. Double again after one week. Continue this until BL falls to less than 15 μg/100 ml. or for 3 months.

DMSA (succimer) 10 mg/kg/dose t.i.d. for 20 days is more effective and less toxic.

SUPPORTIVE MEASURES INCLUDE: (1) Thiamine, 10 to 50 mg/kg to improve neurological manifestations. (2) Calcium gluconate i.v. for colic. (3) Magnesium or sodium sulphate 8 to 12 g. will change unabsorbed lead salts to the highly insoluble lead sulphate and hasten its passage in the stools. (4) Calcium versenate of disodium acts as an ion exchanger in which the calcium is exchanged for the heavy metal ion and a soluble, stable, and unionized chelate of lead is formed. The complex is stable and is a less toxic molecule. The rate of excretion of lead as the EDTA complex in the urine increases fiftyfold above the normal untreated excretion rate. Chelating therapy serves to detoxify the lead, withdraws it from the effector sites and promotes excretion. EDTA 5 ml. of 20% solution is diluted with 250 to 500 ml. of normal saline or 5%

glucose, and given by drip method over a period of one hour, twice daily for 5 days, and can be repeated after an interval of 2 days. (5) B.A.L. 4 mg/kg. of body weight every 4 hours is useful. BAL chelates lead both intracellularly and extracellularly. Two molecules of BAL combine with one atom of lead to form a complex that is excreted in the bile and urine. In the presence of renal impairment, BAL is the chelator of choice, as its main route of excretion is the bile. BAL should be given at least 4 hours before EDTA, as EDTA mobilises lead from tissue stores and aggravates symptoms of lead poisoning. (6) Penicillamine 0.3 to 0.5 g. orally one to 5 times daily is effective in excretion of circulating lead but is not as effective as EDTA. This may be continued for one to two months. (7) DMSA (succimer) is superior to EDTA. It is given in a dose of 10 mg/kg orally every 8 hours for 5 days, followed by the same dose every 12 hours for 14 days. (8) DMPS. (9) A diet poor in calcium, and ammonium chloride one g. ten times daily is given. By this lead deposited in the bones is mobilised into the blood and excreted. High doses of parathormone have similar effects. (10) Treat the symptoms on general lines.

Postmortem Appearances: They are not constant. A blue line may be seen on the gums. Paralysed muscles show fatty degeneration. The stomach and intestines may show ulcerative or haemorrhagic changes and are contracted and thickened. The liver and kidneys are contracted. The brain is very pale and greatly swollen. PAS-positive, pink-staining, homogeneous material may be seen in the perivascular spaces in the brain. The heart may be hypertrophied and there may be atheroma of the aorta and aortic valves. Bone marrow shows hyperplasia of leucoblasts and erythroblasts with a decrease in fat cells. Segmental demyelination of peripheral nerves may be seen. Eosinophilic intranuclear inclusions may be seen in hepatocytes and cells of the proximal tubules of the kidneys.

Cause of Death: In acute poisoning, death is due to gastroenteritis and subsequent shock. In chronic cases, malnutrition, intercurrent infection, failure of liver function, respiratory failure, renal failure and encephalopathy can all be the direct causes.

Absorption: Absorption of inorganic lead compounds from digestive tract is slow. Absorption is greater and more rapid by inhalation. Absorption from skin is poor. **Tetraethyl lead, and other alkylated compounds are absorbed from the skin.** Adults may consume up to 300 μg. of lead every day, but only about 10% of this is absorbed. Children absorb 50% of lead. Bullets or pellets lodged in joints, peritoneum, pericardium, or other soft tissues may result in lead poisoning. Accumulation and toxicity occurs if more than 0.5 mg/day is absorbed. Half life is 32 years in bone and 7 years in kidneys.

DISTRIBUTION: Lead is normally present in almost all tissues. It is a typical cumulative poison. In poisoning, liver, kidney and spleen among the soft tissues, show the highest concentration. The bones contain large amounts, and also hair and nails. Lead crosses the placenta. It is stored in the bones as phosphate and carbonate. The major proportion of lead in blood is found in the red cells. With continued exposure, lead gradually becomes fixed to bone as inert and insoluble lead phosphate and carbonate. High calcium levels favours storage, while calcium deficiency causes lead to be released into blood stream. Lead is drawn to those areas of skeleton that are growing most rapidly, such as femur, tibia, and radius. Dense transverse bands or lead lines extending across the metaphysis of the bones and iliac crest is significant. Lead lines seen on X-rays as densities are due to hypermineralisation. The width of the lead lines is related to the duration of the exposure. These lines reflect "bone growth arrest". They are seen only in heavy chronic poisoning (minimum 4 weeks). Multiple lead lines indicate repeated episodes of toxicity. They are most commonly seen between 2 to 5 years. Normal lead level in blood is <0.03 mg/l.

EXCRETION: Absorbed lead is excreted mostly in urine and also from epithelial tissues and sweat. A urinary excretion rate below 80 micrograms per day is normal.

TEST: Hydrochloric acid produces a white precipitate, soluble in boiling water, and crystallizing on cooling.

The Circumstances of Poisoning: Acute poisoning is very rare. Chronic poisoning is more common and is regarded as an industrial disease. (1) Homicidal poisoning is rare. (2) Accidental chronic poisoning occurs in workers with the metal. (3) It is not used for suicide. (4) Diachylon paste (lead oleate), or red lead is used locally for abortion. (5) Red lead is sometimes used alone or mixed with arsenic as a cattle poison. (6) Lead missiles remaining embedded in the tissues due to gunshot injuries may produce poisonous symptoms in 12 to 48 days.

COPPER

Copper as a metal is not poisonous. **Copper compounds are powerful inhibitors of enzymes.**

Poisonous Compounds: (1) Copper sulphate (blue vitriol) occurs in large, blue crystals. (2) Copper subacetate **(verdigris),** occurs in bluish-green masses or powder.

Absorption and Excretion: Copper is a normal constituent of the body. Copper content of the body is 150 mg. The safe daily intake of dietary copper is 2 to 3 mg. **It is absorbed through the lungs, mucous membranes and raw surfaces. It is excreted more by the bowels than by the kidneys and in traces in saliva, bile and milk.**

Signs and Symptoms: Symptoms appear in 15 to 30 minutes. There is a metallic taste, increased salivation, burning pain in the stomach with colicky abdominal pain, thirst, nausea, eructations and repeated vomiting. **The vomited matter is blue or green. There is diarrhoea with much straining;** motions are liquid and brown but not bloody. Oliguria, haematuria, albuminuria, acidosis and uraemia may occur. In severe cases haemolysis, haemoglobinuria, methaemoglobinaemia, jaundice, pancreatitis and cramps of legs or spasms and convulsions occur. The breathing is difficult, cold perspiration and severe headache occur. In some cases, paralysis of limbs is followed by drowsiness, insensibility, coma and death due to shock. Later deaths occur due to hepatic or renal failure or both.

Acute inhalation of a large dose of copper dusts or fumes can cause upper respiratory irritation resulting in sore throat and cough. Conjunctivitis, palpebral oedema and sinus irritation may also occur. Nasal mucous membrane may show atrophy with perforation. Exposure of the skin to copper compounds may cause an irritant contact dermatitis, and severe exposure may cause a greenish–blue discolouration of the skin.

Fatal Dose: Copper sulphate, 10–20 g.; copper subacetate, 15 to 30 g.

Fatal Period: One to three days.

Treatment: (1) Stomach wash with 1% solution of potassium ferrocyanide. (2) Emetics are contraindicated. (3) Demulcent drinks form insoluble albuminate of copper. (4) Haemodialysis is useful in the early stage of poisoning. (5)

Castor oil is given to remove poison from intestines. (6) Chelation with penicillamine or EDTA or BAL.

Postmortem Appearances: The skin may be yellow. Greenish-blue froth may be present at mouth and nostrils. The gastric mucosa and stomach contents are greenish or bluish. The gastric mucosa may be congested, swollen, inflamed, and occasionally eroded. The liver may be soft and fatty. Spontaneous haemolysis of blood and degenerative changes in proximal tubules of kidney may occur.

CHRONIC POISONING: It may occur in workers with the metal due to inhalation of dust or from food being contaminated with verdigris. Chronic inhalation of copper sulphate spray can cause vineyard sprayer's lung disease characterised by a histiocytic granulomatous lung. Chronic poisoning causes Wilson's disease.

The symptoms consist of gradual anaemia, green line on gums, nausea, vomiting, colic, diarrhoea, malaise, peripheral neuritis, degeneration and atrophy of muscle may occur.

The presence of copper deposits in the tissues is called CHALCOSIS. Copper may be deposited in the cornea resulting in a pigmented ring in the deeper layers. Chronic contact with swimming pool water containing algicidal copper chemicals can cause green hair discolouration.

TEST: Ammonium hydroxide gives a greenish-blue precipitate, which is soluble in excess and forms a blue solution.

The Circumstances of Poisoning: (1) It is rarely used for homicide because of the colour and taste. (2) Suicide cases are rare. (3) Accidental poisoning results from eating food contaminated with verdigris which is formed from the action of vegetable acids on copper cooking vessels which are not properly tinned on the inside. Ingestion of food to which copper has been added to keep the green colour of the vegetables may cause poisoning. Children sometimes swallow copper sulphate attracted by its colour. (4) Sometimes, the salts are taken internally for abortion. (5) Rarely it is used as a cattle poison.

IRON

ACTION: Increased capillary permeability, postarteriolar dilatation, release of hydrogen ions, inhibition of mitochondrial function and corrosive action on gastric mucosa. Unbound iron circulates freely and is distributed within the cells and disrupts physiological mechanisms.

SYMPTOMS: They are divided into four stages. Few hours after ingestion, vomiting, abdominal pain and haemorrhagic gastroenteritis, shock, acidosis and coma occur. The second stage sets in 6 to 24 hours in which patient is symptom free. In the third stage (24 to 48 hours) metabolic acidosis, jaundice, hypoglycaemia, shock, coma with hepatic and renal failure occurs. After one to two weeks, in the fourth stage late complications such as gastric stricture, and pyloric stenosis occur.

FATAL DOSE: 20 to 30 g.

FATAL PERIOD: 24 to 30 hours.

TREATMENT: (1) Stomach wash with 5% sodium bicarbonate solution. Instil 5 to 10 g. of desferrioxamine at the end of lavage. (2) Give plenty of egg and milk to form iron-protein complexes. (3) Magnesium hydroxide 1% solution orally. (4) Desferrioxamine 1g. i.m. followed by 500 mg 4th hourly for 2 doses and finally 500 mg 4 to 12 hourly up to a maximum of 6 g. in 24 hours. It can also be given in infusion 15 mg/kg/hr in normal saline. (5) Haemodialysis or exchange transfusion in severe cases.

P.M. APPEARANCES: In severe cases gastric mucosa shows haemorrhagic necrosis and perforation of the gastric or jejunal wall. The liver may show acute hepatic necrosis and the kidneys degenerative tubular changes.

THALLIUM

Thallium sulphate and thallium acetate are important salts, which are odourless, tasteless and water-soluble. They are used in the dye and glass industries and as rodenticides and insecticides.

SYMPTOMS: They occur after one to 12 days after a therapeutic dose due to overdose or idiosyncracy. In mild cases joint pains in legs and feet, loss of appetite, stomatitis, and drowsiness occur, which pass off in a few days. In severe cases, there is colic, vomiting, pain in muscles, joints and nerves, lethargy, motor and sensory neuropathies, convulsions, psychosis, optic neuritis, tremors, delirium and coma. Hair loss occurs after one to two weeks. Large tufts tend to come away. Loss of outer third of eyebrows is said to be very significant. There may be cardiac manifestations. Maculopapular skin eruption having butterfly distribution on face is characteristic. There may be Mees lines on the nails. Death occurs due to respiratory failure due to paralysis of respiratory muscles. After recovery, the patient may suffer from peripheral neuritis resembling Guillain-Barre polyneuritis. Death appears natural. It can be seen radiologically in the intestines and is deposited in the liver.

FATAL DOSE: 1 g.

FATAL PERIOD: 24 to 36 hours.

CHRONIC POISONING: Thallium triad is characterised by alopecia, skin rashes, painful peripheral neuropathy and mental confusion with lethargy.

TREATMENT: (1) Stomach wash with one percent potassium iodide or Prussian blue. (2) Activated charcoal. (3) Prussian blue (potassium ferric cyanoferrate) 250 mg/kg/day orally in two divided doses. (4) Haemodialysis along with haemoperfusion. (5) Forced diuresis.

P.M. APPEARANCES: Signs of asphyxia are present. Mucosa of stomach may be inflamed with submucous petechial haemorrhages. Alopecia, stomatitis, fatty heart and liver, renal damage, pulmonary and cerebral oedema are seen. It can be detected in the ashes of the burnt body.

MANGANESE

The important compounds of manganese are potassium permanganate and manganese dioxide. Parkinsonism symptoms are produced by inhalation of vapour of manganese for a long time.

POTASSIUM PERMANGANATE

It occurs as dark-purple, slender crystals, and has a sweet astringent taste. It is a powerful oxidising agent and is used as a disinfectant.

ACTION: In strong solution or in the solid state, it acts as a corrosive or strong irritant, while after absorption it causes paralysis of the heart. It causes coagulation necrosis and brown discolouration of mucous membranes.

SIGNS AND SYMPTOMS: Burning pain from the mouth to the stomach, nausea, vomiting, intense thirst, difficulty in speaking or swallowing, dyspnoea, stridor, and a persistent spasmodic cough. The lips, gums, teeth, tongue, tonsils and pharynx are discoloured, inflamed, and superficially corroded. If seen soon after poisoning, the colour is purple-brown, but it becomes brown or dark-brown in few minutes, and later coal-black due to the formation of manganese dioxide. Shock is sometimes severe and there may be immediate collapse.

FATAL DOSE: 5 to 10 g.

FATAL PERIOD: Few hours.

TREATMENT: (1) Gastric lavage should be continued until the washings are colourless; 20% sodium thiosulphate should be used for the initial washings. (2) Demulcents. (3) Medicinal charcoal. (4) Symptomatic.

POISONING: (1) Poisoning is usually suicidal. (2) Accidental poisoning may occur in children who may eat the crystals in mistake for sweets. (3) It is sometimes taken orally as an abortifacient. (4) It is

rarely used to produce fictitious injuries, e.g., to simulate the lesions of tertiary syphilis by applying a tablet to the skin for 10 to 20 minutes. (5) Sometimes, a tablet is inserted into the vagina to procure abortion which causes ulceration of vaginal wall or cervix.

BARIUM

POISONOUS COMPOUNDS: (1) Barium chloride: (colourless rhombic crystals). (2) Barium nitrate. (3) Barium carbonate: It is used as a rat poison. (4) Barium sulphate: It is a heavy, white, tasteless, odourless powder. It is used for the X-ray examination of the gastrointestinal tract. It is insoluble. (5) Barium sulphide (greyish-black powder). It is a deadly poison and used as a depilatory.

ACTION: It acts locally as an irritant of almost corrosive degree. After absorption it acts especially on muscle, including heart muscle.

SIGNS AND SYMPTOMS: The first effects are those of severe gastrointestinal irritation, namely nausea, vomiting and diarrhoea. It causes cramps and stiffness of the muscles, dilation of the pupil, paralysis of the tongue and larynx, and vertigo. The heart is affected early, the blood pressure rises, the pulse is slow and irregular and the heart may stop in systole. The most characteristic changes are an areflexia and paralysis.

FATAL DOSE: About 1 g.

FATAL PERIOD: Usually within 12 hours.

TREATMENT: (1) Wash-out the stomach. (2) 10 ml. of 10% sodium sulphate i.v. every 15 minutes to convert the soluble salt into insoluble sulphate. (2) Repeated bowel wash. (3) Symptomatic.

ANTIMONY

Metallic antimony is not poisonous. Antimony potassium tartrate (tartar emetic), occurs in the form of whitish or whitish-yellow powder, and antimony trichloride (butter of antimony) are poisonous. The mode of action and symptoms of acute and chronic poisoning are similar to those produced by arsenic.

FATAL DOSE: Tartar emetic 0.2 to 0.5 g.; antimony trichloride 0.1 to 0.2 g.

FATAL PERIOD: Usually within 24 hours.

TREATMENT: (1) Stomach wash. (2) Tannic acid 4 g. by mouth forms an insoluble antimony tannate. (3) B.A.L. (4) Symptomatic.

NICKEL: Exposure causes lung cancer.

CADMIUM poisoning causes proteinuria and painful bone lesions known as Ouch-Ouch disease.

METAL FUME FEVER: It is caused by inhalation of fumes of zinc, copper, magnesium, nickel, mercury, lead, iron, silver, chromium, cadmium, cobalt, antimony and manganese. The syndrome resembles a flue-like illness which starts 6 to 8 hours after exposure of fumes, with fever, chills, cough, dyspnoea, cyanosis, myalgia, salivation, sweating and tachycardia. Symptoms subside in 36 hours after stoppage of exposure.

CHAPTER

28 INORGANIC IRRITANT POISONS

FM 9.2: Describe general principles and basic methodologies in treatment of poisoning: decontamination, supportive therapy, antidote therapy, procedures of enhanced elimination with regard to phosphorus, iodine, barium.

PHOSPHORUS (P_4)

Varieties: There are two varieties: (1) White or crystalline. It is used in fertilisers, insecticides, rodenticides, incendiary bombs, smoke screens, fireworks, etc. (2) Red or amorphous Table (28–1).

Action: It is **protoplasmic poison, which affects cellular oxidation**.

Signs and Symptoms:

(1) Fulminating Poisoning: This is seen when more than one gram is taken. These patients usually die within twelve hours due to shock and cardiovascular collapse because phosphorus has a direct action on the heart and blood vessels. Those who survive more than twelve hours are restless, delirious and some maniacal before death. Thirst, severe nausea, vomiting and retching occur.

(2) Acute Poisoning: (A) First Stage: Due to local irritation, symptoms occur within a few minutes to few hours after exposure and last from 8 hours to three days. Ingestion produces burning pain in the throat and abdomen, with intense thirst, nausea, vomiting, diarrhoea and severe abdominal pain. **Breath and excreta have garlic-like odour. Luminescent vomit and faeces are diagnostic.** Skin contact produces painful penetrating second and third degree burns which heal slowly.

(b) Second Stage: This is a symptom-free period lasting for two to three days.

(3) Third Stage: Symptoms of systemic toxicity occur from absorbed poison. There is nausea, vomiting, diarrhoea, haematemesis, **liver tenderness and enlargement, jaundice, and pruritus.** Haemorrhages occur into skin, mucous membrane and viscera, due to injury of blood vessels and inhibition of blood clotting. Renal damage results in oliguria, haematuria, casts, albuminuria and sometimes anuria. **Involvement of central nervous system causes convulsions, delirium and coma.** If the patient survives, symptoms may persist for a long time. Death may result from shock, hepatic failure, central nervous system damage, haematemesis or renal insufficiency.

Fatal Dose: 60 to 120 mg.

Fatal Period: 2 to 8 days.

Treatment: (1) Gastric lavage using 1:5000 solution of **potassium permanganate oxidises phosphorus into phosphoric acid and phosphates, which are harmless.** (2) Activated charcoal adsorbs the poison. (3) Stomach can be washed with **0.2% copper sulphate solution or 0.2 g. of copper sulphate may be given every 5 minutes until vomiting occurs.** It coats the particles of phosphorus with a film of copper phosphide which is relatively harmless. As it has caustic properties and can cause acute copper poisoning adequate care should be taken. (4) **Vitamin K, 20 mg. i.v. in repeated doses** to combat hypoprothrombinaemia or blood transfusion. (5) The bowel should be evacuated with magnesium sulphate. (6) Wash out the bowel and repeat at intervals for several days. (7) Oil and fats should be avoided as they dissolve phosphorus and promote absorption. (8) Transfusion of glucose-saline and plasma with vitamins and noradrenaline is useful to protect the liver and to correct shock and dehydration. (9) If renal

Table (28–1). Difference between white and red phosphorus

	Trait	White phosphorus	Red phosphorus
(1)	Colour:	White or yellow.	Reddish-brown.
(2)	Appearance:	Translucent, waxy cylinders.	Amorphous, solid mass.
(3)	Smell:	Garlicky.	Odourless.
(4)	Taste:	Garlicky.	Tasteless.
(5)	Luminosity:	Luminous in the dark.	Non-luminous.
(6)	Exposure to air:	Oxidises and emits white fumes; ignites at 34°C. and as such kept under water.	Non-oxidised, non-fuming, non-inflammable.
(7)	Use:	Fertilisers, vermin-killers, rodenticide, fireworks, gunpowder, etc.	On the sides of match box.
(8)	Toxicity:	Highly toxic.	Non-toxic.

failure is severe, peritoneal or haemodialysis may be required. (10) Burns should be thoroughly washed with 1% copper sulphate solution in water.

Postmortem Appearances: There may be no obvious changes in fulminating poisoning. However, the oesophagus, stomach and intestines may show signs of irritation and luminous material may be found in the stomach. **In acute poisoning, the body usually shows signs of jaundice. The gastric and intestinal contents may smell of garlic and be luminous.** The mucous membranes of the stomach and intestine are yellowish or greyish-white in colour, and are softened, thickened, inflamed and corroded or destroyed in patches. Multiple smaller or larger haemorrhages are seen in the skin, subcutaneous tissues, muscles, and serosal and mucosal membranes of gastrointestinal and respiratory tract, under endocardium, pericardium, epicardium, peritoneum, in lungs, brain, leptomeninges and uterus. **The liver becomes swollen, yellow, soft, fatty and is easily ruptured.** Small haemorrhages may be seen on the surface and in the substance. **In persons who survive for a week or longer, the appearances of acute yellow atrophy are present Table (28–2).** The kidneys are large, greasy, yellow and show haemorrhages on the surface. The heart is flabby, pale and shows fatty degeneration. Fat emboli may be found in the pulmonary arterioles and capillaries. The blood may appear tarry and its coagulability is diminished. Phosphorus is oxidised in the body.

Chronic Poisoning: The frequent inhalation of fumes over a period of years causes necrosis of the lower jaw in the region of a decayed tooth. **The vapours act on the jaw through a carious tooth or an interspace due to missing tooth where suppurative microorganisms are already present. At first there is toothache, which is followed by swelling of the jaw, loosening of the teeth, necrosis of gums, and sequestration of bone in the mandible. This condition is known as 'phossy jaw'** (glass jaw) **in which osteomyelitis and necrosis of the jaw occurs, with multiple sinuses discharging foul-smelling pus.**

The systemic symptoms are: nausea, vomiting, anorexia, pain in the stomach, indigestion, purging, pain in the joints, loss of weight, bronchitis, jaundice and anaemia.

The Circumstances of Poisoning: (1) Accidental poisoning in children may occur due to chewing of fireworks or by eating rat paste. (2) Phosphorus is occasionally used for homicide mixed with alcohol, coffee, etc. to diminish the taste and smell and administered for the following reasons. (a) There is delay in the appearance of symptoms. (b) Death occurs after few days. (c) Symptoms resemble acute liver disease. (d) The poison is oxidised in the body, if the patient survives long and as such cannot be detected. (3) Sometimes it is taken by mouth or introduced into the vagina to produce abortion. (4) Cases of poisoning may occur during war due to the phosphorus entering the body with fragments of hand grenades, bombs, bullets, etc. (5) For arson, white phosphorus covered with dung or wet cloth is thrown on huts. When the covering becomes dry, the roof catches fire.

IODINE

It occurs as bluish-black, soft and scaly crystals and has a metallic lustre and an unpleasant taste. It gives off a violet-coloured vapour at all temperatures, which has a characteristic odour.

ACTION: It is a protoplasmic poison fixing protein and causing necrosis. Vapours irritate respiratory passages.

SIGNS AND SYMPTOMS: Inhalation produces glottic and pulmonary oedema. Swallowed in the solid form, it acts as an acid corrosive poison. There is burning pain extending from the mouth to the stomach, intense thirst, salivation, vomiting, purging, giddiness, cramps or convulsive movements of the limbs and fainting. The lips and the angles of the mouth are stained brown. The vomited matter and excreta are dark-yellow or blue in colour, contain blood and have the peculiar odour of iodine. The urine is scanty or suppressed, red-brown in colour, contains albumen; metabolic acidosis, nephritis and renal failure occur. Pulse is slow and weak, skin cold and clammy and there may be skin rashes.

FATAL DOSE: 2 to 4 g. (30 to 60 ml. of tincture).

FATAL PERIOD: 24 hours.

TREATMENT: (1) Evacuate the stomach by emetics or wash it out with warm water containing soluble starch and albumen. (2) 1 to 5% solution of sodium thiosulphate will convert tincture of iodine to harmless iodide. (3) Sodium chloride will promote excretion of iodide, as chlorides compete with iodide at the level of the tubules, thereby reducing the effects of iodism. (4) Give alkalis, arrow root, and barley water and treat symptomatically. (5) Activated charcoal binds iodine. (6) Skin lesion can be treated with 20% alcohol.

POSTMORTEM APPEARANCES: The mucosa of the stomach and intestines is inflamed, excoriated and may be brown. The heart, liver and kidneys may show fatty degeneration. There may be oedema of the brain.

CHRONIC POISONING: (Iodism): The symptoms are pain over the frontal sinus, running of the nose, conjunctivitis, bronchial catarrh, salivation, nausea, vomiting, purging, emaciation, lymphadenopathy, parotid swelling (iodide mumps), wasting of breasts, testes, etc., and acne or erythematous patches on the skin, urticaria, etc. (ioderma).

CHLORINE

It is a greenish-yellow gas having an unpleasant irritating odour. Exposure is likely only in laboratories, bleaching-powder factories and other chemical works. It is an oxidising agent and causes destruction of organic tissue.

SIGNS AND SYMPTOMS: When inhaled, it has an irritant and suffocative effect. The symptoms of acute poisoning are intense irritation of the eyes and throat and mucous membrane of respiratory passages, with violent coughing and extreme dyspnoea, nausea, vomiting and spasm of the glottis. Death is caused by cardiac failure following inflammatory oedema of the lungs and pulmonary congestion. Chronic inhalation in repeated small doses may give rise to a chronic condition resulting in anaemia, cachexia, dental caries and progressive wasting.

FATAL DOSE: Exposure to one part in 1000 may prove fatal in five minutes.

Table (28–2). Difference in liver between phosphorus poisoning and acute yellow atrophy

	Trait	Phosphorus poisoning	Acute yellow atrophy
(1)	Size:	Enlarged at first, later may be normal or contracted.	Smaller, irregular, with a wrinkled capsule.
(2)	Colour:	Marbled.	Bright-yellow in earlier stage; deep-red later.
(3)	Consistency:	Soft, greasy and friable.	Very soft and flabby.
(4)	Structure:	Fatty degeneration of liver with some cellular necrosis; small haemorrhages on the surface and in the substance.	Disintegration and necrosis of most cells. Supporting connective tissue is not damaged.

FATAL PERIOD: **Within two days.**

TREATMENT: **The victim should be removed from the poisonous atmosphere. Treat the shock, circulatory collapse and pulmonary oedema.**

POSTMORTEM APPEARANCES: **These are mainly asphyxial. There is inflammation of the respiratory tract, pulmonary oedema, rupture of alveolar walls, haemorrhages and thrombosis in the lung beds and increased viscosity of the blood.**

IRRITANT MECHANICAL POISONS

They are not absorbed into the body, but **they act mechanically and have only local** action, and cause irritation of the gastrointestinal canal when swallowed. Powdered glass, diamond powder, pins, needles, nails, chopped animal and vegetable hair are the examples.

POWDERED GLASS

Symptoms: There is sharp burning pain in the throat, stomach and intestines, nausea, vomiting, usually constipation but rarely diarrhoea. Death may result from shock, if stomach or the intestine is perforated. The fatal dose and fatal period are uncertain.

Treatment: Give bulky food and later emetics and purgatives.

Postmortem Appearances: Erosions may be seen extending from the mouth to the upper part of small intestine. The mucosa of the stomach is covered with sticky mucus and the glass particles may be found in the stomach and intestines. The mucosa of the gastrointestinal tract is congested and may be inflamed.

Medicolegal Importance: It is rarely used for suicide or homicide. It is taken in powdered form mixed with some articles of food. Occasionally, it is used as a cattle poison.

CHAPTER

29

ORGANIC IRRITANT POISONS

FM 11.1: Describe features and management of snake bite, scorpion sting, bee and wasp sting and spider bite.

PLANT TOXINS: Kingsbury has outlined a variety of compounds produced in or absorbed by plants which may cause toxic reactions when ingested by animals.

(1) Alcohols. (2) Alkaloids. (3) Polypeptides. (4) Amines. (5) Glycosides: (a) Cyanogenetic. (b) Goitrogenic. (c) Irritant oils. (d) Coumarins. (e) Steroids and triterpenoids. (i) Cardiac. (ii) Saponins. (6) Oxalates. (7) Resins or resinoids. (8) Phytotoxins. (9) Minerals: (a) Copper. (b) Lead. (c) Cadmium. (d) Fluorine. (10) Nitrogen: (a) Nitrites. (b) Nitrates. (c) Nitroses. (d) Gaseous oxides of nitrogen. (11) Compounds causing photosensitivity: (a) Primary photosensitisation. (b) Hepatogenic photosensitisation.

A **toxalbumens:** Toxalbumens are a group of toxic albumins found in certain plants, bacteria and snake venon. They block protein synthesis by inhibition of RNA polymerase II in ribosomes. They are cytotoxic and vasculotoxic. There may be haemorrhagic tendencies and produce disseminated intravascular coagulation. Phytoxin is a toxin produced by plants. Ricin, cortin and abrin are phytotoxins. Snake and scorpion venoms are animal toxalbumens.

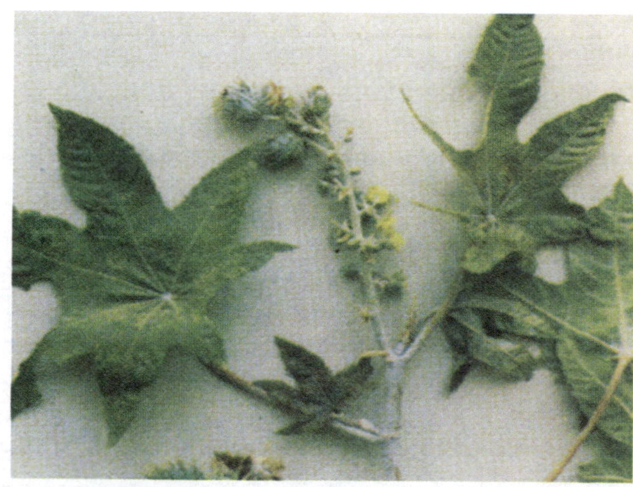

Fig. (29–1). Ricinus communis plant with seeds.

RICINUS COMMUNIS

Physical Characters: The castor plant ***(arandi)*** grows all over India. Fruit is 1.2 to 2.5 cm. long, three-lobed, softly spiny, blue-green or rose-red when immature, brown and bristly when ripe and dry. Seeds are variable, smooth, flattened–oval, mottled, light and dark-brown, or white with yellow-brown or gray markings, or wholly black or red. They are of two sizes, big and small. The small seeds are about 1.2 cm. long and 0.8 cm. broad, and resemble croton seeds **Figs. (29–1 and 29–2)**.

Active Principles: Entire plant is poisonous, though seeds are most poisonous, containing toxalbumen ricin, a water-soluble glycoprotein (highest level in the seeds), and a powerful allergen (CBA). The seeds are rich in a purgative oil, which is pale-yellow with a faint odour and acrid taste.

The unbroken seeds are non-poisonous when swallowed and also when cooked. The 'press cake' contains ricin and is poisonous, whereas **castor oil** contains ricinoleic acid but not toxalbumen and **is not poisonous** as it does not contain ricin.

Action: Ricin has a special binding protein that allows it to gain access to the endoplasmic reticulum in gastrointestinal mucosal cells causing severe diarrhoea. **It can be absorbed through inhalation, ingestion, injection and through skin contact.**

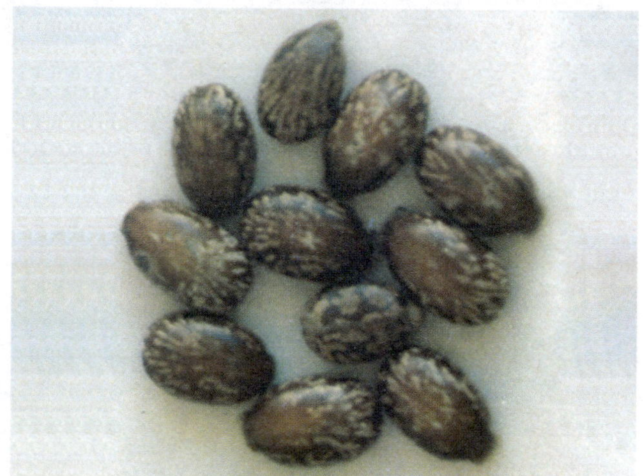

Fig. (29–2). Ricinus communis seeds.

Signs and Symptoms: Dust of the seeds may cause watering of the eyes, conjunctivitis, sneezing, acute nasal inflammation, headache, pharyngitis, asthmatic bronchitis, dermatitis and gastric upset.

Symptoms include burning in mouth, throat and stomach. Burns of the oral mucosa appear similar to an alkali burn. Salivation, nausea, vomiting, bloody diarrhoea, severe abdominal pain, thirst, impaired sight, weak rapid pulse, cramps in calves and abdominal muscles, haemolysis, drowsiness, delirium, convulsions, shallow breathing, uraemia, jaundice, dehydration, collapse and death. It is poorly absorbed, with its full effect taking up to 5 days. **Ricin is excreted by the intestinal epithelium.**

Fatal Dose: 5 to 10 seeds; ricin 60 mg

Fatal Period: Two to five days.

Treatment: Gastric lavage; activated charcoal, whole bowel irrigation, demulcents, cathartics and symptomatic.

POSTMORTEM APPEARANCES: The mucosa of the gastrointestinal canal is congested, softened and inflamed with occasional erosions and submucous haemorrhages. Ricin produces haemorrhagic inflammation of the gastrointestinal tract even when given subcutaneously. Dilation of the heart, haemorrhages in the pleura, pericardium, oedema of the liver, kidneys, spleen and lungs are seen. Fragments of seeds may be found in the stomach or intestines. There may be haemorrhages in the internal organs.

The Circumstances of Poisoning: (1) Accidental poisoning may occur in children from eating the seeds. (2) Rarely the powdered seeds are given for homicide. (3) The powder of seeds causes conjunctivitis when applied to the eye. (4) Its use by terrorists might involve poisoning of water or food, inoculation via ricin-laced projectiles, or aerolisation of liquid ricin or distribution of a powder.

CROTON TIGLIUM

Seeds: **The seeds of croton** *(jamalgota, jaipala, naepala)* **contain crotin, a toxalbumen.** Seeds are oval, dark-brown with longitudinal lines Fig. (29–3). They have no smell. **Crotonoside,** a glycoside, which is less poisonous is also present.

Oil: The oil is brown, viscid, has unpleasant odour and acrid, burning taste but does not contain toxalbumen. The oil contains a powerful vesicating resin composed of **crotonoleic acid,** methyl crotonic acid and several other fatty acids.

Signs and Symptoms: There is hot burning pain from mouth to stomach, salivation, vomiting, purging, vertigo, prostration, collapse and death. **Applied to the skin, the oil produces burning, redness and vesication.**

Fatal Dose: 4 to 5 seeds; one to two ml. oil.

Fatal Period: Six hours to three days.

Treatment: Stomach wash, demulcent drink, and symptomatic.

Postmortem Appearances: There is congestion, inflammation and erosion of the mucosa of stomach and intestines, and congestion of internal organs.

Circumstances of Poisoning: (1) Accidental poisoning results from swallowing croton oil by mistake, or when taken in large doses as a purgative, or by eating seeds or inhaling their dust. (2) Suicide and homicide are rare. (3) The root and oil are sometimes taken internally as an abortifacient. (4) Oil is used as arrow poison.

ABRUS PRECATORIUS

It is also known as jequirity, Indian liquorice, *rosary bead, gunchi or ratti.*

Seeds: The seeds are egg-shaped, bright scarlet colour with a large black spot at one end, 8 mm. long and 6 mm. broad, and weigh 105 mg. on an average. Seeds may be white with black spot, all black, yellow or blue Fig. (29–4).

Active Principles: **The seeds contain an active principle abrin, a toxalbumen, which is similar to viperine snake venom;** also present are **abrine** (N-methyltryptophan), an aminoacid, **haemoglutinin** in the cotyledons; **a lipolytic enzyme, and abralin,** a glucoside. All parts of the plant are poisonous. Seeds are tasteless and odourless. **Abrin inhibits protein synthesis and causes cell death.**

Signs and Symptoms: Symptoms may be delayed from a few hours to two or three days when taken by mouth. They include severe irritation of upper G.I. tract, abdominal pain, nausea, vomiting, bloody diarrhoea, weakness, cold perspiration, trembling of the hands, weak rapid pulse, miosis and rectal bleeding. Delayed cytotoxic effects occur in the CNS, liver, kidneys and adrenal glands 2 to 5 days after exposure.

Animal Poisoning: **When an extract of seeds is injected under the skin of the animal,** inflammation, oedema, oozing

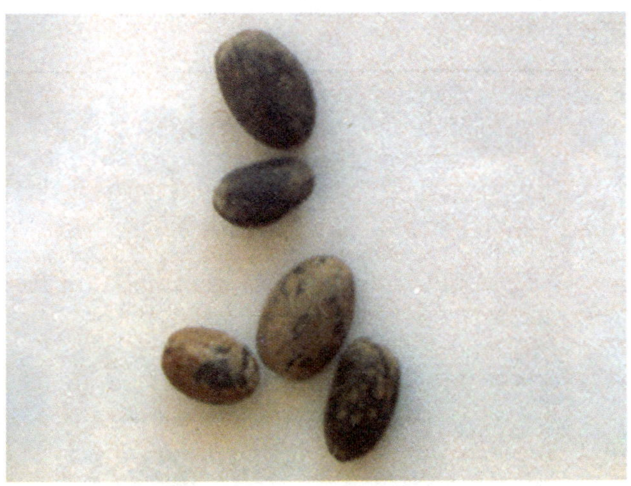

Fig. (29–3). **Croton tiglium.**

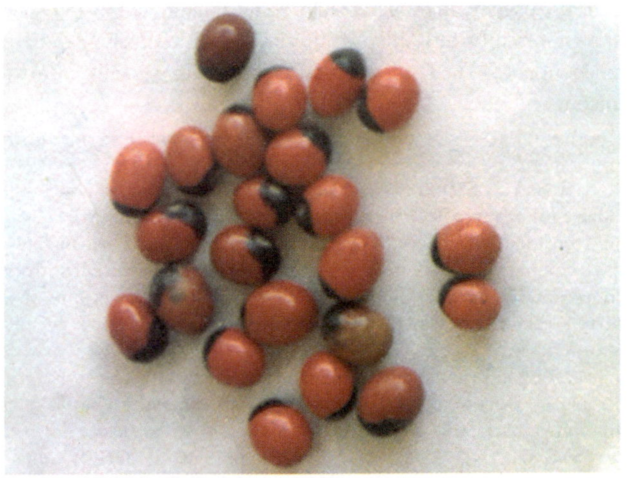

Fig. (29–4). **Abrus precatorius.**

of haemorrhagic fluid from the site of puncture, and sometimes necrosis occurs surrounding the site of injection. The animal does not take food and drops down after three to four days and cannot move. Tetanic convulsions occur or the animal becomes cold, drowsy or comatose and dies. **The symptoms resemble those of viperine snake bite, and as such poisoning is not suspected by the owner.**

Human Poisoning: In man, **at the site of injection, painful swelling and ecchymosis develops, with inflammation and necrosis.** Ingestion of seeds or extract can cause haemorrhagic gastritis. There is faintness, vertigo, vomiting, dyspnoea, and general prostration. Convulsions may precede death from cardiac failure.

Fatal Dose: 90 to 120 mg. (one to 2 seeds) by injection abrin 20–70 µg. **Subcutaneously abrin is 100 times as toxic as by the oral route.**

Fatal Period: Three to five days.

Treatment: (1) Gastric lavage. (2) Activated charcoal. (3) Purgative. (4) Antiabrin is completely ineffective and is not recommended. (5) The needle should be dissected out. (6) Sodium bicarbonate 10 g. orally per day helps in maintaining alkalinity of urine and prevents agglutination of red cells and blocking of renal tubules with haemoglobin G.

Postmortem Appearances: Fragments of the needle may be found. There is oedema at the site of injection, and petechial haemorrhages under the skin, pleura, pericardium and peritoneum. The internal organs are congested and show haemorrhages.

The Circumstances of Poisoning: (1) **The seeds are used for killing cattle and rarely for homicide.** The cattle are poisoned by leather workers to obtain hides cheaply or for revenge. **The seeds are decorticated, and alone or mixed with datura, opium and onion, are made into paste with spirit and water, and small sharp-pointed spikes or needles or *'suis'* are prepared, which are then dried in the sun. The needles are 15 mm. long and weigh 90 to 120 mg. Two needles are inserted by their base into holes in a wooden handle. A blow is struck to the animal with great force which drives the needle into the flesh.** (2) **For homicide, the needle is kept between two fingers, and the person is slapped which drives the needle into the body.** (3) Powdered seeds are used by malingerers to produce conjunctivitis. (4) When taken internally they disturb the uterine function and prevent conception. (5) The seeds are used as an abortifacient and as arrow poison.

ERGOT

CHARACTERISTICS: Ergot is the dried sclerotinum of the fungus Claviceps purpurea, which grows on cereals like rye, barley, wheat, oats, etc. It gradually replaces the grain forming a curved, dark-purple or black compact mass, 0.9 to one cm. long, half cm. thick, with lengthwise ridges, and has peculiar odour and disagreeable taste. It contains about thirty alkaloids, but ergotoxine, ergotamine and ergometrine (ecbolics) are important.

ACTION: Ergot alkaloids exert their primary effect by stimulating adrenergic receptors, both peripherally and centrally. They directly stimulate muscle fibres.

SIGNS AND SYMPTOMS: In acute cases, there is nausea, vomiting, diarrhoea, giddiness, tightness in the chest, difficulty in breathing, marked muscular weakness and exhaustion. There may be tingling and numbness in the hands and feet, paraesthesias, followed by twitchings or cramps in the muscles. Bleeding from the nose and other mucous surfaces is common after large doses. The pulse is rapid and weak, pupils are dilated with dimness of vision, blood pressure is raised.

CHRONIC POISONING (ergotism): There is tingling and numbness of the skin; vasomotor disturbances leading to dry gangrene of the fingers, toes, ears, nose, etc. There is a sensation of insects creeping under the skin. Neurologic disorder characterised by hallucinations, ataxia, and convulsions may occur.

FATAL DOSE: 5 to 10 g.

FATAL PERIOD: One to several days.

TREATMENT: (1) Wash the stomach. (2) Activated charcoal. (3) Syrup of ipecac. (4) Cathartics. (5) Nitroprusside for hypertension and severe ischaemic changes. (6) Diazepam 0.1 mg./kg. i.v. slowly for convulsions. (7) Vasodilators, e.g. nitrites are useful.

POSTMORTEM APPEARANCES: They are not characteristic. The internal organs are congested. There is degeneration of intima of smaller arterioles and thrombus formation.

POISONING: The consumption of bread made with contaminated rye is the chief cause of ergotism. Ergot is commonly used as an abortifacient.

CAPSICUM ANNUM

Capsicum or chillies *(red pepper; lal mirch chili)* have a pungent odour and taste, and are used as a condiment. They are not fatal. The active principles are capsaicin (alkaloid) and capsicin.

SIGNS AND SYMPTOMS: In large doses, it acts as an irritant poison and causes difficulty in swallowing, pain in the stomach and inflammation of oesophagus and stomach. Applied to the skin or mucosa it causes irritation. Powder thrown in the eyes causes severe irritation leading to lachrymation, burning pain and redness.

TREATMENT: (1) Bathe affected skin in vinegar or ice-cold water. (2) If ingested, sucking of ice cubes, or sips of ice-cold water. (3) Demulcents.

Criminal Uses: (1) Powder is thrown into the eyes to facilitate robbery. (2) When theft or confession of some guilt has to be obtained, the person is tortured by introducing the powder into vagina, rectum or urethra or by rubbing on the female breasts.

SEMECARPUS ANACARDIUM

Characteristics: Marking nuts *(bhilwa)* are balck, heart-shaped with rough projection at the base Fig. (29–5). They have a thick, cellular pericarp, which contains an irritant juice which is brownish, oily and acrid but turns black on exposure to air. **The active principles are semecarpol (0.1%) and bhilawanol** (15 to 17%). The juice is commonly used by washermen to put marks on clothes.

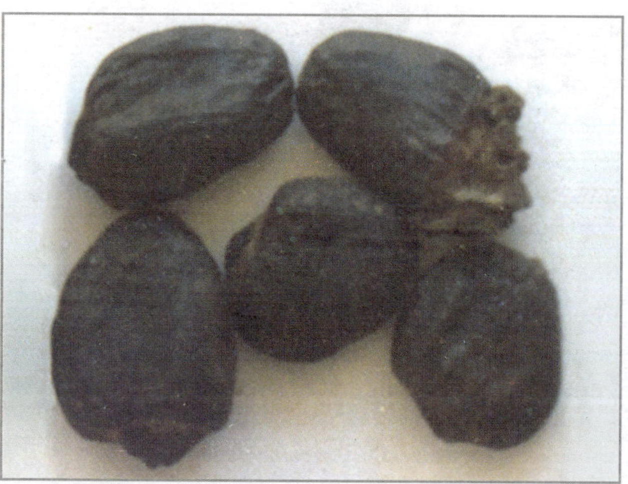

Fig. (29–5). Semecarpus.

Signs and Symptoms: Applied externally, the juice causes irritation and a painful blister which contains acrid serum, which produces eczematous eruptions of the neighbouring skin with which it comes into contact, and there is itching. **The lesion resembles a bruise. Later an ulcer is produced,** and there may be sloughing.

Taken by mouth, the juice causes less irritant action. In large dose, it produces blisters on throat and severe gastrointestinal irritation, dyspnoea, tachycardia, hypotension, cyanosis, absence of reflexes, delirium, coma and death.

Fatal Dose: Five to ten g.

Fatal Period: 12 to 24 hours.

Treatment: (1) Gastric lavage. (2) Demulcent drinks. (3) When applied externally wash with lukewarm water containing antiseptic.

Postmortem Appearances: Blisters are seen in the mouth, throat and stomach which are congested and inflamed.

Circumstances of Poisoning: (1) Accidental poisoning may result from the administration of juice internally by quacks. (2) Homicidal and suicidal poisoning is rare. (3) Sometimes, the juice is introduced into the vagina as a punishment for infidelity. (4) To support a false charge of assault **the juice is applied to skin which produces lesions simulating bruises.** (5) The juice may be thrown on the body to cause injury. (6) For criminal abortion, the bruised nut is applied to the cervical os. (7) Malingerers use the juice to produce ophthalmia.

CALOTROPIS GIGANTEA

Calotropis gigantea *(akdo, madar rakta arka)* has purple flowers and calotropis procera *(shveta arka)* has white flowers. They grow wild throughout India Fig. (29–6).

Active Principles: The active principles are **uscharin, calotoxin, calactin and calotropin** (glycoside). The milky juice in addition contains trypsin. The leaves and stem when incised yield thick acrid, milky juice.

Signs and Symptoms: Applied to the skin, it causes redness and vesication. When taken by mouth, the juice produces an acrid bitter taste, and burning pain in throat and stomach, salivation, stomatitis, vomiting, diarrhoea, dilated pupils, tetanic convulsions, collapse and death.

Fatal Dose: Uncertain.

Fatal Period: 6 to 12 hours.

Treatment: Stomach wash, demulcents and symptomatic.

Postmortem Appearances: Dilated pupils, froth at the nostrils, stomatitis, and inflammation of gastrointestinal tract are seen. The abdominal viscera and brain are congested.

Circumstances of Poisoning: (1) The flowers, leaves, root and juice are used in Indian medicine. (2) The juice is taken by mouth or introduced into uterus on an abortion stick for **criminal abortion**. (3) It is sometimes used for infanticide and rarely for suicide or homicide. (4) Juice is used as a vesicant, depilatory and for chronic skin infection. (5) As a cattle poison, it is smeared on a cloth and pushed into the rectum of the animal, or is given with fodder. (6) It is sometimes used as arrow poison. (7) **The root of calotropis procera is highly poisonous to cobras, and other poisonous snakes, which cannot stand even its smell.**

PLUMBAGO ROSEA *(lal chitra)* and PLUMBAGO ZEYLANICA *(chitra)*

The root contains as an active principle, plumbagin, a crystalline glycoside. All parts of the plant are poisonous.

Fatal Dose: Uncertain.

Fatal Period: Few days.

Symptoms: Applied externally, roots produce irritation and blisters. Taken internally, there is burning pain from mouth to stomach, vomiting, thirst, diarrhoea, collapse and death.

Treatment: Stomach wash, demulcents and symptomatic.

Postmortem Appearances: Signs of gastroenteritis and congestion of internal organs are found.

Circumstances of Poisoning: (1) Roots are taken by mouth or applied as paste to the cervix or to abortion stick for criminal abortion. (2) Roots are rarely used for homicide.

CANTHARIDES

The Spanish fly (blister beetle) is two cm. long, and 0.6 cm. broad Fig. (29–7). The powder of the dried body is greyish-brown and contains shiny green particles. The active principle is cantharidin. It is used externally as an irritant. The Indian fly (beetle) is 2.5 cm. long and 0.8 cm. broad. It contains about 2.9% cantharidin. Cantharidin is readily absorbed from all surfaces including the skin.

SYMPTOMS: Applied to the skin, redness and burning pain are produced after two to three hours followed by vesication. Taken internally, symptoms appear in half to two hours. There is burning

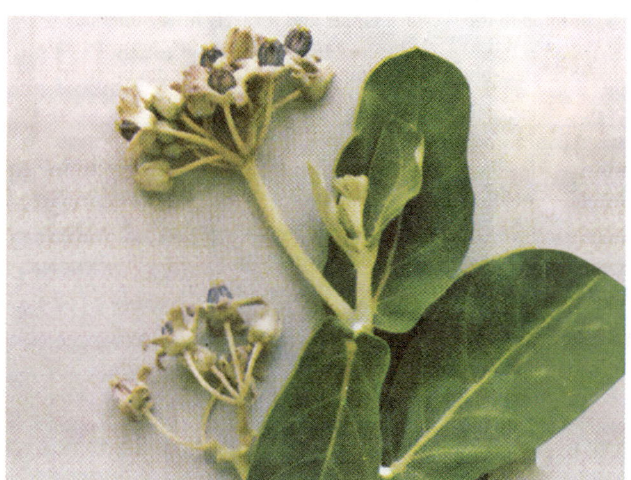

Fig. (29–6). **Calotropis giganta.**

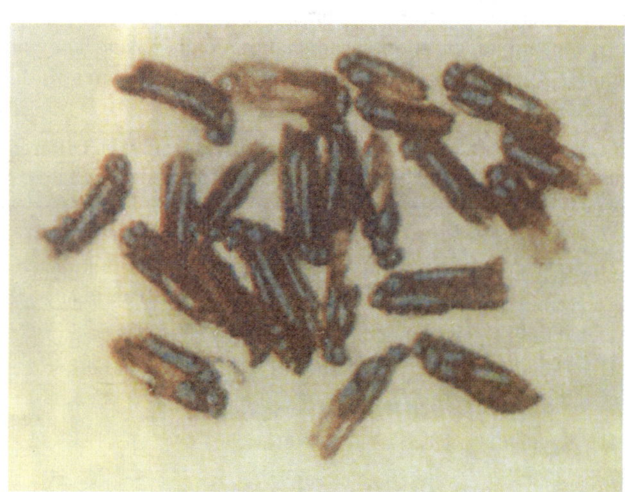

Fig. (29–7). **Spanish fly (Cantharis vesicatoria).**

sensation in the mouth and throat, followed by pain in the stomach, nausea and vomiting of bloody mucus, severe thirst, difficulty in swallowing and speech. Later a dull pain is felt in the loins, the urine is scanty and bloodstained, though there is an increased desire to pass urine. Priapism may occur; there is often tenesmus. Abortion occurs in pregnant women. In severe cases, the patient becomes prostrated, convulsions occur, and death may take place in a condition of coma.

FATAL DOSE: 30 to 50 mg. of cantharidin, or one-and-half to three g. of powdered cantharides.

FATAL PERIOD: 24 to 36 hours.

TREATMENT: Stomach wash, demulcents and symptomatic.

POSTMORTEM APPEARANCES: The mouth shows inflammation and sometimes vesication. The mucous membrane of the oesophagus is often swollen and engorged, and may show patches of ulceration. The mucosa of the stomach is markedly congested and shows petechial haemorrhages with foci of superficial erosion. These changes may extend to the upper portion of the small intestine. Particles of the insects may be found sticking to the mucosa. The kidneys are acutely inflamed and there is haemorrhage in the renal pelvis and bladder. The bladder mucosa is inflamed and ecchymoses may be present. The surface of the heart and endocardium show haemorrhages. The lungs may be oedematous, and the air-passages contain blood-stained mucus.

CIRCUMSTANCES OF POISONING: (1) Accidental poisoning may occur by its external application as counterirritant. (2) It is rarely used for homicidal purposes. (3) It is used as an aphrodisiac, but the action is doubtful. (4) It is taken for criminal abortion.

SNAKES

There are more than 3500 species of snakes, but only **about 250 are venomous. In India about 216 species are found, of which 52 are venomous.** According to WHO, there are more than 2.5 million venomous snake bites world-wide each year with more than 1,25,000 deaths. **In India only five of them are dangerously poisonous to man, i.e., king cobra, common cobra, common krait, Russell's viper and saw-scaled viper.** The most common venomous snake is common krait.

Classification: The venomous snake may be divided into five families. (1) **(A) Viperidae:** Russell's viper, gaboon viper, saw scaled viper, puff adder. They are found in all parts of the world except the Americas. **(B) Crotalidae**: Rattlesnakes, pigmy rattlesnakes, copperheads, cottonmouths (water moccasins), pit viper, and the massasaugas, bushmaster. They are found in Asia and the Americas. The water moccasin is found in swampy areas or along the banks of streams. It is a strong swimmer and can bite under water. (2) **Elapidae:** Cobras, kraits, mambas, tiger snake, taipan, death adder, copperhead snakes, coral snakes. They are found in all parts of the world except Europe. (3) **Hydrophidae or sea snakes:** All sea snakes are poisonous but they seldom bite. (4) **Colubridae:** Boomslangs, bird snake of the African continent. (5) **Atractaspididae:** African and Middle Eastern burrowing asps or stilleto snakes also known as burrowing or mole vipers or adders, or false vipers.

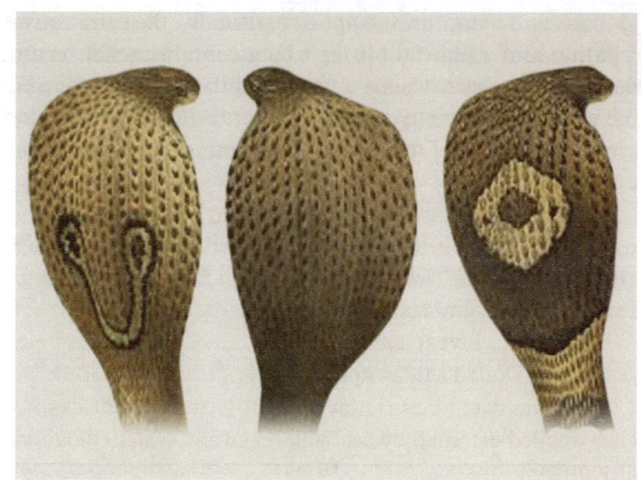

Fig. (29–8). Cobra: (1) Binocellate, (2) Black, (3) Monocellate.

COMMON VENOMOUS SNAKES: (1) THE COBRA *(nag, naja tripudians, naja naja, kala samp)* has a hood, which on dorsal side often bears a double or single spectacle mark, but it has sometimes an oval spot surrounded by an ellipse. Head scales are large and the third labial touches the eye and the nasal shield. The portion of the neck surrounding the spectacle mark is darker than the rest of the back, and is often speckled with small golden spots. The hood cannot be seen in a dead cobra, as the joints and neck become stiff. There are two black spots, and three black bands on the underside of the hood. The caudal scales are double. There is a white band in the region where the hood touches the body region. The colour is brown or dark Fig. (29–8). It grows to a length of about two metres. Maxillary bone extends beyond palate. Poison fangs are followed by one or two small teeth. The neck is dilatable. It is found throughout India. The monocled cobra (N. Kaouthia) is found in Bengal, Orissa, Madhya Pradesh, Uttar Pradesh and Sikkim. A third variety, the central Asian or black cobra (N.Oxiano) is found in J&K, Punjab, Rajasthan and Madhya Pradesh. Difference between cobra and viper is given in Table (29–1). (2) THE KING COBRA *(rajnag, nagraj, naja bungarus, humadryad)*, has a hood but no mark on it, and the length is about three to four metres. The colour may be yellow, green, brown or black and has yellowish or white cross-bands in the body. The tail scales are entirely present in their proximal ends, but divided in the distal ends. It is confined to the Western Ghats and it rarely bites humans. (3) THE COMMON KRAIT *(karayat, bungarus caerulus, manyar, kalotaro, kawriya)* is steel-blue, often shining and has single or double white bands

Table (29–1). Difference between cobra and viper

	Trait	Cobra	Viper
(1)	Body:	Long and cylindrical.	Short, narrow neck.
(2)	Head:	Small; seldom broader than body; covered by large scales or shields of special forms.	Large; broader than body; triangular and covered by numerous small scales.
(3)	Pupil:	Round.	Vertical.
(4)	Maxillary bone:	Carries poison fangs and other teeth.	Carries only poison fangs.
(5)	Fangs:	Grooved, short, fine.	Canalised, long.
(6)	Venom:	Neurotoxic.	Haemotoxic.
(7)	Tail:	Round.	Tapering.
(8)	Eggs:	Lay eggs.	Give birth to young ones.

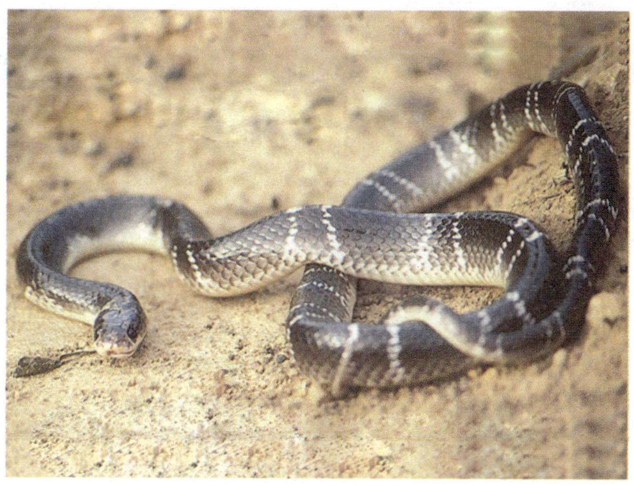

Fig. (29–9). Common krait (Bungarus carruleus).

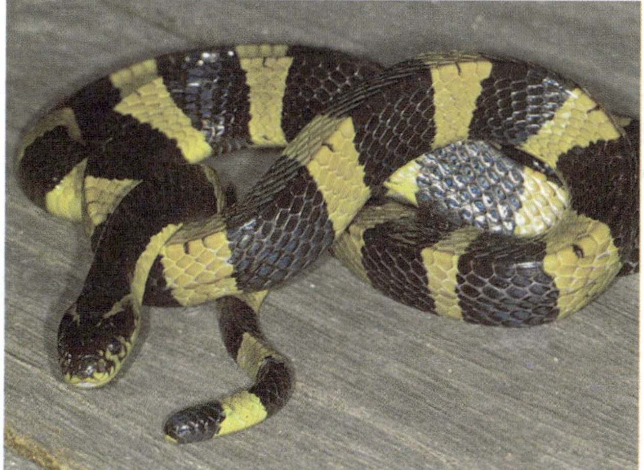

Fig. (29–10). Banded krait.

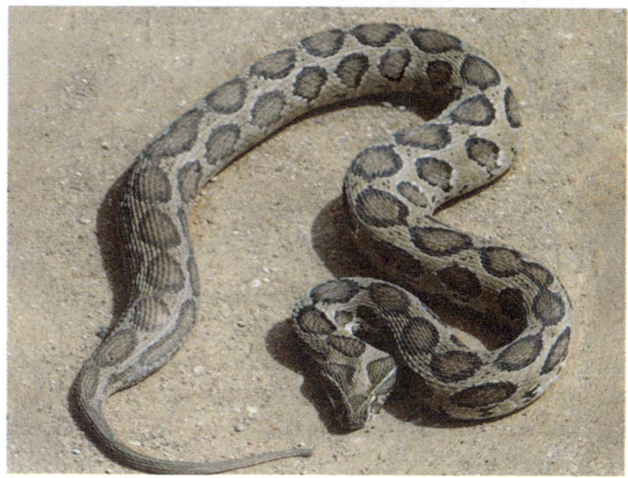

Fig. (29–11). Russell's viper.

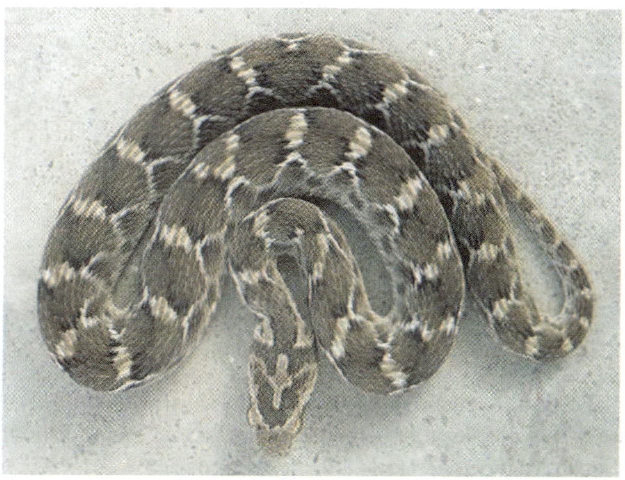

Fig. (29–12). Saw-scaled viper.

across the back, and a creamy-white belly. Its length is one to one-and-half metres. The stripes are not very distinct in the anterior region. The head is covered with large shields. Four shields are found on either side of the lower lip. The scales in the central row down the back are large and hexagonal. The tail is round. The plates under the tail like those on the belly are entire and not divided Fig. (29–9). These snakes are nocturnal in habit. They are seen throughout India. (4) THE BANDED KRAIT *(ahiraj, raj sanp, bungarus fasciatus, koelea krait)* is one-and-half to two metres in length. The tail ends bluntly and is swollen at the tip. It has a jet black five cm. wide cross-band alternating with a deep yellow band of the same size on its back. There is a black mark on the neck which is spread up to the eyes. The scales are hexagonal Fig. (29–10). They are found in Bengal, Orissa, Madhya Pradesh, Andhra, Assam. The newer kraits are Sind krait (B. Sindanus) found in Rajasthan; Wall's Sind krait (B. Sindanus Walli) found in Maharashtra, Bengal, Uttar Pradesh and Bihar and black krait (B. niger) found in North-East States, Sikkim, Bengal and Assam. These kraits have either no markings in the case of black krait or have less obviously paired, equally placed white bands, often with a large spot on the hexagonal scale. The hexagonal scale is a constant key identification throughout the krait species. It is usually found in North-Eastern States. (5) RUSSELL'S VIPER OR DABOIA *(kander, charn viper, khadchitro)* has a flat, heavy and triangular head with a white V-shaped mark, the angle of the V pointing forwards. It has three rows of diamond-shaped black or brown spots along the back, the outer two rows consisting of spots ringed with white edges. Its body is whitish with dark semilunar spots. It narrows towards its tail, which is short. It can be identified by the entire broad plates on the belly, the small scales on the head, and the shield beneath the tail divided into two rows Fig. (29–11). It is heard to hiss loudly and continuously. It is found throughout India. (6) THE SAW-SCALED VIPER *(afai, echis carinate)* is brown, half metre in length, and has wavy white line on each flank of the back with diamond-shaped areas between these two lines. It has a triangular head, the upper surface of which is covered with a white mark resembling a bird's foot-print or an arrow. The tail is short and tapering. The broad belly plates with brown or dark spots, small scales on the head, and entire shields beneath the tail are the distinguishing features Fig. (29–12). It is found in most parts of India. The northern sawscaled viper (Echis Sochureki) is found in Rajasthan, Gujarat and J&K. In the Western Ghats, the hump-nosed pit viper (Hypnale hypnale) is found which is poisonous. (7) PIT VIPERS have a pit located between the nostrils and the eyes.

Banded krait and common green pit viper (*bamboo snake*) are also venomous. Rat snake is not venomous.

Common krait, cobra, Russell's viper, and saw-scaled viper are seen all over India. Banded krait is seen mainly in East India, and King cobra in Western Ghats.

Sea Snakes: Twenty types are seen in Indian waters, all of them being venomous. They have small eyes, prominent nostrils on the top of the head, broad ventrals, small tuberculated dorsal scales and paddle-shaped flat tails. They are black, greenish-black or bluish-black with or without bands. They can be found is estuaries, rivers and even fresh water lakes.

Table (29–2). Difference between venomous and non-venomous snakes

	Trait	Venomous snakes	Non-venomous snakes (Fig. 29-3)
(1)	Head scales:	(1) Small (vipers). (2) Large, and (a) if there is an opening or pit between the eye and nostril (pit viper). (b) Third labial touches the eye and nasal shields (cobra or coral snake). (c) No pit and third labial does not touch the nose and eye and central row of scales on back enlarged; undersurface of the mouth has only four infralabials, the fourth being the largest (kraits).	Large with the exceptions as mentioned, under the poisonous snakes.
(2)	Belly scales:	Large and cover entire breadth.	Small, like those on the back or moderately large, but do not cover the entire breadth.
(3)	Fangs:	Hollow like hypodermic needles.	Short and solid.
(4)	Teeth:	Two long fangs.	Several small teeth.
(5)	Tail:	Compressed.	Not much compressed.
(6)	Habits:	Usually nocturnal.	Not so.

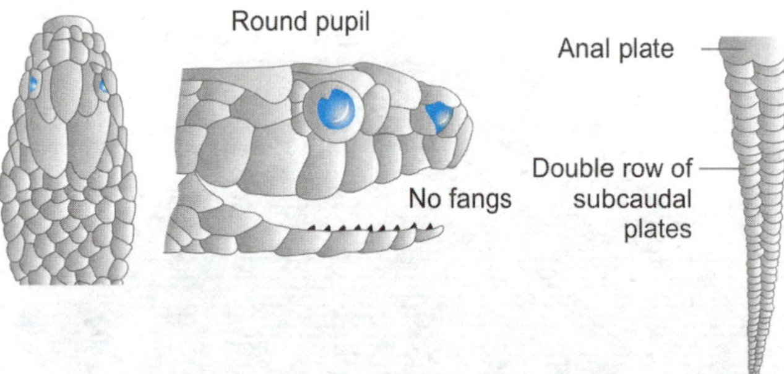

Fig. (29–13). Nonvenomous snake.

Poison Venom Glands: They are the salivary glands of the snake and are situated behind the eyes, one on each side of the head above the upper jaw.

FANGS: All venomous snakes have two fangs. These are curved teeth situated on the maxillary bones and are attached to parotid salivary glands situated behind both eyes and lie along the jaws, and are covered by a flap of mucous membrane. When the snake is about to bite, they become erect and point directly forward. They are bigger than the other teeth and are grooved or canalised in venomous snakes, and are solid in non-venomous snakes. When a venomous snake bites, it normally leaves two deep faint impressions, the distance between them being 8 mm to 4 cm. A side swipe may produce a single puncture and also small marks of other teeth. Many venomous species have more than one set of fangs and can produce multiple puncture marks. Many non-venomous species have two enlarged teeth that can produce two puncture marks. Non-venomous snake bites leave a number of small impressions in a row Table (29–2) and Fig. (29–13).

The discharge orifice of a viper fang is usually well above its tip. The fang can penetrate deeply, but part or most of the venom may be ejected superficially or externally without entering the wound. As such, even a thin layer of clothing may afford great protection. As the venom is injected superficially by vipers, and also by elapids and hydrophids, about 20% of patients bitten by venomous snakes do not show evidence of poisoning, even though the fangs have penetrated the skin, "dry bites". In sea snake bites, symptoms are not produced in about 80% of bites. The exact number of fang marks vary because of glancing blows, multiple fangs, multiple strikes, or from protection of clothing or shoes.

Snake Venom: Venom is the saliva of the snake. **Cobra venom is faint transparent yellow and is slightly viscous.** When exposed to sun, it becomes slightly turbid. **Russell's viper venom is white or yellow.** Venoms of different species of poisonous snakes vary in toxicity, composition and antigenic structure. **It is basically a mixture of toxalbumins and enzymes in varying proportions. The enzymatic components cause local and systemic effects and the non-enzymatic compounds provide lethality.** Venon is water and alcohol soluble.

CONSTITUENTS: (1) Proteolytic enzymes liberate histamine from damaged endothelium leading to dissolution of blood vessel walls with extravasation of blood. They cause digestion of tissue proteins and peptides and produce marked tissue changes, oedema, blistering, bruising and necrosis. They may contribute to hypersensitive action. (2) Fibrin ferments enhance coagulation process. (3) Neurotoxins are found in elapid, hydrophid, vipirid and cortalid venoms. They are neuromuscular non-depolarising blocking agents, which produce a curare-like effect and paralysis, especially of respiratory centre. (4) Cholinesterase is rich in venom of cobra and krait. It causes hydrolysis of acetylcholine to choline and acetic acid leading to impairment of neuromuscular transmission. (5) Haemolysins (mainly in viper venom) cause disruption of endothelial cell functions and alveolar septa and cause pulmonary congestion and increased lung weight. These effects also occur locally at the site of bite, causing haemorrhagic oedema and systemic bleeding leading to shock. (6) Cardiotoxin found particularly in cobra venom is toxic to the heart. It also affects skeletal and smooth muscle membranes and neuromuscular junction. (7) Cytolysins (mainly viper venom) cause lysis of cell structures of blood and tissues. (8) Agglutinins cause agglutination of red cells. (9) Lecithinases act on the lipid layers of endothelial cell linings, producing lysolecithin and helping in increase of fragility and permeability for leakage of cells. (10) Phospholipase A,B,C,D act as catalysts in hydrolysis of lipids. It destroys phospholipids in nervous tissues and alters neuromuscular conduction. It also helps in penetration of neurotoxin into nervous tissue. (11) Phosphotidases cause haemolysis and most of the effects on the heart and circulation. (12) Proteinases have trypsin-like action, causing tissue damage. They catalyse the conversion of prothrombin to thrombin producing coagulant effect. (13) Hyaluronidase helps in rapid spreading of the venom. It is present in all venoms. (14) Ribonuclease and deoxyribonuclease present in all venoms help in rapid spread of venom. (15) Ophioxidase helps in autolysis. (16) Protease causes dissolution of vascular wall. (17) Biological amines, such as histamine and 5-hydroxytryptamine may contribute to local pain and permeability changes at the site of bite. (18) Enzymes include phospholipidase A, proteases, hyaluronidase, cholinesterase, hydrolases, ATPase, transaminase, phospholipase, ribonuclease, deoxyribonuclease, etc. They cause increase in cell wall permeability, with haemolysis, disruption and alteration of connective tissue, muscle and subcutaneous tissue damage leading to necrosis, and promotion of i.v. clotting and fibrinolysis resulting in a defibrinated syndrome. (19) Peptides and polypeptides (lethal compounds) cause systemic effects.

The concentration of venom shows diurnal and seasonal variation. **Bites inflicted at nights and immediately after hibernation are the most severe. Venom travels in the body through lymphatics and superficial veins and spreads rapidly through subcutaneous areolar space.**

Crotalidae venoms are rich in proteolytic enzyme activity. The viperidae venoms have lesser amounts and the elapidae and hydrophidae venoms have little or no proteolytic activity. **Hyaluronidase is found in every snake venom.** L-aminoacid oxidase is found mainly in the viperoid and crotalid venoms. It is not found in sea snake venoms. Cholinesterase is rich in elapid venoms, while it is absent or found only in small amounts in viperid and crotalid venoms.

Types of Venom: **The colubrine and elapidae venom is mainly neurotoxic, and has a primary toxicity for the respiratory and cardiac centres**. Neurotoxic features are due to selective d-tubocurarin-like neuromuscular blockade which results in flaccid paralysis of muscles. It can produce marked cardiac or vascular changes, or have a direct effect on the blood. **The viperine venom is mainly haemolytic and causes intravascular haemolysis and depression of the coagulation mechanism**. It can produce changes in the nervous system or in vascular dynamics. Russell's viper venom contains two proteases which activate the blood clotting cascade. **As a rule, one of the modes of action far exceeds the other. The sea snake venom is myotoxic.**

The venom of rattlesnakes, cotton mouth and copperhead contain enzymes that possess cytotoxic, haemorrhagic and neurotoxic properties. Coral snake venom is neurotoxic causing curare-like effects on the neuromuscular junctions and neurologic symptoms.

Venom may not be detected in dry bite, washing of the area, bite through thick layers of clothing, leakage from superficial bite in mobile parts of body.

Signs and Symptoms: Ophitoxaemia is poisoning by snake venom. Most of the snake bites are from non-venomous snakes. In venomous snake bites, inadequate snake venom is injected in more than half of the cases, producing mild symptoms. The most common symptom following snake bite (venomous or non-venomous) is fright, especially the fear of rapid and unpleasant death. Due to fright, the victim may become semiconscious with cold clammy skin, hypotension, feeble pulse and rapid breathing. These emotional symptoms appear within few minutes of the bite. **Sometimes, it produces psychological shock and even death.** It may also give rise to tetanus or gas gangrene.

The signs and symptoms depend upon: (1) the nature, location, depth and number of bites; 98% of the snake bites occur over the extremities; (2) the length of time the snake holds on; (3) the extent of anger or fear that motivates the snake; (4) the amount of venom injected; (5) the species and size of the snake; (6) the condition of its fangs and venom glands; (7) the age and size of the victim; (8) the victim's sensitivity to the venom; (9) the pathogens in the snake; and (10) the first aid and medical care.

Cobra bite: In cobra bite, **the transfer of venom is not complete. Local symptoms start within 6 to 8 minutes. A small reddish-bluish coloured wheal develops at the site of bite. The bitten area is tender with slight radiating burning pain and oozing of bloodstained fluid.** Swelling may be minimal or even absent. **Systemic symptoms appear after about 30 minutes.** The patient feels sleepy, slightly intoxicated, weakness of legs, and is reluctant to stand or move. Nausea and vomiting are sometimes the early symptoms. Cyanosis is very marked. **Ptosis is the earliest neuroparalytic manifestation followed by ophthalmoplegia.** There may be extraocular muscle weakness and strabismus. **Weakness of the muscles increases, and develops into paralysis of the lower limbs. The paralysis then spreads to the trunk, and affects the head which falls forward.** The eyelids also hang down. After half to one hour, there is excessive salivation and even vomiting, headache, vertigo, paraesthesia around the mouth and myalgia. **This is followed by paralysis of the facial muscles, palate, jaws, tongue, vocal cords, neck muscles.** Muscles of deglutition become progressively flaccidly paralysed due to which there is difficulty in speech and swallowing. **After about two hours, the paralysis is complete. Respiratory arrest may occur** due to obstruction of upper airway by the paralysed tongue or inhaled vomitus, or due to paralysis of intercostal muscles and diaphragm. A basic means of assessing imminent respiratory failure is inability to raise the head in supine position. Though the patient is conscious, **he is not able to speak.** Coma sets in and finally the respirations stop with or without convulsions and the heart stops. In cases of recovery, the skin and cellular tissues surrounding the bite mark undergo necrosis.

Krait bite: **Symptoms resemble those of cobra bite,** but there is no swelling or burning pain at the site of the bite, and the convulsions are milder, while the feeling of drowsiness and intoxication is more intense. Albumin appears in urine.

Russell's Viper and Echis Carinate Bite: A viperid snake merely strikes, discharging the venom the moment the fangs penetrate the skin and then immediately leaves it. **More than 50% of the victims have minimal or no poisoning, as little or no venom is injected. About 25% will develop serious generalised poisoning, but death is rare.** When venom is injected, **the spot develops a severe pain within eight minutes.** The area around the bite is red and painful. Small clots may be present in vicinity of fang marks and blood vessels. **The onset of swelling starts within 15 minutes and there is often blood-stained discharge from the wound. Persistent bleeding from bite site is a constant feature.** Blisters **begin to appear in about 12 hours in and around the bitesite, progressing subsequently to involve the entire limb. When the amount of venom injected is less, pain and swelling restricted to below the elbow or knee,** and some nausea disappear within one to two days. In moderate poisoning, there is a marked feeling of intense pain, vomiting, giddiness, sweating, abdominal pain, dilatation of the pupils, getting insensitive to light and in about one to two hours, there is marked collapse and often complete loss of consciousness. Skin temperature is raised. **Tingling and numbness over the tongue and mouth or scalp and paraesthesia around the wound occur.** These symptoms usually subside within the next few hours. **There is local extravasation of blood, and swelling spreads as far as the trunk in one to two days, without further generalised symptoms.** Though the limb is swollen and red, it is usually not tender. **Haematuria may be seen within a few hours of the bite.** The local swelling and discolouration, and sometimes a few blisters heal without necrosis within one to four weeks. In about 10 to 15% of the cases, extensive necrosis of skin, s.c. tissues and muscles may occur followed by epistaxis, haemoptysis, ecchymoses, intracranial and subconjunctival haemorrhages, and bleeding into the floor of the mouth, tympanic membrane, G.I and G-U tract, retroperitoneum and intraperitoneum. **In severe cases, the main feature is the persisting shock.** Blood may show haemoconcentration early, then a decrease in red cells and platelets, and urine contains blood, sugar and protein. **Bleeding and clotting time are usually prolonged.** A **haemorrhagic syndrome with blood-stained sputum, haemorrhages from the gums, rectum, the site of bite, etc., occur due to the increased coagulation time. Intravascular haemolysis may lead to haemoglobinuria.** In the case of Russell's viper and hump-nosed viper, **renal failure is a frequent complication. Petechial haemorrhages are common. In systemic poisoning, the blood becomes defibrinated and therefore will not clot.** Increasing respiratory depression, blurring of vision, headache, dizziness and weakness often occur. Towards the end, there is an extensive suppuration and sloughing, followed by a malignant oedema of the bitten area. Paralysis does not occur. **Death is usually due to shock and haemorrhage.** In the case of echis, death may not occur, but the secondary symptoms continue for days, and the haemorrhages are severe and the wound shows mild necrosis. The patient should be observed for 12 to 24 hours Table (29–3).

Sea Snake Bites: **Bites cause little or no local reaction. After half to one hour, the patient develops pain, stiffness and weakness of the skeletal muscles. Sea snake bites result in marked polymyositis with a limb-girdle distribution.** Trismus occurs in early stage. Later, **flaccid paralysis develops, beginning with ptosis.** Muscle enzymes and plasma potassium levels are increased and myoglobinuria with renal failure may occur. Marked weakness of muscles persists for several months. **Death may occur due to cardiac arrest or paralysis of respiratory muscles.**

Pythons and boas kill by constricting chest causing traumatic asphyxia.

Fatal Dose: Cobra 12 mg; Russell's viper 15 mg; echis 8 mg; krait 6 mg; of dried venom. The approximate yield in one bite in terms of dry weight of lyophilised venom is: cobra 170 to 325 mg; Russell's viper 130 to 250 mg; krait 20 mg; and echis 20 to 35 mg.

Fatal Period: Cobra half to six hours; viper one to two days.

Diagnosis: (1) **Snake specific venom antigens have been detected** in wound swabs, aspirates or biopsies, serum, CSF, urine and other body fluids. As such, **skin and underlying tissue surrounding the fang punctures, wound and blister aspirates, serum and urine should be collected. Bitten area should be preserved in normal saline. Urinary venom may remain detectable even though the victim is treated with antivenom.** (2) **Radioimmunoassay (RIA) is most sensitive and specific** which can detect venom levels of 0.4 µg/1. Bitten area of skin should be preserved. (3) **Enzyme immunoassay (EIA) is commonly used as it is simple and can detect venom levels of 5 µg/1.** (4) **Cholinesterase and thromboplastin may be detectable in bitten area** of skin if there is no bacterial infection or putrefaction, by radioimmunoassay method. (5) Immunological detection of small amounts of **venom antigens in body fluids can be done by ELISA.** Fang marks tissues should be sent to microbiology department. (6) A swab taken from the wound site or extract from the skin is injected into a frog for evidence of toxicity.

First Aid: (1) **Assure the patient.** (2) Apply firm pressure over the bitten area, which delays absorption of venom. (3) **Pressure immobilisation is recommended for elapid and sea-snake bites, but not for viper bites as it may cause local necrosis.** Immediately apply a broad firm bandage **(Sutherland wrap)** on the bitten area and around the limb. As much of the limb should be bandaged as is possible. It should be tight enough to occlude the superficial venous and lymphatic return, but not the arterial or deep venous flow. A pressure of 50 to 70 mm Hg is maintained. In bites on the trunk, head or neck, apply firm pressure over the bitten area. (4) **Immobilise the limb,** as movement can accelerate the spread of venom. Avoid elevation of an extremity, as it may hasten systemic absorption of venom. (5)

Table (29–3). Difference between Colubrine and Viperine bites

	Trait	Colubrine bite	Viperine bite
(1)	Area bitten :	Reddish wheal; tender with slight burning pain; oozing of bloodstained fluid less.	Pain and oozing of bloodstained fluid are more.
(2)	Swelling:	Minimal or absent in bitten area.	Involves limb and spreads up to trunk.
(3)	Symptoms :	Neurotoxic. Appear after 30 minutes or more.	Haemotoxic. Appear immediately to 15 minutes.
(4)	Speech and deglutition :	Difficult.	Normal.
(5)	Paralysis :	Of lower limbs spreading to trunk and head.	Not present.
(6)	Salivation :	Present.	Absent.
(7)	Pupils :	Normal.	Dilated; do not react to light.
(8)	Blood pressure :	Normal.	Hypotension.
(9)	Bleeding and clotting time :	Normal.	Prolonged.
(10)	Haemorrhagic manifestations :	Not present.	Prominent feature.
(11)	Cause of death :	Respiratory failure.	Circulatory failure due to a haemolysis and haemorrhage.

Local incision and suction should not be done as it can cause local bleeding and nerve injury. (6) **Do not suck venom out of the wound, and do not use chemicals** or medicines on the wound. (7) **The wound should not be cauterised** as it actually seals the poison within the tissues. (8) Cryotherapy is not of much use. (9) Clean the wound with soap and water, or iodine and cover with a sterile dressing. (10) Make patient lie on one side in the recovery position so that the airway is clear, in case of vomiting or fainting.

If a patient is brought after few hours (4 to 6) of snake bite with mild local swelling and no systemic symptoms, he should be kept under observation for 24 hours, closely monitored for vital signs, cardiac system and oxygen saturation, given tetanus toxoid and discharged

Treatment: Polyvalent antisnake venon (PAV) is prepared by hyperimmunising horses against the venom of the four common poisonous snakes, i.e., cobra, common krait, Russell's viper and sawscaled viper.

Antisnake venom (polyvalent): Each ml has capacity of specifically neutralising the venom

(1) 0.60 mg of dried Indian Cobra (Najanaja) venom
(2) 0.45 mg of dried common Krait (Bungarus Caeruleus) venom
(3) 0.60 mg of dried Russell's viper (Daboiarusselii) venom
(4) 0.45 mg of dried Saw-Scaled viper (Echiscarinatus) venom
(Dilute vial with 10 ml liquid or distilled water given with it)

This is mixed with normal saline 5 ml/kg and infused

Plasma obtained from the hyperimmunised horses is concentrated and purified. The serum is lyophilised by drying it from the frozen state under high vacuum. It is prepared in the Haffkine Institute, Mumbai, King Institute, Chennai, Serum Institute, Pune, and at Kasauli in India, and is available in the form of lyophilised powder in an ampoule, which retains potency for about five years. **It is useful when given within four hours of bite.** It is of less value if delayed for eight hours, and is of doubtful value after twenty-four hours. **Each vial of PAV will neutralise about 6 to 8 mg of venom.** Its half-life is about 90 hours. **Test dose of PAV should not be administered** as it is a poor predictor of early anaphylactoid reactions and may presensitise the patient to PAV. **If the swelling involves at least half of the bitten limb within a few hours** of bite in the absence of a tourniquet, or if the swelling rapidly continues or if swelling has crossed a joint within first one or two hours of its starting, **it indicates envenomation.** Swelling that is several hours old is not good evidence of current envenomation. **In case of viper bites, incoagulable blood or evidence of spontaneous bleeding from the gums will indicate envenomation.**

Dose: (1) **Minimal symptoms:** Local swelling but no systemic reactions, 5 vials. (2) **Moderate:** Swelling progressing beyond site of bite with systemic reaction, 10 vials (3) **Severe:** Marked local reaction, severe symptoms, 10 to 15 vials. **Children require the same dose as in adults.** The lyophilised powder is diluted in 500 ml of distilled water or normal saline and infused over a period of one hour. **In neurotoxic poisoning, a second dose of ten vials should be given after one hour. In the case of haemotoxic patients** the initial dose of antiserum will be neutralising unbound, free flowing venom. The liver requires six hours to restore clotting factors, as such **patient will not require further PAV for six hours after the first dose.**

20 minutes blood clotting test: Few ml. of fresh venous blood is put in a clean dry glass tube and left undisturbed for 20 minutes and then gently tilted. If the blood is still liquid, it indicates viper bite. This test is repeated every 6 hours for determining repeat dose requirement. Normalisation of clotting time is taken as endpoint of therapy. After that the test is done at 12 hour intervals for at least 48 hours to detect recurring envenoming. **Repeat dosing is required for recurrence of systemic signs.**

Other measures: At the first sign of any of the following, e.g. urticaria, itching, shivering, chills, nausea or vomiting, hypotension, bronchospasm, angio-oedema: (1) (A) Stop PAV infusion. (B) Administer 0.5 mg. 1:1000 adrenaline i.m. for adults (0.01 mg/kg for children). (C) Give hydrocortisone and antihistamine to provide longer term protection. (D) If there is no improvement after 10 to 15 minutes give a second dose of adrenaline. (E) Once the condition has improved start antiserum infusion. (2) **If the antisnake venom is not available, 40 ml. of antivenene is given i.v. and repeated as required. It is effective for cobra and Russell's viper bites.** (3) When treating viper bite a watch should be kept on prothrombin time. (4) **If there are signs of neuroparalysis, give 1.5 mg neostigmine for adults** (paediatric dose 0.04 mg/kg) i.m. with 0.6 mg atropine i.v. (paediatric dose 0.05 mg/kg) to counteract the muscarinic effects of neostigmine. It is repeated twice at ten minutes interval. If the victim shows improvement give 0.5 mg neostigmine half hourly with atropine. In cases of presynaptic envenoming such as kraits or Russell's viper a positive response does not occur. Before every injection, half mg. atropine should be given to block muscarinic side effects. (5) **Heparin** 1000 to 5000 i.u. may be given i.v. if there are clotting abnormalities. (6) **Inject tetanus antitoxin** or a booster dose of tetanus toxoid. (7) A **broadspectrum antibiotic** should be given if there is severe tissue involvement. (8) In viper poisons, sedatives may be given to relieve pain and nervousness. (9) In case of collapse, general stimulants are of value. (10) Mechanical ventilatory support is necessary in respiratory failure. (11) In severe poisoning, infusion of normal saline or transfusion of blood or plasma are very useful. (12) **Haemodialysis may be necessary. Peritoneal dialysis is better.** (13) Give paracetamol for pain, but aspirin should not be given, as it may make the patient bleed. (14) Surgical debridement of the blebs, bloody vesicles, and superficial necrosis may be necessary.

Postmortem Appearances: Clothing shows amber-coloured fluid, which becomes yellowish needles on drying. Venom over skin will be present as yellow crystals. **Venomous snakes leave two or occasionally one fang mark.** Non-venomous snakes leave a semicircular set of tooth-marks. **The punctures are one-and-half cm. deep in colubrine and two-and-half cm. deep in viperine bites. Sometimes, the bite marks may not be visible. In colubrine bite, the site of bite contains fluid and haemolysed blood causing staining of vessels. In viperine bite, there is discolouration, swelling and cellulitis about the mark and haemorrhages occur from the puncture and mucous membranes.** Haemorrhages into the bowel, purpuric spots on pericardium, and haemorrhages in the lungs and in many tissues may be seen. Kidneys are inflamed and show tubular necrosis, cortical necrosis and interstitial nephritis and marked congestion. Subcapsular pinpoint haemorrhages are seen in most cases of viperine bite. **Acute renal failure is the leading cause of death in**

viper bite. Regional lymph nodes are swollen and haemorrhagic. Internal organs are congested. Washing from the bite area may contain cholinesterase or thromboplastin. The skin and underlying tissue surrounding fang marks should be removed for analysis. ELISA (enzyme-linked immunosorbent assay) can identify the nature of venom from the bite site.

Absorption and Excretion: Snake venom is poisonous only when injected, and is harmless when taken by the mouth, as it will be digested by enzymes in intestinal tract and absorbed as amino acids. It is excreted by kidneys, milk and probably by salivary glands and the mucous membranes.

The Circumstances of Poisoning: (1) Poisoning is as a rule accidental. (2) Occasionally, a murder is committed by throwing a venomous snake on the bed of sleeping person. (3) It is very rarely used for suicide. (4) Cattle are sometimes poisoned by snake venom. For this, a cobra is shut up in an earthen vessel containing a banana and heat is applied to the vessel. The snake being irritated, bites the fruit and the venom is injected to the pulp, which is crushed and smeared on a rag. The rag is thrust into the animal's rectum by means of a split bamboo. (5) **The bodies of animals killed by snake poisoning may be eaten without ill-effects, but their blood is poisonous and is fatal if injected into the human body.**

CASE: Queen Cleopatra is reputed to have committed suicide by getting her self-bitten by a venomous snake.

SCORPIONS

There are more than 1250 species of scorpions. About 100 species are found in India. These are eight-legged arthropods and have a hollow sting in the last joint of their tail, which communicates by means of a duct with the poisonous glands, which secrete poison on stinging Fig. (29–14). The venom is a clear, colourless toxalbumen, and can be classified as either haemolytic or neurotoxic. Its toxicity is more than that of snakes, but only a small quantity is injected. The venom is a potent autonomic stimulator resulting in the release of massive amounts of catecholamines from the adrenals. It has also some direct effect on the myocardium. The mortality, except in children is negligible. Colour of scorpions varies from light yellow to black. Most scorpion stings occur on the extremities.

SIGNS AND SYMPTOMS: If the scorpion has haemolytic venom, the reaction is mainly local and simulates the viper snake bite, but the scorpion sting will have only one hole in the centre of the reddened area. The extremity will have oedema, pain and reddening. This usually lasts for one to two hours. The symptoms produced by a neurotoxic venom is similar to cobra bite. There is usually no marked reaction in the local area. Nausea, vomiting, extreme restlessness, fever, various types of paralysis, cardiac arrhythmias, convulsions, coma and cyanosis, respiratory depression, and death may occur within hours from pulmonary oedema or cardiac failure. The diagnosis is confirmed by ELISA testing.

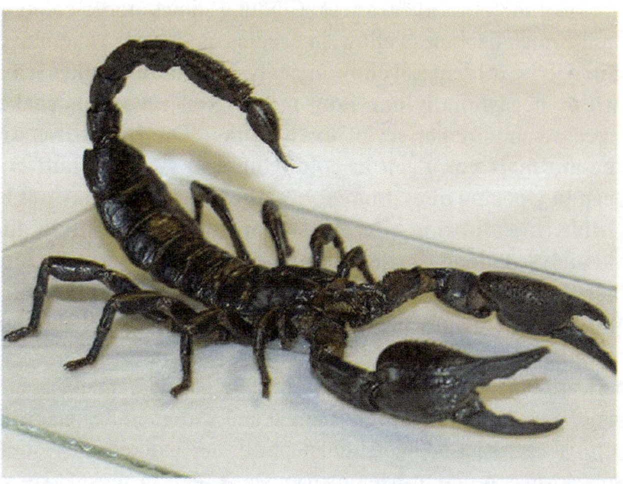

Fig. (29–14). Scorpion.

TREATMENT: (1) Immobilise the limb, and apply a tourniquet above the location of sting. (2) Pack sting in ice, and incise and use suction, and wash the wound with a weak solution of ammonia, borax or potassium permanganate. (3) A local anaesthetic (2% novocaine or 5% cocaine) is injected at the site to lessen pain. (4) A specific antivenin is available for most species. (5) Calcium gluconate intravenously is of value to control local swelling. (6) Barbiturates should be given to reduce excitement and convulsions but morphine is contraindicated. (7) Atropine is valuable in preventing pulmonary oedema.

BEES AND WASPS: Honey bees have a barbed stinger which contain two lancets which become firmly attached to human skin. The stinger of the wasp does not have barbs. Fire ants have well-developed abdominal stingers. They are commonly seen in mango trees. Bees leave their stings behind and can only sting once, but wasps and hornets do not leave their sting behind and can sting many times. Bee venom contains dopamine, histamine, neurotoxin, enzymes and toxic peptides. Wasp venom contains in addition serotonin. Ant venom mainly contains alkaloids and proteins. Painful and sometimes fatal reactions occur in humans. The reactions are usually local. Severe systemic reactions are not common. Venom contains histamine. The local reaction consists of pain, redness, and slight swelling at the site of the sting. Stings of the mouth, throat and sometimes of the face, neck or limbs cause oedema of the larynx or pharynx and obstruction.

Systemic toxic reactions occur due to multiple stings. There is gastrointestinal disturbance and shock. Vomiting and diarrhoea may be accompanied by faintness and unconsciousness. The symptoms last for 24 hours if not fatal.

The anaphylactic reaction may occur immediately or within twenty minutes. There is respiratory distress, faintness, and unconsciousness. A rash may develop. Death may occur in 2 to 15 minutes.

TREATMENT: (1) Apply a ligature above the site of the sting and incise it. (2) The sting should be located and removed by tweezers. (3) Tincture of iodine or local application of antihistamine is useful. (4) Adrenaline is given to combat systemic reactions. (5) ACTH 25 mg. in a litre of normal saline is given by intravenous infusion. (6) Calcium intravenously is useful for urticaria.

CENTIPEDES

They have segmented bodies with a pair of legs on each segment and a pair of claws on the first segment, through which venom is injected. The length is from two to several centimetres. The colour may be greenish-black or black Fig. (29–15). They have powerful jaws and produce relatively large volumes of toxin, which may include histamine, serotonin, hyaluronidase, esterase and proteinases. They produce paired bites of pinpoint type with spacing of up to 12 mm. Fatal bites are rare.

SYMPTOMS: Local swelling, excruciating pain, and necrosis, paralysis and contracture of extremities, cardiac irregularities, arthritis and meningism may occur. Symptoms subside in 2 to 3 days.

LIZARDS: There are no venomous lizards in India Fig. (29–16).

SPIDERS: Spiders are invariably poisonous but majority of species do not pose risk of death. Black widow or hour glass spider (neurotoxic) and violin spider or brown recluse (cytotoxic) produce severe toxicity, and act on the myoneural junction or peripheral nerve endings causing ascending motor paralysis or damage to peripheral nerve endings. Death may occur due to introduced infection (Staphylococus, Penicillium and several species of Bacillus) rather than venom. Spider fangs leave two closely spaced puncture marks on the skin. Nausea, vomiting, sweating, abdominal cramps, chest pain or tightness, difficulty in breathing, tachycardia, hypertension, restlessness, irritability, sweating and swollen eyelids occur. Some spiders may cause local tissue injury and ulcers at the bite site, which

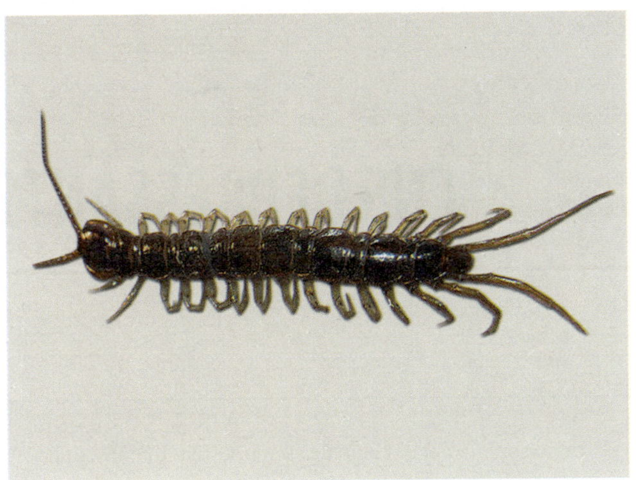

Fig. (29–15). Centipede.

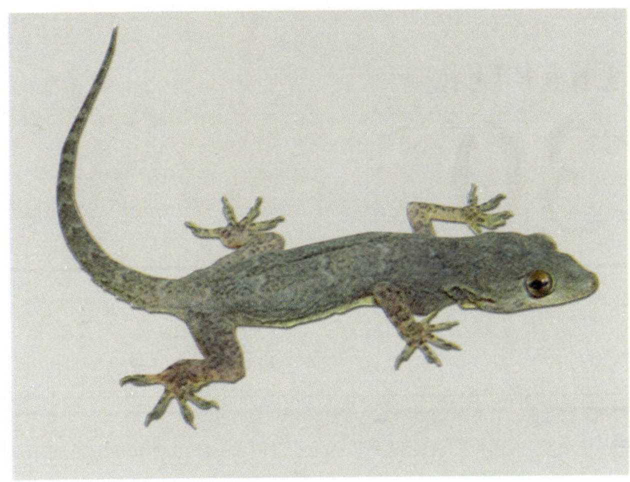

Fig. (29–16). Lizard: Northen house gecko.

may spread over the bitten limb. Local swelling and local painful muscle spasms and tremors appear, which later involve muscles of the back, shoulder, thighs, legs, arms and face. There is circulatory collapse, convulsions and delirium. It may be confused with tetanus and strychnine poisoning.

TREATMENT: (1) Analgesics, antihistamines and antibiotics may be given if indicated. (2) Antivenin. (3) Dapsone 50 to 100 mg. twice daily for 2 to 3 days may halt progression of lesions that are becoming necrotic.

ANTS: They secrete formic acid by certain glands situated in the tail. Ant bite produces pain, irritation and swelling at the site of the bite.

CHAPTER

30

CNS DEPRESSANTS

FM 5.5: Describe and discuss delirium tremens.

FM 9.4: Describe General Principles and basic methodologies in treatment of poisoning: decontamination, supportive therapy, antidote therapy, procedures of enhanced elimination with regard to ethanol, methanol, ethylene glycol.

CNS DEPRESSANTS

CLASSIFICATION: (1) Ethyl alcohol. (2) General anaesthetics. (3) Opioid analgesics. (4) Sedative hypnotics.

SEDATIVE-HYPNOTICS: Sedative drugs are those that decrease activity, moderate excitement, and exert a calming effect. A hypnotic drug produces drowsiness and facilitates a state of sleep, resembling natural sleep.

CLASSIFICATION: (1) Barbiturates. (2) Benzodiazepines: diazepam, chlordiazepoxide, oxazepam, chlorazepate, flurazepam, lorazepam, temazepam, alprazolam, halazepam, prazepam, triazolam. (3) Non-barbiturates: paraldehyde. (4) Alcohols, chloral hydrate. (5) Propanediol carbamates: meprobamate, ethinamate. (6) Piperidinediones: glutethimide, methyprylon. (7) Quinazolines: methaqualone.

ALCOHOL

Inebriant poisons produce intoxication, i.e., light headedness, confusion, disorientation, and drowsiness, e.g., alcohol, barbiturates, chloral hydrate, cannabis, benzodiazepines, paraldehyde, anaesthetics, hydrocarbons, formaldehyde and many pesticides, etc. In most cases there is recovery after prolonged sleep, with some after-effects (hangover), consisting of headache, irritability, lethargy, nausea and abdominal discomfort.

PHYSICAL APPEARANCES: The term alcohol in common use refers to ethyl alcohol (C_2H_5OH). It is a transparent, colourless, volatile liquid, having a characteristic spirituous odour and a burning taste. Absolute alcohol contains >99% alcohol; rectified spirit contains 95% alcohol, and industrial methylated spirit or denatured alcohol is a mixture consisting of alcohol 95% and 5% of wood naphtha.

SOURCES: Ethanol is produced by the fermentation of sugar by yeast. This process stops at an alcohol concentration of about 15% by volume, because of the death of the yeast. Alcoholic beverages are a mixture of alcohol and water with small amounts of congeners, which are simultaneously produced during the fermentation process. The characteristic flavours of alcoholic beverages are due to organic compounds called congeners, such as propyl alcohol, octyl alcohol, glycerin, aldehydes, dimethyl and diethyl esters, acids from acetic to linoleic, ketones, trimethyl amine, allyl mercaptan, diethyl sulphide, pyrozine, etc. The total content of congeners rarely exceeds half percent. The odour may persist in the tissues for several hours after all alcohol has been metabolised.

PROOF SPIRIT: "Proof spirit" is one which at 10.5°C weighs exactly 12/13 part of an equal measure of distilled water. Weaker spirits are termed "underproof" and stronger spirits "overproof". Proof is defined as twice the percentage of the alcohol content of the drink. The amount of alcohol consumed can be expressed in units; one unit being about 8 g. of alcohol.

Concentration: The approximate percentage of alcohol by volume in some of the more common beverages is as follows:

Vodka	: 60 to 65%
Rum, liquors	: 50 to 60%
Whisky, gin, brandy	: 40 to 45%
Port, sherry	: 20%
Wine, champagne	: 10 to 15%
Beers	: 4 to 8%

Consumption of alcohol must not exceed 1 to 2 drinks per day. A standard drink is roughly 45 ml of distilled spirits (15 g. of alcohol) or 150 ml of wine (11g. alcohol) or 350 ml of beer (13 g. alcohol). 210 g. of alcohol in men and 140 g of alcohol in women per week are considered safe limits for drinking, if liver damage is to be avoided.

Arrack: It is a liquor distilled from palm, rice, sugar or jaggery, etc., and has a strength of 40 to 50%. It may be mixed with chloral hydrate and potassium bromide, dhatura, bhang for getting a greater kick.

ABSORPTION: Alcohol requires no digestion prior to absorption. Its small molecular size permits it to pass readily through membranes by simple diffusion. A small amount is absorbed from mouth and oesophagus. Absorption from the stomach and small intestine begins almost immediately upon ingestion. About 20% is absorbed from the stomach and 80% through small intestine. About 60% of diluted alcohol taken on empty stomach is absorbed in 30 to 60 minutes and 90% in 60 to 90 minutes Alcohol can be detected in the blood within 2 to 3 minutes of swallowing a few sips of whisky or beer. The maximum concentration in blood is reached within 45 to 90 minutes after ingestion with majority of persons reaching their maximum one hour after ingestion. Carbonated drinks hasten absorption, as the bubbles greatly increase the surface area carrying alcohol. Food delays its absorption, and the delay is most marked in the presence of fat and protein. A large fatty meal can delay total absorption for a number of hours. A mixed meal can depress the maximum concentration of the blood alcohol by about half. Food ingested with alcohol may prevent 10 to 20% of the ingested alcohol from being absorbed. Warm alcoholic drinks which dilate gastric mucosal capillaries are more quickly absorbed than iced drinks of the same strength. Persons with achloryhydria or chronic gastritis have slower absorption rates. Absorption is most rapid at concentrations of 10 to 20%. Lower and higher concentrations are absorbed more slowly. Dilute drinks, such as beer may take double the time to absorb compared to stronger drinks. Drinks containing more than 40% alcohol are absorbed slowly due to: (1) Pyloric spasm. (2) Irritation of gastric mucosa, and secretion of mucus. (3) Reduced gastric motility. Habituated heavy drinkers absorb alcohol more rapidly than abstainers, probably due to more rapid emptying time of the stomach and thus the rate of absorption. Drugs, e.g., benzine or atropine, may slow the rate of absorption of alcohol probably by retarding the emptying time of stomach. Alcohol is absorbed rapidly in cases of gastrectomy. If the concentration of alcohol in the air is too high, the irritating properties of the alcohol make breathing difficult or impossible. About 60% of alcohol inhaled can be absorbed into systemic circulation. Tolerable concentrations in the air are so low that intoxication by inhaling alcohol vapour is unlikely, since it is eliminated more rapidly than it is absorbed by this route. Alcohol is poorly absorbed through intact skin.

DISTRIBUTION: Some alcohol is lost by diffusion into the alveolar air, as the arterial blood passes through the lungs. In arterial blood, the concentration of alcohol further decreases due to passage through the capillary network. Alcohol is lost from the blood to the tissues in proportion to the water content of the tissues with which it comes in contact, till equilibrium is reached between the blood and tissues, except adipose tissues, as ethanol is insoluble in fat. Red cells contain less alcohol than plasma, so that a whole blood concentration is slightly less than that in separated plasma or serum Table (30–1). A given intake of alcohol will produce a higher blood alcohol level in obese persons as compared to the lean persons of the same weight, as the aqueous compartment is smaller. Ethanol is distributed evenly throughout the body water, passing the blood-brain barrier easily and bathes neurons via the cerebral extracellular fluid. A smaller volume of distribution for ethanol in women, a faster and a more variable absorption from the gut, a lower activity of gastric ADH enzyme, a faster hepatic clearance, a higher concentration of acetaldehyde and poor solubility in body fat are physiological factors due to which females of the same body weight will have a higher (25% higher) blood alcohol concentration for the same amount of drink, as their aqueous compartment is smaller. Venous blood alcohol in the absorption phase is about 10% lower than arterial blood. This accounts for a higher concentration of alcohol in alveolar breath compared to venous blood. One hour or more after drinking, venous blood contains the same concentration of alcohol. Capillary blood alcohol, and the ratio between the concentration of alcohol in arterial blood and brain, becomes constant in one to two minutes. Equilibration in muscle may require one to two hours.

EXCRETION: Alcohol is excreted through all the routes of excretion. About 5% of ingested alcohol is excreted in the breath and about 5% in the urine. Negligible amounts are excreted in the sweat, saliva, milk, tears and faeces. The peculiar odour of the alcohol is due to the excretion of alcohol by the skin glands.

METABOLISM: As soon as ethanol enters the blood, the body starts to dispose it of by metabolism and excretion. About 90% of alcohol absorbed is oxidised in the liver, and the remaining 10% is excreted. In the liver, alcohol is oxidised to acetaldehyde by alcohol dehydrogenase (ADH) and its coenzyme, nicotinamide adenine-dinucleotide (NAD).

Table (30–1). Relative concentration of alcohol at equilibrium

Sample	Relative concentration
Whole blood	1.00
Plasma or serum	1.12 to 1.2
Brain	0.85
Spinal fluid	1.1 to 1.27
Vitreous	1.2
Urine	1.3
Liver	0.85
Alveolar air	0.0021

In the second step, acetaldehyde is transformed into free acetic acid or its activated form, acetyl coenzyme A. Finally the acetate enters the general pool, and undergoes oxidation to CO_2 and water in the citric acid (Krebs) cycle. Acetate can form glycogen, proteins and possibly fats and cholesterol. The diabetic who is ketogenic will produce fat from alcohol, because he cannot use the sugar. Large doses of fructose increase the rate of metabolism. During its oxidation, alcohol is not stored in the tissues. It disappears from the blood at a fairly uniform rate of about 10 to 15 ml. per hour. This is the equivalent of about 15 mg/100 ml. from the blood per hour. Recent research indicates that this should be raised to 18 mg/100 ml. Basically, elimination varies from 12 to 27 mg/100 ml per hour. Larger doses are lost rather faster. Chronic alcoholics are able to metabolise alcohol at a faster rate, 30 to 40 mg./100 ml./hour, than the non-alcoholics, due to an increase in liver enzymes, until they develop severe liver damage. Many chronic alcoholics develop liver damage and their rate of alcohol metabolism is depressed, due to which they remain intoxicated for hours after a few drinks. 10% of metabolised alcohol is deposited in the tissues as lipids in the form of cholesterol and neutral fat.

ACTION: Traces of ethyl alcohol are found in all persons. Endogenous alcohol is partly due to normal metabolism and partly due to bacterial activity in gastrointestinal tract. Alcohol is a well-known stimulant, but is a selective depressant, especially of the higher nervous centres which it inhibits. Ethanol depresses primarily reticular activating system. The frontal lobes are sensitive to low concentrations (resulting in mood changes) followed by the occipital lobe (visual disturbances) and cerebellum (loss of coordination). Alcohol acts on neural cells in a way similar to hypoxia and reduces their activity. In lower concentrations, it causes depression of more specialised and sensitive cells of the cerebral cortex (centres regulating conduct, judgement and self-criticism), with release of their inhibitory tone, and leads to unrestrained behaviour. Increasing concentrations, progressively depress brain functions. Finally, the vital centres in the midbrain and medulla are depressed, which may cause death from cardio-respiratory failure. It causes generalised vasodilatation, especially in the skin and may increase haemorrhage from relatively minor wounds. It is not a true aphrodisiac. It is a hypnotic and diaphoretic. It creates a sensation of warmth, but it increases heat loss. With low concentration heart rate is increased, but when exceeds 300 mg% bradycardia may develop. In moderation, it stimulates appetite as it promotes salivation and the secretion of gastric juice, but the stronger beverages have a reverse effect. A little brandy has a carminative action. Diuresis occurs secondary to inhibition of antidiuretic hormone release from the posterior pituitary. Spirituous liquors on an empty stomach can cause severe, even haemorrhagic gastritis and hypoglycaemia.

TOXIC EFFECTS: Ethanol has toxic effects on almost every organ system. Some of the toxic effects can be related to effects of the metabolite acetaldehyde or to change in the redox potential of cells, but the mechanism by which ethanol causes intoxication is not specifically known. Although every neurotransmitter system is affected by ethanol, there do not appear to be specific receptors for ethanol.

Acute intoxication may block the metabolism of and lead to increased levels of drugs such as aspirin, opioids, benzodiazepines, barbiturates, tricyclic antidepressants, and phenytoin. It has synergistic effects with other sedative-hypnotic agents.

Moderate (15 to 30 g. per day) consumption increases concentration of HDL and decreases LDL. It has favourable effects on haemostatic factors, such as plasma fibrinogen, fibrinolytic activity and platelet adhesiveness.

"Mixing of drinks" is said to produce greater intoxication, than would be expected from the amount consumed. This may be due to the presence or formation of substances which affect the rate of emptying of the stomach, with more rapid absorption of the alcohol. Normal fasting blood alcohol concentration is less than 0.001 mg%. The old Roman saying, "IN VINO VERITAS", which means, "in wine there is truth", has a high degree of accuracy. In other words, the real personality of an individual often will be revealed when he is intoxicated.

Cause of Death: Death is caused either by the direct depressive effects upon the brain stem, mediated via the

respiratory centre, or due to aspiration of vomit. Deaths due to acute overdose of alcohol are not common, but deaths due to the chronic effects of alcohol are common. Death with alcohol blood concentration below 400 mg% may occur in persons with chronic debilitating diseases, especially severe arteriosclerotic heart disease, pulmonary emphysema and varying degrees of hypoxia.

Symptoms: Serious acute alcohol poisoning is usually a consequence of deliberate heavy drinking, either small doses at short intervals, or a large dose at a time. The effects of acute alcohol intoxication are more pronounced when blood level is rising than falling. There are three phases of intoxication Table (30–2).

(1) Stage of Excitement: There is first a feeling of well-being and a certain slight excitation. **The actions, speech and emotions are less restrained** due to lowering of the inhibition normally exercised by the higher centres of the brain. **There is increased confidence and a lack of self-control, which is a constant feature of alcoholic poisoning**. The person may disclose secrets. Normal good manners are forgotten. The neat and orderly are careless in their dress. **At blood alcohol concentrations of 30 mg%, impairment of cognitive function, motor co-ordination and sensory perception occur. Beyond 50 mg%, slurring of speech, unsteadiness, drowsiness, impaired reasoning and memory, reduced perception and decreased concentration occur. Alcohol reduces visual acuity** in concentration as low as 20 mg% in abstainers, 20 to 33 mg% in moderate drinkers, and 40 to 70 mg% in heavy drinkers. **Significant effects on judgement and motor control may occur with blood alcohol concentration (BAC) of 25 to 50 mg%.** The reaction time of individuals becomes impaired at 50 mg%. Strong light is often needed to distinguish objects, and dimly lighted objects may not be distinguished at all. It takes longer to see clearly again after being dazzled by a strong light. It alters time and space perception, e.g., the person may underestimate the speed of objects and distances travelled. The pupils are dilated. Definite deterioration in driving ability occurs. Between 50 to 100 mg%, loss of inhibitions, loquaciousness and laughter occurs. Slurred speech, unsteadiness and nausea are seen between 100 to 150 mg%. **When jerking movement is in the direction of the gaze and independent of the position of the head, it is known** as **alcohol gaze nystagmus.** Positional gaze nystagmus is seen when person is lying down and head is placed sideways. They occur due to effects of alcohol on vestibulochochlear system. **It appears at blood levels of 40 to 100 mg.% (average 80 mg.%).** It is not a constant or common sign. **Mental concentration is poor and judgement impaired.** The faculty of attention deteriorates rapidly. Recall memory is often markedly disturbed, in which the person cannot accurately recall certain situation, or even names of individuals whom he has known for years. Sensitivity to pain decreases at 80 mg%. The emotions are affected. Alcohol increases the desire for sex, but markedly impairs the performance, often resulting in prolonged intercourse without ejaculation. These effects are usual between 50 to 150 mg.% of blood alcohol.

(2) Stage of Incoordination: When the alcohol content of the blood attains a **level of 150 to 250 mg/100 ml., the sense perception and skilled movements are affected.** The increased loss of the inhibitory action of the higher centres causes an alteration in the conduct of the individual. **He may become carefree, cheerful, ill-tempered, irritable, excitable, quarrelsome, sleepy, and so on, according to the dominant impulses which have been released.** There is certain clumsiness and incoordination in the fine and more skilled movements, as shown by slight alteration in speech and in the fine finger movements. Nausea and vomiting are common. The face is flushed and the pulse is rapid. Sense of touch, taste, smell, and hearing are diminished. The temperature becomes subnormal. Heart rate is increased.

(3) Stage of Coma: In this stage, the motor and sensory cells are deeply affected, speech becomes thick and slurring, coordination is markedly affected, causing the patient to become giddy, stagger and possibly to fall. The person passes into a state of coma with stertorous breathing. The pulse is rapid and temperature subnormal. **The pupils are contracted, but stimulation of the person, e.g., by pinching or slapping, causes them to dilate with slow return (Mc Ewan Sign).** This sign occurs at or above 300 mg% of blood level of alcohol.

With recovery, the coma gradually lightens into a deep sleep, and **the patient usually recovers in 8 to 10 hours,** and wakes up with acute depression, nausea, abdominal discomfort, irritability, lethargy, and severe headache **(Hangover).** If coma continues for more than five hours, the prognosis is likely to be worse. Death occurs from asphyxia due to respiratory paralysis, but it may occur from shock. **Most deaths from alcoholic intoxication do not occur at peak blood levels, but occur some hours later after irreversible damage has been done to vital centres.**

Prolonged coma due to alcohol may cause irreversible hypoxic brain damage and death. In such cases blood alcohol level is usually low, as some or even all of the alcohol in the body may

Table (30–2). Physiological effects of alcohol

Blood alcohol concentration	Effects
0 to 50 mg%	No significant effect or mild euphoria.
50 to 100 mg%	Decreased inhibitions, increased self-confidence, decreased attention span, slurring of speech, mild incoordination, alteration of judgement, nystagmus.
100 to 150 mg%	Some mental confusion, emotional instability, loss of critical judgement, ataxia, impaired memory, sleepiness, slowed reaction time.
150 to 300 mg%	Loss of muscular coordination, staggering gait, marked mental confusion, drowsiness, exaggeration of emotions, dizziness, decreased pain response, disorientation; thickened speech.
300 to 400 mg%	Stupor, marked incoordination, marked decrease in responses to stimuli, possibly coma.
400 mg % and above	Anaesthesia, depression of responses, respiratory failure, deep coma, death.

have been oxidised and excreted. Low levels are also seen if the person survives for several hours after excessive drinking.

CAGE questionnaire is an internationally used assessment instrument for identifying alcoholics.

MICTURITION SYNCOPE is a condition which occurs usually after heavy beer drinking. When the person rises from bed in the middle of night to pass urine, he loses consciousness during the act of urination, probably due to sudden upright posture.

MUNICH BEER HEART is a condition in which cardiac dilatation and hypertrophy is seen due to excessive and prolonged beer drinking.

Fatal Dose: 200 to 250 ml. of absolute alcohol consumed in one hour.

Fatal Period: 12 to 24 hours.

Tolerance to Alcohol: It is acquired and may be lost by those 'out of practice'. It is restricted by liver damage. A person in the habit of taking alcohol daily can drink alcohol without getting 'drunk' in quantities which would seriously affect a person unaccustomed to taking it. Tolerance may be a matter of tissue sensitivity, or of the rate of absorption. Barbiturates are metabolised via the same route; however in the presence of alcohol which is preferentially metabolised, they remain active longer.

Consent for Examination: The consent of the detained person to medical examination is necessary. **If the person is unconscious, or otherwise not in a fit condition to give consent, the doctor called by the police should not disclose to the police any information he obtained during his examination, but should wait to get the consent of the patient when he regains consciousness, or is in a fit condition to be asked.** The person can be examined without consent, if requested by Subinspector of police.

Treatment: (1) **Evacuation of the stomach and bowel and gastric lavage** with an alkaline solution usually causes a diminution in the symptoms. (2) The patient must be kept warm, and if there is congestion of the brain, ice bags should be applied to the head. (3) One litre of normal saline with 10% glucose, 100 mg. thiamine and 15 units of insulin are useful. (4) If the coma deepens, nerve stimulants, such as caffeine and strychnine should be used and artificial respiration, if there is difficulty in breathing. (5) **Inhalation of oxygen** is of great value. (6) **Haemodialysis or peritoneal dialysis** is very useful.

POSTMORTEM APPEARANCES: On opening the cavities of the body, alcoholic odour is frequently noted. Acute inflammation of stomach with a coating of mucus is commonly found. The brain, liver and lungs are congested, and the smell of alcohol in the viscera may be noted. The blood is usually fluid and dark. Oedema and congestion of the brain and meninges and cloudy swelling of parenchymatous organs are seen.

CHRONIC POISONING: ALCOHOL ADDICTS are people who cannot stop drinking for long, or who experience withdrawal symptoms, if they do. It results in impaired social or occupational functioning. CHRONIC ALCOHOLICS are those who have reached a state of more or less irreversible somatic or brain changes caused by alcohol. The patient suffers from nausea, vomiting, anorexia, diarrhoea, jaundice, tremors of the tongue and hands, insomnia, loss of memory, impaired power of judgement, hypoproteinaemia and general anasarca. The symptoms of peripheral neuritis and dementia occur in the last stage. Such patients generally die suddenly from coma.

POSTMORTEM APPEARANCES: Signs of malnutrition may be present. The gastric mucous membrane is deep reddish-brown with patches of congestion or effusion and is hypertrophied. The liver is congested and shows fatty infiltration, enlarged and weight may exceed 2 kg., surface is pale and greasy, and patchy yellowish areas may be seen within normal hepatic parenchyma. Later, cirrhosis occurs with 5 to 10 mm nodules, and becomes smaller and contracted to a hard, greyish-yellow block of 800 to 1200g. The kidneys show granular degeneration. Gastritis, oedema of larynx and oedema of intestines without ulceration may be seen. The heart is dilated and shows fatty degeneration and patchy fibrosis. Shrinkage of cerebral cortex and visible accumulation of fluid "wet brain" is seen in chronic alcoholics.

Treatment: (1) **Disulfiram** (Antadict, Esperal) is given in a single daily dose of 250 mg. It inhibits aldehyde dehydrogenase. The dosage is gradually reduced until an adequate daily dosage of 0.125 to 0.25 g. is reached, which should be continued until the patient has been conditioned to accept adequate follow-up therapy. **Antabuse** (tetraethylthiuram disulfide) inhibits the bio-transformation of ethanol beyond the acetaldehyde stage. Ethyl alcohol is metabolised by the liver as two-step process: (a) Conversion of alcohol to acetaldehyde in the presence of NDA (nicotinamide adenine dinucleotide) and alcohol dehydrogenase, and (b) oxidation of the acetaldehyde to carbon dioxide and water or combining of the acetaldehyde as a two-carbon fragment into acetyl COA. Antabuse partially blocks reaction 2, leading to accumulation of acetaldehyde in the blood and tissues and causes unpleasant symptoms, such as flushing, palpitation, anxiety, sweating, headache, abdominal cramps, nausea and vomiting, due to which the patient dislikes alcohol. Disulfiram-like reaction is caused by metronidazole. (2) **Citrated calcium carbimide** (Temposil) 50 mg. tablet once a day can be used with less side-effects. (3) Chlorpromazine 25 to 50 mg. every 4 to 6 hours is also useful. (4) Clonidine 60 to 180 mg/hr i.v. (5) Chlormethiazole.

The Conditioned Reflex Treatment: It consists of giving alcoholic beverages to the patient in surroundings that affect his visual and olfactory senses. With a backdrop of bottles of various alcoholic beverages, the patient is given various types of liquor, together with drugs that will cause immediate and acute nausea and vomiting. After 5 to 8 daily treatments, symptoms are brought on simply by the sight of a bottle, and the patient begins mentally to associate his painful sickness with the alcohol. Hypnosis and psychotherapy are also useful.

Alcoholics Anonymous is an international voluntary organisation which has branches throughout India. The addicts who are desirous to give up alcohol narrate their bad experiences to other alcoholics through group meetings, letters, press and other media. The organisation functions on a self-supporting basis through contribution from the members.

DRUNKENNESS

Drunkenness is a condition produced in a person, who has taken alcohol in a quantity sufficient to cause him to lose control of his faculties to such an extent, that he is unable to execute safely, the occupation in which he was engaged at the particular time.

The clinical diagnosis depends on the combination of a number of symptoms and signs, no single one of them being peculiar to this condition, except the odour of alcohol from the breath. **An individual can react differently under different circumstances, and that the same amount of alcohol can produce different effects on different people under the same circumstances.** Mentally unstable subjects, epileptics and those who have suffered cerebral trauma at some earlier date may show an excessive reaction to small amounts of alcohol.

A Model Scheme of Medical Examination: The scheme of examination of an alleged alcoholic has been suggested by the Special Committee of the British Medical Association, "The Drinking Driver", 1965. The medical examiner's record should include a note of the date and of the time at the beginning and at the end of the examination.

(1) Exclusion of Injuries and Pathological States: The following conditions which simulate alcoholic intoxication should be excluded: (a) Severe head injuries. (b) Metabolic disorders, e.g., hypoglycaemia, diabetic pre-coma, uraemia, hyperthyroidism. (c) Neurological conditions, e.g., disseminated sclerosis, intracranial tumours, Parkinson's disease, epilepsy, acute aural vertigo. (d) Drugs: Insulin, barbiturates, antihistamines, morphine, atropine, hyoscine. Drugs capable of producing sedation or depression of the nervous system (antihistaminics, tranquilisers), will simulate or enhance the effects of alcohol. (e) Certain pre-existing psychological disorders, e.g., hypomania, general paresis. (f) High fever. (g) Exposure to CO.

(2) History: The history of the relevant events should be obtained from the accused person while observing him. The amount and the time of liquor taken should be noted. Enquire whether he suffers from any disease or disability and whether he is under medical treatment.

(3) General Behaviour: (a) General manners and behaviour. (b) **State of dress:** Presence of slobber on mouth or clothing; presence, character and colour of any vomit, soiling of clothes by excretions. (c) **Speech:** Note the type, e.g., is it thick, slurred or over-precise? Slight blurring of certain consonants is one of the earliest signs of incoordination of the muscles of the tongue and lips. Certain test phrases may be used to bring out this difficulty in speech, such as 'British Constitution', 'West Register Street', 'Truly Rural', etc. A sober person will say that he is not good at such phrases; the semi-intoxicated person will often insist on getting them correctly. (d) **Self-control.:** Note whether he is able to control himself in response to the demands made on him by the examiner.

(4) Memory and Mental Alertness: The memory of the person for recent events, and his appreciation of time can be judged by asking suitable questions about his movements during the preceding few hours, and the details of his accident if any. A few very simple sums of addition or subtraction may be asked.

(5) Handwriting: The examinee should be asked to copy a few lines from a newspaper or book. A note should be made of: (a) The time taken. (b) Repetition or omission of words, letters, or lines. (c) Ability to read his own writing. Both the original and the copy should be retained. The examinee should be asked to sign his name. The signature can be compared with that on his driving license if any.

(6) Pulse: The resting pulse should be taken at the beginning and at the end of the examination. The pulse is rapid and is usually full and bounding. A slight increase in B.P. may occur, often in the systolic level.

(7) Temperature: The surface temperature is usually raised.

(8) Skin: Note whether skin is dry, moist, flushed or pale.

(9) Mouth: (a) Record the general state of mouth, teeth and tongue, noting whether the tongue is dry, furred or bitten. (b) The smell of the breath should be recorded.

(10) Eyes: **(a) General appearance:** (1) Whether the lids are swollen or red, and whether the conjunctivae are congested. (2) The colour of the eyes, and abnormalities. **(b) Visual acuity**: Any gross defect should be noted. **(c) Intrinsic muscles: (1) Pupils:** Equal or unequal, dilated or contracted or abnormal in any way(usually dilated in early stages, but may be contracted in later stages or coma). **(2) Reaction to light:** Note whether the action is brisk, slow or absent. They may become unequal, equalising again in response to light, and dilate again slowly even if the light continues to be directed into the eyes. **(d) Extrinsic muscles: (1) Convergence**: Test the degree of ability to follow a finger in all normal directions and to converge the eyes normally on a near object. **(2) Strabismus:** Note whether it is present. **(3) Nystagmus:** The presence of fine lateral nystagmus may indicate alcoholic intoxication. Nystagmus may be produced by fatigue, emotion or postural hypotension.

(11) Ears: Examine for (a) Gross impairment of hearing. (b) Abnormality of the drums.

(12) Gait: The integrity of the nervous and muscular system is tested for the coordination of fine and gross movements, e.g., balance, gait and speech. The examinee should be asked to walk across the room and note: (a) **Manner of walking:** Is it straight, irregular, overprecise, unsteady, or with feet wide apart? (b) **Reaction time to a direction to turn:** Does the examinee turn at once or continue for one or two steps before obeying? (c) **Manner of turning:** Does the examinee keep his balance, lurch forward, or reel to one side? Does he correct any mistake in a normal or exaggerated way? It is undesirable to ask the examinee to walk along a straight line drawn on the floor.

(13) Stance: Note whether the examinee can stand with his eyes closed and heels together without swaying (Romberg's sign).

(14) Muscular Coordination: Ask the examinee to perform the following tests: (a) Placing finger to nose. (b) Placing finger to finger. (c) Picking up medium-sized objects from the floor. (d) Lighting a cigarette with a match. (e) Unbuttoning and rebuttoning coat. (f) Lifting two objects, such as tumblers from the table, and replacing them side by side on the table.

The examiner should not ask the examinee to perform any act which he could not perform easily himself. He should also appreciate the difficulty involved for some people in apparently simple movements, such as picking up small objects from the floor. A chronic alcoholic when sober may not be able to perform tests for coordination as well, as when he has actually consumed alcohol.

(15) Reflexes: Knee and ankle reflexes should be tested which are delayed or sluggish. Plantar reflex may be extensor or flexor.

(16) Pulmonary, Cardiovascular and Alimentary Systems: The heart, lungs and abdomen should be examined, and the blood pressure taken to establish the presence or absence of disease.

(17) Laboratory Investigations: The degree of intoxication can be estimated by the concentration of alcohol in the blood, urine, breath, or saliva. **In fatal accidents with partial body destruction, muscle or the fluid in the eye can be analysed. Vitreous humour and urine are protected from putrefactive processes for a longer period of time and do not contain much glucose. Blood is the most suitable and the most direct evidence of the concentration of alcohol in the brain. The**

disadvantages are: (1) it may be difficult to collect from an uncooperative person, (2) consent of the person is necessary, (3) substances like acetone, ether, paraldehyde, etc. when present in the blood are estimated as alcohol.

Urine: **Urine has about 25% more water than an equal volume of blood, so its concentration of alcohol would be about 25% higher than in blood collected at the same time.** As the urine is secreted, its water will have essentially the same alcohol concentration as the water of the blood passing through the kidney. If the bladder contains urine before drinking began, urine secreted during or after the period will be diluted with the alcohol-free urine. If the bladder was empty when drinking began, urine secreted after some time will reflect the blood concentration of alcohol at that time. **In order to compare the urine and blood, a ratio of 1.3:1.0 is usually accepted when urine and blood are in equilibrium.** Analyses of two urine samples are required. The first sample should be taken as soon as possible following the incident, the bladder being completely emptied. The second sample should be taken 25 to 30 minutes later. The concentration of alcohol in the second specimen reflects the blood alcohol level during the inter-specimen interval. The difference in the alcohol concentrations in the two samples indicates whether the subject was in the absorptive phase, at its peak, or in the elimination phase. Multiplication of alcohol concentration in the second urine specimen by 0.75 (based on a blood-urine alcohol ratio of 1:1.35) gives an approximate value of the blood alcohol level, during the time that this specimen was being secreted. Extrapolation from this blood level back to the time of the incident indicates the extent of the individual's intoxication at the critical moment when the incident occurred. **A urine sample taken postmortem may be more reliable qualitative index of antemortem intoxication, than is blood.** Simultaneous performance of postmortem blood and urine alcohol analyses give useful information. **If the postmortem urine alcohol concentration exceeds that of the blood by more than 25%, it indicates that higher blood alcohol must have existed during life, than was found at autopsy.** If the postmortem blood alcohol level equals or exceeds that of the postmortem urine alcohol concentration, the subject was probably in the absorptive phase at the time of the death, and probably less than two hours had passed since he consumed his last drink.

The disadvantages of urine examination are: (1) A time lag before equilibrium between blood and urine is reached; the maximum concentration is reached about twenty to twenty-five minutes later than in blood. (2) The urine alcohol concentration at any given time after the maximum concentration in blood has been reached will be higher by 20 to 30% than in the blood, because the specimen of urine examined will have been secreted from the blood at some earlier period. (3) Alcohol may pass through the lining of the bladder in either direction both in life and after death, depending on the relative concentration of alcohol in blood and urine.

Collection of Blood: Spirit must not be used for cleaning the skin, and the syringe must be free from any trace of alcohol. The skin is cleaned with a solution of 1:1000 mercuric chloride or washed with soap and water. **Blood samples should be preserved by the addition of 100 mg. of sodium fluoride and 30 mg. potassium oxalate for 10 ml. followed by thorough shaking.** This prevents loss of alcohol by glycolysis and bacterial action. Such samples will maintain their alcohol concentration for several weeks, even at room temperature. 50 mg. of phenyl mercuric nitrate or sodium azide can also be used, as a preservative for 10 ml. of blood or urine.

A screw-capped glass bottle of "universal" size is suitable. The container should be tightly clamped and sealed to prevent loss of alcohol by evaporation and labelled with name, date and time of taking specimens. Rubber stoppers should be avoided, because they may contaminate the sample with oxidisable substances. If they are not transmitted at once to the laboratory, they should be refrigerated but must not be frozen. **Freezing will cause the cells to lyse. When blood is kept in a refrigerator, formation of oxidisable substances is not significant. Analysis is best made within a week. Serum or plasma alcohol concentration is 12 to 20% higher than that of whole blood.**

COLLECTION OF POSTMORTEM SAMPLES: In temperate climates, postmortem blood alcohol determinations are completely valid for 36 hours after death. The best place to obtain blood is from femoral or iliac veins or from axillary veins. Jugular vein is not suitable as it may be contaminated by reflux from the upper thorax. If the concentration of alcohol is same in all these samples the exposure is extraneous, because bacterial and chemical decomposition does not occur at exactly the same rate all over the body. Free blood in the pleural or pericardial cavities should not be used as false high results may be obtained due to gastric alcohol diffusion after death.

In embalmed bodies alcohol can be estimated either in the vitreous or muscle.

Erroneous result can be obtained due to haemolysis, clot formation, postmortem diffusion from other body fluids and tissues, not properly preserved sample, and putrefaction. False blood alcohol levels in excess of 0.1 mg.% may be produced if autopsy blood samples are stored at room temperature for more than a week.

WIDMARK evolved a formula which takes into account the size and sex of the person and the type of alcoholic liquor consumed. The formula is a = prc, where a, is weight of alcohol (in g.) in the body; p, is the body weight (in kg.); c, is the concentration of alcohol in the blood (in mg. per kg.); and r is a constant (0.68 for men and 0.55 for women). The sex difference is due to the different fat-water ratios, men having about 54%, and women 44% water partition by weight.

For urine analysis the formula is a=3/4 prq. q is the alcohol concentration (in mg. per kg.).

BACK CALCULATIONS: The sex, size, obesity, the drinking history, completeness of absorption, timing, amount and nature of meals taken, all alter the parameters of calculation. Wide margins of error (50 to 100 mg%) are possible Table (30–3). Back-calculations are unreliable and inaccurate. The rule of thumb is that 30 ml. of 80° proof liquor will raise blood alcohol concentration by 25 mg %.

If the blood specimen is collected while the intoxication curve was rising, and the level here is insufficient to establish intoxication, an extrapolation backward would result in lower blood alcohol than the known amount. The only way to establish whether or not the specimen was obtained on the upswing or downswing of the alcohol curve is to secure two specimens at spaced intervals and compare their alcohol content.

Methods Used for Determining Blood Alcohol: Presumptive tests which measure the presence of any volatile reducing agent are routinely done. The basic principle is a reduction of potassium bichromate by the test substance. (1) **Kozelka and Hine** test is a macro-method. Alcohol is distilled in a current of steam. The steam is condensed after passing through a reagent which traps interfering substances and the alcohol in the condensate is

Table (30–3). Blood alcohol in relation to alcohol consumed

Amount of ethyl alcohol per 100 ml. of blood	Amount of ethyl alcohol in a man of 70 kg.	Minimum amount of liquor consumed			Time required for complete removal of alcohol from body
		Whisky 40%	Wine 16%	Beer 3.28%	
50 mg.	26 ml.	68 ml.	172 ml.	0.8 Lit.	2.5 hours.
100 mg.	53 ml.	136 ml.	344 ml.	1.6 Lit.	5 hours.
200 mg.	106 ml.	275 ml.	688 ml.	3.2 Lit.	10.5 hours.
300 mg.	159 ml.	411 ml.	933 ml.	4.8 Lit.	16 hours.
400 mg.	212 ml.	550 ml.	1.38 Lit.	6.4 Lit.	21 hours.
500 mg.	264 ml.	687 ml.	1.62 Lit.	8.0 Lit.	26.5 hours.
600 mg.	318 ml.	825 ml.	1.87 Lit.	9.6 Lit.	32 hours.

determined by reduction of dichromate. (2) **Cavett test** is a micro-method. It is modification of Widmark using different chemical reaction to determine the amount of alcohol. Many procedures are employed for determining the values of ethyl alcohol, including ADH (alcohol dehydrogenase) method, head space and direct injection gas chromatography, enzyme-spectrophotometric assays and oxidation techniques. **For medicolegal purposes, the most desirable is gas chromatography in which specificity can be ascertained.**

Test: In a test tube place one ml of unknown solution + one ml of acetic acid + one drop of sulphuric acid and heat gently for one minute. Strong fruity odour is positive.

The amount of alcohol consumed can be determined from the blood alcohol level. In case of blood alchol level of 100 mg%, the amount ingested is roughly one ml. of absolute alcohol per kg of body weight.

BREATH: Breath analysis machines operate on the principle that alcohol absorbs radiation in the infrared region of the spectrum and that the amount of infrared light absorbed by a vapour is proportional to the concentration of alcohol in that vapour. The end portion of a prolonged forced expiration gives correct results. **The concentration of alcohol in deep lung air is dependent on the concentration in arterial blood. 2100 to 2300 ml. of alveolar air contains the same amount of alcohol as one ml. of blood.** This is based on **Henry's law,** which states that when a volatile chemical (ethanol) is dissolved in a liquid (blood) and is brought to equilibrium with air (alverolar air), there is a fixed ratio between the concentration of volatile compound (ethanol) in air (alveolar air) and its concentration in the liquid (blood), and the ratio is constant at a given temperature. (i.e., in alcohol 34°C, i.e., temperature of breathed out air). The converted breath tests are in close agreement with those obtained by direct blood analyses. The person is asked to blow into the apparatus. **Recently developed breath analysers rely on infrared absorption of energy by ethyl alcohol vapour in breath samples. More sophisticated versions based on fuel-cell sensing, electrochemical oxidation and microprocessors have come into use.** They are a direct method which instantly measures breath alcohol quantitatively and provide a printout. **The residual alcohol in the mouth disappears in 20 minutes.** As such, the test should be repeated after 20 minutes.

Plastic, aluminium and other metal flexible bags have been developed, so that breath samples may be preserved for several hours with minimum loss of alcohol. Breath alcohol levels rise faster and fall earlier than venous blood alcohol levels. The estimation of the stage of alcohol absorption, distribution or elimination can be made from analysis of two or more serial specimens from the same individual at known intervals of time.

FALSE VALUES: Many factors can temporarily upset the reliability of breath analysis, such as strenuous hyperventilation, violent physical exercise, emesis and regurgitation of stomach contents, eructation or belching and drinking of liquor within few minutes of the time of the performance of the test. Under these conditions false values are obtained.

Saliva: Mouth should be thoroughly washed with water and about 5 ml. of saliva collected in a test tube containing 10 mg. of sodium fluoride.

Vitreous: At equilibrium, for every unit of alcohol in blood, there are 1.2 units of alcohol in vitreous, as it has a high water content. During the absorptive phase of alcohol, vitreous alcohol levels are lower than in the blood. Vitreous alcohol lags behind blood alcohol by 1 to 2 hours. It does not change after death due to putrefaction.

The Diagnosis: There are usually no difficulties in the diagnosis in extreme cases, i.e., where the person is clearly drunk or clearly sober. Problems arise in the marginal case, and in those with intermediate degree in the disturbance of behaviour. The usual signs of drunkenness are: strong odour of alcohol in breath, loss of self-control and clearness of intellect, unsteady gait, vacant look, congested eyes, sluggish and dilated pupils, dry lips, increased pulse rate, unsteady and thick voice, talks at random and lack of perception of passage of time.

Determination of blood alcohol helps: (1) to know the concentration of alcohol circulating in the body, (2) to determine within fairly wide limits how much alcohol must have been imbibed within a certain period of time. This can be attempted only after equilibrium between the blood and tissues has been attained, which can help the Court in testing the reliability of the statements of the accused, (3) to assist the doctor in confirming his suspicions, (4) enable the Court to accept clinical diagnosis, (5) serve to resolve conflicting reports given by non-medical witnesses.

Susceptibility: There is a large variation in the susceptibility of drinkers to the effects of alcohol. Young persons, or those unused to drinking will be affected by much lower levels of blood alcohol than the average, whereas alcoholics show tremendous tolerance to the effects. The effects of acute alcohol intoxication are more marked when the blood level is rising than falling.

Psychological reaction: The individual psychological reaction to acute alcohol intoxication is variable. It has been established that some individuals remain sober at a very high blood alcohol level. A person may be intoxicated at a low blood alcohol level, but at another time he may be diagnosed as sober at very high levels. A chronic alcoholic with a blood level of 150 mg% may appear sober though there is impairment in the reflexes, visual acuity, memory, concentration, and judgement. Therefore, **the blood alcohol level is only one item in the evidence, which must be considered in relation to other evidence about the behaviour of the person at the material time. This evidence may be medical as well as non-medical.**

Disadvantages of physical examination: (1) The medical examination is extremely subjective, many of the observations made are incapable of objective or quantitative record. (2) There is individual variation from one clinical examiner to another. (3) As the medical examination is usually conducted some considerable time after the accident, it will be very difficult for the doctor to dogmatise about the accused's condition and capacity at the time of accident. (4) If an arrested person suffers from fear or acute anxiety often complicated by fatigue states, the signs may simulate drunkenness. Non-medical evidence about the conduct of the person concerned may be very important, and may be considered by the Court regarding the diagnosis as it may indicate the nature of the behaviour at the time of arrest. **The blood alcohol level is only of value when it is consistent with other non-chemical observations made.**

Medical Terminology: "Under the influence" means that due to drinking alcohol, a person has lost (to any degree), some of the clearness of the mind and self-control that he normally possesses. Loss of judgement and the capacity for self-criticism occur long before the obvious symptoms of intoxication. **All individuals with a blood alcohol level of 140 mg% are intoxicated to the point where they cannot deal with unusual, emergency or non-customary problems.**

Below 10 mg%: Sober.
10 to 80 mg%: Drinking.
80 to 150 mg%: Under the influence.
150 to 300 mg%: Drunk or intoxicated.
300 to 400 mg: Stupor.
400 mg% and above: Coma, and death.

Under the influence: The signs are: flushed face, dilated and sluggish pupils, euphoria, loss of restraint, thickness of speech, carelessness and recklessness, incoordination, stagger on sudden turning.

Drunk: The symptoms are: flushed face, dilated and inactive pupils, rapid movement of eye balls, unstable mood, loss of restraint, clouding of intellect, thickness of speech, incoordination, staggering gait with reeling and lurching when called upon to make sudden turns.

Very drunk: The symptoms are: flushed or pale face, pupils inactive, contracted or dilated, mental confusion, gross incoordination, slurred speech, staggering, reeling gait, tendency to lurch and fall, vomiting.

Coma: The symptoms are: rapid pulse, subnormal temperature, stertorous breathing, deep unconsciousness, contracted pupils.

HAZARDS OF ALCOHOL: Fatal acute poisoning by alcohol is rare, but mild and moderate degrees of intoxication are frequent and create a social and medical problem. Alcohol is associated with domestic violence, child abuse and suicide. The personal risks are: (1) He may die of exposure. (2) Alcohol in the tracheobronchial tree can cause pneumonia. (3) Inhale his vomit or dentures. (4) A bolus of food or meat inhaled into larynx can cause death due to choking. (5) Alcohol reduces man's resistance to the effects of hypoxia. This makes alcohol a hazard to those engaged in mountain climbing, aviation, and in any person who has a cardiac or pulmonary condition with borderline hypoxia. (6) He may fall and sustain a head injury. (7) He may fall into water and be drowned. (8) He may turn on the gas and forget to light the burners. (9) He may electrocute himself when fumbling with a plug or a defective electrical circuit. (10) He may take poison by mistaking it for alcohol. (11) An intoxicated person driving motor vehicle is a grave danger to others. (12) The so-called Saturday Night Paralysis occurs in the stage of coma, and results from pressure on a nerve trunk, as when an arm hangs over a chair (pressure on the radial nerve).

Alcoholic Palimpsests (alcoholic blackout): It is a condition seen among alcoholics, and rarely in the non-addictive drinker, after drinking a moderate amount of alcohol. **The behaviour resembles the 'blackouts' in anoxaemia**. This may result in the loss of memory of a period during a drinking spell, or in some cases, the inability to recall what happened over a period of days. Amnesia can be fragmentary or total. In the latter case, the memory with regard to the "lost time", is unlikely to return. It is a late manifestation of alcoholism. **During such state, the person may perform a criminal act, and may not remember this after he recovers from the effects of intoxication.**

Alcohol and Traffic Accidents: There is progressive loss of driving ability as blood alcohol concentration rises. The safe driving is interfered due to: (1) It increases reaction time. (2) It creates false confidence. (3) It impairs concentration, dulls judgement, and degrades muscular coordination. (4) It decreases visual and auditory acuity.

Below 50 mg.% concentration of blood alcohol, majority of drivers are not affected, as regards road safety. Tasks which require control of speed and sensorimotor coordination in keeping a vehicle on its course and braking is impaired at 50 mg%. The driver experiences an increase in boldness and impulsiveness. This results in a tendency to drive faster and more erratically. At 60 mg%, the driver of a vehicle is twice as likely to be involved in an accident as compared to a sober driver. Risk of accident begins to increase markedly at 80 mg%; by 100 mg% risk is 12-fold and at levels of over 150 mg%, this becomes 20 times more likely. At 100 mg%. all individuals are affected, and accidents are common. Drivers under the influence genuinely believe that they are driving better than they are.

The punishment for first offence is fine up to Rs. **10,000** or 6 months imprisonment or both and for a second or subsequent offence fine up to **15,000** or imprisonment up to 2 years or both.

Alcohol and Driving: In some countries, the law has made it an offence for a person to drive a motor vehicle above a specified blood alcohol level, e.g., 20 mg% in Poland and Sweden, 50 mg% in Norway, 80 mg % in U.K. and France and 100 to 120 mg% in different States of U.S.A. **The statutory limit in India is 30 mg%** (S.185, Motor Vehicle Act, 1988).

Drugs and Driving: Many drugs affect driving, such as tranquilisers, opiates, barbiturates, cannabis, hallucinogens, anti-histaminics, anti-depressants and anti-psychotics.

ALCOHOL WITHDRAWAL: Symptoms appear 12 to 48 hours after reduction in alcohol intake. Most common symptom is tremors or shakes. The essential features are a coarse tremor of the hands, tongue and eyelids in association with at least one of the following: (a) nausea and vomiting, (b) malaise and weakness, (c) hypertension, tachycardia

and sweating, (d) anxiety, depressed mood and irritability, (e) transient hallucinations and illusions, (f) headache and insomnia. Withdrawal seizures are typically single and generalised and usually develop 6 to 48 hours after last drink. About one-third of these patients will develop delirium tremens unless preventive measures are taken.

Treatment: 20 mg of chlordiazepoxide, or 100 mg of diazepam, are given four times a day. Anticraving agents, such as acamprosate, naltrexone and fluoxetine are used. Behaviour therapy, psychotherapy and group therapy. Deterring agents (alcohol sensitising drugs): Disulfiram, citrate calcium carbimide, metronidazole, nitrafezole and methyl tetrazolethiol.

PATHOLOGY: (1) DELIRIUM TREMENS: This results from the long-continued action of the poison on the brain. It occurs in chronic alcoholics due to (1) temporary excess, (2) sudden withdrawal of alcohol, (3) shock after receiving an injury, such as fracture of a bone, or (4) from acute infection, such as pneumonia, influenza, erysipelas, etc.

It typically begins 72 to 96 hours after the last drink. There is an acute attack of insanity in which the main symptoms are coarse muscular tremors of face, tongue and hands, insomnia, restlessness, loss of memory, psychomotor agitation, confusion, disorientation, uncontrollable fear and has tendency to commit suicide, homicide or violent assault or to cause damage to property. Other symptoms are diarrhoea, dilated pupils, fever, tachycardia, tachypnoea, and hypertension. There is disorientation as to time and place, and a peculiar kind of delirium of horrors owing to hallucinations of the sight and hearing. The patient imagines that insects are crawling under the skin, or snakes are crawling on his bed. **It is considered unsoundness of mind, and not intoxication.** Death occurs in about 5 to 15% of cases due to cerebral oedema, cardiac failure or shock. To control agitation diazepam should be given.

(2) WERNICKE'S ENCEPHALOPATHY: This results from neuronal degeneration and haemorrhages in hypothalamus, midbrain and cerebellum lesion due to heavy drinking. Vitamin B_1 deficiency occurs.

Symptoms: Ocular: Coarse nystagmus and ophthalmoparesis, external ocular palsies (involvement of sixth cranial nerve), retinal haemorrhages, papilloedema, pupillary irregularity and impairment of vision.

CNS: Disorientation, confusion, recent memory disturbances, poor attention span, distractibility, peripheral neuropathy, stupor. Apathy and ataxia are early symptoms. It has a high mortality and can cause death in 24 hours. If untreated about 80% cases progress to a more chronic condition which presents as an organic amnestic syndrome known as Korsakoff psychosis, in which impairment of anterograde and retrograde memory, severe disorientation in time, with inability to learn new information and confabulation (recitation of imaginary experiences to fill gaps in the memory) are seen.

(3) ALCOHOLIC POLYNEURITIS AND KORSAKOFF'S PSYCHOSIS: The symptoms of polyneuritis are weakness, pain in the extremities, wrist and foot drop, unsteady gait, loss of deep reflexes and tenderness of muscles of arms and legs.

Treatment: (1) Diazepam 40 to 80 mg/day in divided doses. (2) Chlordiazepoxide 80–120 mg/day in divided doses or haloperidol 20 mg/day. (3) In some withdrawal symptoms cases only restoration of alcoholic drinks helps.

(4) ALCOHOLIC PARANOIA: In this there are fixed delusions but no hallucinations. The person becomes deeply suspicious of the motives and actions of those he meets and of his family members.

(5) ACUTE ALCOHOLIC HALLUCINOSIS: Persistent hallucinations develop within 48 hours after cessation of alcohol intake. The hallucinations may be auditory or visual and their content is usually unpleasant and disturbing. The disorder may last several weeks or months.

(6) ALCOHOLIC EPILEPSY: Seizures occur after a day or more of the termination of a drinking session. Sometimes, the attacks may occur while the patient is actually drinking.

(7) CARDIAC DYSRHYTHMIAS: Episodes of atrial fibrillation may occur after 10 to 12 years of heavy alcohol abuse, especially induced by drinking binges (Holiday Heart syndrome). In alcohol withdrawal, tachyrhythmias are common probably because of high adrenergic nervous system activity, which may cause sudden death.

(8) MARCHIAFAVA'S SYNDROME: Degeneration of the corpus callosum may occur in alcoholics.

(9) MALLORY-WEISS SYNDROME: Ruptured oesophagus with mediastinitis occurs.

(10) Malnutrition.

(11) Gastric and peptic ulcer.

(12) Cirrhosis.

(13) Myocarditis.

(14) Pancreatitis.

(15) Mental illness. Depression and high risk for suicide.

(16) Alcohol creates a disturbance in tryptophane metabolism. Conversion of tryptophane to 5-hydroxyindolacetic acid (the urinary metabolite of serotonin) is depressed in the chronic alcoholic.

ALCOHOL AND CRIMINAL BEHAVIOUR: The frequency of crimes committed by persons under the influence of alcohol is not due to failure to realise the nature and consequences of the acts, but to the repression of those inhibitory influences that in sober persons prevent the commission of such acts. Illegal acts are usually committed while the excitement due to the stimulation of the brain is at or about its height. At this time, the actions of the individuals are purposeful and the likely consequences are generally fully appreciated. Such person has the same intention and knowledge as a sober person performing the same act would have, though he does not have the same power of resisting the impulse towards its performance. A strong relationship exists between the abuse of alcohol and the occurrence of accidents and acts of violence. The crimes most frequently indulged are those activated by the passions. As the suppressed feelings of aggression and hostility are released, the drinker goes into a state of artificial display of bravery. Acute alcohol intoxication is a factor in suicides and homicides.

Alcohol slows the reactions of the victim, and he may not be able to protect himself in time from an assault. He may be struck down with a minimum or no defence injuries. **Alcohol causes dilatation and congestion of blood vessels, so that injuries will result in greater and prolonged bleeding.** If there is chronic alcoholic liver disease which impairs the clotting of blood, the bleeding will be more extensive. If a victim is severely intoxicated, he may die from inhalation of blood or vomit while lying on his back following injuries, especially of the head or face.

S. 510, I.P.C: Misconduct in public by a drunken person is punishable with imprisonment up to 24 hours.

Alcohol and Sudden Death: (1) In some persons alcohol has an effect on the myocardium, predisposing to and producing arrhythmias. Cocaine, amphetamine and toluene also predispose to and can cause cardiac arrhythmias by a direct action on the myocardium. (2) **An intoxicated person during the struggle, or more commonly immediately after it, suddenly becomes unresponsive, develops cardiopulmonary arrest and dies.**

No anatomical cause for the death is found at autopsy. Catecholamines are released during struggle, which in combination with alcohol may produce cardiac arrhythmias and death. (3) Occasionally, the person has a physiological lesion of the conduction system of the heart predisposing to and causing arrhythmias, which can be aggravated by alcohol and release of catecholamines. Peak levels of catecholamines are reached, immediately after cessation of the struggle. (4) After a violent struggle, the victim may be restrained in such a way, that breathing is impaired, producing a relative hypoxia. In some persons, death may result, when this is combined with alcohol and the release of catecholamines. **The cause of death in such cases can be certified as "cardiopulmonary arrest, contributed by alcohol during a violent struggle"**. (5) Intoxicated person who is severely beaten about the face may collapse and die. The autopsy is essentially negative. Death probably occurs from a combination of CNS depression due to alcohol and diffuse axonal injury from beating.

ALCOHOL AFTER DEATH: Alcohol diffuses through the intact stomach wall after death into the surrounding blood and tissues, including the pericardial fluid and pleural fluid. As such, higher blood levels are found than what actually existed during life, if blood samples are taken from parts into which postmortem diffusion has taken place, i.e., heart, or a large vein in the chest.

If death occurs instantaneously from trauma, then a postmortem alcohol estimation will give a true picture of the individual at such time. Subdural blood clot will contain the same concentration of alcohol as that in blood at the time of fatal injury. Such clots will give the exact concentration of alcohol at the time of the fatal injury, even though the victim may survive for several hours. In cases of severe internal injury, gastric contents may collect in the thoracic cavity. This may give rise to the possibility of diffusion of alcohol in the heart blood. No appreciable loss of alcohol from body or blood takes place by evaporation or any other means after death. With advanced putrefaction, the entire contents of the vascular system including alcohol is destroyed. Analysis of brain gives best results.

ALCOHOL IN PUTREFACTION: Endogenous production of alcohol is not seen in all decomposed bodies. Ethanol and other alcohols can be produced during putrefaction by fermentation of the carbohydrates and proteins of the body (usually 20 to 30 mg/100 ml). This may occur due to enzymes, bacteria, yeast or fungi. The commonest organism is E. coli. The longer the interval after death and the higher the temperature, the more is produced. Alcohol produced by advanced putrefaction may be as high as 0.2%. A combination of glucose in urine and Candida albicans reaction can result in the production of large amounts of ethanol. Alcohol concentrations in excess of 0.2% would indicate alcohol consumption prior to death, while levels below 0.2% may be attributed to possible production due to putrefaction. In cases of putrefaction, if alcohol is found in the blood and organs, but not in the urine and vitreous humour, the alcohol reaction in the blood is probably false due to putrefaction.

METHYL ALCOHOL

Types: Pure methyl alcohol (wood alcohol or methanol) is colourless, volatile liquid, with an odour similar to ethyl alcohol, and has a burning taste. Mineralised methylated spirit consists of 90% by volume of ethyl alcohol, 9.5% of wood naphtha, and 0.5% of crude pyridine. It is present in certain home-made beverages, antifreeze, paint removers, dyes, resins, adhesives and varnish.

Absorption: It is rapidly absorbed through the stomach and intestines, and also through the lungs and the skin. Though its action resembles that of ethyl alcohol to a great extent, **its rate of oxidation is one-fifth that of ethanol** and with repeated small doses tends to accumulate in the blood. **80 mg/100 ml. of blood is dangerous level.** It does not completely disappear from the blood for 3 or 4 days. **Methanol is oxidised by the liver to formaldehyde, (which is 33 times more toxic than methanol), which in turn is oxidised to formic acid, which is six times more toxic than methanol, which is responsible for the associated metabolic acidosis and the retinal toxicity.** Formate may inhibit the cytochrome oxidase chain, increasing lactate production and metabolic acidosis. It is distributed in the tissues according to their water content, and a high concentration is found in vitreous body and optic nerve.

Elimination: The liver slowly metabolises methanol. 3 to 5% is excreted through the lungs and up to 12% through kidneys.

Signs and Symptoms: Methyl alcohol produces symptoms of drunkenness in the same way as ethyl alcohol, but inebriation is not prominent, and the effects are more prolonged. Toxicity can result following its absorption through skin or respiratory tract. **Symptoms may appear within an hour, or may not appear for 24 hours.** They consist of nausea, vomiting and pain or severe cramps in the abdomen, headache, dizziness, neck stiffness, confusion, vertigo. There is marked muscular weakness, and depressed cardiac action and hypothermia. There may be dyspnoea and cyanosis. **The odour is usually present in the breath. The effect on the central nervous system is more intense and persistent than with ethyl alcohol. There may be delirium and coma which may last for two or three days.** There is a toxic effect on the liver and kidneys (acute tubular necrosis) and on highly specialised nerve elements. Urine is strongly acid and may contain acetone and a trace of albumin. **Acidosis** is caused by the inhibitory effect on oxidative enzyme systems produced by methanol with the resultant accumulation of lactic and other unidentified acids. **The pupils are dilated and fixed.** Visual disturbances like photophobia and blurred or misty vision (snowfield vision), seeing spots, central and peripheral scotomata, decreased light perception, concentric diminution of visual fields for colour and form, followed by **fairly sudden failure of vision or complete blindness occur due to optic neuritis and atrophy from the effects of formic acid on the optic nerve. 10 to 20 ml. of methanol can cause blindness.** Fundoscopy shows hyperaemia of optic disc followed by retinal oedema. The retinal ganglion cells and optic disc show degenerative changes. In fatal cases, convulsions are usual as a terminal event.

Severe non-diabetic anion metabolic acidosis in unconscious persons is suggestive of methyl alcohol poisoning.

An increased osmolol gap accompanied by visual symptoms suggest methanol poisoning. An anion metabolic acidosis is characteristic of methanol, ethylene glycol diabetic ketoacidosis, lactic acidosis and salicylate intoxication.

Fatal Dose: 60 to 200 ml.

Fatal Period: 24 to 36 hours; may be delayed for 2 to 4 days.

Cause of Death: Death is mainly due to acidosis from production of organic acids, and CNS depression is a minor factor.

Treatment: (1) **Gastric lavage using 5% bicarbonate solution** should be done, and 500 ml. of this may be left in the stomach. (2) **Activated charcoal** reduces the mortality significantly. It acts by reducing the absorption of alcohol from the digestive tract, and by creating a concentration gradient in favour of movement of alcohol and its metabolites back into the gut. (3) **Ethanol is the antidote.** It is given i.v. as a 10% solution, starting with 500 ml. as an infusion and repeated as required, until blood level falls below 25 mg%. Serum ethanol levels must be checked frequently to assure that a level of 100 to 150 mg.% is being maintained at all times. The i.v. route is preferred to avoid gastritis. Methyl alcohol is oxidised to formaldehyde by the enzyme catalase. **This catalase can also oxidise ethyl alcohol to acetaldehyde. In methyl alcohol poisoning, ethyl alcohol by competition for catalase, blocks the formation of formaldehyde and allows the less toxic methyl alcohol to be excreted unmetabolised.** (4) **Alternatively, 60 ml of ethyl alcohol in 200 ml fruit juice can be given orally over a period of 30 minutes.** For maintenance, give 15 ml of 50% ethyl alcohol every hour. (5) **Haemodialysis** is the treatment of choice in severe poisoning. **It reduces the half-life of methanol from 40 hours to about one hour.** There is no role for peritoneal dialysis or haemoperfusion. (6) **4 methyl pyrazole (4MP, or fomepizole).** The usual dose is 15 mg/kg of 4 MP, followed 12 hours later by 10 mg/kg 12th hourly for 4 doses, and then increased to 15 mg/kg 12th hourly for as long as necessary. It is a competitive inhibitor of alcohol dehydrogenase. It blocks formation of formaldehyde and formic acid and can be used instead of ethanol. (7) **Folinic or folic acid 50 to 75 mg. every four hours** is useful to increase the elimination of formic acid, decreasing the metabolic acidosis, and reducing symptoms. (8) Blood sugar should be measured frequently while ethanol is being given, as it may cause hypoglycaemia, especially in children. (9) The basic treatment for alcoholic ketoacidosis is crystalloid therapy, dextrose, thiamine, and phosphate. Correct potassium and magnesium defects. (10) Soda bicarbonate i.v. to correct metabolic acidosis. (11) Place patient in a left lateral decubitus position with head down to avoid aspiration of vomit. (12) Eyes should be kept covered to protect them from light. (13) Keep the airway clear.

Postmortem Appearances: Cyanosis is marked, and there is an absence of postmortem clotting of the blood. **The pyridine may give the skin a purple colour.** The mucous membrane of the stomach and the duodenum is congested and inflamed with small haemorrhages. **Small or large intestine or both are contracted resembling a thick pipe of a very narrow lumen.** The lungs are congested and oedematous. The brain is oedematous and shows local haemorrhages. The mucosa of the bladder is often congested. The liver shows fatty change and sometimes early necrosis, and there is tubular degeneration of the kidneys.

ANALYSIS: Methyl alcohol and formic acid are found in all organs, blood and urine. Formaldehyde cannot be demonstrated probably because of the rapidity with which it combines with protein and its speedy oxidation to formic acid.

Anticoagulants such as EDTA, heparin, methenamine and formalin give a positive test for methanol.

The Circumstances of Poisoning: Poisoning is mostly accidental. Sometimes it is used as an intoxicating beverage, when ethyl alcohol is not available.

ETHYLENE GLYCOL

It is a clear, colourless, odourless, non-volatile liquid with a bitter-sweet taste. It is mainly used as an antifreeze agent. It is not absorbed through skin. It is metabolised to glycoaldehyde, glycolic acid and oxalic acid and inhibits oxidative phosphorylation.

SYMPTOMS: Initial symptoms are vomiting, lethargy, ataxia, inebriation, convulsions and coma. In 12 to 24 hours tachycardia, tachypnoea and circulatory collapse, electrolyte imbalance and metabolic acidosis occur. In one to three days, hypocalcaemia, oliguria, tubular necrosis and renal failure occur. Urine contains crystals of calcium oxalate.

FATAL DOSE: 100 to 200 ml.

FATAL PERIOD: 3 days

TREATMENT: (1) Gastric lavage. (2) Activated charcoal. (3) Ethanol in same dose as for methyl alcohol. (4) 4-methyl pyrazole. (5) Haemodialysis. (6) I.v. sodium bicarbonate. (7) 10% calcium gluconate i.v.

POSTMORTEM APPEARANCES: Cerebral oedema, chemical meningo-encephalitis, liver and kidney damage may be seen. Oxalate crystals are seen in brain, spinal cord and kidneys.

ISOPROPANOL

It is a colourless, volatile liquid with a faint odour of acetone and is slightly bitter. It is used as a disinfectant, paint remover, antifreeze, sterilising agent industrial solvent and for massage. It is absorbed through all routes. It is rapidly metabolised and converted to acetone which is excreted in urine and breath. It is two to three times more potent than ethanol as CNS depressant. Fatal dose is about 250 ml.

SYMPTOMS: Abdominal pain, gastritis, vertigo, headache, lethargy, ataxia, haemorrhagic tracheobronchitis and apnoea.

TREATMENT: (1) Gastric lavage. (2) Activated charcoal. (3) Haemodialysis.

CHLOROFORM

It is a heavy, colourless, volatile liquid, with sweet pungent taste and a characteristic ethereal odour.

SIGNS AND SYMPTOMS: When swallowed, there is burning pain in the mouth, throat and stomach and vomiting. Within ten minutes, unconsciousness and coma with slow stertorous breathing occurs. Pupils are dilated and pulse is feeble, rapid and irregular. When inhaled it causes irritation in throat and burning of eyes. The face is flushed and the patient becomes delirious. In 3 to 4 minutes, patient becomes unconscious and corneal and other reflexes are lost. Pulse and respiration are slow and feeble, temperature subnormal and pupils contracted. All the muscles are relaxed. If the inhalation is continued, the patient passes into a stage of paralysis. Skin is cyanosed and pupils dilate. Death occurs from cardiac or respiratory failure.

FATAL DOSE: Thirty ml. when ingested; a concentration of five percent or more in air when inhaled.

TREATMENT: Stomach wash, artificial respiration, stimulants and symptomatic.

POSTMORTEM APPEARANCES: They are not characteristic except the smell in serous cavities, lungs and brain. There is usually marked congestion.

THE CIRCUMSTANCES OF POISONING: Accidental death may occur during anaesthesia or when liquid chloroform is swallowed accidentally. It is occasionally used for suicide. Homicide by inhalation or by ingestion is very rare. It is extremely difficult to put a person under the influence of an anaesthetic without his consent.

ETHER

It is a colourless, volatile liquid having a peculiar penetrating odour and sweetish pungent taste.

SINGS AND SYMPTOMS: When inhaled, effects are similar to chloroform, but there is more irritation of respiratory tract and more secretion of mucus and saliva. Taken by mouth, effects are similar to alcohol, but is more rapid in onset and shorter in duration.

FATAL DOSE: Thirty ml.

TREATMENT: As for chloroform.

POSTMORTEM APPEARANCES: Brain is slightly oedematous. Trachea contains frothy mucus. Lungs are congested and oedematous.

OPIUM

Characteristics: Opium (afim) is the dried juice of the poppy (Papaver somniferum) which is cultivated in India and other Eastern countries, only under a licence. The plant grows up to one metre in height. Each plant bears 5 to 8 capsules. Flowers are white. **The unripe capsule is incised and the white juice which exudes is collected and allowed to evaporate to obtain opium Fig. (30–1). Ripe and dry poppy capsules contain a trace of opium and are used for their sedative and narcotic action.** Their warm decoction is used locally as a sedative fomentation and poultice. **Poppy seeds (khaskhas) are white, harmless, demulcent and nutritive and are used as food Fig. (30–2).** The oil from the seeds is used for cooking purposes.

Features: Opium occurs in rounded, irregularly formed or flattened masses and has a strong characteristic odour and bitter taste. When fresh, it is soft, flexible and internally moist, coarsely granular or smooth and reddish-brown on keeping.

Active Principles: Crude opium contains a large number of alkaloids, about 25, combined with meconic, lactic and sulphuric acids. These form two chemically different groups: (a) the phenanthrenes: morphine (about 10%), codeine (about 0.5%), and thebaine (about 0.3%), which are narcotic, and (b) the isoquinoline group: papaverine (about 1%), and narcotine (about 6%), which have mild analgesic but no narcotic properties. Thebaine acts as convulsant.

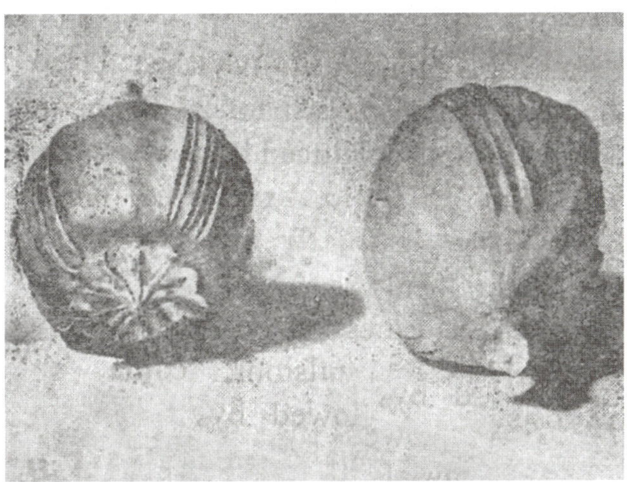

Fig. (30–1). Poppy capsules.

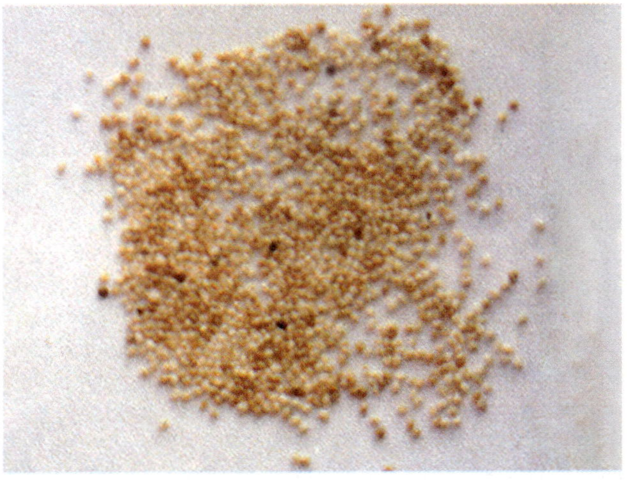

Fig. (30–2). Poppy.

Morphine occurs as white powder or as white shining crystals, has bitter taste and alkaline reaction. The narcotic symptoms of opium poisoning are practically those of morphine poisoning.

Classification: (1) **Natural:** morphine, codeine. (2) **Semi-synthetic:** Substances which are derived by modification of the chemical constituents of opium are called semisynthetic narcotics. They are chemically related to opium alkaloids and are called opioid analogues, e.g., heroin, hydromorphone, oxymorphone, oxycodone. (3) **Synthetic**: Synthetic analogues called designer drugs are manufactured illicitly in calandestined laboratories for recreational use, which are highly potent and addictive, e.g., meperidine, methadone, levarphanol tartrate, paregoric, diphenoxylate, fentanyl, propoxyphene.

Action: Opiates exert their effects because of their chemical similarity to natural substances called endorphins. The opiate drugs activate receptor sites normally occupied by the natural opiates or endorphins. Opium depresses all centres except oculomotor, vomiting and sweating. It is a peripherally acting analgesic. It stimulates non-propulsive rhythmic contraction of small intestine. Opium and its derivatives act synergistically with alcohol and barbiturates.

Absorption: It is absorbed from mucous membranes, raw surface or wounds, hypodermic injection and when smoked in cigarettes.

Elimination: It is destroyed by the tissues, particularly by the liver. **It is eliminated mainly as morphine in urine and faeces,** and also by stomach, intestines, saliva, bile and milk. Morphine can be easily recovered from blood, urine and bile.

Fatal Dose: Opium 2 g; morphine 0.2 g; codeine 80 mg; methadone 100 mg, Propoxyphene 1g. and pentazocine 300 mg. Fentanyl is 50 to 100 times more potent than morphine.

Fatal Period: 6 to 12 hours.

Signs and Symptoms: The contact of morphine with the **skin of sensitive persons may cause erythema, urticaria and itching dermatitis.**

When opium is taken by mouth, symptoms begin within half hour. If the drug is injected, its action is noted within 3 or 4 minutes. **It first stimulates, then depresses and finally paralyses the nerve centres.**

(1) Stage of Excitement: This stage is of short duration, and may be absent if a large dose is taken. There is an increased sense of well-being, increased mental activity, freedom from anxiety, talkativeness, restlessness or even hallucinations, flushing of face and greatly excited or maniacal condition may be seen.

(2) Stage of Stupor: The symptoms are headache, nausea, vomiting, incapacity for exertion, a sense of weight in the limbs, giddiness and drowsiness. The subject lies motionless, with eyes closed as if in a sound sleep from which he may be aroused at first, but soon passes into stupor and coma. The pupils are contracted, face and lips are cyanosed and an itching sensation is felt all over the skin. The pulse and respirations are normal.

(3) Stage of Coma: The patient passes into deep coma from which he cannot be aroused. The muscles become flaccid and relaxed and all reflexes are abolished. The face is pale, and conjunctivae congested. **The pupils are contracted to pinpoint size and do not react to light** but dilate during the agonal asphyxial phase caused by respiratory depression and ultimate paralysis. **All the secretions are suspended except sweat. Perspiration is very much increased.** The skin is cold and often covered with perspiration. **Temperature is subnormal.** Blood pressure is low, the pulse slow and full, the breathing is slow and stertorous and may be reduced to 3 to 4 per minute. **The odour of opium may be present in breath.**

In case of fatal termination, lividity of the surface increases, pulse becomes slow, irregular and imperceptible, the respiration becomes Cheyne-Stokes in type, and finally death occurs in deep coma from asphyxia.

The skin blistering seen in dependent parts of victims of deep coma is due to cutaneous oedema caused by cessation of venous return following muscle flaccidity.

DIFFERENTIAL DIAGNOSIS: (1) OPIUM POISONING: The odour of breath, slow pulse and moist perspiring skin are prominent. The triad of coma, pinpoint, immobile pupils and respiratory depression are diagnostic.

(2) ACUTE ALCOHOLIC POISONING: Odour of alcohol in breath, congested eyes and hyperaemia of face and neck, pupils dilated and reacting, subnormal temperature, slow and stertorous breathing.

(3) BARBITURATE POISONING: Shallow respiration, deep coma, no response to painful stimuli, deep reflexes are depressed, subnormal temperature, low blood pressure, thready pulse, dilated pupils.

(4) CARBOLIC ACID POISONING: Odour of breath, white patches on lips and mouth, and carboluria.

(5) CARBON MONOXIDE POISONING: History of exposure to poisoning with gas, intermittent convulsions, cherry-red colour of skin and carboxyhaemoglobin in blood.

(6) EPILEPTIC COMA: History of characteristic seizures, pupils fixed and dilated, skin flushed, face and lips cyanosed, froth at the mouth and nostrils, tongue may be bitten, slow respiration, rapid recovery.

(7) URAEMIC COMA: Gradual onset, pallor of face, Cheyne-Stokes respirations, ammoniacal odour, general anasarca, epileptiform convulsions, albumin, blood and casts in urine.

(8) DIABETIC COMA: Gradual onset, flushed face, slow and deep respirations, low intraocular tension, subnormal temperature, sweet odour of acetone in the breath, sugar and acetone in the urine.

(9) HYSTERICAL COMA: Usually in females, previous history with convulsive movements, usually occurs in presence of audience, unusual attitude, reflexes are not altered.

(10) CEREBRAL HAEMORRHAGE: Old age, sudden onset, history of hypertension, slow, full pulse, Cheyne-Stokes respirations, paralysis, usually hemiplegia, dilated pupils, raised temperature, bilateral extensor plantar reflexes.

(11) BRAIN TRAUMA: History or evidence of head injury, bleeding from nose, mouth or ears, respirations rapid, irregular or Cheyne-Stokes, pulse rapid, later slow, pupils inactive, often unequal, paralysis of cranial nerves, subconjunctival haemorrhages.

(12) CEREBRAL MALARIA: History of fever with rigors, enlarged spleen, may be hyperpyrexia.

(13) ENCEPHALITIS: Acute onset, fever, involuntary movements, ocular palsies, changes in cerebrospinal fluid.

(14) MENINGITIS: Gradual onset, signs of meningeal irritation, fever, CSF changes.

(15) HEAT HYPERPYREXIA: Prolonged exposure to high temperature or sun, congested conjunctivae with contracted pupils, hyperpyrexia, absence of sweating, dry skin, circulatory collapse, and convulsions.

Treatment: (1) Wash the stomach thoroughly and frequently, with a solution of 1: 5000 **potassium permanganate,** leaving some of the solution in the stomach for oxidising the alkaloid. **Gastric lavage should be carried out even after hypodermic injection of the drug, for the alkaloid is re-excreted into the stomach after absorption.** (2) A tablespoonful suspension of charcoal may be introduced into the stomach. (3) **The intestines should be cleared out by enema twice daily for two days to prevent reabsorption.** 30 g. of sodium sulphate by mouth with large amounts of water is also helpful. (4) Establish adequate airway. Use endotracheal intubation, if necessary. (5) **Atropine is not recommended,** for it can cause death by paralysing the motor and sensory nerves just like morphine. (6) **Naloxone hydrochloride is a specific opioid antagonist.** Unlike levallorphan and nalorphine, it neither causes psychotomimetic effects nor CNS depression. It competes with opioids at receptor sites. It can reverse not only the respiratory depressant, analgesic and euphoric effects of opioids but also the dysphoric, delusional, and hallucinatory properties of the synthetic opioids. **Two mg. is given i.v.** if there is respiratory depression, and repeated every half to one min. up to a total dose of 10 to 20 mg. i.v. It can be given i.m. or sublingually. Both coma and cardiopulmonary depression are reversed. If there is no response in two minutes, endotracheal intubation is necessary, and the same dose should be repeated. In any opioid overdose, a continuous infusion at a rate of 0.4 to 0.8 mg/per hour may be continued up to 48 hours, especially those with long-acting opioids such as methadone. (7) **Nalmefene has longer duration of effect than naloxone.** 0.1mg is given i.v. and if withdrawal reaction does not occur 0.5 mg is given, followed by 1 mg in 2 o 5 minutes if necessary. It can be given i.m. or s.c. (8) **Coma Cocktail:** In comatose patients where the identity of poison is not known, **100 ml. 50% glucose, 100 mg. thiamine, and 2 mg. naloxone** should be given i.v. (9) Nalorphine and levallorphan are not recommended. (10) Dextrose 50 ml. of 50% solution i.v. and thiamine 100 mg. (11) Physostigmine 0.04 mg/kg. i.v. may be given to reverse respiratory depression. if naloxone is not available. (12) Amiphenazole 20 to 40 mg i.v. can be given if necessary. (13) **If the patient is seen in the early stage, he should be made to walk about in the open air to help excretion, but if poison has been absorbed and is acting upon the cells of the cortex, it may do more harm than good by further exhausting the patient.** (14) When coma is deep, artificial respiration should be carried out continuously and oxygen given by inhalation. (15) Analeptics, e.g., amphetamine, caffeine, or ephedrine, may be given. (16) Bupernorphine and LAAM are considered effective in long-term management. (17) Symptoms are treated on general lines.

Postmortem Appearances: They are not characteristic, but **signs of asphyxia are prominent.** The face and the nails are cyanosed. Froth is seen at the mouth and nostrils. Postmortem staining is well-marked and cyanotic (deep blue). The smell of opium is noticed on opening the chest, but it disappears if putrefaction has set in. The stomach may contain small lumps of opium. The trachea and bronchi are congested and covered with froth. The lungs are oedematous and congested. The brain, meninges and abdominal organs are congested. The blood is usually dark and fluid. **Opium disappears rapidly from the cadaver.**

MARQUIS'S TEST: **A drop of a mixture consisting of three ml. of concentrated sulphuric acid, and three drops of formalin added to a fragment of the suspected residue produces a purple-red colour which gradually changes to violet and finally to blue.**

Poisoning: (1) Opium is selected by suicides because death is painless. (2) It is rarely used for homicide because of its bitter taste, characteristic smell and colour. (3) Poisoning may occur in addicts. Drugging of children by opium to keep them quiet, and overdosage of medicines containing opium may result in accidental poisoning. (4) It is rarely used as cattle poison. (5) It is sometimes used for doping race horses. (6) Sometimes opium is used to steady the nerves for doing some bold act requiring special courage.

CHRONIC POISONING: **(morphinism; morphinomania): The mechanism of tolerance is not known, but is thought to reside at a cellular level. The habit is acquired by young people as it is believed to be an aphrodisiac and as it produces a sense of euphoria. Opium addicts can tolerate 3 to 6 g. per day. The morphine addict has a dry skin, and shows scars of healed abscesses or abscesses themselves, and sometimes tattooing from needles. The habitual use first causes a pleasurable feeling of relief and well-being, but as larger doses are taken there is disinterest, and recurring periods of depression follow. The patient becomes restless and irritable and sleep is disturbed by dreams or there is insomnia. Loss of memory, mental fatigue and gradual intellectual and moral deterioration occur. Hallucinations may occur. Constipation, contracted pupils, anorexia, emaciation and weakness and impotence are frequent. Sudden cessation of opioid use in dependent pregnant woman may be life-threatening to the foetus.**

TREATMENT: **(1) Gradual withdrawal of drug. (2) Methadone 30 to 40 mg. daily to be tapered off gradually. (3) Naltrexone combined with clonidine. (4) Propoxyphene, diphenoxylate, buprenorphine, lofexidine are alternative to methadone. (5) Dihydrocodeine or codeine may be suitable for the less severely opiate dependent, not controlled with symptomatic treatment. (6) Propranolol 80 mg. relieves anxiety and craving. (7) Tranquilisers or sedation at bed time. (8) Psychiatric counselling.**

Morphine can sometimes be detected in liver or bile even when none is detectable in blood or urine. Opiate drugs can be identified in the hair.

HEROIN (Brown Sugar): There are three types of heroin, white, brown and black tar. Street heroin is known as "smack, junk, or dope" and is diluted with quinine, lactose, mannitol, etc. **It is not taken orally because it is rapidly hydrolysed in the stomach. It is the most dangerous among all drugs of addiction.** Solid heroin (diacetyl morphine) can be dissolved in a liquid and injected or it can be heated (usually on a piece of silver foil) and the smoke or vapour inhaled (chasing the dragon) or used as snuff. A combination of heroin and cocaine is known as **"Speedballs".** It is four times powerful in action than morphine. Fatal dose is about 50 mg. Fatal period 12 hours.

Metabolism: It is metabolised to monoacetylmorphine or acetylmorphine. Monoacetylmorphine is then hydrolysed to morphine in 30 to 60 minutes. As such, **chemical analysis will detect morphine but not heroin.** After injection, morphine and monoacetylmorphine are found in the urine almost immediately. Tolerance **occurs very rapidly (within days) and can be increased to more than hundred times the initial dose.**

Signs and symptoms are same as in opium, but due to i.v. administration, all stages marge into one. Intense euphoria lasts for several minutes followed by sedation for about one hour, and the **effects are completely lost in 3 to 6 hours.** Heroin and some opiates cause mast cells to release histamine, and can result in intense pruritus. It causes excitation by lifting cortical inhibitions similar to alcohol. **It can cause sudden death, even in persons who have been using it for some time, with the needle still in the vein.** A few deaths may be due to some personal hypersensitivity to the drug. Overdose causes death from a very strong CNS depressant action. In almost all cases, the victims are under the influence of alcohol at the time of death.

Treatment: (1) **Methadone** 40 mg. daily will usually prevent withdrawal symptoms; in a chronic addict 80 mg. will usually prevent heroin-induced euphoria. The dose is gradually reduced by 20% daily. If signs of withdrawal appear, dose reduction should proceed more slowly. Heroin addicts should never be given 20 mg. methadone at one time. (2) Detoxification. (3) Narcotic antagonist, such as naltrexone, naloxone, haloperidol, clonidine and cyclazocine.

Autopsy: Lungs are heavy and congested, Severe pulmonary oedema is the common autopsy finding probably due to sudden ventricular dysrhythmia. Microscopically, lungs show foreign body granulomas. Liver shows chronic triaditis with mononuclear cell infiltrates.

MEPERIDINE (pethidine): Meperidine hydrochloride is a colourless, crystalline powder with a bitter taste. It is administered by the i.m. or i.v. route for its **analgesic, antispasmodic and sedative properties.**

Action: It acts on the cerebrum and produces analgesia and sedation.

Fatal dose: 1 to 2 gm.

Fatal period: 24 hours.

Symptoms: **Effects are similar to those of morphine.** It causes more dizziness than morphine and greater elation. Tolerance to its toxic effects is not complete, and addicts may have twitchings, tremors, mental confusion, hallucinations, dilation of the pupils, dry mouth and sometimes convulsions. The impairment of ability to work is more than with morphine. Abstinence syndrome resembles that of morphine withdrawal and symptoms appear in 3 to 4 hours, and reach maximum intensity 8 to 12 hours later. Then they decline rapidly and disappear in four to five days.

It is a drug of addiction. The addiction is common among doctors and nurscs. Monoamine oxidase inhibitors and phenothiazines can produce severe reactions and even death when taken together with pethidine.

Treatment: Same as for opium.

Opioids: Other opioid drugs of addiction include: codeine, dihydrocodeine, papaverine, pethidine, methadone, dipipanone, dextromoramide, pentazocin, cylizine, diphenoxylate and dextropropoxyphene.

METHADONE: It is a long-acting opioid, with a half-life of about 15 hours, which has all the physiologic properties of heroin. It is an analgesic more powerful than morphine. It can be given orally or parenterally.

Fentanyl is 50 to 100 times more potent than morphine. It can be taken i.v., orally, smoked, snorted or as skin patches.

BARBITURATES

They are white, crysalline, odourless powders, with a faintly bitter taste.

Pharmacological Action: **They have a depressant action on the central nervous system.** Large doses directly depress the medullary respiratory centre.

CLASSIFICATION: (1) Long-acting: (onset of action 2 hours and duration of action 6 to 12 hours): Barbitone, phenobarbitone, methyl phenobarbitone, diallylbarbituric acid, mephobarbital, phenytoin.

(2) Intermediate-acting: (onset of action half to one hour and duration of action 3 to 6 hours): Amobarbitone, butobarbitone, probarbitone, sodium amytal, aprobarbital, vinbarbital, allobarbitone.

(3) Short-acting: (duration of action less than 3 hours): Cyclobarbital, pentobarbital, seconal, ortal, amobarbital, cyclobarbitone, quinalbarbitone.

(4) Ultra-short acting: (onset of action immediate and duration of action about 5 to 10 minutes). Pentothal sodium, kemithal sodium, thiamylal sodium.

ABSORPTION, Distribution and Elimination: They are rapidly absorbed from the gastrointestinal tract including the rectum, and from the subcutaneous tissues. They are concentrated in the liver for a short time, and then evenly distributed in the body fluids. They are partly destroyed in liver and excreted in urine. **Barbiturates, alcohol and CO produce irreversible brain damage and yet the patient survives for a sufficiently long period so that they are completely metabolised or excreted before death occurs.**

Signs and Symptoms: Acute poisoning may result from a single large dose or with repeated small doses. Usually the **first symptom is drowsiness.** A short period of confusion, excitement, delirium, and hallucinations is common. Ataxia, vertigo, slurred speech, headache, paraesthesias, subjective visual disturbances occur. A stupor progressing to deep coma, with inhibition or loss of superficial and deep reflexes, and gradual loss of response to painful stimuli occur. The Babinski toe sign may become positive. **Respirations may be rapid and shallow or slow and laboured, but the minute volume is always reduced.** There is a fall in cardiac output and an increase in capillary permeability leading to an increase in the extracellular fluid. Mild but progressive cardiovascular collapse, evidenced by cyanosis, hypotension, weak rapid pulse, and cold clammy skin occurs. **The pupils are usually slightly contracted but react to light; they may dilate during terminal asphyxia.** Decreased peristalsis may occur in deeply comatose patient and tends to be a bad prognostic sign. The urine may be scanty or suppressed and may contain sugar, albumen and haematoporphyrin. Incontinence of urine and faeces may occur. The body temperature is usually reduced; fever indicates bronchopneumonia. **Respirations become irregular, sometimes Cheyne-Stokes in character and finally stop.** There is delirium, hallucinations, ataxia, paraesthesias, loss of reflexes, hypotension, cyanosis, stupor progressing to coma. **Blisters on the skin, often on an area of erythema, strongly suggest barbiturate poisoning.** Blisters contain clear serous fluid. Rupture of a blister leaves a red, raw surface which later dries to a brown parchment-like area. They are commonly found in sites where pressure has been exerted between two skin surfaces, such as the interdigital clefts and inner aspects of the knees, buttocks, backs of thighs, calves and forearms. Occasionally, an entire side of a forearm or a thigh is blistered. **Blisters occur in about 6% of cases,** and are believed to be due to a direct toxic action on the epidermis. The coma may continue for a few hours to a few days and the patient then makes a gradual recovery. During recovery nystagmus, diplopia and temporary failure of accommodation may occur. Death may occur from respiratory failure or ventricular fibrillation in early stages, and bronchopneumonia or irreversible anoxia with pulmonary oedema in the later stages. **The combination of alcohol and barbiturates causes rapid death.** Phenytoin causes gingival hyperplasia in chronic therapy.

Patients who have taken an overdose of phenobarbitone may remain unconscious for a prolonged period of time, but they tend to remain at a somewhat safer level of unconsciousness than patients who have taken a large overdosage of short-acting barbiturate. Severe shock or respiratory failure are more common and more serious with medium and short-acting barbiturates.

Fatal Dose:

Short-acting: One to two g.

Medium-acting: Two to 3 g.

Long-acting: Three to 5 g.

The lethal blood levels are:

Long-acting: Ten mg. per 100 ml.

Medium-acting: Seven mg. per 100 ml.

Short-acting: Three mg. per 100 ml.

Fatal Period: One to two days.

Treatment: (1) **Gastric lavage should be carried out (up to 8 to 24 hours post-ingestion),** with warm water mixed with potassium permanganate and suspension of activated charcoal or tannic acid. A concentrated solution of magnesium sulphate should be left in the stomach to produce purgation and minimise intestinal absorption. (2) **There is no specific antidote.** Analeptics do not shorten the period of unconsciousness or increase the rate of excretion. **Analeptic therapy should be avoided unless a clear and compelling need exists.** (3) **'Scandinavian method', uses anti-shock measures, maintenance of patent airway, and adequate respiratory support. CNS stimulants have been totally eliminated.** Fluid replacement therapy should be used and not vasopressors. If shock persists dopamine should be given. (4) Normal saline with five percent glucose i.v. increases the rate of excretion. Two-and-half to three litres should be given in 24 hours. (5) Artificial respiration and oxygen is given. (6) The patient should be kept warm and mucus removed from the throat, either by raising the foot of the bed or by aspiration. An endotracheal tube may be left *in situ* for the first 3 days, but after this a tracheostomy should be done. (7) Bowels should be evacuated by enema. (8) Noradrenaline two mg. diluted with 500 ml of 5% glucose in saline i.v. to counteract shock and low blood pressure. (9) **Haemodialysis** and exchange transfusion are sometimes life-saving. (10) **Charcoal haemoperfusion.** (11) **Forced alkaline diuresis** is most useful in poisoning by barbiturates which are not protein-bound like phenobarbitone, allobarbitone and barbitone. Increasing urinary pH interferes with the renal tubular reabsorption of phenobarbitone by increasing the ionic form of the drug in the urine. It is not of much use in cases of poisoning by barbiturates which are more protein-bound, have a large volume of distribution and are less poisonous. Forced diuresis is brought about by mannitol 100 to 200 ml. of 25% solution, followed by an infusion of 500 ml. of 5% solution during the next 3 hours. It can be continued alternating with 5% dextrose solution for the next 24 hours so as to maintain a urine volume of 10 to 20 litres in 24 hours. (12) For deep-vein thrombosis and thromboembolism in patients with prolonged coma, mini-heparinisation, elastic stockings, and inflatable cuffs are useful. (13) Antibiotics to minimise risk of pneumonia. (14) Symptomatic treatment.

Postmortem Appearances: They are not characteristic, but are mainly those of asphyxia. Cyanosis is present. A quantity of white particles of ingested barbiturate may be seen in the stomach. The gastric mucosa may be eroded. The fundus may be thickened, granular and haemorrhagic. The cardiac end and lower oesophagus may be eroded from regurgitation. Haemorrhagic blistering and haemorrhagic necrosis of the gastric mucosa may be seen due to poisoning from seconal and sodium amytal. The lungs are congested, oedematous and almost black. Petechial haemorrhages may be present in the lungs and on the pleura and pericardium. The whole venous system is engorged with dark, deoxygenated blood. The kidneys show degeneration of the convoluted tubules. Other organs are congested. **In delayed deaths, there is symmetrical necrosis of the globus pallidus and corpus callosum, focal areas of necrosis in the cerebrum and cerebellum and a variety of vascular lesions. Putrefaction causes significant decrease in blood barbiturate levels.**

DETECTION: Calorimetric methods have now been superseded by specific gas-liquid and high pressure liquid chromatography methods.

CHRONIC POISONING: Tolerance develops rapidly and is usually marked. There is also a cross-tolerance with alcohol. It occurs when barbiturates are used therapeutically in epilepsy or psychoneurotic patients. The signs and symptoms resemble those of chronic alcoholism with progressive impairment of cerebral function, dysarthria, ataxia and depression. Tendon reflexes may be depressed, or there may be hypertonia and tremors of Parkinsonian type. Addiction is a serious problem. Dependence is both psychic and physical. The impairment of mood, behaviour, and intellectual functions causes social deterioration. Withdrawal symptoms appear within a day and may persist for two weeks. Common features are anxiety, nausea, vomiting, weakness, hypotension, tremors and disturbances of vision. Convulsions may occur.

The Circumstances of Poisoning: Barbiturates are commonly used for committing suicide. Due to the large size of a fatal dose and prolonged unconsciousness, they are rarely used for homicide. **Accidental poisoning may result due to "automatism" (involuntary suicide).**

METHAQUOLONE: "Mandrax" and "melsedine" containing methaquolone are used for insomnia. Some persons are extremely sensitive to this drug and may become unconscious even after one tablet. If it is taken some hours after food, the patient may feel dizzy, sweat and a syndrome similar to hypoglycaemia is produced. Two-and-half g. of the drug produces unconsciousness within half hour.

Fatal Dose: 5 g.

SYMPTOMS: In modest doses, the drug produces an euphoric state, and inhibitions disappear. Excitation, delirium, extrapyramidal signs (hypertonicity, hyperreflexia and myoclonus) and convulsions occur. Muscular twitchings, extensor plantar response, carpopedal spasm and paraesthesia, tachycardia, cardiac arrhythmias ranging from patterns similar to pericarditis, incomplete to complete bundle branch-block, or myocardial infarction, hypotension, hypothermia, hypoprothrombinaemia and gastric bleeding.

Addiction may occur, and some degree of tolerance is seen after prolonged use. Excretion is mainly in the urine.

Treatment: Stomach wash and symptomatic.

CHLORAL HYDRATE: (Dry wine): It is colourless, crystalline substance having peculiar pungent odour, and a pungent bitter taste. **Its principal action is to depress the central nervous system.**

Absorption: It is absorbed rapidly form the stomach and small intestine, and also from the rectum. It is metabolised rapidly in the liver, mainly to trichloroethanol which is also hypnotic. Trichloroethanol is conjugated with glucuronic acid and excreted in the urine.

Signs and Symptoms: They resemble those of barbiturates, but in addition there is retrosternal burning sensation, vomiting, and rarely jaundice. Albuminuria may be found due to renal damage. Sometimes, due to idiosyncrasy, a scarlatinal or urticarial rash may be seen on the skin. Hepatorenal damage may occur. Death usually occurs from paralysis of the respiratory centre. In a few cases, death may occur from failure of the heart soon after swallowing the drug.

Fatal Dose: 5 to 10 g.

Fatal Period: 8 to 12 hours.

Treatment: (1) Wash the stomach with alkaline solution. (2) Forced diuresis or dialysis. (3) Flumazenil 0.1mg. as infusion to a total of 3 mg. produces marked improvement. (4) Symptomatic.

Postmortem Appearances: Gastric mucosa is softened and reddened and eroded, and smells of chloral hydrate. Brain and lungs are congested. Hepatorenal damage is seen.

Chronic poisoning: It occurs after prolonged therapeutic use. Symptoms are those of gastrointestinal irritation with erythematous and urticarial eruptions on skin, tremors and dyspnoea. Convulsions, mental degeneration and liver damage may occur. Habitual use can lead to tolerance and physical dependence with delirium when the drug is withdrawn.

The Circumstances of Poisoning: Accidental poisoning results by taking large doses as hypnotic. Suicidal cases are rare. **It is given in food or drink to render a person suddenly helpless for the purpose of robbery or rape. Its action is so rapid under such conditions that it has been given the name of 'knockout drops'.** A combination of alcohol and chloral is commonly known as **'Mickey Finn'**. It is often added to liquor to increase its potency.

BROMIDES: Potassium and sodium bromide are in constant use in medicine. Acute fatal poisoning is rare and is likely to occur only in circumstances of suicide. Poisoning is usually accidental. Up to ten percent patients exhibit intolerance.

SIGNS AND SYMPTOMS: There may be nausea, colic and vomiting due to the local action, followed by vertigo, staggering gait, mental confusion, fall of blood pressure, feeble pulse, subnormal temperature, shallow respirations, muscular weakness or paralysis, collapse, stupor or coma. It usually appears within a few days of the commencement of taking the drug, though rarely after a long period of tolerance. There may be irritation and oedema of the mucous membranes. The bromides displace chlorides from plasma and cells, and may cause fatal depression of the nervous system. Excessive consumption may lead to clinical picture resembling intoxication.

FATAL DOSE: 30 to 45 g. 50mg/100ml. in blood is a toxic level.

FATAL PERIOD: 6 to 18 hours or more.

TREATMENT: (1) Gastric lavage. (2) Chloride increases the elimination of bromides, and as such, normal saline i.v. by drip method, or 2 g. of sodium chloride in capsules every four hours by mouth are useful. (3) Haemodialysis in severe poisoning. (4) Symptomatic.

Postmortem Appearances are not characteristic.

TEST: They give a whitish-yellow precipitate with silver nitrate, which is not readily soluble in ammonium hydrate, but is soluble in potassium cyanide.

CHRONIC POISONING (bromism): It results from the continued ingestion of bromides. There is blunting of memory, muscular weakness and incoordination, skin rashes, and there may be delusions and hallucinations.

In over 30% of cases of chronic bromide ingestion, a "bromide rash" develops. It begins as an acneiform eruption on the face and may spread to the whole body.

PARALDEHYDE

This is a clear, colourless liquid with an unpleasant ethereal odour, and an acrid nauseous taste. It is used as a hypnotic by mouth, rectum or parenterally and as a basal anaesthetic. Fatal poisoning is uncommon. Poisoning is usually accidental. Suicide is rare. It is a less common drug of addiction.

SIGNS AND SYMPTOMS: When ingested there is nausea, vomiting, eructations, headache and giddiness and the breath smells of paraldehyde. Drowsiness sets in, pulse becomes slow and feeble, shallow breathing, dilated pupils, cyanosis, subnormal temperature and coma and death may occur from respiratory failure. Pulmonary oedema and bronchopneumonia are common.

Fatal Dose: 25 to 50 ml. orally; 10 to 12 ml. parenterally.

FATAL PERIOD: Few hours.

TREATMENT: (1) Gastric lavage with a solution of sodium bicarbonate to be continued until washings cease to smell of the drug. (2) Activated charcoal is useful. (3) High colonic irrigation. (4) Calcium gluconate and dextrose intravenously. (5) Artificial respiration and oxygen inhalation. (6) Symptomatic.

POSTMORTEM APPEARANCES: The body smells of paraldehyde. The mucosa of the stomach is hyperaemic and may be slightly inflamed. The viscera are congested. Pulmonary oedema and bronchopneumonia are usually seen.

CHRONIC POISONING: Symptoms are similar to those seen in chronic alcoholism, such as gastric irritation, muscular weakness, and tremors of the hands and tongue. Hallucinations and delusions may be present.

HYDROCARBONS

Most of the hydrocarbons are derivatives of petroleum distillates. Aliphatic hydrocarbons include gasoline, naphtha, mineral spirits, **kerosene,** butane, propane, turpentine, paraffin wax, petroleum jelly, tars, asphalt and mineral seal oil. **Halogenated (chlorinated) hydrocarbons include organochlorines, methyl bromide, fluorocarbons, methylene chloride, carbon tetrachloride, trichloroethylene and tetrachloroethylene. Aromatic hydrocarbons are benzene, toluene, xylene and naphthalene.** Turpentine and pine oil are products of wood distillation. The toxic substances like gasoline, **kerosene,** naphtha, mineral spirit, light gas oil, and mineral seal oil are poorly absorbed from the GI tract. Benzene, toluene and xylene are highly volatile and well absorbed from the GI tract. Methane and butane are gases and act as simple asphyxiants. **LPG is a mixture of butane and propane.** Lubricating oil and asphalt are non-toxic. Turpentine and pine oil are readily absorbed from the GIT.

Signs and Symptoms: (1) Acute or chronic contact with hydrocarbons causes chronic eczematoid dermatitis, with redness, itching and inflammation. Cutaneous exposure to gasoline and other hydrocarbons can cause second degree burns, and systemic manifestations. Fever may be present. (2) **Pulmonary:** Gasping, coughing and choking indicate aspiration. Nasal flaring, intercostal retractions, dyspnoea, tachypnoea and varying degrees of cyanosis are seen. If severe injury occurs, pulmonary symptoms progress up to 48 hours, with complete resolution in 3 to 5 days. (3) CNS depression, somnolence, dizziness, convulsions and coma. (4) Eye: Photophobia, redness and transient corneal irritation. (5) Cardiac involvement is rare after acute ingestion. **During solvent abuse especially with chlorinated and fluorinated hydrocarbons sudden death secondary to dysrhythmias can occur.**

Methane or butane inhalation causes hypoxia. They can cause CNS symptoms but lungs are spared. Gasoline, turpentine and naphtha are aspirated and can cause CNS depression, but effects of GI absorption are not significant. Petroleum spirits, kerosene, mineral seal oil cause pulmonary complications. Lubricating oils, mineral oil, asphalt are non-toxic but may cause lipoid pneumonias in cases of direct aspiration. CNS toxicity following ingestion appears to be indirect and secondary to pulmonary involvement.

Chronic exposure: Benzene is considered a human carcinogen. Aplastic anaemia, myelocytic and monocytic leukaemia have been reported. Toluene inhalation is associated with renal tubular acidosis, and peripheral sensorimotor neuropathy.

Fatal Dose: 30 to 100 ml. of kerosene. 15 to 20 ml benzene.

Fatal Period: Within one day.

Treatment: (1) Remove contaminated clothing, and wash the affected areas of skin with soap and water. In ocular exposure, prolonged irrigation with sterile solution is to be done. (2) Gastric evacuation is indicated for (a) camphorated products, (b) halogenated products (e.g., methylene chloride, carbon tetrachloride), (c) aromatic hydrocarbons (e.g., benzene, toluene); aniline. Ipecac induced emesis is preferred over lavage. Gastric evacuation for pure petroleum distillate or turpentine ingestion is not recommended. (3) Activated charcoal has limited value. (4) A cathartic may be given. (5) Continuous positive airway pressure (CPAP) or positive- end-expiratory pressure (PEEP), or high frequency jet ventilation is beneficial in severe poisoning. (6) Absorption of ingested kerosene can be slowed by giving 250 ml of liquid paraffin orally. (7) Corticosteroids.

Postmortem Appearances: Signs of asphyxia are present. There may be acute gastroenteritis and the odour may be present in the lungs and alimentary canal. There may be atelectasis, interstitial inflammation and necrotising bronchopneumonia. The pleural and cut surfaces are deep-red and purple, oozing a blood-stained watery and frothy fluid. Petechial haemorrhages, or larger haemorrhages into the mucous membranes and subserous tissues may be found in the trachea, gastrointestinal tract and elsewhere. Cloudy swelling, or fatty degeneration of the liver and kidney may be seen. **In toluene poisoning red cells may show basophilic stippling.**

The Circumstances of Poisoning: Poisoning is usually accidental, especially among children. Adults may be accidentally poisoned by drinking it by mistaking it for country liquor. Suicidal poisoning is very rare. They are not used for homicide. In the siphoning of gasoline from a tank, the mobile liquid can easily be aspirated into the lungs and cause death.

TURPENTINE: It is obtained by the distillation of the oleoresin from various species of pine tree. When fresh it is colourless. It is extensively used to dissolve varnish paint and grease stains. It is eliminated from the lungs, and breath has a characteristic smell. In the

urine it is excreted in combination with glycuronic acid. Some amount is excreted by the skin.

FATAL DOSE: 150 to 200 ml.

FATAL PERIOD: 1–2 days.

SIGNS AND SYMPTOMS: SKIN: redness, itching, vesication. G.I.T.: nausea, vomiting, colic, diarrhoea. R.S.: central depression, pneumonia. C.N.S.: excitement, giddiness, delirium, convulsions, coma, RENAL: albuminuria, haematuria, oliguria, renal failure.

TREATMENT: (1) Gastric lavage with weak solution of sodium bicarbonate. (2) demulcents. (3) supportive therapy.

POSTMORTEM APPEARANCES: Stomach shows haemorrhagic spots and contents smell of turpentine. Lungs, brain and meninges are congested. Kidneys show degenerative changes.

POISONING: (1) Accidental. (2) Suicidal. (3) Abortificient.

NAPHTHALENE: Moth balls contain naphthalene or paradichlorobenzene. Fatal dose is 2 to 5 gm. Symptoms are nausea, vomiting, diarrhoea, abdominal pain, fever, headache, confusion, sweating, dysuria, convulsions and coma. It can cause haemolysis in patients with glucose-6-phosphate dehydrogenase deficiency and acute renal failure. Chronic exposure to naphthalene can result in aplastic anaemia, hepatic necrosis and jaundice.

CHAPTER

31 PSYCHOTROPIC DRUGS

FM 8.4: Describe the laws in relations to poisons including narcotic drugs, psychotropic substances (NDPS)—their abuse, signs, symptoms and management.

Psychotropic drugs are substances that affect psychic function, behaviour or experience. They consist of: (1) Antidepressants. (2) Neuroleptics. (3) Hallucinogens.

Psychoactive Drug Classification: (1) Sedatives: (a) Barbiturates and others. (b) Minor tranquilisers. (c) Alcohol. (2) Stimulants: (a) Amphetamines, methylphenidate. (b) Cocaine. (3) Opiates: Heroin, methadone, morphine, etc. (4) Hallucinogens. (5) Marihuana. (6) Major tranquilisers: chlorpromazine and others. (7) Antidepressants: (a) Tricyclics. (b) Monoamine oxidase inhibitors. (8) Antimania drugs.

METHAMPHETAMINE

Action: Amphetamines increase the synaptic concentration of neurotransmitters dopamine and norepinephrine. It blocks re-uptake of norepinephrine and causes an increase of catecholamine release. **The euphoric effect is similar to cocaine, but last ten times that of cocaine.** It is also a cardiovascular stimulant. **They are powerful stimulants of CNS and CVS.** Use in order of frequency are: oral, injection and smoking. **The effects of single dose may last for 10 to 16 hours. The onset of fatigue is delayed and tasks are more easily completed, but there is a loss of judgement and accuracy.** Designer drugs of amphetamine are abused by youngsters during rave parties for dancing throughout the night.

Symptoms: Acute poisoning: Toxicity is similar to cocaine. (1) **Mild:** Restlessness, talkativeness, insomnia, tremors, sweating, dilated pupils.

(2) Moderate: Hyperactivity, confusion, hypertension, tachycardia, tachypnoea, vomiting, sweating, hallucinations.

(3) Severe: Delirium, hyperpyrexia, convulsions, coma, arrhythmias.

Acute intoxication may present as a paranoid hallucinatory syndrome which closely mimicks paranoid schizophrenia.

It can cause sudden death by stroke, seizure or cardiac dysrhythmia and may cause excited delirium.

Chronic poisoning: (1) Amphetamine psychosis characterised by: (a) Stereotyped, compulsive behaviour, (b) paranoid personality, (c) delusions, usually persecution, (d) hallucinations, usually visual, sometimes tactile. (2) Cardiomyopathy. (3) Intracranial haemorrhage.

Treatment: (1) Gastric lavage. (2) Acidification of urine. (3) Symptomatic. (4) Chlorpromazine for amphetamine psychosis.

Fatal Dose: 150 to 200 mg.

P.M. appearances are those of asphyxia. Myocardial fibrosis is seen in long-term use.

M.L. imp: Long-term use leads to psychological dependence and tolerance. Withdrawal of drug can lead to depression and sometimes suicide.

40% of amphetamine is excreted unchanged in urine. The term **liquid gold** is slang for urine for amphetamine addicts which is collected and sold.

Derivatives: Methamphetamine, dextroamphetamine, fenfluramine, phentermine, mephentermine, methylphenidate and synthetic amphetamines.

Dangers of misuse are: (1) Abusers known as speed freaks who inject the drug, exhibit bizarre and often violent behaviour. (2) Paranoid psychosis. (3) 3Shock and collapse. (4) Risk of suicide during the withdrawal phase.

ANTIDEPRESSANTS

CLASSIFICATION: (1) Tricyclic: (a) Tertiary amines, amitriptyline, doxepin, impramine, trimipramine. (b) Secondary amines: desipramine, nortriptyline, protriptyline. (c) Tetracyclic: maprotiline. (2) Dibenzoxazepine: amoxapine. (3) Trizolphyridine: trazodone. (4) Bicyclic: fluoxetine.

(II) Manoamine oxidase inhibitors (MAOI): nilamide, tranylcypromine. (III) Lithium carbonate. (IV) Miscellaneous: amphetamines, caffeine.

The new group are selective serotonin reuptake inhibitors (SSRIs). These include fluoxetine, paroxetine, fluvoxame, sertraline. They are less toxic than tricyclics, as they do not have the cardiotoxic component.

The toxicity of the antidepressants is due to (1) their anticholinergic effects such as: supraventricular tachycardia, agitation, seizures, coma, hallucinations, and respiratory depression, (2) their ability to block reuptake of norepinephrine at the synapses, resulting in both atrial and ventricular disturbances and hypertension, (3) their quinidine-like membrane depressant effects on the heart by altering sodium influx resulting in conduction delays and myocardial depression, (4) peripheral

alpha blockade causing hypotension, and (5) inhibition of sympathetic reflexes centrally.

STIMULANTS: They include cocaine, amphetamine, methamphetamine, coffeine, nicotine, methyl phenidate, etc. These agents stimulate CNS, induce a sense of well-being, increase alertness, decrease fatigue, suppress appetite and can lead to strong psychological dependence.

CYCLIC ANTIDEPRESSANTS

CLASSIFICATION: (1) First generation: Imipramine, amitriptyline, desipramine, doxepin, nortryptiline, protriptyline, trimipramine. (2) Second generation; Amoxapine, maprotiline. (3) Newer agents: Bupropion, trazadone, netazodone, fluoxetine, paroxetine, sertraline.

ACTION: Inhibition of neurotransmitter reuptake, anticholinergic blockade, a-adrenergic blockade and myocardial depressant effect.

SIGNS AND SYMPTOMS: C.N.S.: Depression of mental state and coma, delirium, altered sensorium, generalised, brief and self-limited convulsions, myoclonus, nystagmus, dysarthria and ataxia. C.V.S.: Sinus tachycardia, conduction delays, ventricular arrhythmias, depressed inotropy, hypotension, atrioventricular block, bradycardia, Parasympathetic: Dry skin and mucosa, ileus, urinary retention, mydriasis and hyperthermia.

FATAL DOSE: 1 to 2 g.

TREATMENT: (1) Stomach wash. (2) Emesis should be avoided. (3) Activated charcoal and cathartic following lavage. (4) Multiple dose activated charcoal. (5) Physostigmine.

MONOAMINE OXIDASE INHIBITORS (MAOI)

They include iproniazid, isocarboxazid, phenelzine, pheneprazine, nialamide and tranylcypromine.

ACTION: They block the action of monoamine oxidase, resulting in alterations of neurotransmitter metabolism.

SIGNS AND SYMPTOMS: Symptoms develop after 12 hours.

Phase-1: CNS excitation. Headache, dilated pupils, tremors, convulsions, hallucinations, confusion, nausea, hyperpyrexia, hypertension followed by hypotension.

Phase-2: CNS and CVS depression: Coma, cardiovascular collapse.

Phase-3: Complications: Haemolysis, rhabdomyolysis, pulmonary oedema, acute renal failure.

FATAL DOSE: 2 to 5 mg/kg.

TREATMENT: (1) Stomach wash. (2) Activated charcoal. (3) Symptomatic.

PHENCYCLIDINE: It is usually smoked, sniffed or injected (i.v. or s.c.)

SIGNS AND SYMPTOMS: Nystagmus, miosis, ataxia, tremors, dysarthria, tachycardia, hypertension, lethargy, catatonia, coma, agitation, violent tendency, bizarre behaviour, acute psychosis with delusions and hallucinations.

TREATMENT: (1) Gastric lavage. (2) Activated charcoal 1 g/kg. (3) Cathartic.

NEUROLEPTICS (TRANQUILISERS): They are antipsychotic agents which therapeutically modify behaviour.

CLASSIFICATION: (1) Phenothiazines: (a) Aliphatic: chlorpromazine, triflupromazine. (b) Piperazine: trifluoperazine, prochlorperazine, perphenazine, fluphenazine. (c) Piperidine: thioridiazine, mesoridiazine. (d) Benzodiazepines: Diazepam, lorazepam, oxazepam. (2) Thioxanthenes: chlorprothixene, thiothixene. (3) Butyrophenones: haloperidol. (4) Indoles: molindone. (5) Dibenzoxazepines: loxapine.

Newer drugs are clozapine, risperidone and remoxipride.

ACTION: The phenothiazines are anticholinergics and antidopaminergics to varying degrees. Other properties are central and peripheral cholinergic blockade, and adrenergic action secondary to the inhibition of reuptake of catecholamines.

FATAL DOSE: 5 to 10 g.

SYMPTOMS: Myocardial depression, hypothermia or hyperthermia, decreased sweating and salivation, amenorrhoea, miosis, decreased intestinal motility and secretions, agranulocytosis, haemolytic anaemia, ventricular tachycardia, orthostatic hypotension, sedation, seizures, gynaecomastia, corneal opacities, cholestatic jaundice, priapism, laryngospasm, urticaria, dermatitis, photosensitivity and gray-blue pigmentation. There are three acute movement disorders occurring between one to 60 days of initiation of therapy. (1) Acute dystonia: oculogyric crisis, jaw, tongue, lip and throat spasms, neck twisting, opisthotonos, facial grimacing and abdominal wall spasm. Symptoms rapidly resolve with parenteral antihistamines, anticholinergics, or benzodiazepines. (2) Akathisia: restlessness and inability to sit. (3) Parkinsonism: shuffling gait, resting tremor, rigidity, pill rolling, a mask-like expression, fine movements, muscle weakness, and bradykinesia are typical symptoms.

TREATMENT: (1) Emesis. (2) Gastric lavage. (3) Activated charcoal in repeated doses. (4) Catharsis. (5) Symptomatic.

BENZODIAZEPINES: They have sedative and tranquilising effects and are used mainly as antianxiety and muscle relaxant agents. The commonly used preparations are: **Diazepam,** flurazepam, chlordiazepoxide, nitrazepam, oxazepam, alprazolam, and lorazepam. They are tranquilisers commonly used to relieve anxiety. They are highly protein-bound and have good CNS penetration. Excretion in the urine may continue for several days. Addiction may occur. **They enhance the inhibitory actions of the neurotransmitter GABA, located in the brain.**

Fatal Dose: 5 to 6 g. Death is rare.

Signs and Symptoms: Symptoms appear in 1 to 3 hours. Acute poisoning causes vertigo, slurred speech, nystagmus, diplopia, dysarthria, ataxia, staggering walk, shallow breathing, sedation and somnolence and coma. **If taken alone they are not toxic, but mixed with alcohol or other drugs, they can contribute to death.**

Chronic Poisoning: High dose, long term therapy (30 to 40 mg of diazepam daily) may produce withdrawal symptoms when stopped suddenly, such as: **C.N.S:** headache, anxiety, insomnia, muscle spasms, tremors, rarely convulsions and psychiatric disturbances. **G.I:** anorexia, vomiting. **R.S.:** respiratory depression is rare.

Treatment: (1) Gastric lavage. (2) Activated charcoal. (3) **Flumazenil** is an imidazodiazepine that selectively blocks the central effects of benzodiazepines by competitive interaction at the benzodiazipine recognition site. It is also useful in poisoning by zolpidem, an imidazopyridine hypnotic. It is given in a dose of 0.2mg/min as infusion to a total of 3.5 mg. If resedation occurs (in 20 to 120 minutes), the dose is repeated. (4) Forced diuresis.

The withdrawal syndrome from benzodizipines includes fits and psychosis. In addition, anxiety symptoms, such as sweating, insomnia, headache, tremors, nausea and disordered perception such as feelings of unreality, abnormal bodily sensations and hypersensitivity to stimuli may be seen. A long-acting drug, such as chlordiazepoxide or diazepam are useful to prevent complications.

Long-term use may possibly cause behavioral disinhibition, which may induce a person to hostile acts, aggressive behaviour and verbal indecency. Many of these drugs are capable of causing anterograde amnesia.

PSYCHEDELICS (Hallucinogens)

Psychedelics are substances that produce an alteration in environmental awareness while the individual maintains the capacity to recognise that what he is experiencing is not real. Such person is usually fully awake, alert and oriented but confronted with varied perceptual abnormalities and varied sensations. Sensory perception and thought processes are grossly distorted, and mood is altered. Reality (space, time, bodily dimensions) is distorted and a feeling of depersonalisation makes the patient feel separated from the situation. Hallucinations produced by drugs usually have some environmental stimulus providing the basis for the illusion. Most of the hallucinations are visual. Often hallucinations take the form of gross somatic distortions. Occasionally blending of sensory modalities (synesthesia) may be noted. Profound philosophical thoughts, deep introspection, self-examination, or religious overtones may be prominent components of the psychological experience. The response to a psychedelic is related to the persons mind-set, emotions, or expectations at the time and can be altered by the setting. The person may experience euphoria or dysphoria, can be emotionally labile but usually realises that he is under the influence of a drug.

LSD, cannabis, mescaline (from the peyote cactus), dimethyl tryptamine (DMT), psylocybin (from mushrooms), psylocin, peyote, phencyclidine (PCP) are important hallucinogenic drugs. Hallucinogenic mushrooms or "magic mushrooms" contain psilocybin and psilocin and are taken orally, raw or cooked.

ACTION: They involve various neurotransmitters in the CNS. LSD involves the serotonin system and tropane alkaloids (atropine, scopolamine and hyoscyamine), have anticholinergic effects. There is psychic dependence only and no abstinence syndrome.

SIGNS AND SYMPTOMS: Both sympathetic and parasympathetic symptoms are produced. Sympathetic symptoms may include dilated pupils, tachycardia, tachyapnoea, hyperthermia, diaphoresis, piloerection, dizziness, weakness, hyperactivity, muscle weakness, ataxia, altered mental status and coma. Parasympathetic symptoms include salivation, lachrymation, diarrhoea, nausea, vomiting, bronchoconstriction and hypertension.

During hallucinations sensory perceptions are intensified; colours seem brighter and more clear, sounds seem excessively loud with an exaggeration of detail. The individual feels a sense of depersonalisation and separation from the environment. The person may perceive that he is observing an event as opposed to being involved in one. The person's body image may become distorted, so also the boundaries of objects in the environment. Alternatively, synesthesias or sensory misperceptions occur such as hearing colours or seeing sounds.

Drugs that may alter mood, such as benzodiazepines, barbiturates and amphetamines can produce perceptual changes during withdrawal. Alcohol in excess (alcoholic hallucinosis), or alcohol deprivation (delirium tremens) can cause hallucinations.

LSD (lysergic acid diethylamide): It is a colourless, tasteless, odourless, semi-synthetic compound, the lysergic acid portion of which is a natural product of the ergot fungus Claviceps purpurea. **It is a powerful antagonist of serotinin, and can also mimic its action. It is taken orally. Rarely, it may be smoked or injected parenterally.** It is absorbed from the gastrointestinal tract and considerable amounts become bound to blood protein. It is rapidly distributed to the body tissues, the highest concentrations appearing in the lungs, liver, kidney and brain. A high proportion of the dose is found in the bile. **The dose required to produce psychotropic effects ("take a trip") is 100 to 200 micrograms. The trip usually occurs after half to one hour, peaking after 2 to 6 hours and fading after 12 hours.** The effects depend very much on the individual and on the circumstances, with the same user having a bad or good "trip" on different occasions, or even within the same trip. **Some users experience bad trip** consisting of an acute panic reaction instead of psychedelic experience which may last for 8 hours. **During this period, paranoid delusions, violent behaviour, automatism or depersonalisation may occur.** Symptoms are dry mouth, sweating, dilated pupils, tachycardia, hypertension, extreme mood change, visual hallucinations, alterations in time perception, etc. **Altered changes in vision and hearing, like floating feeling, illusions, sensation of synesthesia or seeing smells and hearing colours occur.** The action may persist for 12 to 18 hours. The drug is mainly used for self-exploration, to experience varied hallucinations and to get out of day-to-day boredom. In the recovery stage there may be apprehension and distraction that is not immediately obvious to onlookers. **Tolerance develops in 2 to 3 days** with daily dosing but rapidly disappears if the drug is withheld for two days. It is commonly taken as: (1) liquid on sugar, (2) saturated sugar cube, (3) soaked into blotting paper, (4) capsule, and (5) blue pills.

Adverse effects are: depression, panic attacks, schizophrenic episodes and psychosis.

Fatal Dose: About 14 mg.

The after-effects may persist for days or weeks. At the height of the effects of the drug on the mind, **individual becomes violent or panic-stricken and he may attack others (urge to kill) or hurt himself** from disregard of reality, and the normal considerations of the safety. **The feeling of being able to fly under the influence of LSD can lead users to jump out of windows.** In some persons lasting disturbances, depersonalisation, chronic dread, depression, mood swings and paranoid attitudes and beliefs may be found following repeated exposure to LSD. In the recovery stage, there may be apprehension and distraction, that is not obvious to onlookers. Biological half-life of LSD in man is three hours. It does not cause chromosomal breakage and is not teratogenic.

Repeated use by an addict can lead to permanent psychosis.

Flash-back Phenomenon: This may occur days, weeks or even months after the ingestion of a dose, and the person experiences a recurrence of the emotional and psychological aspects of the previous 'LSD' trip. **Flash-back symptoms occur most frequently with abuse of psychotomimetics, such as LSD, STP, tryptamines, mescaline and psilocybin.** These delayed recurring symptoms may lead to eccentric behaviour, suicide or even homicide.

Treatment: (1) **Low doses of anti-anxiety drugs and benzodiazepines, such as diazepam** 10 to 20 mg or 5 to 10 mg i.v. with repetitive dosage are the drugs of choice. (2) Prolonged talking known as "talking the person down" which may extend up to 12 to 18 hours. (3) Psychotherapy.

Amphetamine, cocaine and ecstasy can cause psychological dependence but not a major physical withdrawal syndrome.

KHAT (catha edulis) is chewed for its stimulant effect. Cathinone is the main component, which produces effects similar to those caused by amphetamine.

ECSTASY (3,4, methylene-dioxymethamphetamine-MDMA) is a stimulant with hallucinogenic properties. It is also known as one of the "club drugs" or "rave drug". A dose of 75 to 100 mg. produces

effects within half to one hour. In addition to the general symptoms of stimulants, trismus (spasm of the muscles of mastication) and bruxism (grinding of teeth) may occur.

Anabolic steroids taken orally or by injection produce mood swings, aggressive behaviour, depression and paranoia.

Peyote: It is a cactus. The top of the plant consists of round buttons which are cut, dried and chewed. The active principle is mescaline. The effects last for 8 to 12 hours. It can be prepared synthetically. Taken orally it produces a trance-like state. Overdose will produce psychosis and death.

Psilocybin and psilocin: They are alkaloids present in Mexican mushrooms. Their potency is less than LSD. Psilocybin is made synthetically. The effects last for about six hours. Overdose can cause death.

Alkyl nitrites (poppers) such as amyl nitrite, are used as euphoric relaxants. Inhalation of the vapour causes headache, dizziness and flushing. Excessive use may produce methaemoglobinaemia.

PHENCYCLIDINE: It is taken orally or smoked on tobacco, by injection and inhalation. It can cause acute psychosis and violent behaviour which can lead to death from trauma. Rarely, sudden death may occur.

CHAPTER

32

DELIRIANT POISONS

FM 12.1: Describe features and management of abuse/poisoning with cannabis.
FM 14.17: To identify and draw medicolegal inference from common poisons, e.g., Datura.

DATURA FASTUOSA

Characteristics: Two varieties of this plant exist: (1) Datura alba (safed datura) **Fig. (32–1),** a white flowered plant and (2) Datura niger (kala datura), a deep-purple flowered plant. It grows on waste places all over India. The fruits are spherical and have sharp spines (thorn-apple), and contain up to 500 yellowish-brown seeds **Fig. (32–2)**. The flowers are bell-shaped. Datura stramonium grows at high altitudes in Himalayas. All parts of these plants including nectar (honey) are poisonous, especially the seeds and the fruit.

Active Principles: They contain 0.2 to 1.4% of hyoscine (scopolamine), hyoscyamine, and traces of atropine.

Action: The alkaloids atropine, hyoscyamine and hyoscine first stimulate the higher centres of brain, then the motor centres and finally cause depression and paralysis, especially of the vital centres in the medulla. The respiration is first stimulated, then depressed, and the heart centre is stimulated. Peripheral effects are predominant and result from anticholinergic (parasympatholytic) action.

Signs and Symptoms: Contact with leaves or flowers causes dermatitis in sensitive persons. If the seeds are eaten, symptoms appear within half an hour, if a decoction of the seeds is given within a few minutes and if alkaloids are used almost immediately. A bitter taste, dryness of mouth and throat, with difficulty in talking, dysphagia, burning pain in the stomach and vomiting are first noticed. The voice becomes hoarse. The face becomes flushed, conjunctivae congested, pupils widely dilated with loss of accommodation for near vision, developing in temporary blindness, photophobia and diplopia. Light reflex at first is sluggish and later absent. **The pollen can cause unilateral mydriasis** (cornpicker's pupil). Mental changes include restlessness and agitation and patient cannot recognise relatives or friends. Urinary retention and inability to pass urine occurs. The patient becomes confused, giddy, staggers as if drunk. The skin is dry and hot, the pulse rapid 120 to 140 per minute, full and bounding, but later becomes weak and irregular, and the respirations are increased. **The temperature may be raised by 2 or 3°.** Hyperpyrexia is caused by atropine, amphetamine, dinitro-orthocresol, suxamethonium, and halothane. Muscle tone and deep reflexes are increased, and there may be muscular spasm or convulsions. **A scarlatinal rash or exfoliation of the skin** may be seen over most of the body. **Delirium** is **restless and purposeless; in its earlier stages it is indicated by excitement, talkativeness and incoherence. The patient may be silent but usually he is noisy, tries to run away from his bed, picks at the bed clothes, (carphologia), exhibits typical pill rolling**

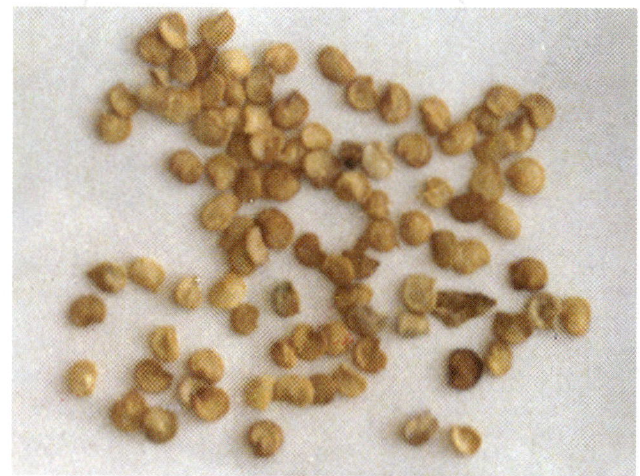

Fig. (32–2). Datura.

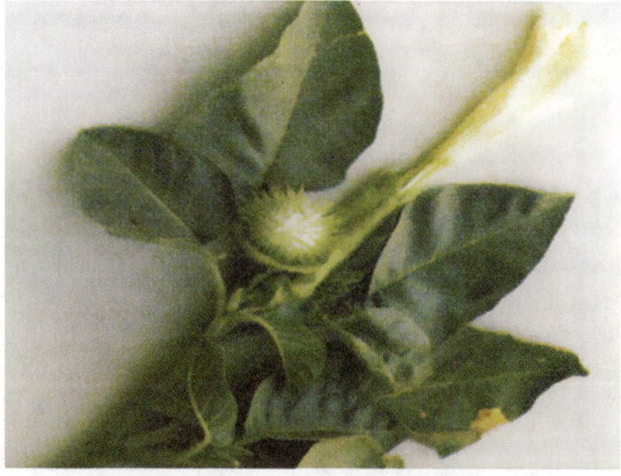

Fig. (32–1). Datura alba.

Table (32–1). Difference between the seeds of datura and capsicum

	Trait	Datura seeds, Fig. (32–3)	Capsicum seeds, Fig. (32–3)
(1)	Size:	Large and thick.	Small and thin.
(2)	Shape:	Kidney-shaped.	Rounded.
(3)	Color:	Dark or yellowish-brown.	Pale-yellow.
(4)	Margins:	Laterally compressed and double-edged at the convex border.	The convex border is simple and sharp.
(5)	Surface:	Numerous small depressions.	Smooth.
(6)	Smell:	Odourless.	Pungent.
(7)	Taste:	Bitter.	Pungent.
(8)	Embryo:	On longitudinal section, embryo is curved outward at the hilum.	Embryo is curved inward like figure 6

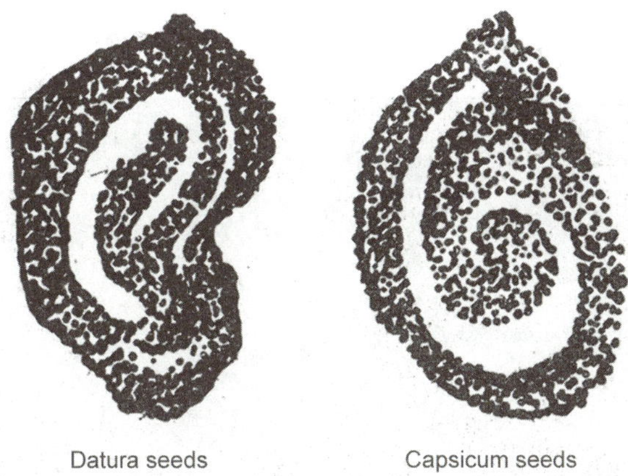

Fig. (32–3). Longitudinal section of datura and capsicum seeds.

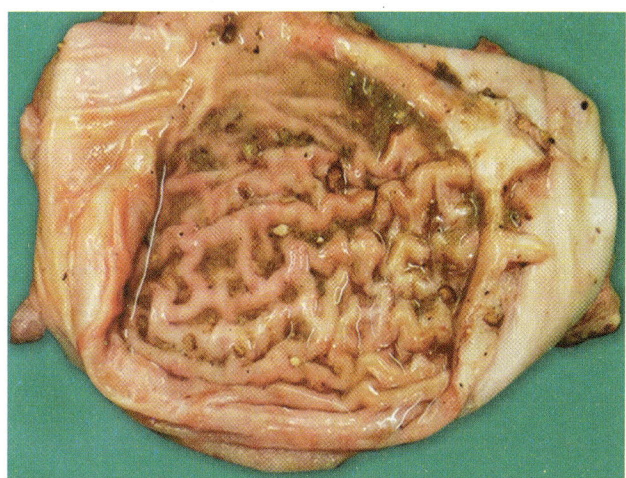

Figs. (32–4). Datura poisoning in a male child of 4 years male who accidently ate Datura fruit. Datura seeds adhered to stomach wall are present at places.

Courtesy: **Dr Radhey Khetre, Associate Professor, GMC, Aurangabad, Maharashtra.**

movements, tries to pull imaginary threads from the tips of his fingers, threads imaginary needles. Hallucinations of sight and hearing and delusions occur. As intoxication advances this excitement passes off in one to two hours, and the **patient passes into deep sleep or coma which may end rarely in death from respiratory paralysis.** The patient may remain in this condition for 2 to 3 days but usually distinct improvement occurs in 24 hours.

8 D's: Dryness of mouth, dysphagia, dilated pupils, dry, hot skin, drunken gait, delirium, drowsiness, death due to respiratory failure.

Fatal Dose: 0.6 to 1 g. 100 to 125 seeds.

Fatal Period: 24 hours.

Treatment: (1) Emetics can be used. (2) Wash-out the stomach repeatedly with a weak solution of tannic acid. (3) Give activated charcoal and a cathartic. (4) Wash-out the lower bowel frequently. (5) **Physostigmine** 1 mg., i.v. or i.m., at hourly intervals. In many cases a single dose is sufficient. (6) **Pilocarpine nitrate,** 5 mg. s.c. is useful, but it does not counteract action of datura on brain. It can be repeated after two hours. (7) Morphine is to be avoided because of the danger of depressing the respiratory centre. (8) Delirium can be controlled by bromides and short-acting barbiturates, but ether or chloroform is more beneficial . (9) Light diet, and free purgation should be carried on for 3 to 4 days to remove the seeds and to increase intestinal motility. (10) Symptomatic.

Postmortem Appearances: They are not characteristic, but are those of asphyxia. Seeds or their fragments may be found in the stomach and intestines **Figs. (32–4 and 32–5)**. The stomach may show slight inflammation and the lungs oedema. The seeds resist putrefaction for a long time.

The Circumstances of Poisoning: (1) Crushed or powdered seeds or an extract is used by criminals for stupefying a victim prior to robbery, rape or kidnapping **(Road poison). It is usually given in food or drink, e.g., *chapatis,* curry, sweets, tea, liquor, etc., to travellers in railway stations, choultries, etc. Sometimes, the seeds are mixed with incense wood, and the victim is exposed to the fumes which cause lethargy.** The victim goes into a temporary twilight phase and soon falls into a deep sleep and later wakes up to find his belongings lost. He does not remember what has happened. (2) It is not taken by the suicide. (3) Homicide is very rare. (4) It is sometimes used as an abortifacient. (5) It is believed to have aphrodisiac properties. (6) Accidental cases occur usually in children by eating the fruits. The seeds and leaves are mixed with tobacco or ganja and smoked in a pipe. (7) A decoction of seeds is sometimes added to liquor or toddy to increase the intoxicating property. (8) It is sometimes used as love philter. **A person suffering from delirium of datura is not criminally responsible for his acts.**

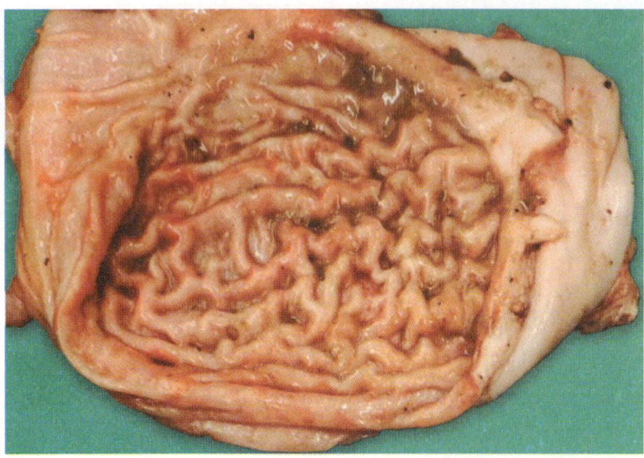

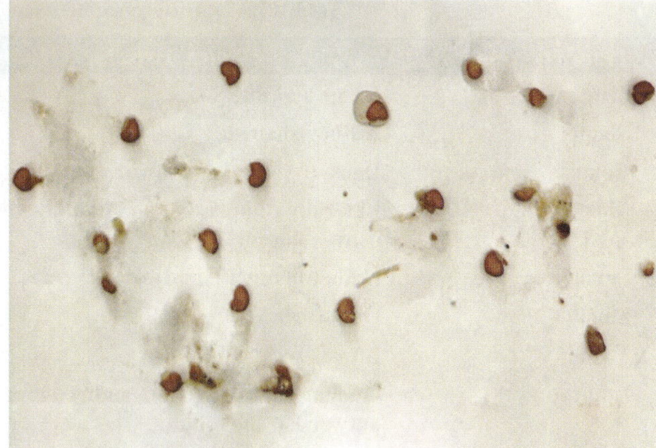

Figs. (32–5). Accidental Datura poisoning in a 3 years old boy showing stomach wall with seeds remanants. A few intact seed are shown on a piece of paper.

***Courtesy:* Dr Radhey Khetre, Associate Professor, GMC, Aurangabad, Maharashtra.**

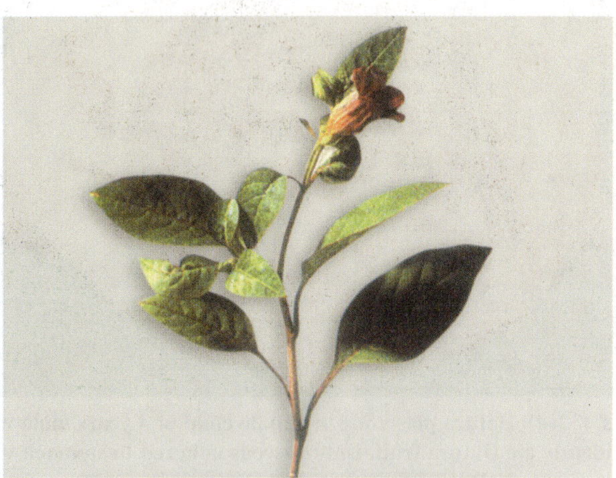

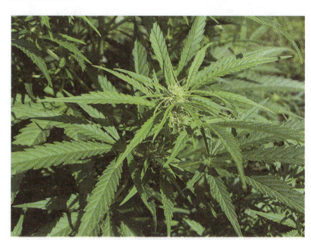

Figs. (32–6). Belladonna plant.

Figs. (32–7). Cannabis sativa.

Mydriatic Test: A drop of the solution to be tested is put into the eyes of a cat. The pupils dilate within half hour if datura is present, due to the presence of atropine.

ATROPA BELLADONNA AND HYOSCYAMUS NIGER (KHORASARI AJWAYAN) Fig. (32–6): **The Atropa belladonna, or deadly nightshade is a plant of Europe and Asia. All parts are toxic, more so in maturity. The active principle is mainly 1- hyoscyamine. The root contains 82 to 97% of hyoscyamine, 3 to 15% atropine, and up to 2.5% scopolamine. This group of compounds acts by inhibiting the muscarine effects of acetylcholine. They are absorbed from skin and from parenteral sites. They are rapidly detoxicated in the liver. The signs and symptoms, treatment and postmortem appearances are similar to datura. 60 to120 mg. of atropine or hyoscyamine and 30 mg. of hyoscine are fatal within 24 hours.**

CANNABIS SATIVA OR INDICA

It is also known as Indian hemp (dope grass). The plant grows all over India, but its cultivation is restricted by law. The female plant is taller, about 4 to 6 metres, and has more darker and luxuriant foliage than the male Fig. (32–7). The active principles are contained in its resin. The principal constituent of the resin are cannabinol, which has no action; cannabidiol is also inert, but on exposure to heat, it is partly converted to the very **active isomeric tetrahydrocannabinols (THC).** THC acts on widely distributed specific receptor regions of brain. **All parts of the plant, male or female, contain the active material, except, root and seeds. It is a CNS stimulant.** It is variously known as pot, grass, dope, weed, hash, mary jone, M.J., hashish or bhang. **It is a psychoactive drug.** THC is metabolised in the liver. THC is lipid soluble and rapidly absorbed after inhalation. About 1% penetrates blood-brain barrier. **About 2/3rd of the drug is excreted in faeces and 1/3rd in urine.** On oral ingestion, 3 to 6% of THC is absorbed. **It is the most widely used illicit drug in the world.**

Common preparations: (1) Bhang *(siddhi, sabji):* **It is prepared from the dried leaves and fruit shoots.** It is used as we use tea to prepare a decoction. **It is the mildest and contains 15% of active principle.** Fresh bhang is highly intoxicating and narcotic. Bhang kept in storage for two to three years is mildly stimulating and pleasure-giving.

(2) Majoon: **It is a sweet prepared with bhang.** It increases the appetite and sexual desire.

(3) Ganja: It is prepared from the flower tops of the female plant. It has a rusty-green colour and a characteristic odour. **It is mixed and smoked with tobacco in a pipe or *hukka*. It contains 15 to 25% of the active principle.** Ganja (pot, grass, weed, maryjone,) also known as marihuana, is used for smoking in cigarettes, which contain 0.3 to 0.6 g. cannabis and are known as **Reefer or Joint.**

(4) Charas or hashish: It is the resin (dope or shit) **exuding from the leaves and stems of the plant, and it contains 25% to 40% of the active principle.** It is dark-green or brown in colour. **It is mixed and smoked with tobacco in a pipe or *hukka*.** The smoke is inhaled deeply into the lungs and retained for as long as possible for potent effects. Persons habituated to cannabis, both drinkers and smokers, prefer to smoke or drink in company.

A concentrate of cannabis is produced by repeated extraction to yield a dark viscous liquid called **hashish oil. One or two drops of oil is added to tobacco of a cigarette and smoked.**

Signs and Symptoms: They appear soon after smoking and last for one to two hours, and within half-an-hour after swallowing and last for 2 to 3 hours. **Taken in small dose, the effects are very slight,** which usually include euphoria, passivity, heightening of subjective experiences, and disorientation. **With moderate doses these effects are intensified by impaired immediate memory function, disturbed thought patterns, lapses of attention, and a subjective feeling of unfamiliarity. High doses produce changes in body image, depersonalisation and marked sensory distortion.**

Symptoms of Intoxication: (a) Psychiatric: (1) Feelings of detachment, clarity, cleverness, disinhibition, depersonalisation, euphoria, elation, relaxation, well-being, dreaminess, sleepiness, self-confidence, jocularity, laughing, silliness, rapidly changing emotions. (2) Thought processes: irrelevant thoughts, altered reality testing, decreased concentration and attention span, altered sense of identity, disorientation. (3) Sensory novelty and increased awareness of stimuli:vivid images, illusions and hallucinations. (4) Feelings of precordial distress and tightness in chest; fear of dying. (5) Altered concepts of time and space. Change in body image, self-confidence, altered sexual feelings. (6) Maladaptive behavioural effects: impaired judgement, failure to meet responsibilities. (7) Speech changes: rapid, impaired, talkative, flighty, poor immediate memory. During the so-called "trip" due to distortion of perception, the users feel that they could fly from high windows or stop passing buses with their bare hands. **(b) Physical:** Increased appetite and thirst, slight nausea, heaviness and pressure in the head, dizziness, dysesthesias, somnolence, paraesthesias, restlessness, ataxia, tremors, dry mouth, tachycardia, urinary frequency, injected conjunctivae. The characteristic odour of cannabis may be perceived if the drug has been smoked, but not if it has been ingested.

Sensitive individuals, particularly persons recovering from a mental illness, may become paranoid after a relatively low dose. The victim becomes drowsy and passes into deep sleep, and wakes with exhaustion and impaired mental function, and recovery occurs in about six hours. Deaths occur with extreme rarity due to respiratory failure.

Fatal Dose: Charas 2 g.; ganja 8 g.; bhang 10 g./ kilo body weight. THC 30 mg/kg.

Fatal Period: Several days.

Treatment: (1) Stomach wash or emesis, activated charcoal and cathartic. (2) 100 ml. of 50% glucose, 2 mg. naloxone, and 100 mg. thiamine i.v. (3) 5 to 10 mg. diazepam, if the patient is violent or aggressive. (4) Assure the patient that he will recover. (5) **If flashbacks occur give anti-anxiety and if necessary anti-psychotic drugs, such as haloperidol.** (6) Psychotherapy.

Postmortem Appearances: These are not characteristic, but are those of asphyxia.

Chronic Poisoning: The use of the drug in small quantities even for long period is not harmful. **Tolerance and psychological dependence develop. Used in excess, it causes degeneration of the central nervous system and insanity.** Chronic use reduces serum testosterone and sperm count, and is associated with gynaecomastia. There is loss of appetite, weakness, wasting, tremors, sleepy facial expression, vacant look, red eyes, impotence and moral and mental deterioration. **Rarely they become insane (hashish psychosis), and may suffer from auditory and visual hallucinations and delusions of persecution.** Heavy marijuana users may develop manic or paranoid psychosis. The person may **run amok,** i.e., he develops a **psychic disturbance marked by a period of depression, followed by violent attempts to kill people (impulse to murder). He first kills a person against whom he may have real or imaginary enemity and then kills anyone that comes in his way until the homicidal tendency lasts. Then he may commit suicide or may surrender himself. Chronic use may lead to amotivational syndrome** with loss of age appropriate behaviour, like lethargy, lack of interest in day-today activities at home and school. **If the abuse is continued for a considerable time, it may lead to behavioural problems, crime and even mental derangement.**

It does not cause physiological dependence or addiction. Cannabis compounds and LSD can be detected in biological specimens by radioimmunoassay procedures. Marijuana is a potential carcinogen.

The Circumstances of Poisoning: (1) Most of the cases of poisoning are due to overindulgence, but there may be accidental ingestion or inhalation. (2) Majun and charas are sometimes used by road poisoners to stupefy persons to facilitate robbery. (3) It is sometimes taken by criminals before committing a criminal act, to strengthen the nerves. (4) It is used as an aphrodisiac and is supposed to increase the duration of coitus.

The experiences of people vary depending on life experiences and personality styles. The environmental and social setting in which it is smoked or ingested as well as the dose can change the effects. It is usually taken only once in a day in the evening when the person feels tired. Ascetics and religious mendicants often take cannabis to overcome hunger and thirst, and believe that it helps in the concentration of mind towards meditation. *Fakirs* often believe bhang frees them from worldly attachments and brings about participation with divine spirit.

COCAINE

It is obtained from the leaves of Erythroxylum coca, which grows wild in South America, India, Java, etc. **The leaves contain about 0.5 to 1% cocaine.** It is a colourless, odourless, crystalline substance with bitter taste. **It contains alkaloids ecgonine, hygrine and cinnamyl cocaine.** It is used as local anaesthetic. It is also known as coke, snow, cadillac and white lady. Crack **is prepared by combining cocaine with baking soda and water, which is suitable for smoking.**

Action: It desensitises the terminal nerves and causes vasoconstriction at the site of application. **It is a powerful stimulant of CNS for a short time, followed by depression. Similar but less marked effect is seen on the spinal cord.** It is an excitant and stimulator of autonomic nervous system. It has sympathomimetic properties. The euphoric effect depends on the release of dopamine, serotonin and other neurotransmitters, especially in the pleasure centre of brain. **Its action is somewhat like that of amphetamine.**

Absorption and Excretion: It is rapidly absorbed from the mucous membranes and from the subcutaneous tissues. The usual routes of intake are by application to the nasal mucous membrane (snorting), and by the i.v. route. It is also smoked. It is rapidly hydrolysed by liver and plasma esterases to ecgonine methyl ester and by non-enzymatic hydrolysis to benzolecognine. **The biological half-life of cocaine is half to one hour.** It appears almost immediately in the urine. It is destroyed in the liver and is excreted in the urine within 24 hours in its metabolised forms. **Cocaine, amphetamine, nicotine and barbiturates can be found in the stomach even when given parenterally.** Cannabis interferes with motor skills and judgement, leading to motor vehicle accidents.

Signs and Symptoms: When inhaled, the onset of action is within one to three minutes; when used i.v. or smoked it acts in seconds and peak action is in 3 to 5 minutes; when applied topically to the nasal mucosa, it peaks in 20 to 30 minutes; when ingested orally it peaks within 60 to 90 minutes. **Its action is short, and as such it has to be taken every half to one hour to maintain a high.**

(1) Stage of Excitement: There is bitter taste, dryness in the mouth, dysphagia, **feeling of well-being and loss of depression and fatigue. The patient may be excited, restless and talkative,** but this passes into a calm, dull condition. The pulse is rapid, respirations rapid and deep, pupils dilated, headache, pallor of the skin, cyanosis, sweating, and the temperature is raised. The reflexes are exaggerated, and there may be tremors or convulsions. Occasionally, the patients may have hallucinations and become maniacal. There is **often a feeling of tingling or numbness in the hands and feet,** and a numb feeling at the place where the drug has touched, e.g., nose and back of throat, when it has been sniffed. With spinal anaesthesia there is an occasional case of post anaesthetic myelitis, which leads to permanent symptoms of cord degeneration.

(2) Stage of Depression: Within an hour or even less, respirations become feeble, profuse perspiration, collapse, convulsions and death occurs. Death is due to respiratory failure, cardiac failure, or vascular collapse. **Sudden death may occur following i.v. injection, and smoking than snorting, due to cardiac arrhythmias due to direct action on myocardium, and cardiopulmonary arrest.**

Cocaine produces hypertension which like amphetamine may lead to cerebral bleeding. Rupture of an aneurysm may occur. It may produce coronary artery spasm. Foetal death and abortion can be caused by maternal use of the drug. The children are born premature and often have developmental, behavioural and learning problems.

Large doses or a "binge" may result in anxiety and panic leading to paranoia. **A combination of cocaine and heroin taken by injection is known as "speedball". The person may die suddenly and unexpectedly during or immediately after a struggle.**

Fatal Dose: 1 to 2 gm. orally. 20 mg i.v. Procaine is about half as toxic as cocaine; butacaine is twice and dibucaine five to ten times.

Fatal Period: Few minutes to few hours.

Complications: Cerebrovascular accidents, subarachnoid or intracerebral haemorrhage, myocardial infarction, skin necrosis, aortic dissection and pulmonary infarcts.

Treatment: (1) If it has been taken by mouth, gastric lavage should be performed with warm water containing potassium permanganate, charcoal or tannic acid. (2) If applied to the nose or throat, wash-out the mucous membrane with water. (3) If injected, apply a ligature above the part. (4) Convulsions should be controlled with chloroform or short-acting barbiturates. (5) **Amyl nitrite is antidote and is given by inhalation.** (6) Airway and circulatory stabilisation. (7) Thiamine 100 mg. i.v. (8) Naloxone hydrochloride 2 mg. i.v. (9) The symptoms should be treated on general lines.

Postmortem Appearances: There may be intense asphyxial signs. Pulmonary congestion and oedema with the lungs weighing 3 to 4 times normal. Heart may show foci of scarring which may be the source of fatal dysrhythmias. Pyogenic infections are common with phlebitis and distant embolic abscesses occur. Injection sites may ulcerate. There may be regional lymphadenitis and endocarditis affecting any of the heart valves. Cocaine decomposes rapidly. **Blood should be preserved by adding fluoride.** Brain should be analysed as it does not hydrolyse cocaine into benzolecognine as in blood.

Cocaine can be recovered from recent injection sites, or by swabs from the nasal mucosa.

Cocaine Habit: It is also known as cocainism, cocainophagia or cocainomania. **Chronic abusers can tolerate ten grams a day.** It causes digestive disturbances, anorexia, salivation, tachycardia, tachyapnoea and insomnia. The face is pale, eyes sunken, pupils dilated, and the gaze 'shifty'. **The tongue and teeth are black.** Over a period of time, the addict loses interest in family, friends, food, sexual activity, etc., and appears emaciated and physically exhausted. **Sometimes, a manic, paranoid or depressive psychosis develops (cocaine psychosis or excited delirium).** Complications include persistent rhinitis, nasal erosions, sinusitis, chronic cough, bronchitis, etc. The sniffing habit leads to ulceration of the nasal septum, but perforation is very rare. Degeneration of central nervous system and profound physical deterioration occurs, and the patient may suffer from hallucinations, convulsions, delirium, delusions of persecution, and insanity. **Magnan's symptom or cocaine bugs** is characteristic, **in which there is a feeling as if grains of sand are lying under the skin or some small insects are creeping on the skin giving rise to itching sensation (formication, tactile hallucination) with resultant excoriation, leading to irregular scratches and ulcers.**

It is a drug of addiction and causes lowering of moral tone and loss of decency and self-respect. The cocaine substitutes are not habit forming.

The Circumstances of Poisoning: (1) It is rarely used for homicide or suicide. The common names of substances used by addicts are: crack, pasta, bazooka, and speed-ball. (2) Accidental cases occur from addiction, hypodermic injection and from urethral, vesical and rectal injection. (3) It is believed to be an aphrodisiac and to increase the duration of sexual act by paralysing sensory nerves of glans penis. (4) Prostitutes sometimes inject cocaine solution into vagina to produce local constriction.

CHAPTER 33

SUBSTANCE (DRUG) DEPENDENCE AND ABUSE

FM 12.1: Describe features and management of abuse/poisoning with following chemicals: tobacco, cannabis, amphetamines, cocaine, hallucinogens, designer drugs and solvent.

A DRUG is any substance, or product that is used or intended to be used to modify or explore physiological systems or pathological states for the benefit of recipients (WHO).

Substance abuse arises out of a maladaptive pattern of substance use, manifested by recurrent and significant adverse consequences related to the repeated intake of the substance.

These problems must occur recurrently during the same 12 month period. The criteria for substance abuse do not include tolerance, withdrawal, or a pattern of compulsive use, and instead include only the harmful consequences of repeated use.

SUBSTANCE INTOXICATION refers to unwanted physiological or psychological effects that cause maladaptive behaviour. It must produce disturbances in the level of consciousness, cognition, perception, affect, or behaviour that are clinically significant.

Drug Addiction is defined as a chronic disorder characterised by compulsive use of drugs (craving) resulting in physical, psychological and social harm, and continued use despite evidence of that harm.

Drug habituation is a condition resulting from the repeated consumption of a drug, in which **there is psychological or emotional dependency on the drug.** Caffeine and nicotine are habit-forming drugs.

Substance dependence arises out of a maladaptive pattern of substance use, leading to a cluster of behavioural, cognitive, and physiological phenomena that develop after repeated intake.

It includes a strong desire to take the drug difficulties in controlling its use, persisting in its use despite harmful consequences, a higher priority given to drug use than to other activities and obligations, increased tolerance, and sometimes a physical withdrawal state.

Drug dependence includes both the terms 'addiction' and 'habituation'.

Physical or physiological dependence is defined as an alteration in neural systems which is manifested by tolerance and the appearance of withdrawal phenomena when a chronically administered drug is discontinued or displaced from its receptor. Psychological dependence is a compulsive need for a drug in order to maintain a state of well-being, and it can occur in the absence of physical dependence.

Substances withdrawal should be restricted to major symptoms resulting from the cessation of substance abuse, accompanied by a maladaptive behaviour change. There should be clinically significant distress or impairment in social, occupational, or other important areas of function.

Designer drugs: They are **synthetic variations of well-known controlled drugs,** such as fentanyl, phencyclidine, mescaline, etc. **with similar pharmacological effects but different molecular structures.** The most commonly known types of synthetic analog drugs available in the illicit drug market **include analogs of fentanyl and meperidine, phencyclidine, amphetamine and methamphetamine.**

Alcohol and tobacco are the commonest substances abused, followed by sedatives and tranquilisers, cannabis, amphetamine, opiates and cocaine. Amphetamines and hallucinogens are less popular.

Pharmacologically, addiction evolves through the following stages: (1) Habituation. (2) Physical dependence, wherein an altered physiological state exists because of the frequent exposure to the drug. Withdrawal of the drug causes physical and emotional illness, known as the abstinence or withdrawal syndrome. (3) Tolerance to many of the pharmacologic effects of the drug Table (33–1).

Most persons use drugs of dependence with a certain discrimination, and in such cases little harm results. Indiscriminate use of any of these drugs becomes dangerous, and produces a gradual mental, physical, and moral deterioration of the individual, and sometimes also sexual perversions or crime. To obtain the money for the drug the addict often turns to prostitution or crime. The majority of drug victims are neurotic individuals who are mentally unbalanced. A normal person has no tendency to become a drug addict and is most unlikely to become one, even when all the facilities are available. Hereditary factors, abnormal mental conditions, frustrations in life, anxiety, chronic tensions, physical inability to do a job, curiosity, etc. are some of the causes of drug addiction. Addicts fall in two groups. (1) Those who originally used the drug for some disease and thus have acquired the habit, and (2) those who use the drug for its narcotic effect alone. The first group are more easily cured than the second. The inability to discontinue the use of drug may be due either to a desire for satisfaction, or an anxiety to avoid the discomfort of withdrawal symptoms, or both. Most drug users appear normal.

Common adulterants for drugs of addiction include quinine, lactose, sucrose, and rarely baking soda, mannitol and magnesium silicate.

Table (33–1). Difference between drug addiction and drug habituation

	Trait	Drug addiction	Drug habituation
(1)	Compulsion:	Present.	Desire but no compulsion.
(2)	Dose:	Tendency to increase.	No tendency to increase.
(3)	Dependence:	Psychological and physical.	Some degree of psychological but not physical.
(4)	Withdrawal symptoms:	Characteristic symptoms.	None or mild.
(5)	Harm:	Both to the individual and society.	If any, primarily to individual.

According to the Narcotics Control Bureau, there are more than 30 million amphetamine addicts in the World. This is more than the total number of heroin and cocaine addicts put together. Another estimate states that 0.5% of world population is addicted to some form of amphetamine drug today.

Drug abuse is a major medical problem with extensive legal, social, moral, ethical and even political problems. A person made tolerant to a large dose of one narcotic is also cross-tolerant to many of the effects of another narcotic.

CLASSIFICATION

(1) Ethanol. (2) Tobacco. (3) Tranquiliser and sedatives: barbiturates, benzodiazepines, chloral hydrate, chlormethiazole, ethchlorvynol, glutethimide, meprobamate, methaqualone, zolpidem, zopiclone. (4) Opiates and opioids. (5) Cocaine. (6) Cannabis. (7) Amphetamines and "Designer drugs". (8) Hallucinogens: Lysergic acid diethylamide (LSD), phencyclidine, psilocybine, bufotenine, mescaline, ketamine, dimethyltryptamine (DMT). (9) Inhalants: Fluorinated hydrocabons (freons), ethers, ketones, aromatic and aliphatic hydrocarbons. (10) Miscellaneous drugs and substances: Caffeine, datura seeds, analgesics, anabolic steroids, cough syrups, laxatives.

Symptoms of Drug Dependency: Drugs of abuse may be taken by injection (intravenous, subcutaneous or rarely intramuscular), by sniffing into the nostrils, through rectum or vagina, by inhalation, smoking or orally. Loss of appetite and weight; clumsy movements, unsteady gait, tremors; reddening and puffiness of eyes, unclear vision; slurring of speech; loss of interest, sleeplessness, lethargy and passivity; acute anxiety, depression, profuse sweating; mood changes, temper tantrums; depersonalisation and emotional detachment; impaired memory and concentration; preference for solitude, especially spending long hours in the toilet. Acute intravenous narcotism is characterised by the appearance of fulminant pulmonary oedema and immediate collapse and death.

Money and articles disappear from home, and needles, syringes, strange packets, etc. are found at home.

Alcohol, cannabis, cocaine, morphine, heroin may produce a variety of mental conditions.

Withdrawal Symptoms: If the drug is abruptly withdrawn, a withdrawal syndrome will occur in a physically dependent person. **The withdrawal symptoms are usually opposite to the effects of the drug itself. They may begin within 6 to 8 hours following stoppage of the drug or they may be delayed for 24 to 48 hours, depending upon the particular drug being used. The length of period of withdrawal symptoms also varies and can last up to ten days.** The intensity of the symptoms depends on the dose and type of the drug used, the duration of addiction, and the suddenness of withdrawal of the drug. Early symptoms are chilliness, sensation of cold, uneasiness, yawning and rhinorrhoea. Later, respirations become laboured, sharp and very rapid. Goose skin, lachrymation, gross tremors and dilated pupils are seen. Anorexia is present in all the stages. The third stage is one of sleep lasting from 8 to 16 hours. Upon awakening, all the previous symptoms become intense. In addition, there is tachypnoea, fever, hypertension, pain and cramps in the legs and abdomen, perspiration, vomiting and diarrhoea.

Newborns of addicted mothers may show withdrawal symptoms from one to 56 hours after birth and require treatment. The symptoms are hyperactivity, twitchings and convulsions.

In the alleged 'rainbow' parties, multiple drugs are mixed and the experimenter selects several at random, and then is asked to explain or describe the effects of the resulting experience.

Narcotic addicts may be murdered by a 'hot shot'. This is a dose of narcotic with poison, such as strychnine in it. In such cases, only signs of anoxia and cerebral depression are present. Another method of accidental or homicidal death is by the use of a purer drug than the addict has been using.

Cocaine, cannabis, LSD, amphetamine, and anti-depressants and anti-psychotics do not produce physical dependence. Alcohol, morphine, cocaine and LSD produce psychosis.

Treatment: (1) The person should be removed to an institution, so as to remove him from the association with which the addiction started. (2) Constant supervision to prevent addict from obtaining secret supplies of the drug. (3) Detoxification: This consists of reduction in dosage of drug over a period of one to 3 weeks. (4) Administration of drugs, such as sedatives, benezidrine, hyoscine. (5) Diverting the mind by engaging him physically and mentally in some occupation. (6) Psychotherapy (group, family or individual). (7) Improving general health. (8) Symptomatic. The treatment is successful only in 10 to 25% of cases.

Rehabilitation: Rehabilitation is a continuous process of weaning away the victims of drug dependency. It requires strong family support and follow up to prevent relapse. Social rehabilitation and training for gainful employment are the most important components after weaning addicts away from drug dependency to prevent relapse.

TYPES OF DEPENDENCE: The World Health Organisation recognises the following types of dependence.

(1) MORPHINE TYPE: It refers to addiction to morphine, heroin, opium or morphine substitutes, such as methadone. In this type, there is overpowering desire or need to continue taking the drug and to obtain it by any means and by a tendency to increase the dose due to the development of tolerance. Morphine is usually taken by i.v. or i.m. injection, or by sniffing up the nose. In opium abuse, there is always a high degree of cross-tolerance to other drugs with a similar

pharmacologic action, even if the chemical composition of the opioids is completely different. Tolerance develops at different rates to different effects of opioids, e.g., heroin withdrawal will usually start within 8 hours, progress to a peak and then gradually improve over 48 to 72 hours, whereas withdrawal from methadone may lead to a longer abstinence syndrome. Morphine and pethidine exhibit a high degree of tolerance and physical dependence.

Withdrawal symptoms occur after withdrawal of the drug for more than 12 hours and last about a week. Yawning is a common feature. MINOR: Dilated pupils, piloerection, yawning, rhinorrhoea, myalgias and cramps, lachrymation, anorexia, perspiration. MODERATE: Restlessness, insomnia, hypertension, tachycardia, tachypnoea, diaphoresis. MAJOR: Vomiting, diarrhoea, hyperactive bowel sounds, hypotension. Death may be so rapid that the needle may still be found in the vein, when the body is discovered. Death is caused by cardiac arrest following an arrhythmia and ventricular fibrillation. A standard therapeutic regime involving a morphine type drug for 10 to 14 days is sufficient to cause dependence on the drug in the majority of patients. Methadone 25 to 50 mg twice daily helps recovery.

(2) BARBITURATE TYPE: In this type, the desire to continue the drug is strong, and the tendency to increase the dose is partly due to tolerance. There is a cross-tolerance between these drugs and alcohol, and together they make a powerful and potentially lethal combination. The withdrawal symptoms reach a maximum in 2 or 3 days and subside slowly. Early signs are: tremor, hyperreflexia, diaphoresis, irritability, restlessness, anxiety, tinnitus, nausea, vomiting, paraesthesias, transient hallucinations, confusion, illusions, insomnia, depression, tachycardia, tachypnoea, hypertension, convulsions. Late signs are: profuse diaphoresis, marked disorientation, persistent hallucinations, extreme agitation, tremors, restlessness, hyperthermia, tachycardia, tachypnoea, orthostatic hypertension. Barbiturates (downers) may be combined with amphetamines (uppers) in the same 'purple heart' tablet.

Withdrawal symptoms in addiction to alcohol, barbiturates and sedative-hypnotics include: confusion, agitation, tremors, fever, bizarre behaviour and convulsions.

(3) COCAINE TYPE: In this the desire to obtain the drug is overpowering, but tolerance is absent. There is psychodependence on the drug and no withdrawal symptoms. It may cause progressively intensive toxic reactions including paranoid psychosis and its use may be combined with that of heroin or some other morphine-like compound. There is profound mental depression, which may lead to severe mental dysfunction. It produces hypertension which may lead to cerebral haemorrhage.

Crack is prepared by heating cocaine with an alkali, such as bicarbonate, which is more potent.

(4) CANNABIS TYPE: In this the need or desire is present, but there is no tolerance and usually no dose increase. There is psychic dependence only, and no abstinence syndrome. The danger of cannabis is not in itself but in the environment in which it may be used, where there may be danger of addiction to other and more dangerous drugs. A person under the influence of cannabis may injure himself or cause harm to others. As the withdrawal syndrome is mild, supportive and symptomatic treatment is given.

(5) AMPHETAMINE TYPE: This may be combined with barbiturates. Here the need or desire is present, and there is a tolerance to the drug, and a tendency to increase the dose. Dependence is psychic and there is no abstinence syndrome, but continuous use of amphetamines may lead to severe hyperexcitement, hallucinations and psychoses. There is hyperpyrexia and hypertension, which can occasionally precipitate a cerebral or a subarachnoid haemorrhage and a risk of cardiac arrhythmias.

Drug Combination: The effects of drug combinations are different from each drug taken singly, and **mixtures of drugs are particularly liable to lead to tolerance and habituation.**

Illicit drugs believed to be transmitted through breast milk include cocaine, heroin, amphetamines, marijuana and phencyclidine.

Loss of Tolerance: There is loss of tolerance following withdrawal during hospitalisation or imprisonment. The addict on being released often goes back into his old environment and resumes his addiction, taking the same dose that he did before, which may cause death.

COTTON FEVER: Fever developing due to injection of a water extract of the cotton remaining after the heroin supply is used in a "bag".

DRUG ABUSER'S ELBOW: Myositis ossificans resulting due to repeated needle punctures near the elbow in the i.v. drug abuser.

BODY PACKER (SURGICAL MULES) SYNDROME: Illegal drugs, such as cocaine, heroin, amphetamine and cannabis are compressed into cylinders of about 25x12 mm size, heat-sealed in plastic film and wrapped again in multiple layers of latex (condoms, balloons, foil, fingers of rubber gloves, etc.) and swallowed. One packet may contain 3 to 7 g. of the narcotic. Drugs such as loparamide or diphenoxylate hydrochloride with atropine may be taken to reduce gut motility and prevent the passage of the packages on a long-distance flight, before the end of journey. **This is done for the purpose of smuggling, termed "body-packing".** They can conceal half kg of drug. **On arrival at his destination, the courier takes a laxative, retrieves the packets and passes them on to the "pusher"** who distributes the drug. The packets may cause bowel obstruction secondary to torsion, intussusception or impaction. Sometimes, packets become unsealed or burst in the small intestine, especially cocaine-filled containers, allowing massive absorption and cause the courier's death from poisoning. **Even if the packets do not rupture, drugs may passively diffuse from the stomach into surrounding organs,** including the lower lobe of left lung, left lobe of liver and heart and appear in the circulation and urine.

BODY STUFFER SYNDROME: Persons arrested swallow illegal drugs for concealing the evidence from authorities. This is termed "body stuffer". Drugs may be concealed in the ears, mouth, nose, vagina or rectum (body pushers). These drugs may not be well wrapped and may result in signs and symptoms within a couple of hours. **Most packets are seen on X-ray, and all are seen with CT scanning or barium contrast studies.**

Treatment: (1) Diazepam 10 mg. i.v. followed by 5 mg. i.v. every 5 min. until the patient becomes calm. (2) Give glucose, thiamine and multivitamins. (3) Fluid and electrolyte balance. (4) Oxygen.

CASE: A 24 year old male who swallowed 80 capsules containing 270 g of heroin (each capsule had 3 to 4 g.) and was to travel to Maldives, was arrested at Chennai airport.

SOLVENT ABUSE: (Volatile substance abuse; glue sniffing) It involves the deliberate inhaling of a variety of substances, such as toluene, gasoline (petrol), xylene, benzene, chloroform, methylene and ethylene chloride, fluorocarbons, carbon tetrachloride, butane, propane, kerosene, isopropane, amyl nitrite, acetone, trichloroethylene, methylene chloride, butyl nitrites, ketones, etc., for their psychotropic and hallucinogenic properties. Volatiles such as paint stripper, typewriting erasure fluid, brush cleaner, household aerosols, fabric cleaner, gasoline and glue solvent are misused. **Huffing refers to inhaling vapours from a cloth that is saturated with the volatile substance and held over or near to the nose and mouth. Bagging refers to inhaling and exhaling into a plastic**

bag that has been filled with a small amount of a volatile substance. The open end is then placed against nose and mouth and the air inside breathed. Clinical manifestations depend on the substance abused. Gaseous substances may be introduced directly into the mouth or nose from either a large cylinder or from the small ampoule cylinders for refilling gas cigarette lighters. Others are used directly from pressurised aerosol cans, including pain-relieving sprays. **Sniffing is done by inhaling directly from the neck of a container, such as jerry cans and petro-fillers of motor vehicles.** The effects vary from a condition resembling alcoholic intoxication, and distortion of perception to actual hallucinations. The person feels powerful dreams, heightened sensation and detachment from reality. **The sufferer often behaves totally irrationally, commits antisocial acts and may injure or even kill himself.** Later, the abuser will often have complete amnesia for the period of intoxication. Most of the abusers are young, usually male teenagers. There is no physical withdrawal syndrome.

Cause of Death: (1) The major cause of death is due to sudden cardiac arrest, following an arrhythmia. Any sudden "flight or fright" stimulus, even some considerable time after sniffing, has the ability to precipitate ventricular fibrillation and sudden death. (2) Hypoxia and hypercapnoea from persistent rebreathing and toxic effects of the solvent. (3) Plastic bag asphyxia. (4) Aspiration of vomit. (5) Reflex cardiac arrest due to inhalation of gaseous substances. (6) Drug ingestion may trigger intravascular sickling in certain haemoglobinopathies resulting in sudden death. (7) Accidents, such as a fall from a balcony, drowning, etc.

Postmortem Appearances: There may be reddening or excoriation of the skin around the nose and mouth from the irritant action of the solvent. There may be severe damage of the liver, kidneys, bone marrow and nervous system. The clothing, blood, fat, brain, and lungs should be sent for chemical examination. Blood should be collected in a Teflon-line screw top bottle, because volatile compounds can diffuse through rubber. Blood samples must fill the container so that the solvent is not lost from the 'head space' when the lid is removed. One lung, urine sample, unfixed tissue from liver and brain samples should be placed in nylon bags. In suspected cases of inhaled drugs, nasal swabs should be preserved. Headspace gas chromatography is used for identifying substances of solvent abuse.

INVESTIGATION OF DRUG ABUSE DEATHS: SCENE: **Death is often the result of drug combinations rather than the abuse and overdose of a single agent. Unexpected coma followed by death or irrational behaviour before a bizarre act resulting in death, especially in younger people, raises the possibility of a drug related death. The dead person's clothes should be examined and described for drugs in the pockets or hidden in seams, belt, shoes, money purse, eye-glasses case, jewellery, etc. The body should be examined for caches of drugs that may be in body orifices, taped to the body between buttocks, toes, under the breasts, or attached to a string tied around a tooth and then swallowed. Rarely, the needle, syringe and tourniquet may be found in place on the body. The tourniquet may contain concealed drug. Sometimes, the clothing and the body may be tampered. Photographs of the scene and surrounding objects should be taken. Psychedelic posters may suggest drug abuse. The surroundings should be searched and any drugs found preserved. A needle and syringe, a cooker, lighter and cracker are usually present. The contents of the cooker should be sent for analysis. Tubes of plastic glue or plastic bags indicate death due to a volatile, such as glue (toluene) or solvent. Aerosol cans and balloons indicate "huffing" death.**

APPARATUS AND PREPARATION OF DRUGS FOR INJECTION: Illicit narcotics are purchased "on the street" as packets of powders, tablets or capsules containing the alkaloid (usually 4 to 8%), which has been diluted (cut) by quinine, mannitol, lactose, etc. The powder is placed with water in a small receptacle, e.g., bottle cap or spoon (cooker), which is heated until the powder dissolves. The solution is then drawn into a standard or improvised syringe, usually through a bit of cotton to filter out insoluble particles. Belts or elastic bands are used as tourniquets.

Addicts may attempt to revive the person by injecting saline, milk or water into the arm, back of hands or buttocks. Sometimes the person may be immersed in a cold shower or tub of water, or putting ice on the genitalia or pouring milk into the mouth.

AUTOPSY: (A) EXTERNAL: There is often wasting and signs of self-neglect. The body may be extensively tattooed to hide scars. Stains may be found on the tips of fingers, indicating the possible type of pill or capsule handled. A callus on the medial aspect of thumb "crack thumb" occurs due to repeated use of butane lighter to heat crack (cocaine). Burns on the lower lip, due to smoking hot glass "crack pipes" are common. Excoriation of anterior chest wall are usually a sign of chronic opiate abuse. Linear needle track scars, often pigmented are usually found overlying fibrosed, cord-like veins of the antecubital fossae, forearms, and dorsa of the hands in "mainliners". Sometimes, needle tracks are found on scalp, neck, sublingual areas, shoulder, inguinal region, penis, vagina, popliteal area, ankle and foot Fig. (33–1). Punctate areas of black discolouration (soot tattooing) are caused by deposition of carbonaceous materials along the track of the needle. Such tattooing is called "TURKEY SKIN", as it resembles the plucked bird. Customary target areas for subcutaneous or intramuscular injection are the upper arms, abdomen and thighs. It can lead to areas of subcutaneous sclerosis, fat necrosis, absccsses and if the injections are deeper into the muscle, to chronic myositis. Rarely there may be necrosis and loss of phalanges from thrombotic or septic emboli. The inflammatory foci may resolve leaving no trace, or may form abscesses or ulceration. Chronic oedema of the hands, secondary to occlusive thrombophlebitis in the forearms, is seen occasionally in long-term addicts. A single fresh needle puncture shows a tiny crusted focus, but may be difficult to identify, but incision through the skin may show a perivenous haemorrhagic track. The subcutaneous heroin users show a higher incidence of abscess. Healing by fibrosis may produce hyperpigmented macules or retracted, circumscribed scars which resemble those from smallpox vaccinations. Additional damage to the skin and subcutaneous tissues results from attempts by the addict

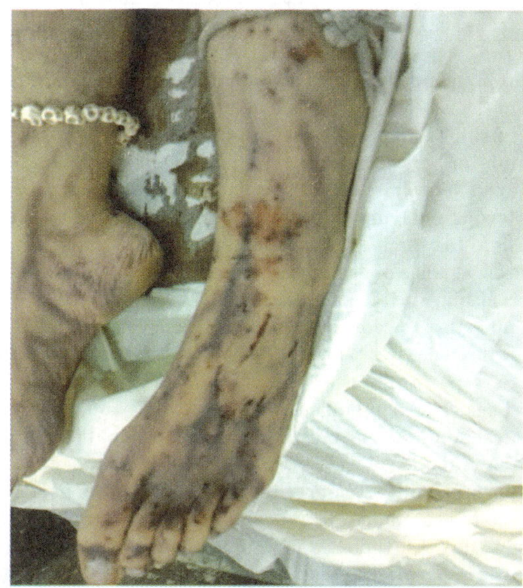

Fig. (33–1). Linear pigmented needle track marks over veins in mainliners in a drug addict.

Courtesy: **Dr Manoj Kumar, BHU, Varanasi**

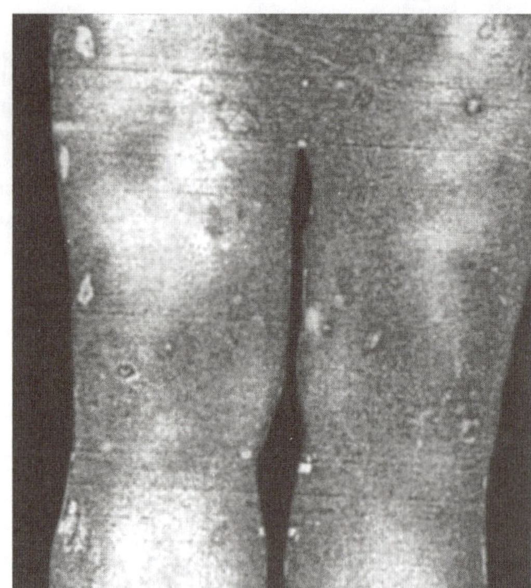

Fig. (33–2). Multiple scars caused by injection of drugs of dependence.

to obliterate the track by overlaying it with a cigarette burn or abrading with pumice stone, sandpaper or using escharotic chemicals. Multiple circular sunken atrophic scars (tissue paper scars), suggest skin popping followed by skin infection Fig. (33–2). The regional lymph nodes may be enlarged. Nasal passages and nasopharynx may reveal irritation or even traces of drugs inhaled through the nose. Habitual inhalation of cocaine or heroin (snorting or sniffing) cause irritation, congestion and atrophy of nasal mucosa perforation of the nasal septum varying in size from a pinhead to several centimetres. They may be round, oval or irregular. Froth may be seen at the mouth and nose. There may be discolouration of lips, tongue, or oral mucosa.

(B) INTERNAL: G.I. tract may contain pills or capsules. Microscopic examination of sections of stomach under polarised light sometimes shows particles of optically active filter material (e.g., starch, talc, cellulose) adherent to the gastric mucosa in victims of fatal drug ingestion and the dye from capsules may colour the mucosa with an unnatural colour. Needle scars show perivenous fibrosis in the intravenous addict and acute or chronic abscesses, or diffuse subcutaneous scarring in the skin-popper. Microscopic examination often shows foreign material in the scar tissues, e.g., fragments of cloth, cotton, talc or unidentifiable matter with surrounding foreign body giant cell reactions. Repeated injections can give rise to a chronic myopathy which is in part due to chronic infection, but is exacerbated by an auto-immune response to damaged muscle. Histologically, affected areas show fibre necrosis, replacement fibrosis and infiltration by polymorphs and lymphocytes which extends far beyond the area of the injection. To examine the veins, make a single longitudinal incision of the flexor surface of each arm from mid-biceps to distal forearm. The incised margins are reflected widely to expose subcutaneous tissues and veins. To reduce artefactual haemorrhage, this should be done after throacic viscera have been removed. There may be phlebitis, phlebosclerosis, thrombosis, and recent and resolving perivenous haemorrhage. The vein and surrounding tissue should be preserved for chemical analysis. The most common internal pathologic changes from parenteral drug abuse consist of hepatic lymphadenopathy, and hepatic portal triaditis. Enlarged lymph nodes at the porta hepatis, adjacent to the common bile duct and at the pylorus of the stomach usually measure 3 to 4 cm. Microscopically, such lymph nodes show non-specific hyperplasia. Dense lymphocytic infiltrates involve all of the portal triads, with or without parenchymal pathologic stigmas of viral hepatitis. Typical visceral anatomic findings include the non-specific pulmonary triad of oedema, bronchopneumonia, and aspiration of gastric contents. Froth is present in the upper respiratory tract, which comes out from the nose and mouth. Lungs are heavy. In mainliners, the crystals lodge in pulmonary capillaries, and produce a foreign body granulomatous reaction. Such granulomas erode the walls of capillaries and unite, forming larger granulomas. In extreme cases, the lungs have a multinodular, gritty texture, and microscopic examination under polarised light shows large quantities of talc, starch or cellulose in these lesions. Pulmonary hypertension with right ventricular cardiac hypertrophy occurs due to extensive microcrystalline pulmonary emboli. Most heroin addicts have a few optically active crystals in their pulmonary capillaries. Pleurae may show petechial haemorrhages. The lungs are usually congested and oedematous with focal haemorrhages. Liver may be slightly enlarged or shows evidence of cirrhosis. The heart may show valvular diseases. Pericardial, pleural and peritoneal effusions may be found. The brain may show oedema and focal areas of necrosis involving the globus pallidus and hippocampus due to hypoxia. Hyperplastic changes in the reticuloendothelial system are common. Splenomegaly and portal lymph node hyperplasia are common. The most constant finding in both spleen and portal lymph nodes is the presence of large germinal centres, but the morphological features are not specific. Birefringent material is present in spleen more often than in portal lymph nodes. Lysozyme containing cells are found in the spleen indicating bacterial contamination. The presence of significantly more IgM and IgE containing cells in spleen and portal lymph nodes indicates acute, subacute and chronic antigen stimulation.

COMPLICATIONS OF INJECTIONS: (1) Self-neglect, malnutrition, dental decay. (2) The veins in the arms, hands, legs and sometimes abdomen, groin or neck are damaged. Overuse of the same veins produces thrombosis and phlebitis, especially if the substance is irritative or unsterile and pulmonary embolism. The veins become dark in colour, may be hard and cord-like due to thrombosis and fibrosis, and may ulcerate. When healed, there may be white or silvery linear scars in the axis of the limb. Fragments may be injected which lead to microemboli in the lungs and liver, where they form granulomas or abscesses. (b) Intra-arterial injection may cause vascular damage and gangrene. (c) Infection: Cellulitis and abscess formation at the injection site, and depressed areas of fat atrophy may be present. Fat necrosis and chronic myositis may be seen. Septicaemia and subacute bacterial endocarditis may occur. (3) Inhalation may precipitate asthma or bronchitis, pneumothorax, pneumomediastinum, and vomiting. (4) Shared syringes and needles can transmit hepatitis B and C, HIV, syphilis and malaria. (5) Acute and chronic liver disease. (6) Kidney problems and amyloidosis. (7) Psychiatric complications. (8) Tuberculosis and pneumonia due to reduced resistance and poor nutrition. (9) They are more commonly involved in various accidents due to impairment of alertness and behaviour. (10) The need to obtain money may lead to squalor, theft and prostitution. (11) Personal violence and murder is more common. (12) Acute myopathy, meningitis, brain and pulmonary abscesses, various neurological abnormalities, acute muscle necrosis with myoglobinuria and renal failure are rare complications. (13) Death can occur due to overdose or from contaminants.

OVERDOSAGE AND HYPERSENSITIVITY: Death can occur rapidly, especially with i.v. use of heroin. Due to hypersensitivity, sometimes a first time user may die rapidly and the needle and syringe may be found in the vein. Death appears to be due to acute left ventricular failure and gross pulmonary oedema. Froth may be seen exuding from the mouth and nose.

CHEMICAL ANALYSIS: Nasal secretions are useful for cocaine, opiates and drugs which are inhaled or "snorted". Blood should be preserved by sodium fluoride and stored at 4°C.

The samples of choice are blood and urine, although nasal secretions, gastric contents, bile, liver, kidneys and lungs may be necessary to definitely identify the type and concentration of drug. If the drug is taken by nasal route, dry swabs from each nostril should be taken. Tissue removed from injection mark should be refrigerated, till it is delivered to the laboratory.

Common methods for detecting drugs of abuse are: gas-liquid chromatography (GLC), thin-layer chromatography (TLC) and spectrophotofluorimetry (SPF).

TOXICOLOGIC RADIOLOGY

In cases of ingestion of hydrocarbons, chest X-ray may show basilar infiltrates, perihilar densities, atelectasis, pleural effusion, etc.

RADIO-OPAQUE POISONS are heavy metals, aspirin, acetazolamide, ammonium chloride, busulphan, carbon tetrachloride, chloral hydrate, enteric-coated tablets, iodides, salicylates, methotrexate, penicillin G & K, phenothiazines, potassium chloride, permanganate, sodium chloride.

DRUG ABUSERS: Heroin or cocaine carriers swallow machine-made condom wrapped, or aluminium-foil wrapped packets (body packers). The abdominal film may show an atypical gas pattern or an unusual number of rounded, cigar-shaped or oblong masses with a complete gas halo. CT scan is better than radiology. Symptomatic patients may have signs of oesophageal, gastric or small bowel obstruction or an ileus resulting from a large number of bags swallowed or the size or position of a particular bag. Typically, obstruction occurs at the ileo-caecal valve.

X-ray of abdomen of an opioid abuser (esp. methadone) may show marked ileus and severe colonic distension due to faecal retention (pseudo-obstruction). Crack (the volatile alkaloidal form of cocaine) is rapidly absorbed by deep inhalation and leads to the rupture of alveolae and produces pneumothorax, pneumo-mediastinum and/or neck and pre-cervical subcutaneous emphysema.

X-ray of chest of a parenteral drug abuser may show diffuse granulomatous changes due to chronic parenteral abuse, and the concomitant injection of the inert, insoluble ingredients of oral preparations or talc. Septic pulmonary emboli appear as round or wedge-shaped densities that may clear later or cavitate. Aspiration pneumonitis or non-cardiogenic pulmonary oedema also occur.

Chest X-ray may show pulmonary abscesses caused by aspiration pneumonitis or after i.v. injection of toxic organic or inorganic materials or bacteria. Aneurysms and pseudoaneurysms may be seen in mainliners. Injections into the internal or external jugular veins, subclavian veins, femoral artery or vein may produce aneurysms, pseudoaneurysms, intrathoracic haemorrhage, vascular obstructions or arteriovenous fistulae. A necrotising angiitis similar to periarteritis nodosa may result from parenteral amphetamine and cocaine associated with microaneurysms, segmental stenoses and thromboses in the kidney, liver, pancreas and small intestine. Intra-arterial injection of amphetamines, cocaine or barbiturates may produce chemical endarteritis.

Hard drugs causes severe physical dependence, e.g., opium, heroin, cocaine, cocaine, methedrin, methamphetamine, alcohol, etc.

Soft drugs do not produce physical dependence but cause psychological dependence, e.g., LSD, antidepressants, antipsychotics, barbiturates, cannabis, mescaline, psilocybin, etc.

GLOSSARY

Acid head = Heavy user of LSD.

Bad or bum or freak out trip = An LSD experience in which the drug effects are unpleasant and sometimes frightening. It usually lasts from 8 to 12 hours.

Bang = To inject drugs.

Bean = Capsule for drugs.

Bombed out = Very much intoxicated by drugs.

Busted = To be arrested.

Connect = To purchase drugs.

Crash = End of drug experience.

Cutting = Mixing a drug, usually a narcotic, with other substances.

Flip = To go psychotic.

Flashback = A transitory, spontaneous recurrence of drug-induced experience in a drug-free state.

Guide = A person who "babysits" for the psychedelic user during a session.

Hangover = Temporary illness usually following recovery from drunkenness.

Hooked up = Made a drug purchase.

Jones = Experience drug withdrawal.

Mainlining = i.v. injection.

Needle freak = A person who prefers to take drugs with a needle.

Shooting = i.v. injection.

Pot = Marijuana.

Physical dependence = Physiologic requirement for a drug to prevent symptoms of withdrawal.

Psychological dependence = The mind's need to continue taking a drug (craving) for its pleasurable effects or to avoid discomfort.

Return trip = Reappearance of LSD-like effects long after the last dose of LSD was taken.

Skin popping (joy popping) = i.m. injection.

Spaced out = Under influence of drugs.

Stoned = Intoxicated.

Trip = Effects of LSD.

Psychotomimetic = Psychosis mimicking.

Tweeking = Prolonged drug use.

CHAPTER

34

SPINAL POISONS

FM 14.17: To identify and draw medicolegal inference from common poisons, e.g., nux vomica.

STRYCHNOS NUX VOMICA

Strychnine *(kuchila)* is a powerful alkaloid obtained from the seeds of strychnos nux vomica, and other species of strychnos, which are found in the jungles in India. Fruit is round, hard, slightly rough, glossy-orange, 4 to 5 cm. wide, with jelly-like white or pale yellow pulp. It has 3 to 5 seeds Fig. (34–1). Strychnine occurs as colourless, odourless, rhombic prisms, having an intensely bitter taste. The bark contains only brucine. The fruit pulp has very low strychnine content. **All parts of the tree are toxic.**

Seeds: The seeds are flat, circular discs or slightly convex on one side, concave on the other, two-and-half cm. in diameter, 6 mm. in thickness Figs. (34–2 and 34–3). They are ash-grey or light-brown in colour, have a shining surface and covered with radiating silky fibres. They are very hard, tough and difficult to pulverize. The seeds of nux vomica contained in the ripe fruit are poisonous. **The seeds contain two principal alkaloids; strychnine and brucine one-and-half percent each. The seeds also contain a glucoside, loganin.** The bark, wood and leaves contain brucine but no strychnine. **Brucine is allied to strychnine in composition and action. Strychnine is 10 to 20 times more poisonous than brucine.** Strychnine is used as a respiratory stimulant, as a rodenticide and for killing stray dogs.

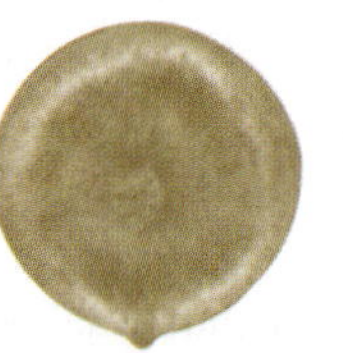

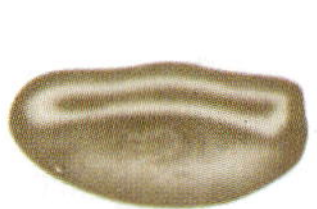

Fig. (34–2). **Nux vomica seeds.**

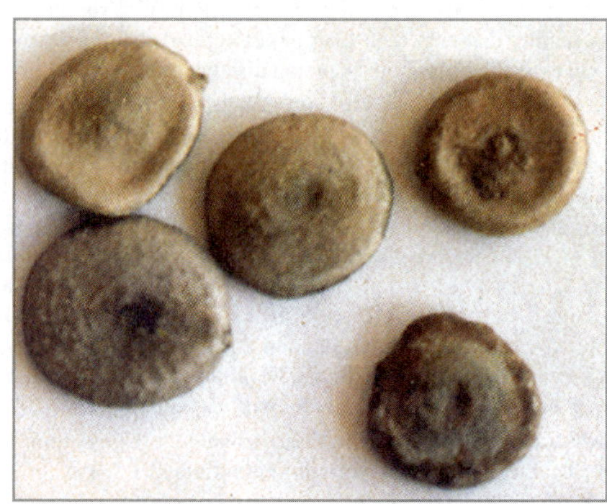

Fig. (34–3). **Nux vomica.**

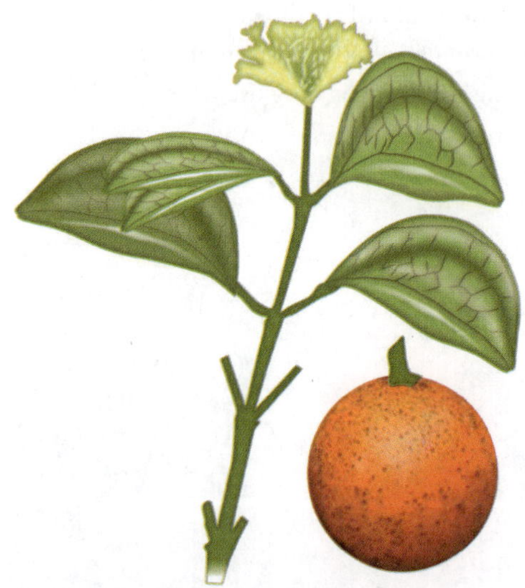

Fig. (34–1). **Strychnos nux vomica.**

Absorption and Excretion: All mucous membranes absorb strychnine. Much is taken up by the liver and muscles to be either released again to blood stream or to be destroyed. **The release of strychnine from the liver and muscles produces convulsions on second or third day of poisoning, after sedation is discontinued.** About 80% is oxidised mainly in the liver. It is excreted slowly by the kidneys and traces in bile, milk and saliva. **It may be found in the cadaver up to four years.**

Action: It competitively blocks ventral horn motor neurone postganglionic receptor sites in the spinal cord and brainstem and prevents the effects of glycine (the presumed inhibitory transmitter). **Widespread inhibition in the spinal cord results in 'release' excitation. The action is particularly**

Table (34–1). Difference between strychnine poisoning and tetanus

	Trait	Strychnine poisoning	Tetanus
(1)	History:	No history of injury.	History of injury present.
(2)	Onset:	Sudden.	Gradual.
(3)	Convulsions:	All muscles of the body are affected at a time.	All muscles are not affected at a time.
(4)	Lower jaw:	Does not start in, nor especially affects the jaw.	Usually starts in, and especially affects lower jaw.
(5)	Muscular condition:	Between fits, muscles are completely relaxed.	Between fits, muscles are slightly rigid.
(6)	Fatal period:	1–2 hours.	More than 24 hours.
(7)	Chemical analysis:	Strychnine found.	No poison found.

noted in the anterior horn cells. It stimulates the cerebral cortex. GABA, the neurotransmitter for presynaptic inhibitory neurons is not affected.

Signs and Symptoms: If swallowed uncrushed, the seeds of nux vomica have no poisonous action, as they are not dissolved in the gastrointestinal tract, and are passed entire in the faeces. When crushed seeds are taken, the symptoms are delayed for an hour or more. If the alkaloid is swallowed, the symptoms occur very rapidly, usually within five to fifteen minutes. Bitter taste in the mouth, sense of uneasiness and restlessness, feeling of suffocation and fear, and difficulty in swallowing occur. **The convulsions are preceded by such prodromal symptoms as increased acuity of perception, increased rigidity of muscles, and muscular twitchings.** Convulsions are produced due to direct action on the reflex centres of spinal cord, and affect all the muscles at a time. These are at first clonic, but eventually become tonic. During the convulsions, the face is cyanosed and has anxious look, eyes are staring, eyeballs prominent and pupils are dilated. **Risus sardonicus results from contraction of the jaws and facial muscles in which the corners of the mouth are drawn back.** The mouth is covered with froth, frequently bloodstained. **The convulsions are most marked in anti-gravity muscles, so that the body typically arches in hyperextension (opisthotonus).** In supine position, the body is supported by the heels and head. The legs are adducted and extended, the arms are flexed over the chest or rigidly extended, and the hands are tightly clenched. The head is bent backwards, and the **whole of the body becomes rigid, often assuming a bow-like form.** Sometimes, the spasm of the abdominal muscles may bend the body forward **(emprosthotonus)**, or to the side **(pleurosthotonus)**. Consciousness is not lost and the mind remains clear till death. The suffering during the spasm is severe, and the patient is conscious of impending danger of death. **The duration of convulsion varies from half to two minutes. In between the convulsions the muscles are completely relaxed, and the patient looks well though somewhat exhausted, and the breathing is resumed.** The cyanosis lessens, cold perspirations cover the skin; dilated pupils may contract. After 5 to 15 minutes or on slightest impulse, e.g. a sudden noise, a current of air, or gently touching the patient, another convulsion occurs. In fatal cases, the convulsions rapidly succeed one another, and increase in severity and in duration, and **death usually occurs after four to five convulsions.** The patient cannot breathe because the diaphragm and thoracic muscles are fully contracted. **Hypoxia causes medullary paralysis and death.** In non-fatal cases the intervals between the convulsions become longer and the spasm less, until these entirely stop within 12 to 24 hours, and recovery takes place in a day or two Table (34–1).

Fatal Dose: 50 to 100 mg.; one crushed seed.

Fatal Period: 1 to 2 hours.

Treatment: (1) The first step is the effective control of convulsions, i.e., **the symptoms treated before the disease.** The patient should be kept in a dark room, free from noise and disturbance. **Convulsions may be controlled initially with diazepam 0.1 to 0.5 mg/kg. i.v. slowly, and then phenobarbital i.v.** If these prove ineffective consider general anaesthesia and/or muscle relaxation immediately by using succinylcholine, curare, gallamine or pancuronium bromide. Inhalation anaesthetics are of little value during convulsion, because of fixation of respiratory muscles and therefore failure of absorption of vapour. **Between convulsions, ether may be administered to the point of unconsciousness. (2) Short-acting barbiturates like pentobarbital sodium, or sodium amytal are antidotes to strychnine** and should be given in dose of 0.3 to 0.6 g. i.v. (3) Wash the stomach with warm water and dilute solution of potassium permanganate, and then introduce a suspension of **activated charcoal to adsorb strychnine,** which should be removed later. Tannic acid may be used if charcoal is not available. (4) Acidifying the urine will increase excretion of strychnine. (5) Treat the symptoms on general lines.

Postmortem Appearances: They are not characteristic. Rigor mortis appears early but is not necessarily prolonged. There may be signs of asphyxia. Extravasated blood may be found in the muscles. Haemorrhages are sometimes found under the peritoneal coat of the stomach. The mucosa of the stomach and duodenum may show patches of ecchymoses or congestion. The lungs, liver, kidneys, brain and spinal cord are congested.

Physiological Test: Injection of an aqueous solution of the suspected material into the dorsal lymph sac of a frog, will produce tetanic convulsions in a few minutes if strychnine is present. Later stimulation of the frog will produce convulsions.

The Circumstances of Poisoning: (1) It is sometimes used for homicide in the form of alkaloid, or as powdered nux vomica seeds, in spite of bitter taste. (2) Suicide is rare because of the painful death. (3) Accidental deaths are more common, due to an overdose of medicinal preparation, or the poison being given by mistake, or in children by eating the seeds. (4) Sometimes, the seeds are used for killing the cattle, and as arrow poison. (5) Sometimes, it is taken as an aphrodisiac.

PERIPHERAL NERVE POISONS

CURARE: This is found in various species of strychnos. Curarine is the active principle. Its action is entirely peripheral and at the myoneural junction, and blocks the postsynaptic nicotinic acetylcholine receptors in muscles, thus causing a flaccid paralysis of skeletal muscles. It is used in the production of muscular relaxation in patients who are lightly anaesthetised. It is not poisonous when swallowed. It is absorbed through wounds or abrasions. It is used as arrow poison.

SIGNS AND SYMPTOMS: It causes gradual paralysis of limbs followed by paralysis of respiratory muscles, and death from asphyxia. There is headache, vertigo, mydriasis, blurred vision and hypotension due to the liberated histamine. The mental faculties are clear till the end. In large dose, there is a definite central action on the nervous system, which may produce a short phase of excitation with muscular movements and even convulsions, followed by depression with loss of consciousness and respiratory failure.

FATAL DOSE: 60 mg.

FATAL PERIOD: 1 to 2 hours.

TREATMENT: Atropine 0.6 to 1.2 mg. followed by neostigmine 5 to 10 mg. i.v. should be given. Physostigmine 3 ml. of 1: 200 solution i.v. is useful. Artificial respiration should be started.

POSTMORTEM APPEARANCES are those of asphyxia. Most deaths are from its use in anaesthesia. It is used as arrow poison.

CONIUM MACULATUM (HEMLOCK)

The plant (Vish Jeera) contains coniine and seven other alkaloids. Coniine content is highest in the unripe fruit and in the seeds, in the leaves especially at flowering time and in the root particularly during the summer. Hemlock was administered to Socrates, the Greek Philosopher in 399 B.C. as a form of execution.

FATAL DOSE: 60 mg of coniine.

SIGNS AND SYMPTOMS: The fresh leaves have a nauseating taste and unpleasant mousy odour. The odour of the dried leaves is strong and narcotic. Ingestion causes burning in mouth and throat, gastric inflammation, vomiting, diarrhoea, slow respiration, increased and later slow pulse, mental confusion, tremors, ataxia, sometimes blindness, progressive motor paralysis extending upwards from the extremities, coma and death from respiratory paralysis.

CHAPTER

35 CARDIAC POISONS

NICOTIANA TABACUM

All parts are poisonous except the ripe seeds. The dried leaves (*tobacco, tambaku*) contain 1 to 8% of nicotine and are used in the form of smoke or snuff or chewed. The leaves contain active principles, which are the toxic alkaloids nicotine and anabasine (which are equally toxic); nornicotine (less toxic). Nicotine is a colourless, volatile, bitter, hygroscopic liquid alkaloid. It is used extensively in agricultural and horticultural work, for fumigating and spraying, as insecticides, worm powders, etc.

ABSORPTION AND EXCRETION: Each cigarette contains about 15 to 20 mg. of nicotine of which 1 to 2 mg. is absorbed by smoking; each cigar contains 15 to 40 mg. Nicotine is rapidly absorbed from all mucous membranes, lungs and the skin. 80 to 90 percent is metabolised by the liver, but some may be metabolised in the kidneys and the lungs. It is excreted by the kidneys.

ACTION: It acts on the autonomic ganglia which are stimulated initially, but are depressed and blocked at later stage. It also acts on the somatic neuromuscular junction, and afferent fibres from sensory receptors.

ACUTE POISONING: G.I.T. Burning acid sensation, nausea, vomiting, abdominal pain, hypersalivation. CARDIOPULMONARY: Tachycardia, hypertension, tachypnoea (early); bradycardia, hypotension, respiratory depression (late). Cardiac arrhythmias may occur. C.N.S.: Miosis, confusion, headache, sweating, ataxia, agitation, restlessness, hyperthermia (early); mydriasis, lethargy, convulsions, coma (late). Death may occur from respiratory failure.

CHRONIC POISONING: Symptoms are cough, wheezing, dyspnoea, anorexia, vomiting, diarrhoea, anaemia, faintness, tremors, impaired memory, amblyopia, blindness, irregularity of the heart with extrasystoles and occasionally attacks of pain suggesting angina pectoris.

WITHDRAWAL SYMPTOMS: Intense urge to smoke, anxiety, impaired concentration and memory, depression or hostility, headache, muscle cramps, sleep disturbances, increased appetite and weight gain, diaphoresis and rapid respirations. A short period (6 to 12 weeks) of maintenance often followed by a gradual reduction in 6 to 12 weeks is adopted.

Nicotine replacement therapy (NRT) includes use of nicotine products including gum, transdermal patch, nasal spray, lozenge and inhaler. Bupropion can be used in those who are motivated to quit. Clonidine and nortryptyline can be used as second line of treatment.

FATAL DOSE: 50 to 100 mg. of nicotine. It rivals cyanide as a poison capable of producing rapid death; 15 to 30 g. of crude tobacco.

FATAL PERIOD: 5 to 15 minutes.

TREATMENT: (1) Wash the stomach with warm water containing charcoal, tannin or potassium permanganate. (2) A purge and colonic wash-out. (3) Mecamylamine (Inversine) is a specific antidote given orally. (4) Protect airway. In mild to moderate poisoning, atropine sulphate 1 to 2 mg. i.m. and hexamethonium chloride 25 to 50 mg. s.c. to counteract peripheral autonomic disturbances and as respiratory stimulant. (5) Vasodilators can be given. (6) Oxygen. (7) Symptomatic.

THE CIRCUMSTANCES OF POISONING: (1) Accidental poisoning results due to ingestion, excessive smoking and application of leaves or juice to wound or skin. (2) For malingering tobacco leaves are soaked in water for some hours and placed in axillae at bed time, which is held in position by a bandage. Poisonous symptoms are seen the next morning. (3) Suicidal and homicidal poisoning is rare.

DIGITALIS PURPUREA

Entire plant is toxic, containing over thirty cardiac and steroidal glucosides Fig. (35–1). The root, leaves and seeds of digitalis contain digitoxin, digoxin, digitalin and digitonin (glycosides).

SIGNS AND SYMPTOMS: GIT: Anorexia, nausea, vomiting, diarrhoea. CARDIAC: Arrhythmias: extrasystoles, ventricular tachycardia and fibrillation, atrial flutter and fibrillation, SA block, AV block. ENDOCRINE: Gynaecomastia. VISUAL: Transient amblyopia, photophobia, diplopia, blurring, scotomata, colour aberration, halos. SKIN: Urticaria. CNS: Headache, fatigue, muscle weakness, neuropsychiatric disorders, confusion, anxiety, depression, disorientation, drowsiness, delirium, hallucinations, trigeminal neuralgia. Death occurs from cardiovascular collapse.

FATAL DOSE: 15 to 30 mg. of digitalin: 4 mg. of digitoxin; digoxin 10 mg; leaf: 2 g.

FATAL PERIOD: 1 to 24 hours.

TREATMENT: (1) Stomach wash with a solution of tannic acid. (2) The bowels should be evacuated. (3) Activated charcoal in repeated

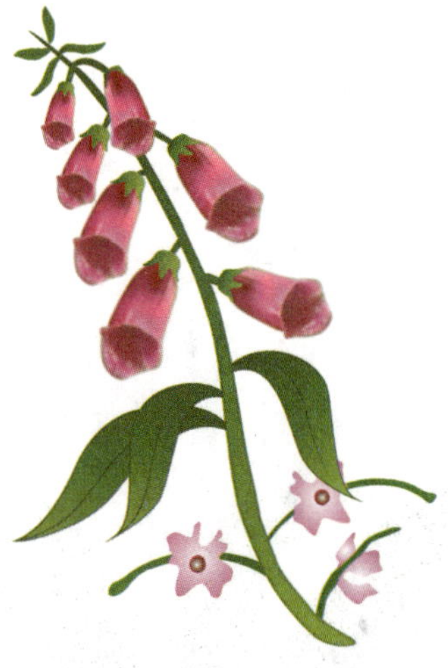

Fig. (35–1). Digitalis purpurea.

doses. (4) Digoxin-specific antibody fragments (Fab) one vial i.v. in 30 minutes. Each vial, contains 38 mg Fab fragments. Total 10 to 20 vials. (5) In the absence of Fab fragments, ventricular irritability can be treated with phenytoin 50 mg/min. i.v. up to 1 g, followed by 300 to 400 mg. daily. Specific antidote for digitalis induced cardiac arrhythmias are: 100 mg. lignocaine i.v. or dilantin or propranolol. (6) Trisodium EDTA may help to lower the serum calcium. (7) Potassium salts to reduce extrasystoles and tachyarrhythmias. (8) Bradycardia should be treated with atropine sulphate 0.6 mg. i.v. repeated as necessary up to four days. (9) Symptomatic.

Poisoning is accidental, due to therapeutic overdose.

NERIUM ODORUM

Characteristics: Nerium odorum *(white oleander, kaner)* **grows wild in India. Flowers usually fragrant, are borne in terminal clusters. They are white, pink, dark-red or rarely pale-yellow. They are two-and-half to five cm. wide and have five petals or in double blooms, many petals. The leaves are narrow, lanceolate, leathery, dark-green on upper surface, lighter beneath, and 10 to 25 cm. long. Seed pod is slim, cylindrical, ribbed, up to 15 cm. long, turns brown, dries and splits, releasing small seeds tipped with brown hairs Fig. (35–2).**

Active Principles: All parts of the plant, including nectar are poisonous, containing several cardiac glycosides, primarily **oleandroside (oleandrin), and nerioside (nerin),** which resemble digitalis in action and **folinerin and rosagenin.** The nector yields poisonous honey.

Signs and Symptoms: The plant is occasionally a source of contact dermatitis. Emanations from flowers, especially when fading cause headache, dizziness, respiratory difficulty and nausea. Ingestion causes difficulty in swallowing and articulation, abdominal pain, vomiting, profuse frothy salivation and diarrhoea. Pulse is first slow and later rapid and weak, blood pressure falls, fibrillation, AV block, respirations are increased, pupils are dilated, muscular twitchings, tetanic spasms, lock-jaw, drowsiness, coma, respiratory paralysis and death occurs. Death usually results from cardiac failure.

Fatal Dose: 15 to 20 g. of the root; 5 to 15 leaves. 8 to 10 seeds.

Fatal Period: 20 to 36 hours.

Treatment: (1) Stomach wash. Activated charcoal. (2) Digoxin immune Fab.

Postmortem Appearances: They are not characteristic. Congestion of organs is seen. It can be detected long after death.

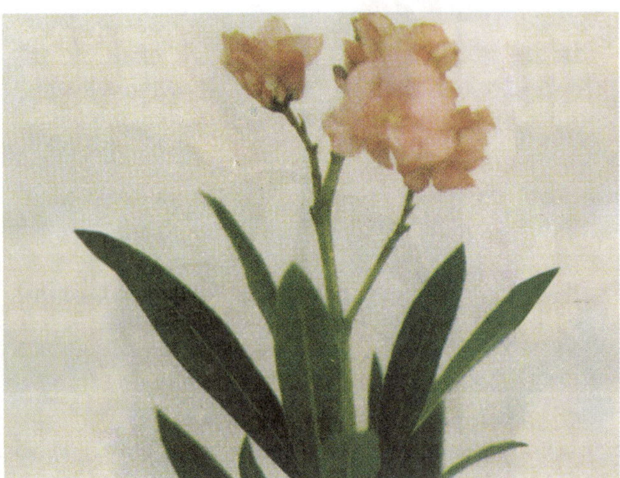

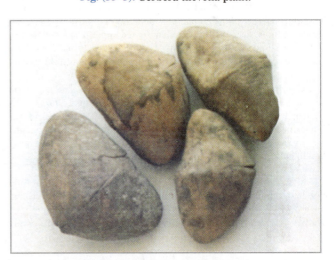

Fig. (35–2). Nerium odorum.

The Circumstances of Poisoning: (1) The root, leaves or fruit are often used as a paste or decoction for suicidal purposes. (2) Homicide is rare. (3) As an abortifacient, root is used either locally or taken internally. (4) Root is taken internally for treating venereal diseases. (5) Root is used for treating cancers and ulcers in the form of paste. (6) The decoction of leaves is applied externally to reduce swelling. (7) As a cattle poison, the juice of root is applied on piece of cloth and inserted into the anus of the animal. (8) **Smoke from the burning plant is toxic. When plant material is used to roast food over a fire, the poisonous sap transferred to the food may be lethal.**

CERBERA THEVETIA

CHARACTERISTICS: All parts of cerbera thevetia (yellow oleander; *pila kaner)* **are poisonous. The flowers are large, bell-shaped and yellow, 5 to 7 cm. long and five cm. wide, the five lobes spirally twisted and spreading, and the leaves are lanceolate. The fruit is globular, light-green, about 4 to 5 cm. in diameter and contains a single nut which is triangular with a deep groove along the edge. Each nut contains five pale yellow seeds Figs. (35–3 and 35–4).**

Active Principles: The seeds contain 4% of the cardiac glycoside **thevetin,** which is one-eighth as potent as **ouabain** and similar to digitalis in action; **thevetoxin** is similar to but less toxic than thevetin; nerifolin (more potent than thevetin); **peruvoside,**

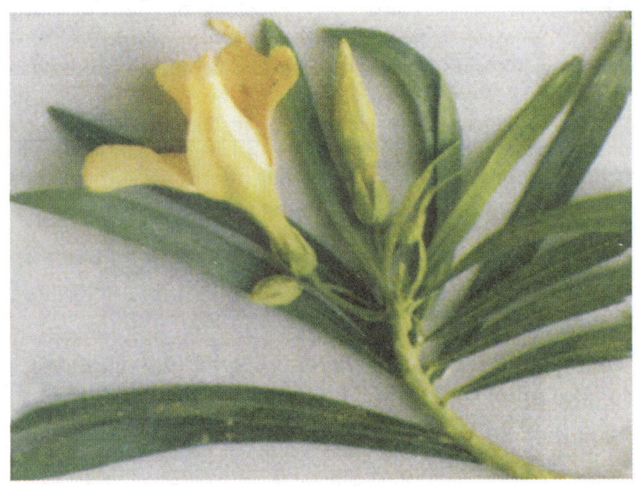

Fig. (35–3). Cerbera thevetia plant.

Fig. (35–4). Cerbera thevetia seeds.

and ruvoside, cerberin and also a bitter principle that acts on the CNS, and produces tetanoid convulsions. All active principles are glycosides. Milky juice exudes from all parts of the plant.

Signs and Symptoms: The sap of the plant may cause inflammation in sensitive individuals. Chewing the bark or seed kernel causes a slight numbing sensation and feeling of heat in the mouth and purging. Ingestion causes burning pain in the mouth, dryness of throat, tingling and numbness of tongue, vomiting, diarrhoea, headache, giddiness, dilated pupils, loss of muscular power and fainting. Pulse is rapid, weak and irregular, blood pressure low. Heart block, collapse and death from peripheral circulatory failure occurs.

Fatal Dose: 8 to 10 seeds; 15 to 20 g. of root; 5 to 10 leaves.

Fatal Period: 2 to 3 hours.

Treatment: (1) Wash out the stomach. (2) Digoxin immune Fab (ovine) is effective in poisoning from digitalis, cerbera thevetia, cerbera odallam, nerium odorum, etc. Each vial contains 38 mg Fab which should be dissolved in 4 ml of sterile water and given i.v. 10 to 20 vials can be given through a membrane filter i.v. in acute poisoning. Sodium molar lactate transfusion with glucose and 1 mg. atropine, 2 ml. adrenaline and 2 mg. noradrenaline is beneficial. (3) Symptomatic.

Postmortem Appearances: They are not specific.

The Circumstances of Poisoning: (1) The root and seeds are used sometimes for suicide or homicide. (2) Root and seeds are taken for criminal abortion. (3) For cattle poisoning, the seeds are crushed and fed to the animal with corn or bread.

CERBERA ODALLAM *(Pilikirbir)*

CHARACTERISTICS: This plant is closely allied botanically to cerbera thevetia. It is a small plant or a shrub that grows wild all over India. The leaves are dark-green, fleshy and lanceolate, 20 to 30 cm. long, and 4 to 6 cm. broad. The flowers are white, like those of jasmine. The fruit resembles a mango, is globular and dark-green and has a thick fibrous mesocarp which encloses usually a single seed. The seed is flattened and ovoid and contains two kernels which are pearly-white but when dry it may have a bluish tinge or it may become gelatinous. Milky acrid juice (toxic) exudes from all parts of the plant. The active principles are cerberin, cerberoside, odollin, odolotoxin, thevetin and cerapain (glycosides) Fig. (35–5).

Signs and Symptoms: They appear within one hour. The initial symptoms are gastrointestinal. Cardiac toxicity may occur within three hours of ingestion. There is bitter taste, nausea, severe retching, vomiting, abdominal pain and in few cases diarrhoea, general weakness, blurring of vision, sinus bradycardia, irregular respiration, collapse and death from heart failure. ECG may show sinus bradycardia, S-A block, atrial fibrillation and other arrhythmias. Hyperkalaemia and depression of transaminase activity are chief biochemical changes.

Fatal Dose: Kernel of one fruit.

Fatal Period: 1 to 2 days or more.

POSTMORTEM APPEARANCES: They are those of asphyxia. Eyes are congested. Lungs are congested and oedematous. Subepicardial, subendocardial and subpleural petechial haemorrhages are found. Stomach mucosa is congested with submucous haemorrhages and gastritis. The internal organs are congested.

Treatment: (1) Stomach wash. (2) Digoxin immune Fab is the specific antidote. Atropine 0.5 mg. i.v. and repeated every 15 to 30 minutes to keep heart rate above 50 per minute. (3) Correct hyperkalaemia.

Circumstances of Poisoning: (1) For suicide, the kernels are taken as such, or after grinding it with jaggery or molasses or by preparing a curry with it. (2) For homicide, the powdered kernel is added to alcohol. (3) Bark, leaves and milky juice are used as emetic and as purgative.

ACONITE

There are several varieties of aconite (monk's hood, blue rocket, *meetha zeher, bish, bikh*), but the roots of Aconitum napellus and Aconitum ferox are commonly used. It grows in the Himalayas. All varieties and all parts of the plant are poisonous; least when young, more so when seeds ripen and most when bloom.

Active Principles: The root and seeds are most potent; contain aconitine and ten or more other alkaloids, such as pseudo-aconitine, indaconitine, bikhaconitine, picraconitine, aconine, mesaconitine, jesaconitine, etc. Aconitine stimulates and then depresses CNS.

Dried roots: The dry root is conical or tapering, and shows scars or bases of broken rootlets, and is arched or shrivelled with longitudinal wrinkles Fig. (35–6). It is usually 5 to 10 cm. long, and 1½ to 2 cm. thick at the upper end. The external colour is dark-brown, and when freshly cut the internal colour is white,

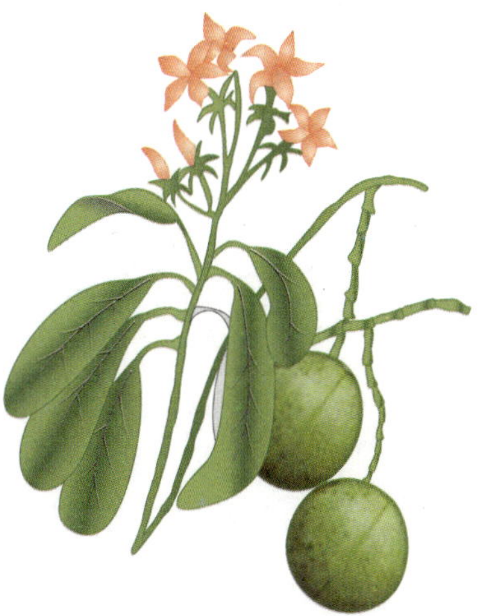

Fig. (35–5). Cerbera odallam.

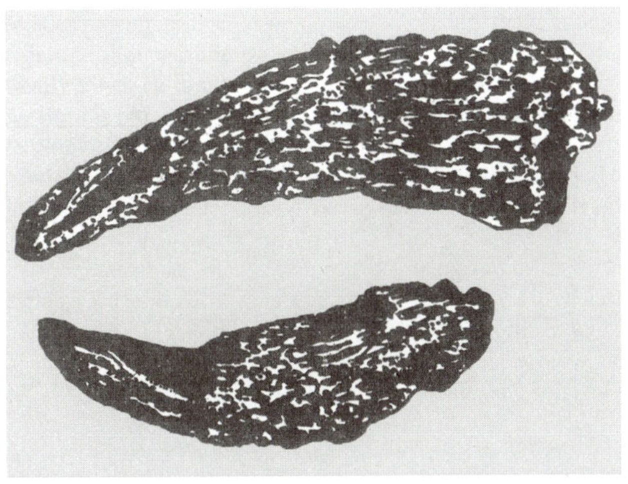

Fig. (35–6). Dried roots of Aconitum napellus.

which becomes pink on exposure to air. It is odourless but the taste is sweet, then acrid. When dried and soaked in oil the root is black, heavy, hard and brittle with a strong offensive odour. The root is mistaken for horse-radish root which is long, cylindrical, yellowish-white externally and whitish internally, does not change on exposure to air and the taste is pungent.

Action: It first simulates sensory nerves. The motor ganglia of heart are paralysed and respiratory centre is slowed.

Signs and Symptoms: **Leaves handled or rubbed on the skin, produce tingling and numbness; so also the root if held for a long time in the hand.** The odour of the plant has a narcotic effect. The pollen causes pain and swelling in the eyes. The symptoms occur immediately or within a few minutes. There is a burning sensation from the mouth to the stomach and **tingling and numbness in the mouth, tongue and pharynx.** This is followed by salivation, nausea, vomiting and diarrhoea. Later the mouth is dry and patient suffers from thirst and is unable to swallow. **Tingling and numbness are then felt all over the body.** There is headache, giddiness, pallor, profuse sweating, subnormal temperature, **the limbs become weak and the patient is unable to walk or stand.** Paraesthesias, ataxia and slurred speech occur. There may be twitching of the muscles with darting pains, and cramps and convulsions may occur. **The pupils alternately contract and dilate (hippus), but remain dilated in the later stages. The vision becomes dim and there may be diplopia.** Hypotension, cardiac arrhythmia with AV block occurs. At first there is tachycardia, but in later stages bradycardia occurs due to AV block. The mind usually remains clear, although there may be hallucinations. There is marked general muscular weakness, oppression in the chest, and **death occurs from paralysis of heart or respiratory centres or both.**

It is eliminated by all routes but mainly in the urine.

Fatal Dose: One g. root; 2 to 5 mg. of aconitine; 250 mg. extract; 10 to 30 ml. tincture.

Fatal Period: Two to six hours.

Treatment: (1) Gastric lavage with warm water, and weak solution of iodine in potassium iodide or tannic acid to precipitate alkaloid, or animal charcoal. **(2) Multiple-dose activated charcoal.** (3) Cathartic. (4) **Atropine** half to one mg. is useful. (5) Symptomatic.

Postmortem Appearances: They are not characteristic, but are **those of asphyxia.** The mucosa of the stomach and duodenum show congestion and occasionally ecchymosis. The lungs, kidneys and brain are congested. Aconitine is extremely unstable and is destroyed by putrefaction.

The Circumstances of Poisoning: (1) Accidental poisoning is due to eating the roots in mistake for horseradish root, by the use of quack remedies containing it, or from taking liquor to which aconite is added to increase intoxication. (2) Suicidal cases often occur. (3) It is given with betel leaf to conceal its taste for homicide. (4) Root is used as an abortifacient. (5) Cattle poison. (6) Arrow poison.

CHAPTER

36 ASPHYXIANTS

FM 9.6: Describe general principles and basic methodologies in treatment of poisoning: decontamination, supportive therapy, antidote therapy, procedures of enhanced elimination with regard to ammonia, carbon monoxide, hydrogen cyanide and derivatives, methyl isocyanate, tear (riot control) gases.

CLASSIFICATION: Henderson and Haggard divided noxious gases into five groups.

(1) IRRITANTS: The gases injure the air passages or lungs or both, and produce inflammatory changes. They are smoke, tear gases, ammonia, formaldehyde, chlorine, phosgene, nitrogen dioxide, sulphur dioxide.

(2) CHEMICAL ASPHYXIANTS: These are gases which by combining with haemoglobin, or by acting on some tissue constituent prevent oxygen from reaching tissue or the tissues from using it. The examples are carbon monoxide, hydrogen sulphide, arsine, carbon disulphide, and cyanide.

(3) SIMPLE ASPHYXIANTS: These are inert gases, which when breathed in high concentration act mechanically by excluding oxygen. They are carbon dioxide, methane, helium, nitrogen and nitrous oxide. Symptoms appear when these gases exceed 20 to 30% of inspired air. When the inspired air contains less than 10% oxygen death may result from slight exertion.

(4) VOLATILE DRUGS: These are gases with little or no irritant effect upon the air-passages, which act after absorption into the blood, either as an anaesthetic, or as agents toxic to the liver, kidneys or other organs including the nervous system. They are aliphatic hydrocarbons, halogenated hydrocarbons and aromatic hydrocarbons.

(5) SYSTEMIC POISONS: These are insecticides, arsine, stibine.

CARBON MONOXIDE

Features: It is a **colourless, tasteless, non-irritative gas which is produced due to incomplete combustion of carbon.** It is insoluble in water. It burns with a blue flame producing CO_2. **It is lighter than** air and significant quantities are present only in the upper reaches in the vicinity of a fire.

In a closed environment, greater concentration is present at 1.5 to 2 metres above the ground. CO seeps through openings around doors or large cracks in walls. It may also rise through a ceiling crack into an attic or from a tight confined space, through plaster board or dry wall, into an adjacent area. In this way it may spread through an entire house and even upstair rooms. A mixture of CO with 2½ times of its volume of air is highly explosive in the presence of a flame.

SOURCES: The common sources of CO include coal gas, smoke from fires and the fumes from defective heating appliances, e.g., furnace, stove, water heater, fire places, burning oil lamps. A yellow flame generates CO, while a blue flame burns completely with no byproducts. It is also found as a component of the fumes of coke kilns, lime kilns, explosion in mines (after damp), choke damp (improperly ventilated collieries at the dead ends), detonation of explosives, and the exhaust fumes of internal combustion engines. Industry accounts for about 20%. In a person smoking one pack of cigarettes per day, CO levels are about 5 to 6% and in a heavy smoker 15 to 20%. Traffic policemen may have up to 10% saturation. The exhaust gas of motor cars contain 1 to 7% of CO, which causes the air of a small garage poisonous in 5 to 10 minutes. "Petrol (gasoline) engines produce up to 5–7% CO in their exhaust fumes and more if engine is idling". Emissions like CO, HC, and smoke opacity depend on both fuel and engine type. Gasoline and CNG engines have 15 to 20 times higher CO emissions as compared to diesel engines.

During haemoglobin catabolism 0.4 to 0.7% COHb is produced in the body endogenously. In haemolytic anaemia, COHb levels may reach 8%. In females CO is twice as great during the progesterone phase of the menstrual cycle as during the oestrogen phase.

Action: CO is readily absorbed across the alveolus and combines with haemoglobin. Normal blood contains 21% of oxygen, with 18 to 19% bound to haemoglobin and 2% dissolved in plasma. About 10 to 21% CO is present in extracellular tissues combined with myoglobin and haemoproteins. **CO affinity to myoglobin is about 40 times greater than oxygen, which may cause direct myocardial depression. CO has 200 to 300 times greater affinity for haemoglobin than that of oxygen. It displaces oxygen from its combination with haemoglobin and forms a relatively stable compound known as carboxyhaemoglobin.** It thus reduces the oxygen content of the blood, and hence that of the tissues. **It acts as a chemical asphyxiant and produces death due to anaemic anoxia.** CO is a potent cellular toxin. It effectively and firmly binds to haemoglobin and myoglobin. **It inhibits the electron transport by blocking cytochrome A_3 oxidase and cytochrome P–450, and therefore intracellular respiration.** It interferes with other ferroproteins such as myoglobin and various enzymes. The presence of COHb in the circulation alters the oxygen affinity of the haemoglobin by shifting oxyhaemoglobin dissociation curve to the left, decreasing the release of oxygen to the tissues. This results in a hypoxia of the tissue greater than what would be produced by an equivalent degree of anaemia. **Normally, after somatic death, the cells near the capillaries continue to function, extract oxygen from oxyhaemoglobin and cause blue staining.** In CO poisoning this cannot occur, because the cells cannot break the COHb compound. Potent cellular poisons, e.g., cyanide, fluoroacetate and freezing, block the metabolism of the cells so fast and completely that they cannot extract oxygen from oxyhaemoglobin. In these cases, the blood under the skin and in the tissues will be cherry-red due to oxyhaemoglobin. Platelet aggregation is inhibited.

ELIMINATION: It is eliminated through lungs; about 1% is metabolised to CO_2. Half-life of CO in a healthy adult breathing 21% oxygen (room air) is 4 to 5 hours. It is not metabolised and is not lost through the skin, bile, perspiration, urine or faeces. CO is not absorbed by a body after death.

Signs and Symptoms: The brain and heart extract the greatest percentage of oxygen, 6.1 and 11 vol%. Therefore, these organs are the earliest and most greatly affected by a reduction in oxygen delivery. **The symptoms of poisoning are often mistaken for symptoms of influenza or illness caused by eating contaminated food.** The development of symptoms has a progression, roughly parallel to the rise in the saturation of the blood by CO Table (36–1). Similarly, regression of symptoms corresponds with the clearance of CO from the blood. **Victims may not notice anything, except a headache, until they lapse into coma and die. The effects of CO are simply those of suboxia.** As most deaths are relatively rapid, **blisters are rare**. Bullae tend to be separate and isolated lesions. The bullous fluid is usually thick and cellular and there is often an inflammatory reaction in the surrounding skin. These bullae are localised by external pressure and are seen in the regions of the calves, buttocks, wrists and knees. They are caused due to skin hypoxia which can be mistaken for second degree burns. They rarely involve fingers and toes. **There is a tendency of the dying victim to wild, erratic swinging movements inside the room, disturbing clothing and furniture which gives an impression of violent struggle (CO automatism).** The saturation required to cause death varies with the age and health of the person. **Death usually occurs when eighty percent of haemoglobin is saturated with CO.** Senility, any disease or the co-existence of any respiratory or circulatory deficiency, or of anaemia or in association with hypnotic drugs and alcohol result in a significant reduction of maximum lethal saturation, and death can occur from as little as thirty percent saturation. **CO can pass from the maternal to the foetal blood, and COHb concentrations are 10 to 15% higher than maternal levels, and can produce intrauterine death, even though the mother survives.** The rate of CO combining with haemoglobin depends on the atmospheric concentration and rate of respiratory exchange. **Physical activity during exposure increases rate of saturation of blood. Children saturate their blood more rapidly than adults** because of their relatively high rates of respiratory exchange. Patients recovering from CO poisoning may suffer neurological sequelae including tremors, personality changes, memory impairment, monoplegia, hemiplegia, psychosis, peripheral neuropathy, visual loss, inability to concentrate and Parkinsonism within 2 to 4 weeks. These effects may be temporary or permanent. Complete recovery after serious poisoning may take many weeks. Sometimes, people become ill again up to 4 weeks after recovery.

Table (36–1). Symptoms of CO poisoning

COHb%	Symptoms
0–10	No appreciable symptoms.
10–20	Breathlessness on moderate exertion, mild headache, weakness.
20–30	Throbbing headache, irritability, emotional instability, disturbed judgement, defective memory and rapid fatigue.
30–40	Severe headache, nausea, vomiting, dizziness, dimness of vision, confusion. cherry-red colour.
40–50	Increasing confusion, sometimes hallucinations, severe ataxia, rapid respirations and collapse with attempts at exertion. Symptoms resemble alcoholic intoxication.
50–60	Syncope or coma with intermittent convulsions, rapid respirations, tachycardia with a weak pulse and pink or red discolouration of the skin.
60–70	Increasing depth of coma with incontinence of urine and faeces.
70–80	Profound coma with depressed or absent reflexes, a weak thready pulse, shallow and irregular respirations and death.
> 80	Rapid death from respiratory arrest.

Chronic Poisoning: Symptoms include headache, confusion, weakness, paraesthesias, visual disturbances, hypertension, hyperthermia, palpitations, atrial fibrillation, bundle branch blocks, AV block, abnormal left ventricular function, decreased cognitive ability, mental retardation, psychosis, Parkinsonism and incontinence.

Delayed Deaths: Coma is accompanied by degenerative changes in brain and capillaries. **Individuals with long term survival following significant exposure may have a Parkinsonian syndrome** or may develop even neurological states.

The Effect of Different Air Concentrations of CO Table (36–1): Humidity, high environmental temperature, and physical activity increase the respiratory rate and thus, the absorption of CO. **The upper limit of safety is 0.01% CO in air. If a person breathes CO in low concentration for a considerable length of time, especially during sleep, he will be poisoned just as effectively as though he were exposed to a high concentration for a shorter period. When low concentrations of gas are inhaled, coma does not occur immediately, but often cause severe muscular incoordination, weakness and confusion, due to which the victim is unable to escape and dies of asphyxia, the body being burnt after death.** A concentration of 0.5 to 1% of CO in the atmosphere can produce carboxyhaemoglobin saturation levels of 75% in 2 to 15 minutes. Exposure to atmosphere containing 0.2% of gas will cause death in about four hours, 0.4% in one hour, and 10% in 20 to 30 minutes. If production of CO ceases after the onset of irreversible coma, individual will gradually eliminate CO from the body, even through irreversible injury has occurred. In such cases, low carboxyhaemoglobin will be seen.

Treatment: (1) Remove the patient to fresh air immediately. If he is conscious and breathing, no treatment is required. (2) Any patient with COHb level greater than 25% should be treated. (3) The most widely accepted treatment is **100% oxygen provided**

by a tight-fitting mask **preferably with rubber seals and endotracheal intubation for patients with a depressed mental status, until COHb falls to 15 to 20%.** (4) CO_2 should not be given. (5) **Hyperbaric oxygen (HBO) therapy has several disadvantages,** such as vomiting, convulsions, agitation, rupture of tympanic membranes, blocked sinuses, etc. (6) Gastric lavage early in the course of treatment may prevent aspiration pneumonitis. (7) A whole blood transfusion is useful. (8) The patient should be kept at complete rest for at least 48 hours. (9) Avoid stimulant drugs. (10) Give antibiotics as a prophylaxis against lung infection. (11) Cerebral oedema should be treated with fluid restriction, steroids, and mannitol.

Postmortem Appearances: **A cherry-red colouration of the skin, mucous membranes, conjunctivae, nail-beds, areas of hypostasis, blood, tissues and internal organs is seen in 15 to 20% of cases only. It is associated with 30 to 40% COHb.** In an anaemic person, the colour may be faint or absent. In dark-coloured victims, the colour may be masked, but may be seen in the inner aspect of lips, nail-beds, tongue, palms and soles, inside the eyelids, but rarely in the sclera. The colour will not be changed by embalming or preservation by formalin. Cyanide poisoning and exposure of the dead body to the cold may cause redness similar to that due to CO. The cherry-red discolouration changes to dark-green, then to brown with the onset of decomposition. **The blood is fluid, hyperaemia is general and serous effusions are common. There may be blistering of the skin of dependent areas, such as buttocks, calves, wrists and knees, due to cutaneous oedema.** Congestion of the lungs with pink fluid blood, and if the victim survived for some time, pulmonary oedema with congestion are found. The lungs may show bronchopneumonic consolidation. In delayed deaths, tiny focal necroses occur in the myocardium. Frank myocardial infarction has been reported after severe exposure and relative hypoxia, usually in the presence of pre-existing coronary disease. Within five days histological changes occur here. Pleural and pericardial anoxial haemorrhages are common. **In persons surviving after severe CO exposure and in delayed deaths bilateral, symmetrical necrosis and cavitation of the basal ganglia in the brain, especially the putamen and globus pallidus is the most characteristic lesion,** though the cerebral cortex, hipppocampus, cerebellum and substantia nigra of brainstem may be affected. **Punctiform and ring-shaped haemorrhages in the white matter of the brain with widespread oedema are common.** Haemorrhages in the meninges and cortex, and selective cellular necrobiosis of ganglion cells in the cortex may be seen.

After death, small quantities of CO are produced due to decomposition of haemoglobin and myoglobin.

The Circumstances of Poisoning: (1) **In India, suicide by CO is very rare.** The person may be seated in his car with a tube leading from the exhaust into the passenger compartment or he may lie on the floor of the garage near the exhaust pipe, with doors and windows closed. (2) Accidental deaths may be caused by use of flueless braziers, exposure to exhaust gas of petrol engines, exposure to gas in mines following underground fires or explosions, and exposure to gas during fires. Accidents may occur in connection with incomplete combustion of wood, charcoal or coal in ill-ventilated room. (3) Homicide is uncommon, unless the victims are adults incapacitated by drink, drugs, disease or infirmity, or they are children.

COLLECTION OF BLOOD: If vapour or gas intoxication is suspected as the cause of death, ten ml. of heart blood should be collected prior to autopsy. CO-blood has very little tendency to clot. The cells tend to separate from the plasma in the blood vessels and organs of the body. Since CO is contained in the cells, care should be taken in removing the sample of blood. If the blood is taken from the heart, this may be done by filling the syringe and flushing it back into the heart, then refilling to take the sample. Fluoride should be added as preservative. It should be placed in a tightly sealed gas-tight container. The blood need not be kept under a layer (2 to 3 mm. thick) of liquid paraffin because the carboxyhaemoglobin molecule is extremely stable. If sufficient blood cannot be obtained from the heart or major vessels, the spleen or muscle should be sent for analysis. Pieces of lungs should also be placed in suitable container tightly sealed and refrigerated. In a badly burnt body CO can be detected in any sanguineous body fluid or bone marrow.

TESTS: (1) In 15 ml. of water in a test tube, place two drops of blood suspected to contain CO and mix. Water turns pink due to COHb. With normal blood, colour is not pink. (2) Kunkel's test or tannic acid test: If tannic acid is added to blood it remains cherry-red in CO poisoning, while oxyhaemoglobin turns deep brown. (3) Hoppe-Seyler's test: Few drops of blood are added to a solution of ten percent sodium hydroxide. Normal blood turns brownish-green, but if CO is present, the colour will remain pink. (4) Spectroscopic examination of blood shows characteristic bands of carboxyhaemoglobin.

If only tissue is available, water is used to extract blood from liver, spleen, kidneys, lungs, bone marrow or other organs. CO persists for many weeks after death, and may be detected even after putrefaction or embalming and prolonged burial. It is preferable to use anticoagulants in specimens for examination.

FAILURE TO DETECT CO: In some cases of fatal CO poisoning, blood analysis may not disclose COHb. This occurs in cases where the victim is shifted to CO free atmosphere, and sufficient breathing had occurred to clear the blood of COHb. But, the poisoned victim may die because of irreversible brain damage sustained while high CO concentration persisted. It is not a product of putrefaction.

Non-dispersive infrared spectrophotometry and gas chromatography are analytical methods.

CARBON DIOXIDE

It is a heavy, colourless gas with a faintly sweet odour. Atmospheric air contains 0.033% CO_2. 21% oxygen and 70 to 80% nitrogen. Carbon dioxide is heavier than air, and therefore it settles when it accumulates in the absence of air movement. Common places which may contain CO_2 in excess include manholes, ship holds, old wells, silos and occasionally cellars.

ACTION: The gas is not toxic, but acts as a simple asphyxiant by preventing the tissue from obtaining oxygen.

SIGNS AND SYMPTOMS: The symptoms vary with concentration of the gas. 5% concentration of CO_2 in air (i.e., above the concentration in alveolar air) causes laboured breathing and mental confusion. Above 10% produces ataxia and unconsciousness. With 40% there is dyspnoea, discomfort, and muscular weakness. With 50% there is dyspnoea, a feeling of tightness in the chest, fullness in the head, ringing in the ears and loss of muscular power followed by drowsiness, unconsciousness, coma and death. 60 to 80% of CO_2 causes immediate unconsciousness with or without convulsive movements and rapid death due to some vasovagal reflex causing cardiac arrest, triggered by a chemoreceptor stimulus.

CO_2 from a well can be collected by using a bottle filled with soda-lime water and putting it inside a well.

TREATMENT: Artificial respiration and oxygen should be given freely. Cardiac stimulants are useful.

POSTMORTEM APPEARANCES: There is marked cyanosis, congestion, suffusion of the eyes, dilation of the pupils and petechial haemorrhages.

Poisoning is usually accidental.

HYDROGEN SULPHIDE (H_2S)

It is colourless, heavy, flammable gas. At exposure to low concentrations (up to 25 ppm), the odour of rotten eggs is detected. At higher concentrations (over 50 ppm), the sense of smell is rapidly paralysed. It is formed during decomposition of organic substances containing sulphur. Hydrogensulphide in combination with methane, nitrogen, hydrocarbons, ammonia and CO_2 formed in sewers is known as **SEWER GAS.** It is often found in large quantities in sewers, septic tanks, coal mines, wells, cess pools, privy vaults and tannery vats. It may also occur in glue factories and gas works, in the distillation of petroleum oil, in the manufacture of artificial silk and in other industries where sulphur compounds are used. It is heavier than air, so it gets accumulated in low lying areas and closed spaces. Normal tolerable limit is 20 ppm and levels more than 100 ppm is dangerous to life. Poisoning by this gas is almost always accidental, especially in sewer workers. It does not combine with haemoglobin but does so with methaemoglobin to form sulphmethaemoglobin. **H_2S interferes with cellular respiration by inhibiting the action of cytochrome oxidase.** A filter paper moistened with lead acetate if exposed to air causes blackening of the paper.

SIGNS AND SYMPTOMS: In great dilution, there is feeling of dullness and sleepiness, and death may occur during sleep without the victim regaining consciousness. In weak concentration, there is cough, giddiness, nausea and feeling of oppression. The breathing is laboured and heart irregular, cyanosis of the face, inflammation of conjunctivae, lachrymation and photophobia, muscular weakness and prostration. In moderate concentration, metabolic acidosis secondary to anaerobic metabolism occurs. This results in CNS, respiratory and myocardial depression. There may be delirium, convulsions or coma, and death occurs from asphyxia. If breathed in a concentration of 0.1 to 0.2%, death occurs immediately from paralysis of respiratory centre. **Its toxicity and rapidity of action are comparable to hydrocyanic acid.**

Chronic low level exposure may be associated with reduced lung function and neurophysiological abnormalities such as headache, depression and personality changes and chronic eye irritation.

Hydrogen sulphide has recently been implicated in suicides in Japan.

TREATMENT: (1) The patient must be removed into the fresh air. **(2) Artificial respiration and 100% oxygen given.** (3) Excretion of sulphide can be accelerated by the formation of sulphmethaemoglobin, which allows for the non-toxic sulphate and thiosulphates to be filtered by the kidney. **(4) Amyl nitrite inhalation and sodium nitrite infusion** in the same dose as for cyanide, will hasten the formation of sulphmethaemoglobin.

POSTMORTEM APPEARANCES: Rotten egg odour is given off. The general signs of asphyxia are present. **The colour of the blood and viscera and bronchial secretions is greenish-purple.**

SULPHUR DIOXIDE (SO_2): It is a direct respiratory irritant causing severe bronchospasm and inhibition of mucociliary transport.

Nitrous oxide is known as laughing gas.

METHANE: The decomposition of organic matter in the well during summer produces methane or marsh gas. In diffused daylight, a series of reactions take place with chlorine successively replacing four hydrogen atoms in methane to form such vapours as chloroform and carbon tetrachloride. In the presence of air and light, the chloroform derived from marsh gas is slowly transformed into carbonyl chloride, an extremely poisonous gas.

METHYL ISOCYANATE (MIC): MIC is fairly stable liquid below 27°C, but becomes gaseous at 31°C. It has a pungent, sweetish smell. It boils at 37°C. It is highly volatile and inflammable. Its vapours are denser than air. It reacts vigorously with water, alkaloids and many solvents. It is used in the manufacture of pesticides, adhesives and plastic. **It is one of the deadliest chemicals** and can kill in very small doses when ingested, inhaled or when absorbed through the skin. It has two actions: (1) the irritant action of the vapour at the biophysical level, and (2) the carbamylation action at the biochemical level. The vapour causes intense irritation of the skin, eyes and mucous membranes.

SYMPTOMS: Acute irritation of the eyes, lachrymation, blurring of vision, severe burning in the throat, chest pain and laboured breathing. Pulmonary oedema causes death. Victims who survive for five to six days experience the above symptoms and also fever, cough with expectoration often bloody, oedema leading to death. About ten percent of the victims have psychiatric symptoms, such as anxiety, depression, sleep disturbances, gas phobia, and a feeling of helplessness. The systemic effects are: liver damage, kidney damage, methaemoglobinaemia and neurological deficits. The isocyanates affect the nucleic acids and thus may be potential teratogenic or mutagenic agents. In females, excessive vaginal discharge, anaemia, stillbirth and foetal abnormalities are seen.

AUTOPSY: Marked pulmonary oedema, increased weight of lungs to two to three times of normal, congestion of organs and effects of severe irritation of the eyes (whitening), nose, trachea and bronchi is seen in deaths occurring within two days. Victims dying between two to four days have pink blood, and those who die 5 days after the accident have dark-red blood, markedly congested organs and toxic necrosis of the gastrointestinal mucosa. Later deaths show parenchymatous degeneration of brain, heart, lung, liver and kidneys.

TREATMENT is purely symptomatic. Sodium thiosulphate is beneficial.

WAR GASES

The term "war gases" includes any chemical (gaseous, liquid or solid) which is used to produce destruction or damage mostly in times of war.

(1) Vesicant or Blistering Gases: These are mainly sulphur, mustard, phosgene, oximes and lewisite (arsenic), which are volatile liquids which continue to give of vapours for days or even weeks. They are discharged in artillery shells so as to saturate the area of attack. Mustard gas causes irritation of the eyes, nose, throat and respiratory passages, skin erythema, blisters, nausea, vomiting and abdominal pain. Bleeding and blistering within the respiratory system, mucous membrane damage and pulmonary oedema are seen. It passes through the clothes into the skin and produces intense itching, redness, vesication, and ulceration especially of the moist areas.

Treatment: (1) Wash the affected parts thoroughly. (2) Eye wash with sodium bicarbonate solution. (3) B.A.L. (4) Bleaching power in the form of a jelly or 0.5% hypochlorite solution rapidly neutralizes mustard gas lewisite. (5) N-acetylcysteine reduces inflammatory response in mustard exposure. (6) Povidone iodine ointment applied within 20 minutes of exposure to mustard liquid protects the skin from vesication. (7) Respirators protect the face and respiratory tract.

(2) Asphyxiants or Lung Irritants: These are chlorine and phosgene which are gases, and can be released from tanks, and gas shells. **Chloropicrin and diphosgene are liquids which are used in gas shells.** Phosgene is ten times and chloropicrin four times more toxic than chlorine. Nitrous oxide, sulphur dioxide, ammonia (choking gases), produce chest tightness and pulmonary oedema. Arsine, cyanogen chloride and hydrogen cyanide are also used. Their action is mainly on the pulmonary alveoli. When inhaled, they cause watering of the eyes, coughing, dyspnoea, tightness of chest, headache, vomiting, restlessness, stertorous breathing, cyanosis and collapse. Death occurs in 24 to 48 hours due to acute pulmonary oedema.

Treatment: (1) Eye wash with boric acid. (2) Oxygen and adrenaline. (3) Anti-tussives. (4) Antibiotics.

(3) Lachrymators or Tear Gases: These are mainly chloracetophenone (C.A.P.) which is solid and ethyliodoacetate (K.S.K.), and bromobenzyl cyanide (B.B.C.) which are liquids.

Other chemicals used are xylyl bromide, 2 chloroacetophenone (CAP/CN) and dibenzoxazepine (CR). Orthochlorobenzylidene malononitrile, 2-chlorobenzal malononitrile (CS). About 15 types of teargases are use. CS is the most popular due to its strong effect and lack of toxicity. The liquid agents become gases at normal temperature and pressure. They are used to disperse riotous mobs. They are fired in artillery shells or pen guns. The vapours cause intense irritation of the eyes with a copious flow of tears, spasm of the eyelids and temporary blindness. They also cause irritation of air-passages. In long-continued exposure there may be nausea, vomiting and blistering of skin. The effects are transitory.

The patient should be removed to the fresh air, and the eyes washed with warm normal saline or boric acid solution. Weak sodium bicarbonate solution is applied to the affected parts of the skin. I.V. aminophylline or salbutamol inhalation.

(4) **Sternutators or Nasal Irritants**: **These are solid, organic compounds of arsenic** and are fired in artillery shells. They are diphenyl chlorarsine (D.A), diphenylaminechlorarsine (D.M), and diphenylchloroarsine (D.C). Diphenylaminechlorarsine (sickening gas) is about six times as heavy as air. It has a specific action upon the vomiting centre in the brain. The vapours cause intense pain and irritation in the nose and sinuses, sneezing, headache, salivation, nausea, vomiting, tightness in the chest and prostration. The symptoms are comparatively short in duration.

(5) **Paralysants**: **These are hydrocyanic acid, sulphuretted hydrogen and carbon monoxide.**

(6) **Nerve Gases**: The term nerve gases is incorrect. The nerve agents are esters of phosphoric acid (liquid) and are identical in their biological activity to organophosphates. **The major agents are GA (Tabun), GB (Sarin), GD (Soman) VE, VM and VX. The vapours are heavier than air, so they tend to sink into valleys, trenches and basements.** All V-agents are oily in consistency and do not degrade or wash away easily and remain on clothes and other surfaces for long periods. They are colourless and odourless volatile liquids. **They are absorbed from the lungs, gastrointestinal canal, skin or conjunctivae. They inhibit acetylcholine esterase. They are the most toxic of the known chemical agents.** Exposure to a large amount of vapour will cause loss of consciousness within seconds, followed several minutes later by convulsions. Absorption of large amounts cause severe bronchospasm, hypotension, bradycardia and cardiac arrest. Muscles become flaccid and breathing stops. Treatment is similar to organophosphates.

Signs and symptoms and treatment is same as that of organophosphates. Full body suit and respirator give protection. Their production and stock piling has been banned.

CHEMICAL WARFARE: The offensive use of non-living toxic products produced by living organisms, (e.g., toxins such as botulinum toxin, saxitoxin and chemical agents) is considered chemical warfare. The agents are chemical substances used to injure or kill enemies during war. They produce physiological changes on the human body. **Some substances are lethal, and some injure or incapacitate people.** These agents are dispersed as tiny droplets through chemical shells, spray tanks, bombs and missiles. Harmful effects are caused when the chemical is inhaled, ingested or when it comes in contact with skin or mucous membrane.

Five types of agents are popular. (1) Sarin, Soman, Tabun and VX (organophosphates). (2) Blister agents: Mustard, Lewisite. (3) Cyanides. (4) Choking agents: Phosgene. (5) Incapacitating agents: Tear gas, pepper spray.

Another group consists of ammonia, chlorine, arsine, hydrogen sulphide, sulphur dioxide, phosphine, methyl isocyanate

Extraction of DNA becomes difficult, such as chloral hydrate, sodium nitrite, cocaine and aconite.

Chemical crowd control agents: The three most commonly used agents are: (1) Orthochlorobenzylidene malanonitrile **(CS, tear gas)**, used by law-enforcement agencies and the military. (2) **CN (Mace), available in devices used for self-protection.** (3) **Oleoresin capsaicin (pepper spray, OC)** is an extract of hot peppers, consisting of capsaicin. The concentration of capsaicin is one percent in canisters sold to the public and 5 to 10% for police. It primarily affects the skin, eyes and respiratory system. Respirations become difficult. It is non-lethal.

These agents are available in varying concentrations and several vehicles, in aerosols or fumes and in particulate form with dispersal device. They are also available in grenades or canisters that can be propelled either by throwing or with a projectile device. Individual spray cans deliver a stream, spray or foam containing the agent. They are used as defensive agents to incapacitate individuals temporarily or disperse groups. They cause: **Eyes:** Burning, stinging or pain, conjunctivitis, tearing, blepharospasm, transient impairment of vision. **Nose and mouth:** Burning, stinging or pain, increased secretions. **Skin:** Burning, stinging or pain, erythema. **Airways:** Burning and irritation, increase secretions, coughing, tightness in the chest. Effects begin within seconds after exposure and usually lost in 10 to 15 minutes. Improvement is usually rapid, and people rarely seek medical attention. Death has been reported after use of CN in enclosed spaces, but not from use in the open air. Absorption of large amount cause severe bronchospasm, hypotension, bradycardia and cardiac arrest.

The patient should be removed to fresh air, and nose and eyes irrigated with 5% sodium bicarbonate.

BIOLOGICAL WARFARE: Biological weapons (B.W.) are defined as microorganisms or their products of metabolism that infect and grow in the target host producing a clinical disease that kills or incapacitates humans or animals. Such microbes may be natural, wild-type strains or may be genetically produced. These include biological toxins and substances that interfere with normal behaviour, such as hormones, neuropeptides and cytokines. **Bacillus anthracis, small pox virus, botulinum toxin and ricin are commonly used. Other agents used are: bacteria causing plague, cholera, typhus, brucellosis, salmonella, Ebola virus, abrin toxin, tularemia, Q fever, etc.** Very small amounts of biological agents or toxins can cause mass casualties. The agents are odourless, tasteless and invisible to the naked eye when aerolised. Dissemination of BW agents occur by aerosol spray, explosives or food or water contamination. Remote control devices can be used. Bioterrorism is the use of biological agents for terrorizing people to settle scores with enemies.

The body should be cleaned with 0.5% hypochlorite or phenol disinfectant and transported to mortuary in an impermeable double bag. Certain bio-agents, such as small pox, tularaemia, viral haemorrhagic fevers, ganders, Q fever, can be transmitted to persons performing autopsies. Collect blood, CSF and tissue samples or swabs for isolation of bacteria and virus.

HYDROCYANIC ACID (HCN)

Sources: Hydrocyanic acid (prussic acid or cyanogen) is a solution of HCN in water either 2% or 4%, the latter being called "Scheele's acid". **It is a vegetable acid found in nature in many fruits and leaves, such as almond, apricot, apple, cherry, peach, plum, pear, bamboo shoots, and in certain oil seeds and beans, where it exists in the form of a glucoside amygdalin, which is harmless, but usually co-exists with the enzyme emulsin, which hydrolyses it and liberates hydrocyanic acid. Amygdalin is converted to cyanide in the small intestine by bacteria in the presence of the enzyme emulsion. All parts of cassava plant contain cyanide.** Hydrocyanic acid is usually obtained from distilling of cyanide by an acid. The pure acid is a colourless, transparent volatile liquid with an odour like bitter almonds and is rapidly decomposed by exposure to light. **About 20 to 40% persons cannot smell the gas,** and the ability to detect it is a sex-linked recessive trait. HCN is the normal constituent of the body (15 to 30 micrograms).

Cyanides: Cyanides are white powders and are in common use in many trades, in metallurgy, photography, electroplating, fumigation of ships and aircraft, in agriculture for spraying to destroy blight. Potassium ferrocyanide and ferricyanide are not poisonous.

Action: **Cyanide inhibits the action of cytochrome oxidase, carbonic anhydrase and probably of other enzyme systems.** It blocks the final step of oxidative phosphorylation and prevents the formation of ATP and its use as energy source. **Cyanide acts by reducing the oxygen carrying capacity of the blood, and by combining with the ferric iron atom of intracellular cytochrome oxidase, preventing the uptake of oxygen for cellular respiration.** There is an interference with the intracellular oxidative processes in the tissues and **it kills by creating histotoxic or cytotoxic anoxia, although the blood may contain a normal oxygen content.**

Absorption and Excretion: Cyanide gas is absorbed rapidly from the respiratory system, and the acid and cyanide salts from the stomach. **The acid is also absorbed through the skin.** Absorption is delayed when cyanide is taken on a full stomach or with much wine. **Alkaline cyanides when ingested are converted by hydrochloric acid in the gastric juice into chlorides, and hydrocyanic acid is liberated.** It has been suggested that those who are achlorhydric cannot therefore be poisoned by cyanides. This is doubtful, if not incorrect, because water in the gastric juice and the tissues of the stomach can hydrolyse cyanide, and liberate hydrocyanic acid. The greater part is converted by an enzyme rhodanase (present in liver and kidney) into thiocyanate. A small amount is excreted unchanged in the breath. It is mainly excreted in the urine.

Signs and Symptoms: **This is the most rapid of all poisons. When inhaled as a gas, its action is instantaneous.** With small doses, the person first experiences headache, confusion, giddiness, nausea and some loss of muscular power. Massive doses may produce sudden loss of consciousness and prompt death from respiratory arrest. If a large dose is taken, symptoms usually occur at once, but in some cases symptoms appear after about one minute, during which the victim may perform certain voluntary acts, such as corking, or throwing away the bottle, or walking a little distance. **All symptoms ultimately reflect cellular hypoxia,** and the symptoms shift rapidly, depending on the extent of the cyanide exposure. **C.N.S.:** Headache, vertigo, faintness, perspiration, anxiety, excitement, confusion, drowsiness, prostration, opisthotonus and trismus, cramps, twitchings, hyperthermia, convulsions epileptiform or tonic, which are sometimes localised but usually generalised, paralysis, stupor, coma, and death. **G.I.T.:** Bitter, acid, burning taste, constriction or numbness of throat, salivation, nausea, rarely vomiting. **R.S.:** **Odour of bitter almonds in breath.** Initially tachypnoea and dyspnoea due to cyanide stimulation of chemoreceptors and the respiratory centre. Later rapid slowing of respiratory rate with severe respiratory depression and cyanosis. **C.V.S.:** Initially hypertension with reflex bradycardia, sinus arrhythmia. Later tachycardia with hypotension and cardiovascular collapse. The heart continues to beat for several minutes after stoppage of respiration. **Skin:** Perspiration, bullae. **Eyes:** Glassy and prominent, pupils dilated, unreactive. **Renal:** Acidosis. Death occurs from respiratory failure.

Inhalation of vapour produces a sense of constriction about the throat and chest, dizziness, vertigo, insensibility, and death from respiratory failure. Inhalation of air containing one part in 2000 of cyanide is fatal almost immediately, 1 part in 1000 within few minutes, and 1 part in 5000 within few hours.

Cyanides: In poisoning by cyanides, the symptoms may not occur for 10 to 20 minutes, because of the delay in the decomposition of the salt by gastric juice, and the liberation and absorption of hydrocyanic acid. **Potassium and sodium cyanide have a corrosive effect on the mouth, throat and stomach,** and cause epigastric pain, vomiting and alkaline burns of the mucosa. Other symptoms are similar to hydrocyanic acid.

Survivors of serious acute poisoning may develop delayed neurologic sequelae, especially in the form of Parkinsonian symptoms.

Fatal Dose: 50 to 60 mg. of pure acid; 200 to 300 mg. of sodium or potassium cyanide.

Fatal Period: 2 to 10 minutes; sometimes immediate. Potassium or sodium cyanide: half an hour. The patient may survive for several hours due to delayed absorption.

Treatment: Treatment should be started immediately. **The principle of the treatment is to reverse the cyanide-cytochrome combination. This is achieved by converting haemoglobin to methaemoglobin by giving nitrites.** Methaemoglobin has a higher binding affinity for cyanide than the cytochrome oxidase complex, and removes cyanide from the cytochrome oxidase. **Cyanides combine with methaemoglobin and form non-toxic cyanmethaemoglobin which in the presence of rhodanase and sulphate donors, such as thiosulphate, converts cyanide to thiocyanate which is excreted in the urine.** Cyanide is directly converted to thiocyanate by the complexing of cyanide with thiosulphate under the influence of the enzyme rhodanase.

Cyanide is also converted to cyanocobalamin (Vit B_{12}) by complexing with hydroxocobalamin (Vit B_{12} A).

Cytochrome oxides + NaCN ⟶ Cytochrome oxidase cyanide.

Sodium nitrite + Hb ⟶ methaemoglobin.

Methaemoglobin + Na CN ⟶ Cyan-methaemoglobin.

Cyanide kit contains 12 amyl nitrite pearls, two 10 ml. vials of 3% sodium nitrite and two 50 ml. vials of sodium thiosulphate.

(1) **Break 0.2 ml. ampoule of amyl nitrite in a handkerchief and hold over the patient's nose for 15 to 30 seconds of every minute, until sodium nitrite infusion is started.** **(2) 0.3 g. of sodium nitrite in 10 ml. of sterile water is given i.v. slowly,** over a period of five minutes. Sodium nitrite forms methaemoglobin (Hb-Fe^{2+}), then competes with cytochrome oxidase for the cyanide ion, thus protecting cytochrome oxidase. Do not remove the needle. (3) Through the **same needle infuse 25 g. of sodium thiosulphate in 50% solution i.v. over a period of ten minutes.** It converts cyanide to non-toxic thiocyanate, which is excreted in urine. (4) Both sodium nitrate and sodium thiosulphate can be repeated at half the initial dose at the end of one hour if symptoms persist or reappear. (5) Other antidotes are: **Hydroxocobalamin (Vit B_{12})** 4 g. i.v. as infusion is given. It detoxifies cyanide by giving a hydroxyl group and then binding a cyanyl group from the cyanide, forming non-toxic cyanocobalamin which is excreted in the urine. It may be used with sodium thiosulphate which reacts with cyanocobalamin in the presence of the enzyme rhodanase, to produce thiocyanate. (6) **Dicobalt EDTA** acts by chelating cyanide to form a harmless product that is excreted in the urine. 600 mg. is given i.v. slowly. It is followed by 300 mg. if recovery does not occur. Cobalt EDTA and aminophenols are more rapid in action, efficacious, and less toxic than nitrites. (7) 4-dimethylaminophenol **(4-DMAP)** 3 mg/kg. i.v. produces a level of 15% metHb within one minute (8) Gastric lavage is then performed on those who have ingested cyanide using activated charcoal, a mixture of 6% sodium carbonate, 15% ferrous sulphate and 3% citric acid, or 3% hydrogen peroxide, or preferably 5 to 10% sodium thiosulphate, or 1:5000 potassium permanganate, and 200 ml. is left in the stomach. Alternatively stomach wash can be done with a mixture of sodium bicarbonate and ferrous and ferric chloride. (9) Methylene blue is not effective. (10) Ventilate with hundred percent oxygen. (11) Methaemoglobin of more than fifty percent is an indication for exchange transfusion or administration of blood. (12) If death is delayed, a mixture of ferrous and ferric sulphate with potassium carbonate may be given as a chemical antidote to form Prussian blue. (13) Keep the airway clear. (14) Patient should be kept under observation for 24 to 48 hours, as cyanide toxicity may recur. (15) In poisoning by inhalation, remove the patient at once to fresh air and start artificial respiration and oxygen.

Postmortem Appearances: Care should be taken to reduce the exposure of individuals in the mortuary to a minimum. **Hydrogen cyanide can be inhaled from the stomach contents when inspecting viscera.** The eyes may be bright, glistening and prominent with dilated pupils. The jaws are firmly closed and there is froth at the mouth. **The colour of the cheeks and postmortem staining may be cherry-red in about half the cases,** because oxygen remains in the cells as oxyhaemoglobin, and due to the formation of cyanmethaemoglobin. **The odour of hydrocyanic acid may be noticed on opening the body.** In cases of suspected cyanide poisoning, the cranial cavity should be opened first, as the odour is usually well-marked in the brain tissues. **All the vessels of the body including the veins contain oxygenated blood.** Blood stained froth may be found in the trachea and bronchi. There is congestion of viscera and oedema of the lungs Fig. (36–1). The serous cavities are ecchymosed. The mucosa of the stomach and intestine is often red and congested. Liver substance is also very shiny to dull radish in colour Fig. (36–2) Degenerative changes may occur in the nervous system.

Potassium or sodium cyanide produce slight corrosion of mouth. Tongue is swollen, grey or black and distorted. Spillage into larynx and air passages cause damage to respiratory mucosa. Aspiration of liquid or vapour into lungs can cause rapid pulmonary oedema and haemorrhages. The mucosa of the stomach may be eroded and blackened due to the formation of alkaline haematin Fig. (36–3). The stomach may contain frank or altered blood from the erosions and haemorrhages in the walls. In less severe cases, the rugae will be streaked with dark red striae. Other findings are same as that of hydrocyanic acid. **The blood concentration of persons dead of cyanide poisoning are usually in excess of 1 mg %.**

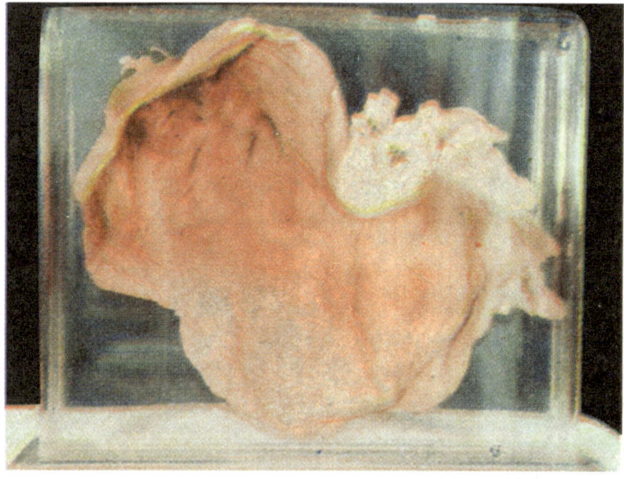

Fig. (36–1). **Stomach in hydrocyanic acid poisoning.**

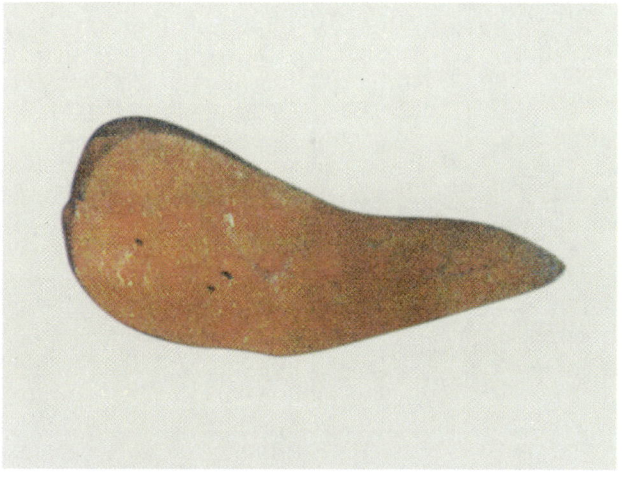

Fig. (36–2). **Liver in hydrocyanic acid poisoning.**

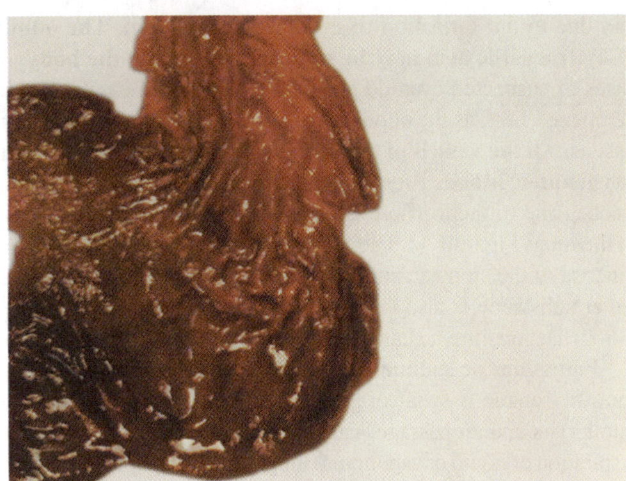

Fig. (36–3). **Stomach in sodium cyanide poisoning.**

Chronic Poisoning: It may be produced by the continued inhalation over long periods of very low concentrations of hydrocyanic acid vapour. The symptoms are headache, vertigo, nausea, vomiting, diarrhoea, chronic cachexia, mental disturbances, visual defects, such as scotomata, optic atrophy, and psychosis.

Viscera preservation: Hydrocyanic acid is an extremely volatile substance. **The blood and viscera should be preserved by adding an alkali and stored in well-stoppered bottles in a refrigerator for analysis. Specimen of blood (fluoride preservative) must be covered with a layer of liquid paraffin to avoid evaporation.** Up to 70% may be lost after some weeks of storage from reaction with tissue components and conversion to thiocyanate. If death is caused by inhalation of hydrogen cyanide fumes, a lung should be sent intact in a nylon bag. **HCN is not produced after death by putrefactive changes.**

HCN retards decomposition like carbon monoxide, and to some extent acts as preservative, because of oxygen binding affinity they possess. Formaldehyde rapidly destroys cyanide and as such embalming should be avoided before autopsy. Cyanide may be formed in stored blood samples at room temperature. By contrast in some positive samples cyanide may decrease on storage.

The Circumstances of Poisoning: (1) Hydrocyanic acid and cyanides are usually used for suicide. **It can be concealed in "suicidal pills", in rings or hollow teeth.** (2) Occasionally, they are taken by accident or the fumes of the acid may be inhaled by those working with it. (3) It is rarely used for homicide and as cattle poison. **Cattle poisoning can occur from eating linseed plant due to the natural development of a cyanogenetic glycoside.**

LEE-JONES TEST: To 5 ml of stomach contents add few crystals of ferrous sulphate and 5 drops of 2% sodium hydroxide. Boil and cool and add 10 drops of 10% hydrochloric acid. Greenish-blue colour indicates cyanide, and purplish colour salicylates.

JUDICIAL EXECUTION: In some countries, hydrocyanic acid gas is used for legal execution. The condemned person is strapped in a metal chair with perforated seat. A bowl with sulphuric acid mixed with distilled water is kept under the chair. Few pellets of sodium cyanide are suspended in a gauze bed just above the bowl. The door is sealed. The executioner seated in an adjacent room operates a lever, which releases cyanide bed into the bowl. This produces large quantity of hydrogen cyanide gas immediately, which rises through the holes in the chair. Unconsciousness takes place very rapidly, although heart continues to beat for 10 to 20 minutes.

CHAPTER

37 MISCELLANEOUS POISONS

FM 10.1: Describe general principles and basic methodologies in treatment of poisoning: decontamination, supportive therapy, antidote therapy, procedures of enhanced elimination with regard to:

i. Antipyretics—paracetamol, salicylates
ii. Anti-infectives (Common antibiotics—an overview)
iii. Neuropsychotoxicology barbiturates, benzodiazepines phenytoin, lithium, haloperidol, neuroleptics, tricyclics
iv. Narcotic analgesics, anaesthetics, and muscle relaxants
v. Cardiovascular toxicology cardiotoxic plants—oleander, odollam, aconite, digitalis
vi. Gastrointestinal and endocrinal drugs—insulin

ANALGESICS AND ANTIPYRETICS

Classification: (1) Salicylates: acetylsalicylic acid, diflunisal. (2) Pyrazolones: Phenylbutazone, oxyphenbutazone. (3) Indoleacidic acids: indomethacin, sulindac, tolmetin. (4) Phenylpropionic acids: carprofen, fenoprofen, ibuprofen, ketoprofen, naproxen. (5) Anthranilic acids: meclofenamate, mefenamic acid. (6) Oxicams: Piroxicam. (7) Phenylacetic acid: diclofenac.

SALICYLIC ACID: Preparations of salicylic acid include: sodium salicylate, methyl salicylate and aspirin. Sodium salicylate is odourless, white, scaly crystals with unpleasant saline taste. Methyl salicylate is colourless liquid with aromatic odour and sweetish taste.

ACETYLSALICYLIC ACID (Aspirin): It is a white, odourless, crystalline powder, having a slight acid taste. It is in popular use as an antipyretic and analgesic. It acts primarily through inhibition of prostaglandin biosynthesis.

They are rapidly absorbed from the stomach, and to a slightly lesser extent from the small intestine. Metabolism occurs chiefly in the liver. Excretion is mainly through urine. The half-life is 2 to 4 hours. They cause extreme irritation of G.I. mucosa.

SIGNS AND SYMPTOMS: A large oral dose of the acid or methyl ester causes mild burning pain in the throat and stomach and causes vomiting. There may be a latent period of several hours following these initial symptoms, during which sweating and slight rise of temperature may occur. The early signs are anorexia, apathy and lassitude. There is nausea, vomiting, thirst and occasional diarrhoea. The respiration is at first fast and deep, and later laboured and dyspnoeic. Vertigo, ringing in the ears, deafness and impaired vision are common and headache may be severe. The temperature is usually raised. Irritability, restlessness, confusion, disorientation, delirium, mania, hallucinations, generalised convulsions and coma are seen. In severe poisoning, a primary respiratory alkalosis due to the central stimulating effect of salicylates on respiratory centre with marked hyperapnoea and loss of CO_2 is caused. Later, metabolic acidosis supervenes due to increased excretion of bicarbonate, potassium and sodium. An increased anion gap metabolic acidosis with respiratory alkalosis, ketosis and tinnitus suggests salicylate poisoning. The urine is strongly acid, contains acetone, albumin and frequently a trace of bile due to mild hepatitis. Hypovolaemia and hypokalaemia and hypoprothrombinaemia may occur. The skin is flushed and moist, pupils dilated and the pulse is rapid and irregular. There may be platelet dysfunction (inhibition of aggregation) and prolonged clotting time. Severe dehydration may occur and in the terminal stages hyperpyrexia of 41 to 42° may occur. Blood levels of over 50 mg% are toxic and over 100 mg% fatal.

REYE'S SYNDROME: It is sometimes seen in children below 15 years on consumption of aspirin. The main features are acute onset of hepatic failure and encephalopathy with residual neurological manifestations.

TREATMENT: (1) Emetics. (2) When a large number of tablets are swallowed, aspirin may form a large dirty grey lump in the stomach, which may not dissolve for a long time. As such stomach should be washed with sodium bicarbonate solution, even after several hours of ingestion. With the advent of soluble aspirin or effervescent preparations, insoluble bolus is not formed. (3) Repetitive activated charcoal is useful. (4) Forced alkaline diuresis will increase the plasma clearance rate to as much as 700% above normal. (5) Peritoneal dialysis and haemodialysis are useful. (6) Exchange transfusions in severe cases. (7) Saline catharsis. (8) Alkali therapy if acidosis is present. (9) Whole bowel irrigation may be useful if salicylate levels are not declining. (10) Vitamin C to control haemorrhage. (11) In idiosyncrasy ACTH and antihistamines. (12) Symptomatic.

CAUSE OF DEATH: Death occurs from acidosis and uraemia with peripheral failure due to shock in the earlier stages or respiratory failure later. About 7 to 8% die. Aspirin can cause sudden cardiac arrest in the absence of any toxic symptoms up to a day or so. Fatal cardiac arrhythmias may supervene.

Idiosyncrasy is seen in 0.2% persons, in whom therapeutic dose produces alarming symptoms which include angioneurotic oedema, urticaria, hypotension, oedema of the mucous membranes with hypersecretion, vasomotor rhinitis, laryngeal oedema, vomiting, excessive salivation, bronchial spasm, cyanosis, maculopapular exanthemata and erythema of the face with oedema of eyelids, haemorrhage in the stomach and intestines due to capillary damage and in severe cases erosion of the mucosa and ulceration.

FATAL DOSE: Sodium salicylate and aspirin: 15 to 20 gm.; Salicylic acid; 70 to 80 gm.; Methyl salicylate: 10 to 20 ml.

FATAL PERIOD: Few minutes to several hours.

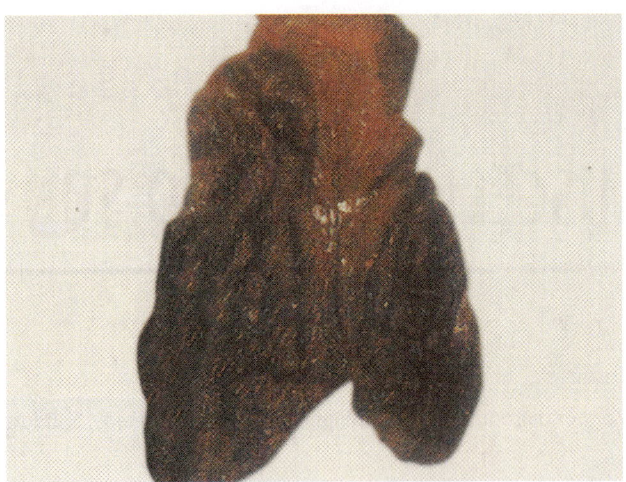

Fig. (37–1). Stomach in aspirin poisoning.

TEST: If few drops of ferric chloride are added to the urine containing aspirin, it turns deep purple.

POSTMORTEM APPEARANCES: The pupils are dilated. Skin rashes may be present. The gastric mucosa is congested and may be eroded Fig. (37–1). This may be localised or spread widely across the fundus and cardia. Black altered blood may be found in the stomach. There is generalised congestion of all the ograns. Subpleural and pericardial petechial haemorrhages are seen. Lungs are congested with some oedema and collapse. If the patient survives for few days, the myocardium, liver and kidneys are usually soft, dirty in appearance and greasy to touch. Hepatitis may be present. Petechial haemorrhages are seen in various organs.

CHRONIC POISONING: Symptoms are confusion, agitation, lethargy, disorientation, slurred speech, hallucinations, convulsions and coma. There may be tinnitus, loss of hearing, dyspnoea, tachycardia and fever.

THE CIRCUMSTANCES OF POISONING: Aspirin poisoning is almost always suicidal. Because of its bitter taste, large quantities are usually not swallowed accidentally.

PARACETAMOL (Acetaminophen)

It is an analgesic and antipyretic without anti-inflammatory properties of aspirin. It is absorbed rapidly from the gastrointestinal tract, and metabolised quickly in the liver. **It is a potent hepatic toxin,** A small part is converted by a liver enzyme into N-acetyl-p-benzoquinoneimine. Glutathione and other sulphydryl compounds detoxify this substance, but in overdose NABP accumulates and causes severe centrilobular liver necrosis. The simultaneous presence of phenobarbitone or phenytoin in epileptics or the presence of chronic alcoholism, greatly worsens the situation. **Large doses act on brain stem and cause rapid death.** Most deaths are delayed for several days, when liver failure occurs. Toxic doses cause depletion of glutathione, which results in hepatic necrosis.

Fatal Dose: 20 to 25 g; 40–50 tablets.

Fatal Period: 3 to 4 days.

Symptoms: Within a few hours, patient experiences anorexia, nausea, vomiting, abdominal pain, diaphoresis, hypotension, tachycardia and dyspnoea. After one to two days, the discomfort disappears. After 2 to 4 days there is vomiting, jaundice, hepatic pain, bleeding, hypoglycaemia, confusion, coma, metabolic acidosis and coarse flapping tremor of hands (asterixis). There may be cardiac arrhythmias, haemorrhagic pancreatitis, disseminated intravascular coagulation, etc. Death usually occurs in 3 to 4 days. **Renal failure due to renal papillary necrosis may occur in 24 to 72 hours even in the absence of hepatotoxicity.** Death from hepatic failure occurs 4 to 18 days post-ingestion. Paracetamol has replaced barbiturates and aspirin in Britain as favourite method of suicide.

Treatment: (1) Gastric lavage. (2) Activated charcoal. (3) **N-acetylcysteine (NAC) is a specific antidote and has maximum efficacy if used within 8 hours.** It is given in a dose of 140 mg/kg. body weight. Then, 70 mg./kg. is given every 4 hours until a total of 18 doses over 72 hours period orally. It can also be given i.v. 150 mg/kg in 200 ml of 5% dextrose over 15 minutes, followed by 50 mg/kg in 500 ml of 5% dextrose over 4 hours, and 100 mg/kg in one litre over 16 hours. (4) Methionine is less effective than NAC. It acts by increasing glutathione synthesis. Initial dose is 2.5 gm. orally, repeated every four hours up to a total of ten gm. Do not give activated charcoal as it will bind methionine. (5) Correct acidaemia. (6) Haemodialysis. (7) Symptomatic.

Postmortem Appearances: They include enlarged, yellowish liver with acute centrilobular necrosis, acute tubular necrosis in the kidney, myocardial necrosis, and cerebral oedema. Liver may be enlarged and may be pale yellow. Renal tubular necrosis and occasionally myocardial fibre damage may be seen.

WATER INTOXICATION

Deaths from water intoxication are very rare. Deaths occur due to ingestion of large quantities of water or the administration of large quantities of i.v. fluids, devoid of electrolytes. Symptoms occur due to sudden expansion of the cell water. There is restlessness, weakness, nausea, vomiting, diarrhoea, polyuria and oliguria, muscular twitchings, convulsions and coma. The victims are usually psychotic. Death occurs due to cardiac arrhythmia produced by electrolyte imbalance.

POSTMORTEM DIAGNOSIS should be based on history and low levels of sodium and chlorides in vitreous fluid. Potassium levels are normal or high, as it is rapidly released from the cells of the body after death, even in the vitreous.

INSULIN

It is a white powder with bitter taste.

SYMPTOMS: Weakness, fatigue, vomiting, dizziness, tachycardia, hypotension, anxiety, confusion, blurred vision, drowsiness, cramps, tremors, profuse sweating, tingling, heavy deep breathing, maniacal behaviour, delirium, shock, coma and death. If severe lowering of blood sugar persists for many hours, brain damage and death will occur.

TREATMENT: (1) Give 10 to 20 g. glucose orally in a solution (or a high carbohydrate food). (2) 50 ml. of 50% glucose i.v. Then continuous infusion of 10% glucose.

TEST: Skin and underlying tissue from the injection site should be preserved with control skin from another site and refrigerated and sent unfixed for assay. Serum should be separated, fluoride added and frozen. Vitreous humour, blood and urine should be preserved by fluoride. Very low vitreous humour glucose levels may strongly suggest hypoglycaemia. Immunoassay and C-peptide assist in distinguishing endogenous from exogenous insulin. Insulin can be recovered from bile by radioimmunoassay.

M.L. IMPORTANCE: (1) Impairment of ability to drive a vehicle. (2) Homicide is very rare. (3) Hypoglycaemia (non-insane automatism).

NITRATES AND NITRITES

(1) Inorganic nitrates: Sodium nitrate, potassium nitrate, bismuth subnitrate, silver nitrate. (2) Organic nitrates: Nitroglycerin, isosorbide

dinitrate, ethyl nitrate, mannitol hexanitrate. (3) Inorganic nitrites: amyl nitrite, isobutyl nitrite, sodium nitrite. (4) Organic nitrites: (a) Bismuth subnitrate in contaminated well water may be converted by intestinal bacteria to nitrites and may cause poisoning. (b) Nitrates in contaminated water in the presence of Bacillus subtilis spores in dried milk powder are transformed to nitrites. Sodium nitrate tastes like and can be mistaken for sodium chloride.

They are available in many houses as medicines. Sodium nitrate is used as a mordant by weavers.

ACTION: Sodium nitrate causes relaxation of smooth muscle, especially of small blood vessels and in toxic doses converts haemoglobin to methaemoglobin by oxidising iron from the ferrous to the ferric state.

FATAL DOSE: Sodium nitrate one to 2 g; nitroglycerine 200 mg; silver nitrate 2 to 10 g. Potassium nitrate 30 g; barium nitrate 15 g.

FATAL PERIOD: Few hours to few days.

SYMPTOMS: Throbbing headache, vertigo, low blood pressure, palpitations, later cold and cyanotic; nausea, vomiting, colick, bloody diarrhoea; syncope, especially when attempting to stand upright; methaemoglobinaemia, cyanosis and anoxia; hyperapnoea and later dyspnoea, slow pulse; disorientation, raised intracranial pressure and intraocular tension; paralysis, coma followed by clonic convulsions; death due to circulatory collapse.

Amyl nitrite and isobutyl nitrates are inhaled (drug abuse) for "getting high". They may be used as an aphrodisiac and to enhance and prolong sexual orgasm and also by some homosexual men to relax anal sphincter.

TREATMENT: (1) Induce emesis with ipecac, if the patient is alert followed by activated charcoal. (2) Gastric lavage with intubation. (3) Magnesium or sodium sulphate or sorbitol. (4) If methaemoglobinaemia is more than 30%, inject methylene blue 1 to 2 mg/kg (1% solution) or 50 mg/kg orally, which converts methaemoglobin to haemoglobin. (5) Exchange transfusion for infants and for patients who do not respond within half to one hour and those with met-Hb level of more than 70%. (6) Symptomatic.

METHAEMOGLOBINAEMIA

Methaemoglobin is haemoglobin in which the normally ferrous iron of the haem moiety has been oxidised to the ferric state, making it incapable of oxygen transport. The shape of oxygen-haemoglobin dissociation curve is altered, aggravating cellular hypoxia. Symptoms associated with methaemoglobin are shown in Table (37-1).

Causes: (1) **Hereditary:** Haemoglobin M, nicotinamide adenine dinucleotide methaemoglobin reductase deficiency. (2) **Acquired:** (a) Direct with nitrites, food high in nitrates, nitroglycerin, nitrous gases, chloroquine, primaquine, silver nitrate, well water (nitrates). (b) Indirect oxidants: aniline dye derivatives, benzocaine, sulphonamides, chlorobenzene, dapsone, naphthalene, nitrophenol, nitroprusside, phenacetin, pyridium, trinitrotoluene, bromates, chlorates, pyrogallol.

Treatment: (1) High-flow oxygen. (2) Activated charcoal. (3) Methylene blue i.v. 1 to 2 mg/kg as one % solution slowly over five minutes. If cyanosis does not disappear within one hour, a second dose should be given.

Table (37–1). Symptoms associated with methaemoglobin concentration

Met Hb Con %	Symptoms
0-3	Normal level.
3-15	No symptoms; slate grey skin.
16-20	Cyanosis, chocolate-brown blood.
21-50	Dyspepsia, exercise intolerance, headache, fatigue, dizziness, syncope, weakness.
51-70	Tachypnoea, metabolic acidosis, dysrhythmias, convulsions, CNS depression, coma.
>70	Severe hypoxic symptoms

NON-STEROIDAL ANTI-INFLAMMATORY DRUGS (NSAIDs)

CLASSIFICATION: (1) Pyrazolones. (2) Propionic acid. (3) Fenamic acids. (4) Heterocyclic acetic acids. (5) Aryl acetic acid. (6) Oxicams. (7) Sulfonanilide.

ACTIONS: Most of these drugs act by inhibiting prostaglandin synthesis.

SYMPTOMS: GIT: Nausea, vomiting, epigastric pain, peptic ulceration. C.N.S.: Drowsiness, lethargy, confusion, vertigo. C.V.S. Hypotension, aplastic anaemia. R.S.: Cyanosis. Renal: Acute tubular necrosis, or acute interstitial nephritis. Hepatitis and hepatic necrosis.

FATAL DOSE: Ten to 20 gm or more.

TREATMENT: (1) Gastric lavage. (2) Activated charcoal. (3) Haemoperfusion in severe cases. (4) Symptomatic.

ANTIHISTAMINICS

The commonly used preparations are: antazoline, (antistine), diphenhydramine (benadryl), alopyramine hydrochloride (synopen), meparamine maleate (anthisan), and promethazine hydrochloride (phenergan). Other preparations are: tripelemamine, chlorpheneramine, cemetidine, ranitidine, nizatidine and famotidine.

SYMPTOMS: In adults CNS depression is the usual dominant reaction characterised by drowsiness, lethargy, fatigue, hypnosis and coma. There is vertigo, ataxia, tinnitus, dilated pupils and blurred vision. The initial sedation is often followed by CNS hyperexcitability; sometimes the excitement is the first evidence of poisoning. This causes tremors, anxiety, insomnia, excitement, delirium and convulsions. Anticholinergic features (mydriasis, hyperthermia and flushing) are seen. Gastrointestinal symptoms are: dry mouth, anorexia, nausea, vomiting, abdominal pain, constipation or diarrhoea. There may be loss of balance, hallucinations, tachycardia, retention of urine and skin rashes. Finally, there is severe central nervous depression, and death results from respiratory failure or cardiovascular collapse.

FATAL DOSE: 25 to 50 mg/kg.

Poisoning is usually accidental and sometimes suicidal. One gram is fatal.

TREATMENT: (1) Stomach wash. (2) Activated charcoal. (3) Diazepam. (4) Physostigmine 0.5 to 2 mg. i.v. every hour, until reversal of symptoms occur. However, it can produce serious adverse effects. (5) Symptomatic.

AUTOPSY: Signs of asphyxia are found.

CAFFEINE

Caffeine stimulates gastric acid, pepsin and secretions from small intestine. Large doses can stimulate directly the myocardium to produce tachycardia, arrhythmias and extrasystoles. It increases cardiac output and stroke volume. It decreases fatigue. Adrenaline and noradrenaline secretion is increased. It can increase the basal metabolic rate by about ten percent. It also increases oxygen consumption. It acts as diuretic. Significant amounts of caffeine are present in tea, cola beverages and chocolates.

FATAL DOSE: One to two gm.

Doses of 50 to 200 mg. result in increased alertness, decreased drowsiness, and lessened fatigue. Doses of 200 to 500 mg. may produce headache, tremors, nervousness, irritability and slight increase of blood pressure. At level of one gram (8 to 10 cups of coffee) per day, a combination of physiological and behavioural symptoms like anxiety-like presentation, insomnia, headache and depressive presentation can appear. With ten grams of caffeine, grand mal seizures, and cardiorespiratory arrest may occur.

Withdrawal symptoms are: headache, yawning, nausea, drowsiness, lethargy, rhinorrhoea, irritability, nervousness and depression.

FORMALDEHYDE

It is a colourless gas having a strong, pungent, irritating odour. 40% solution in water is known as formalin. It is used as disinfectant, for preservation of museum specimens, in plastic, in dyeing, hardening of celluloid and as a reducing agent. It gives off vapour at room temperature. Commercial formalin contains 37% formaldehyde and 10 to 15% methanol. It is readily absorbed in upper respiratory tract. It is metabolised to formic acid in liver and blood.

FATAL DOSE: 30–60 ml.

FATAL PERIOD: One to two days.

SYMPTOMS: Inhalation of vapour causes burning of eyes, lachrymation, coughing, constriction in chest and palpitation. Ingestion produces symptoms similar to strong acid. It can cause contact dermatitis. Chronic exposure can result in allergic contact dermatitis, chronic obstructive pulmonary disease and optic neuritis.

TREATMENT: (1) Wash the stomach with 0.1% solution of ammonia, as it reacts with formaldehyde to form harmless methenamine. (2) Activated charcoal. (3) Mild saline catharsis. (4) Symptomatic.

POSTMORTEM APPEARANCES: Smell is noted on opening the body. Mucosa of the stomach may be red, inflamed and eroded with extravasation of blood, or it may be hard and tough like leather. The intestines and lungs are congested. The liver may show fatty degeneration and the kidneys may be inflamed.

CARBON TETRACHLORIDE

It is used as fire extinguisher, grease remover and for dry-cleaning clothes.

SYMPTOMS: Nausea, vomiting, diarrhoea, burning pain in mouth, throat and abdomen, dizziness, confusion, drowsiness, coma, slow, irregular heart beat which may cause sudden death. Inhalation causes cough, sneezing and mild breathlessness and above symptoms. Skin contamination causes redness, irritation and blisters.

FATAL DOSE: 2 to 4 ml.

TREATMENT: Acetyl cysteine i.v.

CHAPTER

38

FOOD POISONING

Objectives:
- To know common poisoning.
- Signs, symptoms and pathophysiology of different types of poisoning.
- Treatment of food poisoning.
- Postmortem findings in food poisoning.
- Chemical and microbiology investigation.

The term food poisoning in its wider sense **includes all illnesses which result from ingestion of food containing non-bacterial or bacterial products. But the term is usually restricted to acute gastroenteritis due to the bacterial infection of food or drink. WHO defines food poisoning as "diseases usually either infectious or toxic in nature, caused by agents that enter the body through the ingestion of food".**

CAUSES: (I) POISONING DUE TO BACTERIA AND TOXINS.

(II) POISONS OF VEGETABLE ORIGIN **(natural food poisons): (1) Lathyrus sativus. (2) Poisonous mushrooms. (3) Rye, oats, barley, etc. (4) Poisonous berries, such as atropa belladonna. (5) Lolium temulentum. (6) Paspalam scrobiculatum. (7) Argemone mexicana. (8) Cotton seeds. (9) Groundnuts. (10) Vitia fava. (11) Cabbage. (12) Solanine. (13) Soyabean. (14) Sweet clover.**

(III) POISONS OF ANIMAL ORIGIN: **(1) Poisonous fish. (2) Mussel.**

(IV) CHEMICAL: **(1) Intentionally added, such as flavouring agents in processed food, colouring agents, preservatives, extraction of fat by solvents like hydrocarbons. (2) Accidentally added, such as pesticides and insecticides. (3) Products of food processing, e.g. smoking of fleshy foods. (4) Radionuclides.**

S. 272, I.P.C.: **Adulteration of food or drink intended for sale.**

S.273, I.P.C.: **Sale of noxious food or drink.**

S.274, I.P.C.: **Adulteration of drugs.**

S.275, I.P.C.: **Sale of adulterate drugs.**

S.276, I.P.C.: **Sale of drugs as a different drug or preparation.**

The punishment for above offences is imprisonment up to 6 months or with fine or with both.

BACTERIAL FOOD POISONING

Bacterial food poisoning is of the following types. (1) SALMONELLA FOOD POISONING: **It is common form of food poisoning. Salmonellosis is primarily a disease of animals. Man gets the infection from farm animals and poultry through contaminated meat, milk and milk products, sausages, custards, egg and egg products. Rats and mice are another source; they are often heavily infected and contaminate foodstuffs by their urine and faeces. Temporary human carriers can also contribute to the problem. The causative organisms, e.g. S. enteritidis of gaertner, S. typhimurium, S. cholerasuis, and less commonly paratyphoid bacilli, on ingestion, multiply in the intestine and give rise to acute enteritis and colitis.**

(2) STAPHYLOCOCCAL FOOD POISONING: **Enterotoxins of certain strains of coagulase-positive Staphylococcus aureus is the causative agent. These toxins are relatively heat stable and resist boiling for 30 minutes or more. The foods involved are salads, custards, milk and milk products which get contaminated by staphylococci. Incubation period is 1 to 6 hours.**

(3) CL. PERFRINGENS FOOD POISONING: **The organism has been found in faeces of humans and animals, and in soil, water and air. The majority of outbreaks have been associated with the ingestion of meat, meat dishes and poultry. The food has been prepared and cooked 24 hours before at room temperature and then heated immediately prior to serving.**

(4) CEREUS FOOD POISONING: **Bacillus cereus is ubiquitous in soil, and in raw, dried and processed foods. The spores can survive cooking and germinate and multiply rapidly when the food is held at favourable temperatures. B. cereus produces at least 2 distinct enterotoxins, causing 2 distinct forms of food poisoning. (1) The emetic form with a short incubation period of one to six hours.**

THE MAIN DISEASES SPREAD BY INFECTED FOOD: **Food poisoning is common in summer, because the warm temperature favours multiplication of microorganisms. It may occur as isolated cases or small outbreaks. (1) The enteric group. (2) Cholera. (3) Bacillary dysentery. (4) Staphylococcal and other bacterial infections. (5) Amoebic dysentery and other protozoal infections. (6) Acute infective hepatitis. (7) Brucellosis. (8) Various worm infestations. (9) Schistosomiasis. (10) Traveller's diarrhoea (due to pathogenic E. coli).**

E. coli invade intestinal mucosa and elaborate enterotoxin. Infection occurs through water and meat. Incubation period is 1 to 3 days. Symptoms resemble dysentery or cholera.

DIAGNOSIS: **This is made from: (1) History. (2) Clinical features. (3) Isolation of the organism from the remnants of suspected food and from vomit, faeces, blood, etc. from sick person. (4) The injection of portion of left off food into mice or guinea pigs should be performed. If the animals get sick, attempt should be made to isolate organisms from them.**

DIFFERENTIAL DIAGNOSIS: **Food poisoning may be mistaken for cholera, acute bacillary dysentery and arsenic poisoning.**

BOTULISM: In this form of food poisoning there are no or very slight symptoms of gastroenteritis, although poisoning results from absorption of a specific toxin from the alimentary canal. Cl. botulinum does not grow in body, but produces a potent neurotoxin. It is normally present in the soil, dust and the intestinal tract of animals and enters food as spores, especially fruits and vegetables.

Action: Its action is selective being confined to the cholinergic fibres of autonomic nervous system. It affects peripheral cholinergic nerve endings including neuromuscular junction, postganglionic parasympathetic nerve endings and peripheral ganglia without affecting CNS.

Botulism is an intoxication, not an infection. The causative organisum Cl. botulinum multiplies in the food, e.g., sausages, tinned meat, fish, fruits, etc. before it is consumed, and produces a powerful exotoxin under suitable anaerobic conditions. The fatal dose for an adult is 0.01 mg. or even less. The toxin paralyses the nerve endings, by blocking the nerve impulses at the myoneural junctions. It blocks the action of acetylcholine. Its action is selective being confined to the cholinergic fibres of the autonomic nervous system.

VIRUSES: Viral infections usually have 1 to 3 days incubation period and are self-limited and similar to the bacterial type. Norovirus and Rotavirus commonly cause food poisoning.

FOOD ALLERGY: It is not food poisoning, for in this the abnormality is not in the food but in the allergic person. Some persons are hypersensitive to certain types of protein, e.g., meat, fish, eggs, milk, etc. which are ordinarily quite harmless and suffer from gastroenteritis, local urticarial rashes, or asthmatic attack.

PTOMAINES: These are alkaloidal bodies which are formed as the result of bacterial decomposition of protein. When they are formed in the dead tissues, they are known as cadaveric alkaloids. Alkaloids secreted by living cells during metabolism are called leucomaines, which are slightly toxic when injected into an animal but have no action when ingested. They are not bacterial poisons and are not derived from bacteria. They are found only when the food becomes too disagreeable to be eaten. Most of the ptomaines are non-poisonous except neurine and mydalein, which are produced in traces 5 to 7 days after death. The symptoms resemble that of atropine. Ptomaines are not the causative agents of food poisoning.

MYCOTOXICOSIS: The spores of moulds grow on the food of man and animals and release highly toxic mycotoxins. They can remain in meat and be passed into milk or eggs. Mycotoxins are heat stable and survive cooking. The consumption of contaminated food causes poisoning in man. Aspergillus flavus can grow on any food. They produce aflatoxins. It can produce carcinoma of liver and acute encephalitis. The fungus penicillium islandicum growing on yellowed rice produce islandotoxin which is a potent hepatotoxin.

POISONOUS FOODS

Poisonous foods are those which contain poison derived from plants, animals and inorganic chemicals.

LATHYRUS SATIVUS (kesari dal):

This is a variety of pulse which grows under extreme conditions of drought. It is a staple food for the low income groups in some areas of Central India. **Consumption of L. sativus seeds in quantities exceeding 30% of the total diet for more than six months have been known to cause paralysis.** The overall incidence of the disease in the endemic area is about 4%. Men are more susceptible than women.

Active Principle: The active neurotoxic principle is B(N) oxalyl amino-alanine (BOAA), which is present as a free amino acid **in the seed cotyledons** to the extent of about one percent.

Onset is of three types: (1) acute, (2) subacute, and (3) insidious. The continued use of L.sativus produces **neurolathyrism, which is characterised by progressive spastic paraplegia with preservation of sphincters, sensation and mental activity.** It progresses irreversibly into four stages of physical disability.

Symptoms: There may be pain in the back or **weakness of legs, and difficulty in sitting down and getting up. Later the patient is unable to walk without the aid of a stick,** the legs tremble and dragged along with difficulty and spastic gait characterised by a walk on tiptoes with the legs crossing scissor-wise. **Later complete paraplegia occurs.** There is no atrophy or loss of the tone of muscles, and no reaction of degeneration. The knee jerks are increased, ankle clonus is marked and Babinski's sign is present.

Steeping the pulse in hot water and parboiling remove 90% of toxic amino acid. Rich diet with exclusion of the pulse, massage and application of electricity are useful. Death is very rare. At autopsy lateral columns of the spinal cord show sclerosis.

MUSHROOMS

Some species are non-poisonous and are used as food. **Amanita phalloides and Amanita muscaria are the common varieties of poisonous fungi Fig. (38–1).** Poisonous mushrooms usually have a bitter, astringent, acid or salt taste, and on section and exposure change colour; a brown, green or blue colour developing on the cut surface. But there are no easy rules to exclude poisonous varieties. The pileus (top) varies in colour from yellow to orange or red, and is covered by warty scales. It contains an alkaloid **muscarine, the action of which resembles stimulation of parasympathetic post-ganglionic nerves.** Amanita phalloides is also called the deadly agaric or death cap. It is white in colour having an unpleasant taste and when old the odour is offensive. It grows in woody places to a height of 15 to 20 cm. It has a hollow stalk with a prominent bulb at the base, the upper margin of which is formed into a cup. The pileus is usually white, but may be pale yellow or olive, and has gills covered with white spores on its undersurface. The fungus is a powerful poison and contains **phalloidin, phallon, B amanatin, which are cyclopeptides and virotoxins.** These polypeptides are heat stable and insoluble in water. **They are powerful inhibitors of**

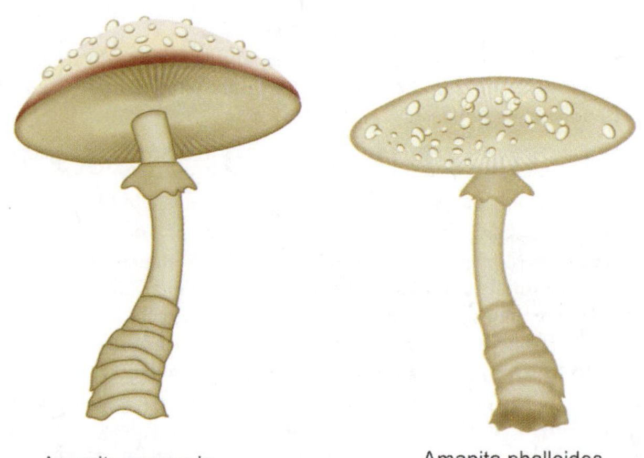

Fig. (38–1). Mushrooms.

cellular protein synthesis. Muscarine stimulates post-ganglionic cholinergic fibres.

Symptoms: In some cases irritant symptoms may be present, and in others neurotic or a combination of both. The irritant symptoms are delayed for 6 to 12 hours. There is constriction of the throat, burning pain in the stomach, nausea, vomiting and diarrhoea followed by cyanosis, slow pulse, laboured respirations, convulsions, sweating, collapse and death. The neurotic symptoms are giddiness, headache, delirium, diplopia, constriction of pupils, cramps, twitching of the limbs, convulsions, salivation, bradycardia and coma. Hepatic and sometimes renal toxicity occurs between 3 to 6 days.

Fatal Dose: One to two mushrooms.

Fatal Period: Usually 24 hours.

Treatment: (1) Stomach wash with potassium permanganate. (2) Activated charcoal. (3) N-acetylcysteine as in paracetomol. (4) Forced diuresis. (5) Benzyl penicillin 3 lakhs to one million units daily. (6) Atropine sulphate. (7) Anti-phalloidin serum. (8) Thioctic acid is obsolete. (9) Haemodialysis. (10) Symptomatic.

Autopsy: Inflammation of the mucous membrane of the alimentary canal, fatty degeneration of the liver, kidneys and heart may be found. In case of neurotic symptoms, congestion of the brain, and petechial haemorrhages in serous membranes are seen.

Poisoning is usually accidental, and rarely homicidal.

ARGEMONE MEXICANA *(Ujarkanta; kutila; sialkanta)*: It grows wild all over India in the cold season. It has sessile, spiny, thistle-like leaves. The flowers are yellow Fig. (38–2). The seeds are contained in prickly oblong or elliptic capsules two to four cm. long. The seeds are dark-brown in colour, globular, smaller than mustard seeds and covered with minute, regularly arranged projections, and depressions. When the seeds are pressed on a slide they burst with a report, whereas mustard seeds collapse quietly. **The plant contains two alkaloids berberine and protopine. The oil contains two alkaloids, sanguinarine and dihydrosanguinarine. All parts of the plant are poisonous. The oil causes** epidemic dropsy. The oil from the seeds is sometimes used as an adulterant of mustard oil, or other edible oil. It causes abnormal permeability of blood vessels.

Symptoms: Symptoms appear slowly with loss of appetite, diarrhoea, **marked oedema of the legs, sometimes generalised anasarca. In severe cases, myocardial damage and dilatation of the heart is seen.** Blood pressure is low and pulse feeble and rapid. **Liver may be enlarged and tender.** Patient becomes breathless. Tingling and hyperaesthesia of skin and tenderness of the calf muscles may be seen. The jerks are feeble or absent. Dimness of vision is seen in about 10% of cases due to increased intraocular pressure of glaucoma. **Bluish mottling of the skin is seen due to dilation of the peripheral vessels.** Some of these areas may develop into subcutaneous telangiectasis or haemangiomata. Death occurs from severe damage to the heart.

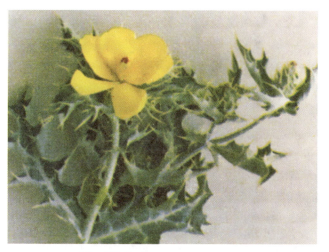

Fig. (38–2). **Argemone mexicana.**

Treatment: Good diet and supportive treatment of heart.

RYE, WHEAT, OATS, BARLEY AND BAJRA: These grains are attacked by the fungus Claviceps purpurea. The ear of the plant contains deep-purple diseased grains, which when dried is called ergot.

Action: Blood vessels become abnormally permeable. The target organs are liver, heart, kidneys and lungs.

LOLIUM TEMULENTUM (DARNEL): This weed grows in wheat fields. The grains are similar to wheat, but much smaller in size. The grains are attacked by a fungus which contains toxin temuline. The symptoms are headache, muscular weakness, tremors, gastrointestinal irritation, stupor and coma. It does not cause death.

PASPALAM SCROBICULATUM *(kodra)*: This corn contains a poison which is destroyed by boiling. The symptoms are similar to those of Lolium temulentum.

COTTON SEEDS: It has toxin gossypol (cake) released by bacteria present in cotton which makes lysine unavailable to the body.

GROUNDNUTS: Groundnuts stored under humid conditions are contaminated with metabolites of strains of Aspergillus flavus to which the collective name "AFLATOXINS' is given. A wide range of domestic and laboratory animals are affected by the toxin. Hepatic damage occurs in almost all cases, and death if the concentration of toxin is sufficiently high. With chronic exposure, the toxic agents have carcinogenic property. In rhesus monkeys, hepatic cirrhosis has been observed.

VITIA FLAVA: It is a legume producing flavism. The toxin is divicine.

CABBAGE: Brassia family has sulphur-containing compounds, which inhibit thyroxine secretion.

SOYABEAN: It has trypsin inhibitor which makes protein unavailable to the body. The toxin is destroyed by heat.

SWEET CLOVER: Cattle fed on spoiled sweet clover develop haemorrhagic disease due to the presence of clover of dicoumarin, which is chemically related to vitamin K and blocks its action.

POTATO: Potato contains solanine 0.002 to 0.01% mainly in the skin. Potatoes that are partly exposed above the soil and 'sunburned' (the skin of exposed part being green) contain considerable solanine, and cause poisoning when not thoroughly cooked. Immature and sprouting potatoes contain up to 0.06% of solanine, and cause severe or fatal poisoning. Raw potato peeling, the plant and its fruit also cause poisoning.

STIGMATA MAYDIS (MAIZE) **causes pellagra when eaten, due to lack of nicotinic acid.**

FISH AND MARINE ANIMALS: Fish poisoning: (Icthyotoxicosis; icthyotoxism): A large number of marine fish are inherently poisonous. Ciguatera poisoning and tetradon (puffer-fish) poisoning are common examples. Ingestion of fish causes two types of poisoning. The first is due to bacterial growth in partially decomposed fish. The other is a primary toxicity caused by eating some types of sea fishes such as toad fish, cat fish, lion fish, dragon fish due to the presence of a neurotoxin. 99% of cases of fish poisoning are **icthyosarcotoxic** (involving toxins from muscles, viscera, skin, gonads and mucous surfaces) characterised by various G.I. and neurological disturbances. Rarely, toxicity involves the fish blood or skeleton.

(1) CIGUATERA POISONING: It is the most common poisoning accounting for 50%. Species involved are: barracudas, sea bass, parrot fish, red snapper, grouper, and amber jack. Ciguatoxin found in certain algae and protozoa are eaten by herbivorous fish, which in turn are eaten by large fish which become poisonous. It affects the gut and nervous system. Poisoning occurs after eating fresh or frozen fish prepared by boiling, baking, frying, stewing or broiling. Symptoms set in one to 12 hours are: abdominal pain with cramps, nausea, vomiting, profuse watery diarrhoea, diaphoresis, headache, trembling, dizziness, dysaraesthesias and paraesthesias, tingling and numbness of the tongue, lips, throat and perioral area, myalgias, arthralgias and weakness. Hot substances feel cold and cold substances feel hot. Death may occur due to respiratory paralysis. Treatment is symptomatic.

(2) SCOMBROID POISONING: The species involved are: mahimahi, tuna, amberjack, albacore, bonito, mackerel, skipjack and canned fish of other types, such as sardines and pilchards. The poison is made by bacteria. All of them have a high concentration of histidine in their dark meat, which is converted to histamine. Symptoms begin in minutes to hours and subside in a few hours include headache, red itching skin over the face and body, nausea, belly pain and diarrhoea. Death is rare.

(3) GYMNOTHORAX POISONING: The moray, conger and anguillid eels carry a ciguatoxin-like neurotoxin in their viscera, muscles and gonads. Symptoms appear in half to thirty hours. They cause neurotoxic symptoms or signs of cholinergic toxicity.

(4) TETRODON POISONING: The species involved are: globe fish, balloon fish, blowfish, toad fish, porcupine fish, puffer fish, sun fish and blue-ringed octopus. They affect gut and nervous system. Symptoms appear in minutes to hours. They contain tetrodotoxin mainly in the skin, liver, ovary, and intestine. They cause neurotoxicity. Effects are similar to those of paralytic shellfish poisoning. Within 10 to 45 minutes muscles become weak, then paralysed. The muscles used in breathing are affected, so that the patient is unable to breathe and dies.

(5) SHELL FISH POISONING: The species include clans, oysters, mussels and scallops contaminated by feeding on poisonous dinoflagellates. This is called paralytic shellfish poisoning because the poison affects the nervous system. They contain saxitoxin, which is a potent paralytic neurotoxin. The symptoms begin in half hour. There is nausea, vomiting, headache, numbness and tingling of the lips and mouth, spreading to the legs, arms and the whole body, muscle paralysis, causing blurred vision, difficulty in swallowing, weakness and dizziness, aching muscles, reversal of hot and cold sensations, so that cold objects feel hot. Less commonly: low blood pressure, paralysis of muscles used in breathing, so that the patient is unable to breathe and death occurs. It acts on the peripheral and autonomic nervous systems. Like curare, it effectively blocks depolarisation at the neuromuscular junction.

VENOMOUS FISH: Some fishes such as cat fish, muraena (eel), dragon fish, lion fish, stingrays, mantas, scorpion fish, stone fish, cat fish, dog fish, sharks, etc. have extremely sharp dorsal spines equipped with large poisonous sacs. Several families of bony fish have venom glands enveloping sharp spines, which may be dorsal, ventral, behind the head or on the tail. They inject venom through their spines. Poisonous fish usually look no different from fish that are good to eat. Cooking does not destroy the poison. The lesions consist of a row of intensely painful rounded punctures with swelling and redness, which may bleed freely. The rare systemic symptoms, such as abdominal pain with cramps, nausea, vomiting, fits, low B.P. respiratory difficulty, circulatory collapse and paralysis are variable. The wound should be cleaned and broken spine removed.

The **BOX JELLYFISH** has been described as the world's most venomous animal. The injected toxin has both dermatonecrotic and cardiotoxic properties.

APPENDICES

APPENDIX-I

GLOSSARY OF LEGAL TERMS

AB INITIO: From the beginning.

ACCOMPLICE: One who aids, abets or encourages the main person in the commission of an unlawful act, though he is not actually present.

ACQUITTAL: Not guilty and can be set free.

ACTION: A proceeding in a Civil Court.

AD DIEM: From the cause to the effect.

AD ORUM: According to the value.

ACTUS REUS: Actual physical act causing death.

AD HOC: For this purpose.

AFFIDAVIT: A written statement in the name of a person, called the deponent by whom it is voluntarily signed and sworn to or affirmed.

AMICUS CURIAE: A person not a party to an action may petition to file a brief to provide special information on matters of law.

APPELLANT: The person who files an appeal.

APPELLEE: The party against whom an appeal is brought.

ASSESSOR: One who assists the Court in trying a scientific or technical question, but who has no voice in the decision.

BAIL: Security on behalf of an accused person for his release from custody.

BATTERY: Intentional and unauthorised physical contact with a person without his consent.

BINDING OVER: Requiring a person to enter into a recognisance to perform some necessary act, e.g., binding over a person to give evidence.

BURDEN OF PROOF: The need or duty to establish proof of the facts at trial.

CASE LAW: That part of the law formulated, developed and based on common custom of country (judge made law) and originally unwritten.

CAUSE OF ACTION: A set of facts, which gives a person a right to file proceedings in a civil court.

CAVEAT: Let him beware; a warning against certain acts.

CHARGE: A formal accusation in writing against a person that he has committed an offence.

CHARGE SHEET: A report stating commission of crime by an accused person, submitted to a magistrate by police on completion of an investigation.

CIVIL CASE: A case between two parties in their private capacity, e.g., money matters, property, etc.

CLAIM: A demand to pay.

CODE: A collection of laws in a jurisdiction or on a specific topic area arranged and indexed by subject, with revisions added to reflect the law currently in force.

COGNISABLE OFFENCE: An offence, in which a police officer can arrest a person without warrant from the Magistrate, e.g. rape, murder, robbery, etc.

COMMITTAL: The sending of a person to prison generally for a short period or temporary purpose.

COMMON LAW: Judge made law as opposed to codified law, i.e., law passed by legislature.

COMPLAINANT: One who makes a complaint to justices.

CONTEMPT: A wilful disregard or disobedience of Court's orders, as well as such conduct as tends to bring the authority of the Court and the administration of law into disrepute, or in some manner impede due administration of justice.

CONTRACT: Agreement by two or more parties to carry out some specific activity.

CONVICT: A person who has been proved guilty of a crime.

CORPUS DEFICTI: That which has constituted a breach of law.

CORPUS DELICT: That which has constituted a breach of law.

CRIME: A social harm which has been defined and made punishable by law.

CRIMINAL CASE: A case between two parties in the public interest, e.g. thefts, murder, assaults, etc. One party is the government through the police.

CRIMINAL LIABILITY: Responsibility imposed when a criminal statute, regulation or ordinance is violated.

CULPABLE: Blamable; censurable indicating a fault or a breach of legal duty which is not necessarily criminal.

DAMAGE: The injury suffered by a party.

DAMAGES: The amount of compensation payable to a party to whom injury has been done.

DECREE: A document under the seal of a Court setting out the relief granted to a party or parties.

DEFAMATION: Intentional communication of false personal or business information that injures the reputation or prospects of another. Spoken defamation is slander; written defamation is libel.

DE FACTO: In fact.

DEFENDANT: The person against whom a civil action is filed.

DE JURE: By right.

DEPOSITION: Evidence given on oath.

DOCUMENT: It means any matter expressed or described upon any substance by means of letters, figures or marks which may be used as evidence for that matter.

ESTOPPEL: A bar or impediment by law which prevents one from alleging or denying the truth in a court of law.

EX GRATIA: As a favour.

EXHIBIT: A document or thing produced for the inspection of Court, or sworn to a witness, giving evidence or referred to in a deposition.

EX OFFICIO: By virtue of his office.

EX PARTE: An application in judicial proceeding made (1) by an interested person who is not a party, (2) by one party in the absence of the other..

FELONY: A category of crimes more serious than a misdemeanor, e.g. murder, manslaughter, burglary, house-breaking, rape, etc. usually punishable by imprisonment or death.

FIAT: An order from a superior to an inferior law officer.

IBID: In the same place.

IDEM: The same.

IN CAMERA: The hearing of a case in private, e.g. in Court, the public being excluded.

INDEMNITY: State or obligation to imburse for losses.

INJUNCTION: Court commanding a person or entity to perform or to refrain from performing a certain act.

INJURY: A wrong done to one's person, property or rights.

INTER ALIA: Among others.

IPSO FACTO: By the mere fact.

MALAFIDES: Bad faith.

MALFEASANCE: The doing of a civil or unlawful act.

MALICE: An act committed with intent to cause injury or harm, without just cause or provocation.

MALICE AFORETHOUGHT: The element of evil in the crime of murder.

MANSLAUGHTER: Unlawful homicide not amounting to wilful murder.

MATERIAL EVIDENCE: Evidence relevant to the case, having a legitimate bearing on the decision.

MENS REA: (guilty mind): An evil intention, or knowledge of the wrongfulness of an act.

MISADVENTURE: An accident or mischance, unexpected and undesigned, arising out of lawful act.

MISDEMENOUR: Any crime or indictable offence not amounting to felony, such as perjury, conspiracy, and public nuisances.

MORAL TURPITUDE: An act of baseness, vileness, or depravity in private and social duties which a man owes to his fellowmen or to society in general, but not such acts as are not of themselves immoral, but whose illegality lies in the fact of their being positively prohibited by law.

MUTATIS MUTADIS: The necessary changes being made.

OBITER DICTUM: A generally accepted view. A Judge's comment.

OFFENCE: Any act or omission made punishable by law.

OVER ACT: An open act.

PARI PASSU: Equally; without preference.

PER SE: Taken alone; by itself.

PLAINTIFF: The person who files the suit.

POWER OF ATTORNEY: A formal instrument by which one person empowers another to represent him, or act in his stead for certain purposes.

PRECOGNITION: A statement or deposition which would form the basis of the oral testimony which a witness would give at subsequent trial.

PRIMA FACIE: At first sight; on the face of it; a fact presumed to be true unless proved otherwise.

PROVISO: A clause in a deed or other instrument beginning "provided always that".

REBUTTAL: Opposing or disproving evidence.

RES GESTAE: Remarks made by the victim at the time of or immediately after the crime are admissible as evidence, e.g. statements made to people at the scene or to the doctor in hospital.

RES JUDICATA: A matter already adjudged and decided.

RESPONDENT: The person against whom an appeal is filed.

SINE DIE: Indefinitely.

STATUTE: A written law enacted by a legislature to achieve a specified legislative object.

STATUTE OF LIMITATION: A statute which defines the period of time within which a suit or cause of action may be instituted.

STATUTORY: Concerning a statute or law of the state.

STATUS QUO: The state in which things are, or were.

SUB JUDICE: In course of trial.

SUIT: A civil proceeding in a civil Court of law.

SUMMONS CASE: A case relating to an offence, and not being a warrant case.

SUBPOENA DUCES TECUM: Subpoena that requires a person to personally present to the court a specified document or property possessed or under the person's control.

SUPRA: Above

TESTATOR: One who makes a will.

TESTIMONY: The oral evidence of a witness in Court.

TORT: A civil wrong. An act which causes harm to determinate person, whether intentionally or not.

TORT-FEASOR: A wrong-doer; one who is guilty of a tort.

TRESSPASS: Injury to the person or property of another, usually by violence.

ULTRA VIRES: An act in excess of the authority conferred by law and therefore invalid.

VERDICT: Court's decision at the end of the trial.

VIVA VOCE: By word of mouth.

VIZ (VIDELICET): Namely,

VOIR DIRE: To speak the truth; the preliminary questioning of a presented witness to determine his competency.

WARD: A minor or child under the protection and care of a guardian.

WARRANT: A written order for the arrest of persons, or for their forcible production in Court as witness.

WARRANT CASE: A case relating to an offence punishable with death, imprisonment for life or imprisonment for a term exceeding two years.

WILL: A document by which a person expresses his desire about the devolution and distribution of his property after his death.

WRIT: A document under the seal of Court, commanding the person to whom it is addressed to do or not to do some act.

WRIT OF SUMMON: A process issued in the High Court at the instance of the plaintiff for the purpose of giving the defendant notice of the claim made against him and of compelling him to appear and answer it, if he does not admit it.

APPENDIX-II

INDIAN AND INTERNATIONAL MEDICAL PROFESSION ACTS AND DECLARATIONS

THE INDIAN MEDICAL COUNCIL (PROFESSIONAL CONDUCT, ETIQUETTE AND ETHICS) REGULATIONS, 2002.

DUTIES AND RESPONSIBILITIES OF THE PHYSICIAN IN GENERAL: (1) A physician shall uphold the dignity and honour of his profession. (2) The prime object of the medical professional is to render service to humanity; reward or financial gain is a subordinate consideration. (3) A physician should be an upright man, instructed in the art of healing. He shall keep himself pure in character and be diligent in caring for the sick; he should be modest, sober, patient, prompt in discharging his duty without anxiety; conducting himself with propriety in his profession and in all the actions of his life. (4) The principal objective of the medical profession is to render service to humanity with full respect for the dignity of profession and man. Physicians should merit the confidence of patients entrusted to their care, rendering to each a full measure of service and devotion. Physicians should try continuously to improve medical knowledge and skills. The physician should practice methods of healing founded on scientific basis and should not associate professionally with anyone who violates this principle. The responsibilities of the physician extend not only to individuals but also to society. (5) A physician should affiliate with associations and societies of allopathic medical professions and involve actively in the functioning of such bodies. (6) A physician should participate in professional meetings as part of Continuing Medical Education programmes, for at least 30 hours every five years, organised by reputed professional academic bodies or other authorised organisations. (7) Every physician shall maintain the medical records pertaining to his indoor patients for a period of 3 years from the date of commencement of the treatment in a standard proforma. (8) He shall maintain a Register of Medical Certificates giving full details of certificates issued, and keep a copy of the certificates. He shall not omit to record the signature and/or thumbmark, address and at least one identification mark of the patient on the medical certificates or reports. (9) Efforts shall be made to computerise medical records for quick retrieval. (10) Every physician shall display the registration number accorded to him by the State Medical Council/Medical Council of India in his clinic and in all prescriptions, certificates, money receipts given to his patients. (11) Physician shall display as suffix to their names only recognised medical degrees or such certificates/diplomas and membership/honours, which confer professional knowledge, or recognise any exemplary qualification/achievements. (12) Every physician should, as far as possible, prescribe drugs with generic names and he shall ensure that there is a rational prescription and use of drugs. (13) Every physician should aid in safeguarding the profession against admission to it of those who are deficient in moral character or education. Physician shall not employ in connection with his professional practice any attendant who is neither registered nor enlisted under the Medical Acts in force and shall not permit such persons to attend, treat or perform operations upon patients wherever professional discretion or skill is required **(covering)**. (14) A physician should expose, without fear or favour, incompetent or corrupt, dishonest or unethical conduct on the part of members of the profession. (15) The personal financial interests of a physician should not conflict with the medical interests of patients. A physician should announce his fees before rendering service and not after the operation or treatment is under way. (16) It is unethical to enter into a contract of "no cure no payment". Physician rendering services on behalf of the state shall refrain from anticipating or accepting any consideration. (17) The physician shall observe the laws of the country in regulating the practice of medicine and shall also not assist others to evade such laws. He should be cooperative in observance and enforcement of sanitary laws and regulations in the interest of public health. (18) A physician should observe the provisions of the State Acts, Rules, Regulations made by the Central/State Governments or local Administrative Bodies relating to the protection and promotion of public health.

INDIAN MEDICAL COUNCIL (Professional conduct, Etiquette and Ethics) (Amendment) REGULATIONS, 2009, Part-I

In the 'Indian Medical Council (Professional Conduct, Etiquette and Ethics) Regulations, 2002, the following additions/modifications/deletions/substitutions, shall be, as indicated therein (Amendment, 2009).

In dealing with pharmaceutical and allied health sector industry, a medical practitioner shall follow and adhere to the stipulations given below:

(a) ***Gifts:*** A medical practitioner shall not receive any gift from any pharmaceutical or allied health care industry and their sales people or representatives.

(b) ***Travel Facilities:*** A medical practitioner shall not accept any travel facility inside the country or outside, including rail, air, ship, cruise tickets, paid vacations, etc. from any pharmaceutical or allied health care industry or their representatives for self and family members for vacation or for attending conferences, seminars, workshops, CME programme, etc. as a delegate.

(c) ***Hospitality:*** A medical practitioner shall not accept individually any hospitality like hotel accommodation for self and family members under any pretext.

(d) ***Cash or Monetary Grants:*** A medical practitioner shall not receive any cash or monetary grants from any pharmaceutical and allied healthcare industry for individual purpose in individual capacity under any pretext. Funding for medical research, study, etc. can only be received through approved institutions by modalities laid down by law/rules/guidelines adopted by such approved institutions, in a transparent manner. It shall always be fully disclosed.

(e) ***Medical Research:*** A medical practitioner may carry out, participate in, work in research projects funded by pharmaceutical and allied healthcare industries. A medical practitioner is obliged to know that the fulfillment of the following items (i) to (vii) will be an imperative for undertaking any research assignment/project funded by industry—for being proper and ethical. Thus, in accepting such a position a medical practitioner shall: (i) Ensure that the particular research proposal(s) has the due permission from the competent concerned authorities; (ii) Ensure that such a research project(s) has the clearance of national/state/institutional ethics committee/bodies; (iii) Ensure that it fulfills all the legal requirements prescribed for medical research; (iv) Ensure that the source and amount of funding is publically disclosed at the beginning itself; (v) Ensure that proper care and facilities are provided to human volunteers, if they are necessary for the research project(s); (vi) Ensure that undue animal experimentations are not done and when these are necessary they are done in a scientific and a humane way; (vii) Ensure that while accepting such an assignment a medical practitioner shall have the freedom to publish the results of the research in the greater interest of the society by inserting such a clause in the MoU or any other document/agreement for any such assignment.

(f) ***Maintaining Professional Autonomy:*** In dealing with pharmaceutical and allied healthcare industry a medical practitioner shall always ensure that there shall never be any compromise either with his/her own professional autonomy and/or with the autonomy and freedom of the medical institution.

(g) ***Affiliation:*** A medical practitioner may work for pharmaceutical and allied healthcare industries in advisory capacities, as consultants, as researchers, as treating doctors or in any other professional capacity. In doing so, a medical practitioner shall always: (i) Ensure that his professional integrity and freedom are maintained; (ii) Ensure that patients interest are not compromised in any way; (iii) Ensure that such affiliations are within the law; (iv) Ensure that such affiliations/employments are fully transparent and disclosed.

(h) ***Endorsement:*** A medical practitioner shall not endorse any drug or product of the industry publically. Any study conducted on the efficacy or otherwise of such products shall be presented to and/or through appropriate scientific bodies or published in appropriate scientific journals in proper way.

OBLIGATIONS TO THE SICK: (1) The health and the lives of those entrusted to his care depend on his skill and attention. A physician should endeavour to add to the comfort to the sick by making his visits at the hour indicated to the patients. (2) In case of emergency a physician must treat the patient. No physician shall arbitrarily refuse treatment to a patient. However when a patient is suffering from an ailment which is not within the range of experience of the treating physician, the physician may refuse treatment and refer the patient to another physician. (3) Medical practitioner having any incapacity detrimental to the patient or which can affect his performance vis-a-vis the patient is not permitted to practice his profession. (4) Patience and delicacy should characterise the physician. Confidences concerning individual or domestic life entrusted by patients to a physician and defects in the disposition or character of patient observed during medical attendance should never be revealed unless their revelation is required by the laws of the State. Sometimes, however, a physician must determine whether his duty to society requires him to employ knowledge, obtained through confidence as a physician to protect a healthy person against a communicable disease to which he is about to be exposed. In such instance, the physician should act as he would wish another to act towards one of his own family in like circumstances. (5) The physician should neither exaggerate nor minimise the gravity of a patient's condition. He should ensure himself that the patient, his relatives or his responsible friends have such knowledge of the patient's condition as will serve the best interests of the patient and the family. (6) A physician is free to choose whom he will serve. He should, however, respond to any request for his assistance in an emergency. Once having undertaken a case, the physician should not neglect the patient, nor should he withdraw from the case without giving adequate notice to the patient and his family. (7) In case of serious illness and in doubtful or difficult conditions, the physician should request consultation, which would be justifiable and beneficial to the patient. (8) Consulting pathologists radiologists or asking for any other diagnostic Lab investigation should be done judiciously and not in a routine manner. (9) All physicians engaged in the case should be frank with the patient and his attendants. (10) Utmost punctuality should be observed by a physician in making themselves available for consultations. (11) All statements to the patient or his representatives should take place in the presence of the consulting physicians, except as otherwise agreed. The disclosure of the opinion to the patient or his relatives or friends shall rest with the medical attendant. (12) Differences of opinion should not be divulged unnecessarily, but when there is irreconcilable difference of opinion the circumstances should be frankly and impartially explained to the patient or his relatives. It would be open to them to seek further advice if they so desire. (13) The attending physician may prescribe medicine at any time for the patient, whereas the consultant may prescribe only in case of emergency or as an expert when called for. (14) When a patient is referred to a specialist by the attending physician, a case summary of the patient should be given to the specialist, who should communicate his opinion in writing to the attending physician. (15) A physician shall clearly display his fees and other charges on the board of his chamber and/or the hospitals he is visiting. Prescription should also make clear if the physician himself dispensed any medicine. (16) A physician shall write his name and designation in full along with registration particulars in his prescription letterhead. **Note:** In government hospitals where the patient-load is heavy, the name of the prescribing doctor must be written below his signature. (17) In consultations, no discussion should be carried on in the presence of the patient or his representatives. (18) When a physician has been called for consultation, the consultant should normally not take charge of the case, especially on the solicitation of the patient or friends. The consultant shall not criticise the referring physician. He shall discuss the diagnosis and treatment plan with the referring physician. (19) Whenever a physician requests another physician to attend his patients during his temporary absence from his practice, the physician acting under such an appointment should give the utmost consideration to the interests and reputation of the absent physician and all patients should be restored to the care of the latter upon return. (20) When it becomes the duty of a physician occupying an official position to see and report upon an illness or injury, he should communicate to the physician in attendance so as to give him an option of being present. The medical officer/physician occupying an official position should avoid remarks upon the diagnosis or the treatment that has been adopted. (21) Physicians as good citizens, possessed of special training should disseminate advice on public health issues. They should play their part in enforcing the laws of the community and in sustaining the institutions that advance the interests of humanity. They should be particularly co-operative with the authorities in the administration of sanitary/public health laws and regulations. (22) Physicians, especially those engaged in public health work, should take measures for the prevention of epidemic and communicable diseases. When an epidemic occurs, a physician should not abandon his duty for fear of contracting the disease himself. (23) Physicians should recognise and promote the practice of different services, such as pharmacy and nursing as professions and should seek their cooperation wherever required. (24) A physician should consider it a pleasure and privilege to render gratuitous service to all physicians and their immediate family dependants.

UNETHICAL ACTS: A physician shall not aid or abet or commit any of the following acts which shall be construed as unethical. **(1) Advertising**: Soliciting of patients directly or indirectly, by a physician, by a group of physicians or by institutions or organisations is unethical. A physician shall not make use of his/her name as subject of any form or manner of advertising or publicity through any mode either alone or in conjunction with others which would ordinarily result in his self-aggrandisement. A physician shall not give to any person, whether for compensation or otherwise, any approval, recommendation, endorsement, certificate, report or statement with respect of any drug, medicine, nostrum remedy, surgical, or therapeutic article, apparatus or appliance or any commercial product or article with respect of any property, quality or use thereof or any test, demonstration or trial thereof, for use in connection with his name, signature, or photograph in any form or manner of advertising through any mode, nor shall he boast of cases, operations, cures or remedies or permit the publication of report thereof through any mode. A medical practitioner is however permitted to make a formal announcement in press regarding the following: (a) On starting practice. (b) On change of type of practice. (c) On changing address. (d) On temporary absence from duty. (e) On resumption of another practice. (f) On succeeding to another practice. (g) Public declaration of charges. (2) Printing of self-photograph, or any such material of publicity in the letterhead or on sign board of the consulting room or any such clinical establishment shall be regarded as acts of self-advertisement and unethical conduct on the part of the physician. However, printing of sketches, diagrams, picture of system shall not be treated as unethical. (3) A physician may patent surgical instruments, appliances and medicine or copyright application, methods and procedures. However, it shall be unethical if the benefits of such patents of copyright are not made available in situations where the interest of large population is involved. (4) A physician should not run an open shop for sale of medicines or dispensing prescriptions prescribed by doctors other than himself or for sale of medical or surgical appliances. It is not unethical for a physician to prescribe or supply drugs, remedies or appliances as long as there is no exploitation of the patient. Drugs prescribed by a physician or brought from the market for a patient should explicitly state the proprietary formulae as well as generic name of the drug. **(5) Dichotomy:** A physician shall not give, solicit, or receive nor shall he offer to give, solicit or receive any gift, gratuity, commission or bonus in consideration of, or return for the referring, recommending or procuring any patient for medical, surgical or other treatment. A physician shall not directly or indirectly, participate in or be a party to act of division, transference, assignment, subordination, rebating, splitting or refunding of any fee for medical, surgical or other treatment. (6) The prescribing or dispensing by a physician of secret remedial agents of which he does not know the composition, or the manufacture or promotion of their use is unethical and as such prohibited. All the drugs prescribed by a physician should always carry a proprietary formula and clear name. **(7) Human Rights:** The physician shall not aid or abet torture nor shall he be a party to either infliction of mental or physical trauma or concealment of torture inflicted by some other person or agency in clear violation of human rights. (8) Practicing euthanasia shall constitute unethical conduct. However, on specific occasion, the question of withdrawing supporting devices to sustain cardiopulmonary function even after brain death, shall be decided only by a team of doctors in accordance with the provisions of the Transplantation of Human Organs Act, 1994.

INTERNATIONAL CODE OF MEDIC AL ETHICS

An International Code of Medical Ethics (derived from the Declaration of Geneva) was originally adopted by the World Medical Association in 1949. The code was amended in 1968 and in 1983 and currently reads:

DUTIES OF PHYSICIANS IN GENERAL

A physician shall always maintain the highest standards of professional conduct.

A physician shall not permit motives of profit to influence the free and independent exercise of professional judgement on behalf of patients.

A physician shall, in all types of medical practice, be dedicated to providing competent medical service in full technical and moral independence, with compassion and respect for human dignity.

A physician shall deal honestly with patients and colleagues and strive to expose those physicians deficient in character or competence or who engage in fraud or deception.

The following practices are deemed to be unethical conduct: (a) Self-advertising by physicians, unless permitted by the laws of the country and the Code of Ethics of the National Medical Association. (b)

Paying or receiving any fee or other consideration solely to procure the referral of a patient or for prescribing or referring a patient to any source.

A physician shall respect the rights of patients, of colleagues and of other health professionals and shall safeguard patient confidences.

A physician shall act only in the patient's interest when providing medical care which might have the effect of weakening the physical and mental condition of the patient.

A physician shall use great caution in divulging discoveries or new techniques or treatment through non-professional channels.

A physician shall certify only that which he has personally verified.

DUTIES OF PHYSICIANS TO THE SICK

A physician shall always bear in mind the obligation of preserving human life.

A physician shall owe his patients complete loyalty and all the resources of his science. Whenever an examination or treatment is beyond the physician's capacity, he should summon another physician who has the necessary ability.

A physician shall observe absolute confidentiality on all he knows about his patient even after the patient has died.

A physician shall give emergency care as a humanitarian duty unless he is assured that others are willing and able to give such care.

DUTIES OF PHYSICIANS TO EACH OTHER

A physician shall behave towards his colleagues as he would have them behave towards him.

A physician shall not entice patients from his colleagues.

A physician shall observe the principles of the Declaration of Geneva approved by the World Medical Association.

DECLARATION OF TOKYO, 1975

The World Medical Association adopted the following guidelines for medical doctors concerning Torture and other Cruel, Inhuman or Degrading Treatment or Punishment in relation to Detention and Imprisonment. (1) The doctor shall not countenance, condone or participate in the practice of torture (physical or mental suffering) or other forms of cruel, inhuman or degrading procedure, whatever the offence of prisoners or detainees may be, and whatever be the victim's motives or beliefs, and in all situations, including armed conflict and civil strife. (2) The doctor shall not provide any premises, instruments, substances or knowledge to facilitate the practice of torture or other forms of cruel, inhuman or degrading treatment or to diminish the ability of the victim to resist such treatment. (3) The doctor shall not be present during any procedure during which torture or other forms of cruel treatment is used or threatened. (4) A doctor must have complete clinical independence in deciding upon the care of a patient. (5) If a prisoner refuses nourishment, and is capable of forming a rational judgement about the consequences, he should not be fed artificially. (6) The doctor shall in all circumstances be bound to alleviate the distress of his fellow men, and no motive shall prevail against this higher purpose.

The General Assembly of the United Nations, 1982, also approved a declaration on principles of "Medical Ethics Relevant to the Role of Health Personnel, particularly physicians, in the protection of the Prisoners and Detainees against Torture, and other Cruel, Inhuman or Degrading Treatment or Punishment".

OTHER IMPORTANT DECLARATIONS of the World Medical Association include: (1) The Declaration of Sydney (1968), concerning the definition of death. (2) The Declaration of Oslo (1970 & 1983), concerning therapeutic abortion. (3) The Declaration of Munich (1973), concerning racial, political discrimination, etc. in medicine. (4) The Declaration of Helsinki (1975), concerning human experimentation and clinical trials. (5) The Declaration of Lisbon (1981), concerning the rights of patient. (6) The Declaration of Venice (1983), concerning terminal illness. (7) The Declaration of San Paulo (1984), concerning pollution. (8) The Declaration of Madrid (1987), concerning professional autonomy and self-regulation. (9) The Declaration of Rancho Mirage (1987), concerning medical education. (10) The Declaration of Hong Kong (1989), concerning the abuse of the elderly. (11) The Declaration of Lisbon (1995), concerning the rights of the patient. (12) The Declaration of Helsinki (1996), concerning biomedical research involving human subjects. (13) The Declaration of Hamburg (1997), concerning support for doctors refusing to participate in torture or other forms of cruel, inhuman or degrading treatment. (14) The Declaration of Ottawa (1998), concerning the rights of the child to health care.

HUMAN EXPERIMENTATION

DECLARATION OF HELSINKI: World Medical Association drew up a Code of Ethics on human experimentation in 1964 which was revised in 1975.

(1) BASIC PRINCIPLES: Bio-medical research involving human subjects must conform to the moral and scientific principles that justify medical research, which should be based on scientifically established facts and animal and laboratory experiments. It must be conducted by qualified medical and other personnel and should be preceded by careful assessment of inherent risks in comparison to expected advantages to the subject or others. Particular care should be taken in research liable to lead to personality changes.

(2) CLINICAL RESEARCH COMBINED WITH PROFESSIONAL CARE: The doctor must be free to use a new therapeutic measure which is likely to save a patient's life, re-establish health or alleviate suffering and may be continued if justified by its therapeutic value for the patient, provided consent has been taken of the patient or his legal guardian.

(3) NON-THERAPEUTIC CLINICAL RESEARCH: A doctor's duty is to remain the protector of the life and health of a person, and as such, in a purely scientific clinical research, the involved risks should be explained and a free written consent should be taken from him or his legal guardian, with a proviso of his right to withdraw from the investigations whenever he likes. The right of parents or guardian to give consent is being questioned.

Human experimentation may be: (1) THERAPEUTIC experimentation is concerned primarily with improving the condition of a particular patient under treatment. (2) RESEARCH experiment is concerned primarily with using a human subject as a means of expanding scientific knowledge for the benefit of humanity. (3) INNOVATIVE experiments are therapeutic procedures that have not yet earned a place in medical practice.

Experimental procedures should not vary too radically from accepted methods, and they must be tried only after the failure of customary methods. The innovator must show that he possessed sufficient prior knowledge of the probability of success of the medical technique and of its collateral risks. He must know whether the probable success of the technique outweighs its collateral risks. Extensive animal research is an absolute pre-requisite to the use of an innovative technique in the treatment of human beings. The most difficult innovative cases

will be those in which prior animal research is impossible or would be uninformative. Any appraisal of an innovative technique's propriety must be made in the light of the patient's interests. The treatment should be given cautiously and its aftereffects should be noted and appreciated. Experiment on volunteers can only be justified if they do no significant harm to the subject and the results are likely to be beneficial.

It would be unethical to do something merely by way of experimentation, i.e. which is not strictly related to the cure of the patient's illness. There must also be no great risk in the proposed experimentation, even if the patient consents to run the great risk. A new experiment should not be undertaken merely to find out its efficacy, if there is already a treatment which is equally efficient. The experimentation should be stopped as soon as ill-effect is noted which should be immediately remedied. In considering whether a new treatment is as efficacious as an old one, side-effects of the two treatments and their cost should be considered.

ICMR GUIDELINES FOR HUMAN RESEARCH, 1995: The ICMR has laid down certain ethical guidelines for biomedical research on human subjects. It states that medical and related research using human beings should necessarily ensure that: (1) Purpose of such research is directed towards the increase of knowledge about human condition in relation to its social and natural environment. (2) Research is conducted under such conditions that the subjects are dealt with in a manner conducive to and consistent with their dignity and well-being. (3) Research must be subjected to a regimen of evaluation at all stages.

GENERAL PRINCIPLES: (i) Principle of essentiality: Whereby the research is considered absolutely essential after a due consideration of all factors and options involved. (ii) Principle of voluntariness, informed consent and community agreement: Wherby, the subjects are fully apprised of the research and the impact and risks to him and others; and he retains the right to abstain from further participation in the research irrespective of any obligation they may have entered, subject to only minimal restitutive obligations of any advance consideration received. (iii) Principle of non-exploitation: Whereby as a general rule the research subjects are remunerated for their involvement in the research or experiment. (iv) Principle of privacy and confidentiality: Whereby, the identity and records of the subjects are kept confidential as far as possible. (v) Principle of precaution and risk minimization: Whereby, due care and caution is taken at all stages of a research to ensure that the subjects are put to minimum risk and generally benefit from the experiment. (vi) Principle of professional competence: Whereby, the research is conducted at all times by competent and qualified persons who act with total integrity and impartiality and who have been made aware of the ethical considerations. (vii) Principle of accountability and transparency: Whereby, the research experiment will be conducted in a fair, honest, impartial and transparent manner after full disclosure of all aspects of their interest. (viii) Principle of maximization of public interest and of distributive justice: Whereby the research or experiment and its subsequent applicative use are conducted and used to benefit all humankind. (ix) Principle of institutional arrangement: Whereby, there shall be a duty on all persons connected with the research to ensure that all the procedures required to be complied with and all institutional arrangements required to be made in respect of the research and its subsequent use or application are duly made in a transparent manner. (x) Principle of public domain: Whereby, the research is brought into public domain so that its results are generally made known through scientific and other publications. (xi) Principle of totality of responsibility: Whereby, the professional and moral responsibility, for the due observance of all the principles, guidelines and prescriptions rests with all those involved in conducting the experiment. (xii) Principle of compliance: Whereby, there is a general and positive duty on all persons, conducting with any research entailing the use of a human subject to ensure that these guidelines are adhered in letter and spirit.

BIOETHICS: Bioethic is the study of ethical, social, and legal issues that arise in biomedicine and biomedical research. It includes medical ethics which focuses on issues in health care, research ethics which focuses on issues in the conduct of research. Bioethics is also moral discernment as it relates to medical policy, practice and research. It also includes the study of the more commonplace questions of values which arise in primary care and other branches of medicine. Bioethics are also concerned with the ethical questions that arise in the relationship among life sciences, biotechnology, medicine, politics, law and philosophy. It has addressed a large swathe of human inquiry, ranging from debates over the boundaries of life (e.g., abortion, euthanasia), surrogacy, the allocation os scarce healthcare resources (e.g., organ donation, healthcare rating) to the right to refuse medical care for religious or cultural reasons. The scope of bioethics can expand with biotechnology including cloning, gene therapy, life extension, human genetic engineering, astro-ethics, and life in space, and manipulation of basic biology through altered DNA, XNA and proteins. These developments will affect future evolution and may require new principles that address life at its core, such as bioethics that values life itself at its basic biological processes and structures and seek their propagation. Bioethecists conduct research on ethical, social, and legal issues arising in biomedicine. Environmental ethics focuses on issues pertaining to the relationship between human activities and the environment and public health issues.

THE WORKMEN'S COMPENSATION ACT, 1923: This Act provides for the payment of compensation to workmen for injuries sustained by them by accident, arising out of and in the course of employment. If a workman is killed, his dependants will be entitled to compensation for his death. Under the Act, if a workman contracts any disease specified therein as an occupational disease peculiar to that employment (anthrax, primary cancer of the skin, pathological manifestations due to X-rays, radium, etc., pneumoconiosis, poisoning by lead, phosphorus, mercury, arsenic), etc., it is deemed to be an injury by accident for purpose of compensation. The amount of compensation depends upon whether the injury has caused death, permanent total disablement, or permanent partial disablement.

Legally, disability is physical defect or impairment and the resulting actual or potential deterioration of social or economic status. Disability amounts to inability or incapacity to meet established standards of efficiency and social, occupational, or economic responsibility. Any reasonable medical sequence that connects a disability or death with an event at work is legally adequate grounds for awarding compensation. The employer will not be liable to pay compensation in respect of any injury which does not result in death or permanent total disablement, caused by an accident if the workman at the time of sustaining injury was under the influence of drink or drugs, or wilfully disregarded or removed any safety guard or other device provided for the safety. The workman is obliged to get himself examined by a qualified medical practitioner free of charge, either on the request of the employer or as directed by the Commissioner.

Medical examination: In all industrial diseases and injuries, medical evidence will be necessary. As such, it is important for a doctor to keep complete records of any injury sustained by an employee during the course of employment. It should be determined whether or not there is any causal relationship between an accident or injury and a death and of acceleration or aggravation of a pre-existing natural disease process. He should diagnose and evaluate the presence and extent of occupational disease. The medical certificate required to be issued in all these cases should be conscientious, accurate and without any favour.

CONSUMER PROTECTION ACT, 2019

Central, state, and district consumer councils to render advice, promote, protect, and enforce the rights of consumers have been established. Central Consumer Protection Authorities regulates matters relating to violation of rights of consumers, unfair trade practices, and false or misleading advertisements which are prejudicial to the interests of public and consumers and to promote, protect, and enforce the rights of consumers as a class.

Consumer Disputes Redressal Agencies: (1) Distric Commission consists of president and not less than two members nominated by State Governments. It entertains claims up to one crore rupees. (2) State Commission consists of president and four or more members. It entertains claims between one to ten crores. (3) National Commission consists of president and four or more members. It entertains claims over ten crores. If both complainant and opposite party agree for mediation, the commissions can refer the matter to Consumer Mediation Cell.

Consumer (E-Commerce rule), Central Consumer Protection Council Rules, Consumer Protection Regulation, and consumer protection mediation rules are framed in 2020. **The Act covers all private, corporate and public sector enterprises.** Services availed for commercial purposes have been excluded, thereby making them oriented only to the disputes of ordinary consumers.

Manner in which complaint shall be made: A complaint, in relation to any goods sold or delivered or any service provided or agreed to be provided may be filed with a District Commission by (a) consumer, (b) recognised consumer association, (c) one or more consumers, (d) Central or State Government. If the consumer dies, the legal heir or a representative can file the complaint. Each complaint made in a District Commission shall be charged a fee fixed by the State Government.

Procedure: Every complaint is heard as early as possible. If the complaint relates to any services, the District Commission shall refer a copy of such complaint to the opposite party within 21 days of the admission date, directing him to give his version of the case within a period of thirty days. Notices can be served even by fax. **It is not necessary for the parties to be represented by lawyers. The dispute is settled on the basis of evidence brought to its notice by the complainant and where** the opposite party denies or disputes the allegations contained in the complaint, or on the basis of evidence brought to its notice by the complainant where **the opposite party omits or fails to take any action to represent his case.** The District Commission has the same powers as are vested in a Civil Court (First Class Magistrate), under the Code of Civil Procedure, 1908. Every proceeding before the District Commission, shall be deemed to be a judicial proceeding within the meaning of S.193 and 228 of the Indian Penal Code, 1860, and the District Commission shall be deemed to be a Civil Court. Ordinarily, no adjournment is granted unless sufficient cause is shown. The reasons for adjournment are recorded and the orders for the costs of adjournment are passed.

Penalty: Whoever fails to comply with any order by District, State, or National Commission may be punished with imprisonment of not less than one month which may extend to three years, or with fine of 25 thousand to one lakh rupees.

Appeals: The aggrieved person can prefer an appeal to the State Commission within a period of 45 days from the date of the order. Further appeals can be made to National Commission and finally to Supreme Court, within a period of 30 days from the date of the order.

RELIEF: To make sure that the complainants get the relief by the Consumer Courts, they can attach the property of the opposite party and subsequently dispose it to recover the amounts due to the complainant. The District Collector will play a vital role for recovery of the amount from the opposite party.

CPA and medical services: The doctors and hospitals who render service as medical practitioners are liable for any act of 'medical negligence' and they can be sued for compensation under the Consumer Protection Act. Service rendered to a patient by a medical practitioner by way of consultation, diagnosis and treatment, both medical and surgical, at a Government hospital, health centre or dispensary, or at a non-government hospital or nursing home where charges are required to be paid by all persons or persons who are in a position to pay, and the persons who cannot afford to pay are rendered free of charge, fall within the purview of this Act. Service rendered at a Government hospital, health centre or dispensary, or at a non-government hospital or nursing home by a doctor attached or employed in a hospital or nursing home where no charge whatsover, is made from any person availing the services and all patients (rich and poor) are given free service is outside the purview of the Act. The payment of token amount for registration purpose only at the hospital or nursing home would not alter the position.

Compensation: No change is brought about in the substantive law governing claims for compensation on the ground of negligence. The principles which apply to determination of such a claim before the Civil Court, would equally apply to consumer dispute before the Consumer Dispute Redressal Agencies established under the Act. The doctors are liable to pay compensation to the patient, if their professional negligence results in injury or death of the patient. As there is no scope for testimony by medical experts, and the District commission or State Commission comes to its own conclusions, there is every likelihood of the justice being miscarried. A large number of frivolous cases are also likely to be filed against the doctors.

THE TRANSPLANTATION OF HUMAN ORGANS ACT 1994 AND RULES 1995 (AMENDED IN 2011 AND 2014)

The Act was amended in 2011, and 2014 and rules were framed in 2014 by the Centeral Government. Appropriate Authority is appointed by each state government. They can grant registration of hospitals for organ and tissue transplantation and establishment of tissue banks. They can remove, suspend, or cancel the registration and specify conditions for the same. If Appropriate Authorities refuse to grant registration, an apperal can be made central or state governments. They investigate any complaint of breach of any provisions of the Act, and periodically inspect hospitals and tissue banks. They have all powers of a civil court. The central and state governments constitute Advisory Commitiees to advice Appropriate Authority. Central governmnent maintains a National Registry of donors and recipients of human organs and tissues.

There are three main aspects of the Act: (1) It aims at putting a stop to live unrelated transplants. (2) In the case of a live related transplant, it defines that the donor and recipient are genetically related, with an exception if the transplant is done with prior approval of the Authorisation Committee on an application jointly made by the donor and recipient. (3) It accepts the brain stem death criterion. Certification of death by a panel of experts consisting of medical officer-in-charge of the hospital, an independent medical specialist, a neurologist or neurosurgeon, and the doctor treating the patient is essential. The Act defined human organ as any part of the human body consisting of a structured arrangement of tissues, which if wholly removed cannot be replicated by the body. Bone marrow transplant is outside the purview of the Act. The organs that can be donated after death are: kidney, heart, liver, lungs, pancreas, eyes, eardrums and ear bones. The organs can be removed from the dead body of any donor at any place. Removal of the organs from the donors may be done on his authorisation or that of the person lawfully in possession of the body. In case of unclaimed bodies in hospital or prison, organs can be removed after 48 hours. The organ removed should be preserved according to current and accepted scientific methods to ensure viability. The human organs cannot be removed for any purpose other than therapeutic purposes. The doctor should not remove organs unless he had explained all possible effects, complications and hazards connected with the removal and transplantation, to the donor and recipient respectively. The Act imposes for compulsory registration of hospitals engaged in the removal, storage or transplantation of human organs. The Central and State Governments are empowered to appoint Appropriate Authority which can grant registration of hospitals, renew, suspend or cancel the registration, etc. and to specify conditions for the same. The Government is also empowered to appoint Authorisation Committee or Committees with nominated members for the purpose of imposing restrictions on the removal and transplantation of human organs, etc.

The Ear Drums, Ear Bones Act, 1982 and Eyes Act, 1982, have been repealed.

Commercial Dealing in human organ and tissues is punishable with imprisonment up to 10 years and fine of Rs. 20 lakhs to 1 crore.

THE PROTECTION OF HUMAN RIGHTS ACT, 1993: Under the Act, regulations were made in 1993, and the Act was arranged in 2019. Human rights are rights of humans, relating to their life, liberty, and dignity. They belong to every person and are moral, pre-legal rights. The Act provides for constitution of a National Human Rights Commission (N.H.R.C.) and State Human Rights Commission (S.H.R.C.). The purpose of the Act is to provide better protection of human rights.

FUNCTIONS AND POWERS OF COMMISSION: (1) Inquire suo motu or on a petition violation of human rights or abetment thereof. (2) Intervene in any proceeding involving violation of human rights. (3) Visit any jail or institution and make recommendations. (4) Review safeguards provided by constitution and recommend for their implementation. (5) Review factors including acts of terrorism, that inhibit enjoyment of human rights. (6) Study treaties and other international instruments. (7) Undertake and promote research. (8) Spread human rights literacy among various sections of society and promote awareness of safeguards available. (9) Encourage the efforts of non-governmental organisations and institutions working in the field of human rights.

NHRC is not a judicial body. It has certain powers of civil courts for inquiry into complaints regarding summoning of witnesses, examine on oath, production of documents, etc. It calls for information or report from Central or State Government or any Authority or Organisation.

It can summon any person to give evidence and cause production of any document before it. It makes its recommendation for action, to the concerned Government, after completion of enquiry. It encourages functioning of different non-governmental organisations for protection of human rights. The functions of S.H.R.C. are similar to N.H.R.C.

In 1993, National Human Rights Commission has required all District Magsitrates/Superintendents of Police to report any instance of custodial death/torture or rape directly to it, within 24 hours of its occurrence, failing which, it will presume that an effort was being made to suppress the occurrence.

In 1995, NHRC has made it clear that the use of third degree methods in investigation constitutes violation of rights of citizens of India. If any person is arrested, the information should be given to the relative or friend about the arrest and place of detention. The compensation due to the next of the kin of those who have suffered custodial death should be the liability both of the State and the erring police officials.

Videography of autopsy is necessary only when the preliminary inquest by the Magistrate raises suspicion of any kind of foul play or where a complaint alleging any foul play has been made to the authorities or there is any other suspicion of foul play. The cassette has to be sent to the Commission along with the P.M. report.

ANIMALS IN RESEARCH: All animal experiments should be carried out for advancement of knowledge that is expected to be useful for saving or prolonging human life, alleviating suffering and combating disease, whether of human beings or animals or plants. Animals lowest on the phylogenetic scale (least degree of awareness), which may give scientifically valid results are to be preferred for experiments. Minimum number of animals should be used to give statistically valid results. Alternatives not involving animal testing should be given due consideration. The researchers should avoid or minimise pain and suffering to animals. All scientific procedures that may cause more than momentary pain should be performed with sedation or anaesthesia. After experimentation, euthanasia can be performed only when the animal is unable to perform its natural functions.

THE PRECONCEPTION AND PRENTAL DIAGNOSTIC TECHNIQUES (PROHIBITION OF SEX SELECTION) ACT, 1994 (AMENDED IN 2003)

It was amended in 2001 and 2003, and rules were made in 1996. Six months training rules were framed in 2014.

Diagnostic techniques cannot be conducted expect for the purpose of detection of any of the following abnormalities: (1) Chromosomal abnormalities. (2) Genetic metabolic diseases. (3) Haemoglobinopathies. (4) Sex-linked genetic diseases. (5) Congenital abnormalities. (6) Any other abnormalities or diseases may be specified by Central Supervisory Board.

Genetic Counselling Centres, Genetics Laboratories, Genetic Clinics, unless registered under the Act, cannot conduct or associate with, or help in, conducting activities relating to prenatal diagnostic techniques. They cannot employ or cause to be employed or take services of any person whether on honorary basis or on payment who does not possess the prescribed qualifications.

No Genetic Counselling Centres or Genetic Laboratories or Genetic Clinic or any person can conduct or cause to be conducted prenatal diagnostic techniques including ultrasonography for the purpose of determining the sex of the foetus. No person can cause or allow to be caused, selection of sex before or after conception.

Advertisement relating to preconception and prenatal determination of sex or sex selection is prohibited. Contravention is punishable with imprisonment up to three years and with fine up to ten thousand rupees.

Any medical geneticist, gynaecologist, registered medical practitioner or any person who owns a Genetic Counselling Centre, a Genetic Laboratory or a Genetic Clinic or is employed therein and renders his professional or technical services there, whether on an honorary basis or otherwise and who contravenes any of the provisions of the Act or rules made thereunder shall be punishable with imprisonment up to five years and with fine up to fifty thousand rupees. The name of the registered medical practitioner shall be reported to the State Medical Council concerned for taking necessary action.

Every Genetic Councelling Centre, Genetic Clinic or Genetic Laboratory, Ultrasound Clinic and Imaging Centre is required to maintain certain records such as names and address of patient and their spouse along with date on which they first reported. This record has to be maintained for a period of 2 years from date of completion of the procedure.

BIOMEDICAL WASTE (MANAGEMENT AND HANDLING) RULES, 1998 (AMENDED IN 2016 AND 2019)

The wastes produced may be of the following categories: (1) General waste. (2) Chemical waste. (3) Clinical waste. (4) Radioactive waste. (5) Pressurised containers.

The amount of waste generated per bed per day varies between 1 to 5 kg and the wastes may be: (1) Noninfectious—80% to 85%. (2) Infectious—10%. (3) Hazardous—5%.

Every State including Union Territory will establish Prescribed Authority with such members as is specified in the Rules, for authorisation and implementation of the Rule.

Government will also constitute an Advisory Committee comprising of experts in the field of medical and health, animal husbandry and veterinary science, environmental management, municipal administration and other related departments or non-Government organisations, along with representative form State Pollution Control Board/State Pollution Control committee. This committee will suggest the government and the prescribed authority for implementations of the Rules.

Rules for management and handling of biomedical wastes: (1) Bio-medical wastes cannot be mixed with any other wastes. (2) The waste should be segregated in separate container with proper leveling at the point of generation of such wastes and colour code of such containers are as follows: (a) Black – For non-infected chemical waste and cytotoxic drugs. (b) Red – For infected soiled waste (Infected dressings, POP casts). (c) Yellow – Infected anatomical waste (Placenta, pathological waste and body parts). (d) Blue – Infected plastics (Syringes, gloves and plastic waste) and (e) White – For Sharps (Needles, cut glasses). (3) No biomedical waste to be kept stored beyond 48 hours without the permission of the prescribed authority. (4) Transportation of such wastes can be done in such vehicles authorized for the purpose by competent Authority specified by the Government. (5) Wastes should be disposed of by: (a) Incineration. (b) Autoclave. (c) Micro-oven system. (d) Common waste treatment facility. And Prescribed authority sets up the standards for autoclaving, incineration, deep burial, micro-ovening for liquid waste and for disposal of treatment of bio-medical waste. (6) Proper recording of such disposal is compulsory.

The prescribed authority/environment pollution control board is conferred with the power of inspection and verification of such acts.

EMPLOYEE STATE INSURANCE ACT, 1948

It was amended in 2010, 2018 and 2019. The Act tries to attain the goal of socioeconomic justice. A machinery is provided for effective administration of Act, the apex body being ESI Corporation, subordinate to which are Standing Committee and Medical Benefit Council. The funds required are raised from contributions of employers, employees, and government. It provide a scheme for compulsory health insurance for industrial workers. It provides for establishment of hospitals, dispensaries, maternity centres and appointment of doctors to treat and certify about the health condition of workers and their dependants. The insured worker is entitled to periodical payment in case of sickness, maternity benefit, disabled benefit (including permanent partial or total disablement, dependants benefit, medical benefit, and funeral expenses. Employment injury means a personal injury to an employee caused by accident or an occupational disease arising out of and in the course of his employment. No other person except an Insurance Medical Officer is competent to medically examine an injured person. The medical certificate is in a prescribed form and there are separate forms prescribed for first examination (intermediate and final examination). The Insurance Medical Officer should fill in such forms as may be necessary with utmost care and accuracy and without favour.

THE PROTECTION OF WOMEN FROM DOMESTIC VIOLENCE ACT, 2005

Protection of Women from Domestic Violence Act passed to shield women from domestic abuse and harassment. It defines domestic violence as any form of physical, sexual, verbal, emotional or economic abuse or any threat of such abuse which is likely to cause injury or harm or endanger the life, limb or wellbeing of the aggrieved person. Offences covered under the act are Physical abuse (causing bodily pain, harm, danger to life, limb or health including criminal intimidation and criminal force to the aggrieved woman), Sexual abuse (conduct that abuses, humiliates, degrades or violates the dignity of a woman), Emotional abuse (any insult, ridicule or humiliation, directed at a woman including ridicule for not having a child or a male child and repeated threats to cause physical pain to the aggrieved or any person in whom the aggrieved person is interested), Economical abuse (depriving the aggrieved person of economic or financial resources to whom she is legally entitled to and restricting continued access to resources or facilities in which she has an interest by virtue of domestic relationship including access to the shared household). The case can be filed only by women against perpetrator with whom they are sharing a household such as daughter, sister, wife, daughter-in-law, widow, partner, granddaughter, etc. The act provides that person in-charge of medical facility shall be bound to provide medical aid to the aggrieved person if requested by her or on her behalf by a protection officer or a service provider.

APPENDIX-III

FORMULAE FOR ESTIMATION OF STATURE

Multiplication factors are based on the results obtained by dividing the average height of the body by the average length of the long bone in question.

Multiplication factors for estimating the stature for an individual of some States of India

		Pan (1924) Hindus of Bengal Bihar and Orissa		Nat (1931) Residents of United provinces (Uttar Pradesh)	Siddiqui and Shah (1944) Punjabis
		Males	Females	Males	Males
(1)	Humerus	5.31	5.31	5.3	5.3
(2)	Radius	6.78	6.7	6.9	6.4
(3)	Ulna	6.00	6.0	6.3	6.0
(4)	Femur	3.82	3.08	3.7	3.6
(5)	Tibia	4.49	4.46	4.48	4.4
(6)	Fibula	4.46	4.43	4.48	4.4

Asian males (cm)	/ (cm
2.68 × Humerus + 83.19	4.25
3.54 × Radius + 82	4.60
3.48 × Ulna + 77.45	4.66
2.15 × Femur +72.57	3.80
2.40 × Fibula + 80.56	3.24

Source: Trotter & Glesser (1952) modified by Jantz (1992) & organised by Byers (2002). Data for Asian females can be calculated from that obtained by Asian males multiplied by 0.92

Trotter and Glesser's Formulae (1952, 1958)

1. For **White Male subjects** –

Stature is equal to –

a) Lengths of (femur + fibula) × 1.31 + 63.05 cm; (error ± 3.63 cm).

b) " (femur + tibia) × 1.26 + 67.09 cm; (error ± 3.74 cm).

c) " (fibula) × 2.60 + 75.50 cm

d) " (femur) × 2.42 + 81.93 cm (error ± 3.94 cm)

e) " (tibia) × 2.42 + 81.93 cm (error ± 4 cm)

f) " (humerus + radius) × 1.82 + 67.97 (error ± 4.31 cm)

g) " (humerus + ulna) × 1.78 + 66.98 cm; (error ± 4.37 cm)

h) " (humerus) × 2.89 + 78.10 cm (error ± 4.57 cm)

i) " (radius) × 3.79 + 79.42 cm (error ± 4.66 cm)

j) " (ulna) × 3.76 + 75.55 cm (error ± 4.72 cm)

2. For **White Female** subjects –

Stature is equal to –

a) Length of humerus × 0.68 + length of femur × 1.7 + length of tibia × 1.15 in cm + 50.12 cm; (error ± 3.51 cm)

b) " (femur + tibia) in cm. × 1.39 + 53.20 cm; (error ± 3.55 cm)

c) " femur in cm × 1.48 + length of tibia in cm × 1.28 + 53.07 cm; (error ± 3.55 cm)

d) " fibula in cm × 2.93 + 59.61 cm (error ± 3.57 cm)

e) " tibia in cm × 2.90 ± 61.53 cm (error ± 3.66 cm)

f) " humerus in cm × 1.35 + length of tibia in cm × 1.95 cm + 52.77 cm; (error ± 3.72 cm)

g) " femur in cm × 2.47 + 54.10 cm (error ± 3.72 cm)

h) " radius in cm × 4.74 + 54.93 cm (error ± 4.24 cm)

i) " ulna in cm × 4.27 + 57.76 cm; (error ± 4.30 cm)

j) " humerus in cm × 3.36 + 57.97; (error ± 4.45 cm)

3. For **Negro Male** subjects –

Stature is equal to –

a) Length of (femur + fibula) in cm × 1.20 + 67.77 cm; (error ± 3.63 cm).

b) " (femur + tibia) in cm × 1.15 + 71.75 cm; (error ± 3.68 cm).

c) " femur in cm × 2.10 + 72.22 cm; (error ± 3.91 cm).

d) " tibia in cm × 2.19 + 85.36 cm; (error ± 3.96 cm).

e) " fibula in cm × 2.34 + 80.07 cm; (error ± 4.02 cm).

f) " (humerus + radius) in cm × 1.66 + 73.08 cm; (error ± 4.18 cm).

g) " (humerus + ulna) in cm × 1.65 + 70.67 cm; (error ± 4.23 cm).

h) " humerus in cm × 2.88 + 75.48 cm; (error ± 4.23 cm).

i) " radius in cm × 3.32 + 85.43 cm; (error ± 4.57 cm).

j) " ulna in cm × 3.20 + 82.77 cm; (error ± 4.74 cm).

4. For **Negro Female** subjects–

Stature is equal to –

a) Length of hemerus in cm × 0.44 + length of radius in cm × 0.20 + lenght of femur in cm × 1.46 + length of tibia in cm × 0.86 + 56.33 cm (error ± 3.22 cm).

b) " femur in cm × 1.53 + length of tibia in cm × 0.96 + 58.54 cm (error ± 3.23 cm).

c) " (femur + tibia) in cm × 1.26 + 59.72 cm; (error ± 3.28 cm).

d) " femur in cm × 2.28 + 59.76 cm; (error ± 3.41 cm).

e) " humerus in cm × 1.08 + length of tibia in cm × 1.79 + 62.80 cm; (error ± 3.58 cm).

f) " tibia in cm × 2.45 + 72.65 cms; (error ± 3.70 cm).

g) " fibula in cm × 2.49 + 70.90 cms; (error ± 3.70 cm).

h) " humerus in cm × 3.08 + 64.67 cms; (error ± 4.25 cm.)

i) " ulna in cm × 3.31 + 75.38 cms; (error ± 4.83 cm).

j) " radius in cm × 2.75 + 94.51 cms; (error ± 5.05 cm).

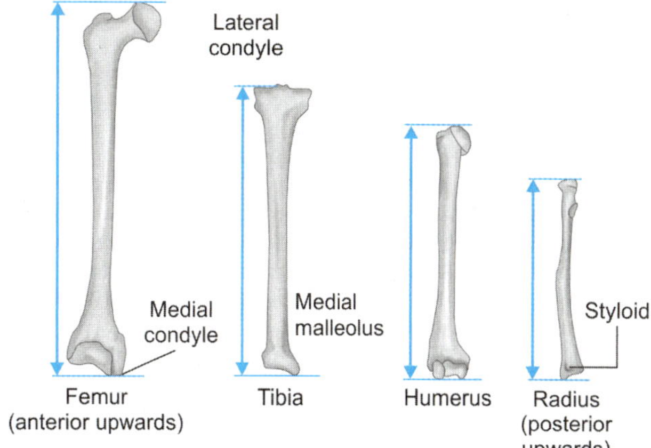

Dimensions of dried bones for estimations of stature (Trotter and Gleser, Dupertuis and Hadden). The right side bone is used for preference. **Femur:** With the bone lying anterior surface upwards, the maximum length is measured from the medial condyle to the most proximal part of the head. **Tibia:** Maximum length between tip of medial malleolus and face of lateral condyle. The intercondylar eminence is not included. **Humerus:** Maximum overall length from the posterior margin of the trochlea to the upper edge of the head. **Radius:** From the tip of the styloid process to the head, lying with the posterior surface upwards. All bones should be measured with an osteometric board. If the bones are not dry, but have articular cartilage in place, the following should be subtracted from the measured length before applying the formulae (Boyd and Trevor): radius and humerus 3 mm each, tibia 5 mm and femur 7 mm.

APPENDIX-IV

ANALYTICAL METHODS IN TOXICOLOGY

CHROMATOGRAPHY: It is a separation technique utilising partitioning characteristics of different chemical substances in different media. It depends upon the ability of a solvent to carry a substance with it as it diffuses in a medium which itself tends to hold back that substance. The substance will have moved a constant distance after a given time, in which the solvent has been allowed to diffuse. The ratio of the distance travelled by the substance to the distance travelled by the solvent is known as the Rf value of the substance for that particular system. Several substances may have the same Rf value in a given set of circumstances, but they can be separated by using different systems. Identification of the substance, then rests on comparing the disclosed Rf values with those which are detailed in reference tables. It is used in the analysis of organic substances.

(1) THIN-LAYER CHROMATOGRAPHY (TLC): It is the simplest analytical technique commonly used for qualitative screening of large batches of (usually organic solvents) samples. A very thin layer of a substance such as permutit, silica gel or aluminium oxide is applied to a glass plate of 20 × 20 × 0.5 cm. as ion exchange resins. Vertical lines are drawn 1.5 cm. apart to allow individual runways for each sample. Purified tissue extracts dissolved in 0.5 ml of methanol are serially spotted with a micropipette and dried in a small circle in the lower centre of a runway 1.5 cm. from the bottom. Other samples are similarly spotted in other runways. A horizontal line (stop point) is drawn 10 or 15 cm. above these starting points. A TLC tank is filled with suitable developing solvents to a depth of about one cm. from the bottom. The plate properly spotted is then dipped into the solvent, the lid is firmly closed and the atmosphere is allowed to saturate with vapour. When the solvent front just touches the 10 cm. horizontal mark, the plate is removed and examined under UV light (at 254 nm and 366 nm) for characteristic fluorescence or absorbance. The separated compounds are stained by using a number of chemical sprays. The compounds are identified based on their staining characteristics and distance of migration when compared to known standards. The test is completed in two hours. This lacks specificity.

Approximate quantitation can be done by comparison with standards similarly prepared on the same plate, for intensity of colour and area size. The order of separation of compounds can be altered simply by changing the nature of the developing agent.

(2) PAPER CHROMATOGRAPHY: Paper is used as the support or adsorbent, but partition probably plays a greater part than adsorption in the separation of the components of mixtures, as the cellulose fibres have a film of moisture around them even in the air-dry state.

(3) COLUMN CHROMATOGRAPHY (HPLC): It is of two types, (a) adsorption chromatography, (b) partition chromatography.

(4) HIGH-PRESSURE LIQUID CHROMATOGRAPHY (HPLC): This is similar to gas chromatography, except that the sample is in a liquid state rather than in a volatile state. This technique can be used to separate and to analyse complex mixtures. This is similar to gas chromatography, except that the sample is in a liquid state rather than in a volatile state. A high pressure (1000 to 6000 pounds per square inch) pump facilitates movement of the specimen through the columns packed with chromatographic adsorbents, e.g. silica gel and alumina. The effluent stream passes through a detector, usually an ultraviolet spectrophotometer, and the appearance of a drug in the solvent is signalled by a recorder peak in the same way as in GC. Again, the size of the peak is proportional to the concentration of drug in the sample. It can quantitate both the drug and its metabolites in a single analysis. This test is not 100% specific.

(5) GAS CHROMATOGRAPHY (GC): It simultaneously separates, identifies and measures drugs and other organic poisons. It is a thermal chamber or oven, in which temperature can be precisely controlled. A long thin spiral tube (column) packed with finely divided solid (carbowax or adiponitrile) coated with a viscous liquid is instilled in it. This liquid is known as stationary phase. About one ml of sample to be analysed is injected by means of a gas-tight syringe into injection port situated at one end of the column. The sample is forced through the column by pressurised streams of carrier gas (helium) known as the mobile phase. At the end of the column, the sample is separated into bands of like molecules, which pass through a flame ionisation detector. The ionised gases generate electrical signal, which is amplified and used to power a mechanical stylus (pen) which produces a chromatogram, into a strip of moving chart paper. This is compared with a known reference standard, to identify a compound present in the unknown mixture. The position of the peak along the chart paper identifies the substance. The area of the peak indicates its approximate concentration. The chromatograph can analyse only liquids and gases, but if a pyrolyser is attached to it, organic solids can also be identified. GC is extremely sensitive and can analyse a number of compounds simultaneously. It is commonly used to quantitate blood levels of volatile liquids, such as ethanol, methanol, ethylene glycol, etc.

Electron capture detector, and the alkali flame detector (nitrogen detector) widen the scope of plasma screening.

(6) SPECTROPHOTOMETRY: The principle involved in spectrophotometry is that there should be no difference between the intensities of the sample and reference beams at all times. Light from the appropriate source which is selected automatically, is passed through the prism. The beam is switched alternatively through the sample and reference beams, produces an electrical signal from the photomultiplier. In spectrophotometer for use in the ultraviolet and visible regions of the spectrum, the sample compartment is placed so that radiation emerging from the monochromator passes through solutions.

(A) MASS SPECTROMETRY: It detects a substance in minute quantity. The testing material in trace amount is placed inside a high-vacuum chamber and is then collided by high energy electrons. This causes loss of electron from the molecules of the testing material which get positively charged. These molecules breakdown instantaneously into numerous fragments, which are then separated according to their mass, by passing them through an electromagnetic field. The graphic presentation of the minute particles of the mass as obtained subsequently, by the same process as applied in case of U.V. or I.R. spectrometry gives a complex pattern with qualitative and quantitative assessment of the material tested. The lines in the graph represent the mass and the height of the lines represent the quantity of each fragmented mass. Thus, the whole graph acts as an unique picture for a material. Mass spectroscopy is applicable only in case of testing some pure material. In case of possible admixture or impurity, the components of the material may first be subjected to fractional separation by gas chromatography and then tested by mass spectrometry for identification and estimation of each type of matter present in the complex. Chemical ionisation mass spectrometry is an easier process to identify components of a mixture without application of gas chromatography beforehand.

(B) INFRARED SPECTROPHOTOMETRY: This instrument is useful for the identification of organic compounds, because each compound has a characteristic spectrum based upon its structure. The use of KBr or KI pelleting process for solids allows accurate determination of drugs and chemicals in the range of 2 to 1000 µg.

(C) ATOMIC ABSORPTION SPECTROPHOTO- METRY (AAS): Here, an element or compound is subjected to the contact of acetylene air flame or a graphite furnace, or a heated strip of metal for vapourisation of atoms of the specimen. Radiation from a light source of similar type is directed towards the vapourised atoms which absorbs the radiation energy with displacement of electrons from the outer circle of the atom. This movement of the electrons emit energy which is passed through a manometer and then the selective radiation is processed through the detector and recorded graphically, which identifies the element's presence in the component. Inductively Coupled Plasma Atomic Emission Spectroscopy (ICP-AES) is a new development that allows simultaneous multi-element analysis. Seventeen elements can be measured from a single sample; aluminium, barium, cadmium, chromium, copper, iron, lanthanum, lead, manganese, molybdenum, nickel, platinum, silver, strontium, tin, titanium and zinc.

(D) SPECTROFLUORIMETRY: Spectrofluorimetry bears the same relationship to fluorimetry as spectrophotometry does to absorptimetry, i.e., the intensity of fluorescence can be measured at different wavelengths to give a fluorescence emission spectrum. The technique provides additional data in the sense that it is possible to reproduce the absorption curve of fluorescent substance as an excitation spectrum at a concentration very much less than those required in spectrophotometry. In spectrofluorimetry on the other hand, a distinction is required between a very weak intensity of fluorescence and that of still weaker fluorescence of blank, and this difference is very smaller than that measurable in spectrophotometry.

(E) ULTRAVIOLET SPECTROPHOTOMETRY (UVS): This technique is based on the principle that many drugs when in solution will absorb UV radiation. The degree of absorption depends on the chemical structure of the drug, its concentration in the solution, and the wavelength of the UVR. The monochromator can select from the light source an ultraviolet ray of any given wavelength ranging from 200 to 340 nm. The sample extract in aqueous medium is placed in a transparent quartz cuvette in the path of the radiation.

The amount of UV radiation which passes through the solution is measured by the photocell. By steady rotation of the monochromator, it is possible to pass sequentially UV rays of all wavelengths from 200 to 340 nm through the extract. The photocell monitors the amount of radiation absorbed at each wavelength and this is transcribed on to a recorded chart. The shape of the spectrum, the wavelength at which absorption is at a maximum, and any changes brought about by changing the pH of the extract are all used as an aid to characterise the agent present. This technique is ideal to quantitate blood levels of paracetamol and salicylates, as well as urine levels of phenothiazines.

(F) EMISSION SPECTROGRAPH : Every element, on being excited appropriately, emits light spectrum. The spectrum can be separated and recorded by photography. The element to be tested is placed in between two carbon electrodes to vapourise and excite the particles of vapour which then emits light, which is then passed through a lens and then through a prism to spread the spectrum which is again passed through another lens to focus it on a screen to be photographed for further study and preserving as record. None of the elements give similar line of spectrum and from the bands of spectrum and dark bands the element can be identified.

In case of a compound, many lines of spectra are recorded having a specific type for each element. From the combination of different lines of spectra, the elementary combination of the component can be assessed and then the compound can be identified and compared with another by similar test. A modification of the process may be adapted by use of laser beam at the initial phase to vapourise the compound. Rest of the test, i.e., exciting of the elements of the compound by carbon electrodes and the subsequent process is same as in the other variety of emission spectroscope.

(7) GAS CHROMATOGRAPHY-MASS SPECTRO- METRY (GC-MS): In this gas chromatography separates the drugs and a mass spectrometer positively identifies them. This method of analysis is 100% specific. It separates the components of biologic extracts and sensitively detects toxic agents in a complex matrix of biochemicals. By means of chemical ionisation and single or multiple ion monitoring techniques, picrogram quantitative analyses are possible.

About one ml sample is injected into the GC and separated on various types of chromatography columns. Syringes, empty capsules and biologic fluids can be analysed for drugs. A column that is selected has good constituent separation, a large range of unstable temperatures and a low background bleed. Helium is used an a carrier gas and is eliminated after chromatography by a jet separator or a diffusion membrane.

As in all mass spectrometers, neutral molecules from the gas chromatograph enter the ion source and are ionised by a stream of electrons, e.g. El-electron Impact Mass Spectrometry. Positively charged ions predominate and are used in the analysis. Ionisation under standard electron energy conditions always occurs at the same bonds in the molecule, thus permitting a reproducible pattern of ions into the quadruple filter, are detected by an electron multiplier, and the amplified signal is displayed as the mass spectrum on an oscilloscope or oscillographic recorder. The total ion current (with a peak for each component separated by the GC and entering the MS represents the usual gas chromatogram and is continuously plotted on a simple potentiometric recorder as the GC-MS analysis proceeds. The output signal can be fed to a computer or data-processing system for storage and manipulation. Both the mass values of the molecule fragments and their relative abundance are qualitatively characteristic of the compound analysed. In the mass spectrum, the most abundant ion is referred to as the base peak and the unfragmented, but positively charged molecule as the molecular ion or parent molecule. The horizontal axis of the spectrum graph represents atomic mass number in which the charge is usually one.

DATA INTERPRETATION: The data that are available following a toxicological analysis of a blood, urine or tissue sample, using GC-MS instrumentation is: extraction characteristics which indicate chemical character (acid, base, neutral) of the compound, the GC retention time relative to a standard compound providing a first presumptive identity, and the mass spectrum which displays the unique molecular fragmentation pattern of the compound. This information must be in consonance before a final specific identification is acceptable. The GC-MS data are compared to libraries of GC retention times and mass spectra of standard compounds to match the unknown to a compound in the library. Following the library search, the teletype prints out the most likely identification according to the least number of mismatches between the unknown and the stored standard. If the library is stored in an inhouse dedicated computer or GC-MS interactive data system, the results can be displayed on a CRT (cathode ray tube) screen very rapidly for comparative inspection, and spectra automatically plotted in normalised form by the computer. A reconstructed gas chromatogram, either total ion display or limited mass search, can also be plotted.

COMPUTER: The dedicated computer or interactive data system expands the instrument capability to an extraordinary degree. No analytical data are lost because the computer can continuously accept, normalise and store 3-second mass spectrum scans as the gas chromatography analysis proceeds in real time. Therefore, in a typical 10 minute GC run, 200 mass spectra will be obtained. The data system is vital to the best quantitative GC-MS analysis and qualitative processing of raw data.

IMMUNOASSAY METHODS: (1) Radioimmunoassay (RIA). (2) Fluorescent immunoassay. (3) Enzyme-mediated immunoassay technique (EMIT). These are convenient methods of screening for a specific drug or group of drugs. The basis for these methods is detection of the reaction between an antibody for the drug and the drug.

RIA is a very sensitive and less specific technique for quantitative analysis. Mixing known quantities of drug-specific antibody and known amounts of radioactive labelled drug to the specimen to be analysed causes a precipitation reaction. The precipitate is removed and measured with a gamma counter. The gamma emittance is inversely related to the quantity of assay drug present in the patient's specimen. It detects very low concentrations of drugs, such as cannabis, digoxin, LSD, paraquat, etc.

EMIT is very useful for quantitative analysis of many popular drugs and substances of abuse. It is specific but less sensitive than RIA and is much easier to use and produces results more rapidly. It works on the principle that the amount of drug present is proportional to the inhibition of an enzyme-substrate reaction. A known quantity of a drug is labelled by chemical attachment to an enzyme. Drug specific antibodies added to the specimen bind the drug-enzyme complex, thereby reducing enzyme activity. Free drug in the specimen competes with enzyme labelled drug and limits the antibody-induced enzyme inactivation. Enzyme activity correlates with drug concentration in the specimen as measured by absorbance change resulting from the enzyme catalytic action on a substrate.

NUCLEAR MAGNETIC RESONANCE (NMR): It can perform both definitive substance identification and screening of body, but sensitivity is much lower than GC-MS.

MELTING POINT APPARATUS: Melting point is determined in a capillary tube and this can be matched with results given in a standard reference book.

BOILING POINT: The boiling point of a liquid is the temperature at which it passes wholly into a gas. Reference to standard boiling points of liquids leads to identity of an unknown liquid.

CRYSTAL STRUCTURE: The identification involves microscopic crystallographic observations of optical phenomenon and measurement of physical constants for positive identification of crystalline compounds.

ULTRAVIOLET SPECTROSCOPY: Many drugs have characteristic ultraviolet spectra, but they must be extracted from body fluids.

REFRACTOMETER: Toxic substances can be readily identified from their index of refraction.

CALORIMETER: It measures the amount of transmitted light of substances.

POLARIMETER: As many drugs and synthetic poisons are optically active, they can be identified through this physical property.

POLAROGRAPHY: This is an electro-chemical method of analysis.

ELECTROPHORESIS : Different protein components of different body fluids are identified by this method. The stationary phase is made of starch or agar gel on a glass slide. The testing material is placed at one end of the stationary phase (gel layer on the slide). Electrodes are attached at both ends of the gel slide. Electrically charged protein component moves on the phase plate and at the end, the gel plate is treated with the colouring agent for the protein which causes appearance of visible characteristic bands depending on the characters of the protein.

NEUTRON ACTIVATION ANALYSIS

It is based on the principle that many substances become radioactive when exposed to bombardment by neutrons which is highly specific of the elements contributing to it. This is a highly sophisticated and expensive method of detection of a variety of inorganic elements at levels well below the limits of conventional analytical techniques. The sensitivity attained is 100 or even 1000 times better than by any other method. The induced radioactivity is highly specific of the elements contributing to it.

When an atom is bombarded with a neutron, isotope of the atom with increased number of neutron develops. However, most of such newly formed isotopes are decomposed and there is radioactive decay of the isotopes. There is radioactivity in the process with liberation of alpha, beta and gamma rays. Alpha rays are positively charged particles, beta rays are electrons and gamma rays are electromagnetic radiation. In a neutron reactor, neutron is bombarded to an atom which enters the nucleus of the atom and during disintegration, the gamma ray radioactivity is liberated. This has characteristic energy value which is assessed by means of either a Geiger counter or a scintillation counter to know the atom of the element.

Many elements can be studied at a time inside a reactor. The characteristic energy value of gamma rays identifies the type of the element and the intensity of gamma ray radiation gives the concentration of the element in a substance.

It identifies an element or compound in one billionth of a gram. Neutron activation analysis can be used for the estimation of any of the 90 naturally occurring elements including antimony, arsenic, cadmium, copper, iron, lead, mercury, phosphorus, selenium, thallium and zinc. Since the trace elements present in hairs, nails, gun powder, drugs, paint, grease, glass, soil, etc. form a unique pattern, characteristics of their source, the method can render valuable aid in identification when comparison samples are available.

APPENDIX-V

FORENSIC MICROSCOPY

MICROSCOPES IN FORENSIC USE

(1) COMPARISON MICROSCOPE: It is basically two microscopes with identical optical system to give the same magnification, joined together by a comparison bridge and eye-piece, and permits the viewing of a portion (usually half) of the field of view from each microscope, side by side with a sharp dividing line in the eyepiece, which may be of either monocular or binocular type. The examiner can view a portion of two different bullets or cartridges simultaneously in a single microscopic field,. Light rays from the surface of both the bullets are reflected and observed through the common eyepiece of the microscope. By adjustment of the positions of the two bullets, the reflected light rays from the primary marks of the two bullets are brought in the same line and observed whether they tally. Similarly, marks on the two bullets are brought closer on the same line. If the marks on the two bullets tally in their dimensions and curvature, it can be opined that the bullet causing the death of the victim was fired from the gun examined.

(2) STEREOSCOPIC MICROSCOPE: It can be used to examine bullets, cartridges, gun powder and other cartridge components, and bullet holes and surfaces around such holes, as well as surfaces of firearms or firearm parts. In this two eyepieces give pictures of two planes of the material examined, giving a 3 dimensional image. It is a reflection microscope which gives surface view of trace elements present on the surface of some other object. The field of view being wider, a wider surface can be examined. The magnification is 15 to 125.

(3) FLUORESCENT MICROSCOPE: By this type only certain specific items can be studied. The specimen treated with fluorescent agent, after absorption of invisible short wavelength, high frequency rays (e.g. U.V. rays), cause emission of rays of longer wavelength and lesser frequency, so as to make the emitted rays visible due to presence of fluorescent agent.

(4) POLARISING MICROSCOPE: In this polariser and analyser are used, the former in between the source of light and the object of study, and the latter (the analyser) in between the object and the eye piece. Though light passes in straight lines in all directions, some materials allow the light (passed through it), to travel in one plane only and not in all directions. This is the function of both polariser and analyser. A polarising lens turns the path of light rays passed through it, to pass in one direction only. The analyser (which is actually another polariser), is used to ascertain, whether the polariser limited the path of light passed through it, in one plane or not. When the analyser is placed in a perpendicular plane, in comparison to the placement of the polariser, then it can be understood if light from the matter tested, was polarised by polariser or not, as in such a case the analyser being placed in the stated manner, will change the pathway of the light rays coming in one plane, after passing through the polariser and will not be visible. Placement of the analyser then, in the same plane of the polariser will cause the light rays to pass in the same direction and the matter will now be visible, if looked through the microscope. By this method, nature of dispersion of light rays by the tested specimen will be known. In this way a polarising microscope identifies the nature of the specimens tested (mostly minerals), from their nature of dispersion.

(5) ELECTRON MICROSCOPE OR SCANNING ELECTRON MICROSCOPE (S.E.M): This is used in the study of surface of some objects, so as to identify it, or any trace material, up to the level of elements. The use of S.E.M. gives highly magnified detail picture of the surface of the material tested for trace element, as well as, a graphic presentation of electrons emitted by the element present in the testing substance which gives clear identification of the trace elements.

Beam of electrons is emitted from a hot tungsten filament. These electron beams are focussed on the surface of the testing material by means of electromagnets. The focussed primary electrons cause emission of electrons from the surface of the testing material. These emitted electrons are scanned, amplified and fed into a cathode ray tube to be converted and focussed on a screen to produce magnified pictures. The magnification of the image may be up to one lakh times than the real dimension of the testing particles. The depth of the picture is about 300 times more than other surface microscopes and the magnified image of surface of the testing material has a 3 dimensional stereoscopic appearance. This helps identification of minute trace elements present on the surface of matter, the exact nature of which is required to be known. Electrons, striking surface of the testing material, also produce X-ray which is deflected from the surface. With the help of an X-ray analyser and recorder, the amount of X-ray emitted, and its character can be known which will identify the elements present on the surface of the examined sample.

It is used to analyse paints, metals, fibres and other similar items. The consistency of a paint layer and its irregularities can best be examined and noted with SEM. It can be used along with X-ray fluorescence. Very small particles can be observed, and elemental constituent data can be obtained. The edges of paint chips can be analysed and the differences in elemental makeup can be identified and compared to other paint chips.

APPENDIX-VI

POSTMORTEM REQUISITION AND POSTMORTEM EXAMINATION

No. .... Date ....
From
To
Sir,

You are requested to hold a postmortem examination on the body of .... sent herewith through (name) .... H.C./P.C.No. Please furnish your report on the attached form.

It is to be particularly noted that the examination should extend to every part of the body.

Place : Station House Officer

REPORT TO BE FORWARDED WITH THE BODY SENT FOR POSTMORTEM EXAMINATION

(1) PRELIMINARY PARTICULARS :

Name :	
Aged about	**years**
Male/Female	**Approximate height cm.**
Colour of eyes:	**Colour of hair:**
Marks of identification: (1)	**(2)**
Village :	**Caste :**
Found/Died at	**A.M./P.M. on**
at (place)	**sent by in-charge**
of P.S.	**with P.C./Head-constable No.**
on at	**A.M./P.M.**

(2) The following wounds are found on the body:

(3) The manner in which and the weapon or instrument (if any) with which the wounds mentioned in item No.2 appear to have been inflicted:

(4) The following articles are sent with the corpse:

Clothes	**:**	**Ornaments - Jewellery :**
Excreta	**:**	**Vomit :**
Weapons	**:**	
Station	**:**	
Date	**:**	**Investigating Police Officer**

POSTMORTEM CERTIFICATE

Postmortem report is also known as **postmortem certificate** in some states while at some places postmortem certificate means a small document which has basic information of the deceased and has name, s/o; w/o; d/o, age, sex, ID, address, date and time of postmortem with main brief cause of death. It is issued along with dead body to relatives for the purposes of transport of body, cremation or burial, and family use. It bears signature and stamp of doctor conducting postmortem. The details of the autopsy are given in postmortem report as given here.

INSTRUCTIONS: (1) It is essential that in all cases, the autopsy should be a complete one. If a complete autopsy is not carried out by the Medical Officer, evidence which later may prove of great medicolegal importance may be irretrievably lost and the course of justice may be impeded. The responsibility of carrying out of complete autopsy must rest solely with the Medical Officer. (2) The identity of the body should be confirmed to the doctor by a police officer. If the identity is not known, all methods of establishing identity must be used. (3) The body should be examined with clothing in place, so that defects caused by trauma can be identified. After removal, clothing must be retained in clean bags and labelled. (4) The body should be photographed clothed, and then unclothed, and then any injuries or other abnormalities should be photographed in closer detail. (5) X-rays are advisable in victims of gunshot wounds and explosions. (6) The surface of the body should be examined for the presence of trace evidence, i.e. fibres, hair, blood, semen, saliva, etc. Fingernail clippings, head and pubic hair, anal and genital swabs, bitemarks, swabs, etc., if necessary should be taken by the doctor. (7) Careful documentation of all external injuries or abnormalities, their type, position, size, shape, etc., is most important and often has much greater value in understanding and in reconstructing the circumstances of injury than the internal dissection. (8) All body cavities should be opened and all the internal organs inspected in situ. All internal organs should then be removed and should be individually dissected and examined to identify injuries and any natural disease. (9) The removal and examination of the organs should be personally carried out by the Medical Officer. (10) All injuries or abnormalities found should be briefly, but fully and accurately described. Abnormal collections of fluid, e.g. pleural, pericardial, peritoneal, etc. should be accurately measured. The relative number, sizes, and distribution of petechial haemorrhages occurring in the substance of or on the surface (pericardial, pleural, etc.) of organs should be noted. When organs appear normal, the appropriate line of report should be endorsed "NOTHING ABNORMAL NOTED". Negative findings should be stated as they may be as important as positive findings. When, for any reason, organs are not examined, the appropriate line of the report should be endorsed "NOT EXAMINED"; it should not be merely left blank, because in court, the absence of a comment may be taken to mean, that it was not examined or specifically looked for. (11) The schedule of observation should be restricted entirely to the recording of facts as found by the Medical Officer at the autopsy. (12) Take the weight of all main internal organs. Tissue samples should be taken as necessary for histopathology and preserved in formalin. (13) Blood should be collected from a large limb vein, preferably from the femoral vein and urine by a syringe through the fundus of the bladder. (14) All signs of recent or old medical and surgical intervention and resuscitation must be described. (15) Make careful notes and drawings and diagrams. (16) In cases of suspected poisoning, the stomach and its contents, 30 cm. of upper part of small intestine and its contents, 500 gm. liver, half of each kidney, 30 ml of blood and 30 ml of urine should be retained for chemical examination. Clean, wide-mouthed, white bottles of one litre capacity fitted with glass stoppers should be used for viscera. Blood should be collected in screw-capped bottle of about 30 ml. (17) Preserve the stomach, and its contents together with a piece of the upper part of small intestine in one bottle; small pieces of the liver and kidney in another bottle, and blood and urine in separate bottles. These viscera are to be preserved in rectified spirit or saturated solution of common salt. Seal and label the bottles. A sample of preservative used should always be sent for chemical analysis. (18) Interpret the overall findings so that the maximum information and opinion can be offered. (19) The report should be full, detailed, legible, comprehensive and objective. The report should be completed as soon as possible after the autopsy and the original postmortem report sent direct to the concerned Magistrate/I.O. in a sealed cover. (20) All forms filled for laboratory investigations should be labelled by the words MLC. (21) Cause of death should be given in the International Classification of Diseases. Where several alternatives for the cause of death exist, and the facts do not allow a differentiation between them, describe the alternatives, and if possible, rank them in order of probability. If this is not possible, then the cause of death should be certified as "UNASCERTAINED". (22) Some standard opinions are: (a) Death is due to shock and haemorrhage as a result of multiple injuries sustained (assault, traffic accident, etc.). (b) Death is due to asphyxia as a result of (hanging, strangulation, etc.). (c) Death is due to respiratory failure secondary to laryngeal oedema as a result of anaphylaxis (drug related deaths). (d) Death is due to (any complication) as a result of burns. (e) Death is due to respiratory failure as a result of consumption of (organophosphate or any other poison).

(f) On perusal of case sheet, postmortem report and chemical analysis report, I am of the opinion that death is due to poisoning by .... (23) After autopsy, evaluation may be provisional, because later findings and later knowledge of other circumstantial facts can necessitate alteration and modifications. Provisional report should not be delayed more than a day or two. (24) The postmortem findings, or any other evidence in the case, should not be discussed by the Medical Officer with any unauthorised person, but he should provide all facilities to the Investigating Officer. (25) Interested parties requiring a copy of the postmortem report should apply to the concerned Magistrate/ police station for such a copy, which should NOT be furnished direct by the Medical Officer.

SCHEDULE OF OBSERVATIONS

Date and hour of receipt of body ....

....

Date and hour of autopsy ....

....

Body identified by (P.C.No..... name ....

P.S. .... and others if any)

Requisition received from (Designation and P.S):

A. GENERAL

PRELIMINARY PARTICULARS:

(1) Name :

(2) Sex :

(3) Apparent Age :

(4) Height :

(5) Weight :

(6) Physique: (State in appropriate terms, e.g. well-built, normal, thin, emaciated, etc.)

(7) Nutritional state :

(8) **IDENTIFYING FEATURES:** (If body is unidentified, describe all identifying features, e.g. skin colour, hair, colour of eyes, scars, moles, tattoo marks, circumcision, amputations, skin diseases, deformities, dental condition, etc. fingerprints and photographs.

(9) **CLOTHES:** (List and describe type of garment, colour, consistency, tears, loss of buttons, etc. Cuts, holes, blackening, etc. should be noted and compared with injuries on the body. Discrepancies in such findings are also to be described. Stains due to blood, semen, grease, etc., poison, vomit, etc. should be described and preserved in clean plastic bags or other containers. List the ornaments and describe the type, design and colour of each (yellow or white metal; white, red or green stones, etc). Pocket contents should be recorded).

(10) **POSTMORTEM CHANGES PRESENT:** (Note body temperature; describe degree (complete, partial, absent) and distribution of rigor mortis. Postmortem lividity (distribution, intensity, colour, reversibility) and putrefactive signs (stained blood vessels, greenish discolouration, odour, softening of eye balls, distention of abdomen and body, exudation from nose and mouth, ova of flies, maggots, blebs over body, peeling of cuticle, loosening of hair, burst thorax and abdomen, sutures of skull, liquefaction of tissues, adipocere, mummification, skeletonization, etc.).

(11) **EXTERNAL APPEARANCES:** (Condition of limbs, shape and abnormal mobility, abnormalities, injection marks, etc.). Describe position of body, stains of blood, vomit, poison, etc., and other trace evidence. In newborn infants note condition of umbilical cord, whether or not the body has been washed, and preserve any wrapping in which it was found. In all cases, examine all external orifices (eyes, ears, nostrils, mouth, anus, vagina, urethra). Note presence of disease, e.g. oedema of legs, dropsy, surgical emphysema, skin disease, eruptions, bed sores, enlarged lymph nodes, and any other pathology).

(12) **INJURIES:** (Briefly but accurately describe all injuries and abnormalities found. State whether injuries are antemortem or postmortem. Note nature, shape, exact measurements, direction, margins, base and extremities, and location relative to anatomical landmarks, signs of vital reaction, foreign particles, discolouration, infection, and healing. Incise locally to demonstrate suspected deep bruises. Bite marks should be swabbed. Sketches, diagrams, or photographs of important injuries are often necessary. Where indicated, take appropriate specimens for histological or bacteriological examinations).

B. HEAD & NECK

(1) SCALP: (Injuries including deep bruising):

(2) TEMPORAL MUSCLES :

(3) SKULL: (Fractures, etc. Note connection between skull and first two vertebrae).

(4) BRAIN, MENINGES AND CEREBRAL VESSELS: (Note presence of any abnormal smell. Note the type and amount of intracranial haemorrhage. Look for cerebral oedema, contusions, lacerations and aneurysms, esp. in circle of Willis).

(5) EYES: (Colour of irises and sclerae, pupils, artificial eyes, conjunctivae, eyelids, opacity of cornea, bleeding, petechiae).

(6) ORBITAL, NASAL, ACCESSORY NASAL, AND AURAL CAVITIES: (Examined only if special indications present).

(7) MOUTH, TONGUE, AND PHARYNX: (Oral mucosa, dentition, oral and nasal discharges, their colour and odour).

(8) NECK, LARYNX, THYROID, AND OTHER NECK STRUCTURES: (If there is suspicion of neck trauma, remove brain and thoracic organs first to achieve a bloodless field. A careful flap dissection of the neck should always be made and all neck structures, esp. hyoid bone, thyroid cartilage and laryngeal cartilages carefully examined to investigate the possibility of being due to acute respiratory obstruction, e.g. strangulation, hanging, etc).

C. CHEST

(1) RIBS AND CHEST WALL: (Shape and stability, fractures, breasts, nipples and pigmentation; demonstrate pneumothorax).

(2) DIAPHRAGM: (Note level on right and left).

(3) MEDIASTINUM AND THYMUS :

(4) OESOPHAGUS: (Open and look for any pathology or foreign bodies).

(5) TRACHEA AND BRONCHI: (All the larger air passages should be opened and carefully examined for the presence of foreign material and any pathology).

(6) PLEURAL CAVITIES: Right: Left:

(7) LUNGS: (Note colour, distended or collapsed: dry, crepitant, soft, oedematous, congested, friable, inelastic, consolidation, emphysematous, atelectoid, exude frothy blood, blood-stained fluid, purulent matter, adhesions, haemorrhages, Tardieu spots, infarction, scars, tubercles on surface, tumours, etc. Look for thrombi and emboli in pulmonary arteries. In newborn infants a full hydrostatic test should be carried out).

(8) HEART AND PERICARDIAL SAC: (Open all chambers of the heart: dissect the coronary arteries and look for thrombi and atheroma; cut into the myocardium. Examine valvular rings and cusps. Examine auricular appendages for thrombi. Measure thickness of auricular and ventricular walls. Look for blood clots and other pathology. In sudden obscure deaths the

possibility of air or pulmonary artery embolism should not be overlooked).

(9) LARGE BLOOD VESSELS: (Abnormalities in the large arteries and veins, e.g., atheroma, aneurysm formation, thrombosis, etc).

D. ABDOMEN

(1) ABDOMINAL WALL: (Bulging, pigmentation, abnormalities).

(2) PERITONEAL CAVITY: (Blood, pus, fluid, adhesions, disease, etc).

(3) STOMACH AND CONTENTS: (Ligate cardiac and pyloric ends of stomach and remove *en masse*. Place in clean tray and slit open along greater curvature of stomach. Note nature of stomach contents, state of digestion, description of identifiable particles, and presence of any abnormal odour, foreign and suspicious matter. Examine mucous membrane for congestion, haemorrhage, ulcers, perforation, etc).

(4) SMALL INTESTINE: (Place in clean tray and slit open along mesenteric attachment. Examine mucous membrane for congestion, inflammation, erosions, ulcers, etc. Examine mesenteric vessels for disease, thrombi or emboli).

(5) LARGE INTESTINE, APPENDIX AND MESENTERY: (Open along anterior taenia; look for findings as in small intestine).

(6) LIVER, GALL-BLADDER, AND BILIARY PASSAGES: (Weight, size, colour, consistency, pathology, injury, etc).

(7) PANCREAS: (Haemorrhage, fat necrosis).

(8) SPLEEN: (Note colour, size, weight, shape, consistency, capsule (wrinkled, thick, adherent), rupture, wounds, etc).

(9) KIDNEYS, RENAL PELVIS, URETERS: Right: Left: (Examine renal arteries for thrombi, emboli and atheroma; strip capsule. Note size and weight. Examine cortex and medulla. Examine renal pelvis for calculi and inflammation).

(10) ADRENALS: (Haemorrhage).

(11) PELVIC WALLS:

(12) URINARY BLADDER AND URETHRA: (Calculi, cystitis, etc).

(13) GENITAL ORGANS: (In suspected sexual assaults, remove external genitalia, rectum and anus, *en block* and dissect. Take relevant swabs prior to this procedure).

E. SPINE

(1) Spinal column and spinal cord: (Palpate and manipulate the spine after the removal of all internal organs for presence of fractures and dislocations. The spinal cord need only be opened and the cord examined if special indications are present).

F. ADDITIONAL OBSERVATIONS

(1) Samples retained for histology, microbiology and other investigations.

(2) Results of ancillary investigations, such as radiology, odontology, anthropology, etc.

E- SPECIMENS REMOVED FOR CHEMICAL ANALYSIS

Sl. No.	Nature of specimen	Nature and quantity of preservative added.
(1)	Stomach and contents :	
(2)	Small intestine and contents :	
(3)	Liver: (Not less than 1/2 kg) :	
(4)	Kidney (Half of each) :	
(5)	Blood 30 ml. from peripheral veins :	
(6)	Urine 30 ml :	
(7)	Any other organ :	

Postmortem concluded at .... A.M./P.M on ....

OPINION AS TO THE CAUSE OF DEATH

(a) The approximate time of death ....

(b) Reserved pending report of ....

(c) The cause of death, ...

Hospital : (Signature)

Date: .... Name :

Designation :

POSTMORTEM CERTIFICATE (Short opinion)

P.M. No. : Date :

Regarding the body of male/female named .... aged about .... years, received on .... at .... A.M./P.M. from .... of police of P.S. .... with his letter No. .... dated .... sent through P.C. No. ....

P.M. was commenced at .... A.M./P.M. and concluded at .... A.M./P.M.

Opinion as to the cause of death:

Place : Signature :

Date : Name :

Designation :

AUTHORISATION FOR PATHOLOGICAL AUTOPSY

I .... bearing the relation of .... and being next of kin to .... a deceased patient, authorise the authorities of the .... to perform an examination of said body with the object of ascertaining the direct and indirect causes of death, and to the retaining of such tissues and organs as the doctor deems necessary for complete examination.

1. Full autopsy.
2. Restricted autopsy.

LETTER FROM MEDICAL OFFICER TO THE DIRECTOR, FORENSIC SCIENCE LABORATORY, REQUESTING FOR CHEMICAL ANALYSIS TO BE DONE.

INSTRUCTIONS: (1) Care should be taken to ensure that all necessary information regarding individual samples submitted is included. (2) The specimen or sample should be well protected against contamination from outside sources. (3) The samples should be wrapped in clean, white glazed paper, or in a cellophane. (4) Small samples, such as hair, fibres, dusts, etc. should be packed in glass tubes or in cellophane card envelopes. (5) Liquid should be packed in clean glass-stoppered bottles. (6) Each specimen must be in a separate package. (7) Each specimen should be sealed and labelled. (8) If any specimen is required to be returned, a note to this effect may be made in the remarks column.

Letter No. Hospital :

Place : Date :

To
The Director,
Forensic Science Laboratory,
Govt. of ....
Sir,

I am forwarding herewith the material objects mentioned below through (name) .... P.C. No. .... of police station .... for chemical examination and certificate. The relevant details of the case are given below. I request you to kindly analyse the materials and forward the report to me at the earliest.

RELEVANT PARTICULARS

(1) Postmortem No. : Date :

(2) Name of deceased : Age :
(3) Crime No. : of Police station :
(4) Material objects :
 (a) Stomach and upper part of intestine with contents.
 (b) Liver 1/2 kg.
 (c) Half of each kidney.
 (d) Blood
 (e) Urine
 (f) Any other material
(5) Method of preservation
 (a) Rectified spirit/saturated saline (for a, b and c)
 (b) Sodium fluoride (for d and e).
(6) Mode of packing: Collected in glass bottles, wrapped with paper, tied and sealed.
(7) Specimen seal used enclosed.
(8) Inquest report enclosed.
(9) Postmortem report enclosed.
(10) Authorisation letter: (enclosed/not enclosed).
(11) Examination required: Detection of poison.

In connection with the examination of trace evidence (hair, stains, etc.), furnish the following information.

(I) Nature of crime:
(II) Facts of medicolegal importance in connection with the case :
(III) List of articles sent for examination :
 Sl.No. :
 Description of exhibits :
 How, when and by whom found :
 Source of exhibits :
 Remarks :
(IV) Nature of examination required :

Place: Signature
Date: Name:
Designation:

LABEL TO BE PASTED ON VISCERA BOTTLE

Hospital : Place :
Cr. No. .... Date .... Police Station ....
Postmortem No. : Date :
Name of the deceased : Age : Sex :
Nature of specimen :
Preservative used: Rectified spirit/saturated saline/sodium fluoride.

Signature of Medical Officer

LETTER TO DEPUTE POLICE CONSTABLE TO TAKE THE VISCERA TO FSL

Office of the .... Dated ....

To,

The Station House Officer of P.S. ....

Sub: Deputation of a police constable to take the viscera to FSL.

Cr.No. .... dated .... of P.S.

P.M. No. .... dated ....

Kindly arrange to depute police constable to take the viscera in the above case to the forensic science laboratory, Govt. of .... for purpose of chemical analysis.

Place : Signature :

Date : Designation :

LETTER FOR AUTHORISATION FOR CHEMICAL EXAMINATION OF VISCERA

Office of the .... Dated :

To: The Principal/First/Second/Additional Judicial First Class Magistrate.

Sir,

Sub: Authorisation for Chemical Examination of viscera.

Kindly authorise the Director, F.S.L. .... Government of .... to examine the viscera of .... P.M. No. .... dated ....

The case has been sent by the Sub-inspector of police of .... police station, vide his letter No. .... dated ....

Place : Yours faithfully,
Date : Signature :
Name :
Designation :

FINAL OPINION OF THE CAUSE OF DEATH AFTER F.S.L. REPORT

To: The Magistrate

Sir,

Sub : Final opinion - Cause of death - Deceased - Furnished.

Ref : (1) Postmortem Certificate No. .... dated ....
 (2) FSL Report No. .... dated ....
 (3) Cr. No. .... of P.S. .... dated ....

On reviewing the case in the light of Forensic Science Laboratory report and postmortem findings, I am of the opinion that the deceased by the name .... aged about .... years, would appear to have died of

Place : Signature :
Date : Name :
Designation :

Copy to: The Sub-inspector of Police of P.S. .... for information.

PROFORMA FOR EXHUMATION

INSTRUCTIONS: (1) Describe clothing. (2) Determine sex, age and stature. (3) Describe identifying marks if any. (4) Conduct autopsy in the routine manner and note all the findings. (5) Preserve viscera for chemical analysis. (6) Collect samples of earth (about half kg) from above, below and from each side of the body and any fluid or debris in the coffin. (7) If only skeleton is present, collect all bones and send them to the expert in sealed and labelled packets (8) The body should be handed over to the police after autopsy.

Requisition from .... Magistrate of .... vide his letter No. .... dated ....

Letter No. .... dated .... from .... of police of P.S. ....

(1) Time of departure :
(2) Time of arrival at the place of burial :
(3) Persons present at exhumation (names and addresses) :
(4) Persons identifying the place of burial (names and addresses) :
(5) Description of the burial place and grave :
(6) Location : Length : Breadth :
(7) Height : Covered with :
(8) Stone inscription if any :
(9) Inquest conducted by :
(10) Grave identified by :
(11) Officers present at the time of exhumation :
(12) Condition of soil of burial place and surrounding area :
(13) Grave digging started at :
(14) Samples of earth from (a) above, (b) below, and (c) within the coffin :
(15) Description of coffin if any :
(16) Body removed from the grave at :
(17) Description of clothes :
(18) Persons identifying the clothes (names and addresses) :
(19) Persons identifying the body (names and addresses) :

P.M. No. .... date ....
P.M. commenced at :
P.M. findings :
P.M. concluded at :
Approximate time of death :
Opinion as to the cause of death :

Place : Signature :
Date : Name :
Designation :

ANNEXURE 1 (A)
FORM NO. 4

MEDICAL CERTIFICATE OF CAUSE OF DEATH

(Hospital inpatients. Not to be used for stillbirths)
To be sent to Registrar along with Form No. 2 (Death Report)

Name of the Hospital ....

I hereby certify that person whose particulars are given below died in the hospital in Ward No. .... on .... at .... AM/PM.

<table>
<tr><td colspan="5">Cr. No. .... Date of Admission ....Name of Deceased .... S/W/D/of .... Address ....</td><td>For use of Statistical Office</td></tr>
<tr><td rowspan="2">Sex</td><td colspan="4">Age at Death</td><td rowspan="6"></td></tr>
<tr><td>If 1 year or more, age in years</td><td>If less than 1 year, age in months</td><td>If less than 1 month, age in days</td><td>If less than 1 day, age in hours</td></tr>
<tr><td>1. Male
2. Female</td><td></td><td></td><td></td><td></td></tr>
<tr><td colspan="4">Cause of Death</td><td>Interval between onset & death approx.</td></tr>
<tr><td colspan="2">I. Immediate cause
State the disease, injury or complication which caused death, not the mode of dying, such as heart failure, asthenia, etc.
Antecedent cause
Morbid conditions, if any, giving rise to the above cause, stating underlying conditions last.
II. Other significant condition contributing to the death but not related to the disease or conditions causing it.</td><td colspan="3">(a) ....
..........due to (or as a consequence of
(b) ....
...........due to (or as a consequence of
(c) ....
....</td></tr>
<tr><td colspan="2">Manner of Death
(1) Natural. (2) Accident. (3) Suicide. (4) Homicide.
(5) Pending investigation</td><td colspan="4">How did the injury occur?</td></tr>
<tr><td colspan="4">If deceased was a female, was pregnancy the death associated with?
If yes, was there a delivery?</td><td colspan="2">(1) Yes (2) No
(1) Yes (2) No</td></tr>
</table>

Name and signature of the Medical Attendant certifying the cause of death
Date of verification ....

(To be detached and handed over to the relative of the deceased)

Certified that Shri/Smt./Kum .... S/W/D/ of Shri .... CR. No. .... R/o .... was admitted to this hospital in ward .... on .... and expired on ....

Doctor's Signature
(Medical Supdt. Name of the Hospital)

MEDICAL CERTIFICATE OF CAUSE OF DEATH
Directions for completing the form

NAME OF DECEASED: To be given in full. Do not use initials. If deceased is an infant, not yet named at time of death, write 'Son of (S/o) or 'Daughter of (D/o), Followed by names of mother and father.

AGE: If the deceased was over one year of age, give age in completed years. If the deceased was below I year of age, give age in months and if below one month give age in completed number of days, and if below one day, in hours.

CAUSE OF DEATH: This part of the form should always be completed by the attending physician personally.

The certificate of cause of death is divided into two parts, I and II, Part I is again divided into three parts, lines (a) (b) (c). If a single morbid condition completely explains the death, then this will be written on line (a) of part I, and nothing more need be written in the rest of Part I or in Part II, for example, smallpox, lobar pneumonia, cardiac beriberi, are sufficient cause of death and usually nothing more is needed.

Often, however, a number of morbid conditions will have been present at death, and the doctor must then complete the certificate in the proper manner so that the correct underlying cause will be tabulated. First, enter in Part I (a) the Immediate cause of death. This does not mean the mode of dying, e.g., heart failure, respiratory failure, etc., These terms should not appear on the certificate at all, since they are modes of dying and not causes of death. Next consider whether the immediate cause is a complication or delayed result of some other cause. If so, enter the antecedent cause in Part I, line (b). Sometimes there will be three stages in the course of events leading to death. If so, line (c) will be completed. The underlying cause to be tabulated is always written last in Para I.

Morbid conditions or injuries may be present which were not directly related to the train of events causing death, but which contributed in some way to the fatal outcome. Sometimes, the doctor finds it difficult to decide, especially for infant deaths, which of several independent conditions was the primary cause of death, but only one cause can be tabulated, so the doctor must decide. If the other diseases are not effects of the underlying cause, they are entered in Part II.

Do not write two or more conditions on a single line. Please write the names of the diseases (in full) in the certificate as legibly as possible to avoid the risk of their being misread.

ONSET: Complete the column for interval between onset and death whenever possible, even if very approximately, e.g., "from birth" several years.

ACCIDENTAL OR VIOLENT DEATHS: Both the external cause and the nature of the injury are needed and should be stated. The doctor or hospital should always be able to describe the injury, stating the part of the body injured, and should give the external cause in full when this is shown. Example: (a) Hypostatic pneumonia; (b) Fracture of neck of femur; (c) Fall from ladder at home.

MATERNAL DEATHS: Be sure to answer the questions on pregnancy and delivery. This information is needed for all women of child-bearing age, even though the pregnancy may have had nothing to do with the death.

OLD AGE OR SENILITY: Old age (or senility) should not be given as a cause of death if a more specific cause is known. If old age was a contributory factor, it should be entered in Part II. Example (a) chronic bronchitis, II old age.

COMPLETENESS OF INFORMATION: A complete case history is not wanted, but, if the information is available, enough details should be given to enable the underlying cause to be properly clarified.

EXAMPLE: Anaemia: Give type of anaemia, if known. Neoplasms: Indicate whether benign or malignant, and site, with site of primary neoplasm, whenever possible, Heart disease: Describe the condition specifically; if congestive heart failure, chronic cor pulmonale, etc., are mentioned; give the antecedent conditions. Tetanus: Describe the antecedent injury, if known. Operation: State the condition for which the operation was performed. Dysentry: Specify whether bacillary, amoebic, etc., if known. Complications of pregnancy or delivery: Describe the complication specifically. Tuberculosis: Give organs affected.

SYMPTOMATIC STATEMENT: Convulsions, diarrhoea, fever, ascites, jaundice, debility, etc., are symptoms which may be due to any one of a number of different conditions. Sometimes nothing more is known, but whenever possible, give the disease which caused the symptom.

MANNER OF DEATH: Deaths not due to external cause should be identified as 'Natural'. If the cause of death is known, but it is not known whether it was the result of an accident, suicide or homicide and is subject to further investigation, the cause of death should invariably be filled in and the manner of death should be shown as 'Pending Investigation'.

ORGAN DONOR CARD
FRONT SIDE

Regn No. ☐☐☐☐

I .... son/daughter/wife of .... in the hope that I may help other, hereby make this anatomical gift, if medically acceptable to take effect upon my brain death. I hereby wish to donate the following organs: Heart, Lungs, Kidneys, Liver, Corneas & .... Special wishes, if any ....

BACK SIDE

Signed by the donor in the presence of two witnesses

....	....
Signature of donor with date	**Date of birth of donor**

....	....	....
Address of the donor	**Telephone No.**	**Blood group**

....	....
Witness	**Witness**

APPENDIX-VII

INTIMATION TO POLICE

Every registered medical practitioner has to perform medicolegal duty during discharge of his/her duty. However, his first priority is to save the life of the patient as held by Supreme Court. A treating doctor should record a proper history, examination including general condition, level of consciousness, vital parameters and report of investigations and the other circumstances of the case and then analyse the injuries to decide if it is an MLC or not. If a case is suspected or registered as medicolegal, then it must be brought to the notice of the nearest police post/station. Reporting a MLC to the nearest police station after giving primary life-saving medical care is one of the legal responsibilities of all doctors according to Section 39 Cr.P.C. Police intimation has to be made in writing and countersignature should be taken from the concerned police official. The name, number of the police official, date and time should be entered in the MLC sheet along with DDR/FIR No. Police must also be intimated whenever a medicolegal case is discharged or absconds or dies while in hospital and the copy of the same should be attached to the case file.

Medicolegal Case (M.L.C) Information

Time______am/pm
Date___________

To

The Officer-in-Charge
Police Post/Station

District_____________________I am to inform you that a patient with the following particulars has been brought to the General Hospital/CHC/PHC____of the district_____________and is being treated/discharged/LAMA has expired in the emergency OPD/___________________________ward of the General Hospital/CHC/PHC Name_______________________S/o. D/o___________________________ __Age______________Sex_________________Hospital Central Registration No.__________________Date and time of admission_____________________ Diagnosis_____________grievous hurt/heated injury/burns__________________________

MLR attached: Yes/No

Signature
(Name of the Medical Officer)
(In block letter)

____

Time and of the receiving the information of the police post.

____

Signature of Police Officer_____________
Name (in capital letters)_______________
Seal of the Police Post________________

APPENDIX-VIII

MEDICAL CERTIFICATES OF DIFFERENT VARIETY

PRELIMINARY PARTICULARS:

(1) Name of patient : Age : sex :
(2) Address and residence :
(3) Brought by :
(4) Place at which the injury or accident occurred:
(5) Nature of injury or accident (simple or grievous):
(6) Alleged cause :
(7) Ward in which admitted/treated as outpatient:
(8) Whether dying declaration necessary :
(9) Hospital/Nursing Home :
(10) Time of despatch of intimation to the Police/ Magistrate.

Place : Signature :
Date : Name :
Designation :

ACCIDENT REGISTER

No .... Date and hour ....

(1) Name ....
(2) Age ....
(3) Sex ....
(4) Caste ....
(5) Occupation ....
(6) Address and residence ....
(7) Identification marks: (1).............. (2).........
(8) By whom brought ....
(9) Consent (signature or thumb impression)
(10) Police informed or not ....
(11) Accompanying P.C.No. and P.S.
(12) Brief history ....
(13) Dying declaration required or not ....
(14) If so, state action taken ....
(15) Examination of clothes ....
(16) Nature of injuries and treatment (State simple or grievous) ....
(17) Signs of intoxication ....
(18) If admitted as inpatient date and time ....
(19) Date of discharge ....
(20) Condition on discharge ....
(21) Date of sending case for radiological examination and P.C.No. ....
(22) Date of receiving the report from radiologist ....
(23) Radiological findings ....

Place : Signature :
Date : Name :
Designation :

WOUND CERTIFICATE

INSTRUCTIONS: (1) Obtain written consent for examination and investigations. (2) Examine without delay at any time of day or night. (3) If treated as outpatient, it should be noted in the report. (4) Admit if injuries are serious. (5) If death is imminent, arrange for dying declaration. (6) Carry out immunisation when necessary. (7) All forms filled for laboratory investigations should be labelled by the words MLC. (8) Inform police before discharging against advice. (9) In case of discharge or death in hospital, inform the police without delay and do not issue death certificate. (10) If a person is brought dead to the hospital, do not examine wounds, inform police and do not hand over the body to the relatives. Fill death certificate form or note on the outpatient ticket without giving cause of death. (11) If the investigating officer gives requisition for any clarifications regarding any points in the report, the answers should be given in writing (S.197, I.P.C. and S.161, Cr.P.C.). (12) Oral statements made to the police and recorded by the police, should not be signed (S.162, Cr.P.C.). (13) If the investigating officer requires any documents regarding the injured person, either original or xerox copy, it should be given and a receipt obtained. (14) The doctor can be summoned to police station for recording a statement if the investigation demands (S.160, Cr.P.C.).

Wounds or injuries found on the person of a male/female calling himself/herself .... aged .... years, an inhabitant of .... who was sent with (letter/memo No.) .... dated .... from P.S. .... and accompanied by (name, number of P.C. of P.S.) .... for report as to certain injuries .... said to have been caused on .... and to be due to ....
Identification marks: (1) .... (2) ....
Consent of the individual for examination ....
Signature or thumb impression of the person
Identified by constable No. .... Name ....
P.S. ....

The injured person was first seen by the undersigned at .... A.M./P.M. on (date) and the examination was commenced at .... A.M./P.M. on (date) when the following injuries were found:

1	2	3	4	5	6	7
Nature of injury, i.e. whether abrasion, cut, bruise, laceration, burn, stab, fracture or dislocation, etc.	Size of each injury in cm, i.e. length, breadth and depth	On what part of the body inflicted	Whether simple or grievous	By what kind of weapon inflicted	Whether the weapon was dangerous or not	Remarks, (age of wound, inpatient or outpatient, etc.)

X-ray and laboratory findings :

OPINION: I am of opinion that (injuries are simple grievous or likely to be fatal) ....

Station: Signature :

Date : Name :

Designation :

DISCHARGE AGAINST ADVICE

Hospital : Reg. No. :

Bed No. : Ward :

Name of the patient :

I am responsible for leaving/taking the above patient out of the hospital against the advice of the doctor.

Date : Signature :

Relationship :

Witness : (1) (Name, Signature) Relationship

(2)

AGE ESTIMATION

INSTRUCTIONS: (1) Obtain written consent for examination and for taking X-rays. (2) For confirmation of age as determined by dental examination, take X-rays of: (a) Between 6 to 12 years: elbow and wrist joints. (b) Between 13 to 16 years: elbow and pelvis. (c) 16 to 17 years: elbow and ankle. (d) 17 to 18: hip. (e) 18 to 19: knee and shoulder. (f) 18 to 20: iliac crest. (g) 21: ischial tuberosity and inner end of clavicle. (3) All forms filled for X-rays should be labelled by the words MLC. (4) Note at least two identification marks, preferably on exposed areas of the person. (a) In the case of mole, note colour, size, shape, hairy or not, raised or not and exact anatomical location. (b) In case of scar, note colour, length, width, shape, fixed or free, smoothness or irregularity of surface, presence or absence of glistening and tenderness, direction and exact location. (c) In case of tattoo mark, note colour, design, size and situation and make a sketch.

Requisition from .... of police of P.S. .... vide his letter No. .... dated .... and accompanied by (name & number of P.C.) of P.S. .... for determination of age.

PRELIMINARY PARTICULARS:

(1) Name of the individual :
(2) Sex :
(3) Parent's or guardian's name :
(4) Address :
(5) Occupation :
(6) Caste :
(7) Married or single :
(8) Age as alleged by :
 (i) Individual to be examined :
 (ii) Person or police accompanying :
(9) Person accompanying or brought by :
(10) Time and place of examination :
(11) Consent of the individual for examination :
(12) Signature of the individual consenting or his/her left thumb impression :
(13) In the case of minors, consent of the guardian and his/her signature or left thumb impression:
(14) Name of female attendant/nurse present at the time of examination :
(15) Date and time of examination :
(16) Marks of identification: (1)................ (2)..................

PHYSICAL EXAMINATION

(1) Height :
(2) Weight :
(3) Chest girth at the level of the nipples :
(4) Abdominal girth at the level of the navel :
(5) General build and appearance :
(6) Voice :
(7) Teeth :

R	(S) 8 7 6 5 4 3 2 1	(S) 1 2 3 4 5 6 7 8
L	(S) 8 7 6 5 4 3 2 1	(S) 1 2 3 4 5 6 7 8

T: Temporary P: Permanent

(S) : Space after teeth

(8) Hair : Scalp :
 Beard : Moustache :
 Axillary : Pubic : Body :
(9) Mammary :
 Development of breasts : milk in :
(10) Generative organs :
 Development of genitals :
(11) Onset of puberty :
 (i) Date of menarche :
 (ii) Regularity of menses :
(12) Date of sending case for radiological examination and P.C.No. :
(13) Number and region of X-rays taken :
(14) Date of receiving the report from the radiologist:
(15) Radiological findings :
(16) Opinion of age :

Station : Signature :

Date : Name :

Designation :

AGE CERTIFICATE

Name of individual: .... Sex .... Cr.No. .... of P.S. .... dated .... accompanied by P.C.No. ....

From physical, dental, and radiological examination of .... bearing the identification marks: (1) .... (2) ....

I am of opinion that the individual is aged about .... years.

Station : Signature :

Date : Name :

Rank :

PROFORMA FOR EXAMINATION OF SEXUAL OFFENCES
EXAMINATION OF THE VICTIM OF RAPE

INSTRUCTIONS: (1) Obtain written consent for examination and collection of specimens of blood, etc. and to supply copies of all medical reports to the police. (2) With a cotton swab take material from introitus, and perineum. Take material from lower part of vagina, posterior fornix and cervical os using separate swabs, and make four slides, and allow them to dry for two to three minutes and fix by heat. (3) Keep one swab in test tube for acid phosphatase determination. (4) Insert a swab in a test tube containing small amount of normal saline, and examine the fluid for motile spermatozoa. (5) Comb pubic hair and place loose hair in labelled envelope. (6) Cut sample of pubic hair (10 to 12 hairs) and place in labelled envelope. (7) Obtain blood 5 ml. (plain) for grouping and DNA profile, and 5 ml. (sodium fluoride) for alcohol and drugs and venereal disease. (8) Obtain fingernail scrapings and place in labelled envelopes. (9) Collect any loose hair or fibres found on the person or clothes. (10) Collect dried bloodstains and indicate the site from which collected. (11) Collect material from cervix for gonorrhoeal infection. (12) Obtain swabs from bite marks. (13) Preserve garments having suspected seminal or blood stains after drying them. (14) In most young women a finger may be passed into vagina although the hymen is intact. (15) If the vaginal opening is enough to admit two fingers easily and the hymen shows old tears, it indicates that the woman is used to sexual intercourse.

Appearances found on the person of female calling herself................ .... age stated .... years, an inhabitant of............................ who was sent with letter/memo No. .... dated .... from .... and accompanied by (name and number of P.C. of P.S.) .... for report as to the result of examination of person for certain injuries or appearances said to have been caused on .... to be due to alleged rape.

Identification marks: (1)..................... (2) ....

The person was seen by the undersigned on (date) .... at (place of exam) .... and the examination was commenced at .... A.M./P.M. on (date) .... when the following were found.

PRELIMINARY PARTICULARS :

(1) Name of the individual :
(2) Parent's or guardian's name :
(3) Address :
(4) Occupation :
(5) Caste :
(6) Age as alleged by the victim :
(7) Person accompanying or brought by :
(8) Consent of the individual for examination :
(9) Signature of the individual consenting or her left thumb impression :
(10) In the case of minor, consent of the guardian and his/her signature or thumb impression:
(11) Married or single :
(12) Name of female attendant/nurse present at the time of examination :
(13) History as given by police :

HISTORY (FROM VICTIM) :

(1) Age : (2) Gravidity :
(3) Age of menarche :
(4) Date of last menses :
(5) Whether pregnant :
(6) Most recent coitus prior to alleged assault :
Date : Time : Condom used or not :
(7) Patient's statement, whether she is a virgin :
(8) Is she suffering from any illness and taking any medicines:
(9) History of any venereal disease (past or present):
(10) History of emotional illness:
(11) Previous vaginal surgical procedure:
(12) Use of alcohol or drugs in twentyfour hours prior to alleged assault. If so amount and time of ingestion:
(13) (a) Date and time when the victim first made complaint to the police :
(b) Date and time when the rape was said to have been committed :
(c) Place where it was committed :
(d) Exact circumstances under which the rape was committed, i.e., whether the parties were standing or lying on the ground:
(e) Whether she was menstruating at the time:
(f) Whether she was sensible during the whole time the offence was committed or under the influence of alcohol or other intoxicants:
(g) Whether she uttered any cries or was she terrified:
(h) Did penis penetrate vulva?
(i) Did assailant wear condom?
(j) Since alleged assault has the victim:
(1) Douched : (2) Bathed :
(3) Defecated : (4) Urinated :
(5) Changed clothes :
(k) General feeling of those accompanying the female towards herself and towards the accused:

PHYSICAL EXAMINATION:

(1) B.P.: Pulse: Temp:
Wt: Height:
(2) General appearance :
(3) (a) Secondary sexual characters :
(b) Breasts: development, areola, nipple, milk in:
(4) Emotional status :
(5) Intelligence :
(6) Gait :
(7) Clothing worn at the time of alleged rape :
(a) Blood stains :
(b) Seminal stains :
(c) Other discharge :
(d) Foreign material :
(e) Hair:
(f) Tears :
(g) Mud, dust, soil, grass stains, etc.
(8) Body surface (injuries to breasts, cheeks, lips, thighs, genitals, etc.):
a) Scratches : b) Bruises :
c) Lacerations : d) Stains :
e) Foreign hair and bodies :
(9) Mouth :
(10) Fingernails (damage, epithelial cells, foreign material, etc.) :
(11) Genitals :
(a) Pubic hair, length, matted or not :
(b) Vulva (injuries and stains) :
(c) Labia minora :
(d) Hymen (tears, recent or old) :
(e) Vagina (digital and speculum exam) :
(f) Fourchette (intact or torn) :
(g) Perineum (tears, stains, scratches, foreign hair):
(h) Cervix :
(12) Is venereal disease present?
(13) Smears taken from vagina, cervix, urethra, sores:

(a) Number :
(b) Number of slides :
(c) Gram's stain :
(d) Stain for spermatozoa :

(14) Any other findings :

(15) Material sent to the laboratory :

(16) Results of laboratory procedures :

(a) Pregnancy test :
(b) Serology :
(c) Gonorrhoeal infection :
(d) Spermatozoa :
(e) Acid phosphatase :
(f) Grouping of blood and semen :
(g) Hair examination :

COLLECTION OF EVIDENCE :

(1) Blood in two tubes for serology and grouping:
(2) Fingernail scrapings :
(3) Loose pubic hair :
(4) Cut pubic hair :
(5) Hair, fibres and blood stains on body and clothing:
(6) Vaginal material for live spermatozoa :
(7) Four slides from vaginal material :
(8) Cervical material for gonorrhoea :
(9) Vaginal secretion on two cotton swabs :
(a) Semen typing : (b) Acid phosphatase :

OPINION: (1) There are signs/no signs of recent vaginal penetration (if hymen is torn and external genitals show injuries). (2) There are signs of recent sexual intercourse (if semen is present in vagina). (3) There are signs of general physical injuries, and / or intoxication.

The signs are consistent/inconsistent with the history given.

Place : Signature:
Date: Name :
Designation:

EXAMINATION OF ACCUSED OF RAPE/SODOMY

INSTRUCTIONS: (1) Obtain written consent for examination, and collection of specimens of blood, etc. and to supply copies of all medical reports to the police. (2) Collect blood for comparison with semen type found in the victim. (3) In the case of accused in a rape case, swab from coronal sulcus, prepuce, penile shaft for blood comparison with the victim's blood. (4) With a cotton swab wipe glans penis, prepare two slides and dry for 2 to 3 minutes for vaginal and cervical cells. (5) Obtain penile washings for vaginal and cervical cells. (6) Look for smegma on corona glandis. It gets rubbed off during intercourse and usually requires about 24 hours to collect. (7) In the case of accused in a sodomy case, penis has peculiar smell of anal glands and may contain traces of lubricant and faecal matter. Fraenum may be torn and abrasion on prepuce and glans. Faecal soiling, blood and foreign hairs may be found on coronal sulcus. (8) In the case of buccal coitus, faint teeth marks and abrasions may be seen on penis. (9) Urethral discharge for gonococcal infection. (10) Comb pubic hair and place loose hair in an envelope. (11) Obtain fingernail scrapings and place in labelled envelope. (12) Preserve garments having suspected seminal stains.

Preliminary particulars and reference, etc. :

As in the case of the victim.

HISTORY :

(1) Brief description of assault: Record general history and omit history of specific incident. Find out how injuries found on body were caused.
(2) Date and time of assault:
(3) Is he suffering from any illness and taking any medicines?
(4) Use of alcohol or drugs in 24 hours prior to alleged assault, if so amount and time of ingestion:
(5) Past illness, surgical operations, serious accidents:
(6) Consenting intercourse with any woman within previous 24 hours :

PHYSICAL EXAMINATION :

(1) B.P.: Pulse: Temp:
Wt: Height: General build:
(2) General appearance and emotional status :
(3) Clothing (changed or not):
(a) Blood stains:
(b) Seminal stains:
(c) Foreign material:
(d) Hairs:
(e) Tears:
(f) Cosmetic contact traces:
(g) Mud, soil, grass, etc :
(4) Fingernails (damage, epithelial cells, foreign material, etc.):
(5) Influence of alcohol or other intoxicant:
(6) Injuries found on body (scratches, bruises, bite marks, etc.):
(7) Genitals (development with special reference to potency):
(a) Pubic hair: length, matted or not:
(b) Penis: Length when flaccid:
Length when erect:
(c) Injuries:
(d) Blood, semen, lubricant, faecal matter:
(e) Smegma :
(f) Prepuce (abrasions, female pubic hair):
(g) Coronal sulcus (faecal soiling, blood and pubic hair):
(h) Circumcised or not:
(i) Fraenum (tears):
(j) Scrotum and testis (development, injuries):
(8) Anal examination:
(9) During alleged assault:
Did penis penetrate vagina / rectum?
Did assailant had orgasm?
Did assailant wear condom?
(10) Since alleged assault:
Bathed : Urinated :
Defecated:
(11) Is venereal disease present?
(12) Material sent to laboratory:
(13) Results of laboratory procedures:
(14) Any other findings:

COLLECTION OF EVIDENCE :

(1) Blood in two tubes for serology and grouping and for drug screening. (2) Perianal swab. (3) Rectal swab. (4) Oral swab. (5) Loose pubic hair. (6) Hair, fibres and blood stains on body and clothing. (7) Urethral discharge for gonorrhoea. (8) Fingernail scrapings. (9) Suspected dried seminal stains on the skin or clothing. (10) Penile washings (presence of vaginal epithelium).

OPINION: (1) There are no signs indicative of recent vaginal/anal penetration. (2) There are signs indicative of recent vaginal/anal penetration (presence of injuries, vaginal epithelial cells, lubricant or faecal stains on penis).

EXAMINATION OF THE VICTIM OF SODOMY

INSTRUCTIONS: (1) Obtain written consent for examination, and collection of specimens of blood, etc. and to supply copies of all medical reports to the police. (2) With a cotton swab wipe the perianal area, and put in a test tube for acid phosphatase determination. (3) Insert a cotton swab into the anal canal without touching the perianal area. Prepare two slides and dry for 2 to 3 minutes. (4) Place the same swab in a tube containing normal saline for acid phosphatase determination. (5) Insert a second swab in a test tube containing small amount of normal saline, and examine the fluid for motile spermatozoa. (6) Cut sample of pubic hair (10 to 12 hairs) and place in labelled envelope. (7) Obtain blood samples (two) for comparison with grouping of the semen and for serological tests. (8) Obtain fingernail scrapings and place in labelled envelopes. (9) Collect any loose hair or fibres found on the person or clothes. (10) Collect dry blood stains and indicate the site from which collected. (11) Collect material from anus for gonorrhoeal infection. (12) In buccal coitus, swab the mouth of the patient, especially the gums and pharynx with a cotton swab, smear on a slide and dry. (13) Place the same cotton swab in a tube containing normal saline for acid phosphatase.

Appearances found on the person of a male/female calling himself/herself .... age stated .... years, an inhabitant of .... who was sent with letter/memo no .... dated .... from .... and accompanied by .... for report as to the result of examination of person for certain injuries or appearances said to have been caused on .... to be due to alleged sodomy.

Identification marks : 1) ....

2) ....

The person was seen by the undersigned on (date and time) .... and the examination was commenced at (date and time) .... when the following were found.

PRELIMINARY PARTICULARS:

(1) Name of the individual:
(2) Parent's or guardian's name:
(3) Address :
(4) Occupation :
(5) Caste :
(6) Age as alleged by the victim:
(7) Persons accompanying or brought by:
(8) Consent of the individual for examination:
(9) Signature of the individual consenting or his/her left thumb impression:
(10) In the case of minor, consent of the guardian and his/her signature or thumb impression:
(11) Name of the female attendant/nurse, present at the time of examination:

HISTORY (from victim)

(1) Is he/she suffering from any illness and taking any medicines:
(2) History of any venereal disease (past or present).
(3) History of emotional illness:
(4) Use of alcohol or drugs in 24 hours prior to alleged assault. If so amount and time of ingestion.
(5) Date and time when the victim first made complaint to the police:
(6) Date and time when sodomy was said to have been committed:
(7) Place where it was committed:
(8) Exact circumstances under which sodomy was committed, i.e. whether the parties were standing or lying on the ground.
(9) Whether he/she uttered any cries or was terrified.
(10) Whether he/she was sensible during the whole time the offence was committed or under the influence of alcohol or other intoxicants:
(11) Details of struggle or resistance :
(12) Use of any lubricant :
(13) Did penis penetrate anus? (degree of penetration):
(14) Did assailant wear condom?
(15) Ejaculation during the act :
(16) Pain experienced at the time of act or subsequently:
(17) Any bleeding :
(18) Since alleged assault has the victim :
  (a) Bathed or washed the anal area :
  (b) Defecated:
  (c) Urinated:
  (d) Changed clothes :

PHYSICAL EXAMINATION:

(1) B.P. : Pulse : Temp :
Wt : Height : Build :
(2) General appearance :
(3) Emotional status :
(4) Clothing worn at the time of offence: (a) Blood stains. (b) Seminal stains. (c) Faecal stains. (d) Mud, dust, soil, grass stains, etc. (e) Foreign material. (f) Hair. (g) Tears.
(5) Marks of violence on the body (scratches, bruises, bite-marks, etc.).
(6) Any type of stains or foreign bodies on the body:
(7) Fingernails (damage, epithelial cells, foreign material, etc.) :
(8) Mouth (in buccal coitus) :
(9) Anal examination: (a) Inspection: Look for recent tears, stains due to semen, blood, faecal matter around the anus, scars, piles, condyloma, shaving of anal hair, smoothness or thickness of anal mucosa, depression of buttocks towards anus, etc. (b) Digital examination (assess tone and degree of dilatation of sphincter, discomfort or pain during examination). (c) Lateral buttock traction test. (d) Speculum examination (look for abrasions, contusions, lacerations, piles, fissures, wrinkles in anal mucosa, etc.).
(10) Any other findings.
(11) **SPECIMENS TO BE COLLECTED:** (1) Blood. (2) Head hair. (3) Pubic hair. (4) Loose hair and fibres found anywhere on the body. (5) Swabs from any soiled areas of the skin. (6) Swabs from the anal and lower rectum. (7) Nail scrapings.
(12) Results of laboratory procedures:

OPINION: (1) Findings are not consistent with entry of a penis into anus. (2) Findings are consistent with entry of a penis into anus. (3) Sodomy has been committed (if semen is present in the anus).

Place: Signature:
Date: Name:
Designation:

PROFORMA FOR EXAMINATION OF CASE OF IMPOTENCY/POTENCY

Appearances found on the person of a male/female calling himself/herself .... age stated .... years, an inhabitant of .... who was sent with letter/memo no .... dated .... from .... of police of P.S. .... and accompanied by (name and No. of P.C. .... of P.S. .... for report as to the result of examination for potency/impotency.

PARTICULARS:

(1) Name of the individual :
(2) Age :
(3) Sex :
(4) Address :
(5) Occupation :
(6) Brought by :
(7) Date, time and place of examination :
(8) Consent of the individual for examination :
(Signature or left thumb impression) :
(9) Marks of identification: (1) (2)
(10) History of the case: (Diabetes, drug addiction, trauma, STD, etc. masturbation, night emissions, homesexual / sexual intercourse).
(11) General examination :
Height : Weight :
Secondary sexual characters :
Physique :
(12) Local examination :
(a) Penis : Length when flaccid :
Length when erect :
Circumference (flaccid and erect) :
Disease / deformity / injury (if any) :
Sensation over glans penis :
Foreskin: Retractable / non-retractable :
(b) Scrotum (pendulous or not) :
(c) Testis: Whether present in scrotum or not; size (small, medium, adult size) :
(13) Systemic examination :
(a) C.V.S. (b) R.S. (c) G.I.S.
(d) G.U.S. (e) C.N.S.
(14) (a) Urine (for sugar) :
(b) Blood/VDRL :
(c) Others :

Place : Signature :
Date : Name :
Designation :

CERTIFICATE OF POTENCY/IMPOTENCY OF MALE

Certified that I examined Sri .... on (date to be given) at (place of examination to be given) and found as follows :

(1) That his genital organs are normal / not of normal development:
(2) That there is evidence / no evidence of disease of testes or epididymes :
(3) That he gives no history / definite history of exposure and had venereal disease :
(4) That there is no evidence of organic disease of nervous system / that his nervous system shows evidence of organic disease :
(5) That there are well-marked secondary sex characters / secondary sex characters are not marked as they ought to be in a man of his age.
(6) That there are psychic causes / no psychic causes:

TESTS FOR IMPOTENCE: (1) Nocturnal Penile Tumescence (NPT) monitoring: During the rapid eye movement phase of sleep, spontaneous penile erections occur 4 to 5 times per night and last about 15 to 20 minutes each. If the man wakes up during one of these phases, he notices erection. This is very important to differentiate organic from psychogenic impotence.

(1) These erections can be detected by wearing a snap gauge around the penis during sleep. This is a simple device with three strings each cutting at a certain amount of penile rigidity. The number of cut strings estimates the strength of erection. (2) The Regiscan is another device that monitors the nocturnal erections precisely and gives a computer printout of the degree of rigidity, duration and number of erectile episodes for both the tip and base of the penis.

(2) Papaverine or Prostaglandin (PGE1) Test: Injection of a vasoactive vasodilating substance like papaverine, phentolamine or PGE1 into the corpora cavernosa leads to dilatation of the cavernosal arteries, sinusoidal relaxation resulting in passive venous occlusion and a full erection in most normal subjects. This test is used to exclude abnormalities in penile haemodynamics. It is a good positive test. The techniques include: evaluation of the penile arteries with duplex ultrasonography during papaverine-induced erection, pudendal arteriography, pharmacocaverno-mosometry, and cavernosography.

OPINION: From all (or some) of the aforementioned objective signs, it can be concluded that (a) There is nothing to suggest that the male examined is not capable of performing sexual act. (b) The person is incapable of performing sexual act.

Place : Signature :
Date : Name :
Designation :

CERTIFICATE OF POTENCY/IMPOTENCY OF FEMALE

Certified that I examined Mrs. .... on (date) at (place) and observed as follows :

(1) That the labia majora and minora were well-developed/ill-developed.
(2) That she has normal vagina / total absence of the vagina, or had a (short) (narrow) vagina with a very small, ill-defined opening.
(3) That her hymen was thick and of a rigid type, not even admitting a small finger, intact / ruptured.
(4) That, at the time of examination, though her genitals were of normal development with an elastic hymen, she complained of excruciating pain and screamed when the inner aspect of the vulva was touched/no vaginismus.
(5) She has/ has no apparent discharge or venereal diseases.
(6) That there are psychic causes / no psychic causes.

OPINION: From the above observations, (1) I am of the opinion that she is incapable of taking part in sexual intercourse (impotent), i.e., she is not apta vira and that she is still a virgin. (2) She is apta vira, i.e., capable of taking part in sexual intercourse.

Place : Signature :
Date : Name :
Designation :

PROFORMA FOR EXAMINATION OF PERSONS FOR DRUNKENNESS

INSTRUCTIONS: (1) Clean the skin with soap and water and collect 5 ml. of blood from antecubital vein. Add 50 mg. of sodium fluoride and 15 mg. of potassium oxalate. The container should be tightly clamped and sealed. Rubber stoppers should be avoided. Refrigerate if sample cannot be sent immediately to the laboratory. (2) The usual signs of drunkenness are: strong odour of alcohol in breath, loss of self-control and clearness of intellect, unsteady gait, vacant look, congested eyes, sluggish and dilated pupils, increased pulse rate, thick, slurred speech, talks at random, lack of perception of passage of time, and defective muscular coordination.

Appearances found on the person calling himself .... age stated .... years, an inhabitant of .... who was sent with letter/memo No. .... dated .... from .... and accompanied by .... for report as to the result of examination of person for certain appearances due to alleged drunkenness.

PRELIMINARY PARTICULARS :

(1) Name of the individual :
(2) Parent's or guardian's name :
(3) Address :
(4) Occupation :
(5) Caste :
(6) Sex :
(7) Age alleged by the person :
(8) Person accompanying or brought by :
(9) Consent (preferably in writing, with signature or left thumb impression) :
(10) Name and number of accompanying P.C. :
(11) Identification marks: (1).................. (2)........................
(12) Date and place of examination :
(13) Time of commencement of examination :

HISTORY :

(1) Has he consumed alcohol? If so at what time and what was the nature and quantity?
(2) What food and drink he took and when?
(3) Is he in the habit of consuming alcohol regularly? If so, since how long and how frequently?
(4) Is he taking any medication or drugs? If so what is the nature and dose?
(5) If diabetic, when the last dose of insulin was taken and how much?

PHYSICAL EXAMINATION :

(1) B.P : Pulse : Temp :
Weight : Height :
(2) General manners and behaviour: (calm, talkative, abusive or obscene) :
(3) State of dress: (decent, soiled or disarranged) :
(4) Speech (normal, thick, slurred, over-precise or incoherent) :
(5) Self-control :
(6) Memory and mental alertness: (memory of recent events, orientation of time and space) :
(7) Handwriting: (note time taken, repetition or omission of words, etc.) :
(8) Pulse: (rapid and bounding, slow, etc.) :
(9) Temperature: (surface temperature raised, lowered, normal) :
(10) Skin: (dry, moist, flushed or pale) :
(11) Mouth: (smell of alcohol, dribbling of saliva, furred tongue, dry lips, etc.) :
(12) Eyes: (lids swollen or red, conjunctivae congested or not, visual acuity, pupils dilated or contracted; nystagmus (present or absent) and reaction of pupil to light and accommodation) :
(13) Gait: (a) Manner of walking (unsteady/steady). (b) Reaction time to a direction to turn. (c) Manner of turning (normal or staggering) :
(14) Stance: (Does he sway when standing erect with his feet together) :
(15) Reflexes: (normal or depressed) :
(16) Muscular co-ordination: (a) Placing finger to nose. (b) Placing finger to finger. (c) Unbuttoning and rebuttoning shirt. (d) Lighting cigarette with a match. (e) Walking along a straight line.
(17) Examination of C.V.S., R.S., and G.I.S. and C.N.S. to rule out any disease:
(18) Laboratory investigations: Blood, urine.

CERTIFICATE OF DRUNKENNESS

Signs of alcoholism found on the person of a male/female called (name) .... aged .... years, an inhabitant of .... who was sent with letter/Cr. No. .... dated from .... of police, of P.S. .... and accompanied by P.C. No. .... for report as to his/her drunkenness.

Identification marks: (1)........................ (2).............................

The person above noted was first seen by the undersigned at .... A.M/P.M. on .... and examination was commenced at .... A.M/P.M. on .... when the following signs were found.

OPINION: (1) Consumed alcohol and is under its influence (intoxicated). (2) Consumed alcohol, but is not under its influence. (3) Has not consumed alcohol

Place : Signature :
Date : Name :
Designation :

(1) Opinion one is given if there is smell of alcohol in the breath, and physical examination reveals abnormal findings. (2) Opinion 2 is given if there is smell of alcohol in the breath, congested conjunctivae and dilated pupils, but other findings are normal. (3) Opinion 3 is given, if there is no smell of alcohol in the breath, and all the findings are normal.

MEDICAL CERTIFICATE RECOMMENDED FOR LEAVE OR EXTENSION OF LEAVE

Signature of applicant or L.T.I.
Identification Marks: (1)........................ (2)...............................

I, Dr. .... after careful examination of the case hereby certify that (name of patient) .... aged ......, sex ...... resident of .... , whose signature is given above is suffering from .... and I consider that a period of absence from duty of .... days with effect from .... is absolutely necessary for the restoration of his health.

Place : Signature, Name & Stamp of Dr.
Date : Reg. No.
Time : State Medical Council of .... State

MEDICAL CERTIFICATE OF FITNESS TO RETURN TO DUTY

To be filled by the applicant in the presence of government doctor/ medical practitioner.

Signature of applicant or L.T.I. .... I,
Identification Marks: 1) 2)

Dr. .... do hereby certify that I have carefully examined .... of the department .... whose signature is given above and find that he has recovered from his illness .... with which he was suffering since .... and is now fit to resume his duties in Govt. services w.e.f. .... I also certify that before arriving at this decision, I have examined the original medical certificates and statement of the case (or certified copies thereof) on which leave was granted or extended and have taken these into consideration in arriving at my decision.

Place : Signature, Name & Stamp of Dr.
Date : Reg. No.
Time : State Medical Council of .... State

HEALTH AND AGE CERTIFICATE

I hereby certify that I have examined Sri .... a candidate for employment in .... office/department, and cannot discover that he/she has any disease (communicable or otherwise), constitutional weakness or bodily infirmity, except .... I do not consider this a disqualification for employment in the office of the .... Sri .... age is, according to his/her own statement .... years, and by appearance about .... years.

Signature of the candidate :	Signature :
Station :	Name :
Date :	Designation :

BIRTH CERTIFICATE

Name: Sex:

Date of birth:

Place of birth:

Name of father:

Name of mother:

Residential address:

Date :	Signature of doctor
Seal :	Name:
	Reg. No.
	State Medical Council of .... State.

APPENDIX-IX

NORMAL WEIGHTS AND MEASURES

USEFUL WEIGHTS AND MEASURES

(Conversion Data)

1 grain = 60 milligrams or 0.06 gm.
1 gram = 60 millilitres or 1.000 mg. or 15.5 grains.
1 ounce = 28.35 grams or 8.5 drachms or 473.5 grains.
1 drachm = 3.5 ml. (approx).
1 pound = 16 ounces or 0.453 kilograms.
1 kilogram = 2.2 pounds.
1 stone = 14 pounds.
10 minims = 0.6 ml. (approx).
1 ml. = 17 minims (approx).
1 litre = 1000 ml. or 35.125 ounces or 1.75 pints.
Teaspoon = 5 ml. (approx). Tablespoon = 15 ml. (approx).
To convert pounds to kilograms (approx), multiply by 5 and divide result by 11.
To convert kilograms into pounds (approx), multiply by 11 and divide result by 5.
To convert feet into centimetres multiply by 30.5.
1 inch = 2.5 cm. (approx).
1 metre = 100 cm.
To convert centimetres into inches (approx), divide by 2.5.
To convert inches into centimetres (approx), multiply by 5 and divide by 2.
To convert feet into centimetres, multiply by 30.5.
Body temperature = 37°C or 98.4°F
Rectal temperature is about 1.5°F more than mouth temperature.
To convert Fahrenheit to centigrade, subtract 32 and multiply by 5/9.
To convert centigrade to Farenheit, multiply by 9/5 and add 32.

WEIGHTS AND MEASUREMENTS OF ORGANS IN ADULTS

BRAIN: 1400 grams (males); 1275 grams (females); 22% body weight.
SPINAL CORD: 27 to 28 grams; length 45 cm.
PITUITARY: 0.5 to 0.6 g; size 2.1 × 1.4 × 0.5 cm.
PINEAL GLAND: 0.1 to o.18 g.
HEART: 300 g. (males); 250 g. (females); 0.4 to 0.45% body weight. Length 12.5 cm; Width 9 to 10 cm. (at atrioventricular groove).
THICKNESS OF WALLS OF ATRIA: 1 to 2 mm.
THICKNESS OF WALLS OF RIGHT VENTRICLE: 3 to 5 mm. (one cm. proximal to pulmonary valve).
THICKNESS OF WALLS OF LEFT VENTRICLE: 10 to 15 mm. (one cm. below atrioventricular valve)
CIRCUMFERENCE (at highest level, usu. near valves): 24 to 25 cm.
CIRCUMFERENCE OF AORTIC VALVE: 7.5 cm. (6 to 7.5 cm.)
CIRCUMFERENCE OF PULMONARY VALVE: 8.5 cm. (7 to 9 cm.)
CIRCUMFERENCE OF MITRAL VALVE: (One cm. below atrioventricular valve). 10 cm. (8 to 10.5 cm.)
CIRCUMFERENCE OF TRICUSPID VALVE: 12 cm. (10 to 12.5 cm.)
AORTA: Length 42–50 cm.
THYROID: 20 to 40 g; size 5 to 7 × 3 to 4 × 1.5 to 2.5 cm.
PARATHYROIDS: 0.12 to 0.18 g.; THYMUS: 15 to 40 g.
RIGHT LUNG: 360 to 570 g; mean 450 g.;
LEFT LUNG: 325 to 480 g; mean 375 g.
BOTH LUNGS: 1% of body weight.
TRACHEA: 11 to 12 cm.; RIGHT BRONCHUS: 2.5 cm.; LEFT: 3.5 to 5 cm.
LIVER: 1400 to 1500 g; 1.8% of body weight. Size: 30 × 18 × 9 cm.
SPLEEN: 150 to 200 g; 0.16% of body weight.
KIDNEY: 130 to 160 g. (males); 120 to 150 g. (females); size 11 to 12 × 5 to 6 × 3 to 4 cm.
PANCREAS: 90 to 120 g; size: 23 × 4.5 × 3.8 cm.; 0.1% body weight.
TESTIS: 20 to 27 g; size: 4 to 5 × 2.5 to 3.5 × 2 to 2.7 cm.
PROSTATE: 15 to 20 g; size: 3.6 × 2.8 × 1.9 cm.
UTERUS: virgin: 30 to 40 g; size: 7.8 to 8 × 3.4 to 4.5 × 1.8 to 2.7 cm. Parous: 100 to 120g; 8.7 to 9.4 × 5.4 to 6.1 × 3.2 to 3.6 cm.
OVARY: 7 g; size: 2.7 to 4.1 × 1.5 to 0.8 cm.
SUPRARENALS: 5 to 6 g.
PHARYNX: 11 to 12 cm; OESOPHAGUS: 25 cm.
STOMACH: length 25 to 30 cm. Weight: 300 g; capacity 1100 to 1200 ml.
SMALL INTESTINE: length 550 to 650 cm; weight 800 to 900 g.
DUODENUM: 25 to 30 cm; JEJUNUM: (upper 2/5); ILEUM: (lower 3/5)
BILE DUCTS: 7.5 cm.
LARGE INTESTINE: length 150 to 170 cm; weight: 600 g; APPENDIX 7.5 to 10 cm.
CAECUM: 6 to 7 cm long; ASCENDING COLON: 20 cm; TRANSVERSE COLON: 50 cm.
DESCENDING COLON: 12 to 15 cm;
PELVIC COLON: 40 to 45 cm; RECTUM: 12 to 15 cm.
ANAL CANAL: 2.5 to 4 cm.
INGUINAL CANAL: 3.5 cm.
THORACIC DUCT: 40 to 45 cm.
BLADDER CAPACITY: 250 ml; URETER: 25 cm.
MALE URETHRA: 20 to 25 cm; prostatic 2.5 to 4 cm; membranous 2 cm; spongy and penile 15 to 20 cm.
FEMALE URETHRA: 2.5 to 4 cm.
VAS DEFERENS: 40 to 45 cm.
UTERINE TUBES: 10 to 12 cm.
VAGINA: anterior wall 7.5 cm; posterior wall 10 cm.
PLACENTA: 500 g; size: 16 to 20 × 2.5 to 3 cm.
BONES: 11.6% of body weight.
SKELETAL MUSCLE: 28.7% of body weight.
FAT: Males: 20 to 25%; Females: 25 to 30% of body weight.
SPECIFIC GRAVITY: Human body: 1.08; Bone: 2.01; Fat: 0.92; Brain 1.04; Muscle 1.08.
The child's brain attains mature size and weight at about six years of age.

APPENDIX-X

MAHARSHI CHARAK SHAPATH

Health Service न त्वहं कामये राज्यम् न स्वर्गम् नापुनर्भवम् । कामये दुःखतप्तानां प्राणिनाम् आर्तिनाशनम् ।। Nation Service

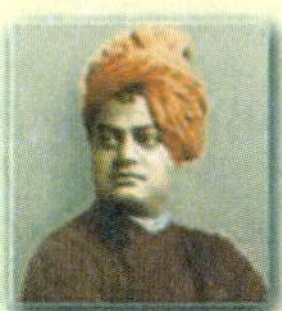

MAHARSHI CHARAK SHAPATH

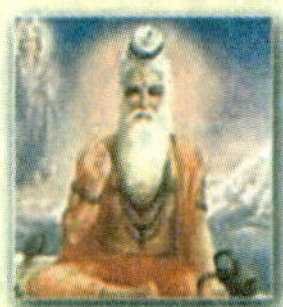

O Dwij (twice born)*! facing the east in presence of the holy fire and the learned people take the oath that :

- During the period of study I shall live a life of self control, piety and discipline. Submitting myself to my Guru (teachers) with complete dedicated feeling. I shall act like a son / daughter for his/her welfare and happiness. My action shall be guarded, service oriented and free from indiscipline and envy. In my dealings I shall be patient, obedient, humble, constantly contemplative and calm. I shall aim my full efforts and ability towards the desired goal of my Guru. As a physician, in order to gain success and fame and earn money I shall always use my knowledge for the welfare of living mankind.
- I shall always be ready to help patients, even when I am extremely busy and tired. I shall not harm any patient for the sake of money or selfish gain nor shall I entertain a desire for other women / men or wealth. Immorality should not figure even in my thoughts.
- My dress ought be decent yet impressive and personality confidence inspiring. I shall always use sweet, pure, appropriate, pleasant, truthful, beneficial and polite words and using my past experience, I shall act keeping in mind the time and the place.
- I shall constantly endeavour to accomplish the newest development of knowledge.
- I (especially a male doctor) shall treat a women only in the presence of her husband or a near relative.
- When examining a patient, my discretion, attention and senses shold be concentrated on the cure of the disease. I shall not make propaganda about the confidential matters regarding patients and their family.
- Though an authority (on my subject), I shall not display my knowledge (and skill) egoistically as by it even near ones may feel insulted.

** A Dwij Means twice born because for the first time one takes birth bodily from his / her mother and second time takes birth spiritually with the education and publication influenced by Guru.*

Any person of any caste or sex, can become aDwij and a doctor. Considering it appropriate amendments have been made in this main substance of the original exiensive Orth of Charak. Every medical student and doctor should take this Oath and put it on his/her working table. Charak Oath is far more extensive.

INDEX

A

B

C

D

E

F

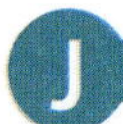

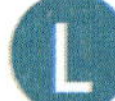

N

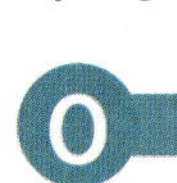

Q

R

S

T

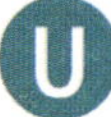

U

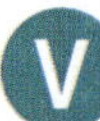

V

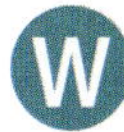

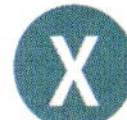

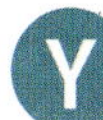

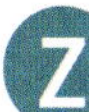